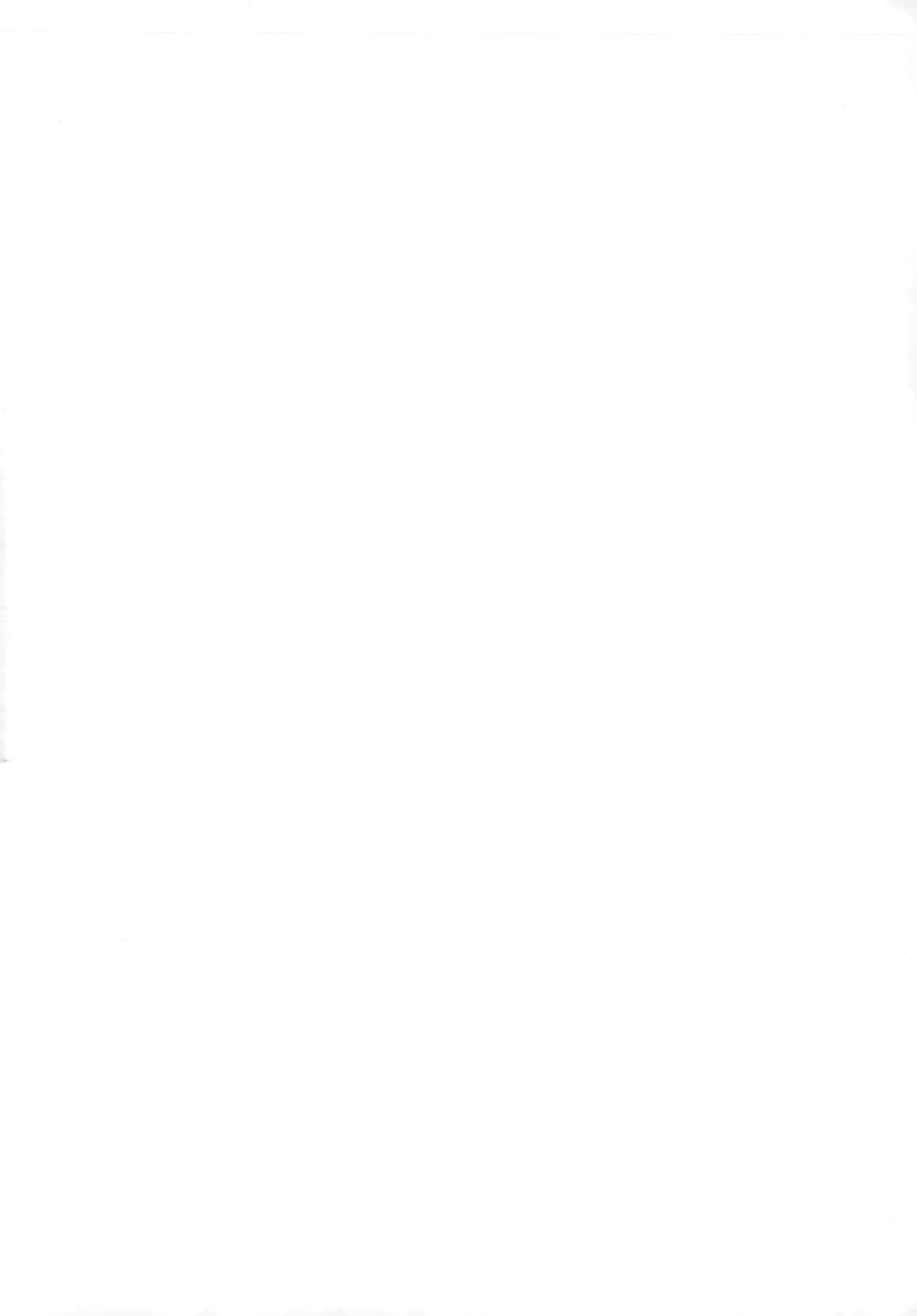

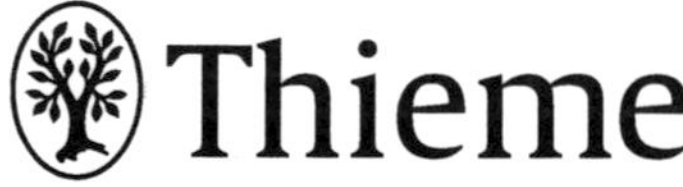

# Functional Anatomy for Physical Therapists

**Jutta Hochschild**
Physical Therapist
Former Head, Physical Therapy School
Department of Orthopaedics
Academic Teaching Hospital
University of Frankfurt
Frankfurt, Germany

1000 illustrations

Georg Thieme Verlag
Stuttgart · New York · Delhi · Rio de Janeiro

**Library of Congress Cataloging-in-Publication Data**

Hochschild Jutta, author.
[Strukturen und Funktionen begreifen. English]
Functional anatomy for physical therapists / Jutta Hochschild.
p. ; cm.
ISBN 978-3-13-176861-2 (alk. paper) –
ISBN 978-3-13-176871-1 (eISBN)
I. Title.
[DNLM: 1. Physical Therapy Modalities. 2. Anatomy. 3. Physiological Phenomena. WB 460]
QM 26
612-dc23

2015034186

This book is an authorized translation of the 2-volume 3rd German edition published and copyrighted 2005 and 2008 by Georg Thieme Verlag, Stuttgart. Title of the German edition: Strukturen und Funktionen begreifen : Funtionelle Anatomie : Therapierelevante Details – T.p. verso.

Translator: Alan Wiser, MD, Ambler, PA, USA
Illustrator: Malgorzata & Piotr Gusta, Champigny sur Marne, France

1st Italian edition 2003
1st Japanese edition 2011



Thieme Publishers Stuttgart
Rüdigerstrasse 14, 70469 Stuttgart, Germany
+49 [0]711 8931 421, customerservice@thieme.de

Thieme Publishers New York
333 Seventh Avenue, New York, NY 10001, USA
+1-800-782-3488, customerservice@thieme.com

Thieme Publishers Delhi
A-12, Second Floor, Sector-2, Noida-201301
Uttar Pradesh, India
+91 120 45 566 00, customerservice@thieme.in

Thieme Publishers Rio, Thieme Publicações Ltda.
Edifício Rodolpho de Paoli, 25° andar
Av. Nilo Peçanha, 50 – Sala 2508
Rio de Janeiro 20020-906 Brasil
+55 21 3172 2297 / +55 21 3172 1896

Cover design: Thieme Publishing Group
Typesetting by Druckhaus Götz GmbH, Ludwigsburg, Germany

Printed in Germany by CPI, Leck

ISBN 978-3-13-176861-2 5 4 3

Also available as an e-book:
eISBN 978-3-13-176871-1

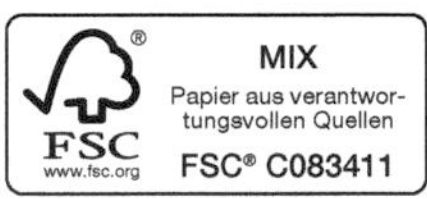

# Contents

# Preface

Anatomy, with all its fascinating facets to investigate and teach, has been and continues to be my calling. To probe more deeply into the interconnections between structures and, through that, to clarify many functional problems that patients have never ceases to engage me.

My students have always had a great deal to learn, but it is important to me that they understand anatomy, not merely memorize it. I dedicate my book to them. Based on 25 years and approximately 7,000 hours teaching functional anatomy—this book evolved from an instructional manual after many years of work.

My book should not and cannot replace the classical anatomy texts. Rather, it is a supplement to them. Thus, I delve thoroughly into joint surfaces and the formation of joints, while only briefly describing the bones. While I have assumed a background knowledge of muscle origins and insertions, I feel it is important to describe the functional aspects of the muscles.

Palpation of the various structures makes up a large portion of the book. It remains an important component of examination and treatment in physical therapy.

I hope that my references to pathology and the practical tips are useful for all my colleagues in everyday practice.

I especially wish to thank the illustrator, Piotr Gusta and his wife, who immersed themselves deeply in their work. The superb, detailed figures found in this book are the result.

I would like to thank Dr. Alan Wiser for his excellent translation. I would also like to extend thanks to Angelika-Marie Findgott and Gabriele Kuhn-Giovannini for their excellent support, and to all the other associates at Thieme Publishers who participated in the production of this book.

I also thank my colleagues at the School of Physical Therapy at the University Hospital Frankfurt. They have always assisted me in gathering important data.

*Jutta Hochschild*

# Chapter 1

## Fundamentals of the Spinal Column



1

# 1 Fundamentals of the Spinal Column

## 1.1 Development and Structure of the Spinal Column (Fig. 1.1)

Viewed laterally, the spinal column develops from being totally kyphotic in the early embryonic phase to the normally curved spine with two areas of kyphosis and two areas of lordosis within the first 7 years of life.

The following events occur **during growth**: Cervical lordosis develops when the infant attempts to lift its head from the prone position while trying to move on all fours. The lordosis in the lumbar spine develops during the process of standing upright. Because of the lack of flexibility of the hip flexors, any extension of the hip joints causes an inclination of the pelvis, which further accentuates the lordosis of the lumbar spine. This process is not complete until near the end of the 6th year of life.

### 1.1.1 Ideal Curvature (Fig. 1.2)

The ideal spinal curvature has been determined with the help of computer analysis. In the erect position, the plumb line cuts through the anterior tubercle of the atlas (**a** in **Fig. 1.2**), the sixth cervical vertebra (**b**), the ninth thoracic vertebra (**c**), the third sacral vertebra, (**d**) and the tip of the coccyx (**e**).

**Practical Tip**

Assessment of the statics of the spine is an important part of the physical therapy record. Among other things, the characteristics of the curvature in the sagittal plane are recorded. Deviations from the norm are the hollow round back with increased lumbar lordosis and thoracic kyphosis, and the flat back with attenuation of the physiologic curvatures.

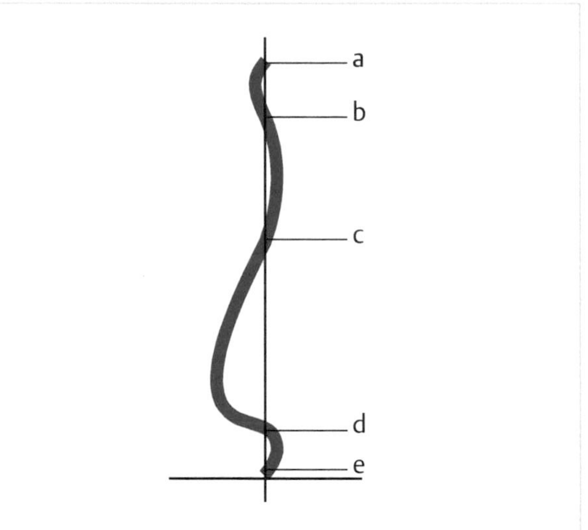


**Fig. 1.2** The ideal curvature of the spine and its intersections with a center of gravity plumb line.

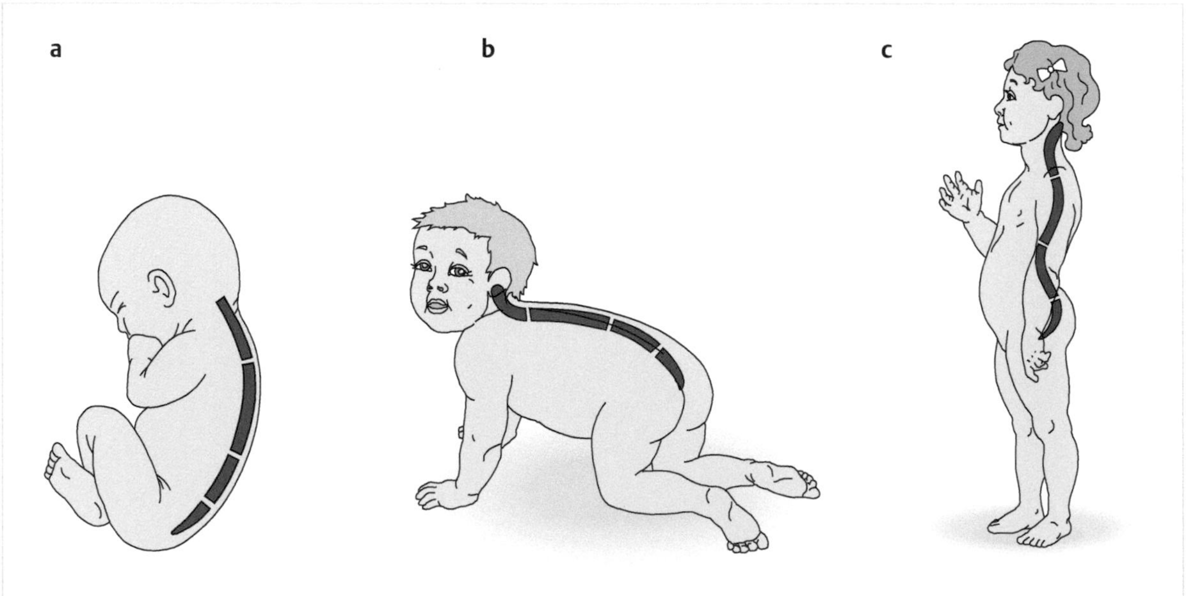


**Fig. 1.1** Development of the spinal curvatures. **(a)** Embryonic period. **(b)** Infancy. **(c)** Early childhood.

## 1.1.2 Architecture of the Cancellous (Trabecular) Bone (Fig. 1.3)

Mechanical stress influences the structural arrangement of trabecular bone. Because of this stress distribution, zones of varying density develop.

A sagittal section through the vertebral body demonstrates an area that is less dense anteriorly. This is caused by lines of stress that run in a fan-shaped curve from the superior edge of the vertebral body to the upper articular processes and the spinous process, as well as from the inferior edge of the vertebral body to the lower articular processes and the spinous process.

In a frontal section, one can also identify fan-shaped stress lines running vertically and horizontally.

The arrangement of the trabecular structure of bone depends on the tensile and compressive load and can adapt to changing forces.

Changes occur if load limits are over- or undershot for a prolonged period of time.

*Examples:*

- Bone structure changes due to poor posture and after fractures that do not heal in the correct axis.
- The skeletal structure becomes fragile if load limits are over- or undershot for a prolonged period of time.
- Structural disorders lead to characteristic vertebral body shapes such as fish vertebrae in osteoporosis and wedge-shaped vertebrae in spondylitis.

### Practical Tip

Eliminating muscle imbalances, reducing excessive weight, and improving the awareness of body posture lead to balanced tensile and compressive stresses on the bone. The strength and configuration of the trabecular structure can be positively influenced and maintained to accommodate long-term weight-bearing and alterations in weight-bearing status.

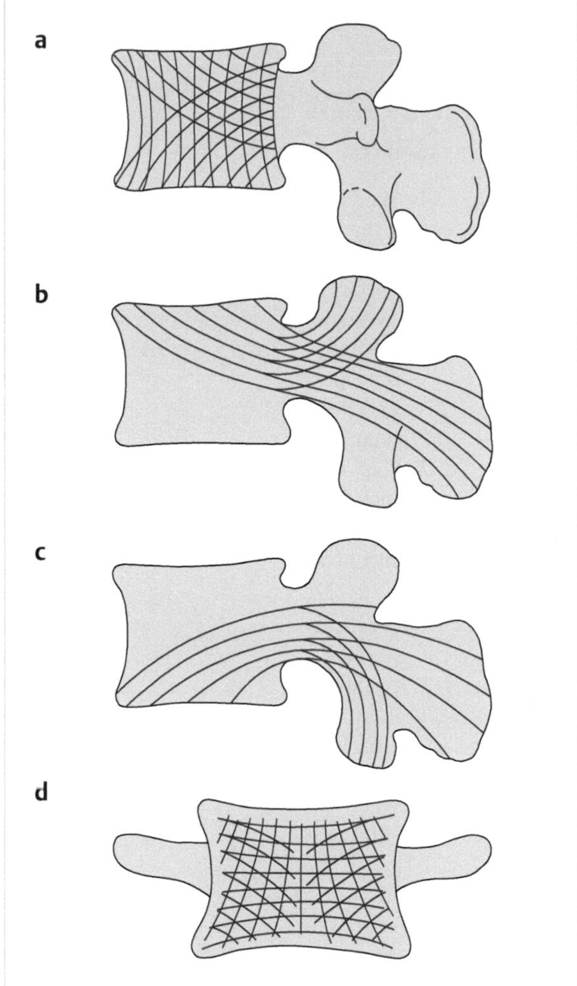


**Fig. 1.3** Architecture of cancellous bone. **(a–c)** In sagittal section. **(d)** In frontal section.

# 1.2 Motion Segment (Fig. 1.4)

The motion segment is a functional unit that corresponds to the movement space between two vertebrae, including the following structures (**Fig. 1.4**):

- **Zygapophysial joints:**
  1 = Joint capsule
  2 = Ligamentum flavum
- **Spinal canal and intervertebral foramen:**
  3 = Spinal nerve
  4 = Meningeal branch of the spinal nerve
  5 = Blood vessels
- **Disk space:**
  6 = Cartilage plate
  7 = Marginal ridge of the vertebral body
  8 = Nucleus pulposus
  9 = Anulus fibrosus
  10 = Anterior longitudinal ligament
  11 = Posterior longitudinal ligament

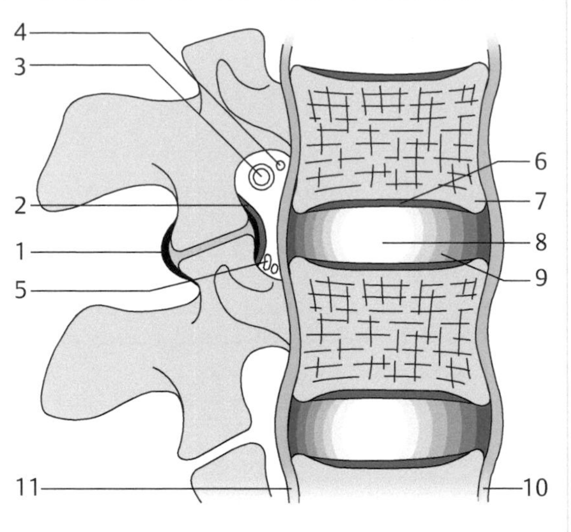


**Fig. 1.4** Motion segment.

The spaces between the overlying vertebral arches, the spinous and transverse processes and all the ligaments and muscles are also included.

This movement complex is anatomically and functionally coordinated. It can be divided into anterior and posterior sections (**Fig. 1.5**). The anterior area, made up of the vertebral bodies and disk spaces, is the support element, absorbing the direct axial compressive forces and passing them on. The posterior area (the facet joints and all that lies between the vertebral arches), determines the direction of motion, i.e., allows certain movements and blocks others. The ligamentous structures and the position of the zygapophysial joints (intervertebral facet joints) and the anulus fibrosus together set the limits of the range of the movement.

The motion segment functions as a unit. An irritation of one part of the segment always has an effect on the other structures.

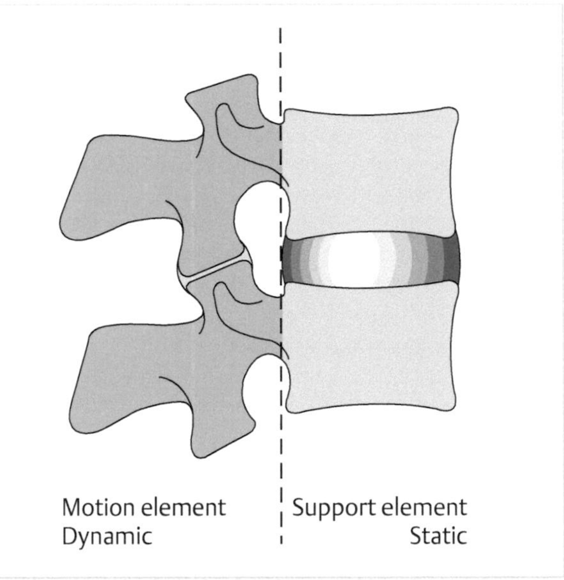


**Fig. 1.5** Division of the motion segment.

## 1.2.1 The Structure of a Vertebra

### Vertebral Body (Fig. 1.6)

The vertebral body consists of a core of cancellous bone that is bounded at the sides by compact bone. The cortical bone is very strong posterolaterally, where the vertebral arches branch off.

The superior and inferior end plates form the transition between the vertebral body and the intervertebral disk. They consist of cartilage and are surrounded by a bony marginal ridge.

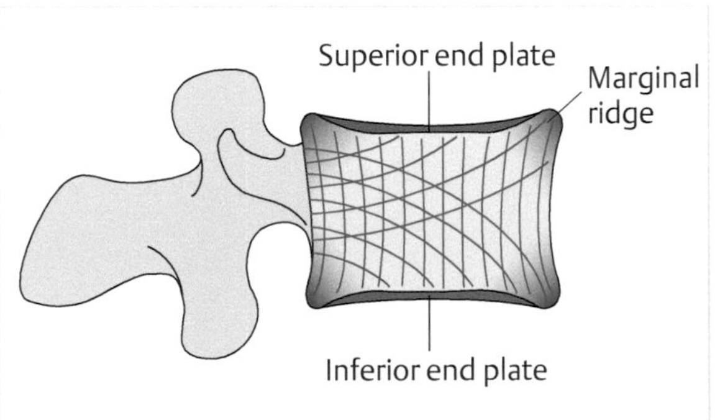


**Fig. 1.6** Vertebral body.

## Vertebral Arch (Fig. 1.7)

The vertebral arches consist of two symmetrical halves that are fused together. In this way, they form the vertebral foramen.

A distinction is made between the anterior section of the vertebral arch (**pedicle**) and the posterior section (**lamina**).

Each vertebral pedicle has bilateral superior and inferior articular processes.

## Transverse Process (Fig. 1.7)

The transverse processes are shaped differently in each section of the spine.

In the **cervical spine**, they come together with the rib rudiment to form the transverse foramen for the vertebral artery.

In the **thoracic spine**, they are very pronounced and articulate with the ribs.

In the **lumbar spine**, they are only present as rudimentary structures, the accessory processes.

## Spinous Process (Fig. 1.7)

The vertebral arches merge posteriorly to form the spinous process, which is an important area for the origin and insertion of the muscles. Its appearance is quite variable. For example, it is split in the cervical spine, while it is very long and projects obliquely downward in the thoracic spine, and is very strongly developed in the lumbar spine.

## Vertebral Foramen (Fig. 1.8)

The size and shape of the vertebral foramina vary from segment to segment. In transverse section, the foramen exhibits a clearly triangular shape in the lumbar spine and a rounded triangle in the cervical spine. In the thoracic spine, it is round and smaller than in the lumbar or cervical areas.

When the vertebrae are stacked one on top of the other, this forms the vertebral canal, within which the spinal cord runs.

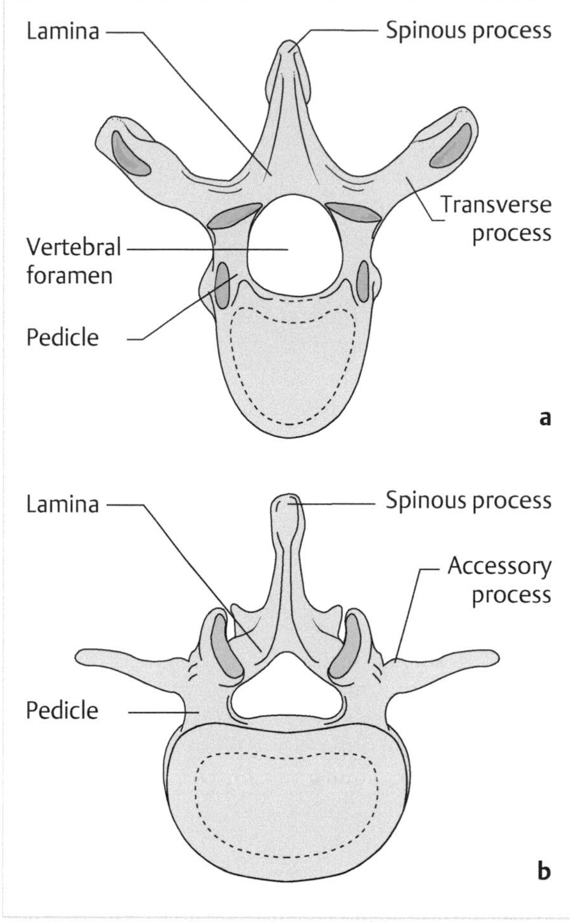


**Fig. 1.7** Vertebral arch, spinous process, and transverse process. **(a)** In the thoracic spine. **(b)** In the lumbar spine.

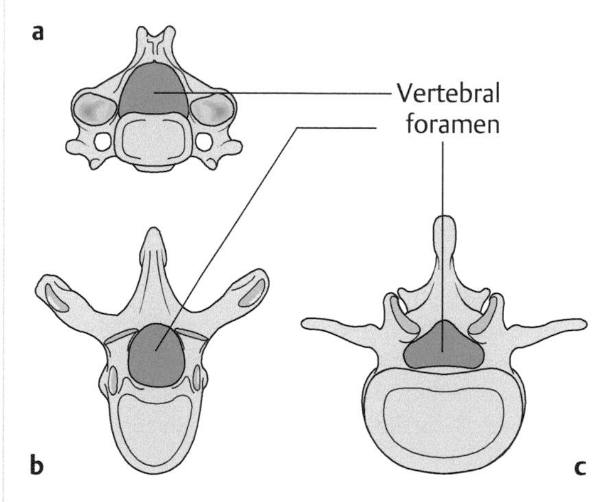


**Fig. 1.8** Vertebral foramen. **(a)** Cervical spine. **(b)** Thoracic spine. **(c)** Lumbar spine.

## Intervertebral Foramen (Fig. 1.9)

The intervertebral foramina lie between two adjacent vertebrae. The superior and inferior borders are formed by the pedicles of both vertebrae. Anteriorly, the borders are the lateral sides of the vertebral bodies and the posterior surfaces of the intervertebral disks. The articular processes form the border posteriorly.

The dura mater of the nerve root sheath merges into the periosteum within the foramen and thus fixes the nerve root. The meningeal branch of the spinal nerve extends back through the foramen into the spinal canal.

During lateral flexion, the ipsilateral foramen narrows and the contralateral foramen widens by one-third. Flexion causes widening, while extension causes narrowing.

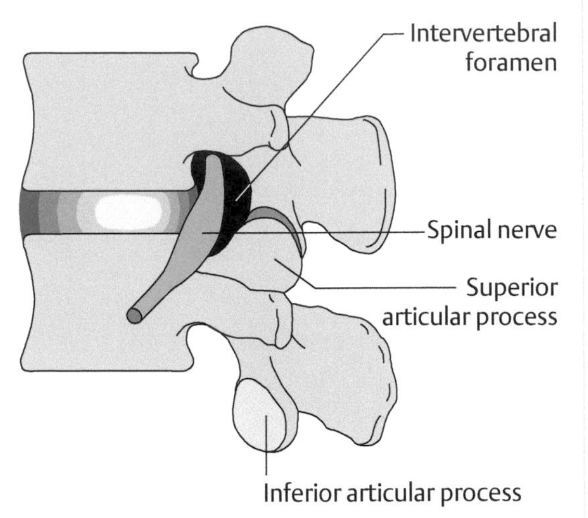


**Fig. 1.9** Intervertebral foramen.

## Articular Process (Fig. 1.9)

Four articular processes (two superior and two inferior) extend from the vertebral arches: two superior and two inferior articular processes. Thus, an inferior articular process of the upper vertebra and the corresponding superior articular process of the lower vertebra form the zygapophysial joint.

# 1.2.2 Zygapophysial Joints (Intervertebral Facet Joints) (Fig. 1.10)

## Joint Surfaces

The zygapophysial joints have the task of absorbing the compressive forces and passing them on. They also help to guide movement, depending on the structure of the joint surfaces and the capsule–ligament apparatus.

**Cervical spine (Fig. 1.10a):** Because the joint surface is inclined, it forms an angle of approximately 45° from the horizontal. The superior articular surface faces posteriorly and superiorly.

**Thoracic spine (Fig. 1.10b):** The articular surfaces lie at an angle of 80° to the horizontal and are rotated 20° outward from the frontal plane, so that the superior articular surface faces posteriorly and slightly superiorly.

**Lumbar spine (Fig. 1.10c):** The articular surfaces form an angle of 90° to the horizontal plane. In the sagittal plane and seen from above, they are oriented 15° toward the anterior, so that the superior articular surface faces medially and slightly posteriorly. This angle increases as one moves down the spine, so that the inferior articular surface of the fifth lumbar vertebra forms an angle of 75° with the sagittal plane.

The spatial position of the joint surfaces determines the range of motion and movement combinations.

*Example:* In the lumbar spine, the position of the joint surfaces allows rotation only if the joint surfaces move apart from each other through flexion. Only then is there leeway for minimal rotation in combination with lateral flexion in the same direction. Therefore one can see that the extent of rotation is very limited when compared with the other directions of movement.

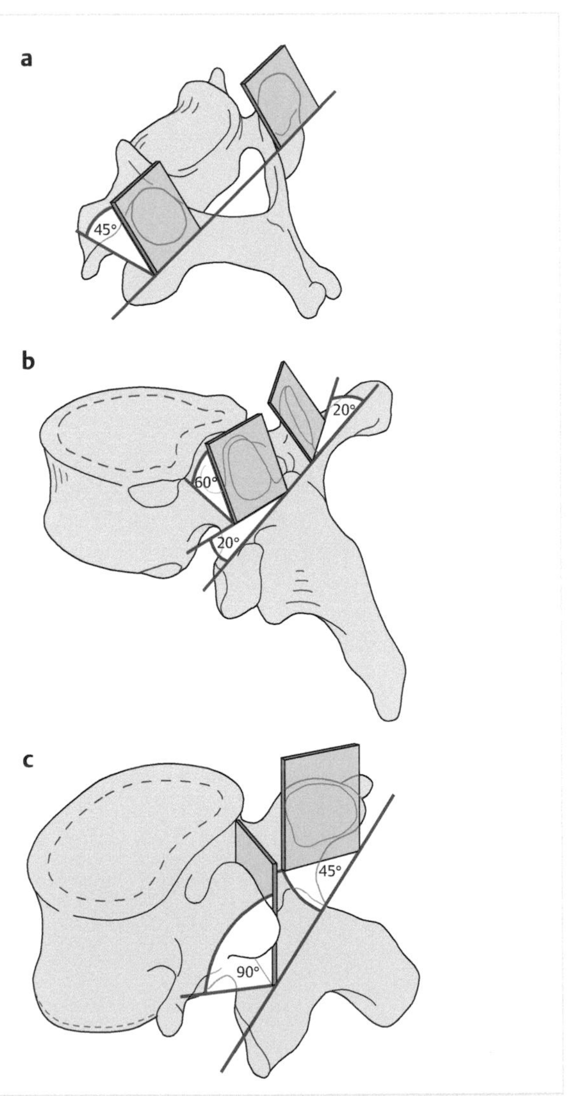


**Fig. 1.10** Position of the zygapophysial joints. **(a)** Cervical spine. **(b)** Thoracic spine. **(c)** Lumbar spine.

## Joint Capsule (Fig. 1.11)

### Synovial Membrane

The synovial membrane extends into the periosteum of the articular process at the bone–cartilage border. It forms recesses or bulges toward the fibrous layer, which represent reserve spaces for extreme movements.

In addition, the synovial membrane forms many eversions that protrude into the interior of the joint. It is assumed that these play a role in so-called blockages of the vertebral joints. These bulges, the synovial folds and villi, are more common in the lordotic sections of the spinal column. In the lumbar spine area, they can protrude up to 6 mm into the joint space. Because of their appearance, they are sometimes termed disks or meniscal folds. They are composed of very thick connective tissue with only a minimal incorporation of fatty tissue. They can become frayed, resulting in small torn pieces of these folds lying within the joint.

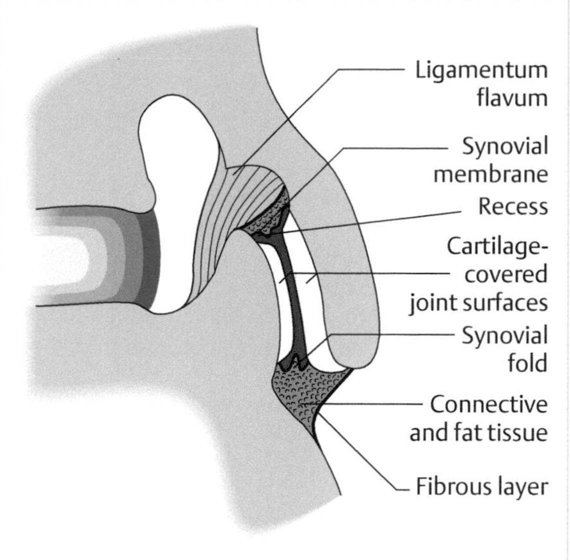


**Fig. 1.11** Joint capsule.

## Fibrous Layer (Figs. 1.11 and 1.12)

Part of the joint capsule arises from the corresponding periosteum. It inserts onto the base of the articular process well away from the edge of the joint surface because of the connective and fatty tissue that is enclosed between the fibrous layer and the synovial membrane.

The fibrous layer has reinforcing bands, which, in the **lumbar spine**, run transversely on the outer edge of the inferior articular process to the mammillary processes and the superior articular processes, which lie inferiorly. The multifidus muscles track onto the reinforcing bands and can tense the capsule.

The orientation of the reinforcing bands is vertical in the **thoracic and cervical spine** areas. In all the vertebral sections, the ligamenta flava lie with their lateral edge against the joint capsule and extend into the joint capsule with a few fibers. The same applies to the intertransverse ligaments with their medial fiber tracts.

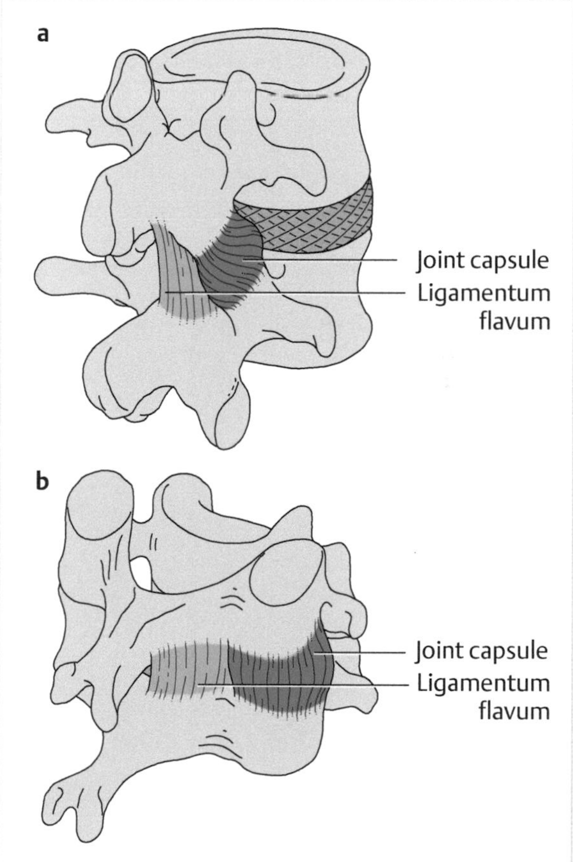


**Fig. 1.12** Course of the fibrous layer. **(a)** In the lumbar spine. **(b)** In the cervical spine.

## Vascular Supply (Fig. 1.13)

The arterial supply of the zygapophysial joints varies depending on the particular region of the spine. In the **thoracic and lumbar spine**, the segmental arteries provide the primary supply:

- Posterior intercostal artery.
- Lumbar artery.
- Iliolumbar artery.

Articular retia form, which also supply the bordering periosteum.

In the **cervical spine**, the primary supply is from the vertebral artery.

### Practical Tip

The large supply channels lying anterior or lateral to the vertebral body give an indication that perfusion of the motion segment can be stimulated by means of *lift-free mobilization* of the entire vertebral section.

### Pathology

Two adjacent segmental arteries provide the blood supply for each of the zygapophysial joints. Thus, if one supply channel is blocked or constricted due to edema forming within the tissues or other causes, the other artery can provide the blood supply.
In the cervical spine area, constriction of the vertebral artery can lead to a unilateral decrease in the perfusion of the capsule–ligament apparatus over several segments.

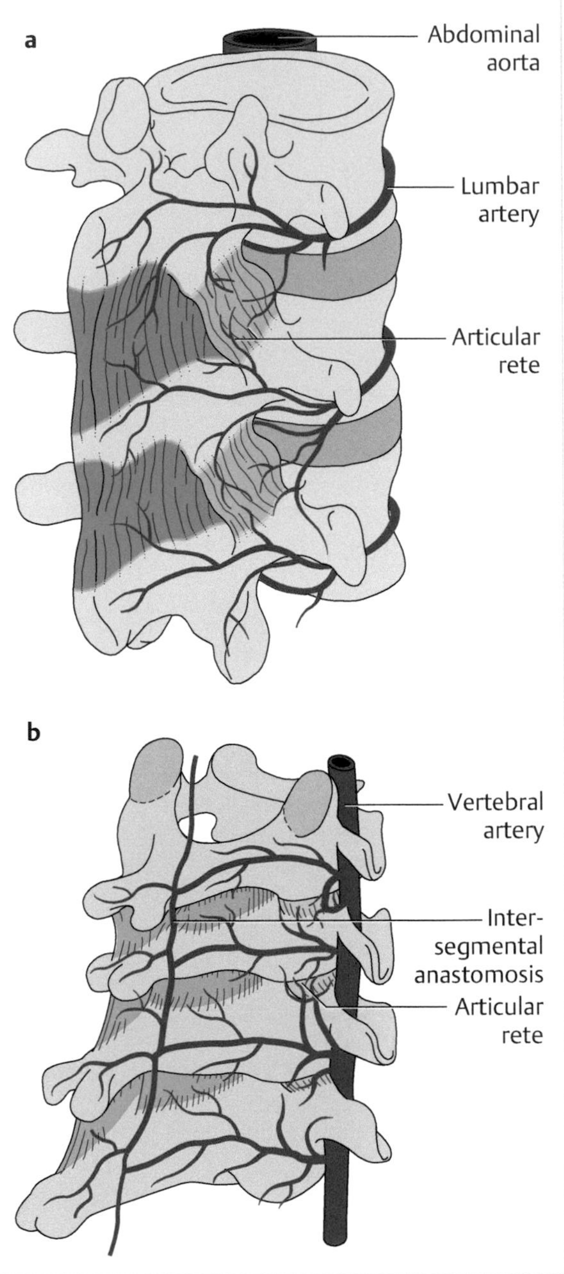


**Fig. 1.13** Vascular supply of the joint capsule. **(a)** In the lumbar and thoracic spine. **(b)** In the cervical spine.

## The Joint as a Sensory Organ

The joint capsule and the bordering ligaments and tendons are densely provided with receptors. The following receptors can be found in the area of the joint capsule.

### Proprioceptors (Fig. 1.14)

*Golgi-type receptors* lie at the transition to the capsule–ligament apparatus. They are encased in a capsule of connective tissue and are myelinated. They have a high conduction velocity.

*Ruffini's receptors* are found primarily in the fibrous layer of the capsule. These receptors are a plexiform structure with low conduction velocity.

These receptors register the tension of the joint capsule and have a reflexive tonic and phasic effect on the muscles, which is transmitted via the motor neurons.

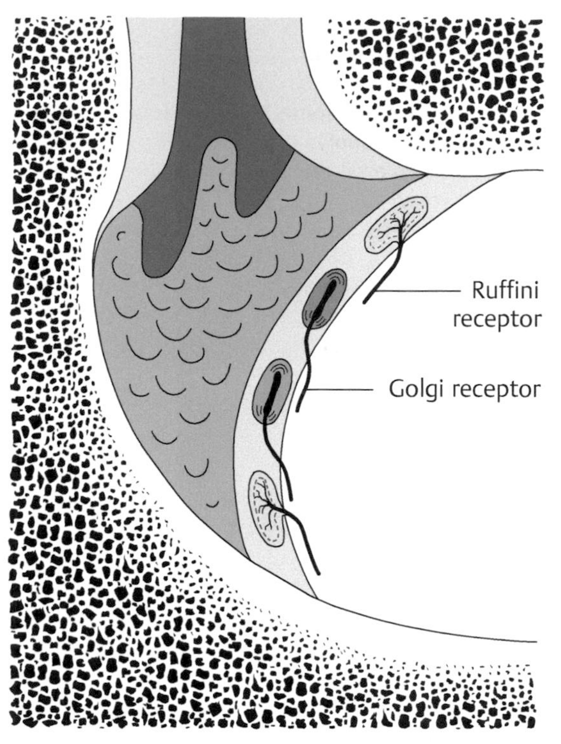


**Fig. 1.14** Proprioceptors in the joint capsule.

### Nociceptors (Fig. 1.15)

Nociceptors are also known as pain receptors. These are free nerve endings that, for the most part, are not myelinated. They spread out like a plexus and have a very slow conduction velocity. They are located in the fibrous layer of the capsule and react to mechanical and chemical stimuli, for instance to inflammatory substances such as polypeptides, serotonin, histamine, etc., which are formed in the body and released secondary to edema or other acute or chronic pressure effects. These chemicals trigger pain sensations and, through the motor neuron, lead to tensing of the muscles in the vicinity of the joint.

The dense network of proprioceptors and nociceptors in the zygapophysial joints explains why they are the dominant cause of movement disturbances.

*Example:* The nociceptive blocking effect is a protective mechanism that prevents harmful movements from injuring joints that are inflamed.

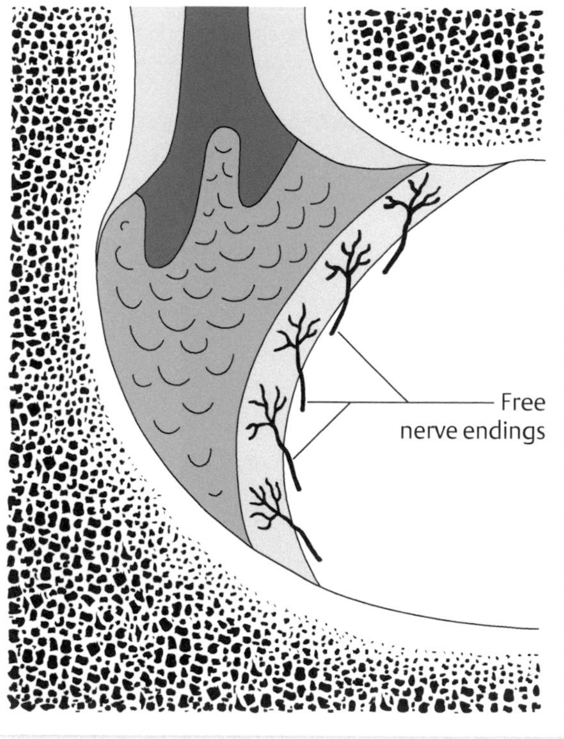


**Fig. 1.15** Nociceptors in the joint capsule.

### The Arthromuscular Vicious Cycle (Fig. 1.16)

The receptors, in conjunction with the motor neurons and the motor centers of the brain, cause a change in muscle tone that is transmitted over the spinal connection. In normal circumstances, there is muscular equilibrium, the capsule unfolds without a problem, and the joint is freely mobile.

Distension of the capsule, as might occur with faulty loading of the joint, causes stimulation of the receptors. This information is transmitted to the brainstem and cortex over the afferent pathway, and, through direct synapsing, to the motor center in the anterior horn of the spinal cord. The efferent nerves leaving here act on both the α and γ motor neurons. This can lead to, for example, shortening of the intrafusal fibers, which in turn results in an increased resting muscle tone.

As long as the joint is disturbed, the muscles dedicated to that joint will demonstrate a chronically increased tone, which will subside only when the arthrogenic disturbance has been rectified.

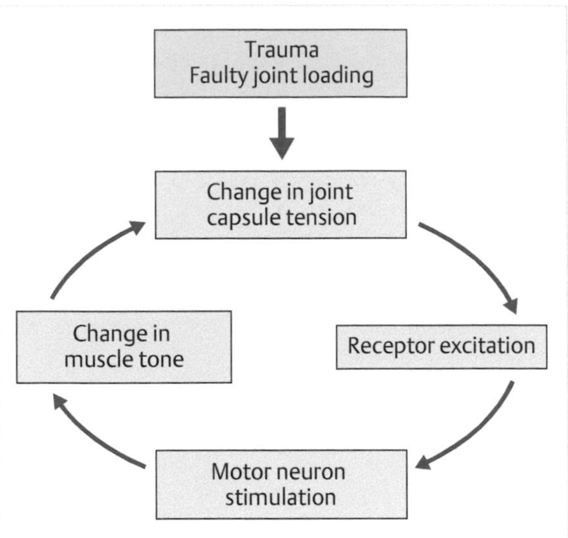


**Fig. 1.16** The arthromuscular vicious cycle.

**Practical Tip**

Treatment techniques in physical therapy influence movement, movement coordination, and posture by way of the receptors.
Using special techniques such as *Contract Relax* and *Rhythmic Stabilization*, proprioceptive neuromuscular facilitation influences muscle tone through proprioceptive stimulation by means of relaxing and stretching a muscle group. Because muscle tone is designed as a protective mechanism, the timing of these procedures must be carefully planned.
To some degree, manual therapy has an effect on the receptors of the capsule–ligament apparatus in that malalignment is corrected by traction and mobilization techniques.
The cycle can therefore be broken in various places. To permanently eliminate a disturbance, however, the cause must be found and treated.

## 1.2.3 Innervation of the Motion Segment

The anterior and posterior sensory nerve roots combine to form the spinal nerve. In the intervertebral foramen or shortly thereafter, the meningeal branch forks off from the spinal nerve and turns back parallel to it, running back into the spinal canal, which is why it is also known as the recurrent branch.

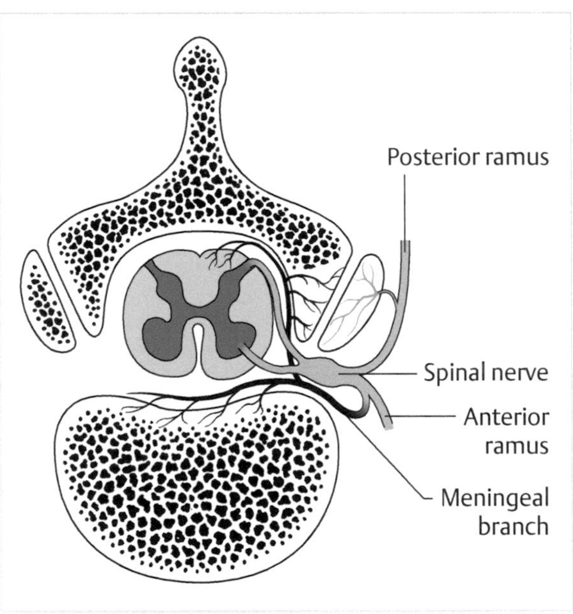


**Fig. 1.17** Area of supply of the meningeal branch of the spinal nerve.

### Meningeal Branch of the Spinal Nerve (Fig. 1.17)

This carries pure sensory-sympathetic nerve fibers and supplies the following structures with anterior and posterior branches:

- Inside the spinal canal: the periosteal, meningeal and epidural blood vessels.
- The posterior longitudinal ligament.
- The outermost layers of the anulus fibrosus.

The terminal fibers form a network with those of the meningeal branch from the adjacent segments. Thus, the segments overlap.

After giving off the meningeal branch, the spinal nerve divides into anterior and posterior rami.

## Posterior Ramus (Fig. 1.18)

Here, too, branching occurs. The medial branch, via the articular branch, supplies the joint capsule of the same segment and gives off collateral branches to the one or two next higher and lower zygapophysial joints. That means that every posterior ramus supplies at least two or three motion segments. The articular branch also supplies the adjoining ligaments and the periosteum. A few branches of the medial branch track into the muscles near the joint.

The lateral branch supplies the autochthonous back muscles and the skin.

## Anterior Ramus (Fig. 1.18)

The anterior rami form the lumbar, sacral, brachial, and cervical plexuses and supply the corresponding muscles and other structures.

## Ramus Communicans (Fig. 1.18)

Shortly after the intervertebral foramen, the ramus communicans establishes a connection to the sympathetic trunk. It carries both afferent and efferent fibers.

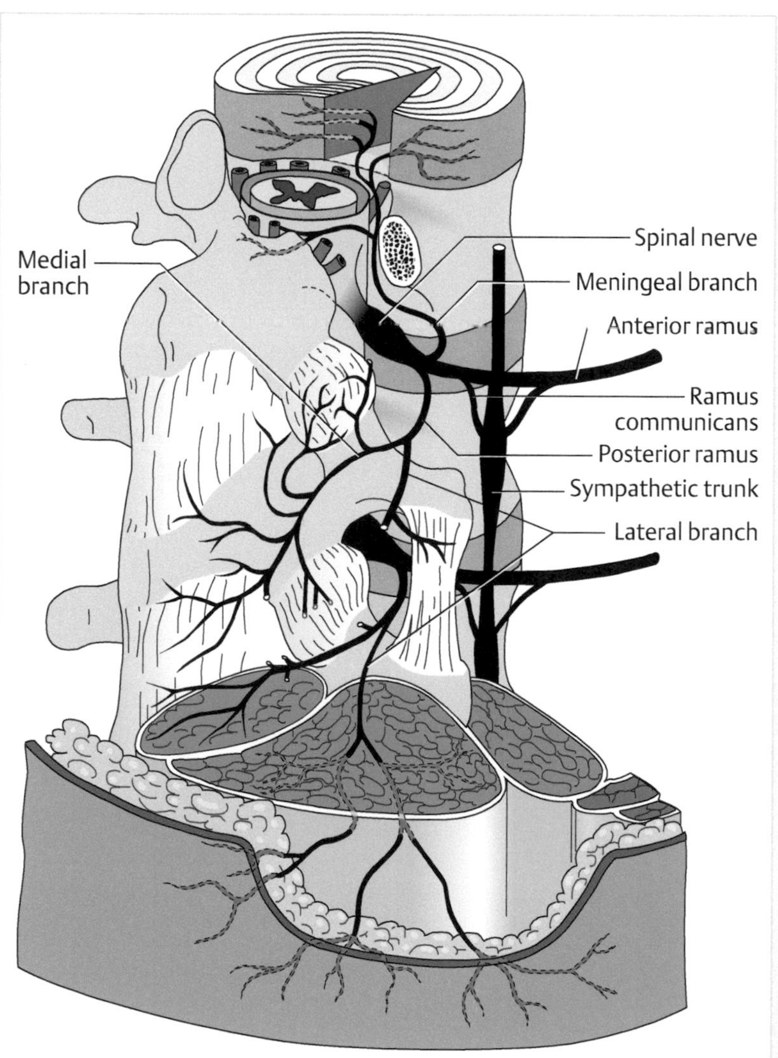


**Fig. 1.18** Innervation of the motion segment.

## 1.2.4 Ligaments of the Spinal Column

### Interspinous Ligament (Fig. 1.19)

This ligament occupies the space between two adjacent spinous processes. Its tensile direction is from posterosuperior to anteroinferior. It merges with the fibrous layer of the capsule of the zygapophysial joint.

### Supraspinous Ligament (Fig. 1.19)

The supraspinous ligament connects the tips of the spinous processes and consists of very strong, vertically running ligamentous bands. The ligament extends from the seventh cervical vertebra to the sacrum. In the cervical section, its place is taken by the ligamentum nuchae.

### Ligamentum Flavum (Fig. 1.19)

The ligamenta flava are stretched out segmentally on the posterior margin of the spinal canal between the vertebral lamina, and thereby close the spinal canal posterolaterally. In the thoracic and lumbar spines, they merge laterally with the zygapophysial joint capsules.

Each ligament is thick and powerfully built, and consists of more than 75% elastic fibers, which is why it appears a yellowish color. This high proportion of elastic components ensures that the ligament is taut in any possible position, and that there is no position in which folds could develop to constrict the spinal canal. The ligamenta flava are subject to large variations in length. At maximum flexion, for instance, they experience an increase in length of 50%.

Because of their proximity to the joint capsule, the ligamenta flava exert pressure posteriorly during flexion and thereby stabilize this part of the zygapophysial joint.

### Intertransverse Ligament (Fig. 1.19)

This ligament runs between the transverse processes.

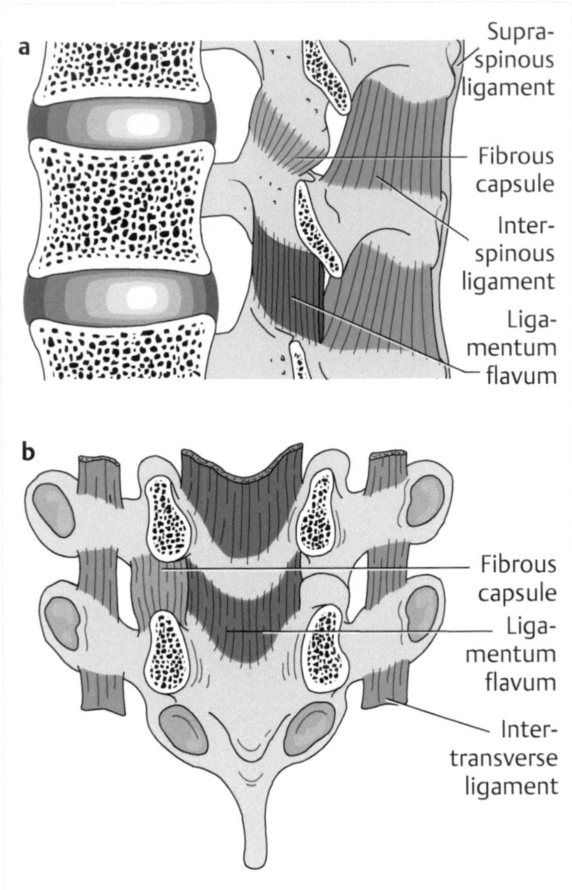


**Fig. 1.19** Ligaments of the spinal column. **(a)** Lateral view (left vertebral arch removed). **(b)** Posterior view (vertebral arches removed).

## Posterior Longitudinal Ligament (Fig. 1.20)

The ligament lies on the posterior side of the vertebral body. It is very narrow in the area of the vertebral body but becomes wider at the level of the disk space, taking on a rhombic shape. It is attached to the intervertebral disks, and some of its fibers extend obliquely downward to the vertebral pedicle, leaving the superior parts of the disk uncovered. A venous plexus (the internal vertebral venous plexus) lies between the bone and the ligament. The ligament extends from the occipital bone to the sacral canal and is wider superiorly than inferiorly.

## Anterior Longitudinal Ligament (Fig. 1.21)

This lies on the anterior surface of the vertebral bodies and extends from the anterior tubercle of the atlas to the first sacral vertebra. Inferiorly, it is broad and strong. The ligament merges with the vertebral bodies but spans over the disk spaces.

This ligament consists of long, superficial bundles of fibers that extend over four or five vertebrae, and shorter, more deeply laid bundles that join two adjacent vertebrae.

The ligaments secure the motion segment in all directions.

*Example:* Lateral flexion to the left creates tension in the intertransverse ligaments and the capsule–ligament apparatus on the right as well as in the right-sided sections of the ligamentum flavum and the posterior longitudinal ligament. These structures thus become vulnerable. Because these components lie deep within the tissues, it is not feasible to use palpation to delineate an irritated structure.

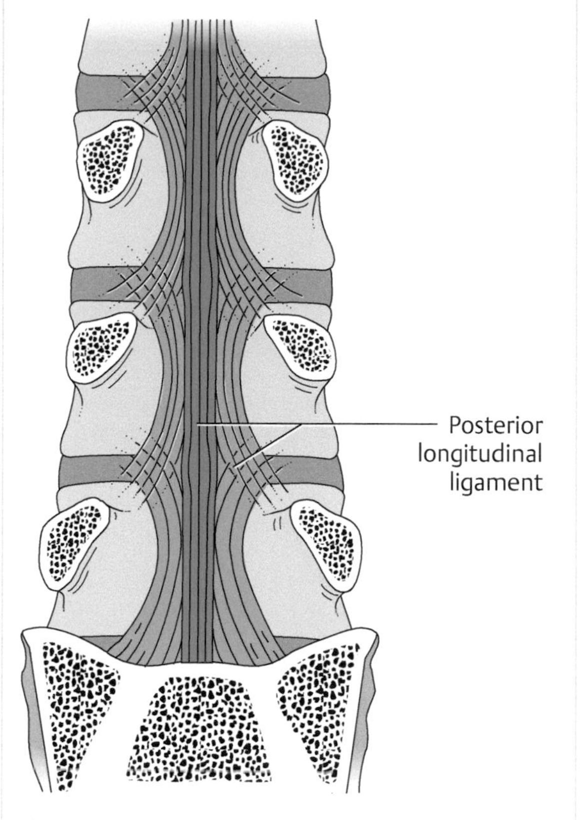


**Fig. 1.20** Posterior longitudinal ligament (posterior view, vertebral arches removed).

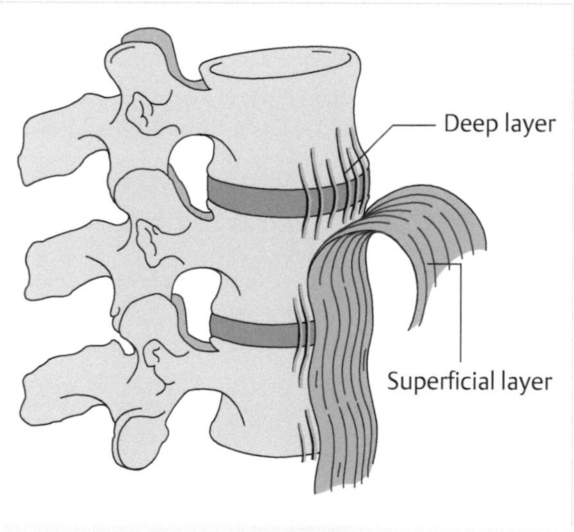


**Fig. 1.21** Anterior longitudinal ligament.

## 1.2.5 Intervertebral Disks

There are 23 intervertebral disks. Only the occiput–atlas and the atlas–axis articulations lack a disk. The disks increase in height from the cervical spine down toward the lumbar spine. They consist of a nucleus pulposus, an anulus fibrosus, and cartilage plates (end plates).

### Anulus Fibrosus (Fig. 1.22)

The outer layers consist of type I collagen fibers, which are geared to handle tensile loads. Thick fibrils are found, which are combined into fibers and arranged parallel to each other. Lesser amounts of elastic fibers are also present. The lamellae are arranged in rings, although these are not always complete, as they do not necessarily circle the entire disk, but rather merge into the adjacent lamellae. The layers are arranged in varying strengths. Anteriorly and laterally, the lamellae are thick; posteriorly, they are more subtle. Therefore the anulus is narrower posteriorly than anteriorly, and the nucleus pulposus does not lie right in the center.

The outermost lamellae of the anulus are fixed to the bony marginal ridge of the vertebral body by means of perforating fibers called *Sharpey's fibers.*

Posteriorly, the outermost layer of the anulus fibrosus merges with the posterior longitudinal ligament. Small blood vessels grow into this area, but they stay in the superficial layers and are only present in small numbers.

The nerve supply to the posterior lamellar layer is provided by the meningeal branch of the spinal nerve of the same and adjacent segments. There are no nerves within the remainder of the intervertebral disk.

### Nucleus Pulposus (Figs. 1.23 and 1.24)

Known as the core of the intervertebral disk, the nucleus pulposus is a gel-like substance that lies inside the disk. It does not have a clear-cut border with the anulus fibrosus because the outer parts of the nucleus pulposus merge with the inner elastic lamellar layer of the anulus. In the lumbar spine, it is located at the transition between the midpoint and the posterior third of the disk. It contains no blood vessels or nerves and consists of thin, elastic collagen fibrils that appear as a three-dimensional network under the microscope.

The nucleus serves as a hydroelastic buffer because its macromolecular composition, primarily of mucopolysaccharides, has the ability to bind water. In young people, the water content makes up approximately 88% of the nucleus. Over a person's lifetime, however, the fluid content diminishes, and with it the inner elasticity as well. The nucleus pulposus exerts its internal pressure outward as a force in all directions. This keeps the space between two vertebral bodies straight, but they are also clamped together by the pressure of the vertically running lamellae in the anulus.

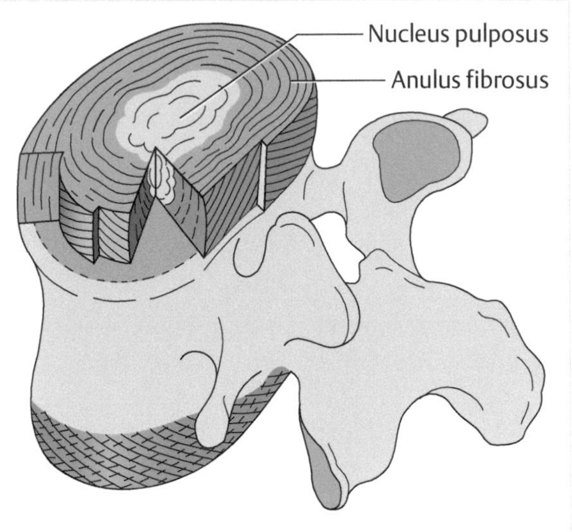


**Fig. 1.22** Fiber layers of the anulus fibrosus.

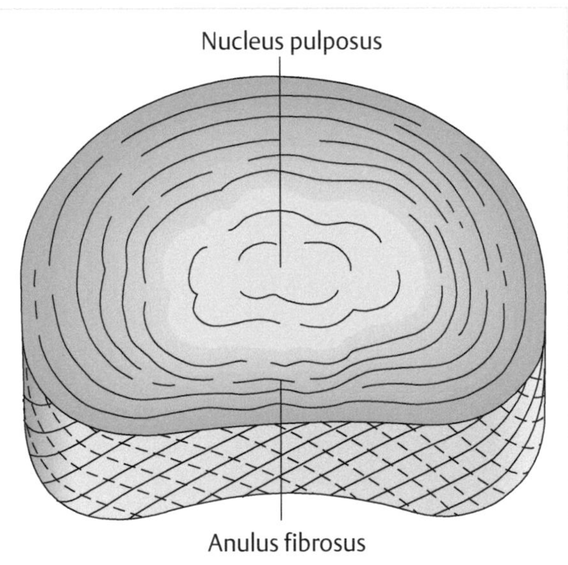


**Fig. 1.23** Intervertebral disk in transverse section.

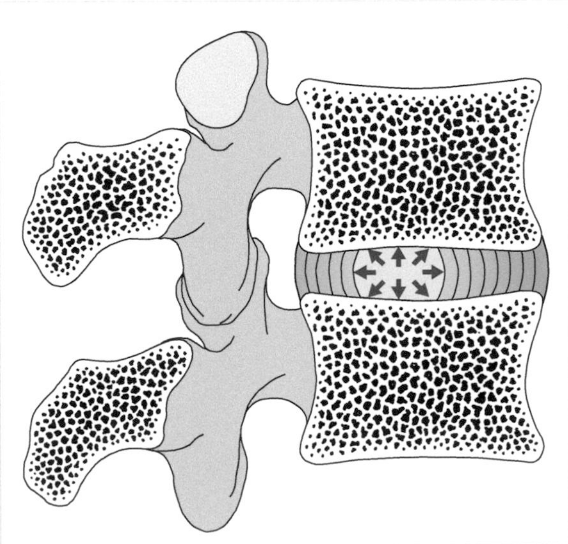

**Fig. 1.24** Nucleus pulposus. ▶

## Cartilage Plates (Fig. 1.25)

Anatomically, the inferior and superior end plates are part of the vertebral bodies, but functionally they are part of the intervertebral disks. The lamellae of the anulus continue on into the cartilage plate, adopting a horizontal course, which is why this part of the cartilage plate consists of fibrocartilage.

Extending out from the vertebral body, the end plate consists of hyaline cartilage. It is approximately 1 mm thick and ends at the inner edge of the marginal ridge of the vertebral body. In the fetus and in early childhood, the plates are heavily vascularized, but the blood vessels regress around the time that growth stops.

The cartilage plates are an important site for the diffusion of minerals from the vascularized spongiosa into the center of the disk and for the evacuation of metabolic waste products. In the center, the plate is slightly thinner—this is where most of the exchange occurs.

### Pathology

During growth, the superior end plates can undergo changes. In Scheuermann's disease, there are small gaps in ossification in the area of the vascular channels, forming a defect in the superior end plate through which the disk tissue can intrude toward the spongiosa of the vertebral body. Radiologically, these intrusions are seen as nodules known as Schmorl's nodes.

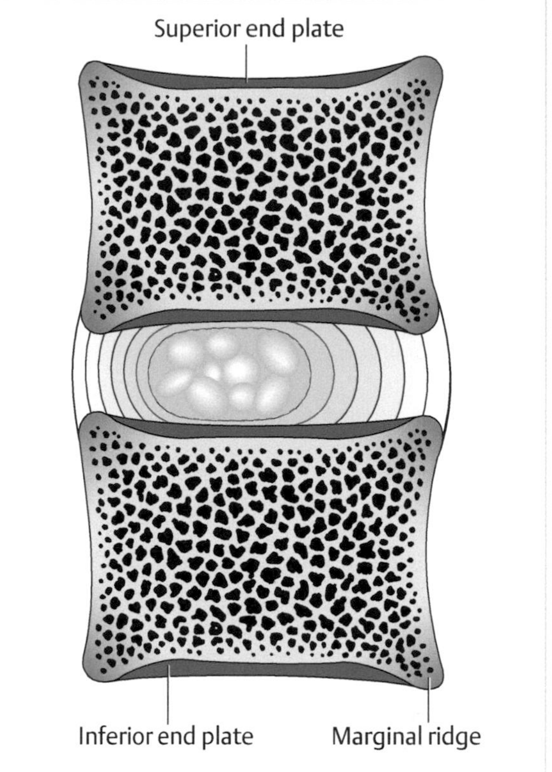


**Fig. 1.25** Cartilage plates.

## Nutrition of the Intervertebral Disks (Figs. 1.26 and 1.27)

The fluid and nutritional exchange between the intervertebral disk tissue and its surroundings occurs for the most part through the bony and cartilaginous end plate, and only minimally through the blood vessels of the outermost lamellar layer. These structures have the characteristics of a semipermeable membrane, which means that they are permeable only to certain substances.

The basic component of the ground substance of the nucleus pulposus is a macromolecular mixture of protein, carbohydrate, sodium, and calcium. This possesses a strong affinity for water and thus has a strong influence on the elasticity and degree of swelling of the nucleus pulposus. This mixture is responsible for the osmotic pressure in the disk, which counters the loading pressure that is exerted on the disk space from the outside. If the pressure acting from outside predominates, the disk releases fluid and metabolic waste products. When the pressure is reduced, the disk absorbs fluid along with important nutrients.

Because the macromolecular mix is diluted by the absorption of fluid, the absorbency of the disk decreases, and an equilibrium develops. This constitutes a protective mechanism to prevent excessive swelling of the disk. On the other hand, increasing the concentration of the mixture provides protection from its being absolutely squeezed out—here the absorbency increases and counteracts the loading pressure.

### Practical Tip

The change from disk loading to relief of loading facilitates the exchange of metabolic products, and movement distributes them to the less loaded side. Both these processes are of great importance for nourishing the disk. In the management of intervertebral disk problems, appropriate treatment measures must be selected to meet these requirements.

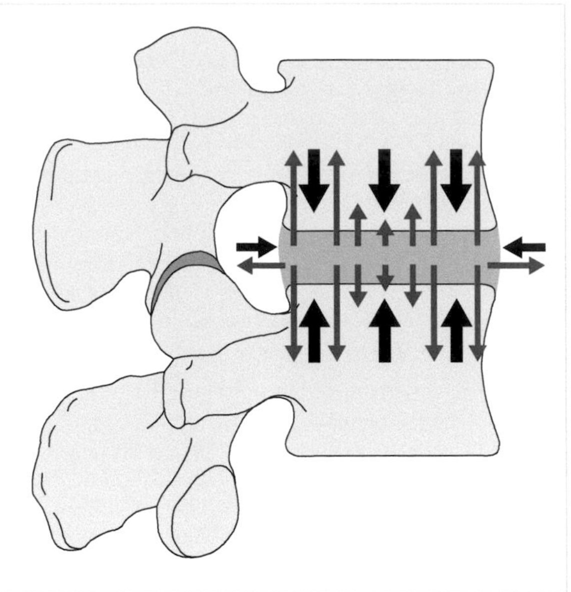

**Fig. 1.26** Release of fluid by the intervertebral disk (red arrows) when the loading pressure is high (black arrows).

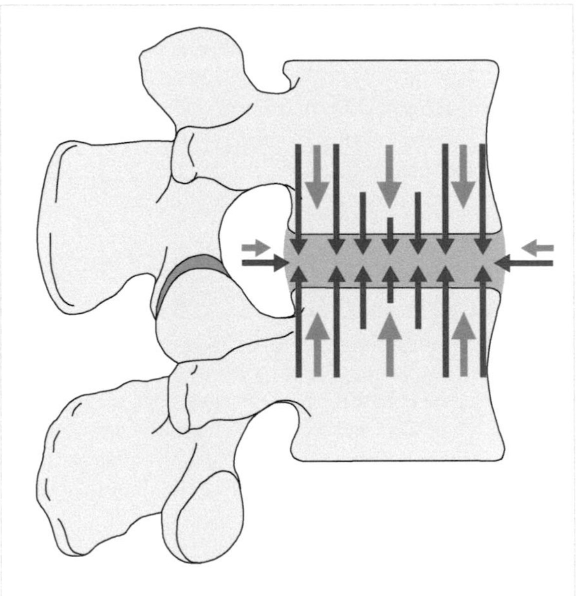

**Fig. 1.27** Absorption of fluid by the intervertebral disk (red arrows) when the loading pressure is low (gray arrows).

## Intradiskal Pressure

### Boundary Between Hydration and Dehydration (Fig. 1.28)

The boundary between fluid absorption and release lies at a disk-loading pressure of 800 N (400 kPa), the so-called intradiskal pressure. The release of fluid is termed dehydration, while the absorption of fluid is hydration. The intradiskal pressure is significantly influenced by certain body positions and exercises.

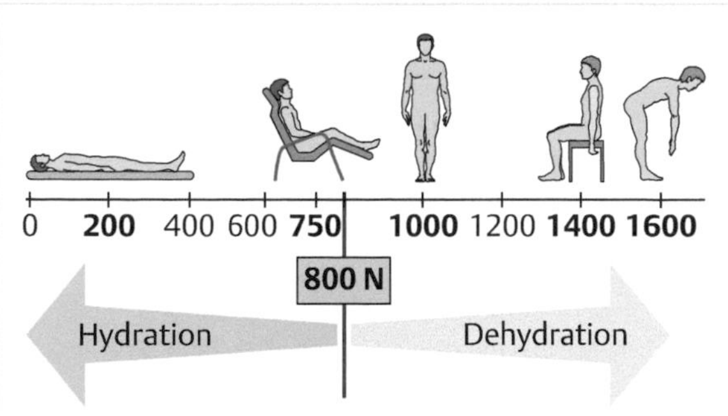


**Fig. 1.28** Boundary between hydration and dehydration.

### Pressure in Various Positions (Fig. 1.29)

Nachemson (1966) provided the first description of the interdependence between body position and intradiskal pressure ratio. His in vivo measurement of the third lumbar vertebra still has validity today. For example:

**Supine** = 250 N (125 kPa).
**Standing** = 1000 N (500 kPa).
**Sitting** = 1400 N (700 kPa).

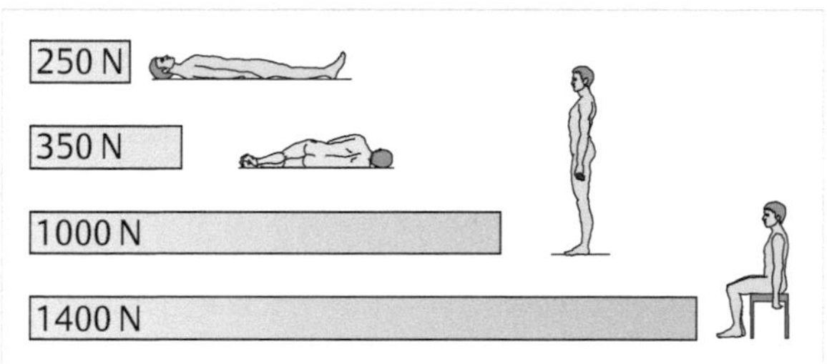


**Fig. 1.29** Intradiskal pressure in various positions.

### Pressure in Various Loading Situations (Fig. 1.30)

With a sudden tightening of the muscles when sneezing, coughing, or laughing, for example, there is a significant increase in pressure, which implies an accelerated release of fluid. The same applies to some back and abdominal muscle exercises.

The intervertebral disk has a high adaptability to mechanical pressure, so that a short increase in pressure has no significant consequences for a healthy disk.

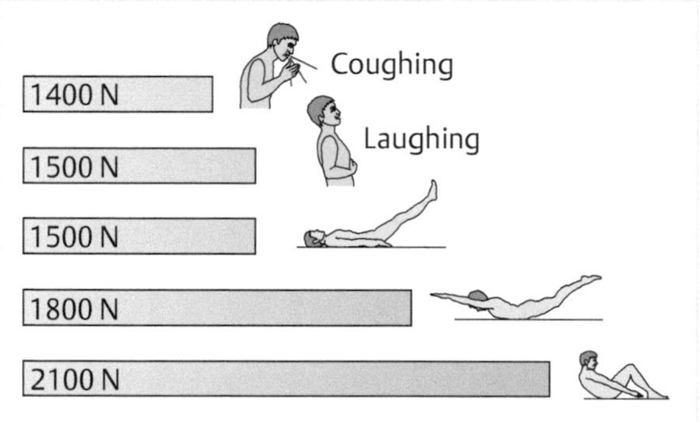


**Fig. 1.30** Intradiskal pressure increase in various loading situations.

### Changes in Disk Height

The height of the disk changes through fluid shifts, which can be demonstrated by measuring the body length in the morning and the evening. Standing, walking, and sitting during the course of the day cause a release of fluid—a loss of up to 2 cm in body length can be observed. The extent of this is dependent on the loading situation and is more pronounced in a young person than in an old person. Overnight, because of the load relief from lying down, the disk reabsorbs fluid, and the height increases.

## Loading During Lifting and Carrying (Figs. 1.31 and 1.32)

Loading of the disk can be very high during lifting and carrying. Leaning forward only 20° with a straight back raises the intradiskal pressure by 1400 N. If a weight is carried in this position, the pressure rises to three or four times the body weight.

If lifting is carried out with a rounded back, the pressure rises by seven- or eightfold. This means that posture plays a significant role during lifting. To avoid exceeding the tolerable load limit, the spinal column must be optimally positioned, i.e., with its normal physiologic curvature.

### Practical Tip

**(Fig. 1.33)**

To avoid an increased compressive load, the factors mentioned above must be considered when choosing treatment methods. As an example, when treating a person to eliminate a muscular imbalance, when the muscles are weakened, one should consider treatment modalities such as segmental stabilization using manual therapy techniques, stabilization and reversion techniques as used in PNF (proprioceptive neuromuscular facilitation) or functional abdominal and back muscle training in line with Klein-Vogelbach.

A further important goal is the acquisition of suitable behavior patterns in everyday life, such as monitoring and, if necessary, correcting the sitting posture and bending mechanics.

*Traction* of the disk space facilitates hydration. For instance, for the lumbar spine, 10–15 minutes of traction suffices to bring about significant widening and thus decompression of the disk space. Not every patient reacts positively to hydration, however. In such patients, appropriate therapy must be sought through a trial of treatment, based on historical information from the patient regarding previous relief of pain in the lying or standing position.

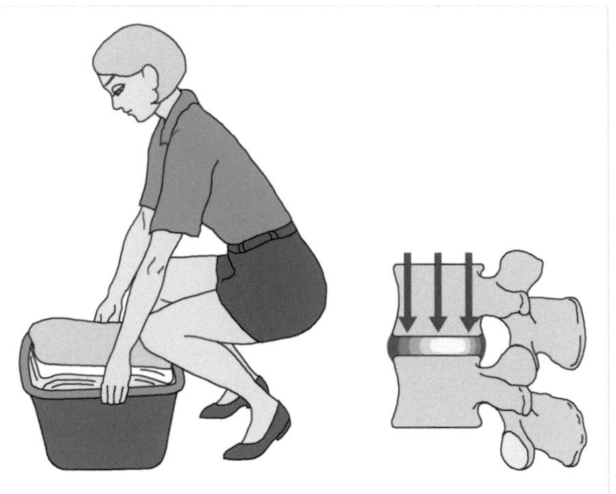

**Fig. 1.31** Loading while lifting in the physiologic position.

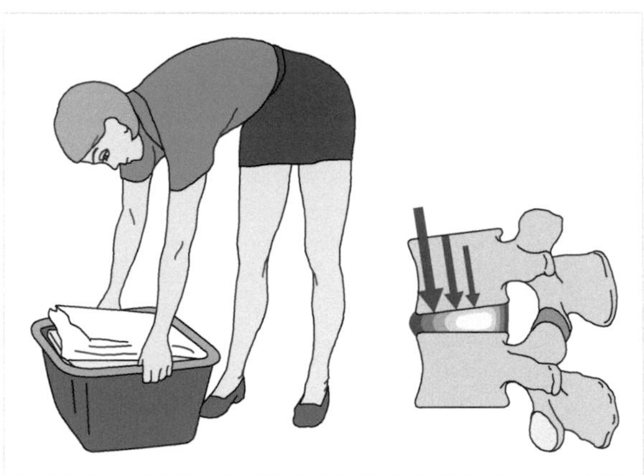

**Fig. 1.32** Loading when lifting with a rounded back.

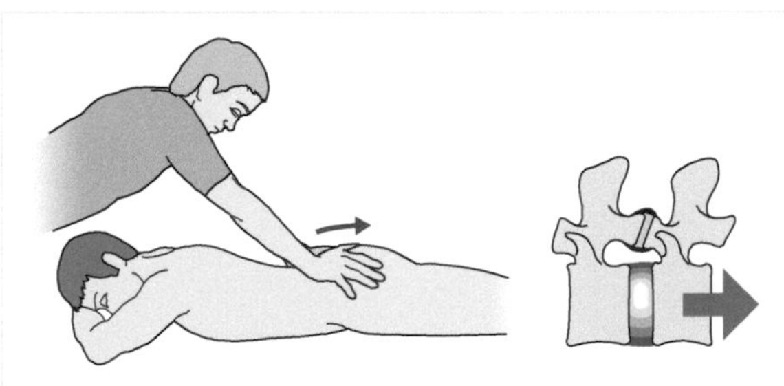

**Fig. 1.33** Traction of the disk space.

## Behavior of the Intervertebral Disk During Movements (Fig. 1.34)

Within certain limits, the inner elastic parts of the disk can shift during movement.

During flexion, the vertebral bodies tilt anteriorly, resulting in a wedge-shaped widening of the disk space posteriorly. The outer collagen fiber layers become taut posteriorly and compressed anteriorly, where they bulge out slightly. The nucleus pulposus adapts to this wedge shape and displaces posteriorly, taking the inner elastic fibers of the anulus fibrosus along with it. This displacement takes up a certain amount of time as a consequence of the viscosity and therefore the sluggishness of the nucleus pulposus. Because the posterior vertebral bodies move apart, the outer layers of the anulus quickly reach the limits of their extensibility, and the displacement process slows down. This tension therefore not only holds the vertebrae together, but also impedes any pronounced tilting, thereby slowing the movement.

During rotation, the fibers become taut, orienting themselves obliquely against the direction of rotation.

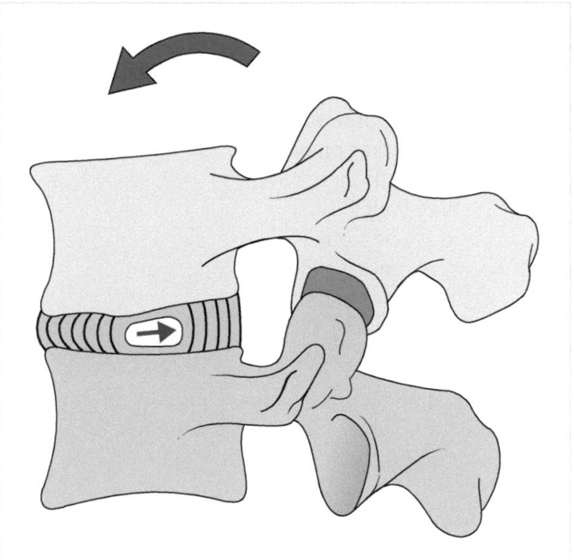

**Fig. 1.34** Behavior of the intervertebral disk during flexion.

## Axes of Motion (Fig. 1.35)

The axes of motion are dependent on how much the nucleus pulposus can be displaced, and therefore cannot be determined exactly. The axis of flexion lies within an oval in the anterior area of the disk, and that for extension lies in the posterior area. The axis for left lateral flexion is situated in the left disk section, and that for right lateral flexion in the right section of the disk. The axis for rotation lies almost in the center of the disk or possibly slightly anterior to it.

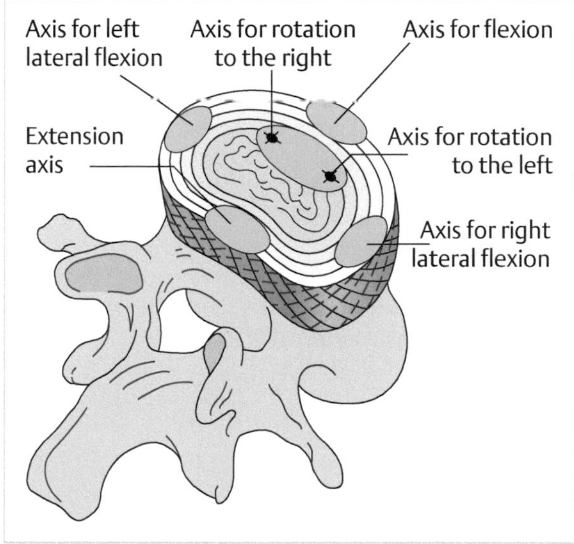


**Fig. 1.35** Axes of motion.

## Pathologic Changes

### Protrusion (Fig. 1.36)

Degeneration of the vertebral disk originates in the collagen fibers of the anulus fibrosus. Constant overloading produces tears, into which the nucleus pulposus can intrude when it is asymmetrically loaded, thus shifting the intact outer layers of the anulus fibrosus. The protrusion is the disk, which bulges out over the posterior edge of the vertebral body. The prospects for healing of a protrusion are favorable because the tissue that has bulged out can shift back again.

The pain of a protrusion is comparable to that of a prolapse because the outer layers of the anulus and the posterior longitudinal ligament are being overstretched; there are, however, no motor symptoms.

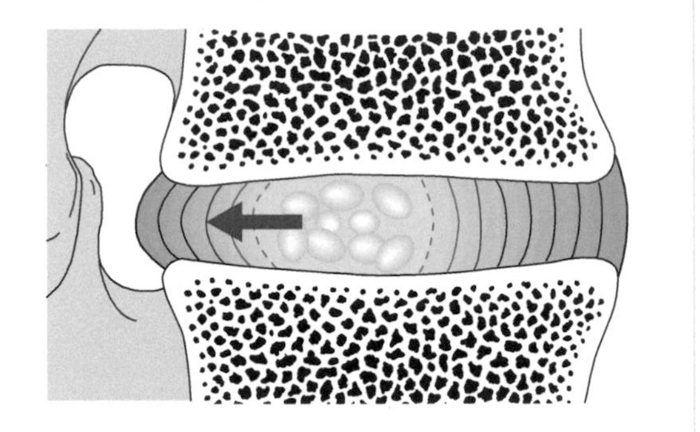

**Fig. 1.36** Protrusion.

### Prolapse (Figs. 1.37 and 1.38)

If all the fiber layers of the anulus are torn, the nucleus can penetrate toward the spinal canal or a spinal nerve. It takes part of the anulus and possibly the cartilage with it, and this constitutes a prolapse.

A medial prolapse compresses the inferiorly running nerve strands of the cauda equina, disrupting very important motor functions. The patient might lose control of bowel and urinary function. Therefore immediate surgery is required if cauda equina syndrome is present.

Prolapse in a posterolateral direction presses against the spinal nerve and, depending on the position of the prolapse, can push the spinal nerve either medially or laterally. To decrease the pressure on the nerve root and thus decrease the pain, the patient assumes a position in which least compression occurs. This is a "forced posture," which the patient can abandon only at the cost of severe pain.

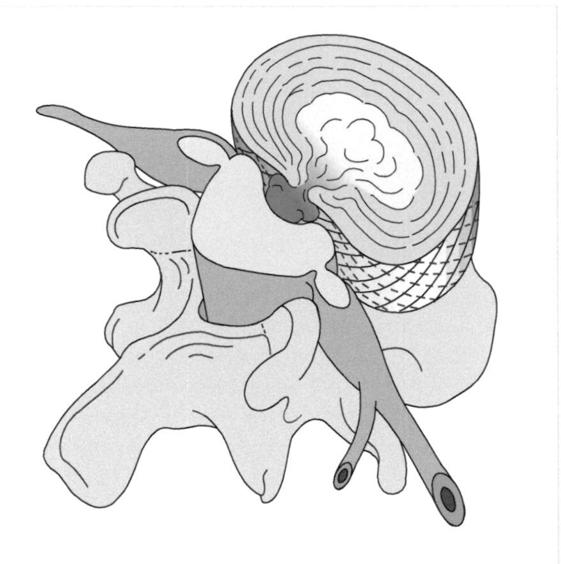

**Fig. 1.37** Medial prolapse.

> **Practical Tip**
>
> In the case of a prolapse, the position of comfort should never be corrected in the acute phase.

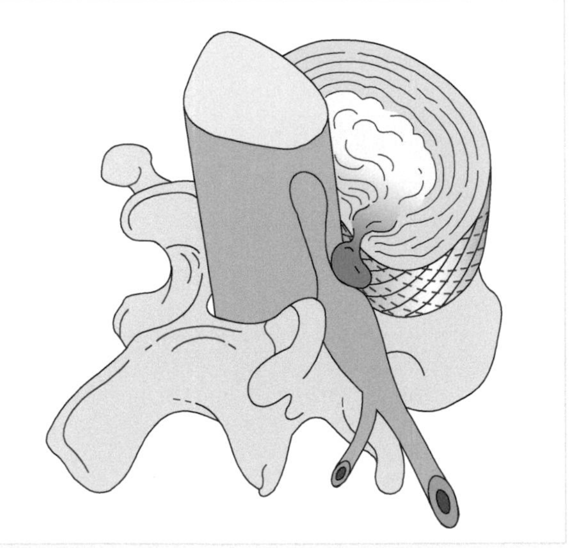

**Fig. 1.38** Posterolateral prolapse.

### Pain Patterns in Localizing a Prolapse

If the prolapse lies beneath the nerve's point of exit, in the "axilla" of the nerve, the pain increases on lateral flexion to the opposite side. Therefore the patient will tilt toward the side of the prolapse to relieve the pressure on the nerve and decrease the pain (**Fig. 1.39**).

If the prolapse lies above the nerve's exit point (on its "shoulder"), the pain is worsened by bending to the side of the prolapse, while bending to the opposite side brings relief of the pain (**Fig. 1.40**).

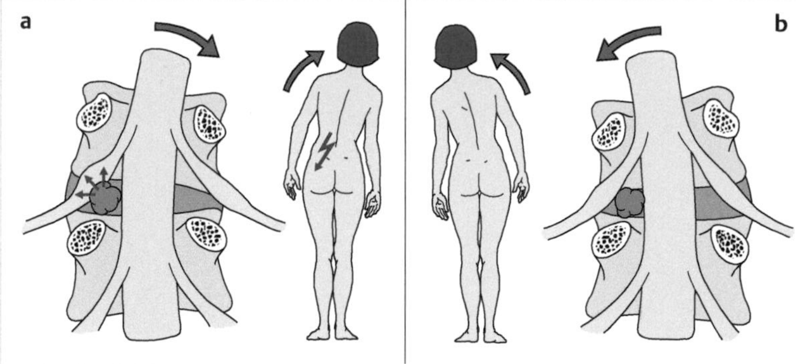


**Fig. 1.39** Prolapse localized inferior to the nerve's exit point. **(a)** Provocation of pain. **(b)** Alleviation of pain.

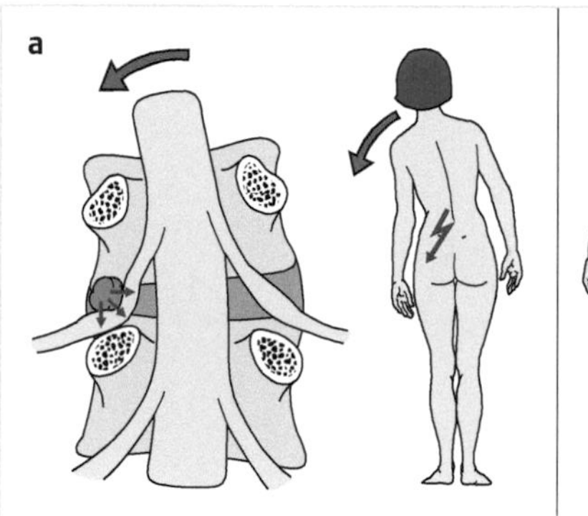


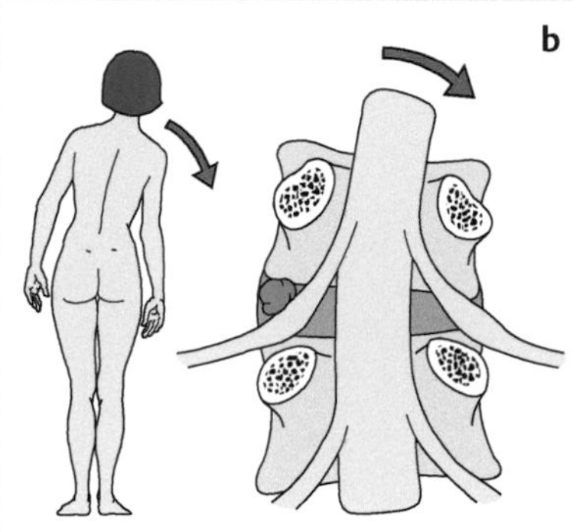


**Fig. 1.40** Prolapse localized superior to the nerve's exit point. **(a)** Provocation of pain. **(b)** Alleviation of pain.

## Results of Intervertebral Disk Degeneration (Fig. 1.41)

In a disk with degenerative changes, the diffusion process is disturbed, the turgor of the nucleus pulposus decreases, and the uniform distribution of pressure and with it the adaptability to the varying loading situations are lost. The results are narrowing of the disk space, increased pressure on the zygapophysial joints, and the formation of marginal osteophytes (spondylophytes, marginal bone spurs) that are more or less prominent and extend from the margins of the vertebral bodies.

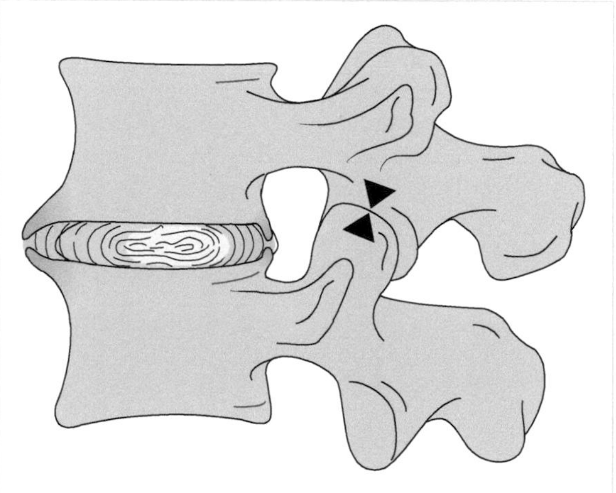

**Fig. 1.41** Results of intervertebral disk degeneration.

### Practical Tip

After the intervertebral disk tissue has torn, regeneration begins, which conforms to the usual process of wound healing. Final healing should be expected to take 1 year. During this time, it should be noted that, in the acute phase, which lasts about 1 week, the disk must be unburdened, meaning bed rest. After that, because of the positive effect of motion on nutrition, cautious mobilization is started. Over time, and with careful observation of the patient's symptoms, alternating load-bearing is incorporated to stimulate diffusion activity.

# Chapter 2

## Cranium and Cervical Spine



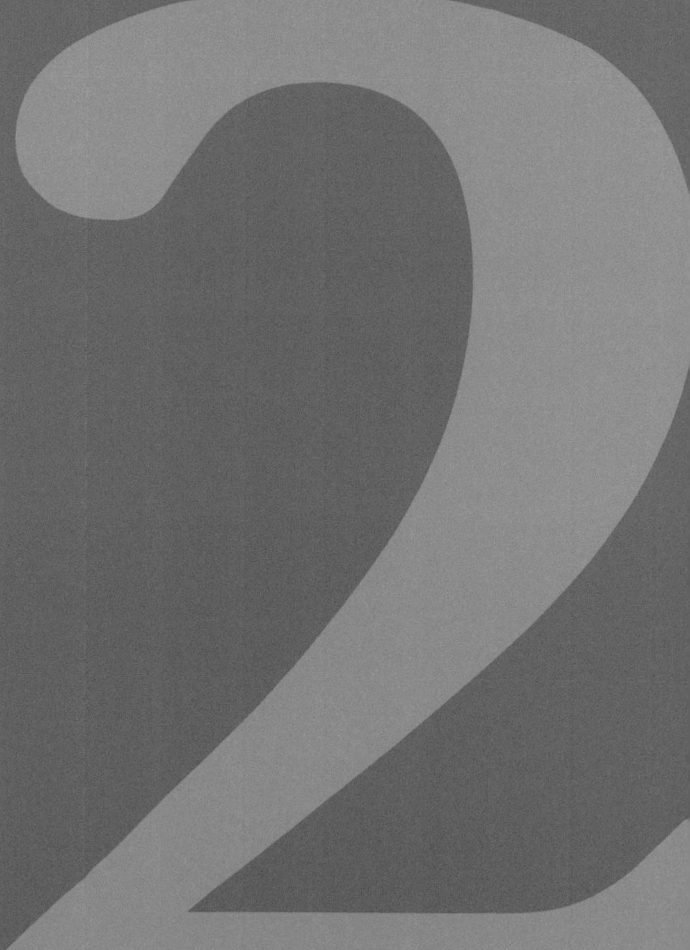

# 2 Cranium and Cervical Spine

## 2.1 Palpation of Landmarks on the Cranium (Skull) and Cervical Spine

▷ Bones, Ligaments, Joints

### External Occipital Protuberance (Fig. 2.1)

This can be found as a distinct prominence in the midline in the occipital region.

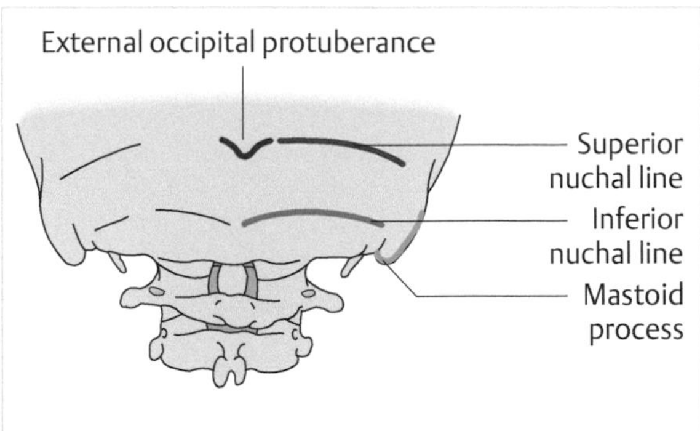


**Fig. 2.1** Palpation of the cranium: bony structures.

### Superior Nuchal Line (Fig. 2.1)

From the protuberance, the superior nuchal line extends to the right and left. It is a small ridge that runs laterally on both sides and is slightly curved, with the convex side upward.

It serves as the origin or insertion point for the superficial neck muscles:

- Medially: trapezius muscle.
- Laterally: sternocleidomastoid muscle.

### Mastoid Process (Fig. 2.1)

The mastoid process is found as a clearly projecting prominence at the lateral end of the superior nuchal line. It serves as the insertion site for the sternocleidomastoid muscle. The ear serves as a further point of reference: the mastoid process is located immediately posterior to the earlobe.

### Inferior Nuchal Line (Figs. 2.1 and 2.2)

The inferior nuchal line runs parallel to and about two fingerbreadths inferior to the superior nuchal line. It is the origin or insertion for the following muscles:

- Medially and slightly superiorly: the semispinalis capitis muscle.
- From medially to laterally: the rectus capitis posterior minor, rectus capitis posterior major, and obliquus capitis superior muscles.
- At the lateral end, toward the mastoid process: the longissimus capitis and splenius capitis muscles.

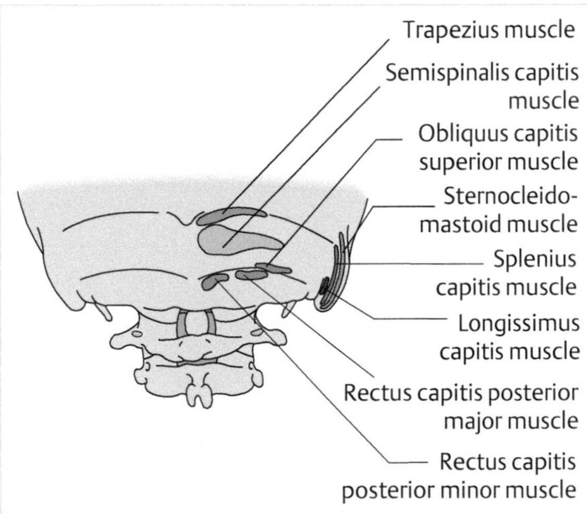


**Fig. 2.2** Palpation of the cranium: muscle insertion points.

> **Practical Tip**
>
> When palpating over the lateral aspect of the nuchal line, trigger points in the upper cervical spine must be differentiated from tendinitis. These trigger points are indicators of a malposition of the C0–C1 zygapophysial joints.

## Temporomandibular Joint (Fig. 2.3)

One can palpate the head of the mandible anterior to the external auditory canal, especially with the mouth closed, because the mandibular head disappears anteriorly when the mouth is opened. Direct comparison of the right and left joints with the mouth opened and closed and during side-to-side movement of the jaw provides information on any asymmetries.

## Coronoid Process (Fig. 2.3)

With the mouth closed, the coronoid process is located behind the zygomatic arch and is therefore not palpable. When the mouth is open, it moves anteriorly out from under the outer part of the zygomatic arch. The insertion site for the temporalis muscle is located here.

## Masseteric Tuberosity (Fig. 2.4)

The insertion site of the masseter muscle is located on the outside of the angle of the mandible and can be palpated at its lower margin when the mouth is closed.

## Transverse Process of C1 (Fig. 2.5)

The transverse process of the first cervical vertebra lies slightly below the mastoid process and directly posterior to the ascending ramus of the mandible. As the transverse process is the origin and insertion point for many muscles, it can be felt as a distinct bulge when palpating deeply.

The transverse processes of the other cervical vertebrae are palpable only by using considerable pressure because of the overlying soft tissue.

### Practical Tip

Palpation of the transverse process allows the position of C1 to be determined and pain and swelling to be assessed. In cases of rotational malalignment, the transverse process on one side is very thick and is palpable further posteriorly than usual, while on the other side it is displaced anteromedially behind the ramus of the mandible.

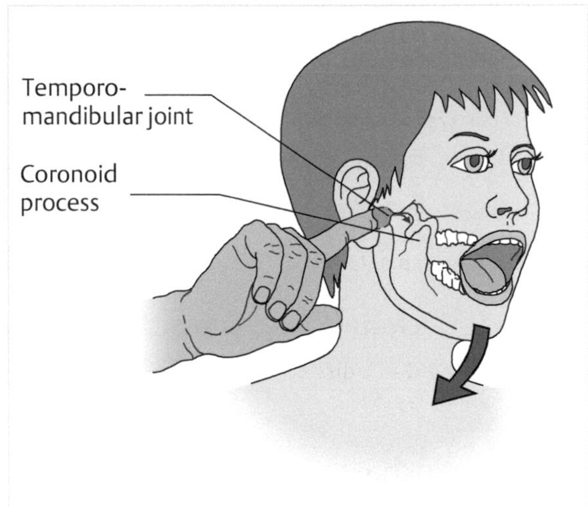


**Fig. 2.3** Palpation of the temporomandibular joint.

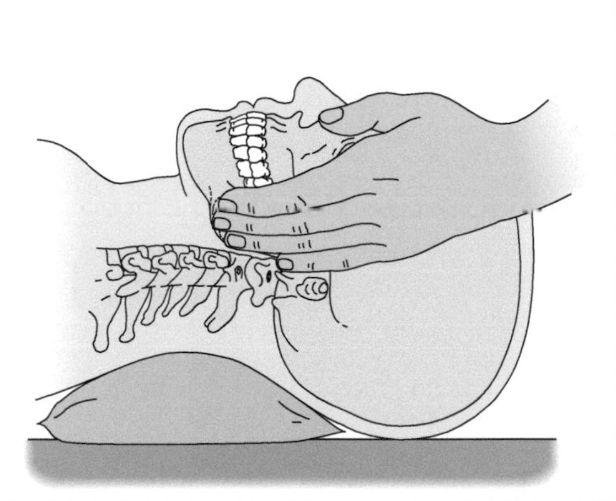

**Fig. 2.4** Palpation of the masseteric tuberosity.

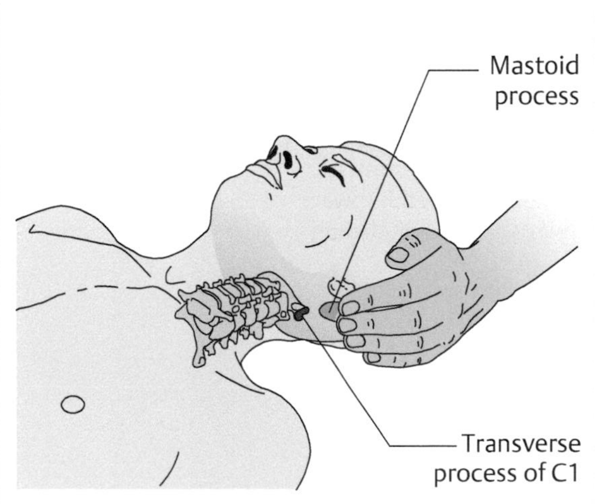


**Fig. 2.5** Palpation of the transverse process.

## Spinous Process (Fig. 2.6)

Inferior to the external occipital protuberance and just below the skull lies a concavity in which a distinct elevation can be palpated—the spinous process of C2.

The other spinous processes are split and more difficult to find. Only that of C7 protrudes prominently, as implied by its name—vertebra prominens.

When in doubt as to which of the protruding spinous processes is C7, place the index, middle, and ring fingers on three adjacent spinous processes at the cervicothoracic junction, and have the patient move very slowly through maximal extension. The spinous process of C6 disappears under the palpating finger, while the one that remains palpable is C7.

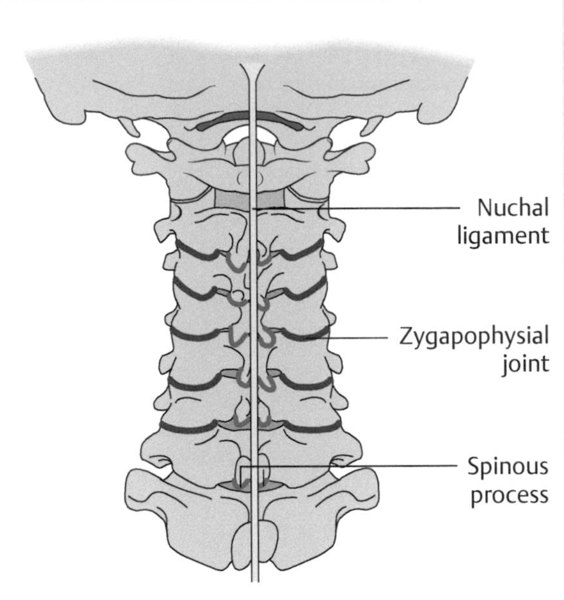


**Fig. 2.6** Palpation of the spinous process and nuchal ligament.

## Nuchal Ligament (Fig. 2.6)

This ligament extends from the external occipital protuberance to C7 and can be clearly felt between the spinous processes. Flexing the neck stretches the ligament, facilitating its palpation.

## Intervertebral Joints (Fig. 2.7)

The C2–C3 zygapophysial joint can be palpated as a small elevation at the same height as the spinous process of C2 and about two fingerbreadths laterally. The other zygapophysial joints can be found at the level of the corresponding spinous processes.

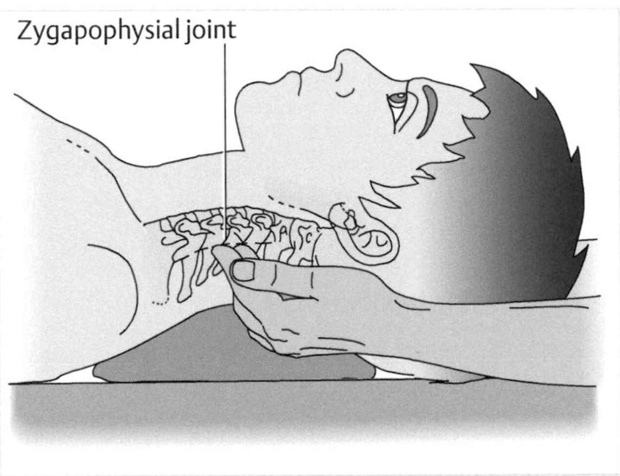


**Fig. 2.7** Palpation of the zygapophysial joint.

### Practical Tip

Tenderness and swelling are often found on the side that is blocked.

## Hyoid Bone (Fig. 2.8)

The hyoid bone with its paired *greater horns* is palpable directly below the mandible toward the neck and feels like a horseshoe clasp. It should be movable to the same degree to right and left.

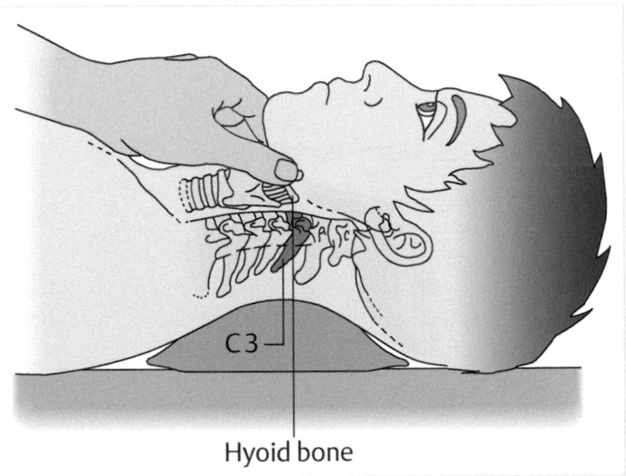


**Fig. 2.8** Palpation of the hyoid bone.

## Carotid Artery (Fig. 2.9)

The carotid pulse can be felt at the anterior border of the sternocleidomastoid muscle, approximately at the midpoint of the muscle.

▷ Muscles

The entire length of a muscle, from its origin to its insertion, should be palpated. The following are evaluated:

- Circumscribed points of pain.
- The presence of sites of tension.
- Areas of swelling.

Palpation is carried out with two or three fingers, both along and across the course of the fibers, using more or less pressure, depending on the location of the muscle.

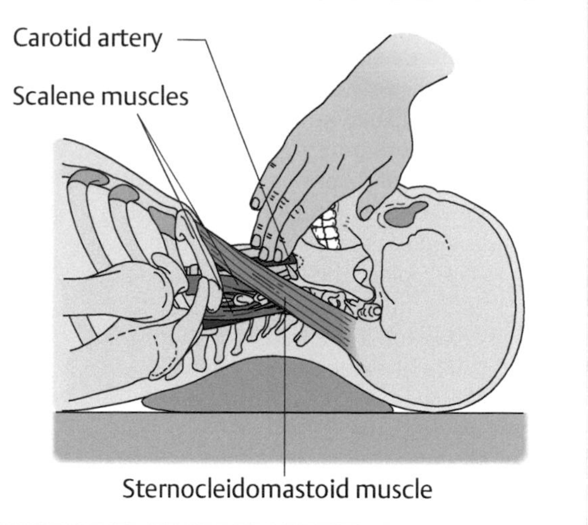


**Fig. 2.9** Palpation of the carotid artery.

## Trapezius Muscle (Fig. 2.10)

This muscle extends from the external occipital protuberance, the superior nuchal line, the nuchal ligament, and the tips of the spinous processes of T1–T12 to the lateral third of the clavicle, the acromion, and the spine of the scapula.

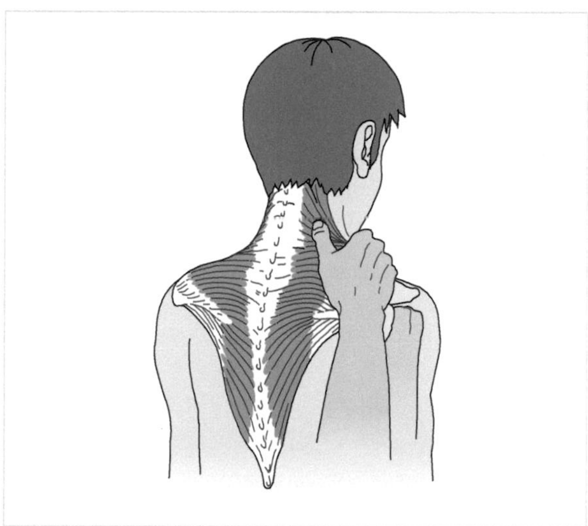

**Fig. 2.10** Palpation of the trapezius muscle.

## Levator Scapulae Muscle (Fig. 2.11)

The point of origin of levator scapulae on the transverse process is not palpable. It is only clearly definable at its insertion site on the superior angle of the scapula, where it often demonstrates trigger points and areas of tension.

## Splenius Capitis Muscle (Fig. 2.11)

Although the muscle belly is for the most part covered by the trapezius muscle, it can be defined in the depths through its course from the mastoid process and the superior nuchal line inferomedially toward the spinous processes of C3–T3.

## Splenius Cervicis Muscle (Fig. 2.11), Semispinalis Capitis Muscle, Longissimus Cervicis Muscle, Longissimus Capitis Muscle, Iliocostalis Cervicis Muscle

These muscles lie deep within the tissues and are not accessible for detailed palpation; instead, they are felt as a cord of muscle that, for the most part, runs parallel to the spinal column.

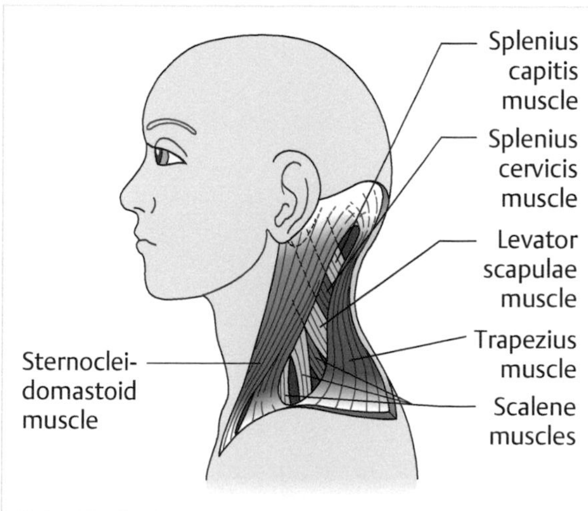


**Fig. 2.11** Palpation of the deep muscles of the neck.

## Sternocleidomastoid Muscle (Fig. 2.12)

From its wide insertion site on the mastoid process and the superior nuchal line, this muscle runs inferiorly and anteriorly toward the sternum. Its sternal origin is located medial to the sternoclavicular joint. The clavicular origin occupies the medial third of the clavicle, and a gap can be felt between the two insertions.

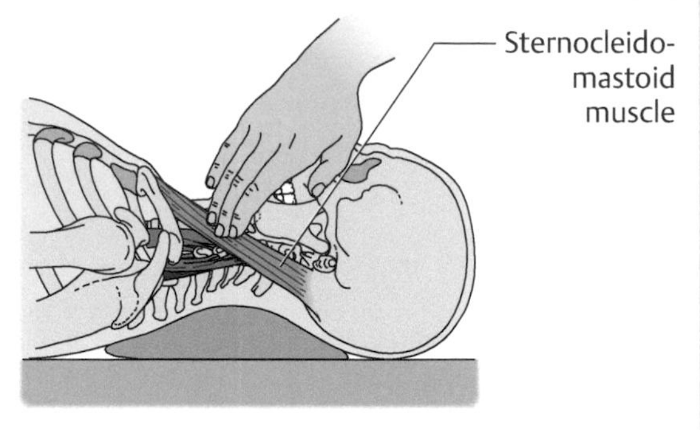


**Fig. 2.12** Palpation of the sternocleidomastoid muscle.

## Scalene Muscles (Fig. 2.13)

The origins of the anterior and middle scalene muscles on the transverse processus of C3–C7 are accessible from an anterior approach by palpating deeply to the right and left of the trachea while the patient tenses toward lateral flexion. The insertions on the first rib are palpable posterior to the clavicle and the sternocleidomastoid muscle.

The posterior scalene muscle runs directly in front of the border of the trapezius and is in part overlain by it.

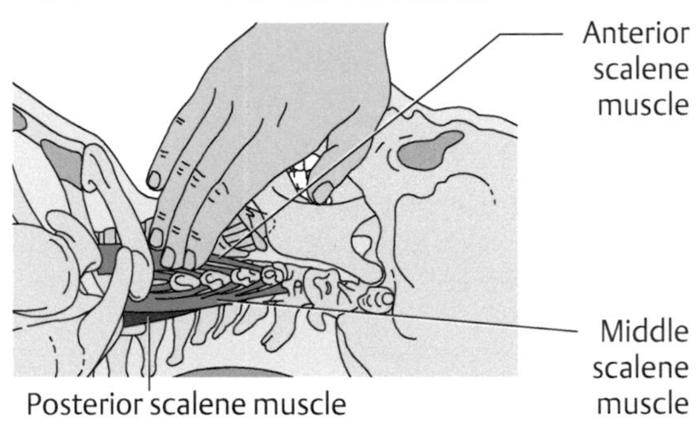


**Fig. 2.13** Palpation of the scalene muscles.

## Longus Colli Muscle

The upper part is potentially palpable superiorly between the sternocleidomastoid muscle and the larynx. The other parts run posterior to the larynx and trachea and are overlain by the scalene muscles.

## Temporalis Muscle (Fig. 2.14)

This runs from the temporal fossa to the coronoid process of the mandible. It can be palpated at its insertion when the mouth is opened, and in the fossa when the mouth is firmly closed.

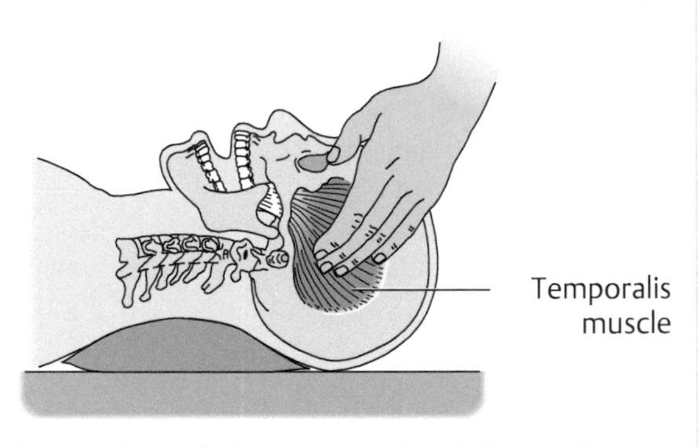


**Fig. 2.14** Palpation of the temporalis muscle.

## Masseter Muscle (Fig. 2.15)

This is a thick, almost rectangular muscle bundle in the area of the angle of the mandible that is easy to palpate, even with a slightly open mouth. When the mouth is closed, it protrudes as a thick muscular bulge.

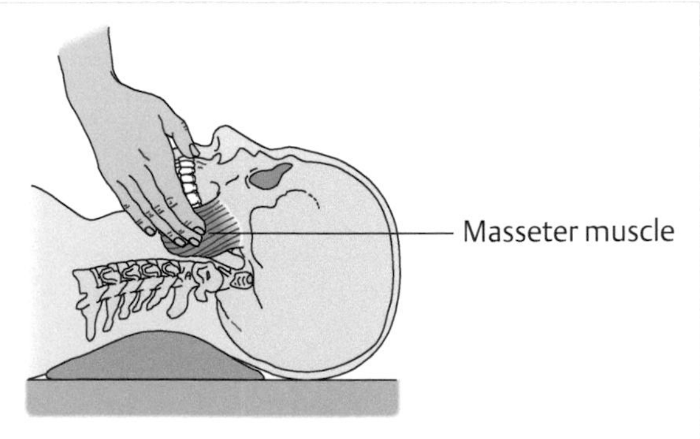


**Fig. 2.15** Palpation of the masseter muscle.

## Digastric Muscle (Fig. 2.16)

This muscle can be palpated on the mastoid process in front of the sternocleidomastoid muscle while opening the mouth. It is also palpable further toward the inner side of the tip of the chin, parallel to the lower jaw.

## Mylohyoid Muscle (Fig. 2.16)

This muscle occupies the entire mandibular floor and can be located while opening the mouth while palpating upward toward the floor of the mouth from below.

## Medial Pterygoid Muscle (Fig. 2.16)

This muscle is palpable during mouth closure at its insertion site on the inner surface of the angle of the mandible. Further palpation superomedially is not possible.

## Lateral Pterygoid Muscle (Fig. 2.17)

Palpation is possible only from within the mouth. The procedure is as follows: palpate from behind the upper molar toward the neck of the mandible, and have the patient open the mouth a little more and then gently open and close it slightly. The tightening of the muscle can be felt as the mouth opens.

### Practical Tip

A functional disturbance in the upper cervical spine region is suggested by the occurrence of trigger points in the neck and throat muscles with pains radiating toward the occiput and temporal area that intensify with pressure on the trigger points.

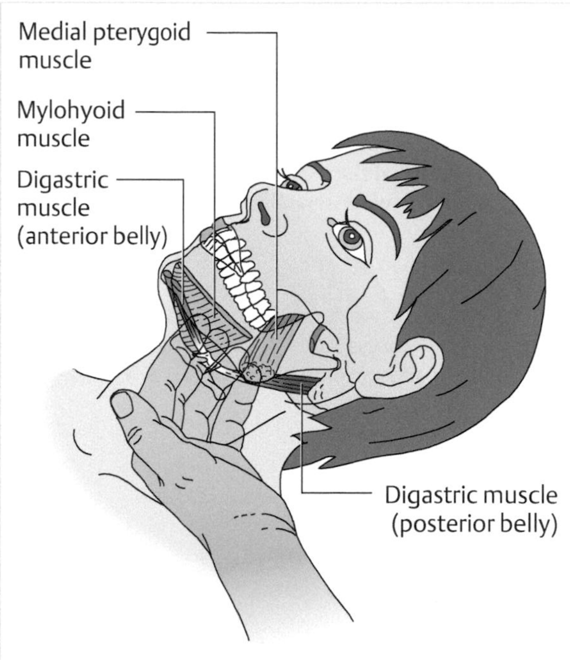


**Fig. 2.16** Palpation of the mylohyoid, medial pterygoid, and digastric muscles.

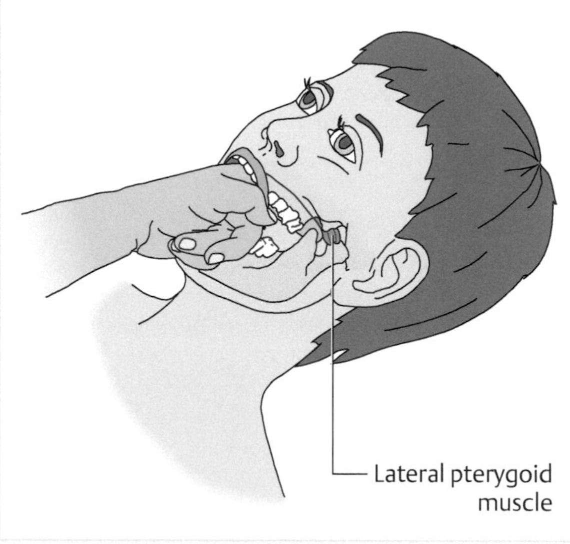


**Fig. 2.17** Palpation of the lateral pterygoid muscle.

# 2.2 Functional Anatomy of the Cranium

## 2.2.1 Bony Components

The cranium is divided into facial and cerebral parts, the *viscerocranium* (facial skeleton) and the *neurocranium* (brain box) respectively.

### Viscerocranium (Fig. 2.18)

1 = Nasal bones
2 = Lacrimal bones
3 = Ethmoid
4 = Zygomatic bones
5 = Maxillae
6 = Mandible
Vomer
Palatine bones
Hyoid bone

### Neurocranium (Fig. 2.18)

7 = Occipital bone
8 = Parietal bones
9 = Temporal bones
10 = Sphenoid
11 = Frontal bone

The cranial base joins the viscerocranium to the neurocranium as well as forming the connection to the cervical spinal column.

### Cranial Sutures (Fig. 2.19)

The bony parts of the cranium are joined together by the cranial sutures. Collagen fibrils, which are found in the gaps between the sutures, form the outer layer and merge with the periosteum of the cranium. Moving inward, there is fibrous connective tissue as well as individual bony bridges, blood vessels, nerves, and receptors.

The sutures are variable in form:

- The **sagittal suture** between the parietal bones is wide and has very pronounced serrations.
- The **lambdoid suture**, which joins the occipital bone to the parietal bones, has shorter serrations.
- The **temporoparietal suture** runs obliquely inward. It is also called the *squamous suture*.

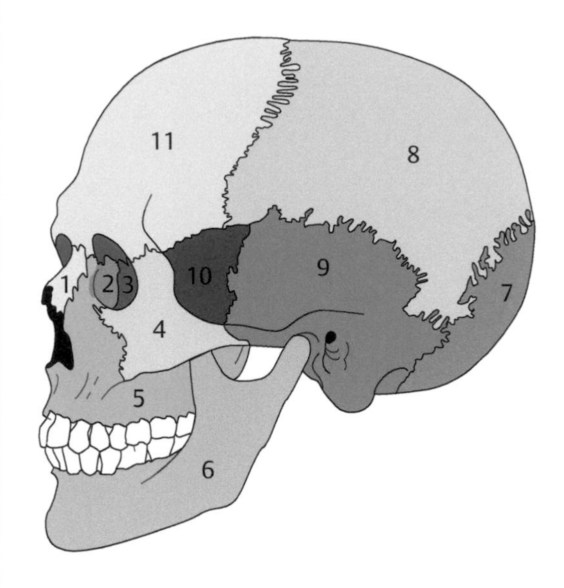


**Fig. 2.18** Bones of the cranium.

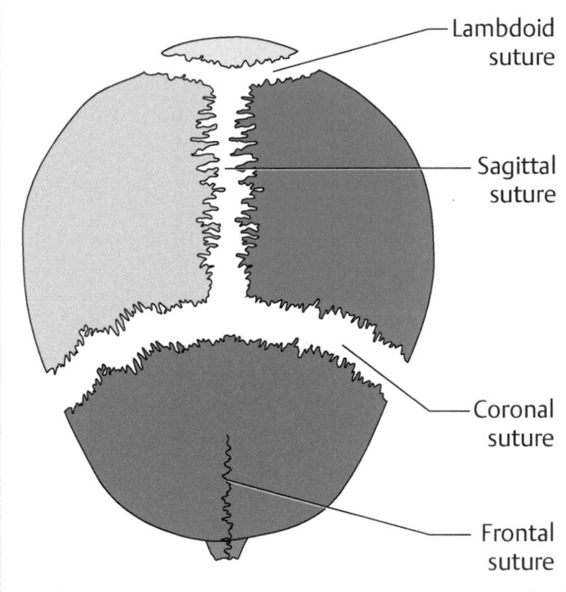


**Fig. 2.19** The sutures.

## 2.2.2 Meninges of the Brain

### Cranial Dura Mater (Fig. 2.20)

- The dura mater is a "tough skin for the brain."
- It lines the inner surface of the cranial cavity and consists of two layers. The outer layer also serves as the periosteum of the cranium. The inner layer follows the contours of the brain and is duplicated in various areas.
- Duplications include the **falx cerebri** between the two cerebral hemispheres, the **falx cerebelli**, as a continuation of the falx cerebri in the furrow between the cerebellar hemispheres, and the **tentorium cerebelli**, which divides the occipital lobe from the cerebellum. These consist of firm bundles of collagen fibers whose alignment in part follows the outline of the cranium and in part is longitudinally oriented.
- The falx and the tentorium represent an important support system not only in a longitudinal direction, but also transversely.
- The **dural venous sinuses** are found within the dura mater. They conduct the venous blood away from the brain to the internal jugular vein.
- The dura contains receptors to monitor pain sensitivity and changes in pressure.

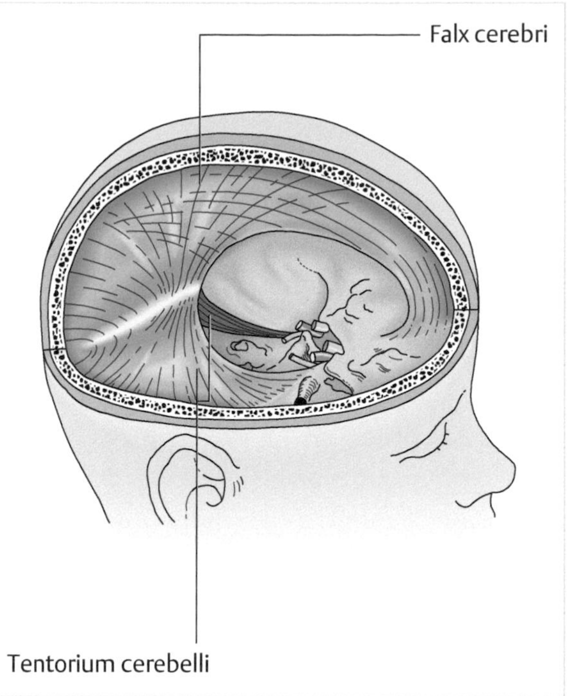


**Fig. 2.20** Cranial dura mater.

### Leptomeninx

- This is "a soft skin for the brain."
- It consists of an outer layer, the **arachnoid mater**, and an inner layer, the **cranial pia mater**.
- It rests on the surface of the brain and follows all its convolutions and recesses.
- The **subarachnoid space** lies between the two layers and is filled with cerebrospinal fluid (CSF). In several locations, there are large openings, the subarachnoid cisterns.

## 2.2.3 Cerebrospinal Fluid (Fig. 2.21)

- There is approximately 100–150 mL of CSF in total.
- Produced in the choroid plexus, it renews itself up to three times per day.
- Resorption occurs through the semipermeable membranes of the arachnoid granulations (villi). The pressure of the CSF plays a part here, and is itself influenced by the venous pressure.
- The CSF pressure is approximately 150 mm $H_2O$. It varies with position (e.g., lying or sitting) and by location (cranial or caudal).
- It contains only about five cells per mL but no protein.

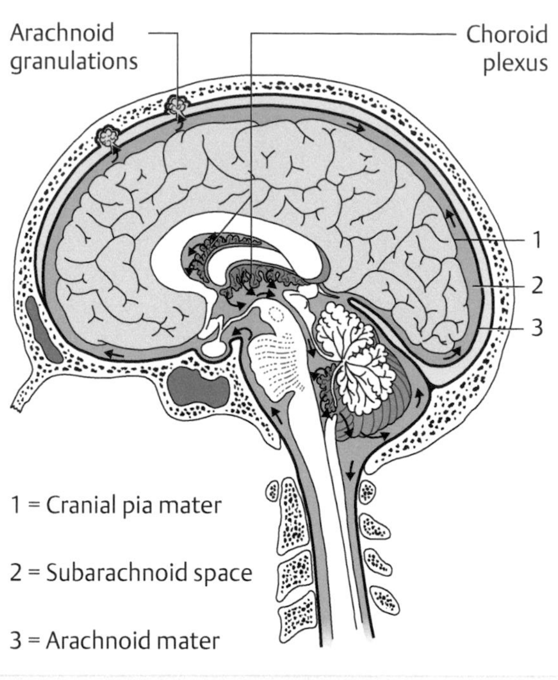


**Fig. 2.21** Dynamics of the cerebrospinal fluid.

## 2.2.4 Mobility of the Cranium (Skull)

The cranium is not a rigid structure but an elastic tissue. Each bone of the cranium has a minimal specific movement with a rhythmic impulse; the normal frequency is about 10 to 14 impulses per minute. The sutures function here as expansion joints. The direction of movement is dependent on the orientation and shape of the suture, in that the bones diverge and converge.

**Practical Tip**

(**Fig. 2.22**)
When there is restriction in the movement of the sutures, osteopathic mobilization of the cranium revives the innate mobility of the structure.
The cranial dura mater is fixed circumferentially to the foramen magnum and transitions here to the spinal dura mater, which attaches to the posterior aspects of the vertebrae from C1 and C2 downward. It first attaches to the anterior side of the vertebrae from S2. This sacral–cranial connection substantiates the treatment of both areas when there are disturbances.

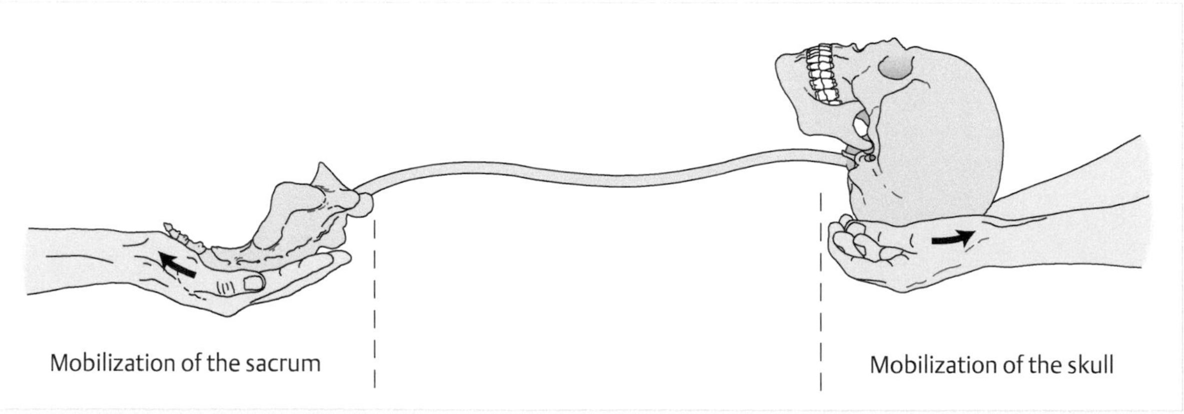


**Fig. 2.22** Mobilization of the cranium and sacrum.

## 2.2.5 Temporomandibular Joint

### Mandible (Fig. 2.23)

#### Ramus of the Mandible

- The *coronoid process* serves as an insertion for the temporal muscle.
- The *condylar process* and the neck of the mandible, on the inner side of the pterygoid fovea, serve as the insertion for the lateral pterygoid muscle.
- The joint surface on the *head of the mandible* is cylindrical and convexly formed in both axes. The axis runs from anterolateral to posteromedial.

#### Body of the Mandible

- The *alveolar part*, with the dental alveoli to anchor the roots of the teeth, forms in the areas where there is less functional strain, such as in the gaps between the teeth.
- The *base of the mandible* contains the mental foramen for passage of the mental nerve and vessels.
- The *digastric fossa* on the inner side is the insertion point for the digastric muscle.

#### Angle of the Mandible

- The *masseteric tuberosity* on the outer side serves as the insertion for the masseter muscle.
- The *pterygoid tuberosity* on the inner side is the insertion point of the medial pterygoid muscle.
- In infants, the angle of the mandible forms an angle of 140°. This decreases secondary to loading from chewing to approximately 120°, and in toothless jaws it can increase again.

### Joint Surface on the Temporal Bone

#### Mandibular Fossa (Fig. 2.24)

- The joint surface on the temporal bone is concave. It is bordered anteriorly by the *articular tubercle*.
- The posterior part lies outside the capsule and forms the lateral wall of the external auditory canal.
- The fossa is 2 to 3 times larger than the joint surface on the head of the mandible.
- The shape of the joint that is formed depends on its loading. In infants, it is flat. It deepens when the permanent teeth erupt, and flattens again in toothless jaws.

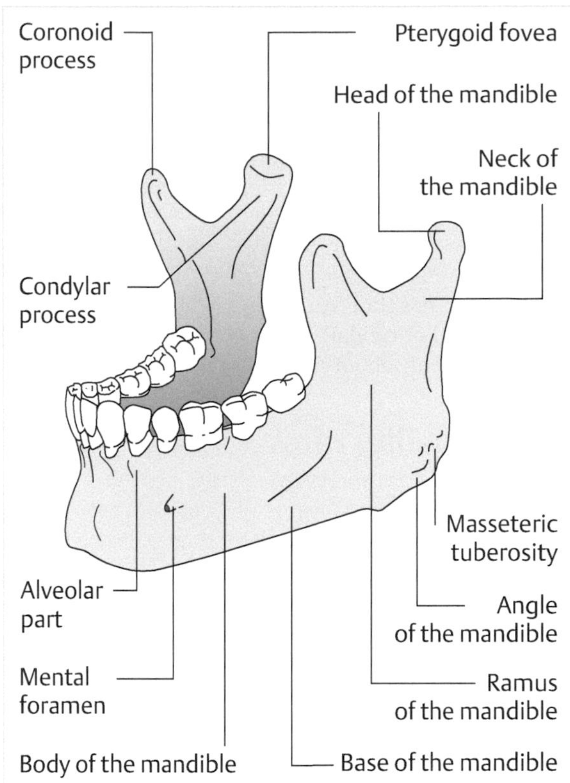


**Fig. 2.23** Mandible.

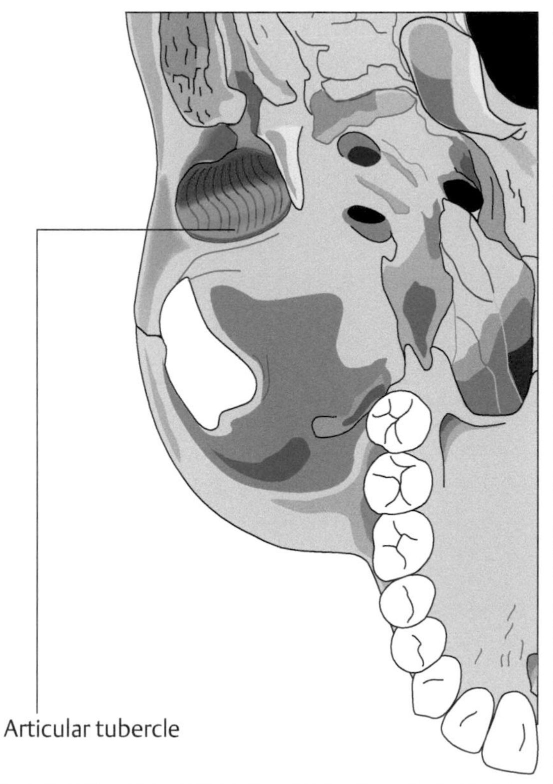


**Fig. 2.24** Mandibular fossa.

## Articular Disk (Fig. 2.25)

The disk consists of firm collagenous connective tissue and fibrocartilage. The fibers are aligned three-dimensionally in the anteroposterior, mediolateral, and superoinferior directions. Because of this, the disk can absorb significant force.

The disk lies between the mandibular fossa, the posterior part of the articular tubercle, and the head of the mandible. Its anterior portion is thin. Fibers of the lateral pterygoid muscle track into it at this point. In contrast, it is significantly thicker posteriorly. The two sections are separated from each other by a connective tissue constriction that is shaped like an hourglass. The posterior portion of the posterior disk is called the **bilaminar zone.** Superiorly, this consists of elastic connective tissue, while the part extending to the head of the mandible consists of fibrous tissue. A retroarticular pad attaches to this zone posteriorly, and only beyond that does the fibrous layer close the joint.

The disk is merged circumferentially with the joint capsule and thus divides the joint cavity into two compartments, the upper **diskotemporal joint chamber** and the lower **diskomandibular chamber.**

The disk contains hardly any vessels or nerves. Only the retroarticular pad contains a few arteries and veins. A few terminal branches grow into the disk in the areas where it attaches to the joint capsule. Otherwise, the disk is nourished from the synovial fluid. Because there are no nerve receptors in the disk, problems first manifest themselves when significant changes in dynamics occur, or when there is a perforation or narrowing of the disk.

The disk improves the congruence of the joint surfaces and transmits pressure onward. When the mouth opens, the disk displaces anteriorly.

The disk is dynamized not only by its fixation to the mandible, but also by its connection with the lateral pterygoid muscle. The superior part of the muscle attaches to the disk and pulls it anteriorly when the mouth opens.

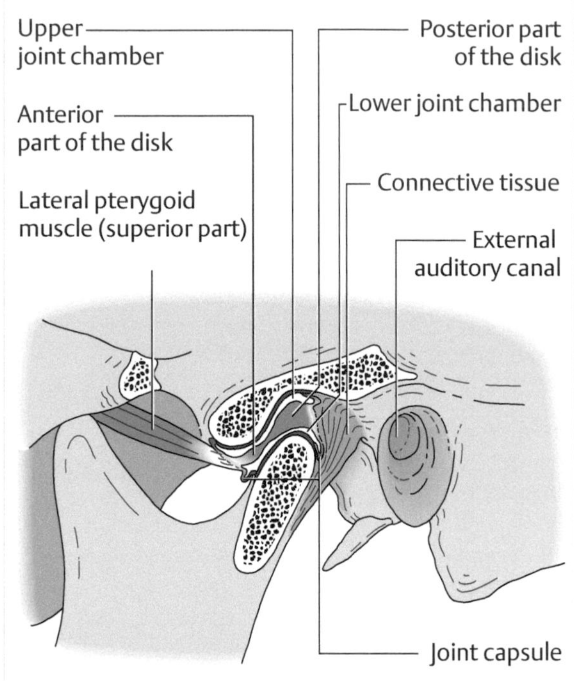


**Fig. 2.25** Temporomandibular joint.

## Joint Capsule (Fig. 2.25)

The joint capsule encloses the joint, including the articular tubercle, leaving the posterior region of the fossa uncovered. Inferiorly, it is attached to the neck of the mandible. The superior part of the lateral pterygoid muscle extends into the anterior capsule.

The capsule is loose and therefore allows large movements without tearing. The lateral, sphenomandibular, and stylomandibular ligaments strengthen the capsule. It is innervated by the auriculotemporal, masseteric, and deep temporal nerves.

## Movements of the Temporomandibular Joint

Movements must occur in both temporomandibular joints simultaneously. The movements are symmetrical when opening and closing the mouth, but asymmetrical when chewing.

### Opening and Closing the Mouth (Fig. 2.26)

When opening the mouth, a combination movement consisting of translation and rotation occurs in the lower joint chamber. In the upper chamber, the disk shifts anteriorly against the temporal bone.

#### *Mouth Closed (Fig. 2.26a)*

The mandibular head and posterior disk lie in the anterior part of the mandibular fossa.

#### *Opening Phase (Fig. 2.26a, b)*

When opening and closing the mouth, the movements are bilaterally symmetrical. A combination rolling-gliding movement starts at the beginning of the opening phase. The head of the mandible turns within the depression between the posterior and anterior parts of the disk. Movement therefore occurs first in the diskomandibular joint chamber.

When opening the mouth further, the head of the mandible shifts the disk anteriorly and inferiorly opposite to the fossa and the rising tubercle. Therefore, in addition to the movement in the lower chamber, translation in the diskotemporal joint chamber now occurs as well. Through this displacement, the posterior part of the disk is stretched. The anterior parts also undergo stretching from the contraction of the lateral pterygoid muscle.

#### *Maximal Opening of the Mouth (Fig. 2.26c)*

When the mouth is open maximally, the head of the mandible turns out of the fossa, and the disk shifts so far anteriorly that its hourglass constriction occurs at the level of the articular tubercle. The bilaminar zone and the posterior parts of the capsule are clearly tightened by this anterior displacement.

When the mouth is closed, the whole complex relocates posteriorly.

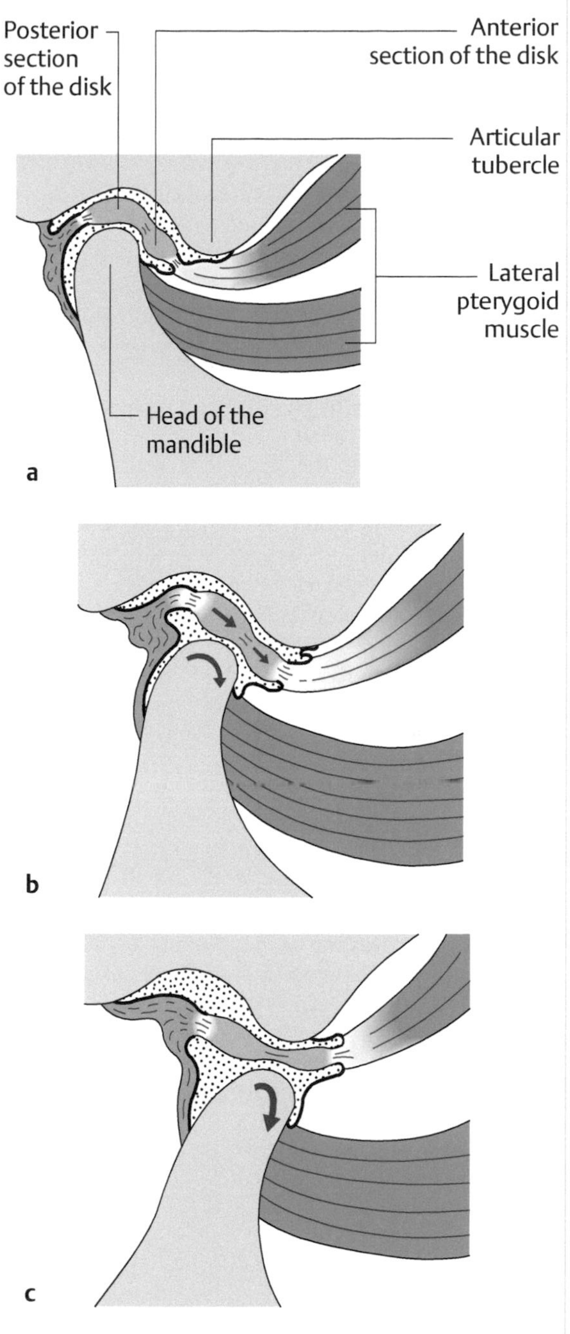


**Fig. 2.26** Position of the temporomandibular joint. **(a)** With the mouth closed. **(b)** In the opening phase. **(c)** In maximal opening of the mouth.

### Protrusion/Retrusion

**Protrusion** describes the shifting of the lower jaw anteriorly; **retrusion** implies its posterior movement. These movements take place primarily in the diskotemporal joint chamber and only minimally in the diskomandibular chamber. A total displacement of 1.5 to 2 cm is expected, of which only 0.2 to 0.5 cm is in a posterior direction. To allow movement of the lower jaw, the mouth must be slightly open. Protrusion and retrusion are gliding movements that are seldom seen in isolation. When opening the mouth, they more often occur in combination with rotation around the frontal axis.

## Laterotrusion/Mediotrusion

Laterotrusion is the movement of the lower jaw away from the midline. Mediotrusion is movement toward the midline. The movements always occur simultaneously in the right and left joints—laterotrusion on one side and mediotrusion on the other. This is not a straight-line movement, but instead takes a course that is a slight arc because it is a combination of translation to the side and rotation around the sagittal axis.

These sidewise displacements are relevant for chewing. The extent of the displacement amounts to approximately 10 to 13 mm in each direction.

## Grinding Movements during Chewing (Fig. 2.27a, b)

During grinding movements, the two joints demonstrate a different motion sequence. On one side, the **working side**, rotation around a vertical axis and a slight laterotrusion occur. The movement is minimal and is stabilized by the muscles of mastication and the ligaments. This is what generates the masticatory pressure.

On the other side of the jaw, the **balance side**, there is a combination of protrusion and mediotrusion. In addition, the head of the mandible shifts inferiorly. In total, the movements on this side are more pronounced than those on the working side.

### Practical Tip

Most dislocations of the disk occur anteriorly. As a result, in the neutral position, the entire disk is located in the anterior area of the joint, so that a translation movement is not possible. Opening of the mouth occurs only through rotation and is very limited.
The blocked joint can be released through relaxation of the anterior structures using tone-reducing measures and translational joint techniques.

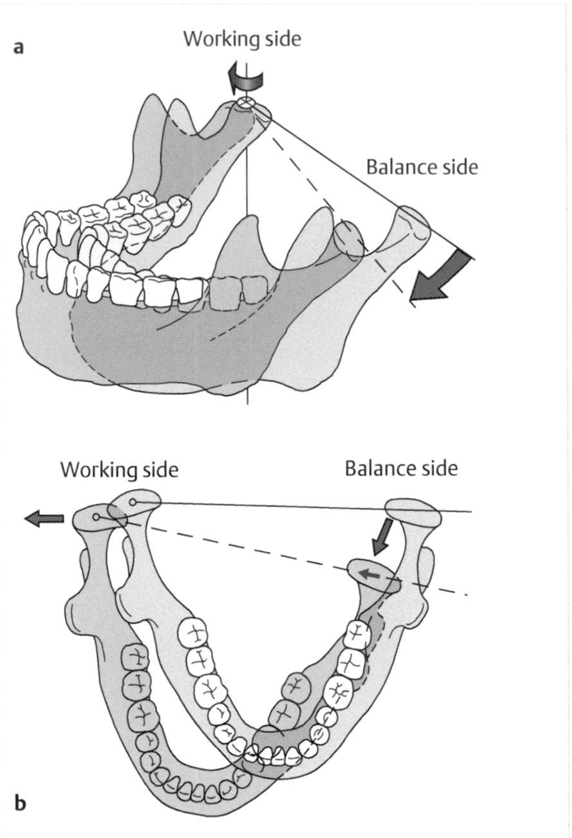


**Fig. 2.27** Grinding motions in the temporomandibular joint. **(a)** Lateral view. **(b)** Transverse view.

## 2.2.6 Jaw–Cervical Spine Functional Unit (Fig. 2.28)

The skeletal sections here—cranium, mandible, shoulder girdle, and cervical spine—together form a functional unit. Therefore problems in the temporomandibular joint, acting through connections with the muscles and joints, also lead to disturbances in the shoulder girdle and cervical spine.

Positional changes in the cervical spine, for instance, have an impact on occlusion. During anterior translation, the dental occlusion will no longer be correct if the mandible is held back by the infrahyoid muscles. Flexion of the cervical spine shifts the mandible anteriorly, while extension shifts it posteriorly, which is significant in, for example, dental treatment.

**Practical Tip**

(**Fig. 2.29**)
In the case of malocclusion secondary to a high crown or a similar condition, it does not make much sense to correct the faulty position of the head because the patient will continue to try to get the best jaw closure. Conversely, the dentist should not get his or her grinder ready right away if there is a change in occlusion—the cause could be malpositioning in the cervical spine region.

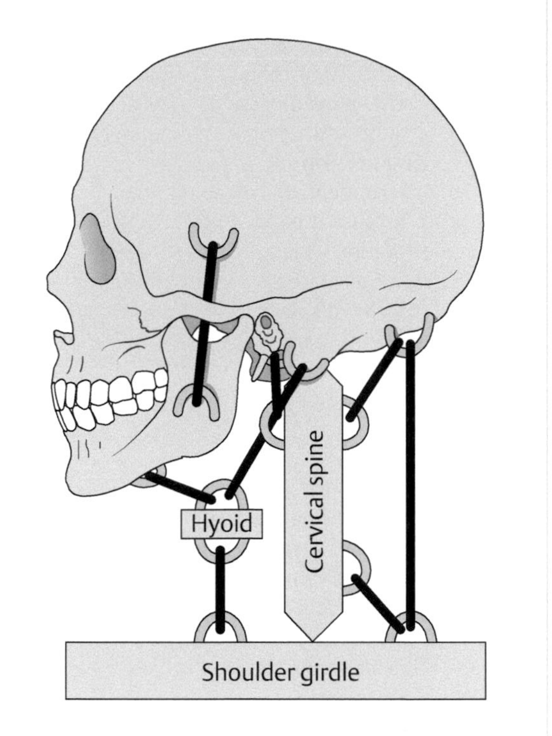


**Fig. 2.28** The functional unit: jaw–cervical spine.

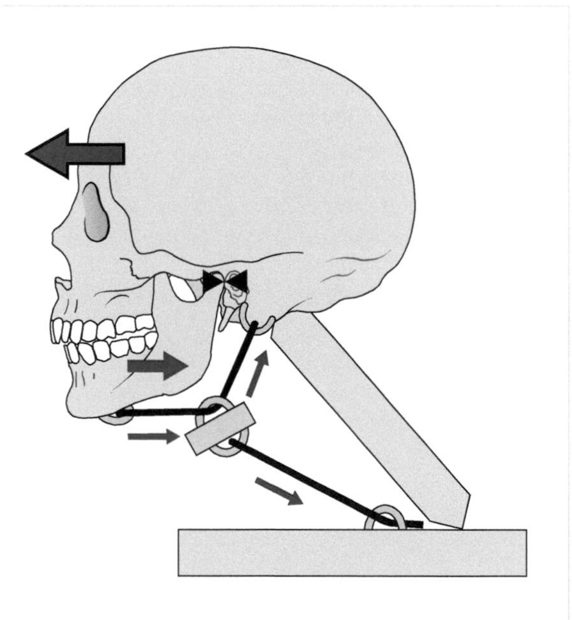

**Fig. 2.29** Positional changes in the cervical spine and the effect on occlusion.

## 2.2.7 Muscles of Mastication

### Temporalis Muscle (Fig. 2.30)

**Functions:**
- All parts: mouth closure.
- Posterior parts: retrusion.

### Masseter Muscle (Fig. 2.31)

**Functions:**
- Powerful jaw closure.
- Through its oblique course from superoanterior to inferoposterior, it can advance the lower jaw.

### Medial Pterygoid Muscle (Fig. 2.32)

**Functions:**
- Mouth closure.
- Protrusion.
- Support of the balance side during grinding movements.

### Lateral Pterygoid Muscle (Fig. 2.33)

**Functions of the inferior part:**
- The onset of mouth opening (after which the suprahyoid muscles supervene).
- Protrusion.
- Grinding movements (balance side).

**Functions of the superior part:**
- Mouth opening.
- Shifts the disk anteriorly during mouth opening.
- Stabilizes the mandibular head by pressing it against the articular tubercle.
- Stabilizes the working side during grinding movements.

**Pathology**

Faulty occlusion, constantly chewing gum, grinding the teeth at night, and emotional problems all lead to increased tone of the masticatory muscles and thus impair the dynamics of the temporomandibular joint. In addition, through the muscular connections of the mandible and maxilla to the sphenoid and temporal bones, the dynamics of the cranium can be influenced, which can compress the sutures.

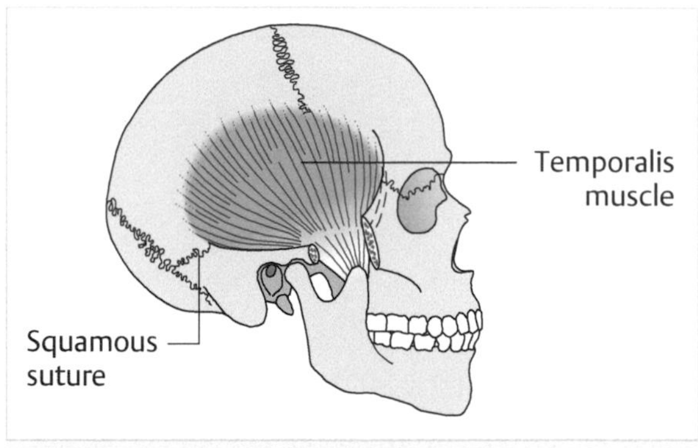


**Fig. 2.30** Temporalis muscle.

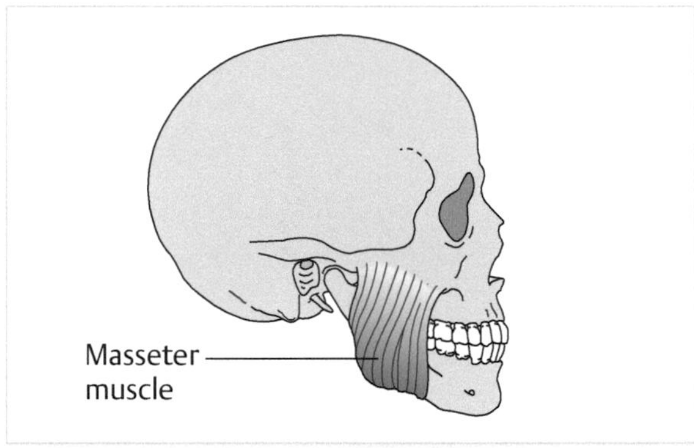


**Fig. 2.31** Masseter muscle.

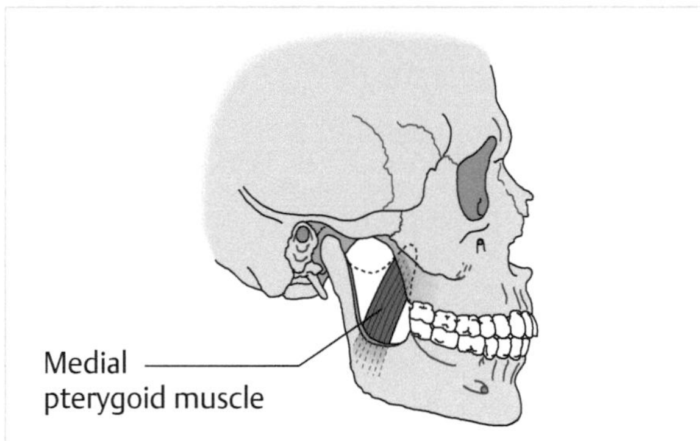


**Fig. 2.32** Medial pterygoid muscle.

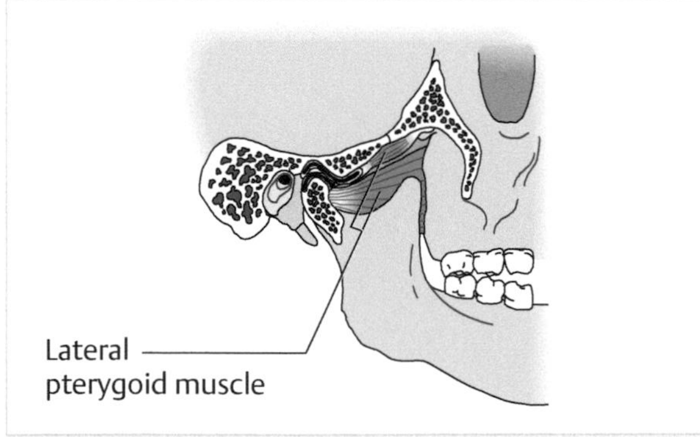


**Fig. 2.33** Lateral pterygoid muscle.

## 2.2.8 Suprahyoid Muscles (Fig. 2.34)

### Digastric Muscle (Fig. 2.34)

*Distinctive feature:* It is divided by an intermediate tendon into the posterior belly and the anterior belly. The tendon is attached to the hyoid bone by a loop of connective tissue.

### Stylohyoid Muscle (Fig. 2.34), Mylohyoid Muscle (Diaphragm of the Mouth) (Fig. 2.35), Geniohyoid Muscle (Fig. 2.35)

**Functions of the suprahyoid muscles:**

- With the fixed ends of the muscles on the lower jaw and skull, they shift the hyoid bone in a superior direction, which is of importance in swallowing movements as well as sucking and blowing.
- With the fixed end on the hyoid bone, they help with opening the mouth. The muscles of the floor of the mouth are active in grinding movements (working side) and raise the floor of the mouth.

## 2.2.9 Infrahyoid Muscles (Figs. 2.36 and 2.37)

### Sternohyoid Muscle (Fig. 2.36), Sternothyroid Muscle (Fig. 2.36), Thyrohyoid Muscle (Fig. 2.37), Omohyoid Muscle (Fig. 2.37)

*Distinctive feature:* At the level of C6, where this muscle crosses the sternocleidomastoid muscle, an intermediate tendon divides the omohyoid into superior and inferior bellies. Through its insertion on the scapula, it creates the connection cranium–hyoid-bone–shoulder.

**Function of the infrahyoid muscles.** These muscles pull the hyoid bone and larynx posteriorly. Because of this, and because of the stabilization of the larynx by the sternothyroid muscle sling, they influence phonation.

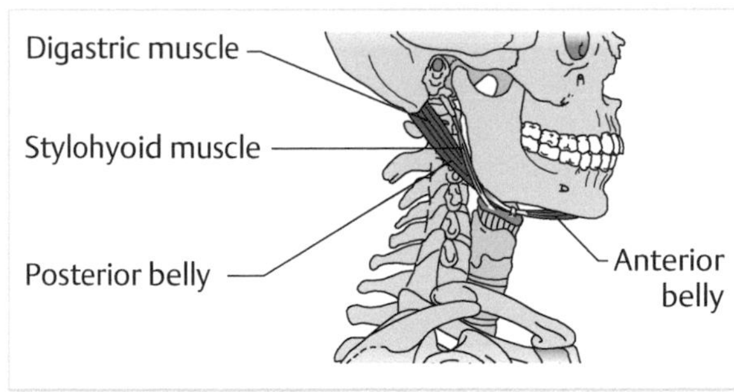


**Fig. 2.34** Suprahyoid muscles.

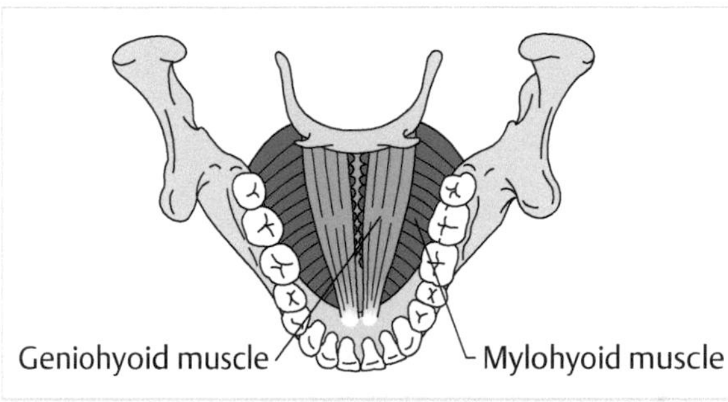


**Fig. 2.35** Muscles of the floor of the mouth.

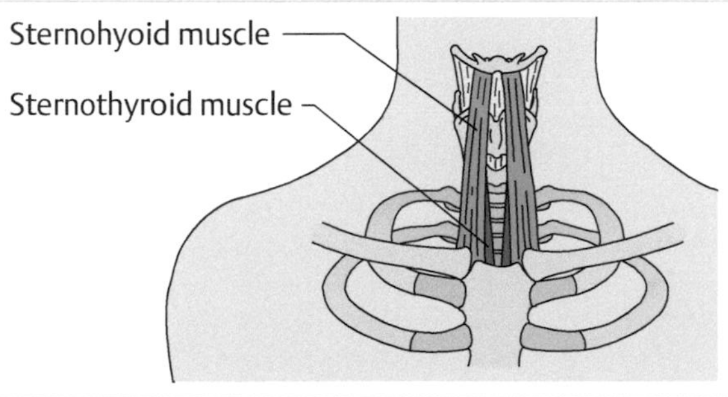


**Fig. 2.36** Infrahyoid muscles: sternohyoid muscle, sternothyroid muscle.

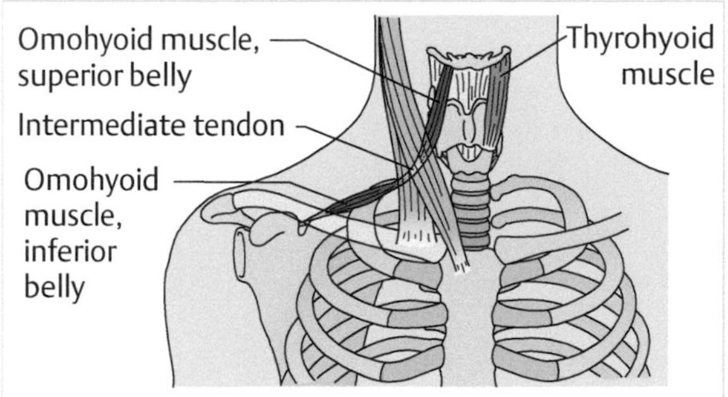


**Fig. 2.37** Infrahyoid muscles: thyrohyoid muscle, omohyoid muscle.

## 2.2.10 Interaction between the Muscles of Mastication and the Suprahyoid and Infrahyoid Muscles (Fig. 2.38)

The suprahyoid and infrahyoid muscles can be viewed as a muscle sling in which the hyoid bone is considered as a fixed point. This sling has a special function. When the muscles of mastication stabilize the temporomandibular joint, insuring firm jaw closure, the suprahyoid and infrahyoid muscles have a flexing effect on the cervical spine, reducing its lordosis. Thus, the sling has significance for cervical spine statics.

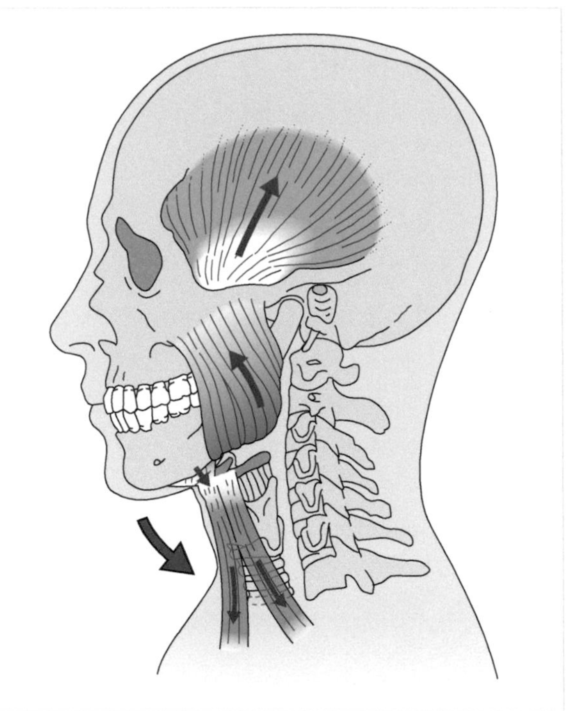

Fig. 2.38 Flexion of the cervical spine by the suprahyoid and infrahyoid muscles when the jaws are closed tightly.

**Practical Tip**

All the muscles that insert onto or arise from the hyoid bone can influence the position of the hyoid. In the case of hoarseness, and perhaps even aphonia and globus hystericus, it is important to evaluate tension in these muscles as a possible cause.

## 2.2.11 Muscles of the Calvaria (Epicranius Muscle) (Fig. 2.39)

### Temporoparietalis Muscle

**Function.** This pulls the ears posteriorly and superiorly.

### Occipitofrontalis Muscle

**Functions:**
- It shifts the skin of the scalp minimally anteriorly and posteriorly over the epicranial aponeurosis.
- With the fixed end of the muscle on the epicranial aponeurosis, the frontal belly raises the eyebrows and eyelids, and wrinkles the forehead.

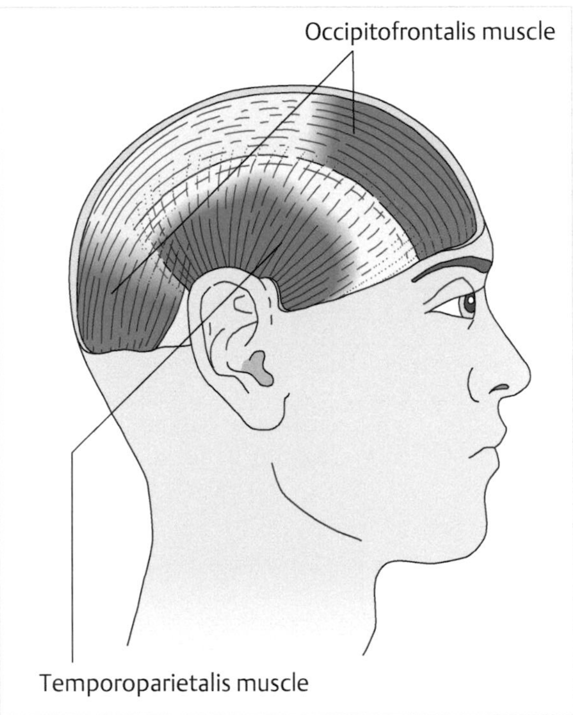


Fig. 2.39 Muscles of the cranium: temporoparietalis muscle, occipitofrontalis muscle.

## 2.2.12 Mimic Muscles (Fig. 2.40, Table 2.1)

**Table 2.1** outlines the functions of these muscles.

**Table 2.1** Muscle functions

| Muscle | Function |
|---|---|
| 1. Corrugator supercilii | Wrinkles the eyebrows |
| 2. Procerus | Pulls the skin between the eyebrows together |
| 3. Nasalis | Narrows and widens the nasal opening |
| 4. Levator anguli oris | Raises the corner of the mouth |
| 5. Buccinator | "Trumpeter muscle": blows out air collected in the cheeks |
| 6. Mentalis | Elevates the bulge of the chin, producing the upwardly convex chin–lip furrow |
| 7. Depressor anguli oris | Depresses the corner of the mouth |
| 8. Depressor labii inferioris | Pulls the lower lip downward |
| 9. Risorius | Draws the corner of the mouth laterally and generates a dimple |
| 10. Obicularis oris | Purses the lips |
| 11. Zygomaticus minor and major | Raise the corner of the mouth upward and outward, and expose the upper row of teeth |
| 12. Levator labii superioris and levator labii superioris alaeque nasi | Pull the nasal alae and the upper lip upward |
| 13. Obicularis oculi | Squints the eyes and distributes lacrimal fluid in the eyes |

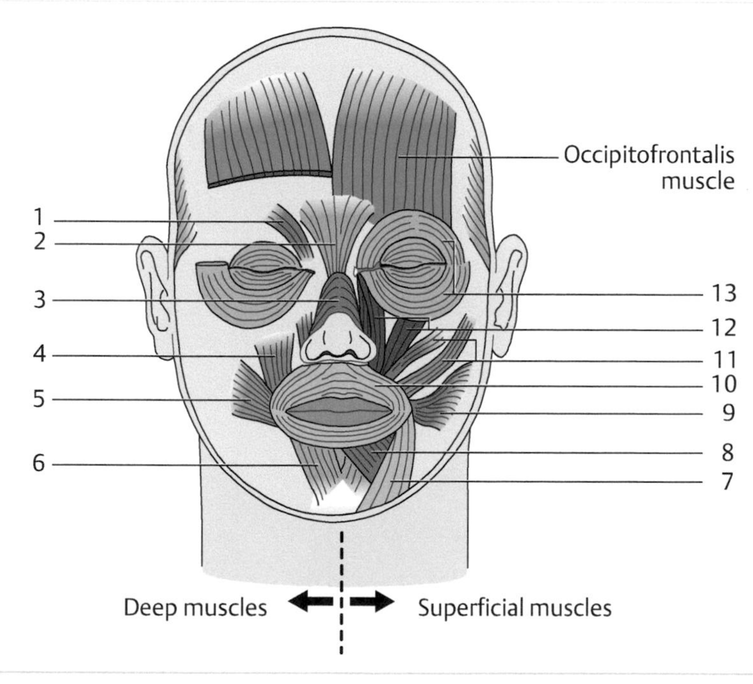


**Fig. 2.40** Mimic muscles.

# 2.3 Functional Anatomy of the Cervical Spine

## 2.3.1 X-Ray of the Cervical Spine

### Anteroposterior View of the Upper Cervical Spine (Fig. 2.41)

- The axis of the dens and the spinous process of C2 lie in the midline, with the atlas in the middle of the foramen magnum.
- The occipital condyles and the lateral masses of the atlas appear upright, parallel, and symmetrical.
- The transverse processes of C1 are the same distance from the occiput and are the same length.
- Lines through the lower border of the occipital condyles (*transverse condylar line*) and through the lower edges of the lateral masses of the atlas (*transverse atlas line*) run parallel to each other.
- The joint surface interval between the lateral masses of C1 and C2 is symmetrical. The joint gap is of the same width bilaterally.
- The inclination of the joint surfaces of C1 and C2 is the same.
- The atlantodental interval is approximately 3 mm and is symmetrical.

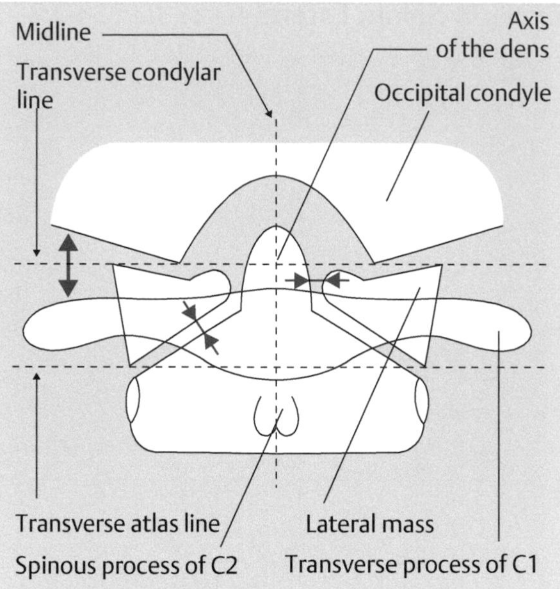


**Fig. 2.41** X-ray image: anteroposterior view of the upper cervical spine.

### Anteroposterior View of the Lower Cervical Spine (Fig. 2.42)

The following are consistent with normal findings:

- The inferior and superior end plates of the vertebral bodies are horizontal and parallel.
- The height of the disks gradually increases from C2 to C7.
- The spinous processes are upright along the plumb line (midline).
- The arches of the pedicles lie directly one on top of the other and are symmetrically distant from the midline bilaterally.
- The uncinate processes are pointed and sharply defined with no protrusions.
- The width of the spinal canal is approximately 24 to 33 mm (from measurement of the interpedicular distance).

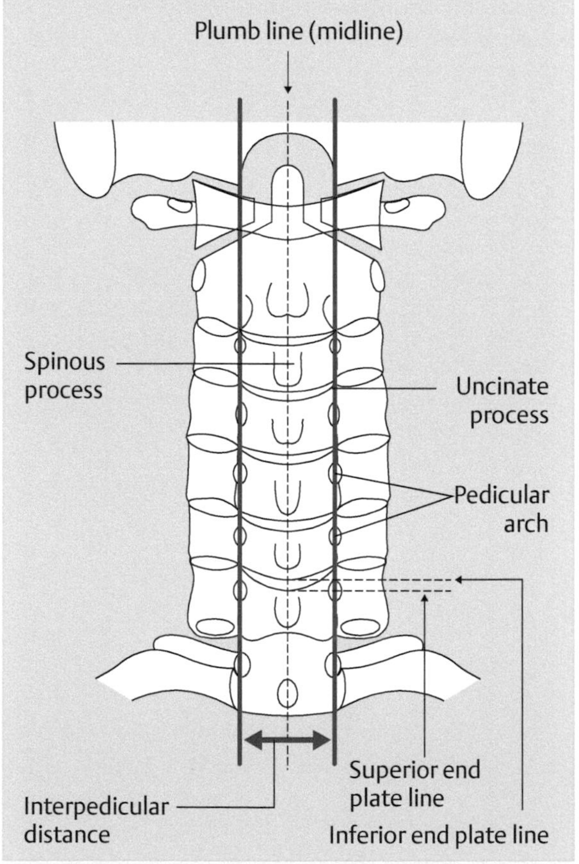


**Fig. 2.42** X-ray image: anteroposterior view of the lower cervical spine.

## Cervical Spine, Lateral View (Fig. 2.43)

- Parallel lines in a harmonious arc are formed by the:
  - Anterior vertebral body line.
  - Posterior vertebral body line.
  - Spinolaminar line.
- The posterior vertebral line and the spinolaminar line form the borders of the spinal canal. The diameter is 16 to 18 mm.
- The horizontal line through the center of the atlas (the atlas plane line) and a line from the lower edge of the pedicle of the vertebral arch to the lower edge of the end of the arch of the axis (the axis plane line) are parallel in the neutral position.
- The intervertebral joints can all be seen.
- The atlantodental interval is approximately 3 mm. The joint surfaces are parallel.

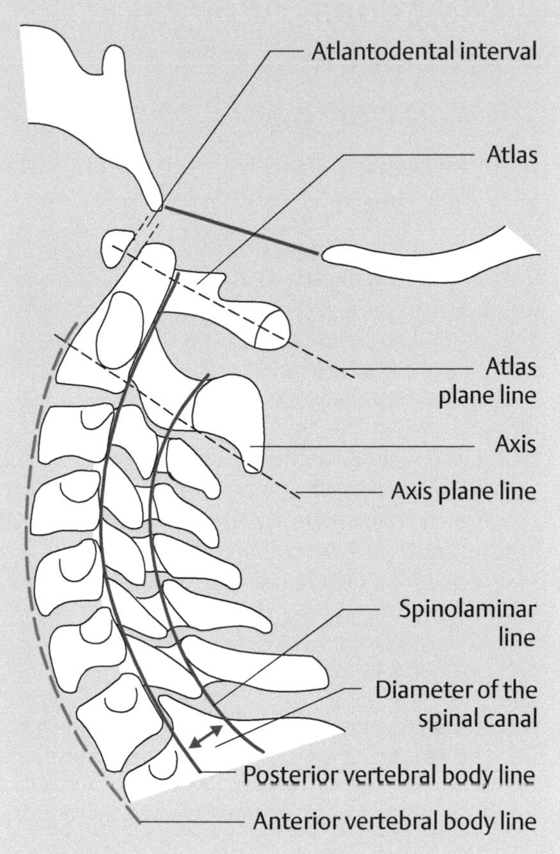


**Fig. 2.43** X-ray image: cervical spine, lateral view.

### Practical Tip

For the precise implementation of manual therapy mobilization and manipulation techniques, it is desirable to have a knowledge of any changes in joint position and clarify any possible contraindications. This information can only be obtained from an X-ray image.
If instability is suspected, functional imaging should be obtained and evaluated.

### Pathology

In an acute cervical syndrome, the typical position is a distinct decrease or reversal of the lordosis above the disk lesion (Güntze's sign).
Patients' complaints do not necessarily correspond to the changes that are seen on X-ray. Thus, patients could have large marginal osteophytes extending from the vertebral bodies without developing any symptoms. On the other hand, there can be obvious clinical findings with scarcely anything to see on X-ray.

## 2.3.2 Upper Cervical Spine

### Atlas (Fig. 2.44)

- It has no vertebral body.
- The lateral parts (**lateral masses**) are connected anteriorly by the anterior arch and posteriorly by the posterior arch.
- The **anterior arch** features an anterior tubercle.
- The **posterior arch** possesses a posterior tubercle, a rudiment of the spinous process. Superiorly, there is a **groove for the vertebral artery** near the branching point of the anterior arch. Here the vertebral artery bends posteriorly out of the **foramen transversarium** and extends superiorly into the foramen magnum.
- Joint surfaces:
  - On the superior side: the **superior articular surfaces of the atlas** for the connection with the occiput.
  - On the inferior side: the **inferior articular surfaces of the atlas** for the connection with the axis.
  - Inward: a **facet for the dens** for the connection with the dens.

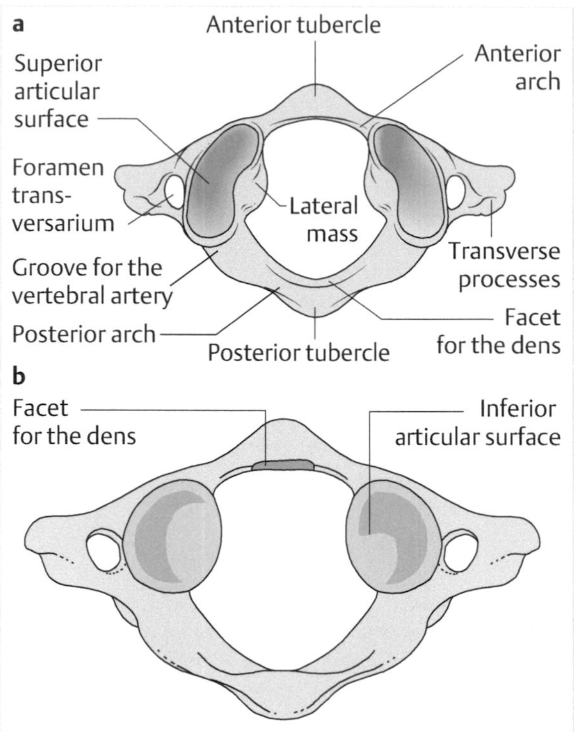


Fig. 2.44 Atlas. (a) Superior view. (b) Inferior view.

### Axis (Fig. 2.45)

- A tooth-shaped process, the **dens of the axis**, arises from the vertebral body. Its tip—the **apex of the dens**—is blunt.
- The spinous process is substantial, and is possibly divided into two cusps.
- The axis has a short transverse process, oriented in an inferolateral direction, with a **foramen transversarium** for the vertebral artery.
- Joint surfaces:
  - Anterior surface of the dens: an **anterior articular facet** for the atlas.
  - Posterior surface of the dens: a **posterior articular facet** for the connection with the transverse ligament of the atlas.
  - The **superior articular facet** of the axis and the inferior articular surface of the atlas form the articular connection to the lateral mass of the atlas.
  - The **inferior articular process** articulates with the superior articular facet of C3.

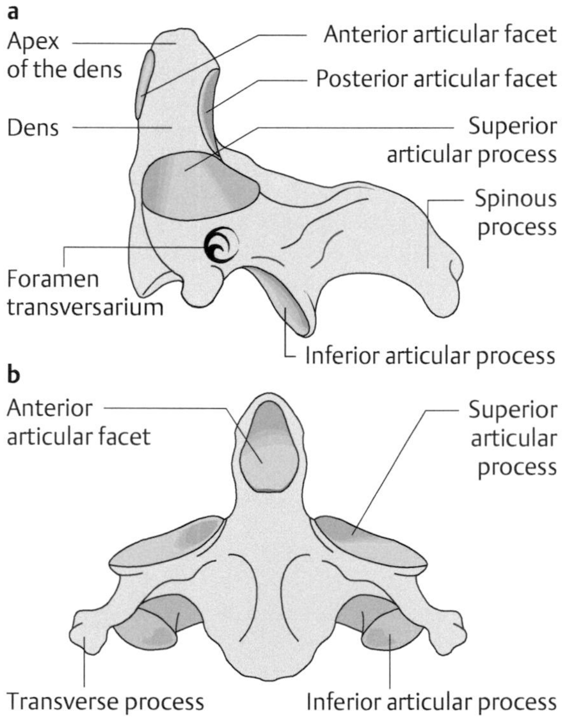


Fig. 2.45 Axis. (a) Sagittal view. (b) Frontal view.

## Atlantooccipital Joint (Figs. 2.46 and 2.47)

- The **occipital condyles** on the occiput at the edge of the foramen are elongated, oval, and convex. The joint axes form an angle of approximately 120° with each other.
- The **superior articular surfaces of the atlas** are oval and concave. The longitudinal axis is oriented anteromedially.
- The joint capsule is relatively wide and is reinforced laterally by the lateral atlantooccipital ligament.

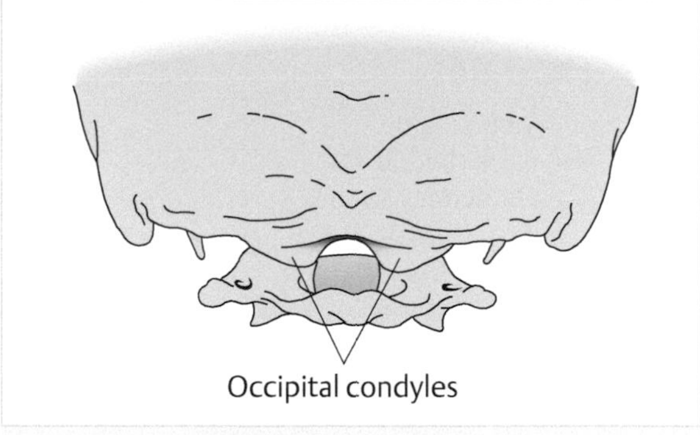


**Fig. 2.46** Atlantooccipital joint.

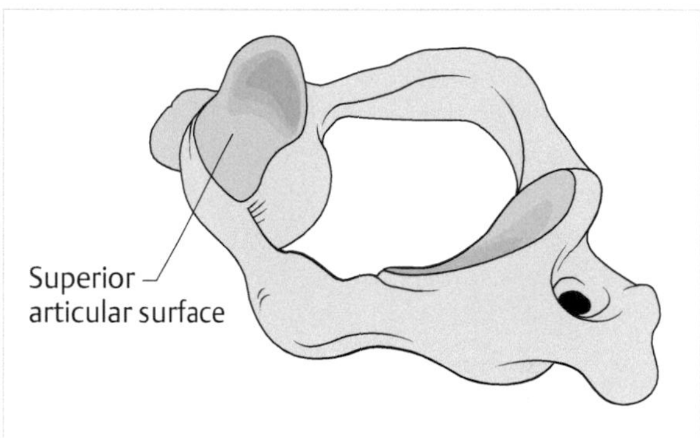


**Fig. 2.47** Superior articular surfaces of the atlas.

## Median Atlantoaxial Joint (Fig. 2.48)

Anterior aspect:
- The **anterior articular facet** on the dens has as oval shape and is convex.
- The **facet for the dens** on the anterior arch of the atlas is slightly concave.

Posterior aspect:
- The **posterior articular facet** on the dens is somewhat saddle-shaped.
- The **transverse ligament of the atlas** has chondrocytes deposited in the area of the articular connection. The ligament arises on the medial surfaces of the lateral masses of the atlas. The joint cavity is closed by the deposition of fatty and connective tissue.

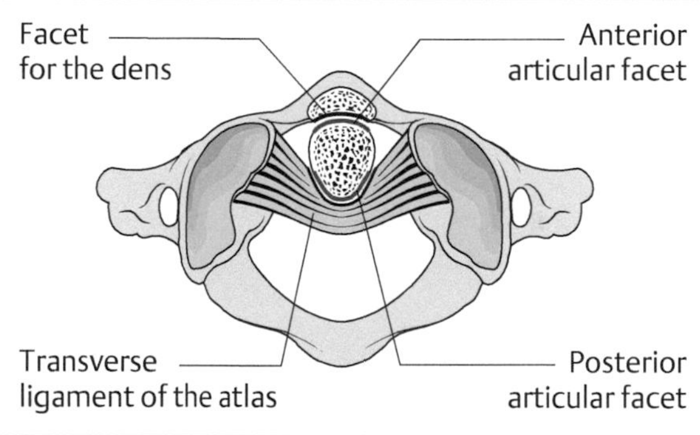


**Fig. 2.48** Median atlantoaxial joint.

## Lateral Atlantoaxial Joint (Fig. 2.49)

- The **inferior articular surface** of the atlas runs from slightly convex to flat.
- The **superior articular facet** of the axis is tilted posterolaterally and is convex. The joint surfaces are somewhat incongruent. The capsule is wide and loose, with synovial folds that project into the joint space, especially anteriorly and posteriorly. The tectorial membrane reinforces the capsule medially and posteriorly.

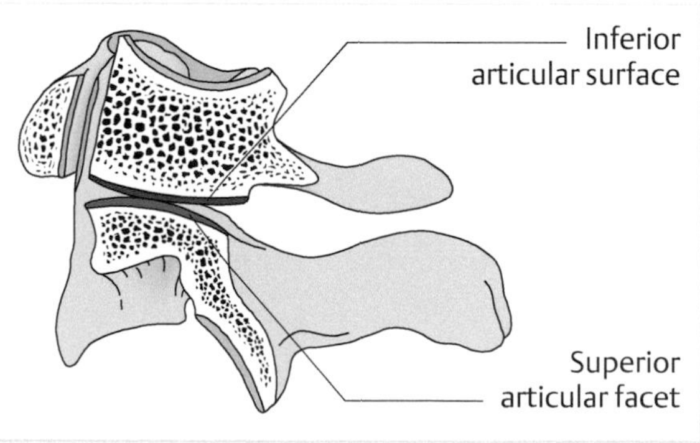


**Fig. 2.49** Lateral atlantoaxial joint.

### Pathology

The atlantooccipital and atlantoaxial joints are richly provided with proprioceptors. In this way, there is a connection to the vestibular nuclei and the reticular formation. The proprioreceptors play a role in orientation in space and in maintaining equilibrium. They also influence the tonic neck reflexes. A functional disturbance in these joints can lead to disturbance in afferent impulses, such as dizziness, and can also be the cause of disturbances in coordination and delayed motor development in early childhood.

## Ligaments of the Upper Cervical Spine (Figs. 2.50–2.53)

### Anterior Ligaments (Fig. 2.50)

#### *Anterior Atlantooccipital Membrane*

This extends from the anterior arch of the atlas to the lower margin of the occiput and, with a long fiber bundle, to the transverse process of the atlas. The membrane consists of a deep layer, which lies directly on top of the atlantooccipital joint capsule, and a superficial layer, which corresponds to the anterior longitudinal ligament.

#### *Anterior Atlantoaxial Ligament*

This connects the atlas and axis anteriorly. Lateral bands reinforce the joint capsule.

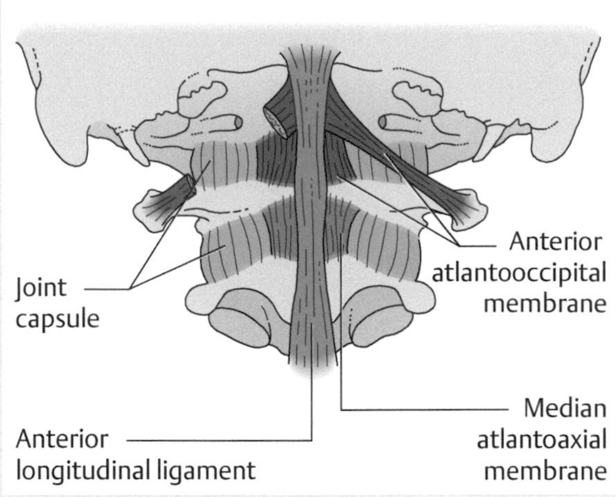


**Fig. 2.50** Anterior ligaments of the upper cervical spine.

### Posterior Ligaments (Fig. 2.51)

#### *Nuchal Ligament*

The nuchal ligament runs from the external occipital protuberance to C7. Below C7, it transitions into the supraspinous ligament. It is fixed to the tips of the spinous processes and merges with the interspinous ligaments.

#### *Posterior Atlantooccipital Membrane*

This runs from the posterior arch of the atlas to the posterior margin of the foramen magnum. The vertebral artery and vein and the suboccipital nerve break through the membrane shortly above its origin. Anteriorly, it merges with the dura.

**Pathology**

Changes in tension in this membrane can compromise the artery as well as the nerve.

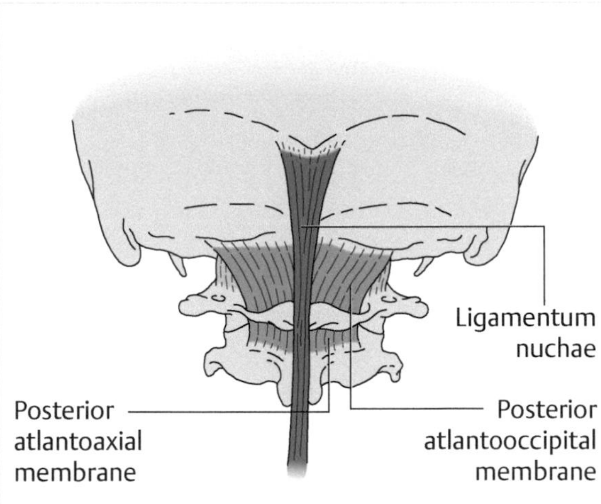


**Fig. 2.51** Posterior ligaments of the upper cervical spine.

#### *Posterior Atlantoaxial Membrane*

This spreads out between the posterior arch of the atlas and the axis.

▷ Superficial Layer after Removal of the Vertebral Arches (Fig. 2.52a)

#### *Tectorial Membrane*

This runs from the clivus to the vertebral body of the axis and borders the vertebral canal posteriorly.

#### *Posterior Longitudinal Ligament*

In the areas C0–C3, this combines with the tectorial membrane.

▷ Middle Layer (Fig. 2.52b)

#### *Cruciate Ligament of the Atlas*

This consists of two parts:

- Transverse part = *transverse ligament of the atlas*. This arises from the inner side of the lateral masses and forms the main part of the cruciate ligament. The ligament widens in its midsection. Chondrocytes are embedded here, so that a thin layer of cartilage forms, thus creating a joint surface for the dens.
- A weaker longitudinal part = *longitudinal bands*. These extend from the body of the axis to the margin of the foramen magnum.

▷ Deep Layer (Fig. 2.52c)

### *Apical Ligament of the Dens*

This extends from the tip of the dens to the midanterior margin of the foramen magnum.

### *Alar Ligaments*

- These extend from the posterolateral surface of the tip of the dens to the anteromedial edge of the occipital condyles.
- The right and left ligaments form an angle of approximately 150 to 170° with each other.
- Inferior fibers insert on the lateral mass of the atlas.

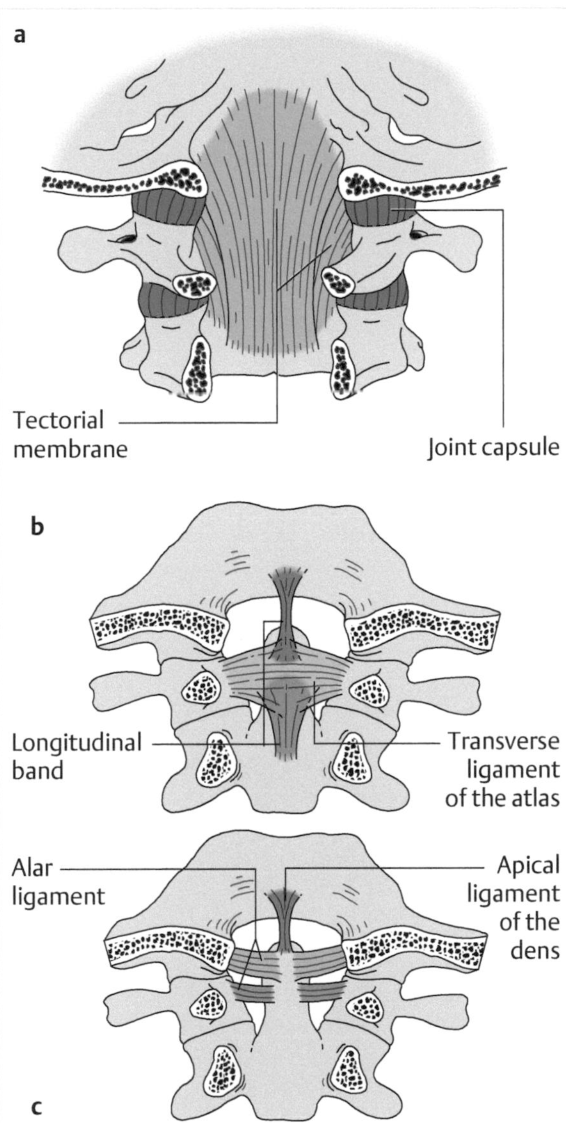


**Fig. 2.52** Posterior ligaments of the upper cervical spine after removal of the vertebral arches. **(a)** Superficial layer. **(b)** Middle layer. **(c)** Deep layer.

## Functions of the Ligaments

Their primary functions are braking and support:

- **Inhibition of flexion** occurs through the posteriorly lying ligaments that have a longitudinal course. The ligamentum nuchae, posterior longitudinal ligament, tectorial membrane, posterior atlantooccipital membrane, posterior atlantoaxial membrane, and longitudinal bands all have a braking effect on flexion.
- **Inhibition of extension** occurs through the anteriorly lying structures: the median atlantoaxial membrane, anterior atlantooccipital membrane, and anterior longitudinal ligament.
- **Inhibition of rotation** occurs through contralateral parts of the posterior atlantooccipital membrane, the tectorial membrane, and the alar ligaments.

The *transverse ligament of the atlas* stabilizes the dens within an osteoligamentous ring, but it is deformable, a necessity for movements such as nodding the head. It also protects the spinal cord from the dens.

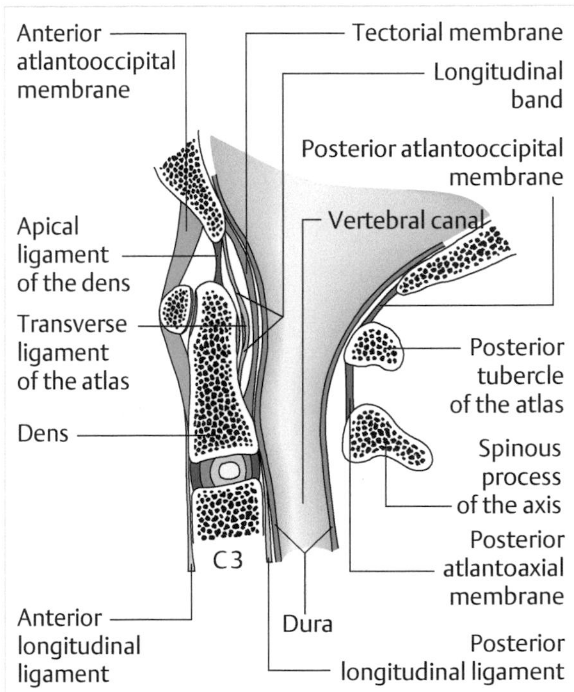


**Fig. 2.53** Ligaments of the cervical spine: sagittal view.

### *Alar Ligaments (Fig. 2.54)*

- In the neutral position, some fiber parts are tensed and others relaxed.
- These ligaments limit flexion and axial rotation between C0 and C2. During rotation to the left, the right ligament tenses because its insertion on the right anteromedial occipital condyle and on the lateral mass of the atlas moves further from the insertion on the dens.
- At maximal rotation to the left, the left ligament turns around the dens and also comes under tension.

#### Pathology

The fiber composition of the ligaments varies depending on their functional demands. The transverse ligament of the atlas and the alar ligaments contain a large proportion of firm fibers with little flexibility. In a whiplash injury, for example, the extreme momentary rotational stress combined with either flexion or extension can overstretch and tear the ligaments. In this situation, the alar ligaments, with a tensile strength of 220 N, are less durable than the transverse ligament, at 350 N. Ligaments with higher proportions of elastic fibers, such as the tectorial and atlantooccipital membranes, are very flexible and very resilient.

#### Practical Tip

Because the ligaments of the atlantooccipital and atlantoaxial joints primarily stabilize the joints between C1 and C2, they should be examined with regard to their stability before a mobilization treatment.

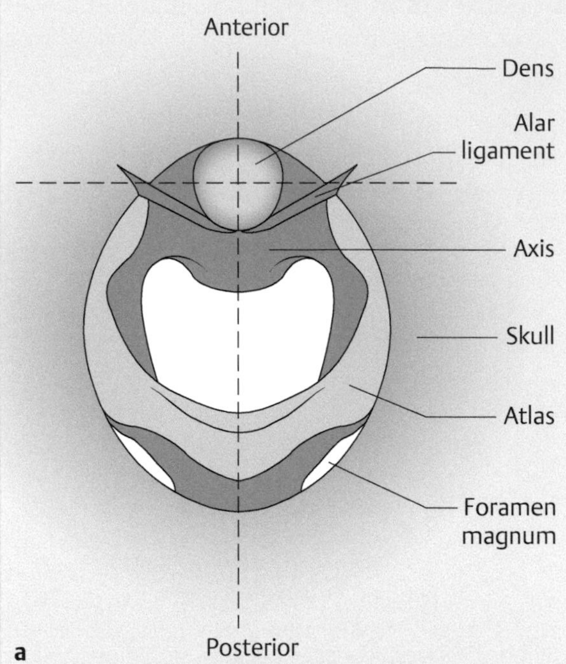


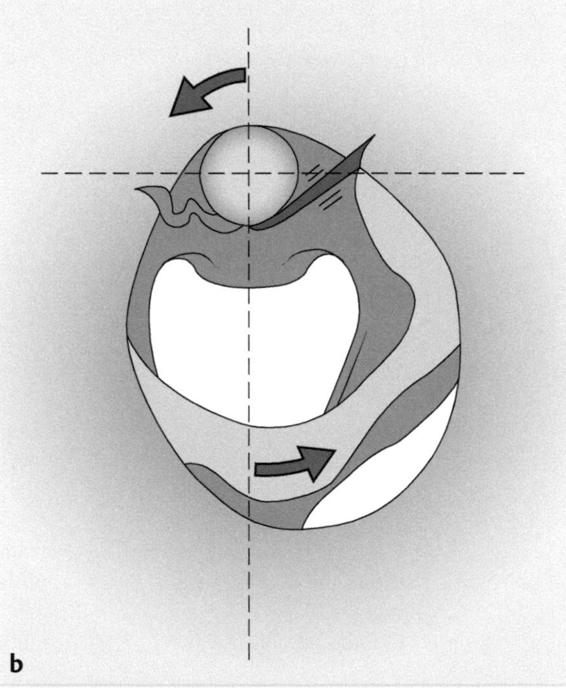


**Fig. 2.54** Course of the alar ligaments. **(a)** In the neutral position. **(b)** During rotation to the left. (Superior view through the foramen magnum.)

## Movements in the Upper Cervical Spine

The atlantooccipital and atlantoaxial joints form a functional unit.

### Flexion (Inclination) C0/C1 (Fig. 2.55)

The occipital condyles glide posteriorly on the superior articular surfaces of the atlas.

The gap between the occiput and the posterior arch of the atlas becomes larger.

### C1/C2 (Fig. 2.56)

- The inferior articular surface of the atlas glides posterosuperiorly.
- The facet for the dens slides inferiorly. Limits to this movement are set by the narrow space between the dens and the anterior arch. As a result, the anterior arch moves further anteriorly from the dens and, at the end of the movement, a gap develops in the superior part of the joint. At the same time, compression occurs in the inferior portion.
- The gap between the posterior arch of the atlas and the spinous process of C2 becomes larger.

The movement is limited by tension in the posterior parts of the capsule, the tectorial membrane, the longitudinal bands, and the nuchal ligament, as well as by the short neck muscles.

### Extension (Reclination) C0/C1 (Fig. 2.57)

- The occipital condyles glide anteriorly.
- The occiput nears the posterior arch of the atlas.

### C1/C2 (Fig. 2.58)

- The inferior articular surfaces of the atlas glide anterosuperiorly.
- The facet for the dens slides superiorly against the dens, during which a small tilting movement occurs: superiorly, the facet and the dens approach each other, but inferiorly, they move apart.

Inhibition of the movement occurs through the anterior capsule and ligamentous structures, such as the anterior atlantooccipital membrane and the anterior longitudinal ligament.

*Range of Motion (Fig. 2.59)*

The range of motion of flexion/extension amounts to 30° in all. Of this, the potential for flexion is greater than it is for extension.

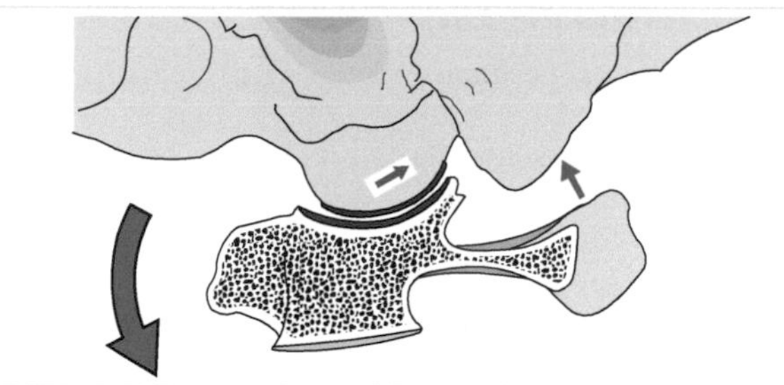

**Fig. 2.55** Flexion in the atlantooccipital joint.

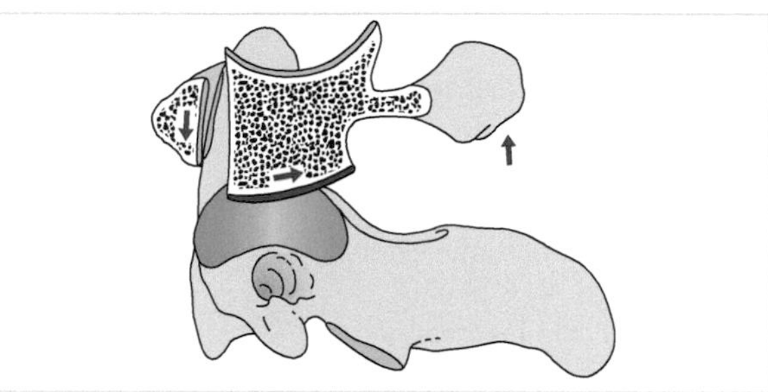

**Fig. 2.56** Flexion in the atlantoaxial joint.

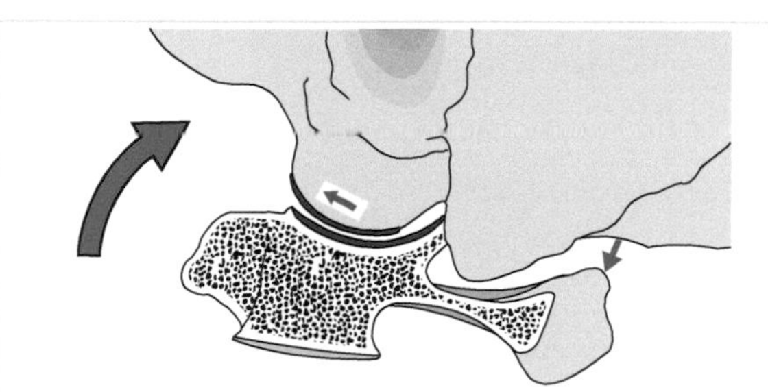

**Fig. 2.57** Extension in the atlantooccipital joint.

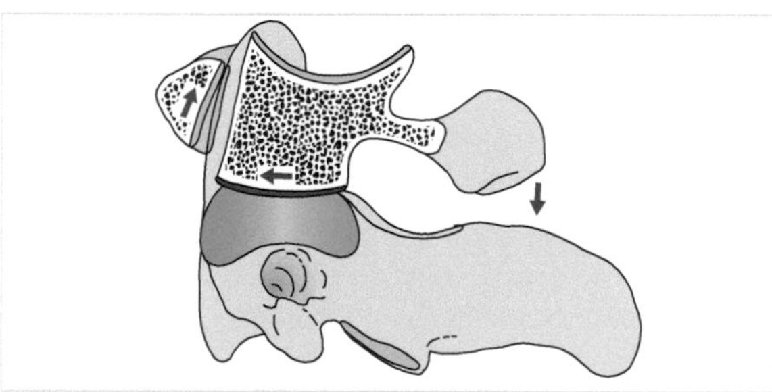

**Fig. 2.58** Extension in the atlantoaxial joint.

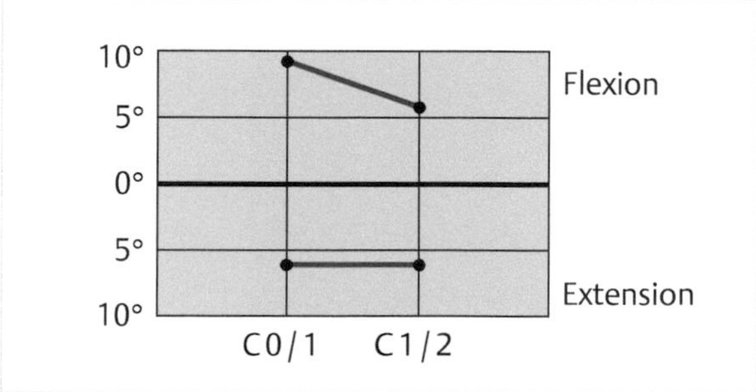


**Fig. 2.59** Movement diagram: flexion/extension in the upper cervical spine.

## Lateral Flexion C0/C1 (Fig. 2.60)

The occipital condyles can glide slightly medially or laterally.

The *range of motion* amounts to only 3 to 5° in each direction.

## C1/C2 (Fig. 2.60)

Because of the interposition of the dens in the osteoligamentous ring, a scarcely measurable lateral flexion is possible. This occurs as a movement that accompanies rotation.

## Rotation C0/C1 (Fig. 2.61)

During rotation to the right, the following occurs:

- The occiput rotates to the right on the atlas as the left condyle glides anteriorly and the right posteriorly.
- The left alar ligament tenses and pulls the left condyle towards the dens, and the head inclines minimally to the left.

The *range of motion* is barely noticeable—only 5°.

## C1/C2 (Fig. 2.62)

During rotation to the right:

- The osteoligamentous ring turns around the dens, which remains fixed.
- The right lateral mass of the atlas glides posteriorly, and the left anteriorly.
- From 20° of rotation onward, the atlas descends on the axis because of the slightly convex joint surface.

The *range of motion* is very extensive: approximately 40° is possible in each direction, which is almost half of the total rotation of the head (**Fig. 2.63**).

### Practical Tip

To assess the mobility of the upper cervical spine, movement of the lower section must be prevented. This can be accomplished either by palpation or by bringing the lower cervical spine into maximal flexion and then testing the ability of the upper cervical spine to rotate in this position. To test reclination and inclination, the lower cervical spine can be placed in maximal rotation.

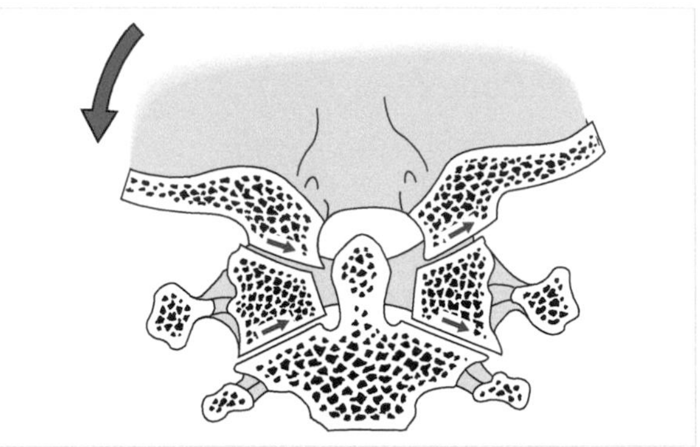

**Fig. 2.60** Lateral flexion in the atlantooccipital and atlantoaxial joints.

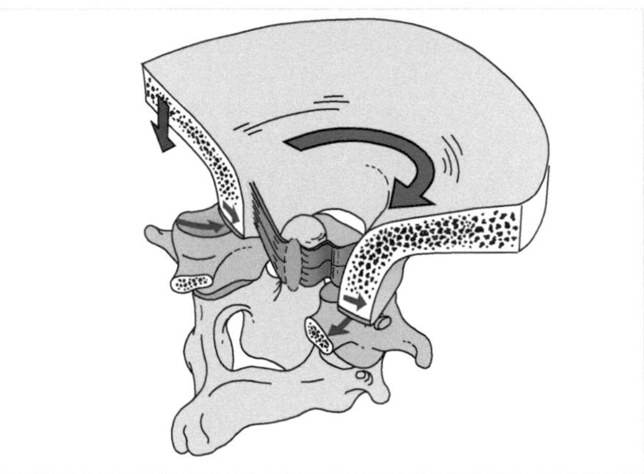

**Fig. 2.61** Rotation combined with lateral flexion in the atlantooccipital joint.

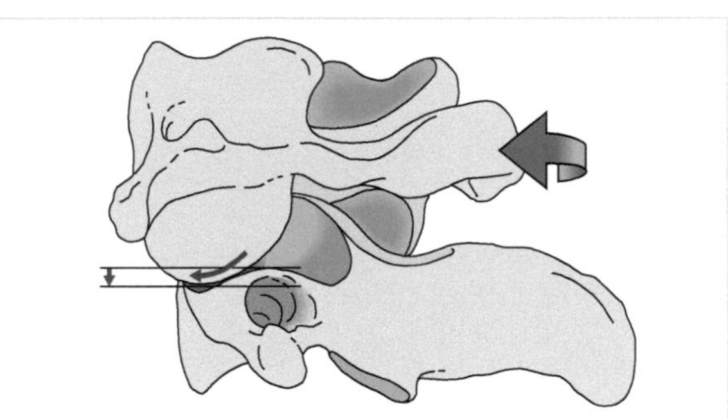

**Fig. 2.62** Rotation in the atlantoaxial joint.

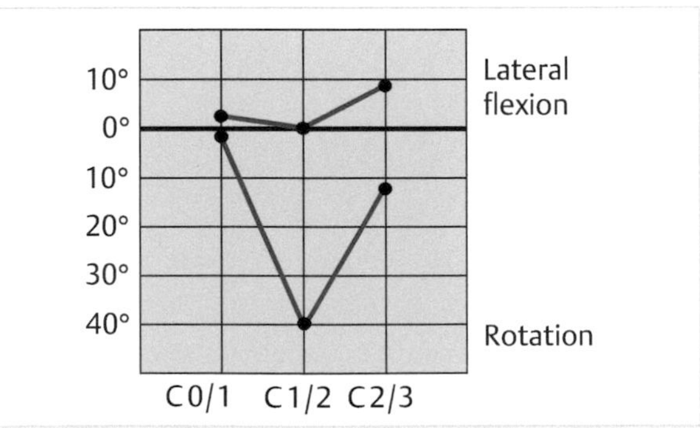


**Fig. 2.63** Movement diagram: lateral flexion/rotation in the upper cervical spine.

## 2.3.3 Lower Cervical Spine

### Vertebral Body (Fig. 2.64)

Clearly exhibited on the lateral margins of the vertebrae are superiorly oriented protrusions, the *uncinate processes.*

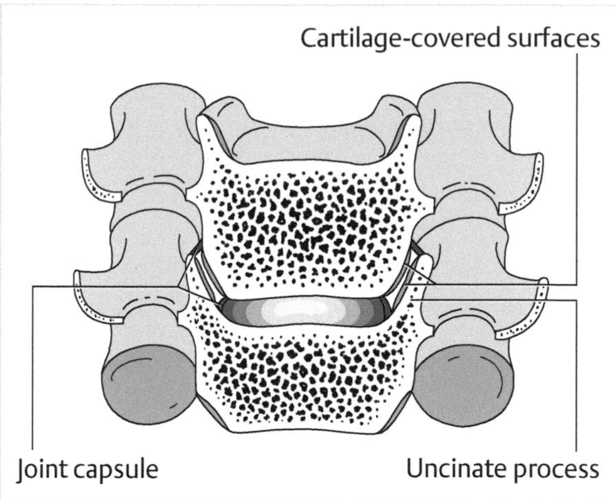


**Fig. 2.64** Cervical vertebra: frontal view.

### Uncinate Process (Fig. 2.64)

- These articulate with the small, oblique margin of the next vertebra. The articulating surfaces are coated with cartilage, and the connective tissue accumulated there forms a type of joint capsule.
- The vertebral artery runs immediately laterally to the joint, and the spinal nerve passes posterolaterally. The shape of the uncinate processes protects the artery and nerve from herniated disks protruding in their direction.

**Pathology**

(**Fig. 2.65**)
Degeneration in the area of the disk with its associated height loss leads to the exertion of a higher pressure on the uncinate processes, which react with osteophyte formation. These osteophytes can narrow the foramen transversarium and with it the artery, or the intervertebral foramen with the spinal nerve. This narrowing is relatively common without the occurrence of significant symptoms because the nerve and artery have plenty of space and are flexible. Symptoms first occur when the spurs are very large or certain morphologic conditions of the vessels exist, such as arteriosclerotic changes.

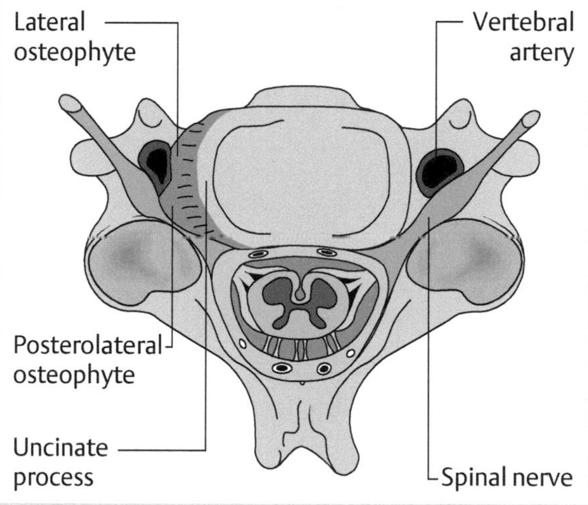


**Fig. 2.65** Formation of osteophytes on the uncinate process.

### Transverse Process (Fig. 2.66)

- The transverse process consists of an anterior part (the rib rudiment) called the *anterior tubercle* and a posterior (true) transverse process called the *posterior tubercle.* Within the transverse process is an opening, the *foramen transversarium,* for the vertebral artery and its accompanying vein.
- From the third cervical vertebra down, the superior surface has a furrow between the two tubercles, the *groove for the spinal nerve.*
- On the anterior tubercle of the sixth cervical vertebra, the *carotid tubercle* protrudes anteriorly.

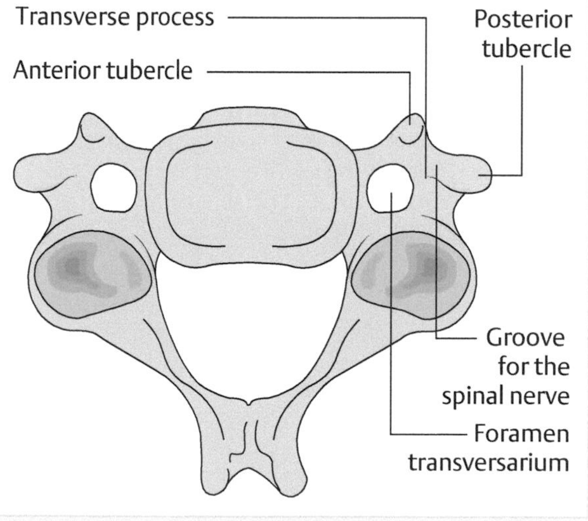


**Fig. 2.66** Cervical vertebra: transverse view.

## Spinous Process (Fig. 2.67)

- This is slanted slightly inferiorly, relatively short, and forked.
- Exception: The seventh spinous process—the *vertebra prominens*—is significantly thicker and longer, and runs almost horizontally.

## Intervertebral Foramen

- This is narrower in the inferior than the superior sections.
- An hourglass-shaped constriction is caused by the uncinate process.

## Articular Process (Fig. 2.67)

- The superior and inferior articular processes are very flat and wide.
- The joint surfaces are inclined 40–60° from the horizontal, so that the superior articular facet is aligned on the posterosuperior side of the joint.
- In addition, the articular facets of the third and fourth cervical vertebrae are turned minimally inward, and those of the fifth to seventh cervical vertebrae slightly outward.

See Chapter 1.2.1, The Structure of a Vertebra.

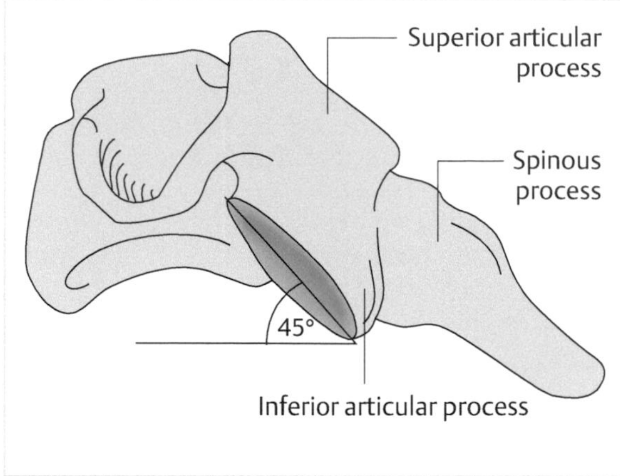


**Fig. 2.67** Cervical vertebra: sagittal view.

## Intervertebral Disks

The intervertebral disks often have horizontal gaps. During aging, the disks can regress and incorporate chondrocytes, so that a proper joint then develops.

## Ligamentous Connections of the Lower Cervical Spine

- Posterior longitudinal ligament.
- Anterior longitudinal ligament.
- Ligamentum flavum.
- Intertransverse ligament.
- Ligamentum nuchae (made up of the interspinous and supraspinous ligaments).

See Chapter 1.2.4, Ligaments.

## Vertebral Artery (Figs. 2.68 and 2.69)

- This arises from the subclavian artery.
- It extends through the foramina transversaria of the second through sixth cervical vertebrae, and passes alongside the uncinate process and anterior to the spinal nerve.
- After passing through the foramen transversarium of the atlas, it bends posteriorly and runs on the posterior arch of the atlas as the *atlas loop*.
- It then extends through the foramen magnum into the posterior cranial fossa, where it ascends along the anterior aspect of the medulla oblongata.
- Both vertebral arteries unite at the level of the pons–medulla border to become the basilar artery.
- The basilar artery then supplies the cerebellum, parts of the midbrain, and the brainstem as well as the organs for hearing and equilibrium, the posterior parts of the cerebrum, the cervical spinal nerves, and the ganglia.
- In its cranial section, the vertebral artery has only a few elastic fiber components and is not very resilient with regard to stretching.

### Pathology

Because two vertebral arteries unite to form the basilar artery and supply important areas of the brain, one of the arteries can, given sufficient time to adapt, supply adequate perfusion through formation of collateral vessels and anastomoses if the other artery becomes constricted. However, this is not possible when a sudden failure of an artery occurs.

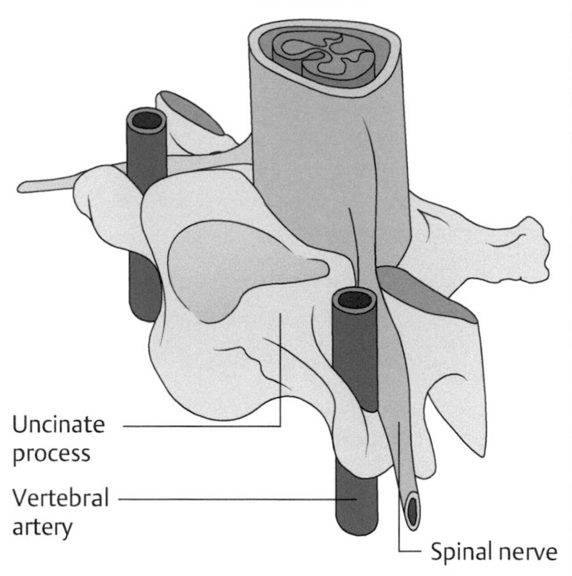


**Fig. 2.68** Course of the vertebral artery in the area between the vertebrae.

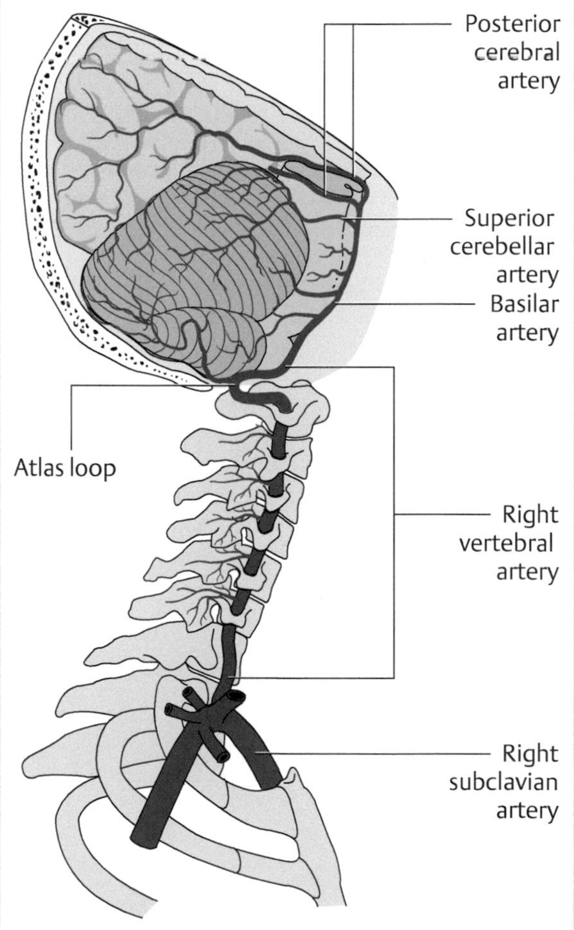


**Fig. 2.69** The complete course of the vertebral artery.

## Influences of Movements on the Vertebral Artery (Fig. 2.70)

Data on the influences of movements on the lumen of the artery are very inconsistent. Basically, one can assume that all extreme movements decrease blood flow on one or both sides. However, pathologic changes to the vessel must take place before symptoms occur because the artery is basically very flexible.

**Extension/flexion:** These movements have hardly any impact on perfusion. The arteries are in fact stretched, but are only significantly narrower if impeded by osteophytes.

**Right lateral flexion:** There is only a minimal influence on the right vertebral artery.

**Rotation:** During rotation to the left, the right artery narrows.

**Combination movements:** Extension or flexion, together with lateral flexion and rotation in the opposite direction, significantly narrow the artery on the side opposite to the direction of rotation.

### Practical Tip

Malalignment of the atlas in rotation, for instance, can cause overstretching of the vertebral artery during a traction treatment.

In the known provocation tests to check the patency of an artery, such as the De Kleyn test, the examiner uses extreme extension with lateral flexion and rotation to the opposite side to constrict the artery on the side opposite to the direction of the rotation. It is questionable whether the artery itself is narrowed, or whether it undergoes constriction as a result of the mechanoreceptors in the adventitia of the artery that are stimulated by too much tension. If pathologic narrowing exists in the artery on the contralateral side, hearing and sight disturbances, nausea, and headache develop as a result of decreased perfusion of the brain, since the artery on the ipsilateral side is narrowed by the position adopted.

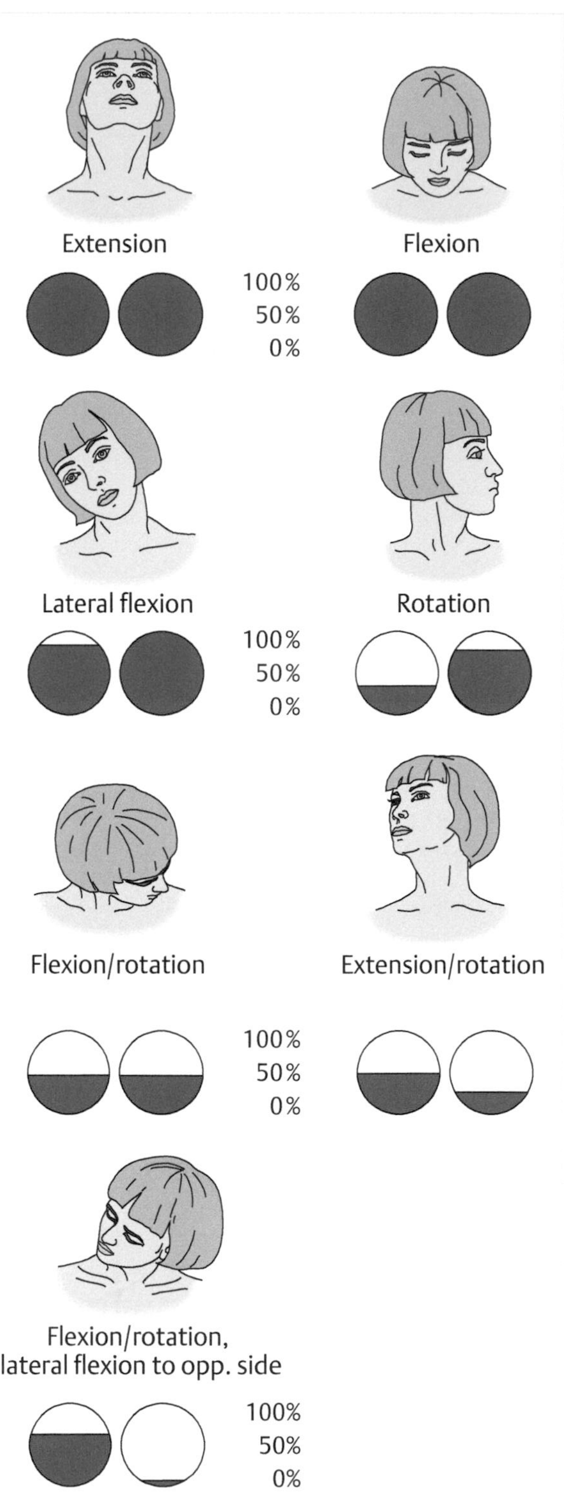


**Fig. 2.70** Influence of movements on the vertebral artery.

## Movements in the Lower Cervical Spine

### Flexion (Figs. 2.71 and 2.73)

- During flexion, the superior joint facets glide superiorly and anteriorly.
- At the end of the movement, the upper joint facet slips over the superior edge of the lower facet. A slight tilting effect occurs, because the joint facets separate in the inferior section of the joint while compression develops in the superior aspect.
- During this **divergence movement**, as the facets glide apart, the area of joint-surface contact decreases.
- As a result, a small step formation is created between the vertebral bodies, which can be seen well on an X-ray at the vertebral body margins.
- The posterior parts of the intervertebral disks, the posterior parts of the joints, and the posteriorly running ligaments inhibit this movement. The end-feel is firm to elastic.
- Maximal *range of motion*: With the mouth closed, two fingerbreadths should fit between the chin and sternum. Passive movement increases the mobility by about 2° per segment.

### Extension (Figs. 2.72 and 2.73)

- In extension, the superior joint facets glide in an inferior, posterior direction.
- During this **convergence movement**, they telescope together, so that compression of the facets develops in the inferior part of the joint at the end of the movement. The superior parts move apart from each other, resulting in a gap.
- The end-feel is firm to elastic because of the compression in the inferior section of the joint. In addition, the anterior parts of the intervertebral disks, the capsule, and the anterior longitudinal ligament inhibit the movement.
- In hypermobility, the spinous processes can come into contact with each other.
- Maximal *range of motion*: The chin–nose line forms an angle of approximately 30° to the horizontal.

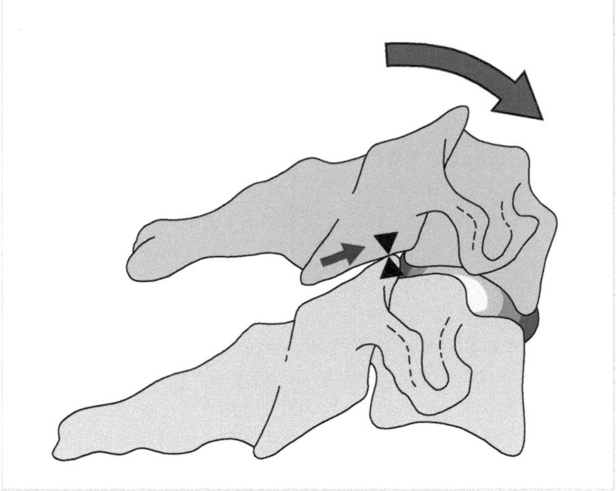

**Fig. 2.71** Flexion in the lower cervical spine.

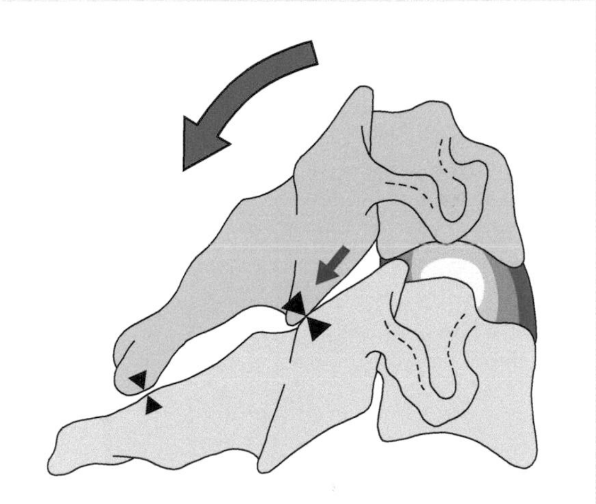

**Fig. 2.72** Extension in the lower cervical spine.

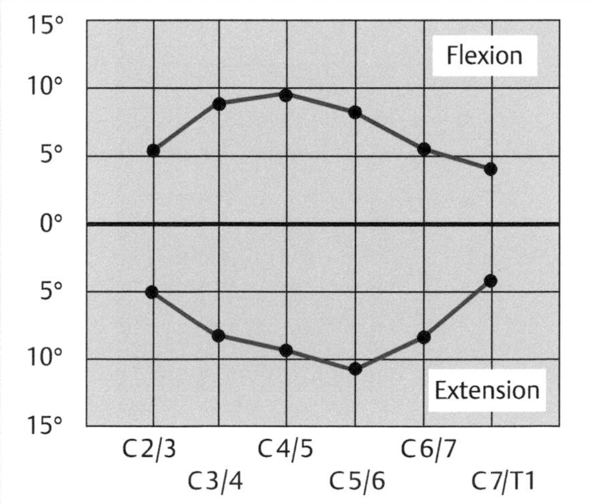


**Fig. 2.73** Movement diagram: flexion/extension in the lower cervical spine.

## Lateral Flexion and Rotation (Figs. 2.74–2.76)

- Pure **lateral flexion** does not occur because of the oblique position of the joint surfaces and the orientation of the uncinate processes. It is always coupled with rotation, which means that the primary lateral flexion always accompanies a secondary ipsilateral rotation. The degree of this concomitant rotation decreases as one moves from superior to inferior. For instance, the concomitant rotation between the third and fourth cervical vertebrae amounts to approximately 7°, with only about 2° of rotation in the C7–T1 segment. Maximal *range of motion*: about 50° of lateral flexion with approximately 30° of concomitant rotation.
- Primary **rotation** is coupled with ipsilateral lateral flexion. This concomitant flexion decreases as one moves inferiorly. For example, it amounts to about 6° between C4 and C5 and only 2° between C7 and T1. Maximal *range of motion*: 40° rotation with 28° of coupled lateral flexion.
- With coupled movements, the following gliding events occur in the zygapophysial joint. On the concave side, the inferior articular facet glides in an inferior–posterior–medial direction and thereby creates a convergence movement. On the convex side, it glides superior–anterior and also slightly medially, which instead corresponds to a divergence movement.

## Cervicothoracic Transition

From a functional viewpoint, the movements of the cervical spine do not end until the level of the fifth thoracic vertebra. The cervicothoracic transition vertebra is the seventh cervical vertebra.

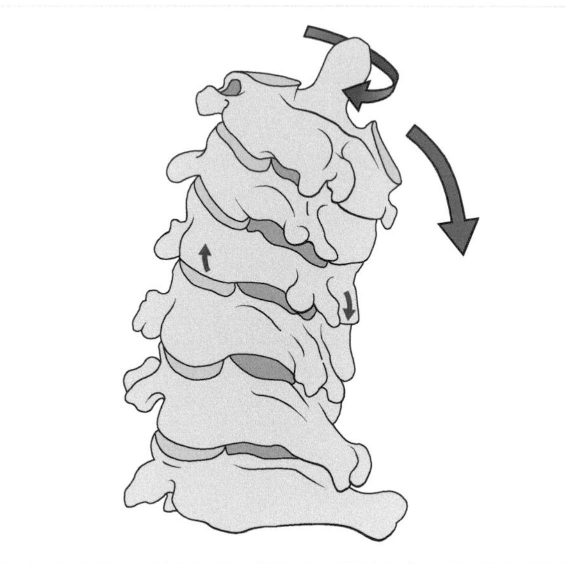

**Fig. 2.74** Combination movement: lateral flexion and simultaneous rotation in the lower cervical spine.

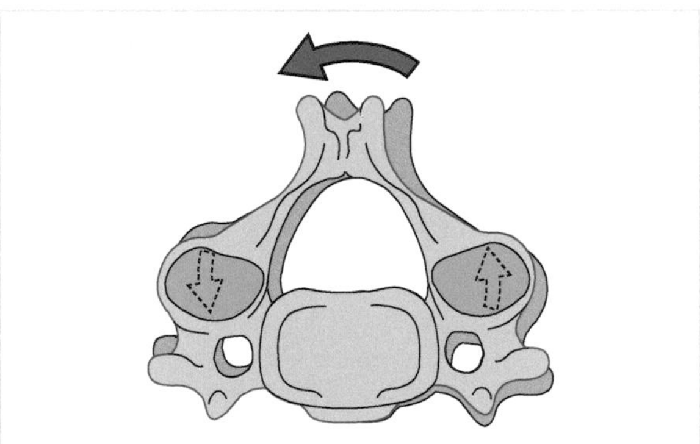

**Fig. 2.75** Rotation in the lower cervical spine.

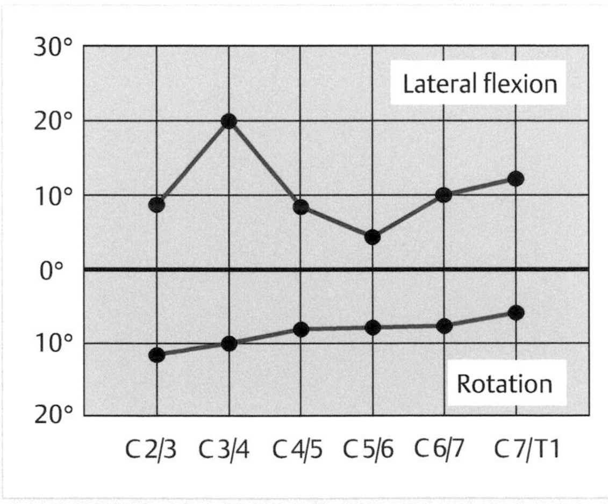


**Fig. 2.76** Movement diagram: lateral flexion/rotation in the lower cervical spine.

## 2.3.4 Prevertebral Muscles

▷ Deep Layer (Fig. 2.77)

### Longus Colli Muscle,

### Longus Capitis Muscle,

### Rectus Capitis Anterior Muscle,

### Anterior Cervical Intertransversarii Muscles

**Rectus capitis lateralis:** This muscle merges with the joint capsule of the atlantooccipital joint.

**Pathology**

The rectus capitis lateralis muscle extends immediately next to the jugular foramen, and, if strongly tensed, can lead to a disturbance of the following structures that run through the foramen: cranial nerves IX, X, and XI and the superior bulb of the jugular vein. This can compromise venous drainage, which in turn can result in diminished fluid resorption.

**Functions of the deep layer:**

- With unilateral contraction: *lateral flexion* on the same side.
- With bilateral contraction: *flexion.*
- These are the most important anterior stabilizers.

▷ See also Functions of the Sternocleidomastoid Muscle below

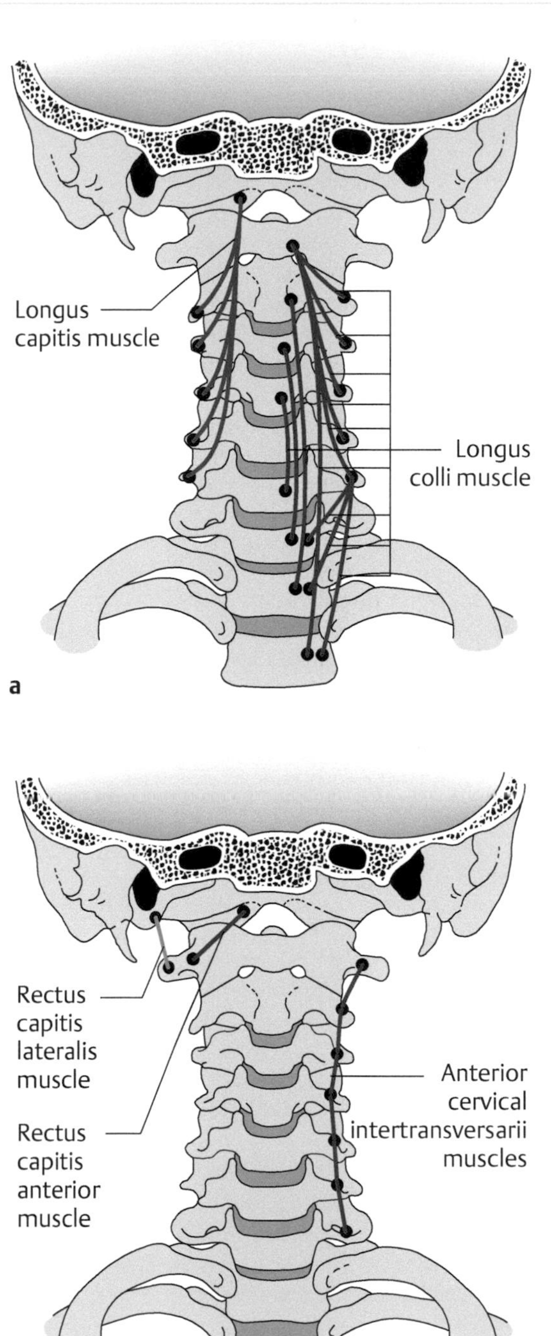


**Fig. 2.77** Deep layer of the prevertebral muscles. **(a)** Longus colli and longus capitis muscles. **(b)** Anterior intertransversarii and anterior and lateral rectus capitis muscles.

▷ Middle Layer (Fig. 2.78)

## Anterior Scalene Muscle, Middle Scalene Muscle, Posterior Scalene Muscle

**Functions:**

- When their fixed end is on the cervical spine, the scalene muscles raise the first ribs bilaterally. They are also activated by normal *inspiration.*
- When their fixed end is on the ribs, bilateral contraction of the anterior and mid parts of the muscles cause *flexion of the entire cervical spine*, while the posterior parts cause *extension of the lower cervical spine.*
- With unilateral contraction, there is *lateral flexion* on the same side and *rotation* to the contralateral side.

## Scalene Hiatus (Fig. 2.79)

*Posterior scalene hiatus:* This is a gap between the anterior and middle scalene muscles with the first rib as the inferior border. The brachial plexus and subclavian artery run through here.

*Anterior scalene hiatus:* This opening is formed by the sternocleidomastoid muscle and anterior scalene muscle. The subclavian vein runs here.

### Pathology

A cervical rib or muscular imbalance, for example from an increase in turgor of the scalene muscles, can cause narrowing of the posterior scalene hiatus.

With a drooping arm, especially when carrying a heavy load, this space narrows further. The existing pain becomes worse, and paresthesias occur in the entire arm. Narrowing of the subclavian artery can also occur, leading to diminished circulation and resultant ischemic events in the hand.

Compression of the anterior hiatus can occur secondary to very tense scalene and sternocleidomastoid muscles, as might happen in individuals with asthma. Symptoms such as bluish, swollen fingers develop, because in this case venous compression is involved, which impedes the return flow.

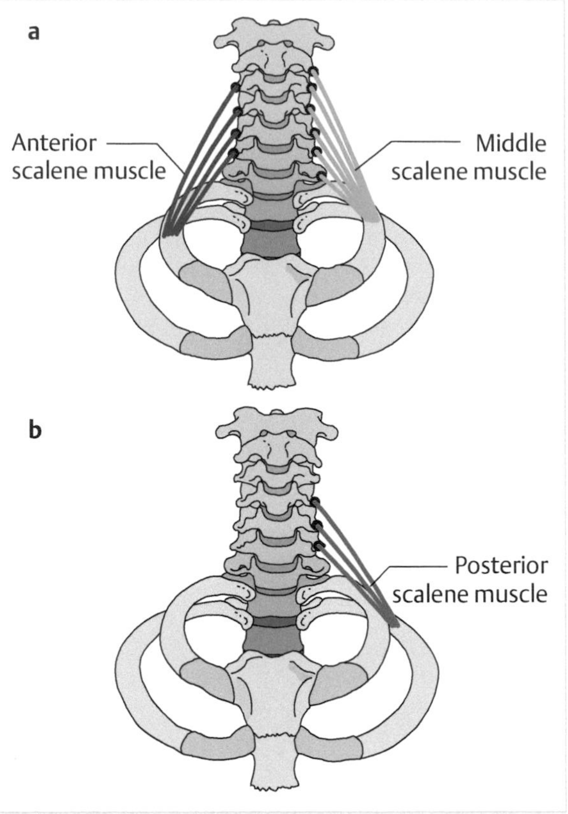


**Fig. 2.78** Scalene muscles. **(a)** Anterior and middle scalene muscles. **(b)** Posterior scalene muscle.

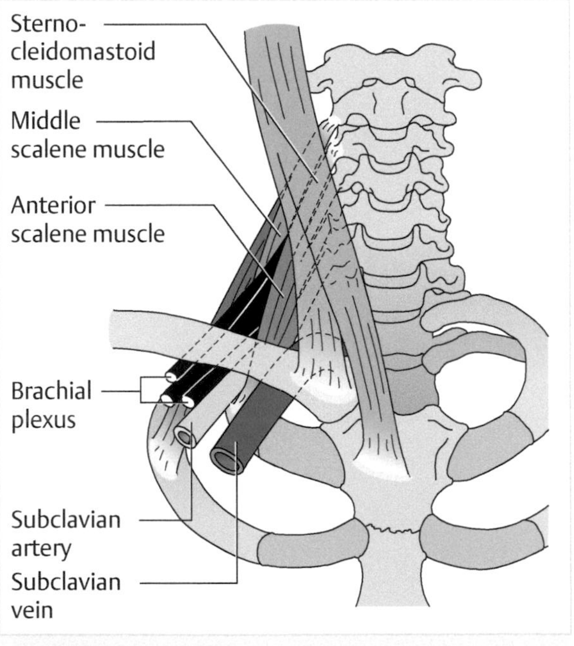


**Fig. 2.79** Scalene hiatus.

▷ Superficial Layer (Figs. 2.80 and 2.81)

## Sternocleidomastoid Muscle

This is covered by part of the *platysma muscle*, a superficial muscle that merges with and tenses the skin.

**Functions:**

- In unilateral contraction, it produces ipsilateral lateral flexion and rotation to the contralateral side.
- With the fixed end on the cervical spine, bilateral contraction raises the thorax, thereby helping with *inspiration.*

The function in the sagittal plane depends on the position of the cervical spine and on anterior stabilization. If the cervical spine is stabilized anteriorly by the deep prevertebral muscles, the sternocleidomastoid muscles produce inclination of the upper cervical spine. If this stabilization is missing, both the scalene and the sternocleidomastoid muscles produce reclination of the upper cervical spine.

**Pathology**

The sternocleidomastoid muscle runs over the occipitomastoid suture, so increased tension in the muscle can influence the dynamics of this suture.

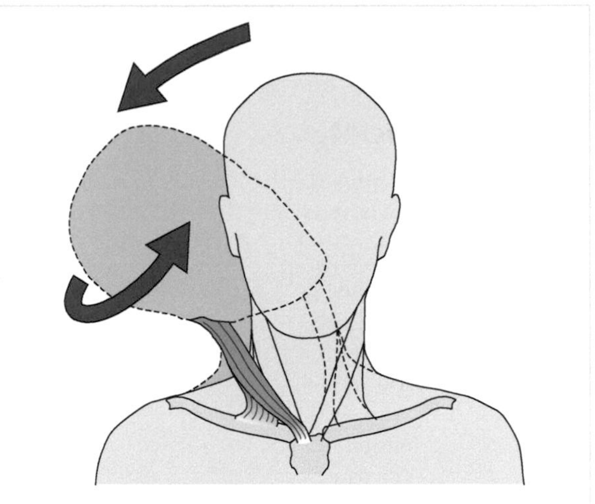

**Fig. 2.80** Function of the sternocleidomastoid muscle: ipsilateral lateral flexion, contralateral rotation.

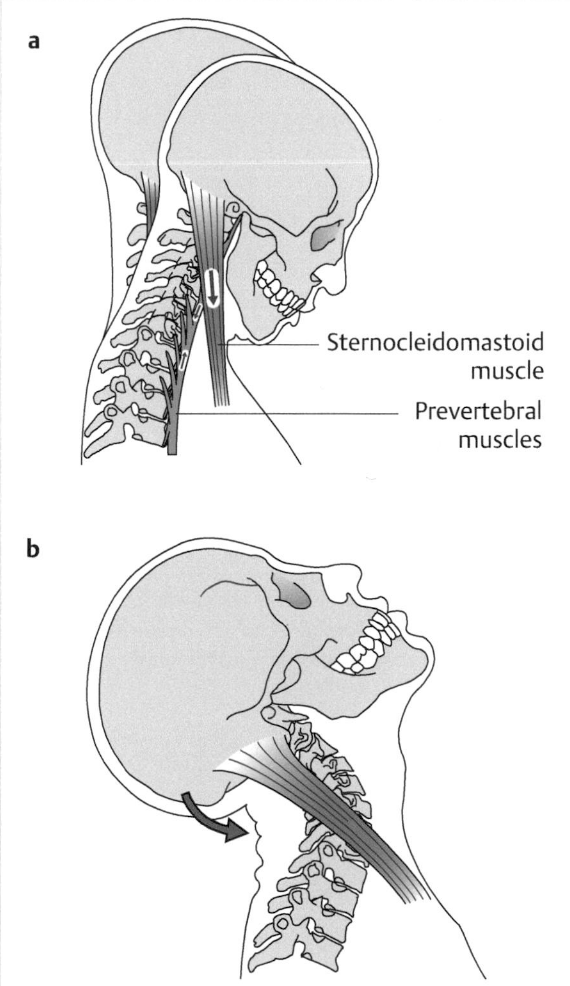


**Fig. 2.81** Function of the sternocleidomastoid muscle. **(a)** With anterior stabilization. **(b)** Without anterior stabilization.

## 2.3.5 Posterior Neck Muscles

▷ Superficial Layer (Fig. 2.82)

### Trapezius Muscle

**Function.** If the fixed end of the muscle is on the shoulder girdle, it produces extension with bilateral contraction. Unilateral contraction causes lateral flexion to the same side and rotation to the contralateral side.

**Practical Tip**

The presence of trigger points over muscle insertions allows conclusions to be drawn on segmental dysfunction in the thoracic spine. For example, the painful point for T6 lies at the insertion sites of the trapezius muscle on the clavicle and acromion.

▷ Middle Layer (Fig. 2.82)

### Longissimus Cervicis Muscle, Longissimus Capitis Muscle, Spinalis Cervicis Muscle, Splenius Cervicis Muscle, Splenius Capitis Muscle

Because of its insertion on both the mastoid process and the occipital bone, the splenius capitis muscle runs obliquely over the occipitomastoid suture. It can therefore influence the mobility of the temporal and occipital bones when it undergoes changes in tension.

### Iliocostalis Cervicis Muscle, Interspinales Cervicis Muscles, Levator Scapulae Muscle

**Function of the levator scapulae muscle.** When the fixed end is on the scapula, unilateral contraction produces lateral flexion and rotation to the same side. Bilateral contraction produces extension.

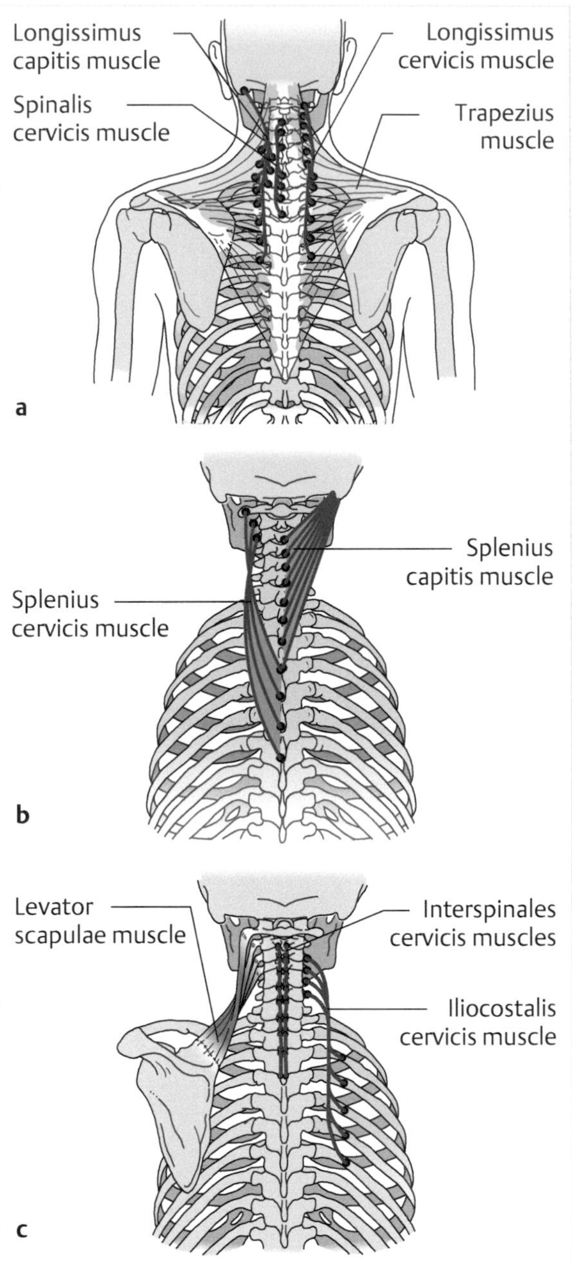


**Fig. 2.82** Superficial and middle layer of the posterior neck muscles. **(a)** Trapezius, longissimus cervicis, Longissimus capitis, and spinalis cervicis muscles. **(b)** Splenius cervicis and splenius capitis muscles. **(c)** Iliocostalis cervicis, interspinales cervicis, and levator scapulae muscles.

▷ Deep Layer (Fig. 2.83)

## Semispinalis Cervicis Muscle,

## Semispinalis Capitis Muscle,

## Posterior Cervical Intertransversarii Muscles,

## Multifidus Muscles,

## Rotatores Cervicis Muscles (Short and Long)

**Functions of the posterior neck muscles:**

- When all the posterior neck muscles contract together bilaterally, they produce *extension* of the cervical spine.
- With unilateral contraction, *lateral flexion* on the same side occurs.
- The muscles of the middle layer, especially the splenius muscles, *rotate* the cervical spine *to the same side.*
- The muscles of the deep layer produce *rotation to the contralateral side.*

Because the center of gravity lies anteriorly, in the area of the sella turcica, the posterior neck muscles act as a stabilizing factor to keep the head in equilibrium. If this stabilization lapses, the head sinks forward, which one can often observe during a train trip or in other public places (**Fig. 2.84**).

**Practical Tip**

The stabilizing tone of the muscles also lapses at night during sleep, so that unfavorable positions of the head can occur, overstretching the capsule–ligament apparatus and causing headaches and functional disturbances in the spinal segments. Therefore extreme positions of the head, such as occur when lying prone, for instance, should be avoided during sleep.

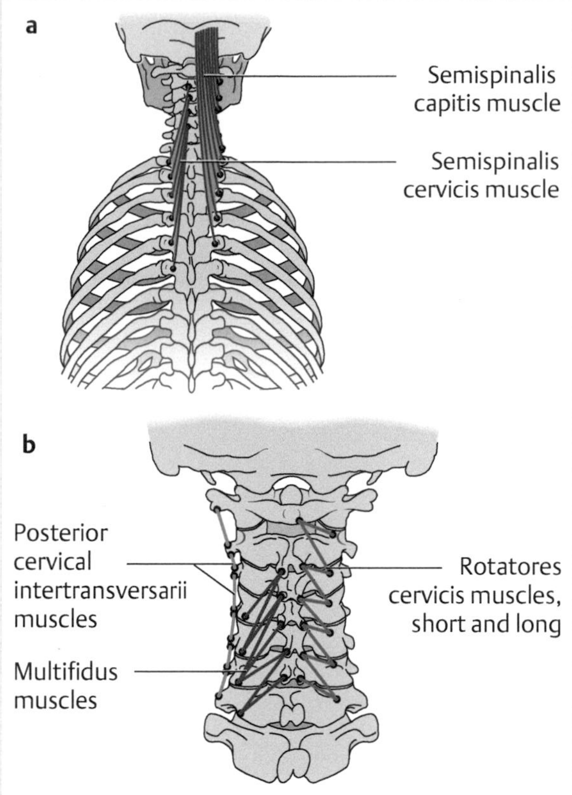


**Fig. 2.83** Deep layer of the posterior neck muscles. **(a)** Semispinalis capitis and semispinalis cervicis muscles. **(b)** Posterior cervical intertransversarii muscles and rotatores cervicis muscles, short and long.

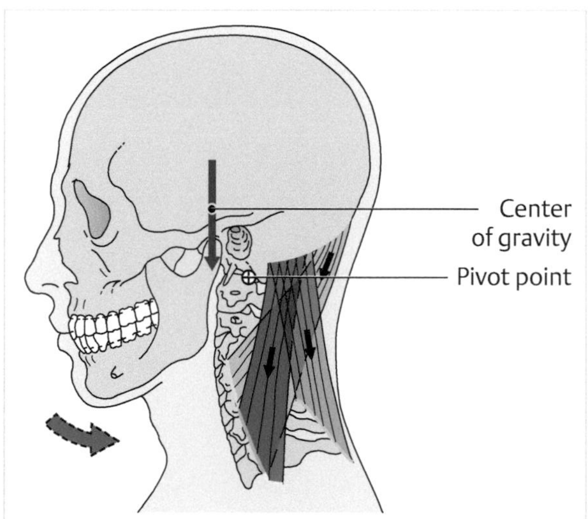


**Fig. 2.84** Stabilizing function of the neck muscles.

## Short Neck Muscles (Fig. 2.85)

- Rectus capitis posterior major muscle.
- Rectus capitis posterior minor muscle.
- Obliquus capitis superior muscle.
- Obliquus capitis inferior muscle.

**Functions (Fig. 2.86):**

- *Bilateral contraction:*
  Extension of the atlantooccipital and atlantoaxial joints = reclination.
- *Unilateral contraction:*
  - *Lateral flexion* to the same side.
  - *Rotation to the same side* by the obliquus capitis inferior and rectus capitis posterior major muscles.
  - *Rotation to the contralateral side* by the medial fibers of the obliquus capitis superior muscle.

Together with the long muscles of the neck, the short neck muscles are an important integral part of the support system for the spinal column.

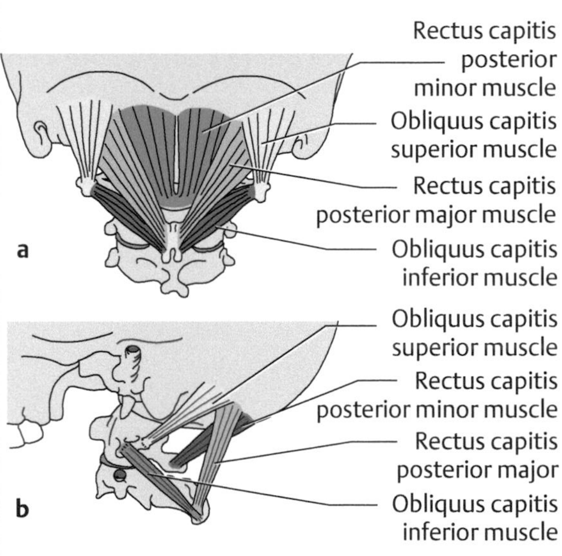


**Fig. 2.85** The short neck muscles. **(a)** Posterior view. **(b)** Lateral view.

### Practical Tip

Strong tension in the short neck muscles can influence the gliding motion between C0 and C2 in a posterior direction and thereby inhibit inclination. Stretch tests of these muscles, along with the usual joint tests, are therefore important in evaluating physiologic motion sequences.

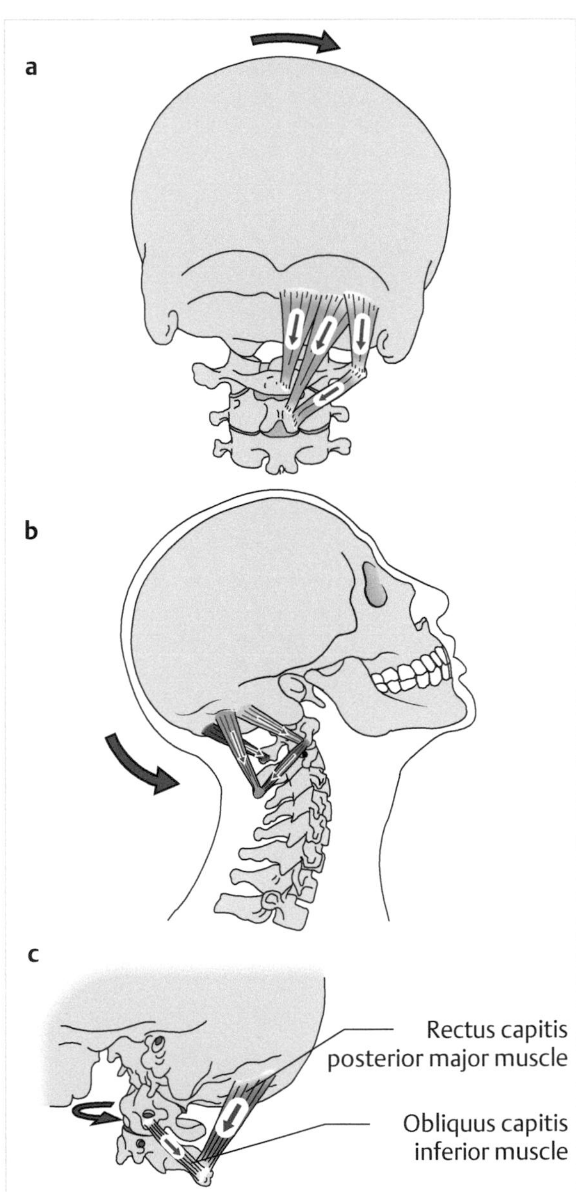


**Fig. 2.86** Function of the short neck muscles. **(a)** Lateral flexion. **(b)** Reclination. **(c)** Rotation to the same side.

## 2.3.6 Brachial Plexus (Fig. 2.87)

The *anterior rami* of spinal nerves C5–T1 combine to form *trunks*, which transition to divisions. There, a branching takes place, from which the *cords* originate. They arrange themselves around the axillary artery in the following manner:

- The posterior cord runs posterior to the artery.
- The lateral cord run superior and anterior.
- The medial cord runs medial and inferior.

The nerves of the arm arise from the cords:

- The axillary and radial nerves from the posterior cord.
- The musculocutaneous and median nerves from the lateral cord.
- The median and ulnar nerves from the medial cord. Note that the median nerve arises from two cords, forming the "*M structure*."

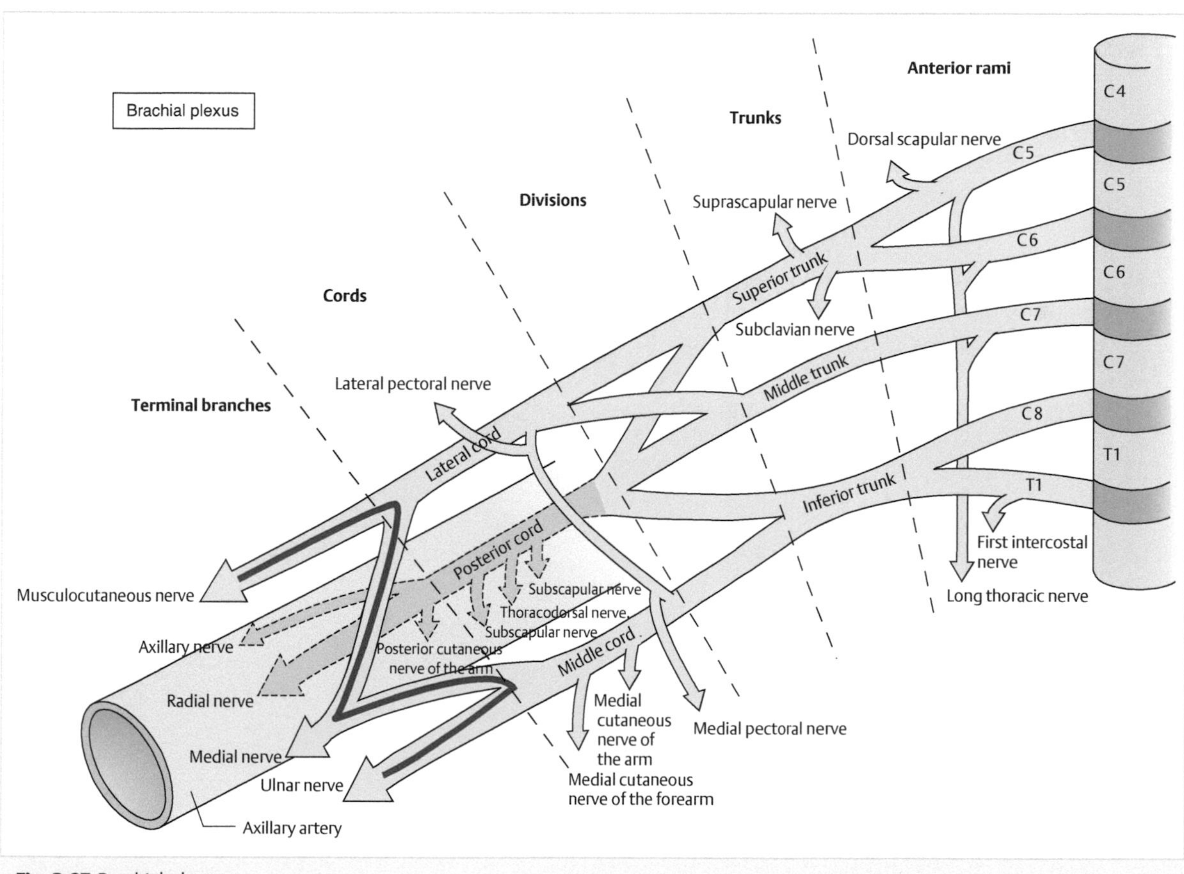


**Fig. 2.87** Brachial plexus.

## Pathology

**Brachial plexus compression syndrome (Fig. 2.88):** There are a few places where the plexus can experience compression after it leaves the intervertebral foramen. The arrangement of the muscles leads to narrow points, such as in the area of the scalene muscles. Other areas in which the plexus can be compressed are as follows.

In the **clavicular area** (costoclavicular space):

This opening is formed by the clavicle and the first rib. Together with the subclavian artery and vein, the plexus runs through here toward the axilla. The costoclavicular space is narrowed by lowering and retracting the shoulder girdle.

The causes of narrowing can be a prominently flat back with retracted shoulders, constantly carrying heavy weight on the shoulder, or a clavicular fracture with subsequent step formation.

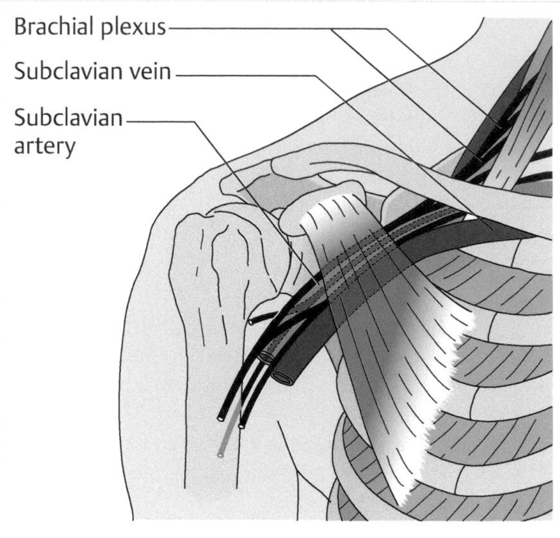


**Fig. 2.88** Brachial plexus compression syndrome.

## Practical Tip

To establish whether a narrowed costoclavicular space is responsible for radiating pain, apply sustained downward pressure on the shoulder girdle to further narrow this space. If the radiating pain is triggered or reinforced, the cause lies in this area.

## Pathology

In the **pectoralis minor** muscle area (hyperabduction syndrome):

Along with the subclavian artery and vein, the brachial plexus passes under the pectoralis minor muscle and the coracoid process toward the axilla. Maximal abduction stretches the plexus, because the tendinous part of the pectoralis minor muscle loops around it. If the pectoralis minor muscle is very tight, raising the arm stretches the plexus. Holding this position for a prolonged time, while sleeping or for other reasons, can cause symptoms.

## Practical Tip

As a provocation test, raise the arm superiorly and posteriorly and hold it in this position. After 1 to 2 minutes, if all is normal, the radial pulse can still be clearly felt and there will be no complaints of radiating pain.

# Chapter 3

## Thoracic Spine and Thorax



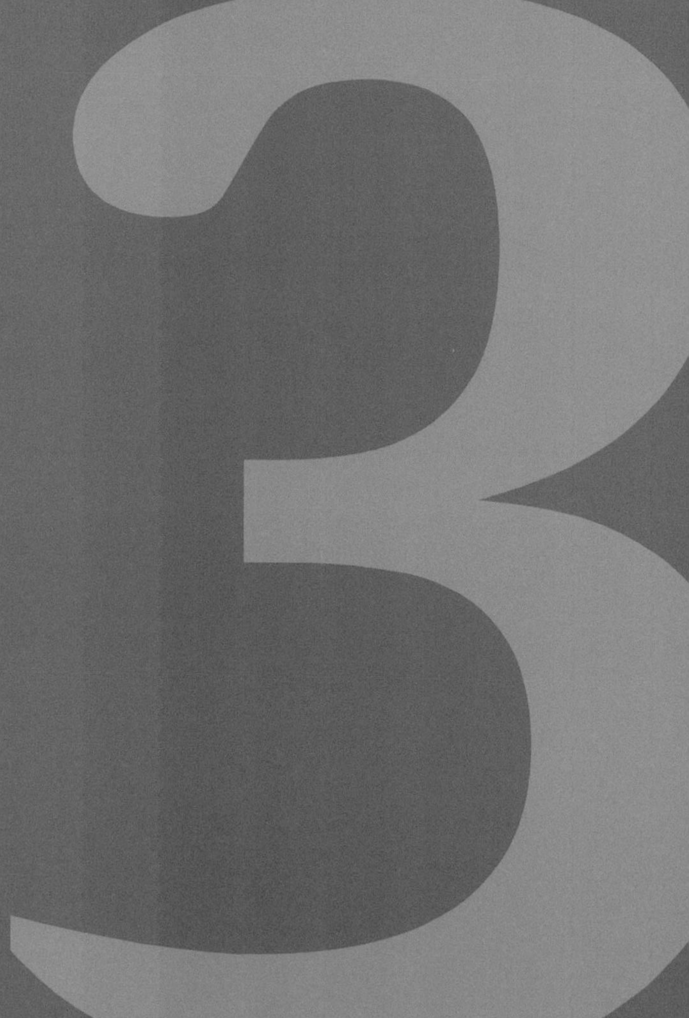

# 3 Thoracic Spine and Thorax

## 3.1 Palpation of Landmarks of the Thoracic Spine and Thorax

▷ Bones, Ligaments, Joints

### Spinous Process (Fig. 3.1)

The spinous processes have numerous muscle insertion sites, which lie very close to each other. Exact identification is barely possible.

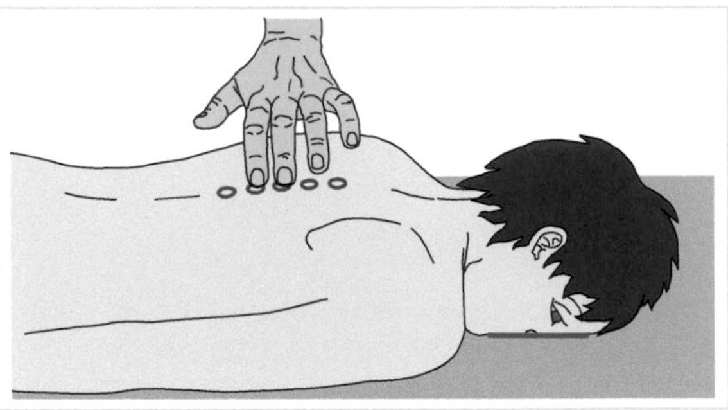

**Fig. 3.1** Palpation: spinous process.

### Muscle Insertion Sites (Fig. 3.2)

1 = Trapezius muscle
2 = Rhomboid major muscle
3 = Multifidus muscle
4 = Splenius cervicis muscle
5 = Rotator muscles
6 = Spinalis muscle
7 = Semispinalis thoracis muscle

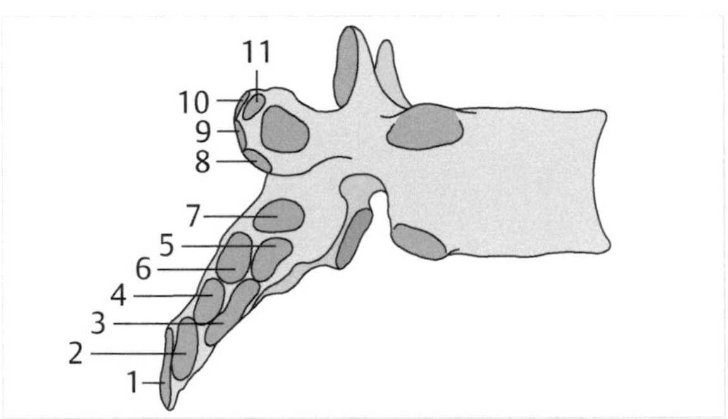


**Fig. 3.2** Muscle insertion sites on the spinous and transverse processes.

### Connecting Ligament

The *supraspinous ligaments* extend from the tip of one spinous process to the next. In flexion, they are stretched by the divergent movement of the spinous processes, and they can then be palpated by approaching from below.

### Transverse Process (Figs. 3.3 and 3.4)

Orientation starts with the spinous processes. The tips of the transverse processes of T1–T4 and T10–T12 lie about two fingerbreadths superior to the corresponding spinous processes. They can be located at the lateral border of the erector spinae muscle, which can be palpated about 2 to 3 fingerbreadths lateral to the spinous processes. For T5–T9, they are about three fingerbreadths superiorly, because the spinous processes run more steeply downward in this area.

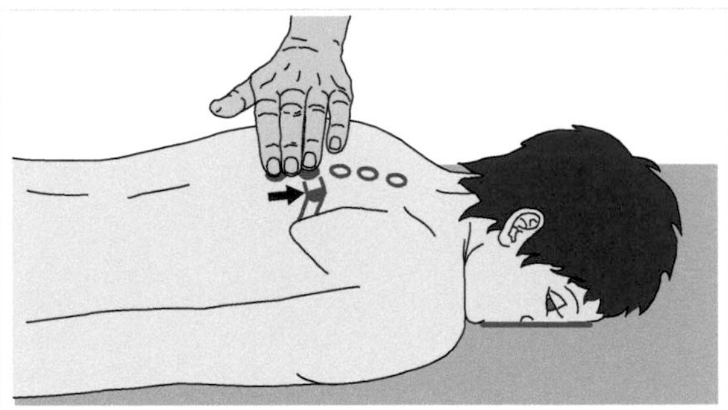

**Fig. 3.3** Palpation: orientation guide for finding the transverse processes in the mid-thoracic spinal region.

### Muscle Insertion Sites (Fig. 3.2)

8 = Levator costae muscle
9 = Iliocostalis muscle, thoracic part
10 = Longissimus thoracis muscle
11 = Longissimus cervicis muscle

Palpation of the deeper lying muscle insertions is barely possible because of the overlying erector spinae muscle.

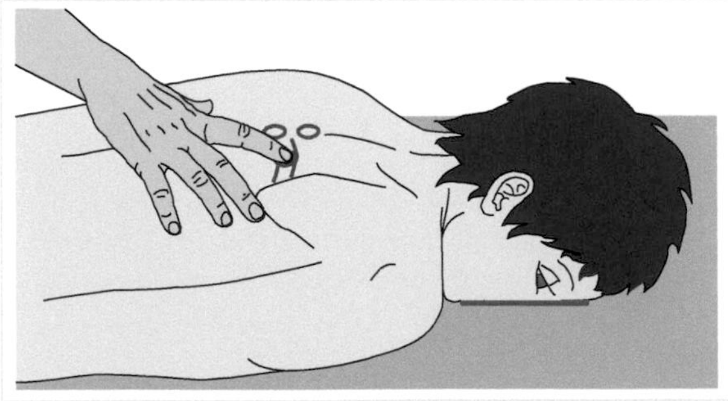

**Fig. 3.4** Palpation: transverse process.

## Costotransverse Joint (Fig. 3.5)

The lateral costotransverse ligament extends from the tip of the transverse process to the rib and can be palpated immediately lateral to the tip. The longissimus thoracis muscle lies above it and must be shifted slightly to the side. The joint gap of the costotransverse joint lies deep under the ligament and cannot be felt.

### Practical Tip

Decreased mobility of a rib can be evaluated by palpating in this area while the patient is taking deep breaths. In the case of functional blockage of a rib, the lateral costotransverse ligament is very painful.

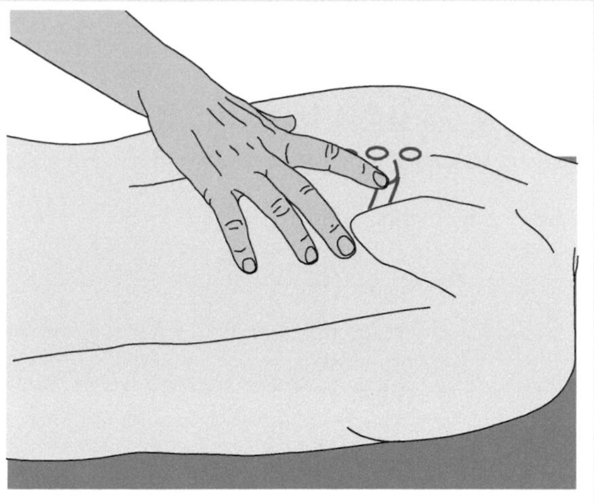

**Fig. 3.5** Palpation: costotransverse joint.

## Angles of the Ribs (Fig. 3.6)

The angle of the rib is located about a handbreadth lateral to the costovertebral joints. It can be felt as a distinctive kink in the rib.

### Practical Tip

Because the angles of the ribs form prominent projections, the heel of the hand can be used to mobilize a rib in an anterolateral direction.

### Pathology

In functional disturbances of the costovertebral joint, the corresponding angle of the rib can be tender to palpation.

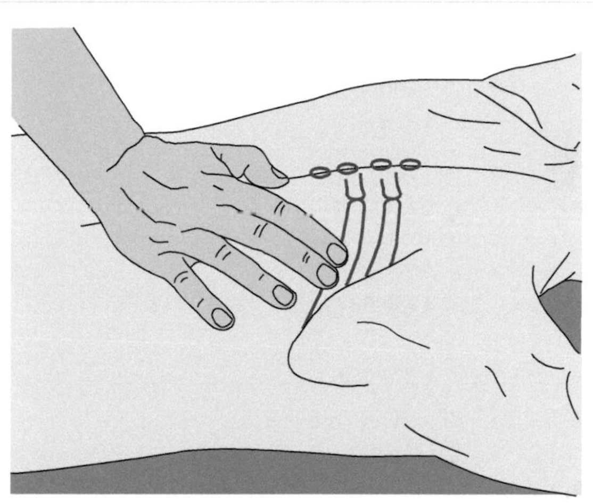

**Fig. 3.6** Palpation: angle of the rib.

## Sternocostal Joints (Fig. 3.7)

To evaluate the interface between the rib and the sternum, use palpation in a direct side-to-side comparison in both the supine and sitting positions. The load on the sternocostal joints is greater in the sitting position than in the supine position.

### Practical Tip

Significantly more pain is felt in the sternocostal joints when a poor posture is adopted, such as sitting with a rounded back and sagging thorax, than when the patient is in an upright sitting position or supine. When the symptoms are pronounced, traction over the ribs can produce a significant improvement. Over time, however, this treatment is not sufficient because the underlying cause will persist as long as the poor posture has not been corrected.

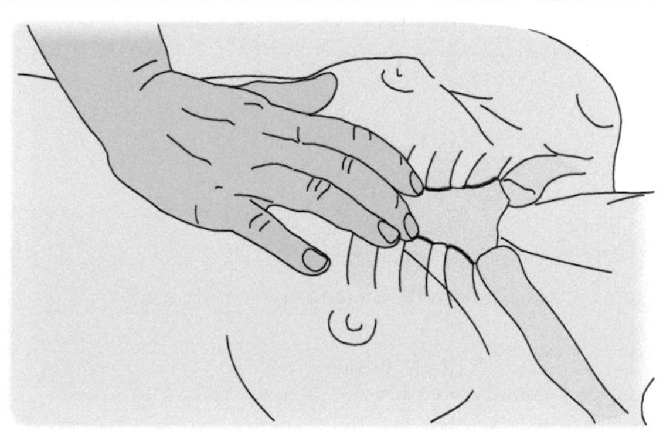

**Fig. 3.7** Palpation: sternocostal joints.

▷ Muscles

## Diaphragm (Fig. 3.8)

Place the thumbs of both hands inferiorly under the lowest costal arch and press the ribs in a superolateral direction.

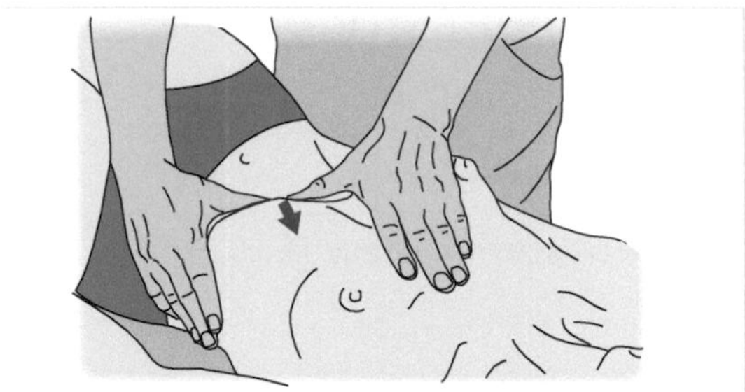

**Fig. 3.8** Palpation: elasticity of the diaphragm.

### Practical Tip

Palpation of the diaphragm provides information about its elasticity, any evasive movements, and painful muscle guarding. The ribs can usually be shifted a considerable distance without resistance, and the movement should also be bilaterally symmetrical.

### Pathology

Muscle tension in the diaphragm can occur as a result of dysfunction in the thoracic area or abdominal cavity.

## Intercostal Muscles (Fig. 3.9)

Use a finger between the ribs to palpate the intercostal muscles by placing it anteriorly and slowly moving it posteriorly within the intercostal space.

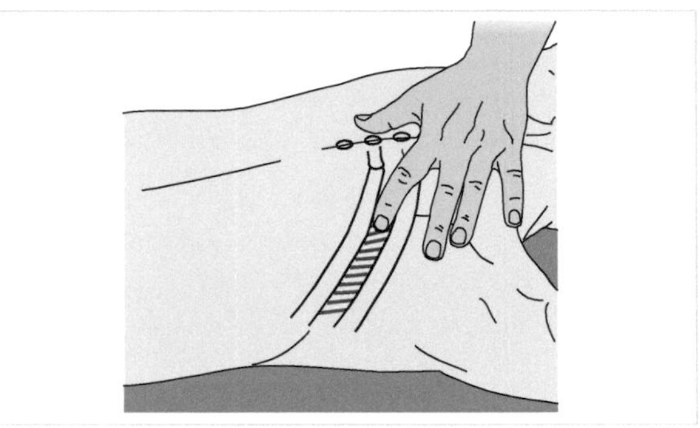

**Fig. 3.9** Palpation: intercostal muscles.

## Erector Spinae Muscle (Fig. 3.10)

The erector spinae muscle lies alongside to the vertebrae. Palpate it as a longitudinally running strand of muscle about 2 to 3 fingerbreadths wide.

Evaluate all the muscles that extend from the thorax and thoracic spine to the arm, head, or pelvis to evaluate their state of tension and possible points of irritation.

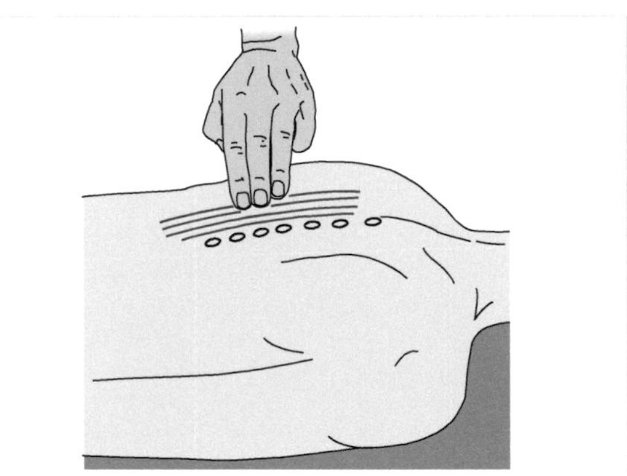

**Fig. 3.10** Palpation: erector spinae muscle.

## Rhomboid Muscles (Fig. 3.11)

The rhomboid muscles run obliquely from the lower cervical spine and upper thoracic spine to the medial border of the scapula. They can be palpated between the shoulder blades.

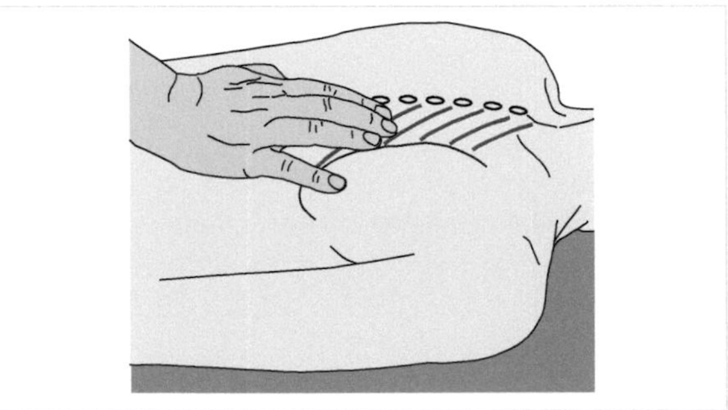

**Fig. 3.11** Palpation: rhomboid muscles.

## Trapezius Muscle/Latissimus Dorsi Muscle,

## Pectoralis Major Muscle/Pectoralis Minor Muscle,

## Sternocleidomastoid Muscle/Scalene Muscles

▷ See Chapters 2.1, Palpation of the Cervical Spine and 4.1, Palpation of the Shoulder

# 3.2 Functional Anatomy of the Thoracic Spine

## 3.2.1 X-Ray of the Thoracic Spine

### Anteroposterior View (Fig. 3.12)

#### Pedicular Arches

These are seen as bilaterally symmetrical oval rings.

#### Spinal Canal Width

The width of the spinal canal increases as one moves inferiorly.

### Thoracic Spine, Lateral View (Fig. 3.13)

#### Kyphotic Angle

If the perpendiculars to the lines through the superior end plate of the T3 vertebral body and the inferior end plate of the T11 vertebral body are connected, the upper (or lower) angle should measure approximately 25°.

#### Intervertebral Disk Spaces

- Parallel end plates.
- Width:
  - Upper thoracic spine 3 to 4 mm.
  - Mid-thoracic spine, approximately 4 to 5 mm.
  - Lower thoracic spine, approximately 6 mm.

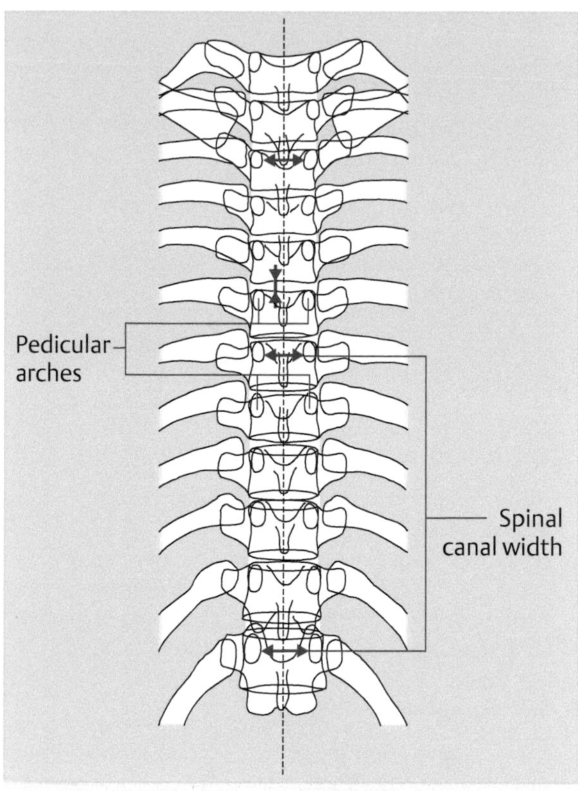


**Fig. 3.12** X-ray image: thoracic spine (anteroposterior view).

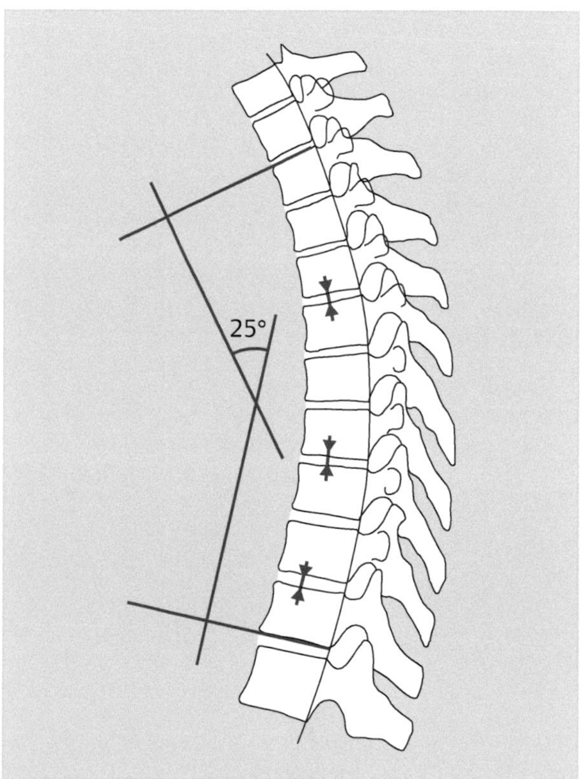


**Fig. 3.13** X-ray image: thoracic spine (lateral view).

## 3.2.2 Thoracic Vertebra

### Vertebral Body (Figs. 3.14 and 3.15)

- The height of the vertebral bodies gradually increases from T1 to T12.
- Joint surfaces for the costal head:
  - A **superior costal facet** on the upper margin of the vertebral body.
  - An **inferior costal facet** on the lower margin of the vertebral body.

From the T9 vertebra downward, the joint surfaces migrate toward the middle of the vertebral body.

### Spinous Process

- This is very long and runs obliquely downward. In most sections, the tip of the spinous process lies about two fingerbreadths inferior to the transverse process.
- In the T5–T9 section, the tip of the spinous process is about three fingerbreadths inferior to the corresponding transverse process.
- The spinous process of T1 is similar to that of the cervical vertebrae.

### Transverse Process

- This is well built and posterolaterally oriented. In the upper thoracic spine, the longitudinal axis through the transverse process forms an angle of approximately 35° with the frontal plane. In the lower section, this angle can reach 55°.
- The **transverse costal facet** on the anterior end of the transverse process forms a connection to the rib.
- The joint surfaces lie in the middle in the superior sections of the thoracic spine, while they have a more superior position on the transverse processes of the lower thoracic spine. They are absent on the 11th and 12th thoracic vertebrae.

### Articular Process

- The **superior articular process** represents the connection to the next vertebra above, and the **inferior articular process** the connection to the one below.
- Position:
  - 20° to the frontal plane.
  - 60° to the horizontal plane in the upper section. Moving inferiorly, the angle increases slightly, so that at T12 it is approximately 80°.

▷ See Chapter 1, Fundamentals of the Spinal Column

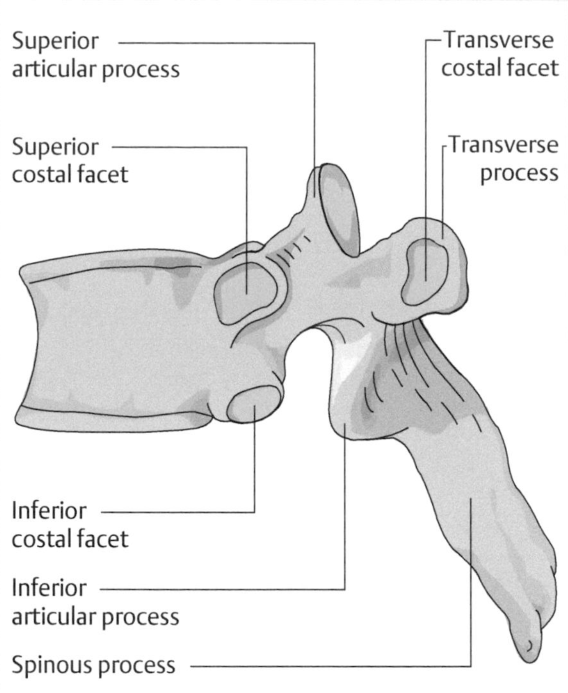


**Fig. 3.14** Thoracic vertebra (lateral view).

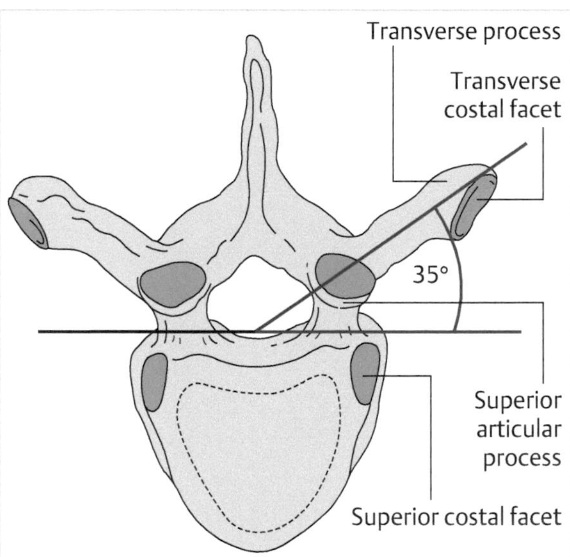


**Fig. 3.15** Thoracic vertebra (horizontal view).

### Distinctive Features of the 12th Thoracic Vertebra (Fig. 3.16)

- The shape of the spinous process conforms to that of a lumbar vertebra.
- The inferior articular process is oriented facing anterolaterally.
- The transverse process is shorter and has an accessory process, like the lumbar vertebrae.

### Intervertebral Disk

The disk space is very narrow in relation to the vertebral bodies and indicates the limited mobility of the thoracic spine.

## 3.2.3 Ligaments of the Thoracic Spine (Fig. 3.17)

### Posterior Longitudinal Ligament,

### Anterior Longitudinal Ligament,

### Ligamentum Flavum, Intertransverse Ligament,

### Interspinous Ligament, Supraspinous Ligament

▷ See Chapter 1, Fundamentals of the Spinal Column

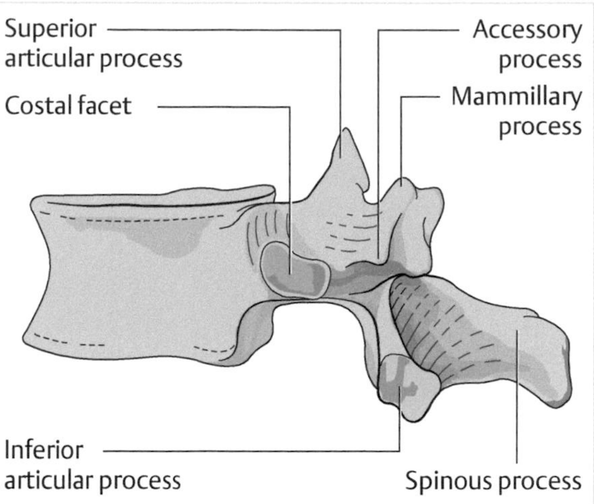


**Fig. 3.16** Twelfth thoracic vertebra (lateral view).

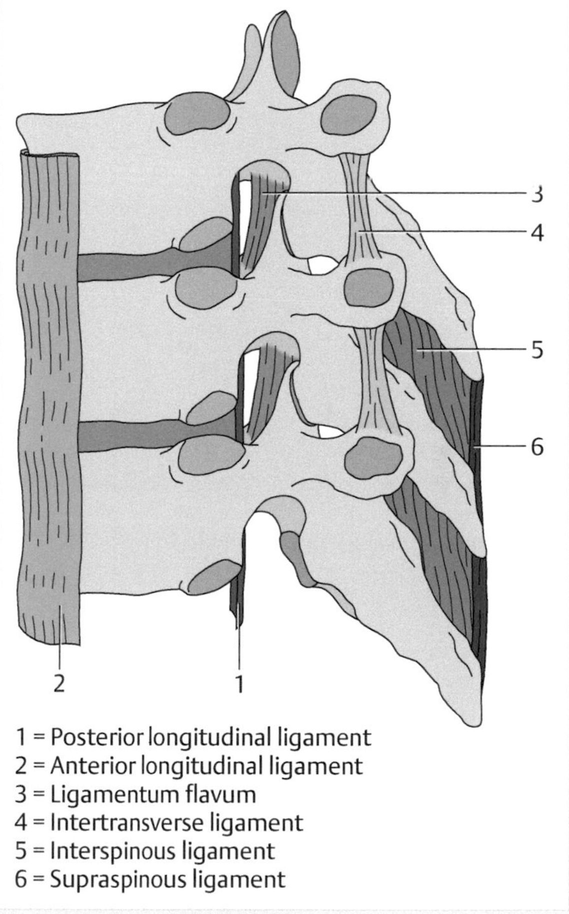


**Fig. 3.17** Ligaments of the thoracic spine (lateral view).

## 3.2.4 Movements in the Thoracic Spine Area

The connection with the thorax sets limits on the mobility of the spine, although the costal cartilage has an elastic give. Because there is a very high proportion of cartilage in the inferior section (T9–T12), this has marked plasticity and thus the best possible mobility.

### Flexion (Figs. 3.18 and 3.20)

A small gap develops in the lower parts of the joint and compression in the upper parts. The movement is limited by the posteriorly lying ligaments and the anulus fibrosus.

*Mobility*

- Lower thoracic spine: good.
- T1–T8: minimal.

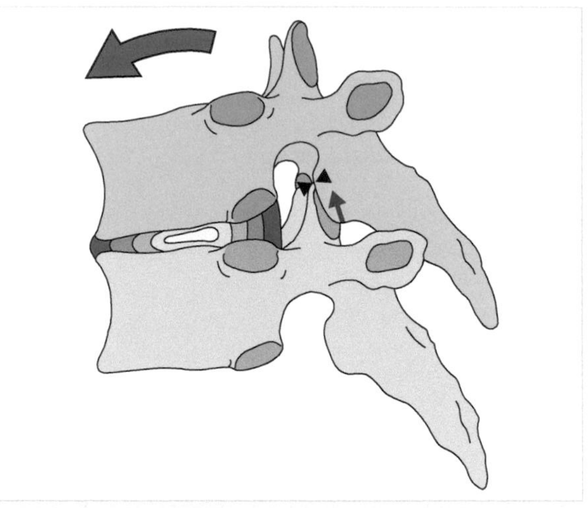

**Fig. 3.18** Flexion in the thoracic spine.

### Extension (Figs. 3.19 and 3.20)

There is negligible gapping in the upper part of the joint and slight compression in the lower part. Extension is limited by the superior reinforcing bands of the capsule, the anterior longitudinal ligament, the anulus fibrosus, and possibly the bony “stop” as the spinous processes come into contact with each other.

*Mobility*

- Lower thoracic spine: good.
- Mid-thoracic spine: very minimal.
- Upper thoracic spine: minimal.
- Overall: very minimal.

Movement testing, normal result: reversal of kyphosis.

Because the exact measurement of mobility is only possible by means of functional X-ray views, the range of motion is estimated.

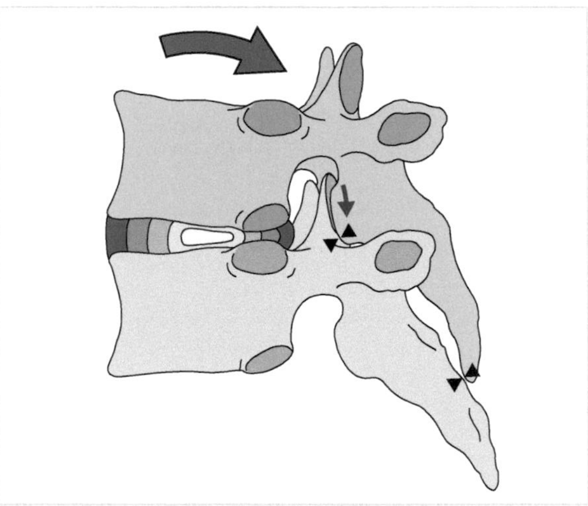

**Fig. 3.19** Extension in the thoracic spine.

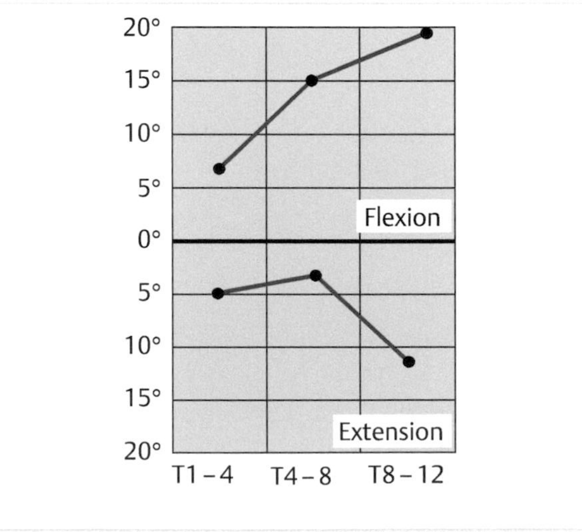


**Fig. 3.20** Movement diagram: flexion/extension.

## Lateral Flexion (Figs. 3.21 and 3.23)

A sliding movement in a superior direction takes place in the joint facets on the contralateral side. On the ipsilateral side, the sliding movement takes place in an inferior direction (see also **Fig. 3.23**).

*Mobility*

- Lower thoracic spine: very good.
- Lower thoracic spine: good.
- Upper thoracic spine: minimal.

During this movement, the intercostal spaces widen on the convex side and narrow on the concave side.

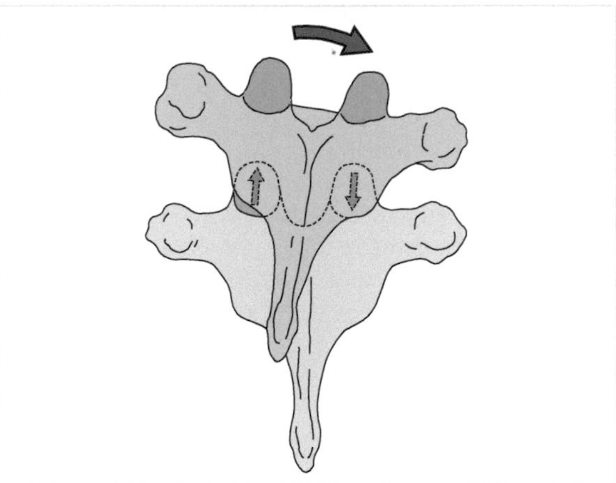

**Fig. 3.21** Lateral flexion in the thoracic spine.

## Rotation (Figs. 3.22 and 3.23)

Rotation may or may not be coupled with lateral flexion owing to the slightly circular curvature of the joint surfaces.

In the thorax, the ribs on the side toward which rotation is occurring are more strongly bent superiorly, while they straighten out somewhat inferiorly. The converse occurs on the side away from the rotation. This deformation of the thorax places the sternum at an angle.

*Mobility*

- Lower thoracic spine: limited mobility.
- Mid-thoracic spine: good mobility.
- Upper thoracic spine: limited mobility.

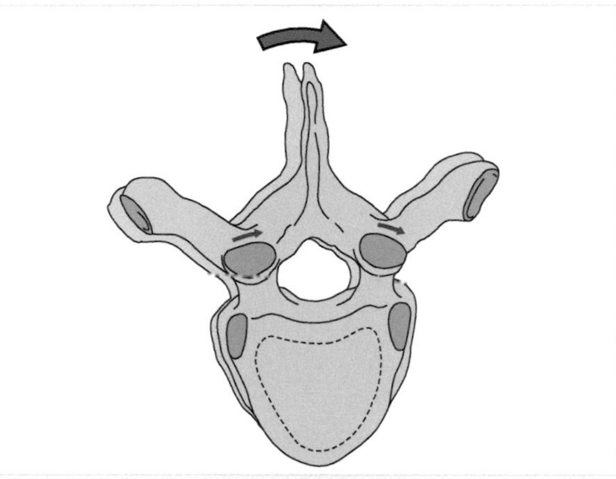

**Fig. 3.22** Rotation in the thoracic spine.

**Practical Tip**

From a functional point of view, the upper thoracic spine belongs to the cervical spine, and it can be well palpated as a continuation movement in the mobility assessment of the cervical spine. For this reason, functional disturbances in the upper thoracic spine have an influence on head movements and can cause radiating pain to the neck, shoulder, and arm.

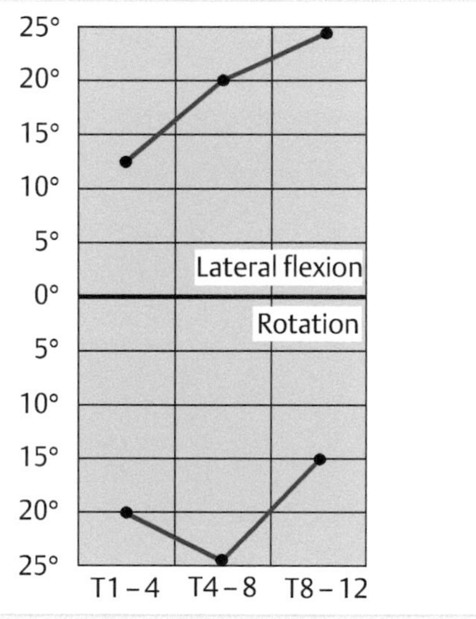


**Fig. 3.23** Movement diagram: lateral flexion/rotation.

## Movement Tendencies of the Thoracic Spine during Breathing

In the upright sitting position or in standing, there is a tendency toward extension of the thoracic spine during inspiration and flexion during exhalation.

Supporting the arms in front of the body fixes the shoulder girdle. This prevents the thoracic spine from straightening and produces an increase in kyphosis (flexion movement) during inspiration.

# 3.3 Functional Anatomy of the Thorax

## Ribs (Fig. 3.24)

- The ribs have bony sections (**body**, **angle**, **neck**, and **head**) and collagenous sections (costal cartilage).
- **True ribs**: The first seven pairs of ribs form a ring, which includes the sternum and the thoracic vertebrae.
- **False ribs**: The 8th to 10th rib pairs are connected by cartilage.
- **Floating ribs**: The last two pairs of ribs remain unattached at their free end.
- Rib position: inclination of 45°.

## Costotransverse Joint (Fig. 3.25)

- The **articular facets of the tubercle** are located on the tubercles of the rib body and are slightly convex in shape in the upper thorax.
- The **transverse costal facet of the transverse process** of the same level has a corresponding concave joint surface.
- The joint surfaces become increasingly flat in the inferior section of the thorax.
- The ribs from T1 to T7 lie directly anterior to the transverse processes. From T8 down, they shift more superiorly on the transverse processes. In the lower region, they lose contact with it.
- The **joint capsule** is thin and has recesses of varying sizes. Meniscoid synovial eversions are also present.

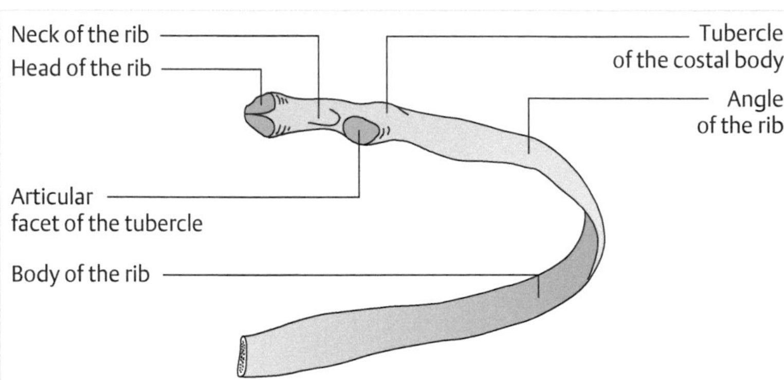


**Fig. 3.24** Rib (posterior view).

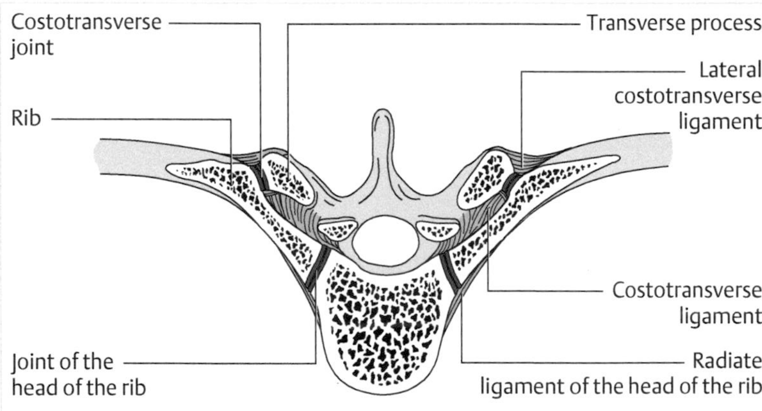


**Fig. 3.25** Costotransverse joint.

## Joint of the Head of the Rib (Fig. 3.26)

- The **inferior and superior costal facets** of two adjacent vertebrae together with the intervertebral disk that lies between form the joint socket for the head of the rib. They lie at the superior and inferior margins of the vertebral body. Exceptions are the joint surfaces of the 1st, 11th, and 12th ribs. Here the joint surfaces lie more toward the middle of the vertebral body.
- The **articular facet on the head of the rib** is divided into two facets by the crest of the head. The lower one is somewhat larger and articulates with the vertebral body of the same level. The smaller, upper facet has contact with the next higher vertebral body. Exceptions are the 1st, 11th, and 12th ribs. They have only one facet and articulate with the vertebral body of the same level.

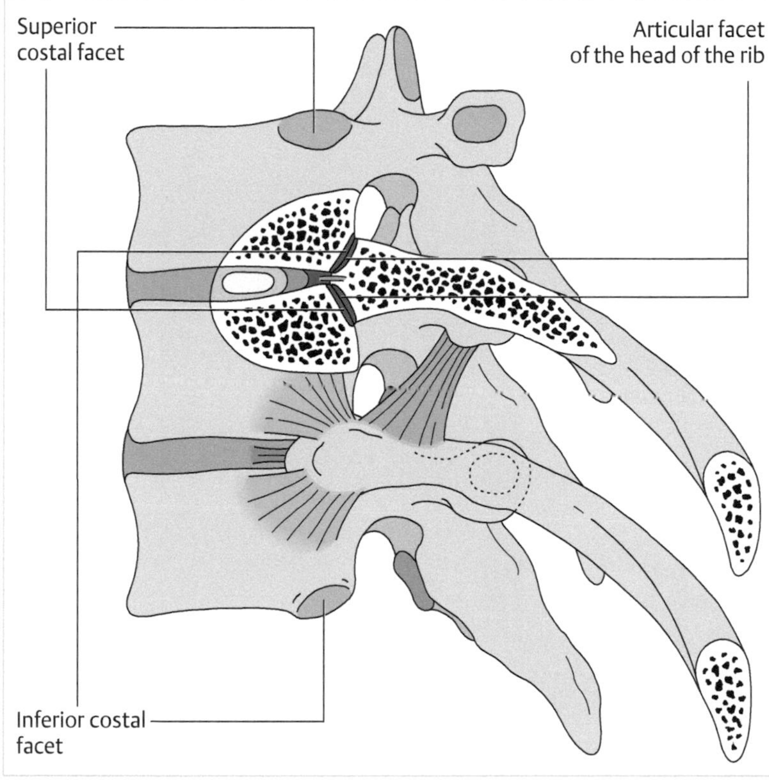


**Fig. 3.26** Joint of the head of the rib.

## Ligaments of the Costovertebral Joint

### Lateral Costotransverse Ligament (Fig. 3.27)

This ligament joins the tip of the transverse processes with the rib and lies directly over the capsule. It is strongest in the area of the second to seventh ribs and is weaker in the inferior area.

### Costotransverse Ligament (Fig. 3.27)

This extends from the neck of the rib to the transverse process of the same level.

### Radiate Ligament of the Head of the Rib (Fig. 3.28)

This merges with the joint capsule and divides into three fibrous bands. The superior and inferior bands extend to the vertebral body and the middle band to the intervertebral disk.

### Intra-articular Ligament of the Head of the Rib (Fig. 3.28)

This ligament lies between the two facets of the joint and divides the joint into two chambers. It extends from the crest of the head of the rib to the outer zone of the anulus fibrosus.

### Superior Costotransverse Ligament (Fig. 3.28)

The ligament runs from the lower margin of the transverse process of the next superior vertebra to the neck of the rib.

**Function of the ligaments.** They stabilize the costovertebral joints.

**Practical Tip**

The joint between the head of the rib and its surrounding ligaments represents a very narrow connection to the motion segment of the thoracic spine.
This means that, when faced with the functional blockage of a rib, it is imperative that the motion segment lying at the same level be treated so that there are no recurrences. Conversely, when there are functional disturbances in the thoracic spine area, the ribs must also be treated.

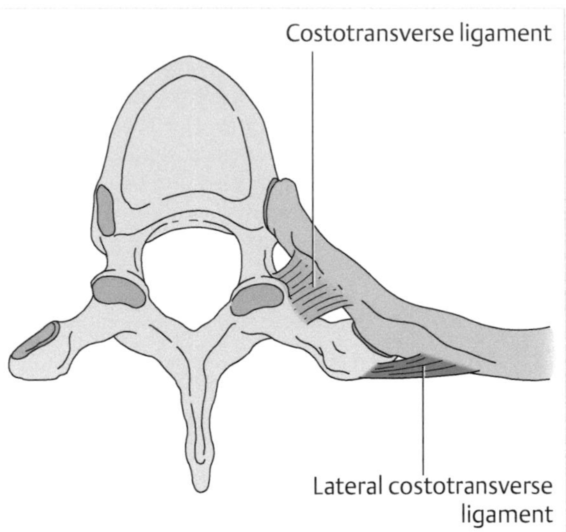


**Fig. 3.27** Ligaments of the costotransverse joint (superior view).

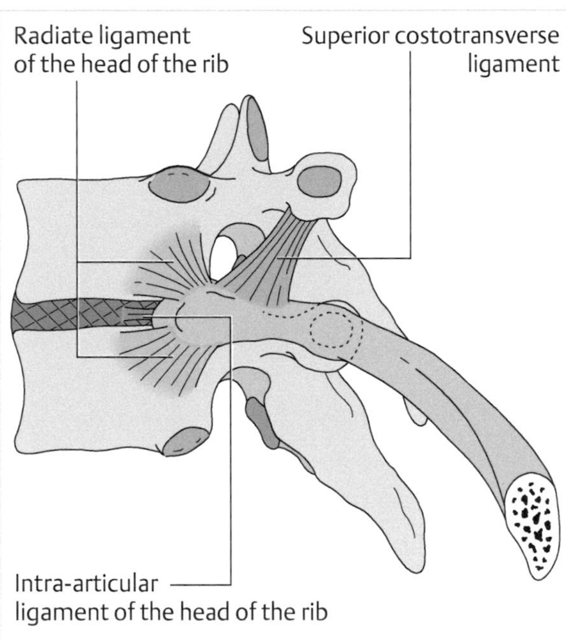


**Fig. 3.28** Ligaments of the costovertebral joint (lateral view).

## Sternocostal Joints (Fig. 3.29)

- The **costal notches** on the sternum and the sternal ends of the costal cartilage articulate with each other.
- A distinct joint space usually develops only in the area of the second to fifth ribs. A fibrocollagenous plate, the intra-articular sternocostal ligament, may divide the joint space into two chambers.
- The **radiate sternocostal ligament** strengthens the joint capsule. It extends from the costal cartilage to the anterior surface of the sternum, where it spreads out like a fan.
- The first, sixth, and seventh ribs form a synchondrosis and are bound directly to the sternum. The **costoxiphoid ligament** extends from the costal cartilage of the sixth and seventh ribs to the xiphoid process.
- The **interchondral joints** join the 8th to 10th ribs together.

### Pathology

A constant kyphotic posture ("sternal load posture") can lead to inflammatory processes in the sternocostal joints because of their constant compression.

### Practical Tip

As a result of the stability of the thorax, disk problems occur rarely in the thoracic spine. However, its connections to the ribs and sternum (and thereby to the clavicle as well), represent disturbance variables, so these structures must be examined when functional disturbances and radiating pain occur.
The thorax is also the insertion site for many peripheral muscle slings, especially for the upper extremity. Transmitted pains can have their origin here.

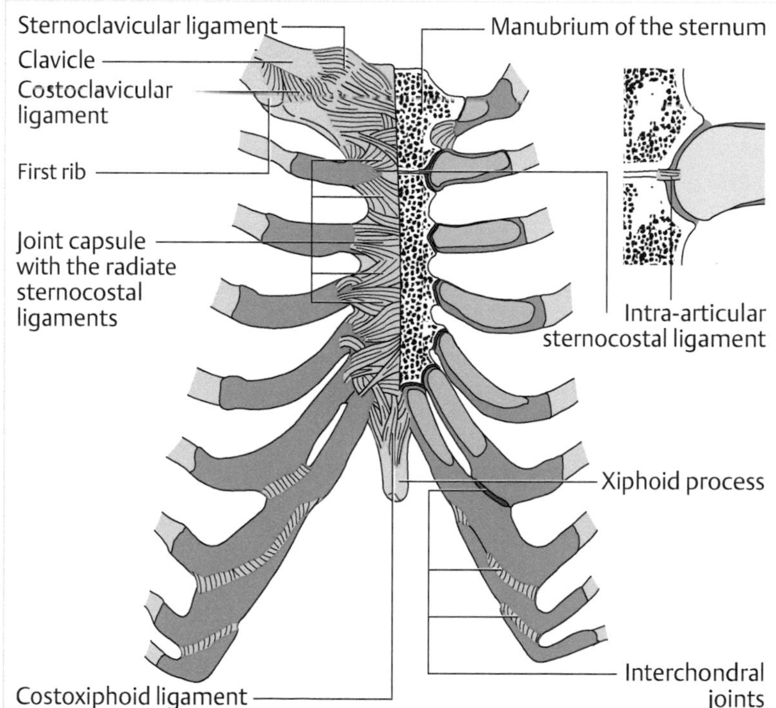


**Fig. 3.29** Sternocostal joints.

## 3.3.1 Movements of the Ribs

### Costovertebral Joints

The rise and fall of the ribs occurs because the ribs rotate around an axis drawn through both costovertebral joints. This represents the longitudinal axis of the neck of the rib, and its position determines the directions of rib motion.

The lateral costotransverse ligament plays a very important role. The axis runs through this ligament almost at right angles to its course. In the upper ribs, the ligament is exposed to strong tensile forces from the rotary motion that takes place because of the shape of the joint surfaces (concave–convex).

In the lower ribs, because of the flat joint surfaces and the position of the joints on the transverse process, tilt and sliding torque develop instead, which means that there is less load on the ligament, but an increased compressive load on the joint.

### Movements of the Upper Ribs (1–5) (Figs. 3.30 and 3.31)

The axis deviates from the frontal plane at an angle of 35°. When the ribs rise—a movement upward and to the front—the sagittal and transverse diameters of the thorax increase.

In the costotransverse joint and in the joint of the head of the rib, a gliding movement occurs in an inferior direction combined with rotation around the intra-articular ligament of the head of the rib.

The arrows shown in **Fig. 3.31** correspond to the movement of the ribs superiorly and anteriorly during inspiration.

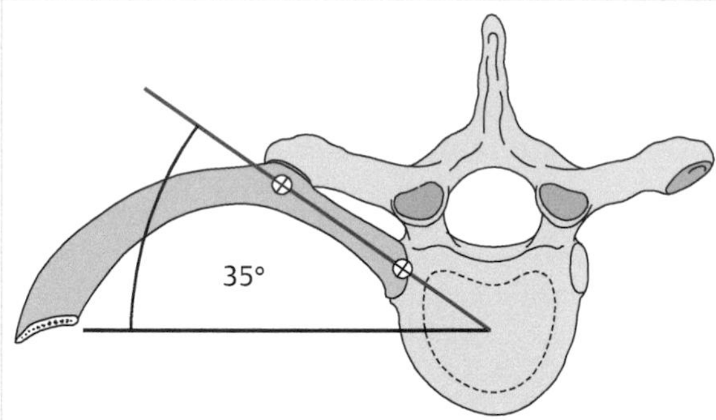


**Fig. 3.30** Angularity of the axis of movement in the upper thorax.

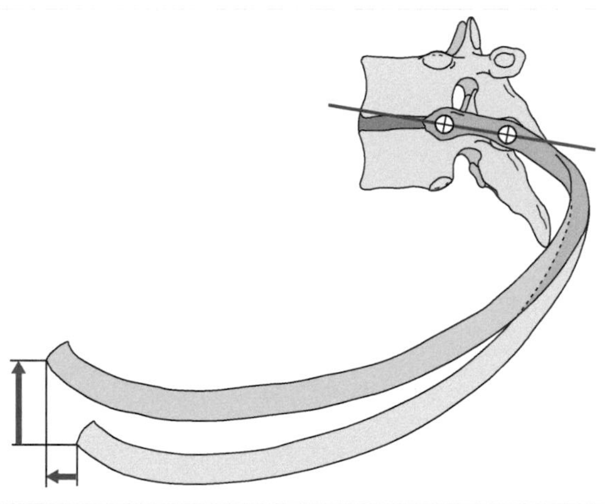

**Fig. 3.31** Movements of the upper ribs during inspiration (gray: initial position; red: position during inspiration).

## Movements of the Lower Ribs (6–10) (Figs. 3.32 and 3.33)

The axis deviates from the sagittal plane at an angle of 35°. When the ribs rise—a movement upward and laterally—the frontal (transverse) diameter of the thorax increases.

In the costotransverse joint, a gliding movement occurs in a superior–posterior direction. In the joint of the head of the rib, a gliding movement in an inferior direction takes place.

The arrows shown in **Fig. 3.33** demonstrate the extent and direction of the rib movements superiorly and laterally during inspiration.

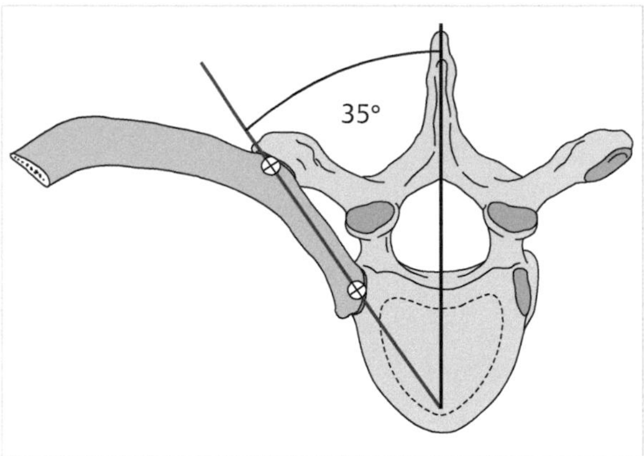


**Fig. 3.32** Angularity of the axis of movement in the lower thorax.

### Pathology

Because of the tensile load on the lateral costotransverse ligament, insertion ligamentopathies tend to develop in the superior region of the thorax, whereas arthritic changes occur in the inferior region due to the increased joint load.

Poor posture changes the course of the ribs and their axes:

- Flat back: a rib slope of approximately 30°.
- Round back (kyphosis): a rib slope of approximately 60°.

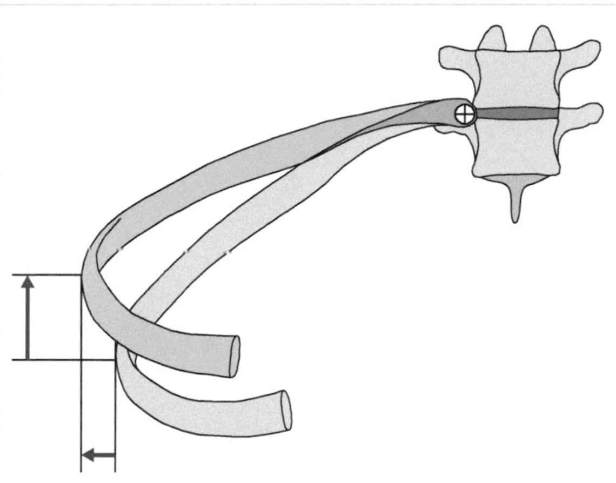

**Fig. 3.33** Movements of the lower ribs during inspiration (gray, initial position; red, position during inspiration).

## Sternocostal Joints

The axis of motion runs in the sagittal plane. During inspiration, a minimal inferior gliding motion occurs in the sternocostal joints. The costal cartilage shifts superiorly and twists; this is reversed in exhalation.

Because of the relatively fixed state of the ribs in the area of the costovertebral and sternocostal joints, the torsion and elasticity of the costal cartilage are significant for movements of the thorax.

## 3.3.2 Muscles of the Thoracic Spine: Lateral Tract

▷ Sacrospinales (Erector Spinae) Muscle Group (Fig. 3.34)

**Iliocostalis muscle, thoracic part:** Connects the lower ribs with the upper ribs.
**Longissimus thoracis muscle:** Connects the pelvis and lumbar spine with the ribs and thoracic spine.

▷ Intertransversarii Muscle Group (Fig. 3.34)

Each **intertransversarii lateral muscle** connects two adjacent transverse processes.

## 3.3.3 Medial Tract

▷ Spinalis Muscle Group (Fig. 3.34)

The **interspinales thoracis muscles** connect pairs of spinous processes.
The **spinalis thoracis muscle** connects the lower thoracic spine and upper lumbar spine with the upper thoracic spine.

▷ Transversospinales Muscle Group (Fig. 3.35)

The **semispinalis thoracis muscle** extends from the lower thoracic spine to the upper thoracic spine and lower cervical vertebrae.
The **multifidus muscles** extend over two to four vertebrae.
The **short rotator muscles** join two adjacent vertebrae.
The **long rotator muscles** join three vertebrae together.

### Function of the Back Muscles

In the thoracic section of the spinal column, the muscles have many functions:

- Stabilization of upright posture.
- Torso and head movements.
- Control of the scapula during arm movements.
- Support for breathing.

Because of the varying lengths of the fiber tracts and their course, which is partly horizontal and partly oblique, they can optimally stabilize the segments. Muscles that fix the scapula on the thorax support the function of the back muscles. They initiate movements to attain the upright position (e.g., the transverse part of the trapezius muscle, the serratus anterior muscle, and the rhomboid muscles).

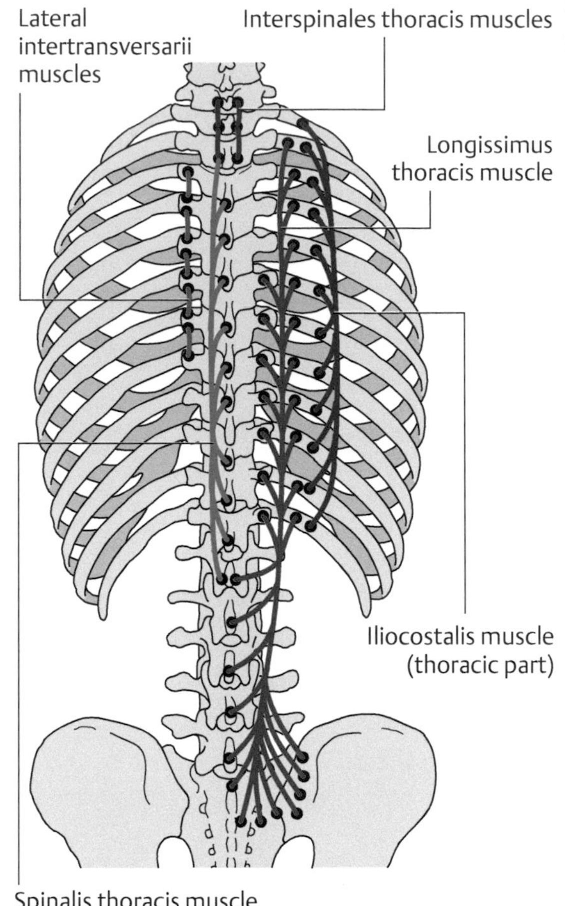


**Fig. 3.34** Muscles of the thoracic spine: sacrospinales, intertransversarii, and spinalis groups.

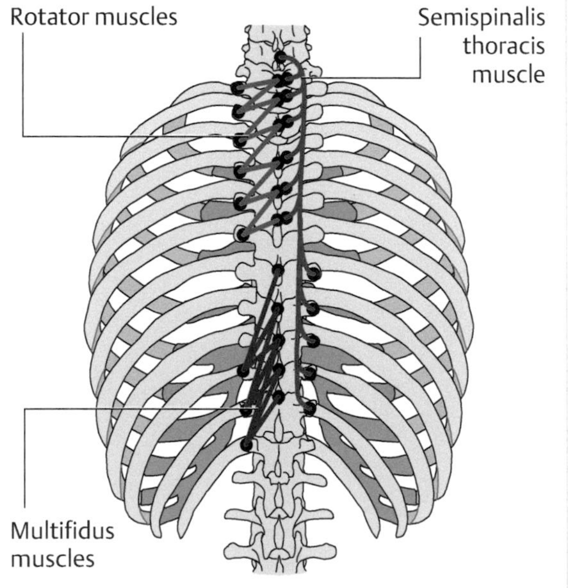


**Fig. 3.35** Muscles of the thoracic spine: transversospinales group.

## Viscero–vertebral Interdependence (Fig. 3.36)

Many internal organs have a neurophysiologic relationship to the thoracic region. This arises from embryologic development and the resultant areas supplied by the spinal nerves. In addition, the organs are primarily supplied by the thoracic segments.

### Practical Tip

In gastric disorders, the following symptoms may be seen:

- A superficial radiation of pain into the left half of the thorax anteriorly and posteriorly from the lower quarter of the scapula to the level of T10, with smaller zones of pain on the left shoulder–neck line, over the left acromion, and above the superior angle of the scapula.
- A hyperalgesic zone corresponding approximately to the superficial pain radiation.
- Muscle tension in the longissimus thoracis muscle, the abdominal muscles, and the iliopsoas muscle.
- Trigger points in the above-mentioned muscles.
- Functional blockage of the fourth to fifth rib bilaterally.
- Functional blockage in the T4–T5 and T7–T8 motion segments.

This viscero–vertebral chain means that disturbance of an internal organ could be the cause of muscle tension, the development of trigger points, and functional disturbances of one or more motion segments with the corresponding rib connections. This can usually be determined from the history. However, if the organ disturbance is silent, a failure of intensive therapy of these functional disturbances indicates a hidden cause. In the case of an acute disease of an internal organ, intensive mobilization treatment of the vertebral and rib connections should be avoided because of the reflective transmission of the stimulus. If the functional disturbances remain even after the illness has faded away, they must be treated with appropriate therapy.

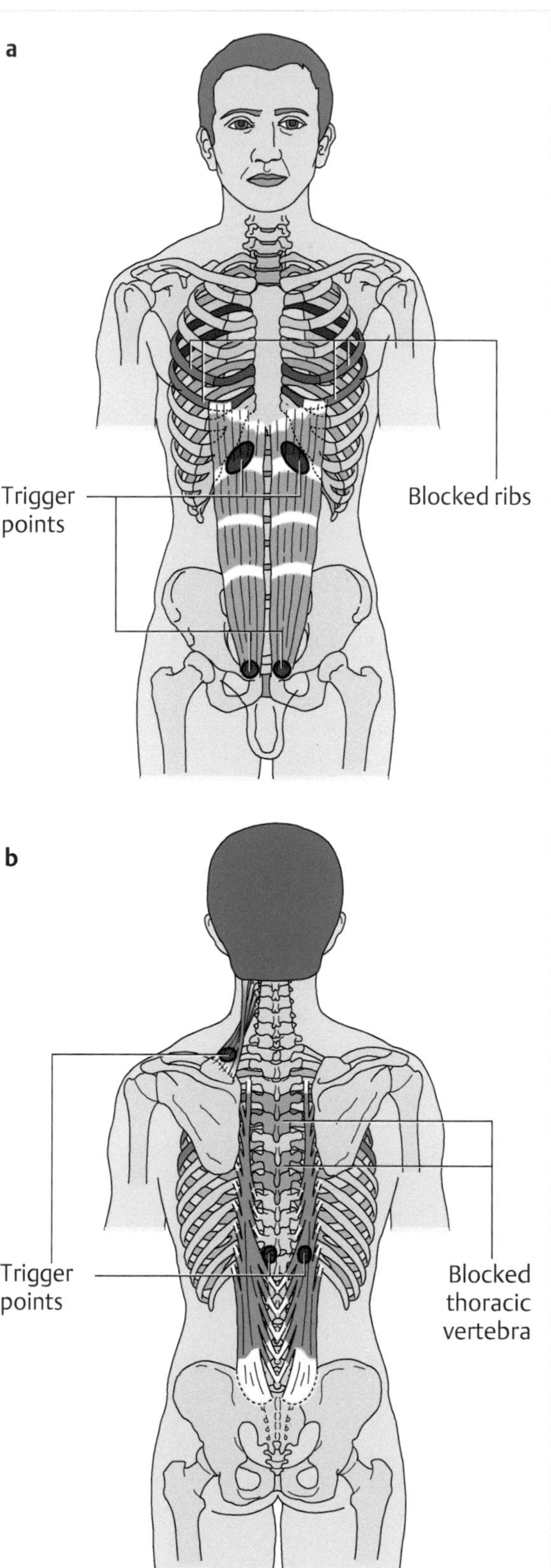


**Fig. 3.36** Viscero–vertebral interdependence: functional disturbances in the stomach–thoracic spine area. **(a)** Anterior view. **(b)** Posterior view.

## 3.3.4 Muscles of Inspiration

### Diaphragm (Fig. 3.37)

- The diaphragm is divided into sternal, costal, and lumbar parts.
- There is a large aponeurosis in the center, the **central tendon** of the diaphragm.
- The **lumbar part** consists of two sections: the right and left crura of the diaphragm.
- The **medial** and **lateral arcuate ligaments** span over the psoas major and quadratus lumborum muscles as tendon arches and merge with the fascia of these muscles.
- Superiorly, the diaphragm connects with the diaphragmatic pleura and, through the pericardiacophrenic ligament, with the parietal layer of the pericardium.
- Inferiorly, the diaphragm connects to the peritoneum. The liver, for example, is fixed to the lateral end of the diaphragm by means of the right and left triangular ligaments.
- Openings in the diaphragm include the **esophageal hiatus** in the superior area for the esophagus to pass through. The **aortic hiatus** for the aorta lies further inferiorly between the two lumbar parts at about the level of L1. The **caval opening** lies the furthest superiorly and anteriorly in the central tendon for passage of the vena cava. The **sternocostal triangle** is located between the sternal and costal parts of the diaphragm. The **lumbocostal triangle**, between the costal and lumbar parts, is filled with connective tissue, through which small blood vessels pass.

**Pathology**

Disturbances in the elasticity or position of the diaphragm can have consequences for the function of the kidneys, liver, and stomach due to its close connection to these organs. Conversely, disturbances of these organs can impair the function of the diaphragm.

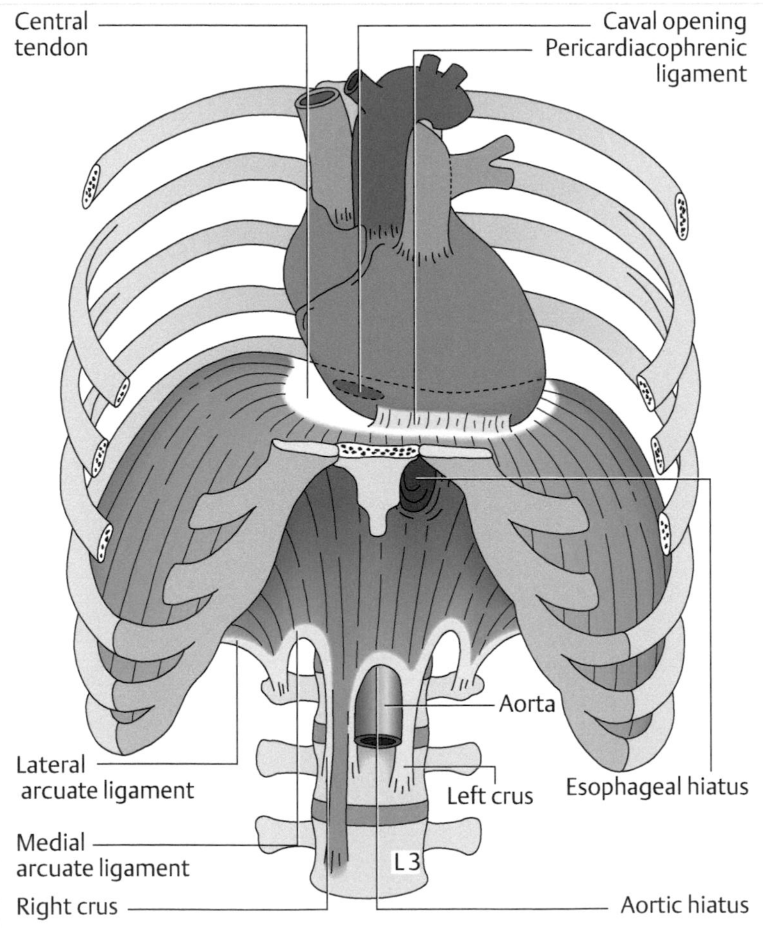


**Fig. 3.37** Diaphragm.

## Function of the Diaphragm (Fig. 3.38)

During inspiration, the central tendon travels up to 5 cm more deeply, taking with it the domes of the diaphragm, which flatten in the process. Through this, the space within the thorax enlarges, facilitating the inflow of air.

Due to the diaphragm's downward movement, the abdominal organs are compressed and move out of the way, primarily anteriorly, but somewhat laterally and posteriorly as well.

> **Pathology**
>
> Pathologic changes that are associated with swelling of the organs, such as an abdominal abscess or ascites, or with swelling of the intestines, can hinder the diaphragm from shifting inferiorly and lead to an elevated diaphragm. This results in dyspnea and possible cardiac symptoms.

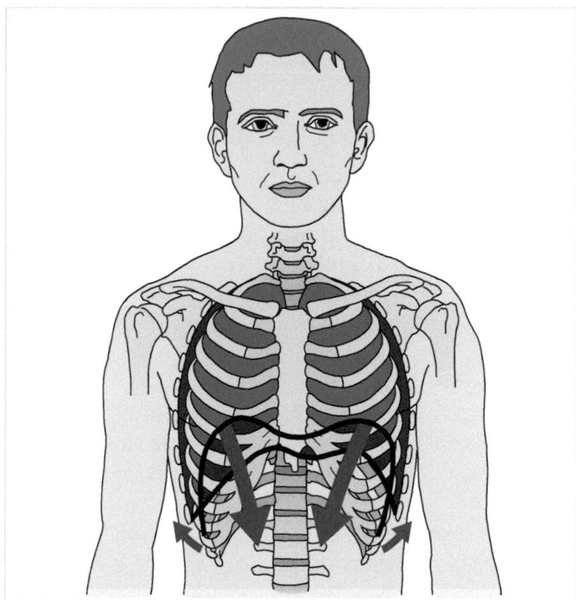

**Fig. 3.38** Shift of the diaphragm with inspiration.

## Levatores Costarum Muscles (Fig. 3.39)

These connect the transverse process with the next lower rib and thus raise the ribs.

## External Intercostal Muscles (Fig. 3.39)

- These have an oblique course from posterosuperior to anteroinferior and raise the ribs.
- The external intercostal membrane is the continuation of the external intercostal muscle from the bone–cartilage interface to the sternum. Its course runs in the same direction as the muscle.
- Electromyographic evaluations show that the external intercostal muscles only become active if they are stretched first.

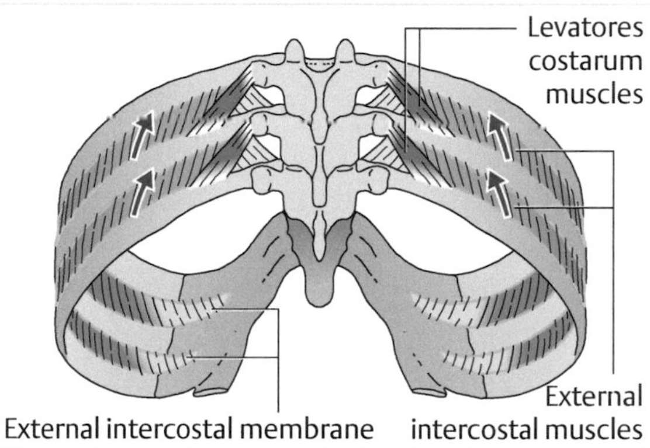


**Fig. 3.39** Muscles of inspiration: external intercostal muscles and levatores costarum muscles.

## Scalene Muscles

- These join the cervical spine to the first ribs.
- If their fixed end is in the cervical spine area, the scalene muscles raise the upper ribs and support inspiration. They contract not only in quiet breathing, but also in forced inspiration.

▷ See Chapter 2.3, Functional Anatomy of the Cervical Spine

## Serratus Posterior Superior Muscle (Fig. 3.40)

This connects the lower cervical spine and the upper thoracic spine with the ribs.

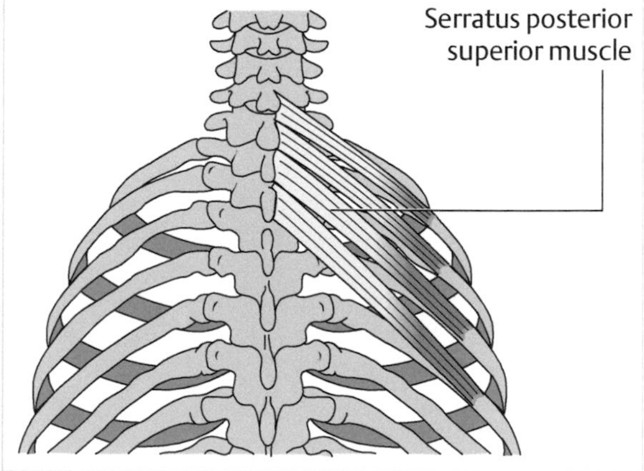


**Fig. 3.40** Serratus posterior superior muscle.

## 3.3.5 Muscles of Exhalation

Exhalation is primarily passive.

### Internal Intercostal Muscles (Fig. 3.41)

- Their course is from posteroinferior to anterosuperior. They lower the ribs.
- Posteriorly, they merge into a membrane (the internal intercostal membrane), which extends to the costal tubercles. It runs in the same direction as the internal intercostal muscles.

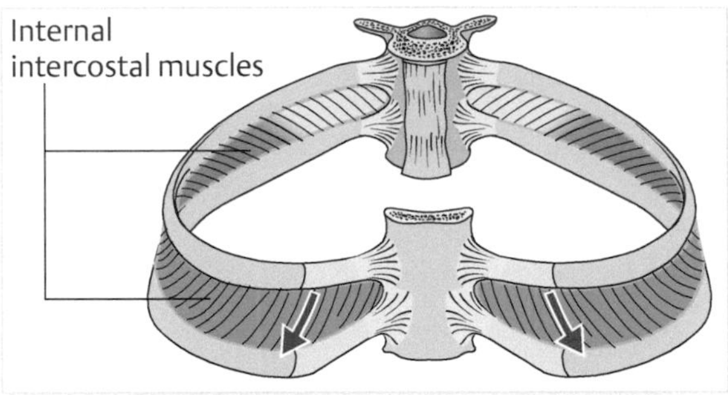


**Fig. 3.41** Muscles of exhalation: internal intercostal muscles.

### Transversus Thoracis Muscle (Fig. 3.42)

- This lies retrosternally and extends from the costal cartilage in an obliquely inferior direction to the sternum.
- When it contracts, it shifts the costal cartilage inferiorly (tending toward exhalation).

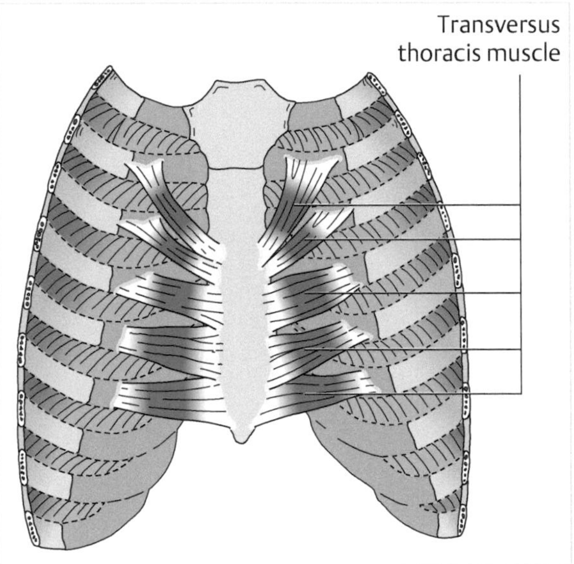


**Fig. 3.42** Transversus thoracis muscle.

### Subcostales Muscles (Fig. 3.43)

These connect the ribs over two or three consecutive levels, and lie on the posterior inner side of the thorax.

### Serratus Posterior Inferior Muscle (Fig. 3.43)

- This joins the thoracolumbar fascia of the lower thoracic spine and the upper lumbar spine with the ribs.
- It supports exhalation because the ribs extend inferiorly.
- Because it stabilizes the inferior ribs, and thereby provides a fixed end for the costal section of the diaphragm, it can possibly be allocated to the inspiratory muscles.

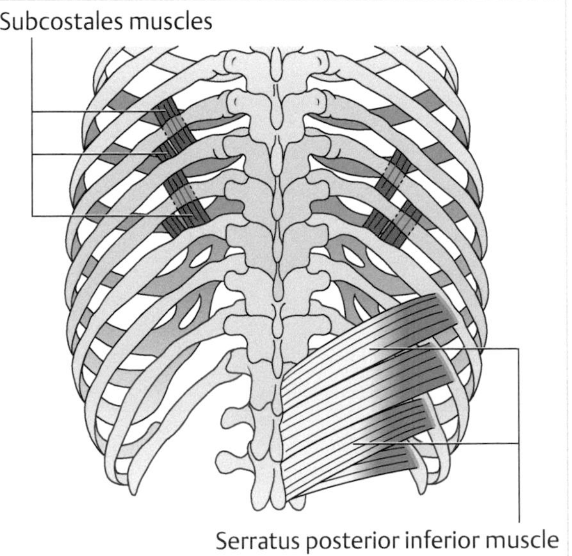


**Fig. 3.43** Subcostales muscles and serratus posterior inferior muscle.

## 3.3.6 Muscles That Assist in Respiration

This group of muscles comes into play only when deep breaths of air are needed, such as after physical exertion or in respiratory problems. *Inspiration:* The muscles that extend from the spinal column to the upper extremity sustain a distal fixed end for inspiration, aided, for example, by bracing with the arms in front. They can thus raise the ribs and sternum (pectoralis major and sternocleidomastoid muscles). *Exhalation:* When the abdominal muscles contract, they push the abdominal contents against the diaphragm, and the thoracic space gets smaller. A few back muscles, the iliocostalis and longissimus muscles, also support exhalation.

## 3.3.7 Course of the Nerves in the Thoracic Spine Region

### Intercostal Nerves (Fig. 3.44)

- These arise from the anterior rami and run in the corresponding intercostal space.
- They are composed of motor fibers that innervate the intercostal muscles as well as the serratus posterior superior, subcostales, and transversus thoracis muscles. The inferior intercostal nerves also supply the abdominal muscles.
- Sensory fibers extend to the diaphragm and supply the anterior thorax and abdomen as cutaneous branches.

### Sympathetic Trunk Ganglia (Fig. 3.44)

- These are also known as paravertebral ganglia.
- The trunks run from C8 to L2 in the immediate vicinity of the heads of the ribs and extend through a gap in the lumbar part of the diaphragm.
- They consist of 10 or 11 paired ganglia that are interconnected, one on top of the other, by the interganglionic branches.
- They are connected to the spinal nerve of the same level over the gray and white rami communicantes.
- They supply the organs in the thoracic cavity: cardiac nerves to the heart and aortic arch, and splanchnic nerves for the abdominal organs.

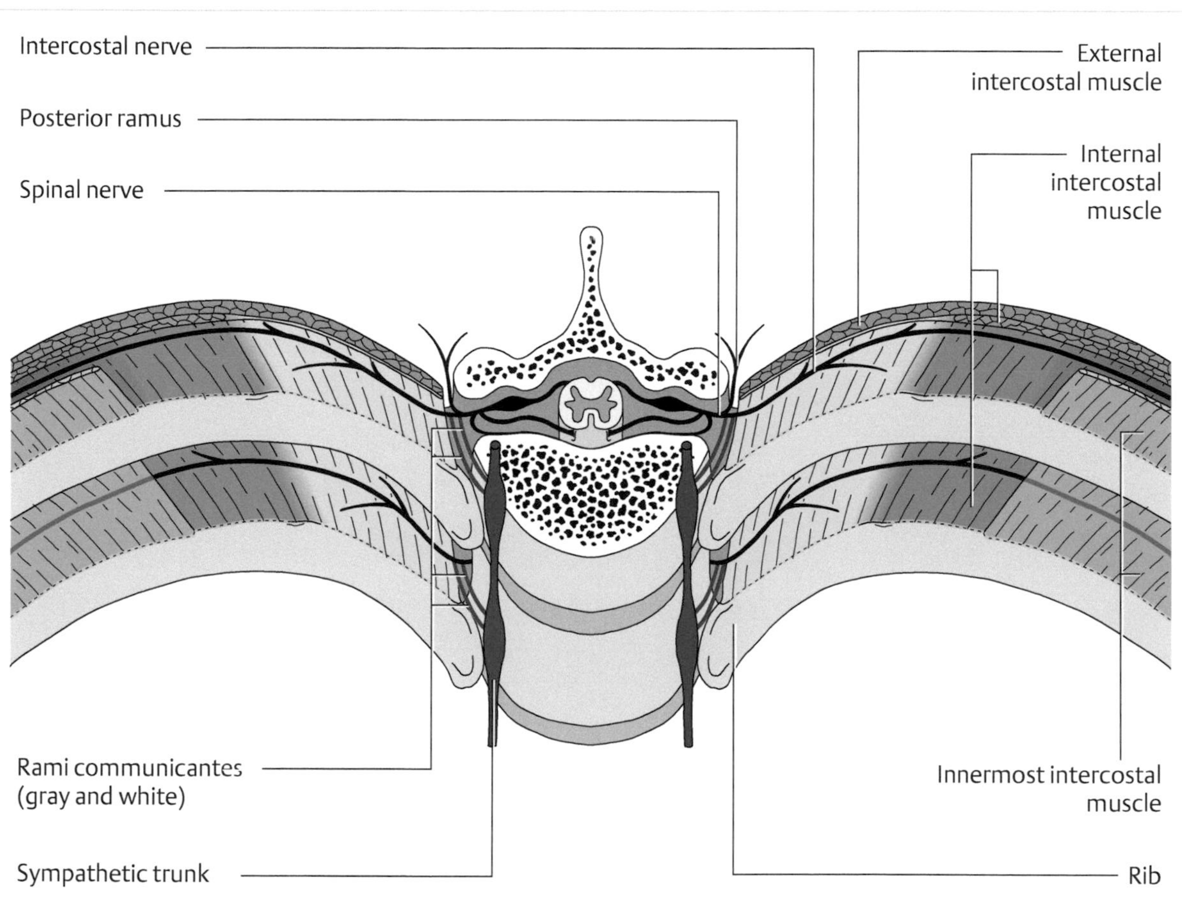


**Fig. 3.44** Course of the intercostal nerves and the sympathetic trunk ganglion in the thoracic spine.

## Phrenic Nerve (Fig. 3.45)

- The phrenic nerve emerges primarily from the C4 level, partly from C3, and sometimes from C5.
- It leaves the plexus very early, and, approaching from posteriorly, extends over the anterior scalene muscle. From there, it tracks between the subclavian artery and vein and runs further inferiorly in the anterior region between the mediastinal pleura and the pericardium. Here it delivers branches into the fibrous pericardium and the pleura. It branches to supply the superior portions of the diaphragm, and then pierces the central tendon with a branch to supply the inferior side. As phrenicoabdominal branches, it travels further toward the liver, stomach, and kidneys and supplies a portion of their sensory innervation.
- It has motor, sensory, and sympathetic fibers.

### Pathology

Bilateral nerve irritation is very unusual. A functional disturbance in segment C4 or constriction in the mediastinum (potentially caused by the thymus, heart, or lungs) can cause unilateral compression of one of the phrenic nerves. This can in turn lead to unilateral elevation of the diaphragm and impaired inspiration.

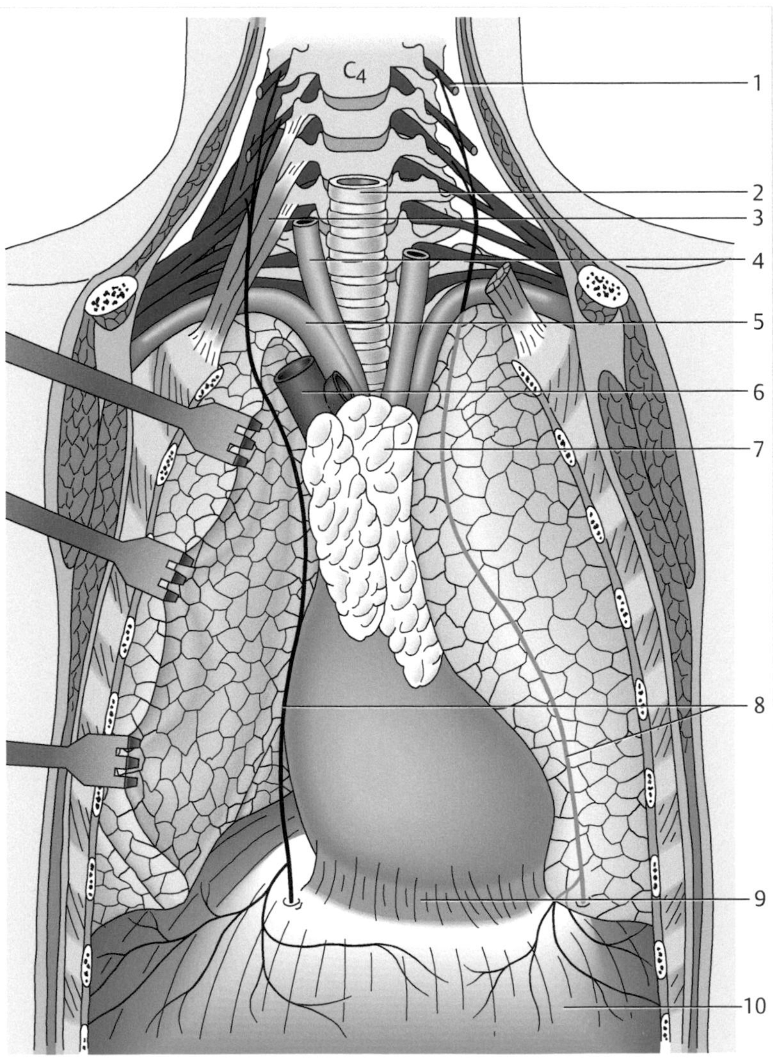


**Fig. 3.45** Course of the phrenic nerve.
1 Anterior ramus $C_4$
2 Trachea
3 Anterior scalene muscle
4 Carotid artery
5 Subclavian artery
6 Superior vena cava
7 Thymus
8 Phrenic nerve
9 Pericardiacophrenic ligament
10 Diaphragm

# Chapter 4

## Shoulder

# 4 Shoulder

## 4.1 Palpation of Landmarks in the Shoulder Area

### Acromion (Fig. 4.1)

Track the spine of the scapula laterally to palpate the angular posterior border of the acromion as an extension. From there, follow the lateral edge of the acromion anteriorly to palpate the slightly rounder anterior border. Pulling on the arm brings it out more clearly.

The acromion serves as an orientation guide for locating the highly diverse structures in this area.

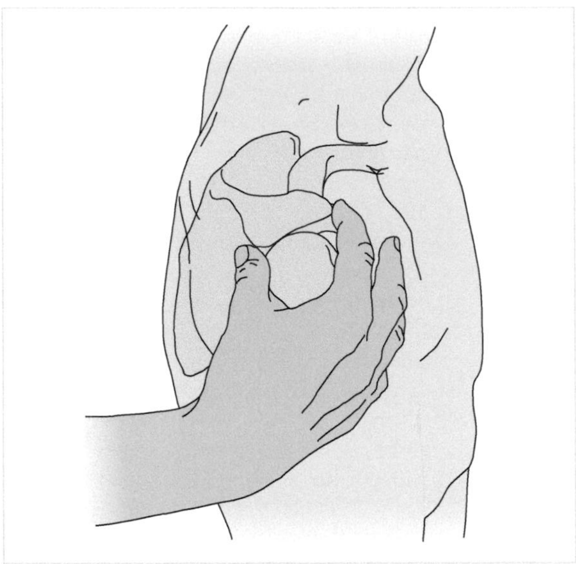

**Fig. 4.1** Palpation of the acromion.

### Acromioclavicular Joint (Fig. 4.2)

The joint space of the acromioclavicular joint can be felt as a small **V**-shaped indentation about one fingerbreadth medially from the anterior neck of the acromion. This is the anterior part of the joint. To accurately gauge the course of the joint, locate the posterior part of the joint space as well. Follow the upper margin of the spine of the scapula laterally to the clavicle. These two structures form a triangle, at the tip of which another small, anteriorly oriented **V**-shaped indentation be felt. The line joining these two locations indicates the course of the joint. Under normal conditions of the shoulder girdle and the thoracic spine, it runs from posteromedial to anterolateral.

Small circular movements of the shoulder girdle confirm the correct localization.

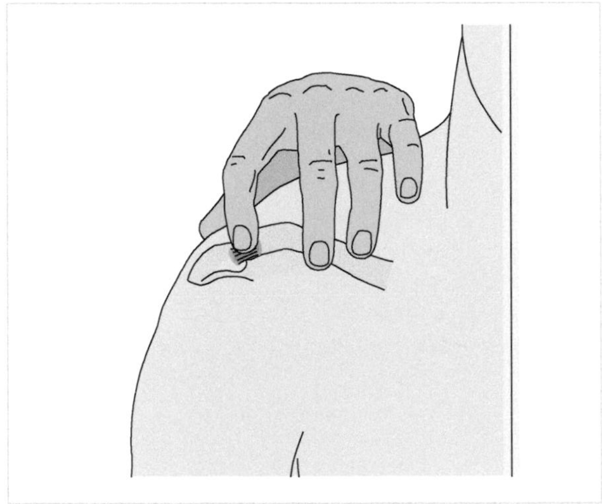

**Fig. 4.2** Palpation of the acromioclavicular joint.

### Sternoclavicular Joint (Fig. 4.3)

Moving laterally from the jugular notch, palpate the protruding sternal end of the clavicle. The joint space lies at the inferomedial margin. It is usually very easy to palpate. Small, circular movements of the shoulder girdle may help.

The course of the joint space is from superomedial to inferolateral.

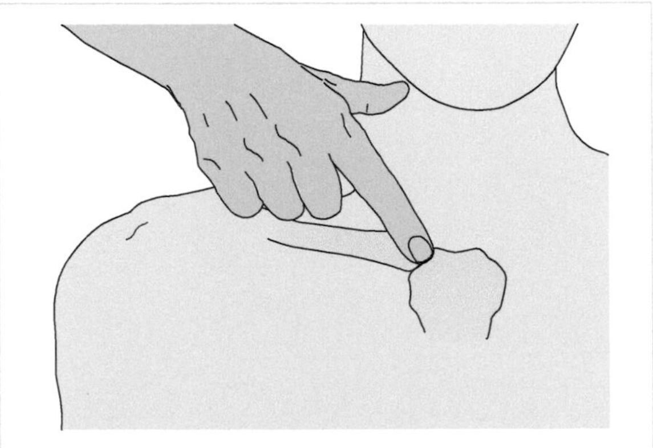

**Fig. 4.3** Palpation of the sternoclavicular joint.

## Coracoid Process (Fig. 4.4)

Palpate the tip of the coracoid process as a broad bulge laterally in the infraclavicular fossa.

The short head of the **biceps brachii muscle** and the **coracobrachialis muscle** extend inferolaterally from its tip. Localize their tendons by palpating crosswise directly under the tip of the coracoid process. The coracobrachialis muscle lies partly under the biceps muscle. These two muscles can only be differentiated by tensing the biceps muscle as if to flex the elbow, because the coracobrachialis muscle spans only one joint.

The **pectoralis minor muscle** extends from an inferomedial direction to the medial border of the coracoid process. Isometrically tensing the muscle toward protraction verifies the localization.

The **coraco-acromial ligament** (**Fig. 4.5**) extends from the superolateral margin of the coracoid process to the anterior neck of the acromion. Palpate across the course of the fibers. Pulling the arm downward facilitates the palpation.

## Lesser Tubercle of the Humerus

The medial margin of the lesser tubercle of the humerus is located immediately inferior to the anterior neck of the acromion, about one fingerbreadth lateral to the coracoid process. In the proximal area, it is about 1 to 1½ fingerbreadths wide and narrows distally. It has the shape of an upside-down pear and is about two fingerbreadths in length.

The insertion area of the **subscapularis muscle** (**Fig. 4.6**) has exactly the same width and length. Palpate the tendon across the fiber orientation both when the muscle is relaxed and when it is tensed in internal rotation. The upper fibers run horizontally, while the lower fibers track upward with an oblique course.

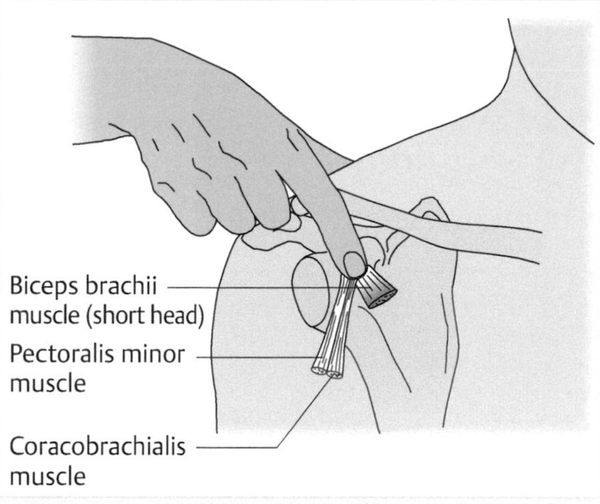


**Fig. 4.4** Coracoid process.

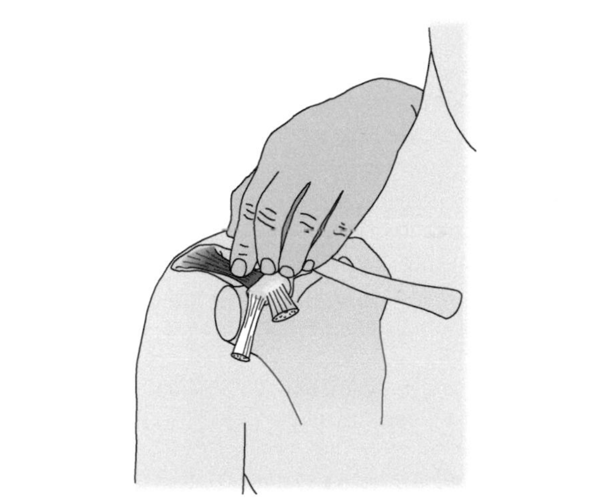

**Fig. 4.5** Palpation of the coraco-acromial ligament.

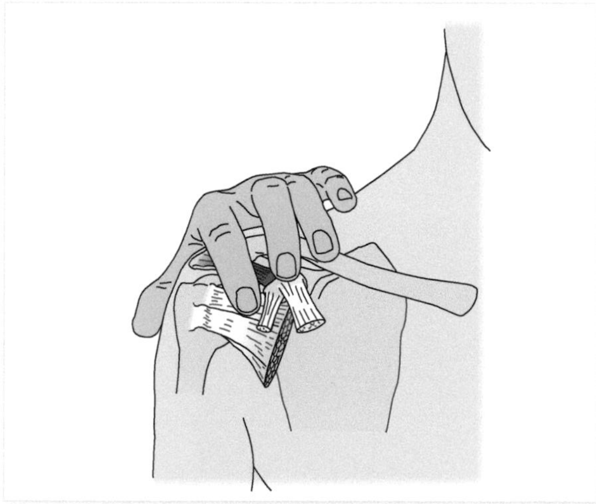

**Fig. 4.6** Palpation of the subscapularis muscle.

## Intertubercular Sulcus (Fig. 4.7)

The intertubercular sulcus is located directly lateral to the lesser tubercle. It cannot be felt it as a distinct groove because it is filled with the tendon of the biceps brachii muscle.

The edges of the lesser and greater tubercula and the biceps tendon between them can be felt using passive external and internal rotational movements.

In the superior area, the transverse humeral ligament and parts of the subscapularis muscle tendon run over the sulcus.

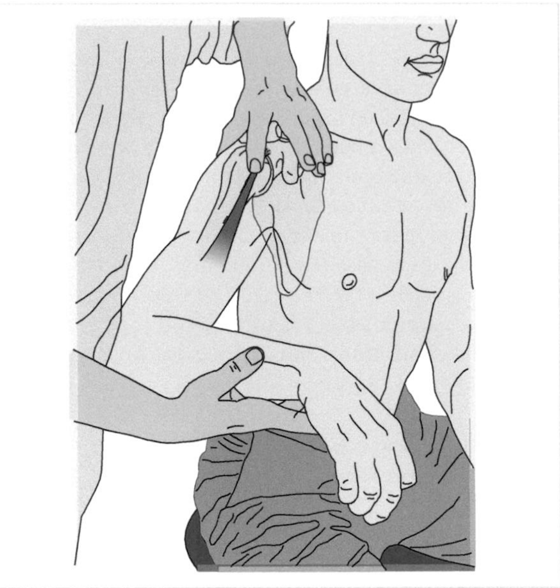

**Fig. 4.7** Palpation of the intertubercular sulcus.

## Greater Tubercle of the Humerus (Fig. 4.8)

The greater tubercle lies lateral to the sulcus. The tendon insertions of the rotator cuff muscles on the humerus lie immediately anterolateral and lateral to the acromion. The position of the arm should be altered to palpate the insertion sites optimally.

## Supraspinatus Muscle (Fig. 4.8)

As the arm extends, the superior facet of the tubercle moves anteriorly. The typical site for a lesion on the supraspinatus tendon lies directly anterior to the neck of the acromion and is confirmed by tensing the muscle as if abducting the arm. Adding maximal internal rotation shifts the greater tubercle medially. The insertion site is about 1 cm wide and 1 cm long.

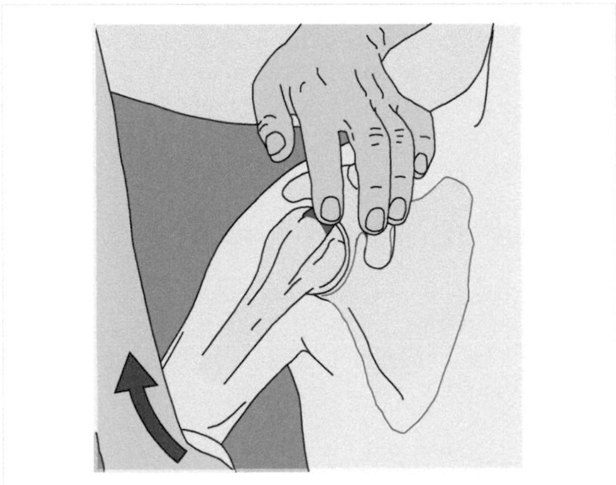

**Fig. 4.8** Palpation of the insertion of the supraspinatus muscle on the greater tubercle.

## Infraspinatus Muscle (Fig. 4.9)

Place the patient's hand on the opposite shoulder and hold it there. This combination of flexion, adduction, and internal rotation brings the middle facet of the greater tubercle from under the posterior neck of the acromion in an inferolateral direction. Using the posterior neck of the acromion as a reference point, feel about two fingerbreadths inferiorly to locate its tendon as a hard strand as it passes over the joint space. It can then be tracked about two fingerbreadths laterally until a bony structure is felt, which is its insertion. Now tense the muscle from this position (external rotation against resistance). It is 2 to 3 cm wide.

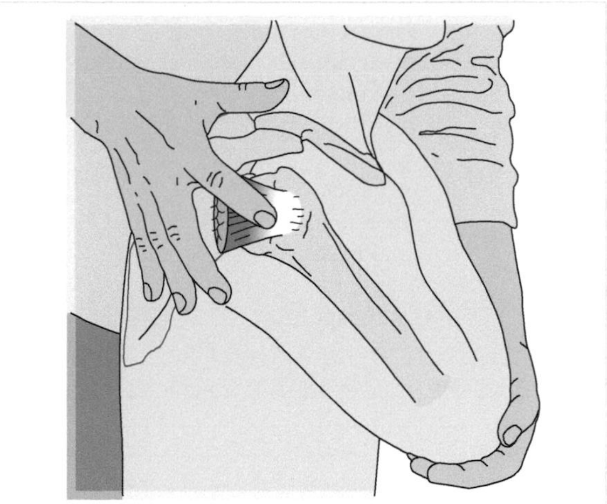

**Fig. 4.9** Palpation of the insertion of the infraspinatus muscle on the greater tubercle.

## Teres Minor Muscle

Somewhat further inferiorly to the insertion of the infraspinatus muscle lies that of the teres minor muscle on the inferior facet of the greater tubercle. An exact differentiation between the two muscles is not possible as they are frequently intertwined.

**Pathology**

Swelling (up to 1 cm thick) and significant soreness indicate a tendon lesion. Further provocation testing by tensing and stretching the muscle confirms the diagnosis.

## Subacromial Space (Fig. 4.10)

A portion of the space can be palpated lateral to the acromion. To assess it better, abduct the arm by 60° and use the fingertips, approaching from laterally, to feel under the acromion.

Evaluate the area for soreness, swelling (which can narrow the space) and the ability of structures to glide within the space with arm movements.

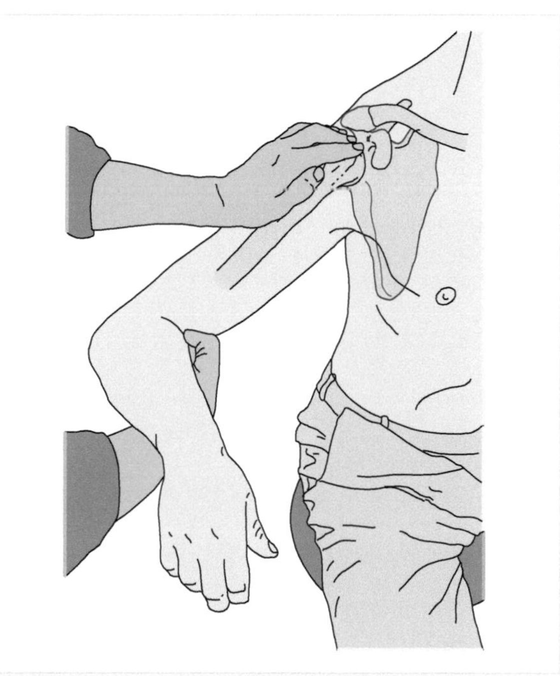

**Fig. 4.10** Palpation of the subacromial space.

**Pathology**

Adhesions in the bursal area limit the ability of the humeral head to glide within the subacromial space.

## Deltoid Tuberosity

The insertion of the deltoid muscle is located about one thumb to index finger span from the acromion on the lateral humerus. It is easy to find by abducting the patient's arm against resistance because all the muscle fibers converge onto the tuberosity. There is a small bursa there, which can become swollen.

Starting from its insertion, palpate the deltoid muscle up to its origins on the clavicle, acromion, and spine of the scapula.

## Scapula

### Superior Angle of the Scapula (Fig. 4.11)

The superior angle points superomedially and is difficult to palpate. The levator scapulae muscle inserts here—palpate it across the fiber orientation just above the angle. Its insertion is about two fingerbreadths wide. Raising the scapula toward the occiput verifies the localization.

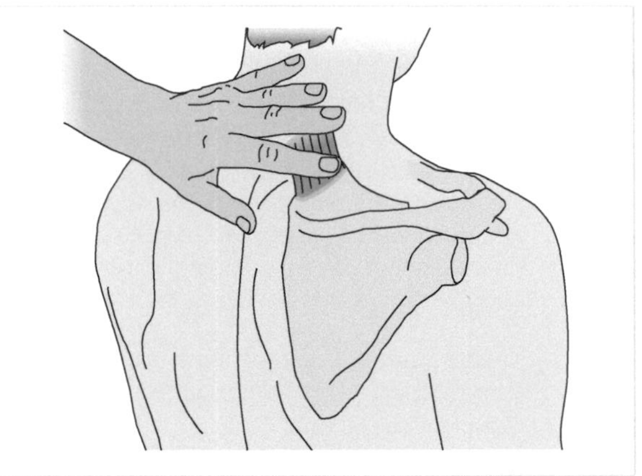

**Fig. 4.11** Palpation of the superior angle of the scapula.

### Medial Border (Fig. 4.12)

This medial border runs downward from the medial area of the spine of the scapula. The rhomboid muscles insert along the border under the trapezius muscle. Palpate them from here to the vertebral column, both across the fiber orientation and along it. Tensing the muscles as if to move the scapula toward the opposite ear demonstrates an increase in tension along the course of the muscle.

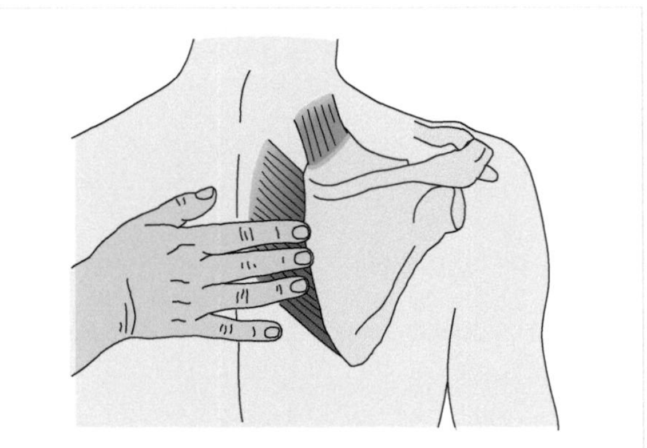

**Fig. 4.12** Palpation of the medial border of the scapula.

### Inferior Angle

The teres major muscle arises from the lower angle of the scapula and can be traced laterally toward the axilla. Tensing in the direction of extension/adduction facilitates its palpation.

### Lateral Border (Fig. 4.13)

The lateral border extends superolaterally away from the inferior angle. This edge is difficult to palpate because several muscles lie over it. Minimal scapular movements medially and laterally help to identify the border. From inferior to superior, the following muscles can be palpated:

- **Latissimus dorsi muscle:** The latissimus dorsi muscle forms part of the posterior axilla, where its superior border can be palpated.
- **Teres major muscle (Fig. 4.13):** The teres major muscle can be traced from the inferior angle along the lateral border toward the posterior axilla. By tensing the muscle in internal rotation, it emerges more fully and can be identified as a quadrilateral, firm pad in the posterior axilla.
- **Teres minor muscle (Fig. 4.13):** Palpate the teres minor muscle in the infraspinous fossa immediately superior to the teres major muscle.

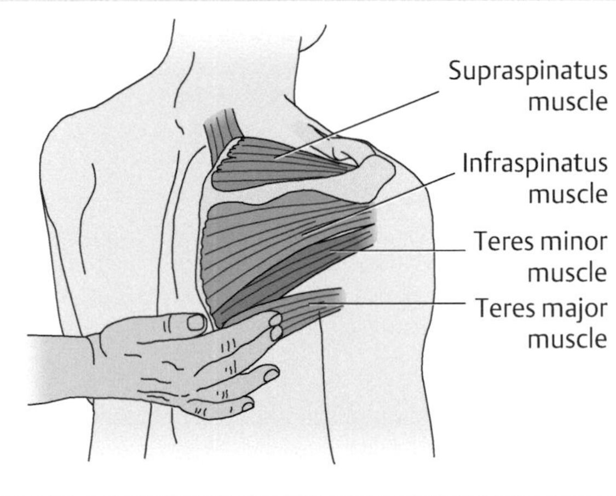


**Fig. 4.13** Palpation of the lateral border of the scapula.

## Supraspinous Fossa (Fig. 4.14)

Palpate the supraspinatus muscle in the fossa above the spine of the scapula through the trapezius muscle. The transition between the muscle and the tendon occurs in the lateral part of the angle formed by the spine of the scapula and the clavicle. Tightening the muscle in abduction in the neutral position confirms the localization.

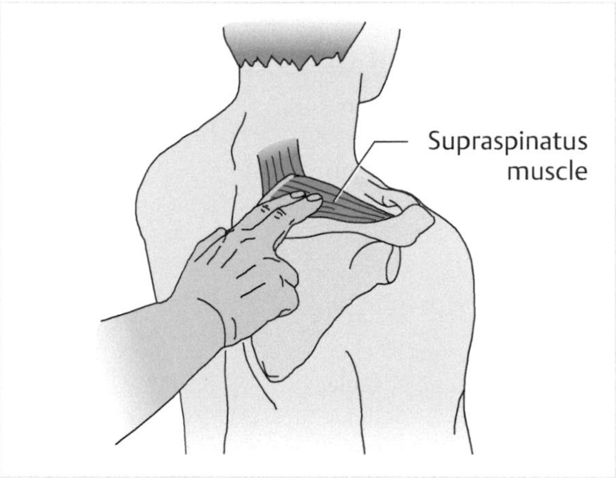


Fig. 4.14 Palpation of the supraspinous fossa.

## Infraspinous Fossa

Palpate the infraspinatus muscle in the large fossa below the spine of the scapula. It can be palpated here very well when the muscle is tensed in external rotation.

## Costal Surface of the Scapula (Fig. 4.15)

Maximally flex or abduct the patient's arm to identify the lateral part of the costal surface. In this position, it swings outward and away from the thorax. As a result, a portion of the subscapularis muscle becomes accessible to palpation.

To approach the costal surface from the medial side, push the fingertips under the medial border of the scapula. Place the patient's arm in internal rotation to facilitate this.

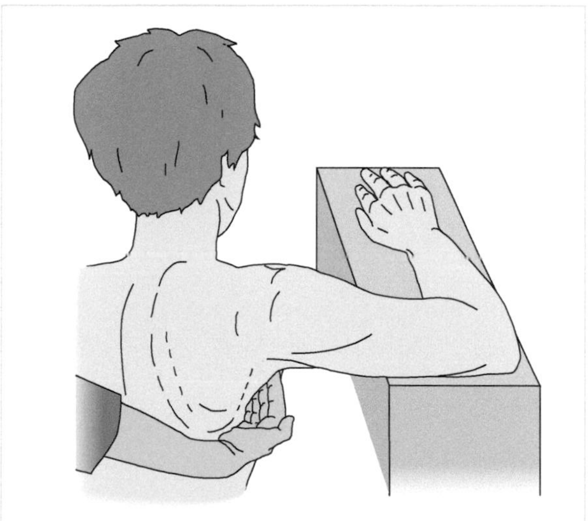

Fig. 4.15 Palpation of the costal surface of the scapula.

## Anterior Axilla (Fig. 4.16)

This is formed by the **pectoralis major muscle**. With the arm slightly abducted, trace the muscle from the clavicle and sternum toward the crest of the greater tubercle.

Palpate the origin, insertion, and course of the following arm, shoulder, and neck muscles:

- Biceps brachii muscle.
- Triceps brachii muscle.
- Trapezius muscle.
- Serratus anterior muscle.
- Sternocleidomastoid muscle.
- Scalene muscles.
- Subclavian muscle.

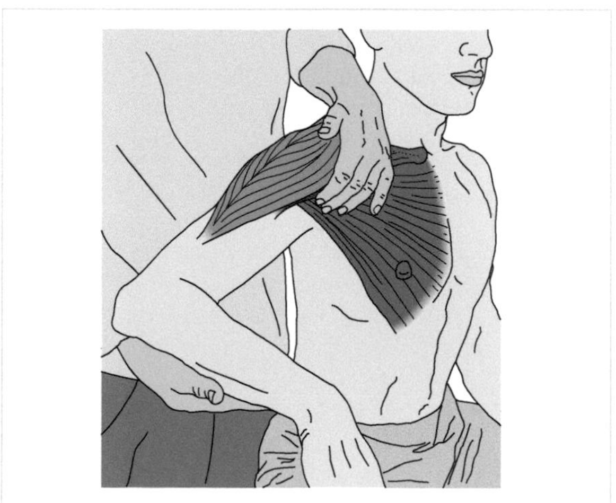

Fig. 4.16 Palpation of the anterior axilla.

# 4.2 Functional Anatomy of the Shoulder

## 4.2.1 X-Ray of the Shoulder

### Anteroposterior View (Fig. 4.17a)

Evaluate the skeletal structures involved in the joint in terms of their normal anatomical shape—the harmoniously rounded head of the humerus, the regular arrangement of the trabecular structure, and a cortical bone thickness of 2 to 4 mm.

Check the following relationships of the joint:

- Acromion–humerus gap: about 9 mm.
- Glenohumeral joint space width: 4 to 6 mm; acromioclavicular joint: 2 to 4 mm.

> **Pathology**
>
> Accumulations of calcium often occur in the supraspinatus tendon and appear as distinct thickenings between the acromion and the greater tubercle in the anteroposterior view.

### Transaxillary View (Fig. 4.17b)

This inferior view at 90° abduction delineates the relationship of the joint socket to the humeral head.

Using this view into the glenohumeral and acromioclavicular joints allows judgments to be made on joint narrowing and osteophyte formation.

> **Pathology**
>
> In the case of osteoarthritis of the shoulder, bony osteophytes form on the anterior rim of the acromion towards the coraco-acromial ligament, thus causing narrowing of the subacromial space.

### Arthrography (Fig. 4.18)

Filling the joint with contrast medium delineates the joint cavity and its communicating recesses.

The anteroposterior image shows the axillary recess, the subscapularis recess, and the synovial sheath that enfolds the tendon of the long head of the biceps. The intertubercular sulcus divides the image into two strips of contrast media.

> **Pathology**
>
> If the supraspinatus tendon ruptures, a connection forms between the bursa and the joint cavity, so the contrast medium is distributed more diffusely.

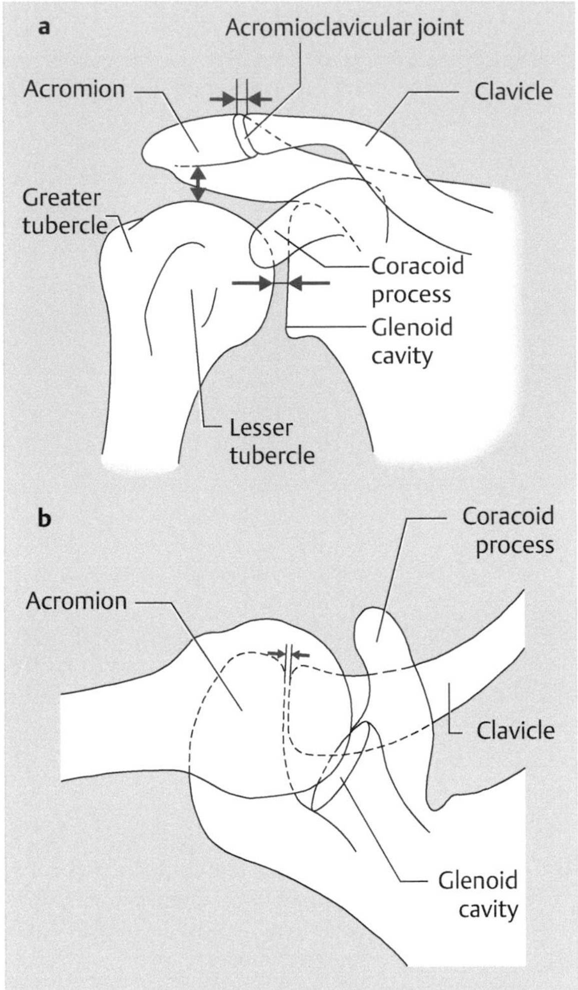


**Fig. 4.17** X-ray of the right shoulder area. **(a)** Anterioposterior view. **(b)** Transaxillary projection.

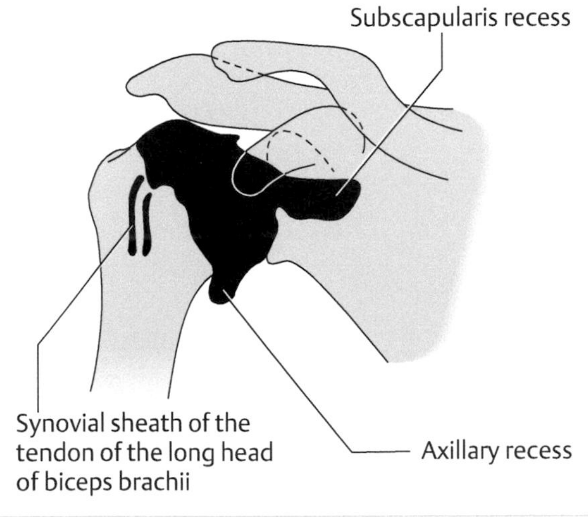


**Fig. 4.18** Arthrogram of the shoulder.

## 4.2.2 Range of Motion of the Arm: Participating Joints (Fig. 4.19)

The extensive range of motion of the arm is only possible through the interaction of several joints. The torso and arm are connected by three true anatomical joints and two "false" (physiologic) joints:

- The *glenohumeral joint* (true joint) and subacromial space.
- The *acromioclavicular joint* and *sternoclavicular joint* (true joints) and the *scapulothoracic physiologic joint (gliding surface)*.
- In addition to the shoulder joint complex, the *flexibility of the ribs* and an upright and *flexible spinal column* are also important if the arm is to achieve full end-range movements.

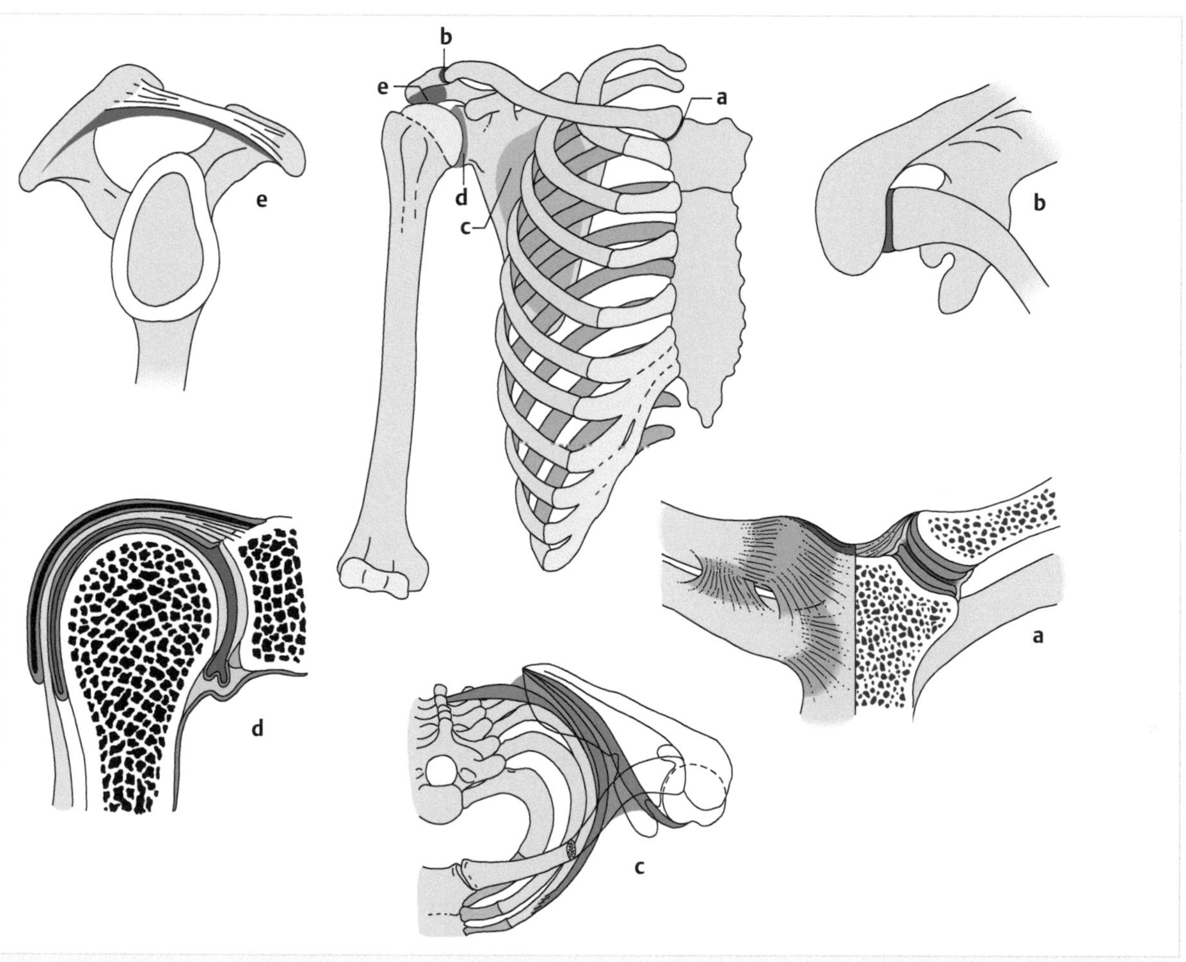


**Fig. 4.19** Joints of the shoulder. **(a)** Sternoclavicular joint. **(b)** Acromioclavicular joint. **(c)** Scapulothoracic joint. **(d)** Glenohumeral joint. **(e)** Subacromial space.

## 4.2.3 Glenohumeral Joint

The glenohumeral joint is a force-locking joint, which means that the muscles and ligaments running over the joint stabilize it.

### Head of the Humerus (Figs. 4.20–4.22)

- The cartilage layer is the thickest in the center.
- The *angle of inclination* is 45° from the axis of the shaft.
- The humeral head is *retroverted* 40° compared with the condylar axis of the distal humerus.

### Glenoid Cavity (Fig. 4.23)

- The cartilage layer is thin in the center and becomes thicker toward the outside.
- The *glenoid labrum* is attached to the bony rim of the cavity, thus enlarging the joint surface.
- Its *inclination* from the vertical is 15°.
- There is a *retroversion* of 10°.
- It is four times smaller in area than the joint surface on the humerus.

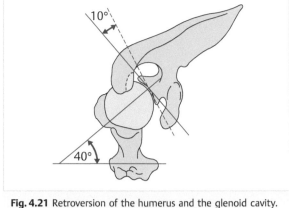

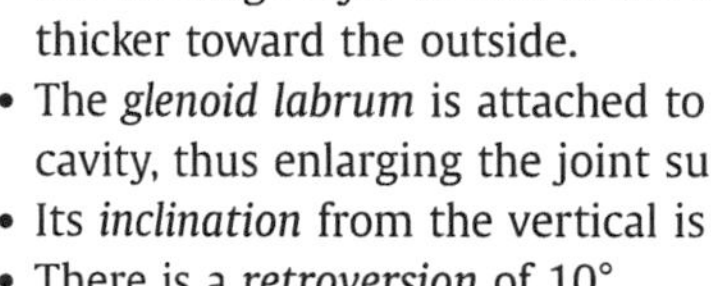


**Fig. 4.21** Retroversion of the humerus and the glenoid cavity.

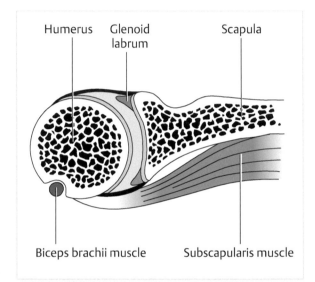

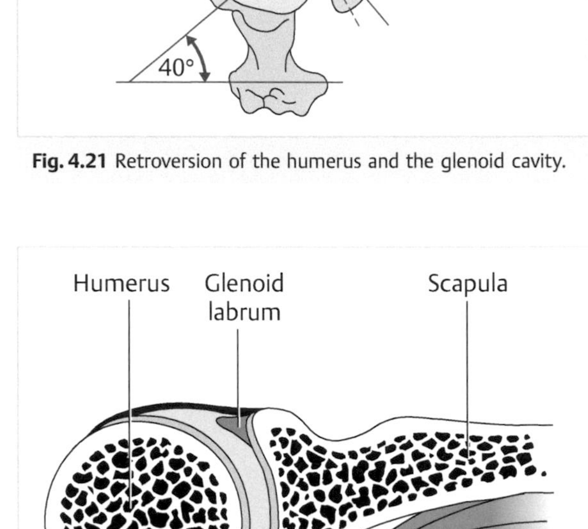


**Fig. 4.22** Glenoid labrum.

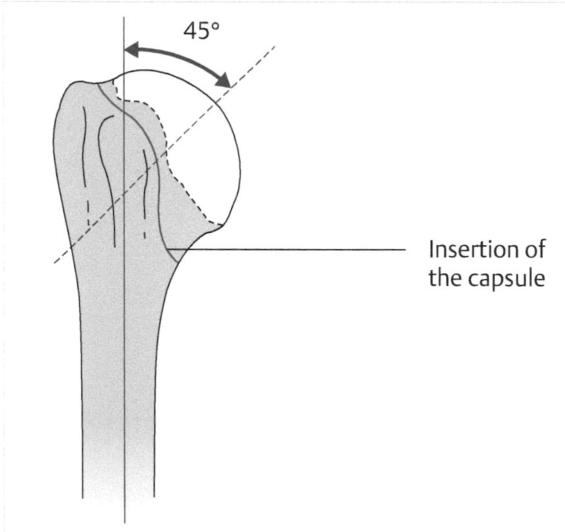


**Fig. 4.20** Angle of inclination of the head of the humerus.

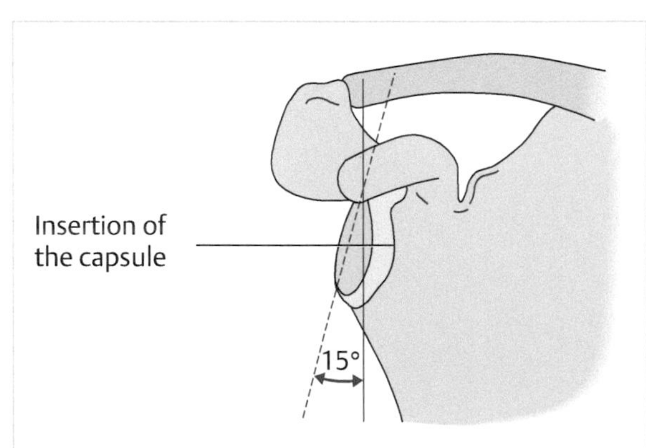


**Fig. 4.23** Inclination of the glenoid cavity.

## Joint Capsule (Fig. 4.24)

The large range of motion needed calls for a loose capsule, which is further expanded by its recesses. The **subscapularis recess** (**Fig. 4.25**) lies as an anterior reflection over the subscapularis muscle and usually connects with the capsule. The **axillary recess** (**Figs. 4.26–4.28**) lies inferiorly.

On the scapula, the capsule merges with the glenoid labrum: the synovial membrane merges onto the free tip of the labrum, and the fibrous layer onto its base.

On the humerus, the joint capsule attaches to the anatomical neck. Anteriorly, it merges with the subscapularis tendon, superiorly with the supraspinatus tendon, and posteriorly with the tendons of the infraspinatus and teres minor muscles:

- In the neutral position (0°), the superior parts of the capsule are tensed, while the axillary recess forms folds.
- At about 45° abduction, both the superior and inferior parts of the capsule are relaxed.
- At 90° abduction, the superior parts are clearly relaxed while the inferior parts are taut.

### Pathology

Inflammation can cause adherence of the axillary recess. This can also occur if the arm is held in one position for a prolonged time in an attempt to relieve pain. The result is a substantial restriction of movement, especially of flexion and abduction, since the recess must be fully relaxed for these movements to occur.

### Practical Tip

The adherent parts of the capsule can be released by intensive glide mobilization, for instance using the inferior glide mobilization technique to treat restricted abduction and flexion.

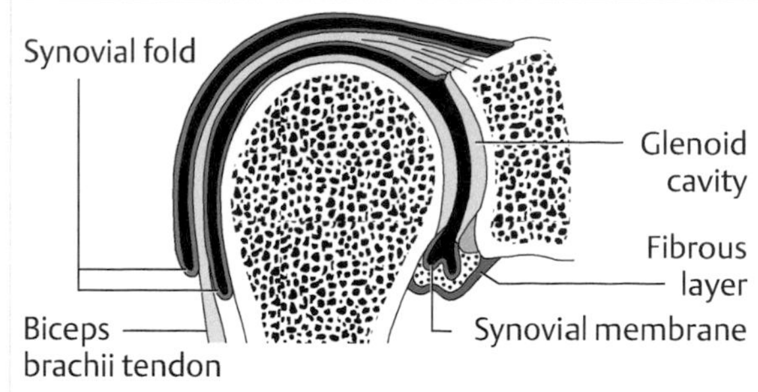


**Fig. 4.24** Joint capsule.

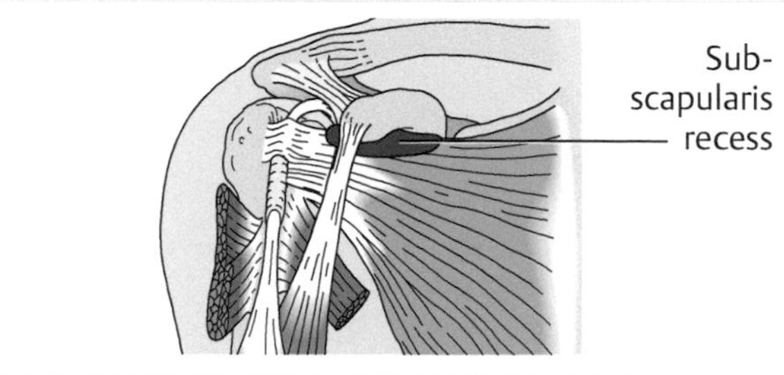


**Fig. 4.25** Subscapularis recess.

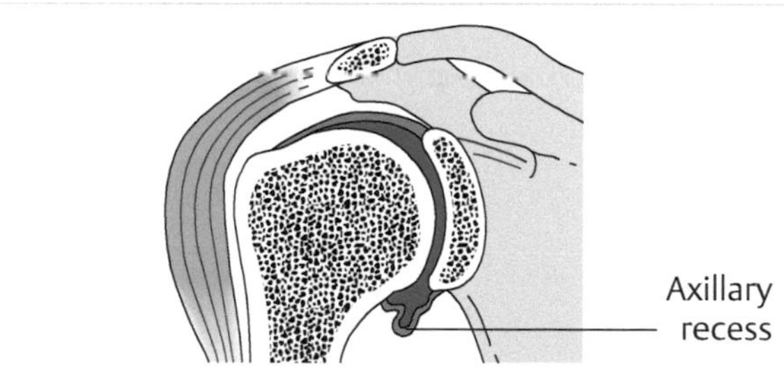


**Fig. 4.26** Axillary recess.

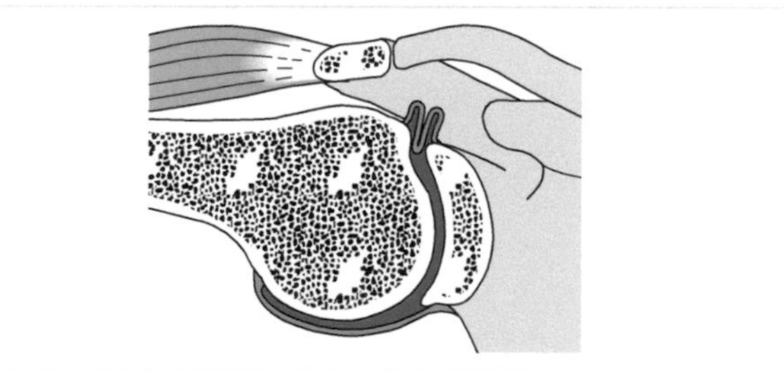

**Fig. 4.27** Unfolding of the axillary recess.

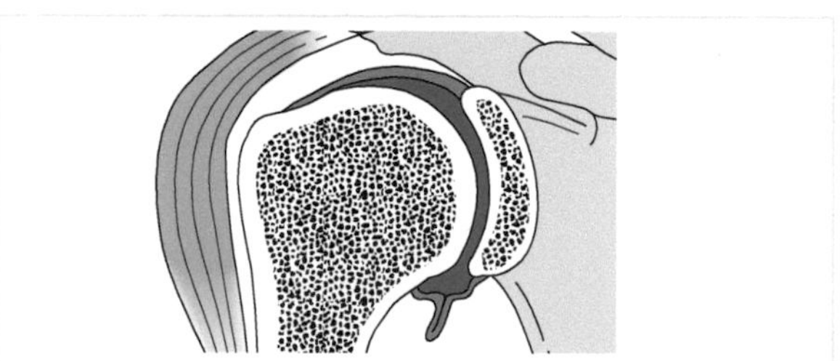

**Fig. 4.28** Adhesion of the axillary recess.

## Arterial Supply (Fig. 4.29)

The arterial supply to the capsule is primarily from the *anterior and posterior circumflex humeral arteries*, which also supply the rotator cuff. They form numerous anastomoses.

## Innervation (Fig. 4.30)

The joint capsule and the surrounding ligaments and muscles are innervated by a network of nerve fibers that stem from the C5–C7 nerve roots, primarily the **axillary** and **suprascapular nerves**.

The **musculocutaneous nerve** gives off small branches into the anterosuperior area, and the **subscapular nerve** provides branches to the anterior capsule.

The fibrous layer contains numerous receptors, primarily mechanoreceptors and free nerve endings.

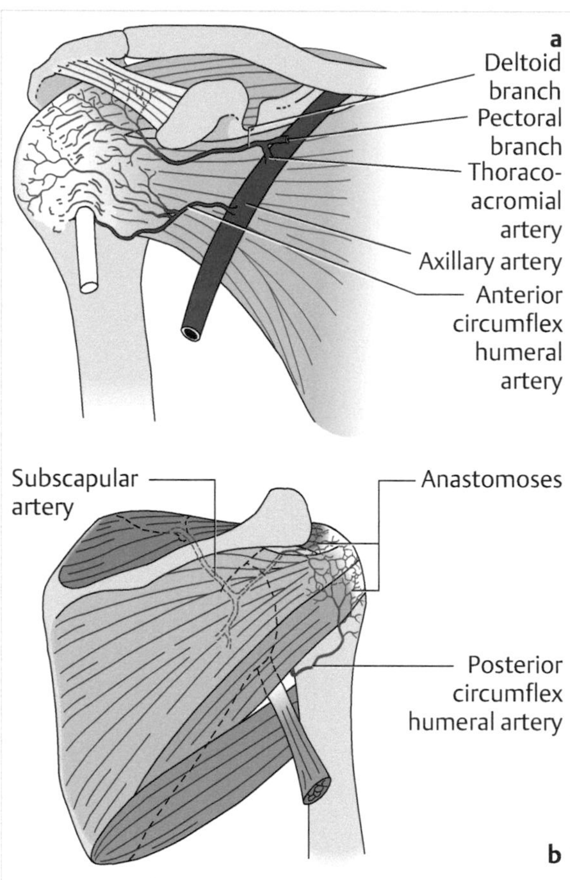


**Fig. 4.29** Arterial supply of the joint capsule and the surrounding area. **(a)** Anterior view. **(b)** Posterior view.

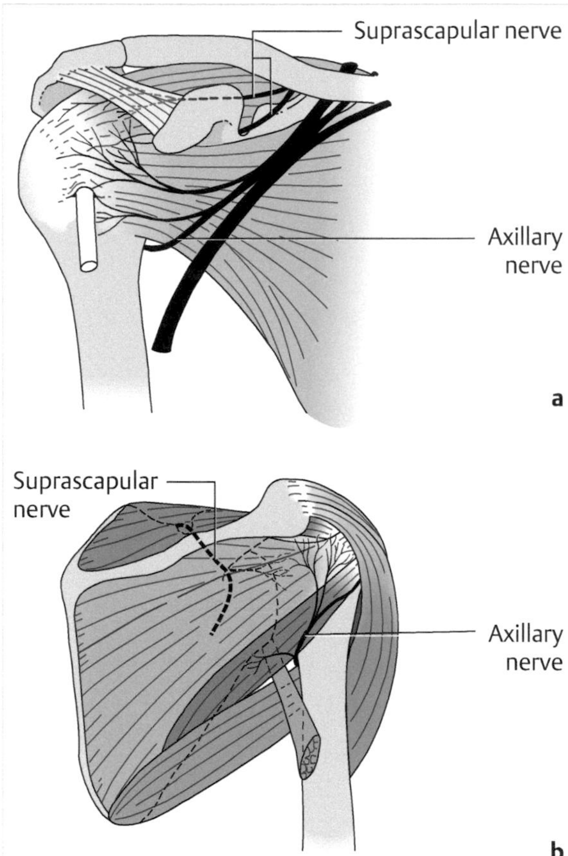


**Fig. 4.30** Innervation of the joint capsule. **(a)** Anterior region. **(b)** Posterior region.

## Ligaments

Superiorly and anteriorly, the capsule receives reinforcement from ligaments, which merge with the fibrous layer.

### Coracohumeral Ligament (Fig. 4.31)

Two parts of this ligament can be distinguished. One part extends from the lateral edge of the base of the coracoid process to the lesser tubercle of the humerus. The second extends from the greater tubercle of the humerus into the coraco-acromial ligament. Offshoots of this section span the proximal portion of the intertubercular sulcus.

The coracohumeral ligament closes the gap in the capsule between the supraspinatus muscle and the subscapularis muscle.

**Function.** The ligament has a stabilizing function in that it prevents the head of the humerus from descending when the arm is hanging down. In addition, it limits flexion, adduction and external rotation when in a 90° abducted position.

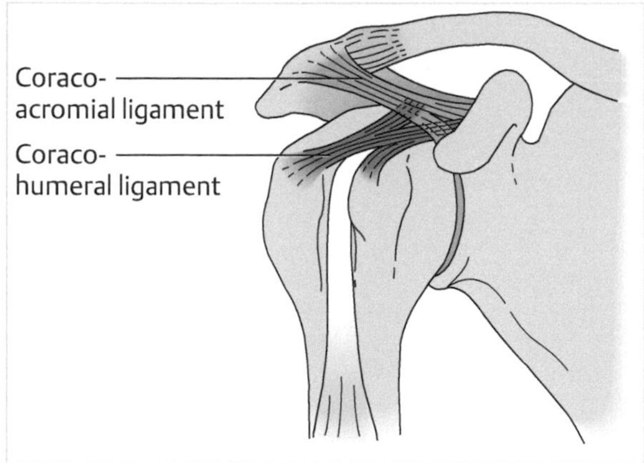


**Fig. 4.31** Coracohumeral ligament.

### Glenohumeral Ligament (Figs. 4.32 and 4.33)

The glenohumeral ligament is very thin and merges with the capsule. It consists of three parts:

- The *superior part* comes from the bone–cartilage border of the cavity, runs directly anterior to the tendon of the long head of the biceps, and inserts on the superior margin of the lesser tubercle. The subscapularis tendon lies over it.
- The *middle part* is usually less well formed and extends from the labrum next to the superior part to insert on the humerus medial to the lesser tubercle under the subscapularis tendon.
- The *inferior part* runs beneath the middle part and strengthens the capsule between the subscapularis muscle and the triceps brachii muscle.

**Function.** The glenohumeral ligament limits external rotation through the tension that develops in all three parts of the ligament. It prevents inferior subluxation of the head of the humerus, and the inferior part plays a role in anterior stabilization, primarily in abduction and external rotation.

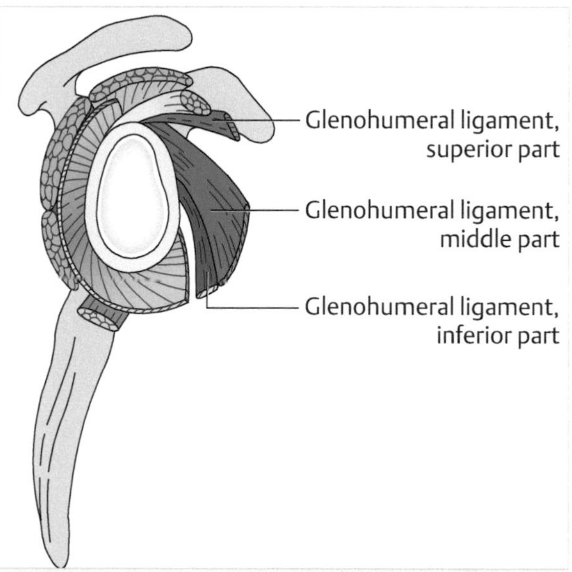


**Fig. 4.32** Glenohumeral ligament.

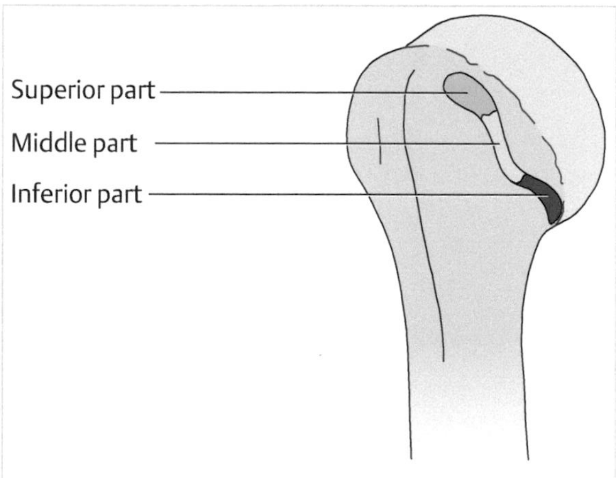


**Fig. 4.33** Insertion of the glenohumeral ligament on the humerus.

**Pathology**

The ligaments that enfold the capsule are not very well developed. In the dissection of an older subject, they can sometimes scarcely be differentiated from the fibrous layer. It also stands to reason that the shoulder becomes unstable if there is a tendency toward laxity of the ligaments and in certain types of sports, such as throwing events.

In the case of chronic shoulder subluxation, the anteriorly lying ligaments and tendons usually need to be surgically gathered and tightened to stabilize the joint.

**Practical Tip**

In an unstable shoulder, the rotator cuff, which has a direct connection to the capsule–ligament apparatus, must undergo an intensive training program to stabilize the joint.

## Coraco-acromial Ligament (Fig. 4.34)

The coraco-acromial ligament extends from the lateral surface of the coracoid process to the anterior neck of the acromion and, to a degree, to the underside of the acromion as far as the acromioclavicular joint. It is very wide in the area of the coracoid process, where there is a small longitudinal gap in the middle.

A few fibers of the short head of the biceps muscle extend into the ligament.

**Function.** It forms part of the "roof of the shoulder" (coraco-acromial arch), and, through its connection to the coracohumeral ligament, prevents inferior subluxation.

**Pathology**

To treat a chronic impingement syndrome with narrowing of the subacromial space, the surgeon splits or divides the coraco-acromial ligament to create space for the thickened structures.

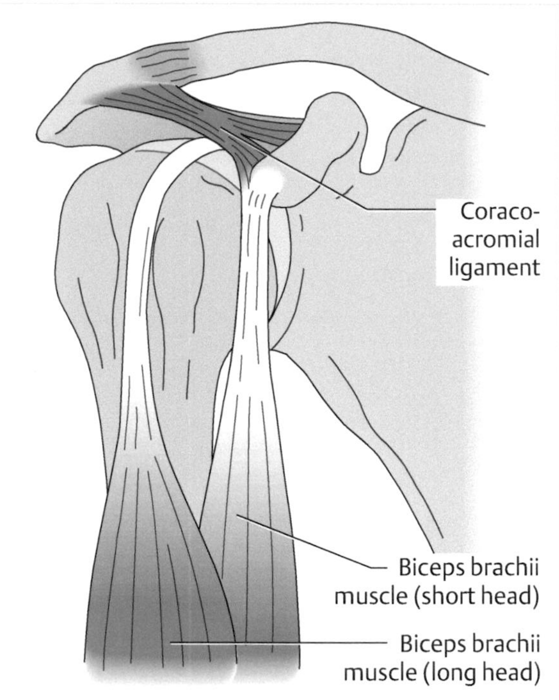


**Fig. 4.34** Coraco-acromial ligament.

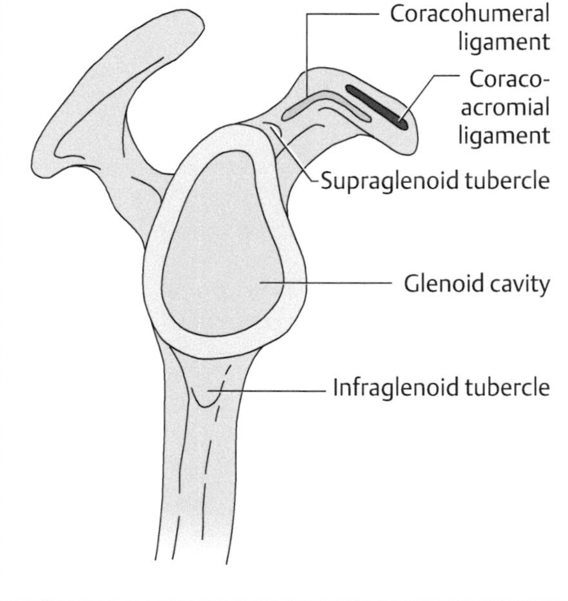


**Fig. 4.35** Insertions of the ligaments on the coracoid process.

## 4.2.4 Subacromial Space (Fig. 4.36)

The space between the head of the humerus and the coraco-acromial arch is not a true joint. It is significant that many degenerative processes occur in this area.

The "roof of the shoulder" (coraco-acromial arch) consists of:

- The **acromion**.
- The **coracoid process**.
- The **coraco-acromial ligament**.

The subacromial space contains the following: the subacromial bursa, the tendons of the supraspinatus muscle, part of the infraspinatus muscle, the tendon of the long head of the biceps, and superior parts of the capsule and ligaments.

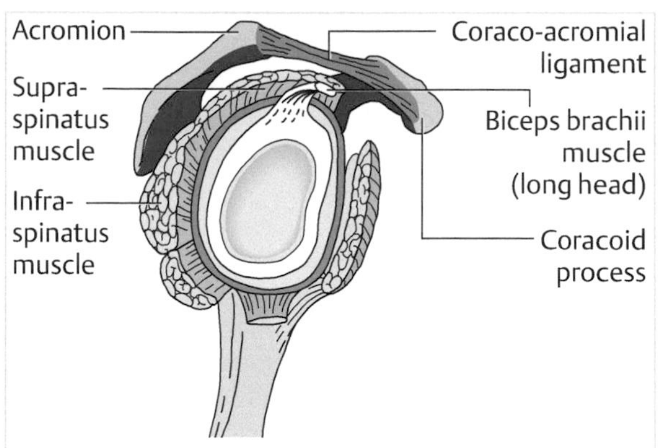


**Fig. 4.36** Subacromial space.

### Subacromial and Subdeltoid Bursae (Figs. 4.37–4.39)

The **subacromial bursa** lies under the coraco-acromial arch and extends up to the acromioclavicular joint.

The **subdeltoid bursa** lies between the deltoid muscle and greater tubercle and the insertion tendons of the infraspinatus and supraspinatus muscles. The two bursae communicate with each other.

The outermost layers of the bursa are known as *leaves*. The superficial leaf merges superiorly with the acromion, and the deep leaf with the rotator cuff and the humerus. A thin film of liquid lies between them. The bursae prevent friction from occurring between the coraco-acromial arch and the tendon sheets. During arm movements, the superficial leaf is fixed and the lower layer slides over it.

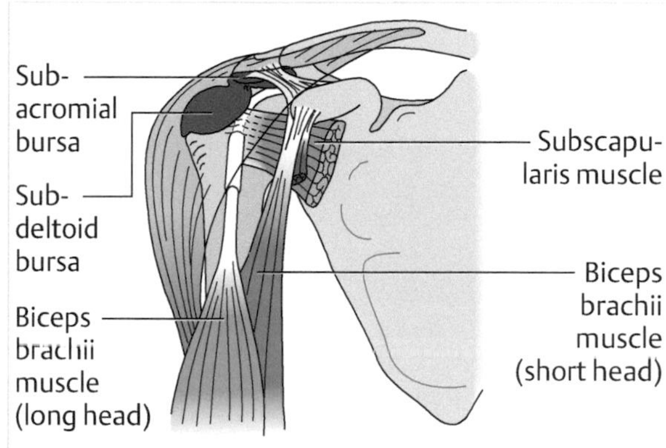


**Fig. 4.37** Bursae in the subacromial region.

#### Pathology

Movement presupposes that the bursal leaves can slide freely over each other without difficulty. Narrowing the subacromial space leads to compression of the bursal tissue and microtrauma caused by movement. The reaction—bursal irritation → formation of edema → further narrowing of the subacromial space—is a vicious cycle. A significantly thickened bursa can cause episodes of impingement.

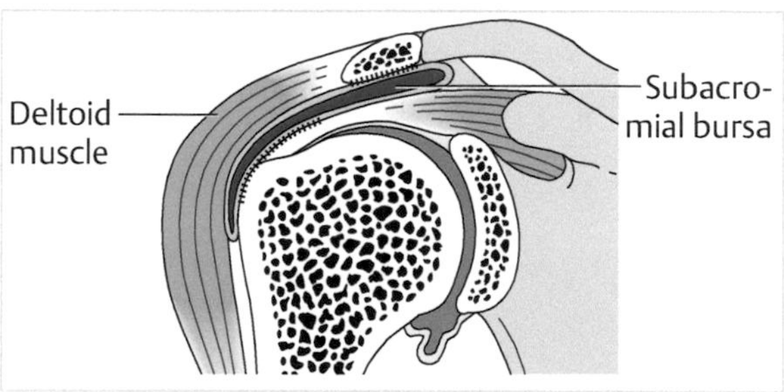


**Fig. 4.38** The attachment areas of the subacromial bursa.

#### Practical Tip

Treatment with inferior traction unburdens the subacromial structures and reduces pain.

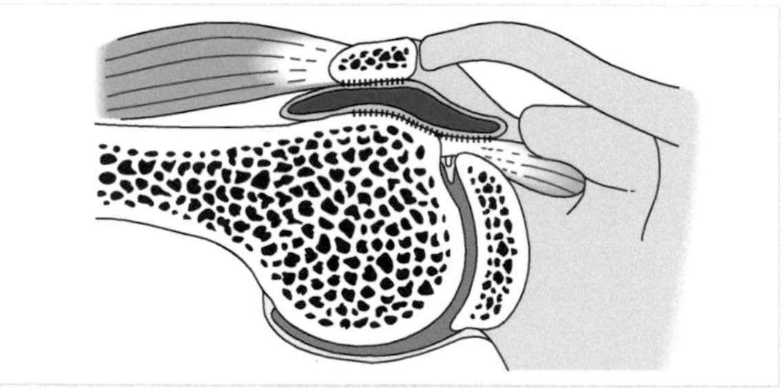

**Fig. 4.39** Shifting of the bursal leaves during abduction.

## 4.2.5 Scapulothoracic Gliding Plane (Figs. 4.40 and 4.41)

In the neutral position, the scapula reaches from the second to the seventh ribs, and the spine of the scapula lies at the level of T3.

Viewed from posteriorly, the scapula is tilted slightly laterally. Its medial border runs at an angle of 3 to 5° to the line formed by the row of spinous processes (**Fig. 4.40a**).

Depending on the thorax, the scapula is aligned somewhat anteriorly in its resting position. That means that, viewed from above, it forms an angle of 30° with the frontal plane. The clavicle forms an angle of 60° with the scapula (**Fig. 4.40b**).

Viewed from laterally, depending on the thorax, the scapula is tilted 20° forward (**Fig. 4.40c**).

**Pathology**

The angle changes when there are changes in the position of the shoulder girdle. For example, when the shoulders are protracted, this scapular angle, viewed from laterally, can amount to more than 20°, so that the inferior angle of the scapula visibly protrudes from the thorax. In the same way, the angle between the clavicle and the scapula can amount to less than 60°.

The scapulothoracic gliding plane is divided into two **gliding zones**:

- The gliding zone between the subscapularis muscle and the serratus anterior muscle is open laterally.
- The gliding zone between the serratus anterior muscle and the thoracic fascia has its entrance from the medial border.

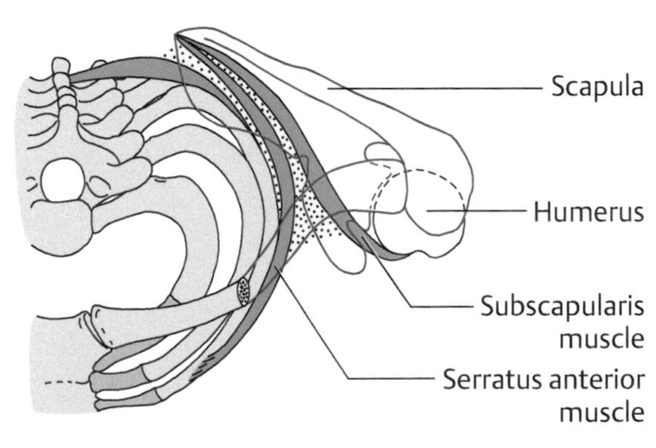


**Fig. 4.41** The scapulothoracic gliding surface.

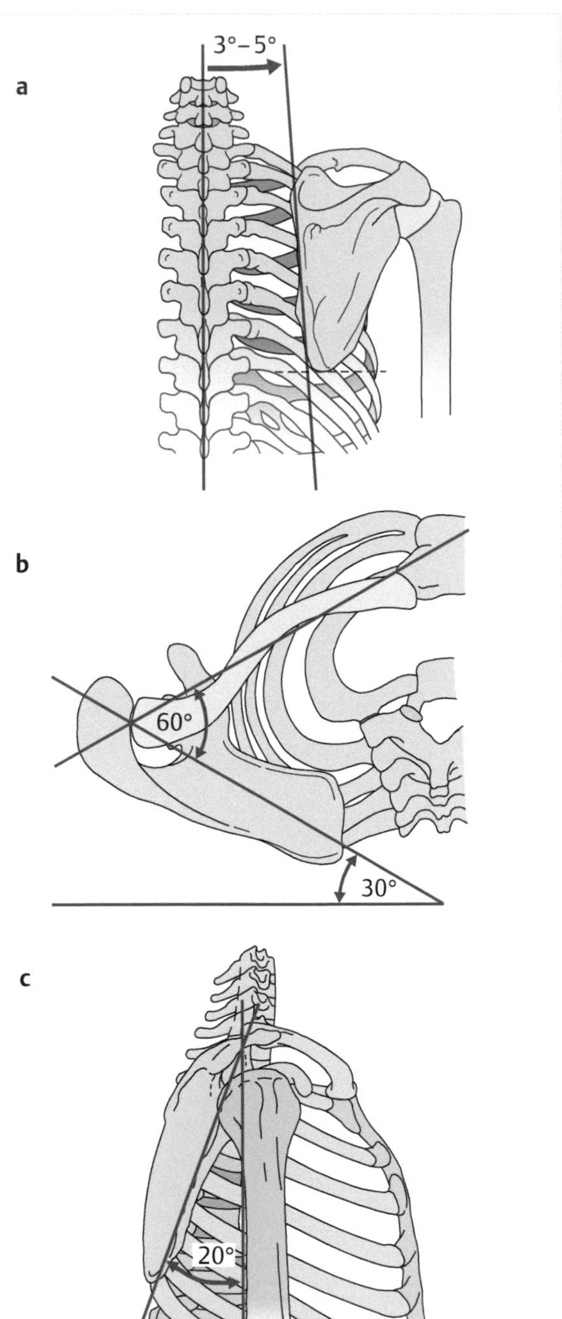


**Fig. 4.40** Position of the scapula. **(a)** In relation to the ribs and the thoracic spine (viewed from posterior). **(b)** In relation to the thorax and clavicle (transverse view). **(c)** In relation to the thorax (seen from laterally).

## Movements of the Scapula (Fig. 4.42)

### External Rotation (Fig. 4.42a)

The lateral swiveling movement of the scapula is termed external rotation. The corresponding axis is aligned at right angles to the scapular plane. It lies approximately in the middle, beneath the spine of the scapula, and migrates inferiorly during the movement.

The entire capacity of the swiveling movement is 60°. During the course of this movement, the inferior angle travels about 10 cm laterally. The superior angle travels only a quarter the distance inferomedially.

External rotation is the most important movement of the scapula, and it occurs along with both abduction and flexion of the arm.

### Elevation/Depression (Fig. 4.42b)

The elevation movement is the shift of the scapula in a superior direction and amounts to about 10 cm. Depression corresponds to a movement in an inferior direction, which is limited to only about 3 cm.

### Adduction/Abduction (Fig. 4.42c)

In adduction, the medial border of the scapula approaches the spinal column. This movement corresponds to retraction of the shoulder girdle. The angle between the clavicle and scapula increases slightly.

Abduction of the scapula corresponds to protraction of the shoulder girdle.

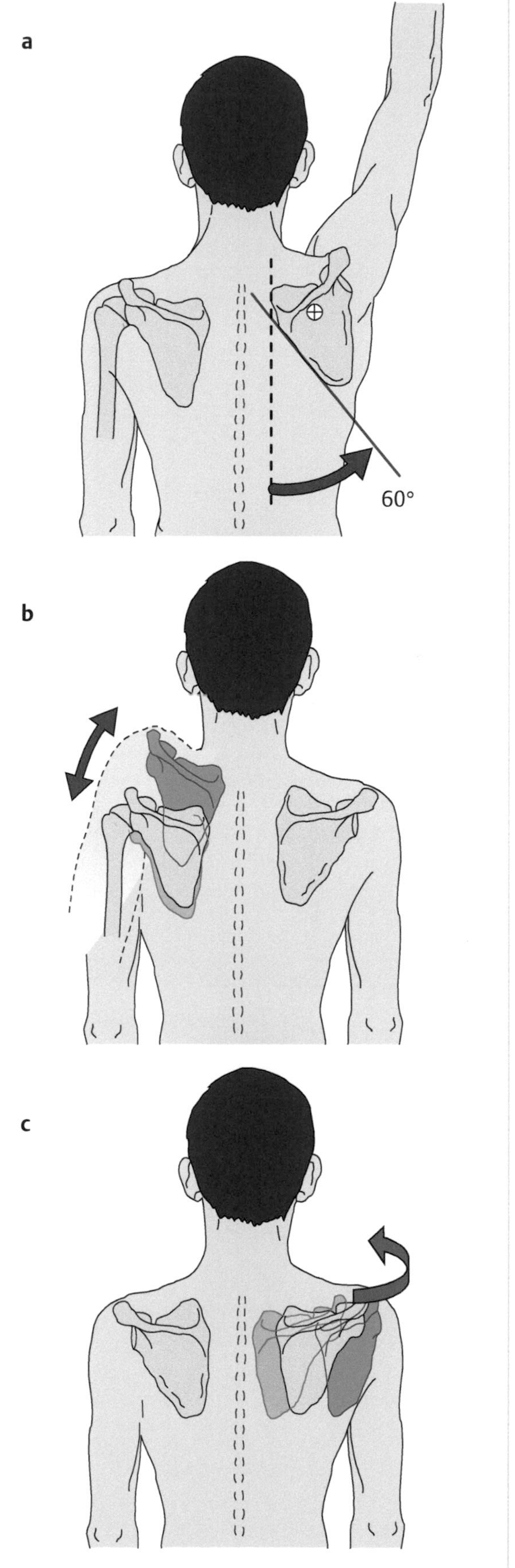


**Fig. 4.42** Movements of the scapula. **(a)** External rotation. ▸ **(b)** Elevation/depression. **(c)** Adduction/abduction.

## 4.2.6 Muscles of the Scapula

### Trapezius Muscle (Fig. 4.43)

- **Descending part**: This pulls the acromion in a superomedial direction, which produces external rotation of the scapula and a shift of the glenoid cavity upward and outward.
  Cervical spine: With the shoulder girdle fixed, the muscle causes extension of the cervical spine and lateral flexion to the same side, and turns the head to the opposite side.
- **Transverse part:** This presses the scapula to the thorax and pulls the medial border toward the vertebral column.
- **Ascending part:** This pulls the medial area of the spine of the scapula in an inferomedial direction, thus acting as a type of fixed end for the lateral swiveling movement of the scapula.

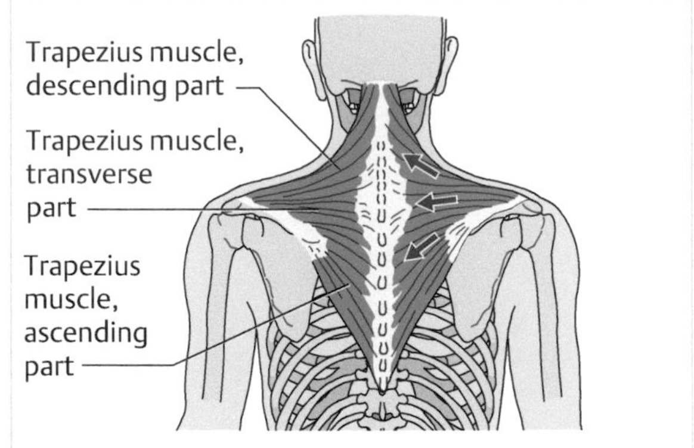


**Fig. 4.43** Trapezius muscle.

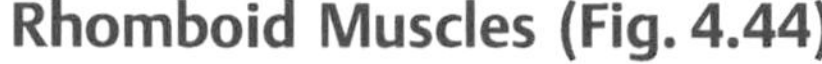

### Rhomboid Muscles (Fig. 4.44)

These pull the scapula in a superomedial direction and help in fixing the scapula to the thorax.

### Levator Scapulae Muscle (Fig. 4.44)

This pulls the medial scapular area upward. When the scapula externally rotates, the muscle must give way eccentrically. This presents a fundamental problem because it is one of the muscles that is inclined toward shortening. It also holds the scapula back toward internal rotation when it is externally rotated.

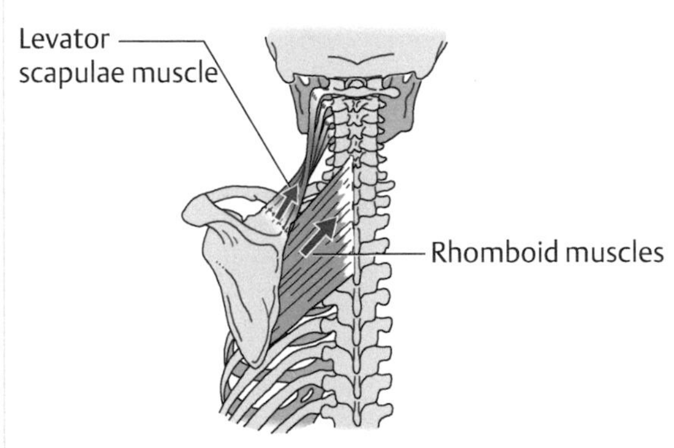


**Fig. 4.44** Rhomboid muscles and levator scapulae muscle.

### Serratus Anterior Muscle (Fig. 4.45)

- The **superior part** is the upper section of the serratus anterior and extends to the superior angle of the scapula. This part, with its thicker muscle belly, is to be differentiated from the flat lower sections. It causes internal rotation of the scapula.
- The **middle part** is very wide with an almost horizontal course to the medial border of the scapula. This portion of the muscle takes on primary responsibility for fixing the scapula to the thorax.
- The **inferior part** consists of obliquely running fibers that extend superiorly to the inferior angle. It acts antagonistically to the superior part, pulling the scapula into external rotation.

When all the parts contract together, they pull the scapula laterally.

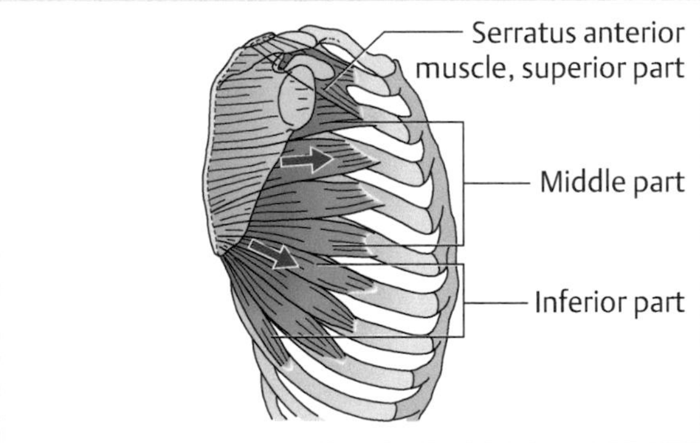


**Fig. 4.45** Serratus anterior muscle.

### Pectoralis Minor Muscle (Fig. 4.46)

This pulls the scapula in an anterior, inferior direction, so that the inferior angle sticks out from the thorax.

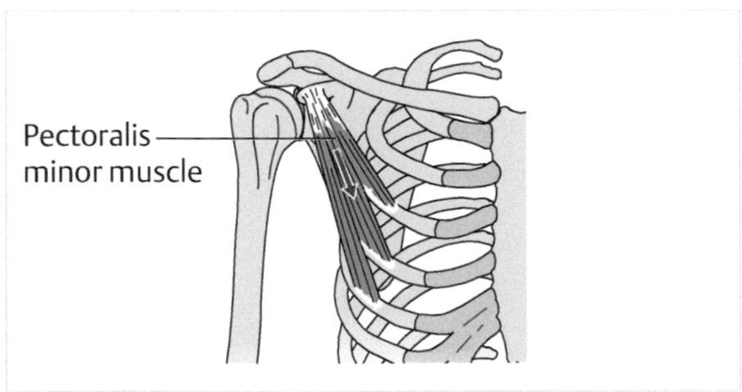


**Fig. 4.46** Pectoralis minor muscle.

## Muscle Slings (Fig. 4.47)

Between the scapula and the torso, there are eight muscular connections that play a pivotal role in positioning the scapula and coordinating its movements. These eight connections can be divided into antagonistic pairs, which are called *muscle slings*. If one muscle contracts, its partner must be able to relax:

- The *levator scapulae–trapezius* (ascending part) *sling* coordinates the movements of elevation and depression.
- The *serratus* (superior and middle parts)*–trapezius* (transverse part) *sling* coordinates the movements of abduction and adduction.
- The *pectoralis minor–trapezius* (descending part) *sling* controls the anterior–inferior and posterior–superior shifts of the scapula.
- The *rhomboid–serratus* (inferior part) *sling* controls the rotational movements of the scapula.

Only when these muscle slings are in equilibrium, i.e., when there are no slackening or contracting tendencies, is the scapula optimally located on the thorax, and can the arm–shoulder girdle movements proceed in a coordinated manner.

### Practical Tip

A weakened muscle is not capable of working against a hypertonic antagonist. With a hypertonic levator scapulae muscle, for instance, the tone in this muscle must first be reduced before its antagonist in the muscle sling can be rehabilitated.

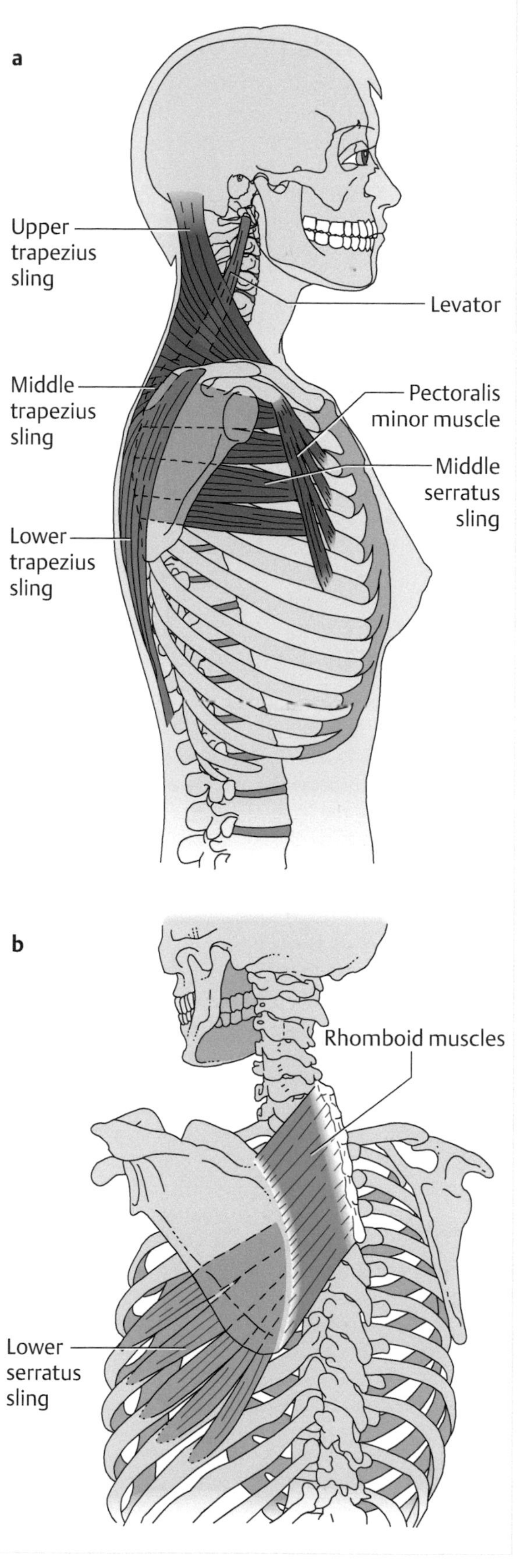


**Fig. 4.47** The muscle slings of the scapula. **(a)** Levator–trapezius sling, pectoralis minor–trapezius sling, and serratus–trapezius sling. **(b)** Rhomboid–serratus sling.

## 4.2.7 Acromioclavicular Joint (Fig. 4.48)

- The **joint surface** on the acromion is flat to slightly convex, as is that of the clavicle.
- A **disk**, usually incomplete, provides for optimal joint closure and transfer of force.
- When viewed from above, the **joint space** runs from posteromedial to anterolateral; viewed from the front, it runs inferomedially.
- Except for its inferior part, the **capsule** is thick and firm. It merges with the acromioclavicular ligament. A few fibers of the deltoid and trapezius muscles extend into the capsule.

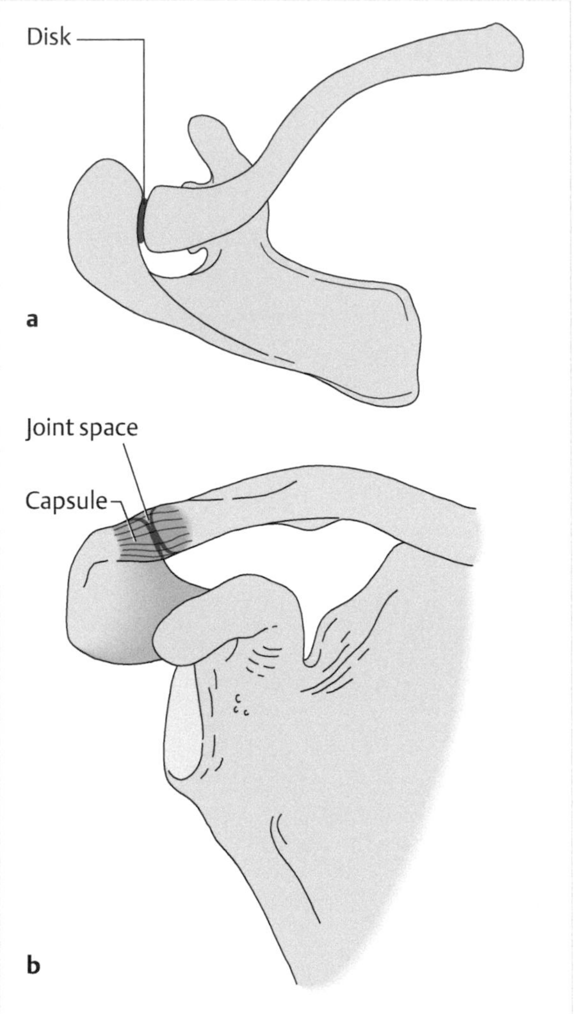


**Fig. 4.48** Acromioclavicular joint. **(a)** Superior view. **(b)** Anterior view.

**Practical Tip**

Kyphosis (a rounded back) changes the course of the joint toward the sagittal plane because the scapula adjusts toward abduction. Therefore, it is important to establish its actual course before applying glide mobilization.

### Ligaments (Fig. 4.49)

The **acromioclavicular ligament** joins the clavicle to the acromion.

The **coracoclavicular ligament** extends from the lower border of the clavicle to the base of the coracoid process. It consists of two parts:

- The *conoid ligament* is fixed on the posteromedial side of the coracoid process and extends to a roughened area, the conoid tubercle, on the underside of the clavicle.
- The *trapezoid ligament* inserts anterior to the conoid ligament on the inner side of the process and extends anterolaterally to the trapezoid line, a linear area of roughness on the underside of the clavicle. This ligament is longer and stronger than the conoid ligament.

These ligaments stabilize the clavicle, meaning that they hold it onto the scapula. They prevent shifts in the frontal and transverse planes.

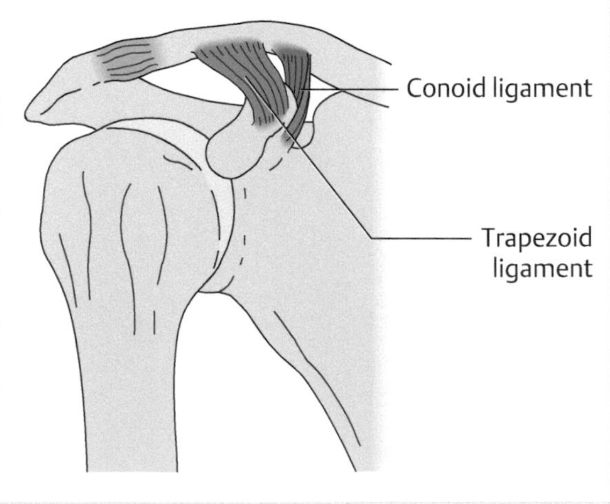


**Fig. 4.49** Ligamentous connections in the lateral clavicular area.

### Movements

Movement is limited by the coracoclavicular and acromioclavicular ligaments. Movement can occur around three axes:

- Anterior–posterior movements: protraction and retraction of the shoulder girdle.
- Superior–inferior movements: elevation and depression (not very pronounced).
- Rotation around its longitudinal axis.

## 4.2.8 Sternoclavicular Joint (Fig. 4.50)

- **Joint surfaces:** The sternal end of the clavicle is saddle-shaped, with the longer axis lying in the superior–inferior direction and the shorter axis from anterior to posterior. Corresponding congruent joint surfaces occur on the sternum. In addition, there is a small joint surface for the first rib on the lower border of the clavicle.
- **Articular disk:** This attaches all around the joint capsule. Its congruence changes so that rotational movements around the clavicle's own axis are possible.
- **Orientation** of the joint: The joint line rises at an angle of about 40° from the horizontal plane and tilts about 20° from the sagittal plane. The course of the joint line is therefore from superior–medial–posterior to inferior–lateral–anterior.

### Ligaments

- The **anterior and posterior sternoclavicular ligaments** strengthen the capsule anteriorly and posteriorly. The anterior ligament is stronger.
- The **costoclavicular ligament** extends from the first rib, lateral to the joint space to the underside of the clavicle. Posterior fibers join with the posterior sternoclavicular ligament. The ligament limits elevation.
- The **interclavicular ligament** joins the two clavicles to each other above the sternum.

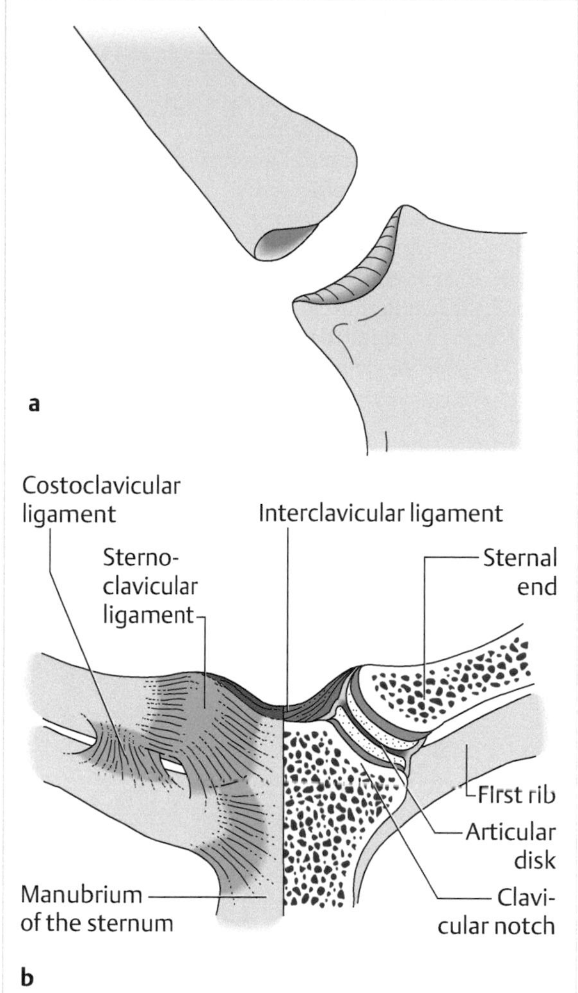


**Fig. 4.50** Sternoclavicular joint. **(a)** Shape of the joint surfaces. **(b)** Section through the joint (anterior view).

## Movements

### In the Frontal Plane (Fig. 4.51)

When the shoulder girdle elevates, the acromial end moves superiorly, so that the clavicle is more steeply oriented. During this process, the clavicle glides inferiorly within the sternoclavicular joint.

The first rib, which lies directly under the clavicle, sets a limit on this movement, thus diverting the sternal end anteriorly. The *range of motion* is about 30°.

With further elevation, the clavicle rotates a short distance around its longitudinal axis. Because of this rotation, and contingent on the S-shape of the clavicle, the acromial end assumes a steeper position. Because the clavicle is taller than it is wide, a gliding movement also occurs in an anterior direction. Through this rotation, the clavicle assumes a still steeper position and gains another 30° beyond the elevation position.

During depression, it glides superiorly and somewhat posteriorly because of the minimal rotation associated with the movement.

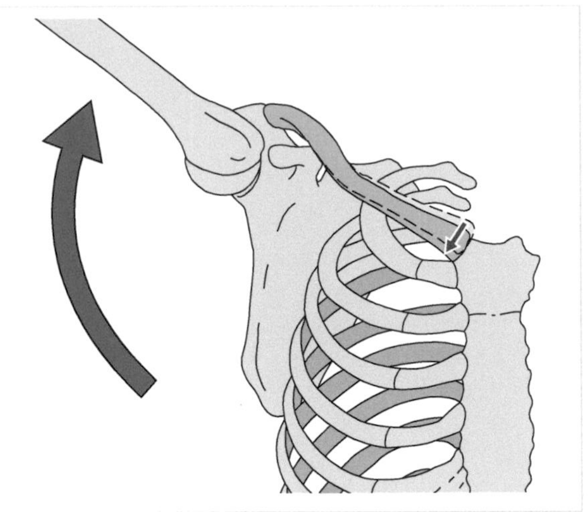

**Fig. 4.51** Gliding movements of the clavicle during elevation.

### In the Transverse Plane (Fig. 4.52)

During shoulder retraction, the concave sternal end of the clavicle glides posteriorly.

During protraction, the clavicle glides anteriorly.

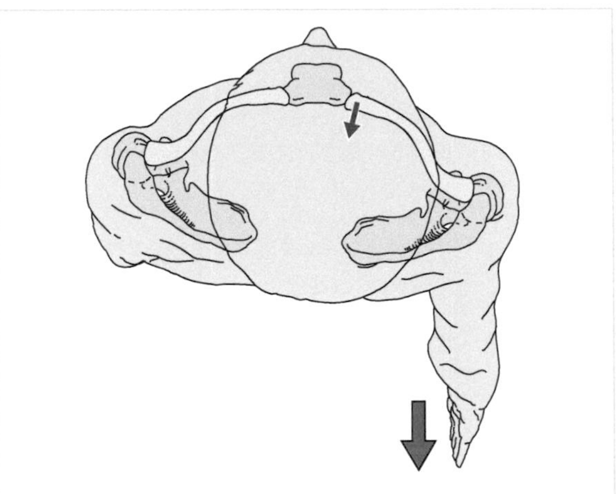

**Fig. 4.52** Gliding movements of the clavicle during retraction.

### Interaction between the Acromioclavicular and Sternoclavicular Joints (Fig. 4.53)

The acromioclavicular and sternoclavicular joints are jointly involved in all movements of the shoulder girdle. Recording the position of the acromial end of the clavicle during the end-range movements of the shoulder girdle in all directions and connecting the points produces an oval shape that is higher than it is wide, representing an elevation movement of about 60°, a depression of 5°, and protraction and retraction of 30° each.

The scapula takes part in all movements of the clavicle.

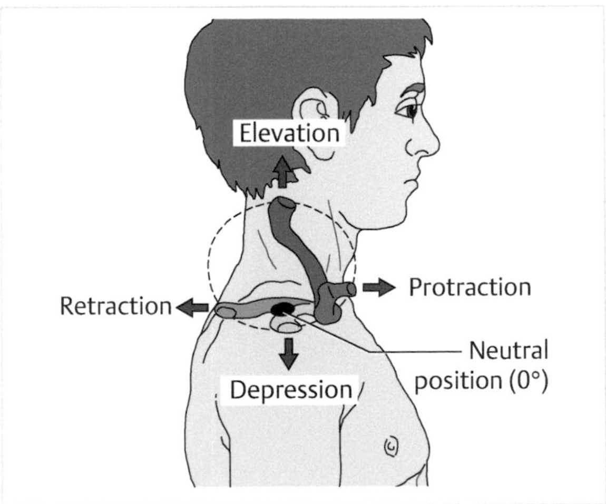


**Fig. 4.53** Direction and extent of movements of the clavicle (lateral view).

## Combination Movements of the Clavicle during Abduction and Flexion (Fig. 4.54)

The following events occur in the shoulder girdle during flexion and abduction of the arm:

- The scapula externally rotates, and the glenoid cavity turns upward and outward.
- Because the mobility in the acromioclavicular joint is limited, the scapula pushes the acromial end of the clavicle approximately 30° in a superior direction, which corresponds to elevation. The movement of the clavicle is then stopped by the sternoclavicular and costoclavicular ligaments. In addition, the gliding movement inferiorly is limited by the first rib.
- To reach the maximum external rotation of the scapula of 60°, the acromial end of the clavicle must move another 30° superiorly. This occurs through rotation of the clavicle around its longitudinal axis and is due to its S-shape.

This rotation does not wait for 30° of elevation to occur, but occurs significantly sooner. There are also individual differences in how frequently these combination movements occur. The extent of the rotational movement of the clavicle cannot be exactly determined, but is probably less than 45°.

The following muscles that insert onto the clavicle (**Fig. 4.55**) can influence the position of the shoulder girdle:

- Trapezius muscle, descending part.
- Deltoid muscle, clavicular part.
- Pectoral muscle, clavicular part.
- Subclavius muscle.

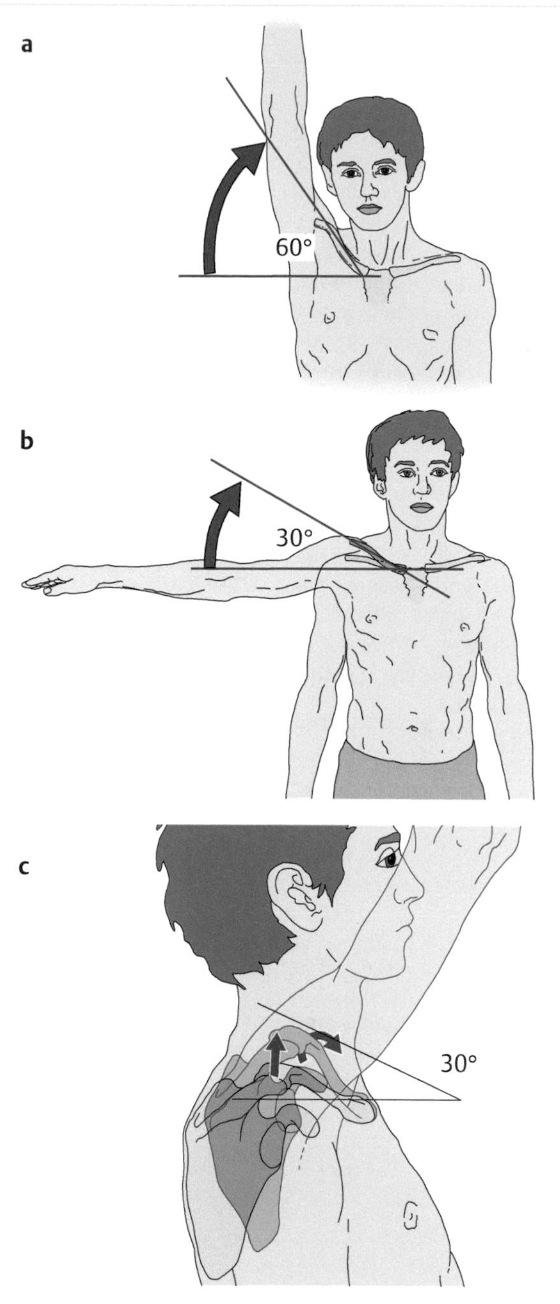


**Fig. 4.54 (a)** The final position of the clavicle at maximal abduction or flexion. **(b)** Elevation of the clavicle. **(c)** Rotation of the clavicle.

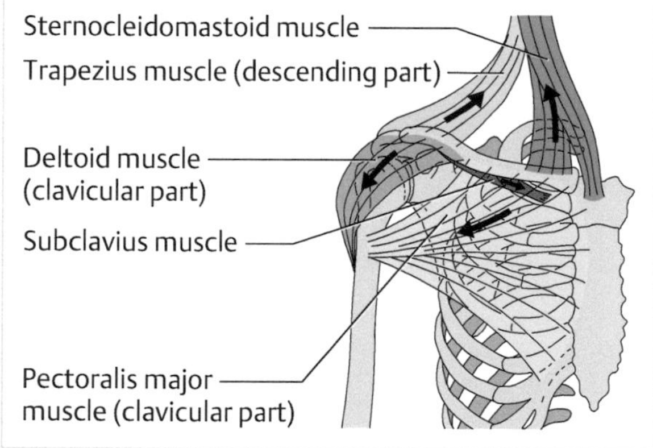


**Fig. 4.55** Muscles that insert onto the clavicle.

# 4.3 Movements of the Arm

## 4.3.1 Movement: Abduction (Fig. 4.56)

The *range of motion* for abduction is 180°. It is made up of three phases:

**Phase 1.** The arm abducts at the glenohumeral joint, meaning that the muscles that extend from the arm to the scapula are active:

- Supraspinatus muscle.
- Infraspinatus muscle, superior fibers.
- Biceps brachii muscle, long head.
- Deltoid muscle, acromial part.

**Phase 2:** From about 30° to 50°, the scapula accompanies the movement. The amount of this varies from individual to individual, so the patient's healthy side will serve as the normal for comparison. The movement is always coupled with movement in the acromioclavicular and sternoclavicular joints. In addition to the muscles mentioned above, the following shoulder girdle muscles become active:

- Trapezius muscle, descending part.
- Trapezius muscle, ascending part.
- Serratus anterior muscle, inferior part.

**Phase 3:** The vertebral column performs the last 20° of the movement: extension of the spine occurs primarily with bilateral abduction. Rotation to the same side and lateral flexion to the opposite side is associated with unilateral abduction. The ribs rise on the same side. These movements do not wait until the 160° level to occur, but start much earlier.

In addition to the above muscles, the following is now added:

- Erector spinae muscle.

### Preconditions for End-Range Motion

Complete abduction mobility is dependent on several factors, of which the following are described in more detail:

- The ability of the joint capsule to "unfold," and the ability of the tendons to glide within the subacromial area.
- The functional interaction of the rotator cuff and the deltoid muscle.
- The humeroscapular rhythm as well as the mobility in the acromioclavicular and sternoclavicular joints.
- The automatic external rotational movement of the humerus.
- The mobility of the spinal column.

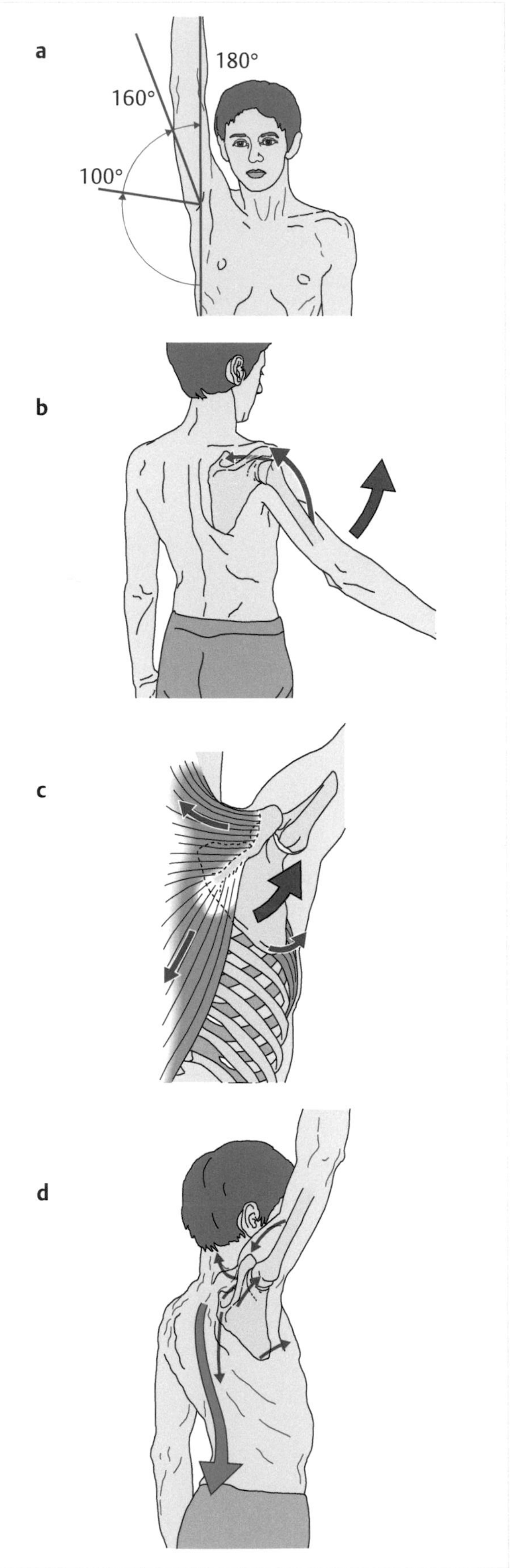


**Fig. 4.56** Abduction. **(a)** Range of motion. **(b)** First phase of the movement. **(c)** Second phase of the movement. **(d)** Third phase of the movement.

## Rotator Cuff (Fig. 4.57)

The shoulder joint is predominantly stabilized by muscles. Especially important is the rotator cuff, to which the following belong:

- Anteriorly: subscapularis muscle.
- Posteriorly: infraspinatus and teres minor muscles.
- Superiorly: supraspinatus muscle.

The tendons of these muscles are broad, lie directly on the capsule–ligament apparatus, and merge with the capsule. The fibers of the rotators form a firm connective tissue plate, the subdeltoid fascia, which attaches to the spine of the scapula, the acromion, and the lower edge of the coracoid process, and extends to the deltoid tuberosity of the humerus.

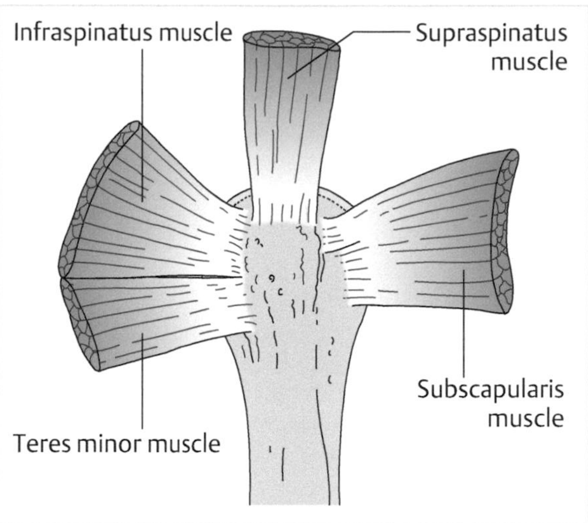


**Fig. 4.57** The rotator cuff.

## Subscapularis Muscle (Fig. 4.58)

- This muscle produces internal rotation.
- The upper, horizontal fibers help with abduction, while the lower, obliquely running fibers help with adduction.
- In the neutral position (0°), the tendon covers a large part of the head of the humerus and thus serves as an important stabilizer in preventing anterior dislocation.
- The subscapularis helps to center the head of the humerus. At 90° abduction, the inferior part of the head is uncovered; the muscle loses its joint-protective function in this position, showing only minimal activity.
- If the fixed end is on the arm, the muscle pulls the scapula laterally.

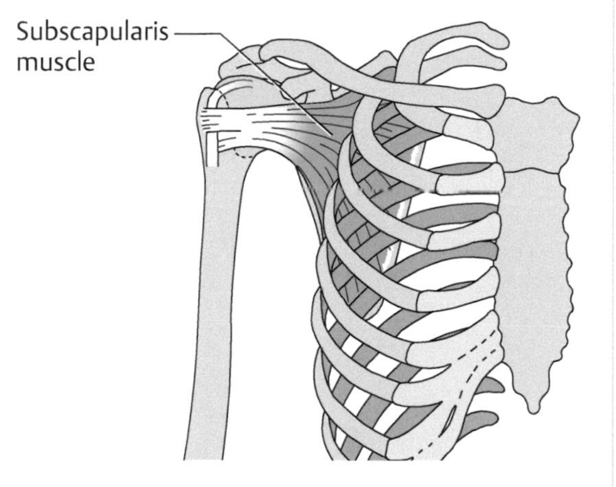


**Fig. 4.58** Subscapularis muscle.

## Infraspinatus Muscle (Fig. 4.59)

- This is the most important external rotator. It accounts for about 90% of the total force of external rotation.
- It causes extension.
- It helps to center the head of the humerus.
- Because of its broad area of origin from the infraspinous fossa, the superior, horizontally running fibers can be differentiated from the oblique fibers arising from the inferior area. The superior fibers help with abduction, while the inferior fibers adduct the arm.

## Teres Minor Muscle (Fig. 4.59)

- This muscle produces external rotation and extension.

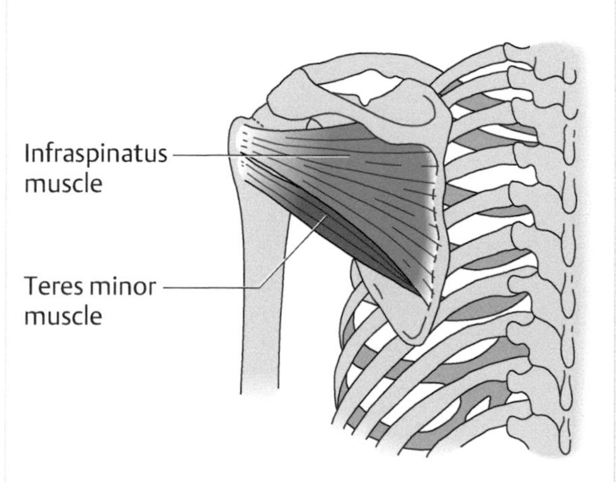


**Fig. 4.59** Infraspinatus and teres minor muscles.

## Supraspinatus Muscle (Fig. 4.60)

The tendon of the supraspinatus muscle is about 2 cm long, equally as wide, and about 3 mm thick. During arm movements, it glides within a compartment bordered by the supraspinous fossa and the acromion.

In addition to its insertion on the greater tubercle, it can also give off a small offshoot to the lesser tubercle.

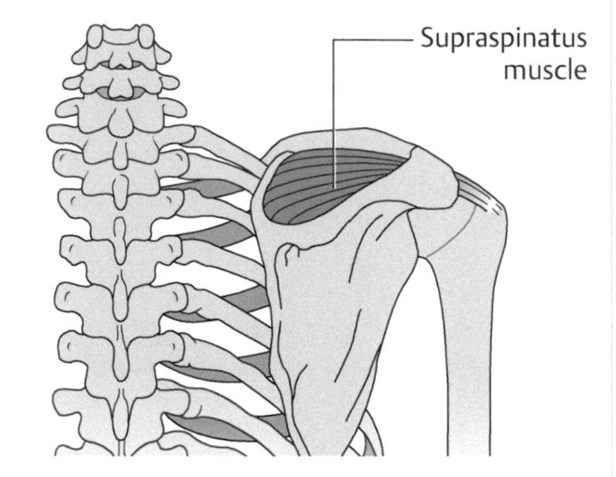


Fig. 4.60 Supraspinatus muscle.

## Perfusion (Fig. 4.61)

The tendon is supplied distally by the deltoid branch of the thoraco-acromial artery and from the circumflex humeral artery, and proximally by the suprascapular and subscapular arteries. These are all terminal branches of their arteries, which form anastomoses shortly before the tendon insertion. Therefore, there is a hypovascular zone in this region.

The vessels can be felt well when the patient's arm is slightly abducted.

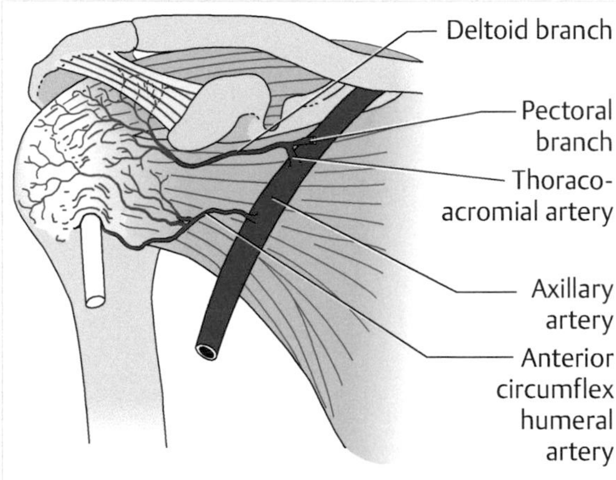


Fig. 4.61 Perfusion of the supraspinatus tendon.

## Function (Fig. 4.62)

Because of its direct course laterally over the head of the humerus in the neutral position, the supraspinatus causes depression of the humeral head and centers it toward the glenoid cavity. The muscle also has an abduction component. With increasing abduction, it no longer causes depression but continues to produce abduction and to center the head.

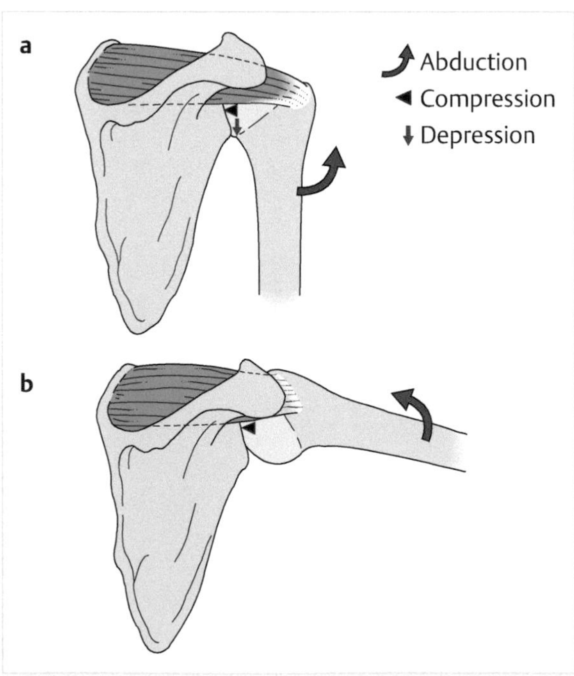


Fig. 4.62 Functions of the supraspinatus muscle. **(a)** In the neutral position. **(b)** In the abduction position.

## Pathology

### Tendinitis

If the tendon is thickened because of inflammation or scarring (as at times it can swell up to 1 cm), it becomes entrapped, and, with further movement, is forced through the compartment with a jerky motion.

### Diminished Perfusion

Strong traction, such as carrying heavy items, produces unfavorable effects on perfusion—no further blood is supplied to the area. The same occurs when adduction is very actively performed, such as in swimming.

Most of the degenerative changes, such as calcification and rupture, occur in the area that is hypoperfused.

### Rupture of the Supraspinatus Tendon (Fig. 4.63)

Small tears with intact sections of tendon on both sides of the tear can heal, again allowing abduction of the arm, but muscle endurance is disturbed.

If no intact parts of the tendon remain around the tear, as in a complete rupture, abduction is only possible using evasive movements, such as flexion. This defect can heal if the bursa has not been lacerated. If the bursa is also torn, there is an ongoing migration of fluid between the bursa and joint, and the tendon cannot heal. In unfavorable cases, the tear can extend and include the upper parts of the subscapularis or infraspinatus muscle, so that the centering function of these muscles fails.

## Practical Tip

Because tears occur in tissues that have undergone degenerative changes, the chances of recovery are understandably unfavorable. In evaluating the patient for treatment, it is important to note the use of evasive mechanisms in raising the arm, such as using flexion in place of abduction. Another consideration is whether the deltoid muscle is completely taking over this abduction function. In this case, patients train themselves to rotate the scapula before raising the arm. Through this movement, the arm goes into slight abduction, and the deltoid muscle can then more favorably develop force for abduction.

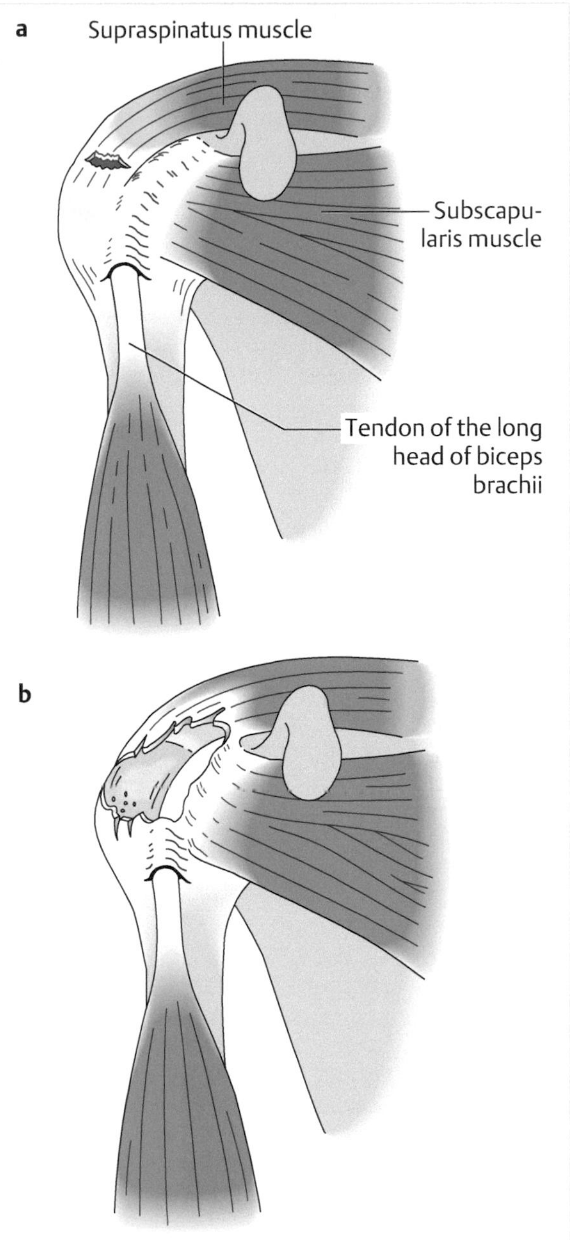


**Fig. 4.63** Ruptures. **(a)** Partial rupture of the supraspinatus tendon. **(b)** Total rupture of the supraspinatus tendon and parts of the subscapularis tendon.

## Deltoid Muscle (Fig. 4.64)

The deltoid muscle forms the contour of the shoulder, so that the shoulder appears angular if the muscle is atrophied. It consists of three parts, named for their origins:

### Spinal Part

The spinal part arises from the upper edge of the spine of the scapula and extends as obliquely descending fibers to the posterior border of the deltoid tuberosity. The fibers are very long and run parallel to each other.

**Function.** Extension/external rotation/adduction.

### Clavicular Part

Functionally, this is the most significant part, because most of the arm's activities take place in front of the body. With its insertion fibers, it extends under the acromial part.

**Function.** Flexion/internal rotation/adduction.

### Acromial Part

This is the most powerful section of the muscle. It arises from the outer edge of the acromion. Numerous septa subdivide it into many muscle fiber bundles containing a greater or lesser number of short fibers.

**Function.** Abduction.

*Analysis of the forces* (**Fig. 4.65**): In terms of its force components, the acromial part of the deltoid muscle can be differentiated into two force vectors in the neutral position. The first is a longitudinal vector that goes from the point of contact through the pivot point. This causes a translational shift of the humeral head in a superior direction against the coraco-acromial arch, which here takes effect as compression. This force is about twice the magnitude of the second force component. The second vector is the force, perpendicular to the longitudinal force, that produces torque. In this case, it is the outwardly oriented, abducting force component.

The further the arm abducts, the more the relative forces reverse, in as much as the abducting force becomes larger. From about 60° on, the superiorly oriented force decreases considerably and changes to a more joint-centering force.

At maximal abduction, the action line of the longitudinal vector points in an inferior direction, which depresses the head of the humerus against the coraco-acromial arch.

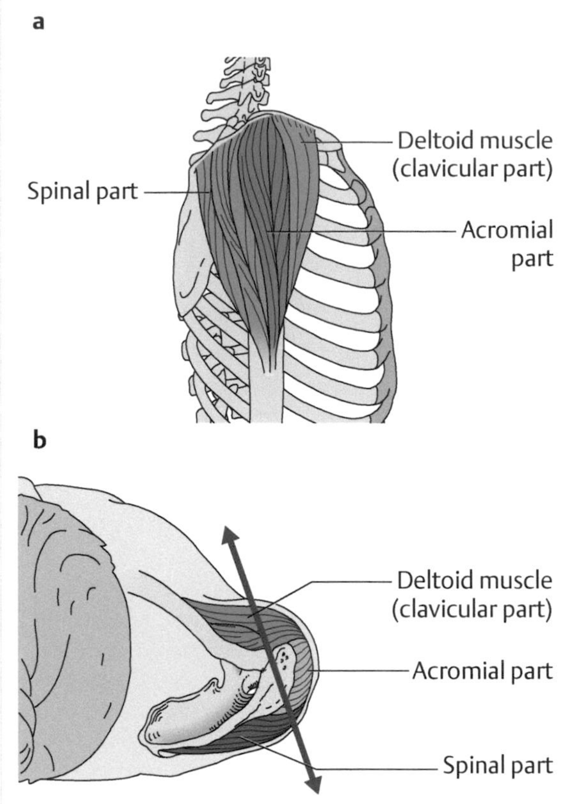


**Fig. 4.64** Deltoid muscle. **(a)** Lateral view. **(b)** Superior view.

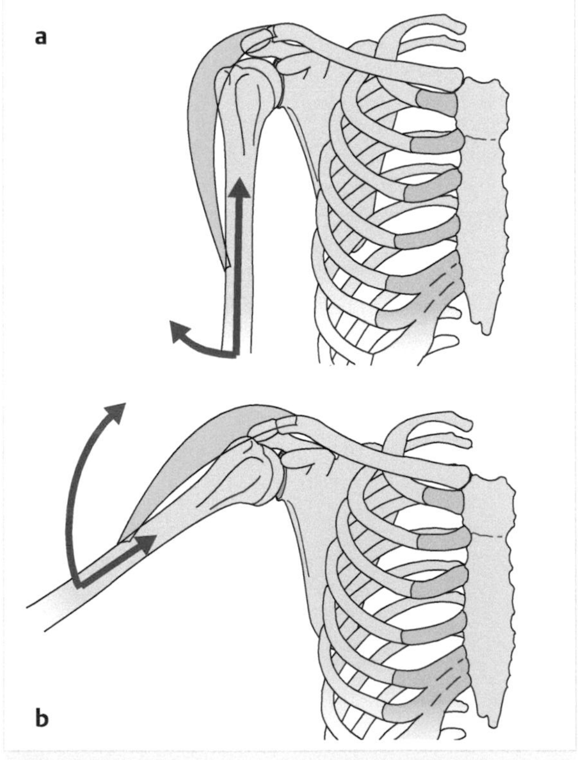


**Fig. 4.65** Force components of the deltoid muscle. **(a)** In the neutral position. **(b)** In abduction.

## Biceps Brachii Muscle (Fig. 4.66)

### Short Head

In addition to the fibers extending to the coracoid process, there is also a connection to the coraco-acromial ligament through fibers growing into it.

**Function in the shoulder.** Flexion/adduction/internal rotation.

### Long Head (Figs. 4.66 and 4.69)

- The long head arises intra-articularly on the supraglenoid tubercle. A few fibers extend to the labrum.
- It passes horizontally through the joint, and then bends round, almost at right angles, into the intertubercular sulcus.
- The *transverse humeral ligament* (**Fig. 4.67**) consists of obliquely running fibrous regions of the capsule and of superior fibers from the subscapularis muscle. It holds the tendon within the sulcus.
- The sulcus (**Fig. 4.68**) forms an angle of 30° to a line on the sagittal plane going through the center of the humeral head.
- The distance from the anchoring point on the supraglenoid tubercle to the entrance of the sulcus is 5 cm when the arm is hanging down and 1.5 cm in abduction. Because of its firm anchoring, the biceps tendon does not shift; instead, the humerus shifts opposite to it.
- In its further course, the long biceps tendon lies between the latissimus dorsi muscle and the pectoralis major muscle, which can exert pressure on the tendon or muscle–tendon transition, which is located at this level.

**Functions in the shoulder region:**

- Abduction/flexion/internal rotation.
- Through its course over the head of the humerus, it helps the rotator cuff in depressing the humeral head.

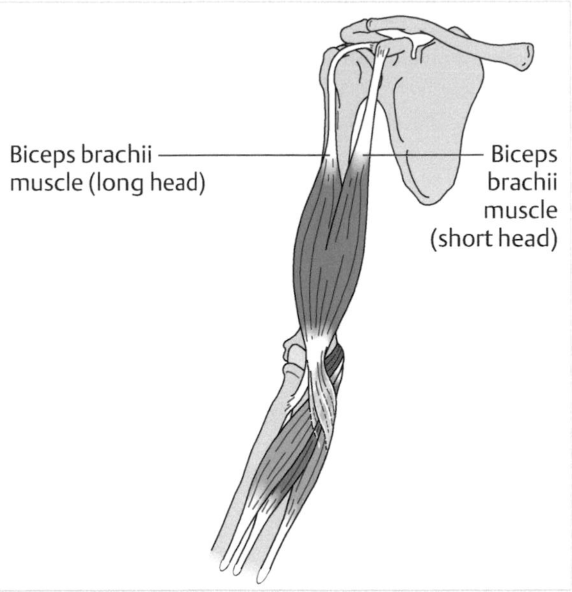


**Fig. 4.66** Biceps brachii muscle.

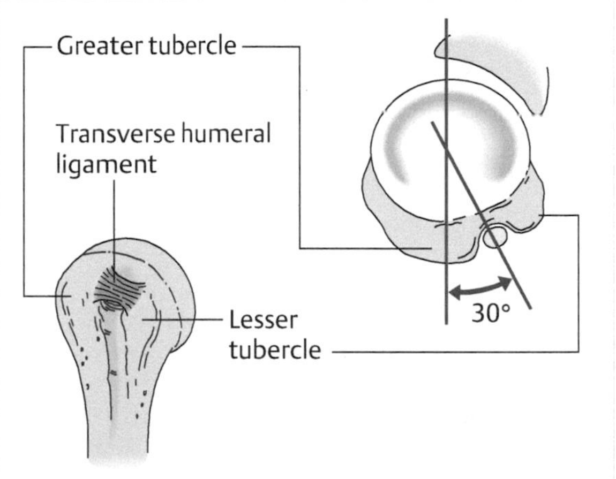


**Fig. 4.67** Transverse humeral ligament.
**Fig. 4.68** Position of the sulcus in relation to the sagittal plane.

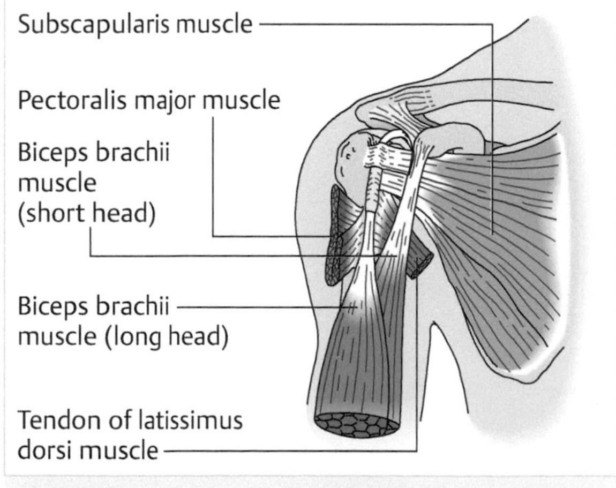


**Fig. 4.69** Course of the tendon of the long head of the biceps.

Pathology

### Tendinopathy of the Tendon of the Long Head of the Biceps

In *pitcher's shoulder*, seen in sports such as team handball, the anterior parts of the capsule and the tendon of the long head of the biceps are overstretched due to the back swing of the arm (horizontal extension of the shoulder). Over time, this can lead to tendinopathies or subluxation of the tendon out of the sulcus.

### Rupture (Figs. 4.70 and 4.71)

A kink in the tendon indicates a bending stress and, with it, an increased load on the tendon. This point is prone to degenerative changes such as calcification or rupture.

Before the tendon actually tears, it frequently attempts to heal itself by forming a new fixation to the bone by growing into the periosteum. This can occur at various sites, such as at the entrance to the sulcus or deeper within it. This new ingrowth can be established by the level of the muscle belly, which slips significantly distally.

When total rupture occurs, there is a resultant decrease in the strength of abduction of about 20%. However, building up the other abductors can compensate for this within a reasonable time frame.

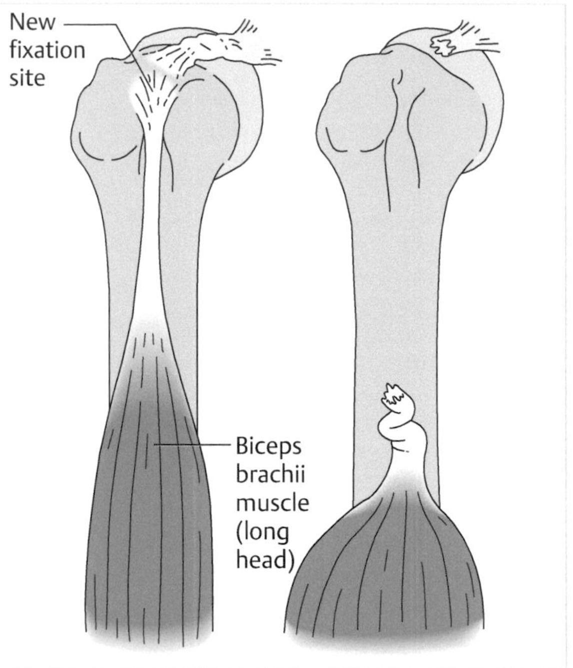


**Fig. 4.70** Rupture of the long head of the biceps tendon.

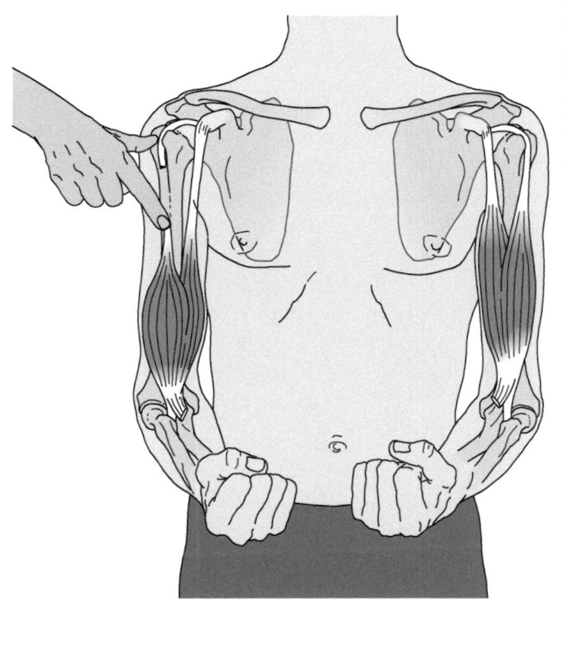

**Fig. 4.71** Comparative palpation of the biceps brachii muscle to determine the rupture.

## Functional Interaction between the Rotator Cuff and the Deltoid Muscle

In abduction, the deltoid muscle does most of the work. Because its force component is primarily oriented superiorly at the onset of abduction, it is dependent on its interaction with the rotator cuff. The rotator cuff counteracts this force, preventing compression against the coraco-acromial arch. Contraction of these muscles causes centering of the humeral head in the joint socket and minimal depression, thus countering the superiorly directed force component of the deltoid muscle (**Fig. 4.72**).

This stabilizing factor is demonstrated by determining the forces acting on the joint (**Fig. 4.73**). In the neutral position (0°), only the deltoid muscle is active, and the resultant joint force, computed by means of the force parallelogram, is directed outside the socket and in a superior direction.

Due to the contribution of the rotator cuff, however, the direction of the resultant force changes. It is now oriented inferiorly and toward the cavity.

In the abducted position, here about 120°, it extends almost at right angles to the cavity.

Because of its course directly over the head of the humerus, the long head of the biceps muscle helps to depress the humerus (**Fig. 4.74**).

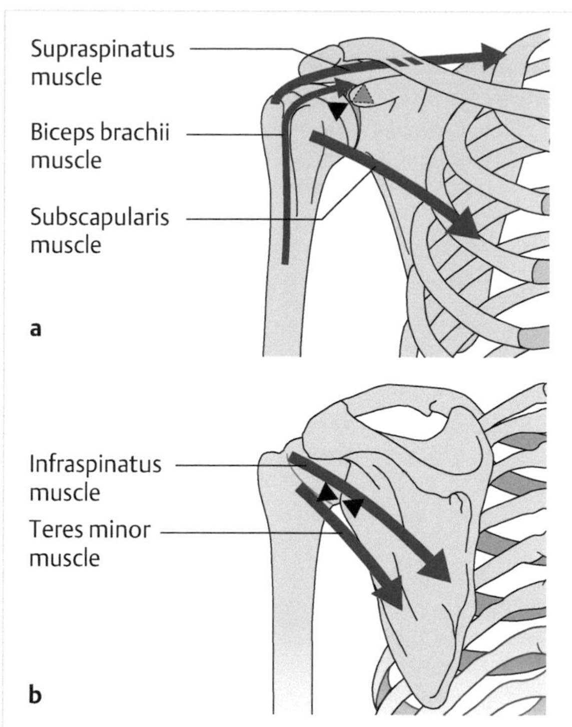


**Fig. 4.72** Rotator cuff: mode of operation. **(a)** Anterior view. **(b)** Posterior view.

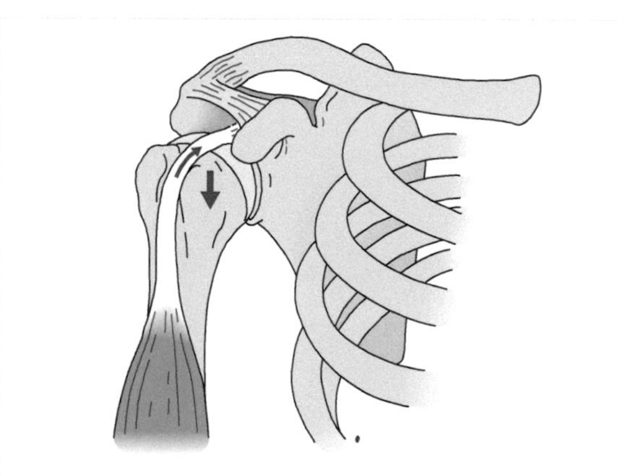

**Fig. 4.74** Depressive effect of the long head of the biceps tendon.

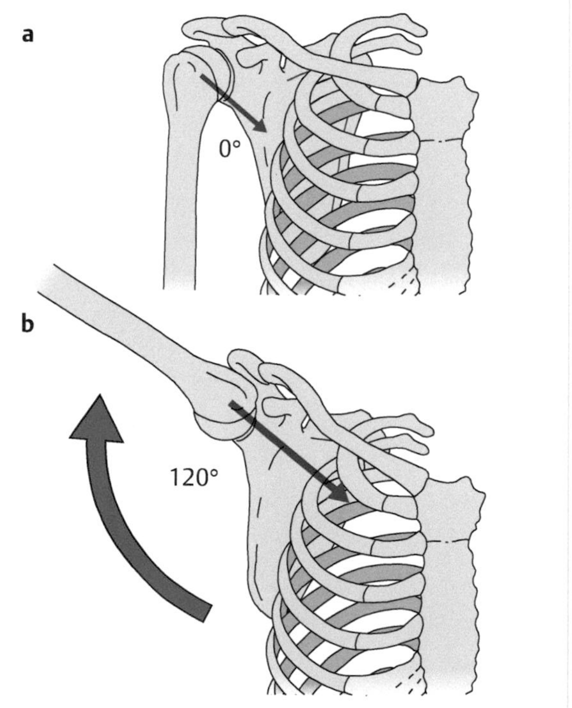


**Fig. 4.73** Direction and magnitude of the force in the glenohumeral joint. **(a)** In the neutral position (0°). **(b)** At about 120° of abduction.

## Automatic External Rotation Associated with Adduction

An arm that is raised in abduction and then returned to the body is always externally rotated. This movement occurs automatically to prevent compression of the greater tubercle of the humerus against the roof of the shoulder. As a rule, an external rotation of about 30 to 50° occurs with an angle of abduction of between 45° and 80°. There are, however, slight individual differences.

From the **neutral position for rotation** (0°), an abduction of 80 to 90° is possible (**Fig. 4.75a**). This can be increased by another 20 to 30° if the arm is maximally externally rotated because the greater tubercle slides under the coraco-acromial arch in a posterior direction, thus freeing up more room within the subacromial space (**Fig. 4.75b**).

When the arm is **internally rotated** and abducted, only 60° of abduction is possible because in this position the greater tubercle presses the structures within the subacromial space up against the coraco-acromial arch, thus blocking any further abduction (**Fig. 4.75c**).

### Practical Tip

If there is restricted movement with respect to external rotation, maximal abduction should not be expected. In this case, the external rotation must be improved in order to extend the potential abduction.

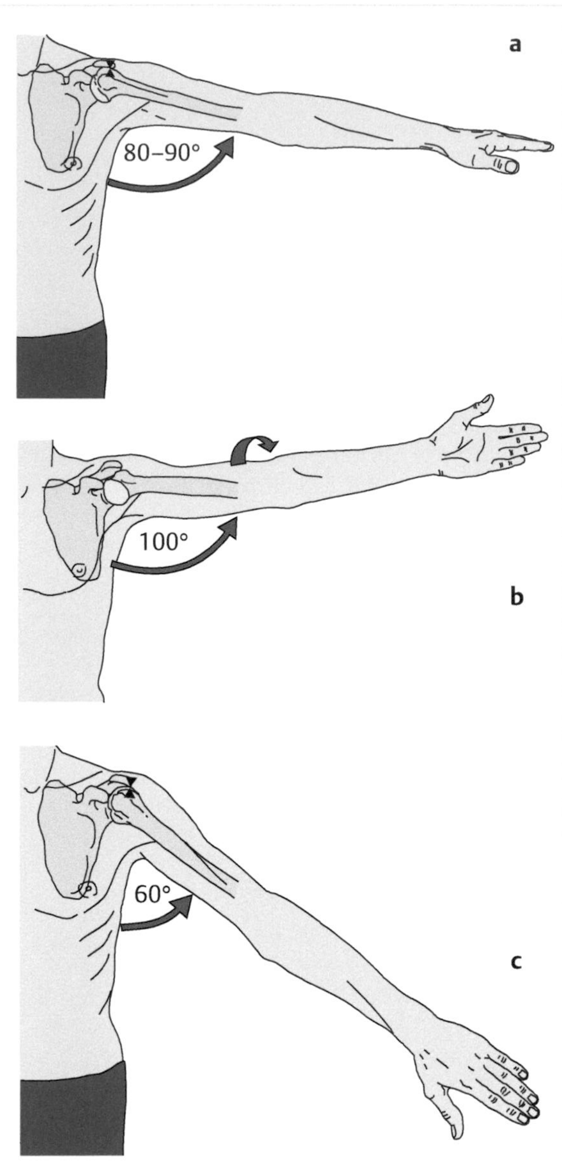


**Fig. 4.75** Abduction. **(a)** At 0° rotation. **(b)** With external rotation. **(c)** With internal rotation.

## Humeroscapular Rhythm (Figs. 4.76 and 4.77)

The arm and the scapula move with each other in a relationship of 2:1 during abduction. For example, for 60° of arm abduction, 40° of the movement occurs in the glenohumeral joint and 20° through shoulder girdle movement. This process only occurs if the scapula is included in the abduction movement. With a minimal range of motion, this rhythm is not noticeable.

### Practical Tip

The humeroscapular rhythm is disturbed by disorders of the shoulder, often with reversal of the relationship. In addition, evasive movements such as elevation take place. Moreover, the scapula moves too early, usually right away. The cause can lie in increased muscle tone in the adductors in the posterior axilla and/or in defective unfolding of the axillary recess. Significant weakness of the abductors can also influence the rhythm.

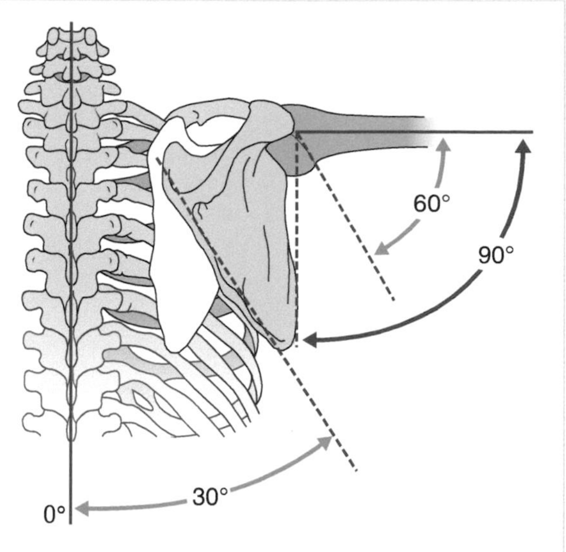


**Fig. 4.76** Movement shares of the humerus and scapula during 90° of abduction.

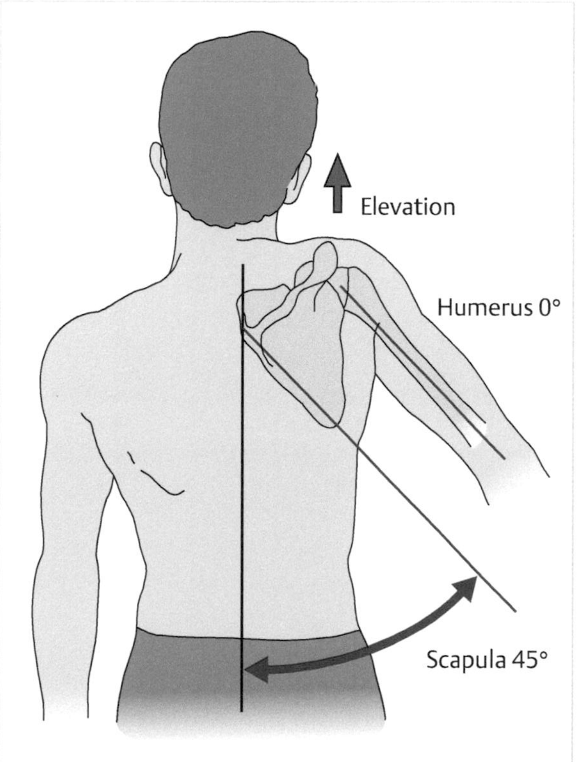


**Fig. 4.77** Defective movement in a humeroscapular rhythm disturbance.

## 4.3.2 Adduction (Fig. 4.78)

The *range of motion* is 40 to 50°. In the neutral position, adduction is not possible because the torso is in the way. Therefore, depending on the patient's anterior abdominal girth, the standard measurement is made in front of the body at either 45° or 90° of flexion (horizontal flexion).

The muscles that perform anterior adduction are (**Fig. 4.79**):

- Pectoralis major muscle.
- Subscapularis muscle.
- Coracobrachialis muscle.
- Biceps brachii muscle, short head.
- Deltoid muscle, clavicular part.

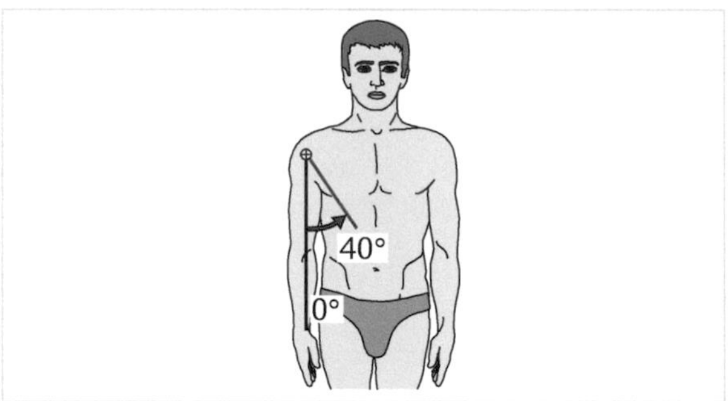


**Fig. 4.78** Range of motion, adduction.

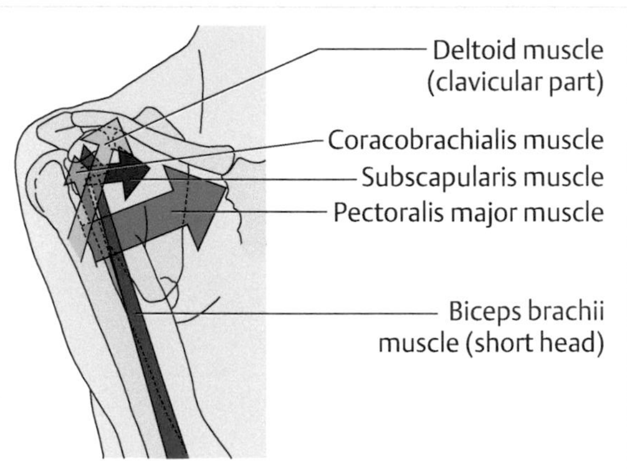


**Fig. 4.79** The adductors.

### Pectoralis Major Muscle (Fig. 4.80)

- This has three parts: the clavicular head, sternocostal head, and abdominal part.
- It forms the anterior axillary fold.
- Its fibers twist around 180° in the anterior axillary region, so that the abdominal part lies furthest posteriorly and superiorly on the crest of the greater tubercle, and the clavicular head lies inferoanteriorly.

**Functions:**

- Adduction and internal rotation
- The clavicular head causes flexion. The abdominal part acts antagonistically; it brings the raised arm back against resistance.
- With the fixed end on the arm, it pulls the shoulder girdle in an anteroinferior direction.
- With the fixed end on the arm and shoulder girdle, the two lower parts of the muscle help with inspiration.

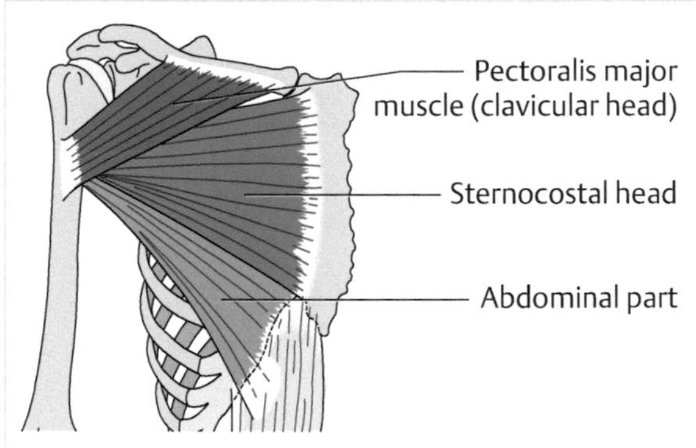


**Fig. 4.80** Pectoralis major muscle.

### Coracobrachialis Muscle (Fig. 4.81)

In its origin and further course, coracobrachialis lies under the short head of the biceps muscle and therefore has the same function in the shoulder region: abduction/flexion/internal rotation.

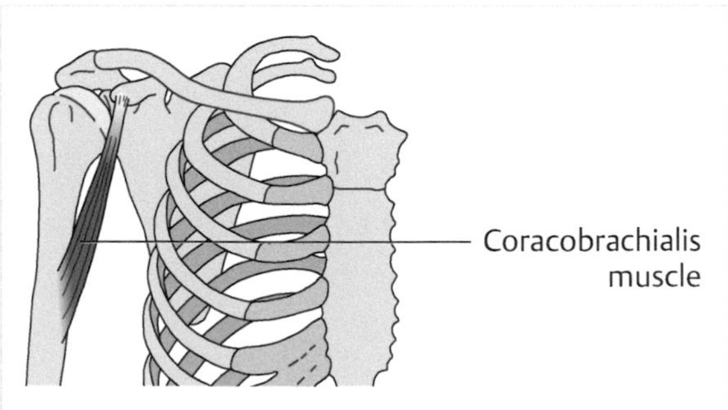


**Fig. 4.81** Coracobrachialis muscle.

The following muscles are active in carrying out posterior adduction:

- Teres major muscle.
- Latissimus dorsi muscle.
- Teres minor muscle.
- Infraspinatus muscle.
- Triceps brachii muscle, long head.
- Deltoid muscle, spinal part.
- Rhomboid muscles.

## Teres Major Muscle (Fig. 4.82)

- This twists at its insertion, similar to the latissimus dorsi muscle.
- It inserts on the crest of the lesser tubercle directly behind the latissimus dorsi.

**Functions:**

- Adduction/extension/internal rotation.
- With the fixed end on the arm, external rotation of the scapula occurs.

## Latissimus Dorsi Muscle (Fig. 4.82)

- This has four parts: scapular, vertebral, costal, and iliac.
- At the insertion site on the humerus, a few fibers extend to the intertubercular sulcus.
- It forms the posterior axillary fold.
- Shortly before its insertion, it twists 180° so that the iliac part inserts furthest anteriorly and superiorly.

**Functions:**

- Adduction/extension/internal rotation.
- With the fixed end on the humerus, it produces external rotation of the scapula, and the costal part helps with inspiration. During the process of coughing, the ribs are fixed and serve as the fixed end for the diaphragm.

## Triceps Brachii Muscle, Long Head (Figs. 4.83 and 4.84)

- The origin is on the infraglenoid tubercle, but the muscle is not intra-articular.
- A few of its fibers extend into the capsule.
- In the posterior axilla, the latissimus dorsi and teres major muscles cross anterior to it, and the teres minor muscle crosses posterior to it.

**Function in the shoulder region.** Adduction/extension.

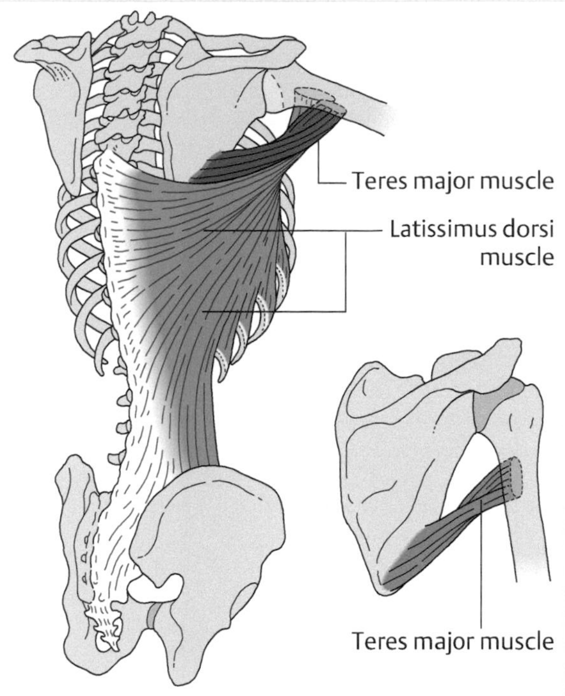


**Fig. 4.82** Teres major and latissimus dorsi muscles.

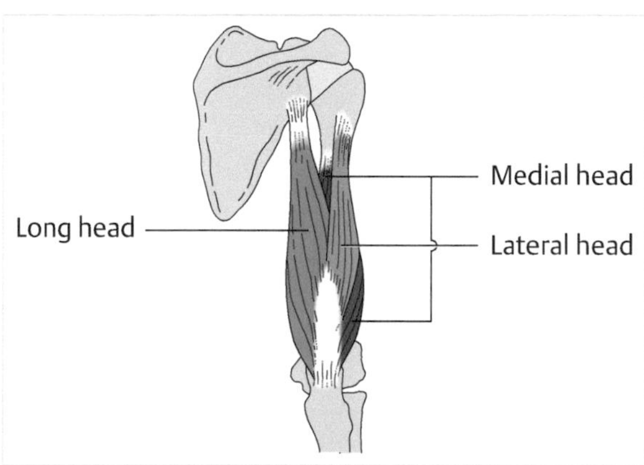


**Fig. 4.83** Triceps brachii muscle.

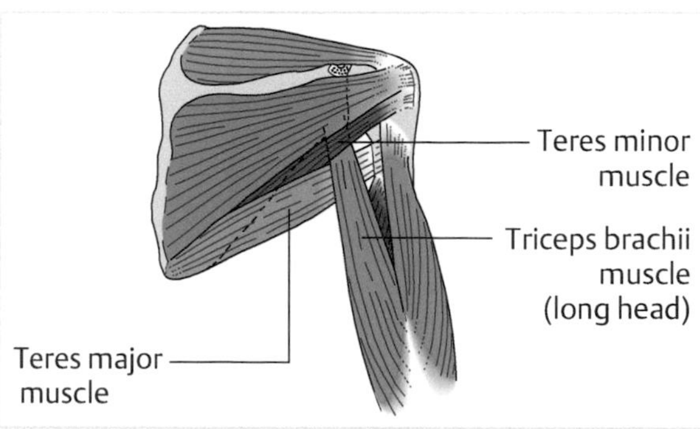


**Fig. 4.84** Course of the long triceps tendon in the axilla.

## Synergism between the Triceps Brachii and Latissimus Dorsi Muscles (Fig. 4.85)

Tension caused by the long head of the triceps brachii muscle pulls the humeral head superiorly against the coraco-acromial arch. This compression effect opposes the latissimus dorsi muscle, which pulls the humeral head inferiorly. These muscles function as important synergists in terms of their effect on the shoulder.

**Practical Tip**

In an impingement syndrome, tensing the muscles isometrically as if to extend the elbow can be painful because there is compression in the subacromial space. Tension directed toward extension and adduction of the shoulder is not painful because, in this instance, the latissimus dorsi muscle is active and the humeral head moves inferiorly at the same time.

## 4.3.3 Extension (Fig. 4.86)

The *range of motion* is 40 to 50°.

The muscles that extend the shoulder are (**Fig. 4.87**):

- Latissimus dorsi muscle.
- Teres major muscle.
- Teres minor muscle.
- Deltoid muscle, spinal part.
- Triceps brachii muscle, long head.
- Trapezius muscle, ascending and transverse parts.
- Rhomboid muscles.

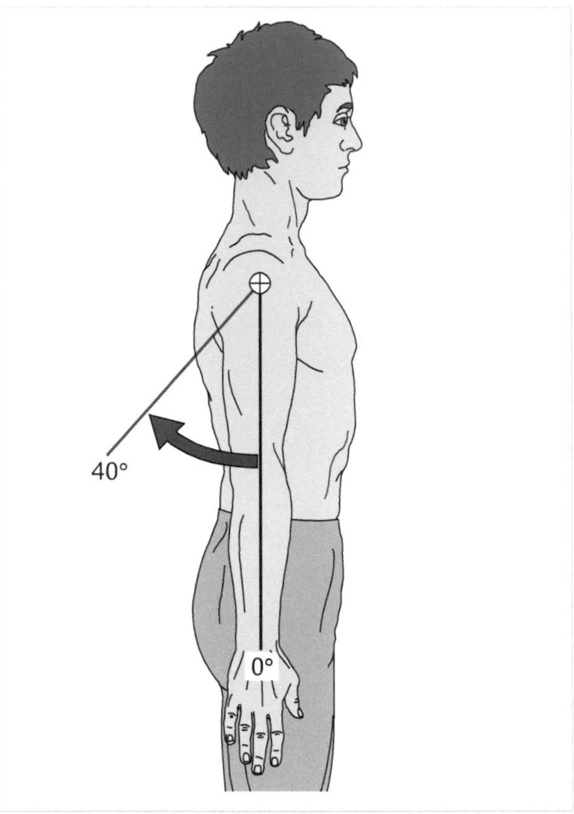


**Fig. 4.86** Range of motion: extension.

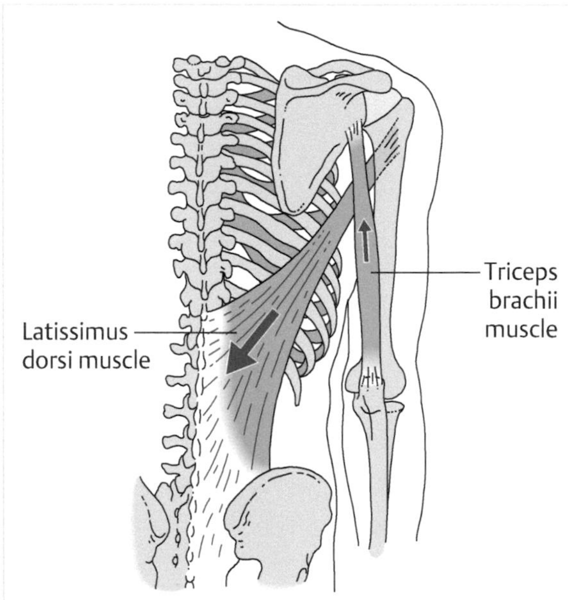


**Fig. 4.85** Synergism between the triceps brachii and latissimus dorsi muscles.

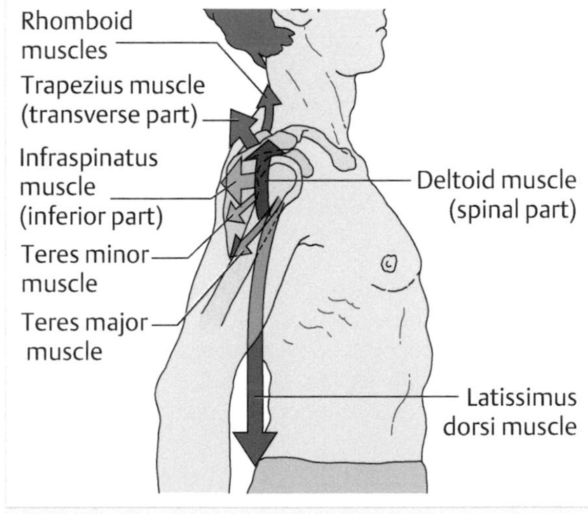


**Fig. 4.87** Extensor muscles.

## 4.3.4 Flexion (Figs. 4.88 and 4.89)

The *range of motion* is 180°.

As with abduction, the entire movement is divided into three phases, but these are not as clearly defined. The transitions take place much earlier, the scapula takes part in the movement right away, and movement can be noted in the ribs and thoracic spine when 100° of flexion is reached.

If the scapula is fixed, flexion is limited to 100–110°. If continuation of the movement into the spine is impeded, flexion is limited to 160°.

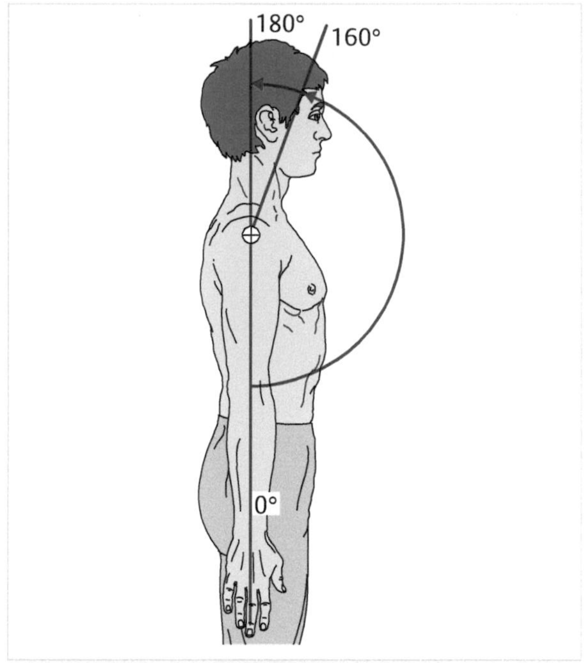


**Fig. 4.88** Range of motion: flexion.

| Muscles that move the arm (a) | Muscles that move the shoulder (b) | Muscles that move the the spinal column (c) |
|---|---|---|
| Deltoid muscle, clavicular part<br>Pectoralis major muscle, clavicular part<br>Biceps bracii muscle<br>Coracobrachialis muscle | Trapezius muscle, descending and ascending parts<br>Serratus anterior muscle | Erector spinae muscle |

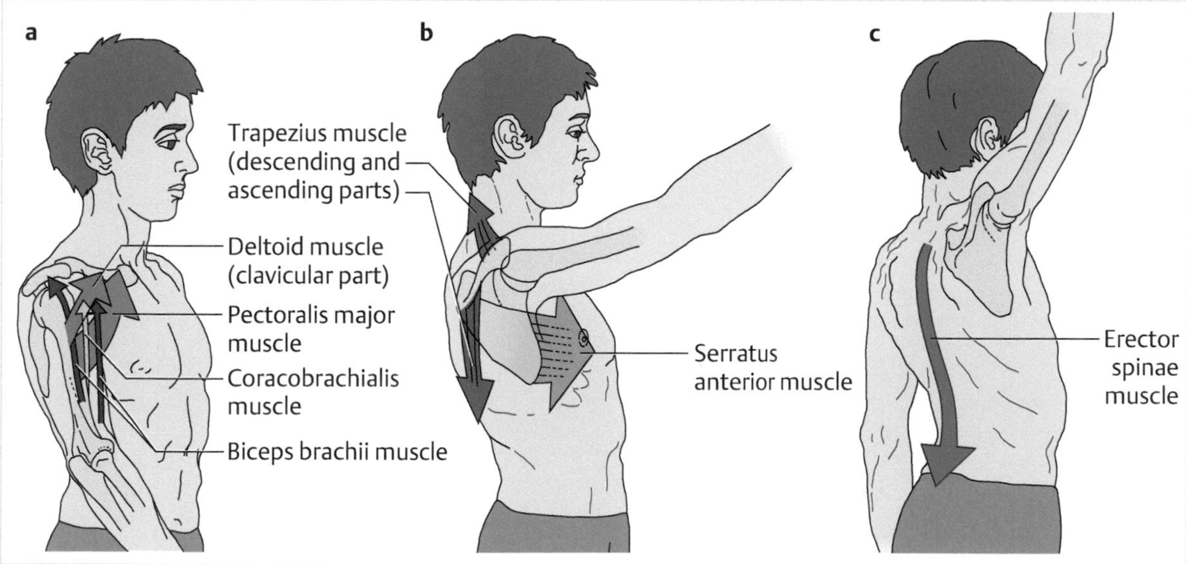


**Fig. 4.89** Flexion. **(a)** through movement in the glenohumeral joint. **(b)** through external rotation of the scapula. **(c)** Through movement of the spinal column.

## 4.3.5 Rotation (Figs. 4.90 and 4.91)

The *range of motion* is measured from the neutral position (0°): external rotation/internal rotation = 60°/95°.

If the forearm is placed behind the back, this corresponds to 95° of internal rotation.

By relaxing and tensing the ligamentous structures of the capsule, the range of motion changes: external rotation/internal rotation = 90°/60°, respectively, when the arm is placed in a position of 90° abduction.

The axis of rotation corresponds to an axis that passes through the medullary space of the humeral shaft.

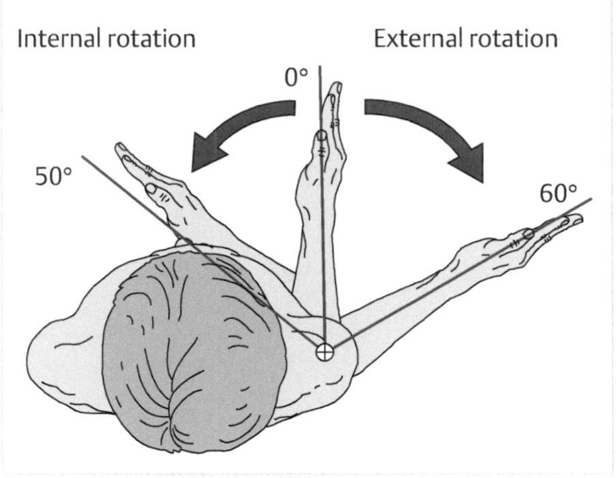


**Fig. 4.90** Range of motion: external and internal rotation.

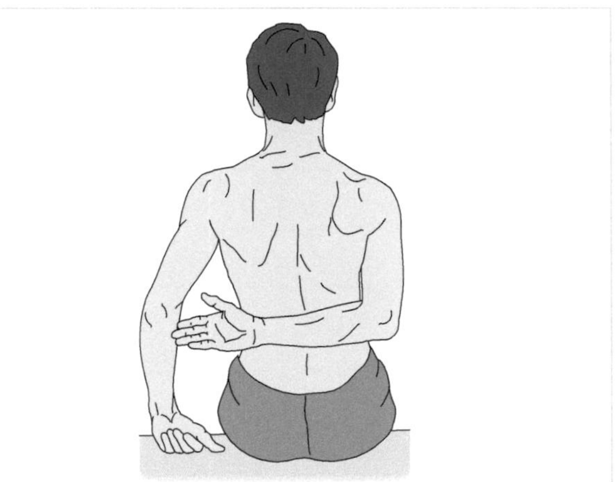

**Fig. 4.91** Maximal internal rotation.

### External Rotators (Fig. 4.92)

- Infraspinatus muscle.
- Teres minor muscle.
- Deltoid muscle, spinal part.
- Triceps brachii muscle, long head.

### Internal Rotators (Fig. 4.93)

- Subscapularis muscle.
- Latissimus dorsi muscle.
- Teres major muscle.
- Pectoralis major muscle.
- Biceps brachii muscle.
- Coracobrachialis muscle.
- Deltoid muscle, clavicular part.

**Pathology**

In the case of a frozen shoulder, external rotation is most severely limited very early in its course. When the arm is held in the position of comfort (internal rotation against the body), the subscapular recess is no longer open and can become adherent. Another reason for the limitation of movement is the dominance of the internal rotators over the external rotators.

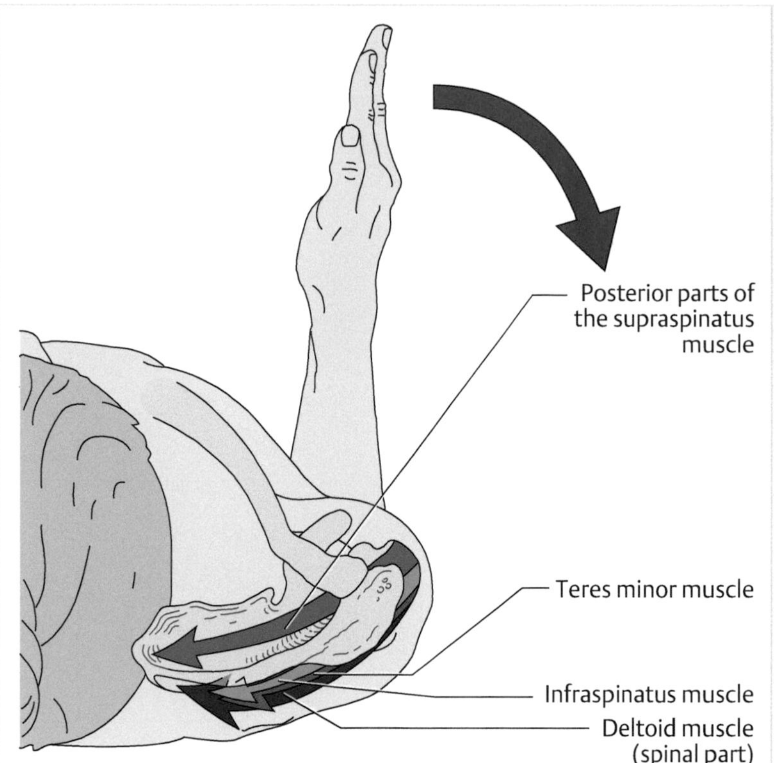


**Fig. 4.92** The external rotators.

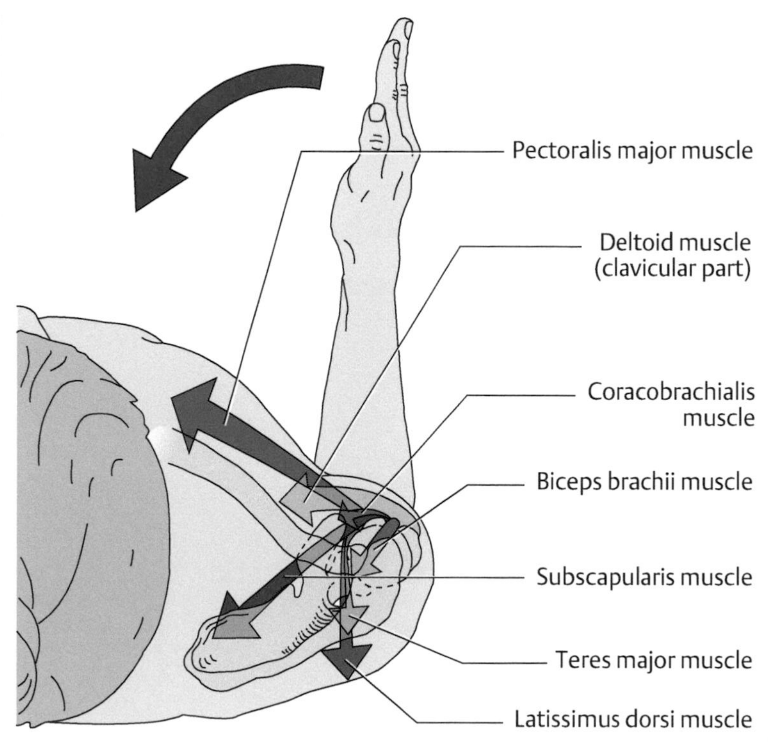


**Fig. 4.93** The internal rotators.

# 4.4 Course of the Nerves in the Shoulder Region

## Dorsal Scapular Nerve (C3–C5) (Fig. 4.94a)

- This pierces the scalenus medius and runs along the levator scapulae muscle and the medial border of the scapula under the rhomboid muscles.
- It innervates the levator scapulae and rhomboid muscles.

## Suprascapular Nerve (C4–C6) (Fig. 4.94a)

- This branches off at the level of the scalene hiatus and runs through the suprascapular notch under the superior transverse scapular ligament to the supraspinous fossa. It bends laterally around the base of the spine of the scapula and into the infraspinous fossa.
- It innervates the suprascapularis and infrascapularis muscles.

**Pathology**

Pressure, as from the carrying strap of a heavy backpack, can damage the suprascapular nerve. Radiating pain extends toward the posterior scapula, and the function of the innervated muscles can be disturbed.

## Thoracodorsal Nerve (C6–C8) (Fig. 4.94b)

- This extends from the scapula toward the axilla and then inferiorly on the anterior border of the latissimus dorsi.
- It innervates the latissimus dorsi muscle and possibly the teres major muscle.

## Subscapular Nerve (C5–C6) (Fig. 4.95)

- Two separate branches of the subscapular nerve are given off from the posterior cord of the brachial plexus toward the thoracic surface of the scapula.
- These branches innervate the subscapularis and teres major muscles.

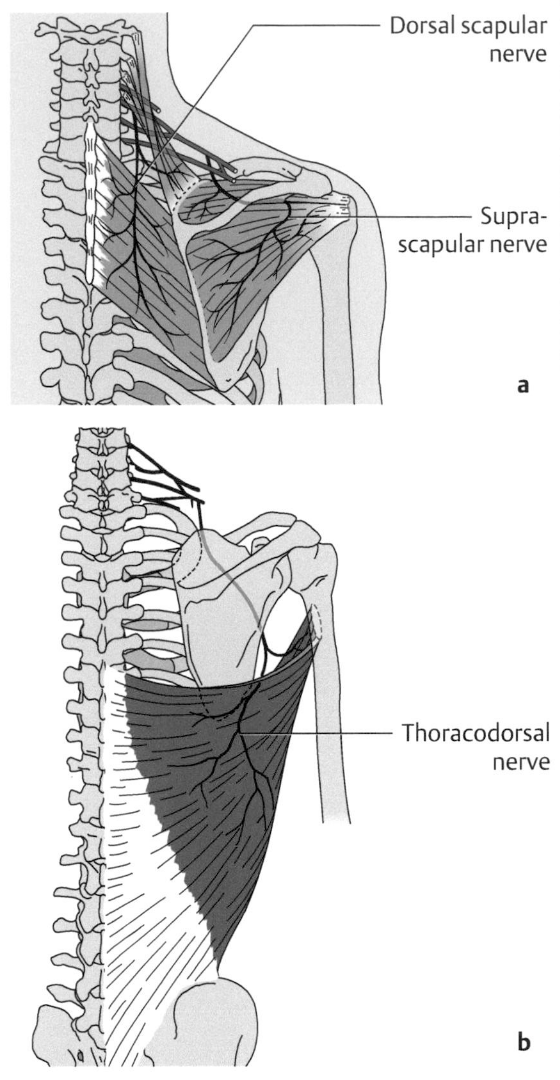


**Fig. 4.94 (a)** Dorsal scapular nerve, suprascapular nerve. **(b)** Thoracodorsal nerve.

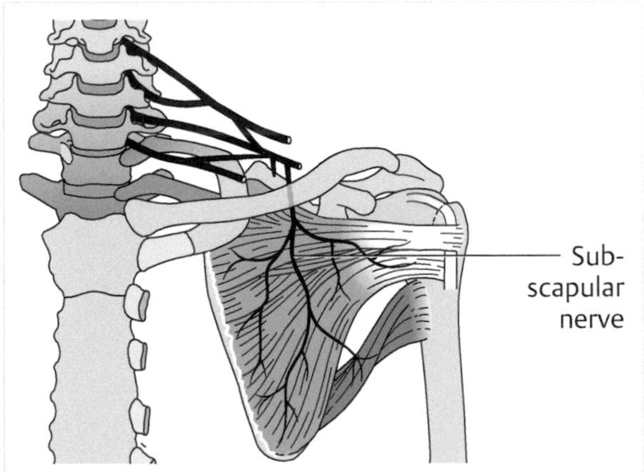


**Fig. 4.95** Subscapular nerve.

## Long Thoracic Nerve (C5–C7) (Fig. 4.96)

- This runs posterior to the plexus, pierces the scalenus medius muscle, and extends steeply in an inferior direction to the lateral ribs.
- It innervates the serratus anterior muscle.

**Pathology**

Maximal flexion combined with external rotation, with the addition of considerable force and speed, as in weight-lifting or in swimming back stroke, can damage the nerve.

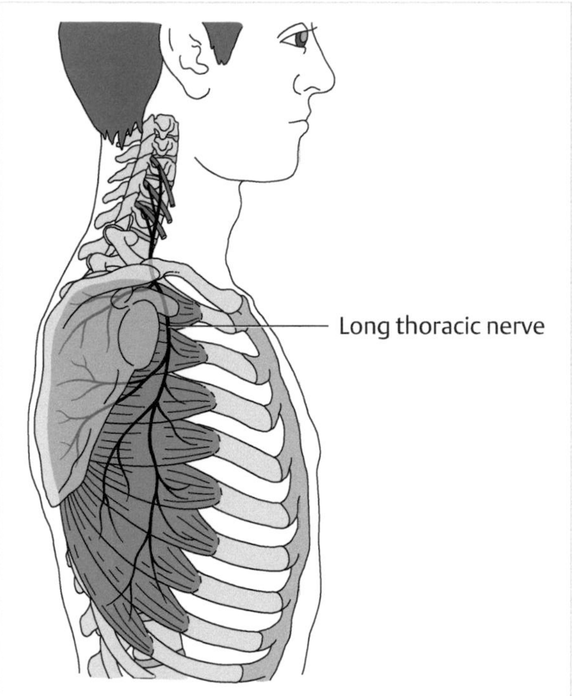


**Fig. 4.96** Long thoracic nerve.

## Medial and Lateral Pectoral Nerves (C5–T1) (Fig. 4.97)

- These arise from the lateral and medial cords of the brachial plexus and extend over the subclavian artery and vein to the anterior axilla.
- They innervate the pectoral muscles.

## Axillary Nerve (C5–C7) (Fig. 4.97)

- This nerve extends with the posterior circumflex humeral artery through the lateral axillary space and around the surgical neck of the humerus toward the deltoid muscle.
- Branches:
  - Articular branches go to the shoulder joint.
  - The superior lateral cutaneous nerve of the arm goes laterally between the deltoid muscle and the long head of the triceps muscle, supplying an area over the deltoid muscle and the outer side of the upper arm.
- It innervates the teres minor and deltoid muscles.

**Pathology**

In a subcapital fracture of the humerus, the displaced, fractured ends of the bone can damage or even sever the axillary nerve.

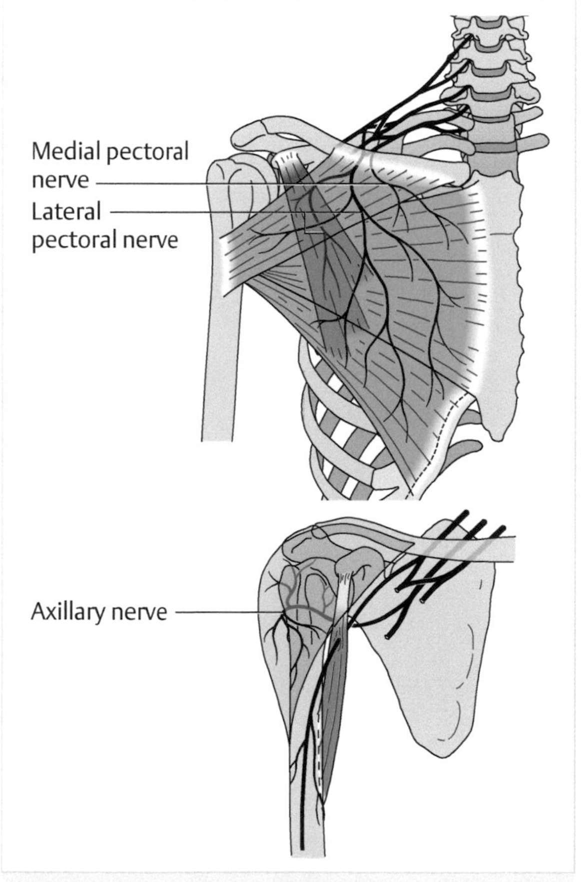


**Fig. 4.97** Medial and lateral pectoral nerves and axillary nerve.

## Musculocutaneous Nerve (C5–C7) (Fig. 4.98a)

- This exits the lateral cord at the level of the lateral border of the pectoralis minor muscle, extends through the anterior axilla, and pierces the coracobrachialis muscle. It runs further distally between the biceps and brachialis muscles.
- Branches:
  - At the level of the musculotendinous transition of the biceps muscle, the *lateral cutaneous nerve of the forearm* extends through the fascia and supplies the skin of the radial side of the forearm.
- It innervates the coracobrachialis, biceps, and brachialis muscles.

## Radial Nerve (C5–T1) (Fig. 4.98b)

- This extends out from the posterior cord posterior to the axillary artery, with which it travels toward the posterior side of the upper arm before running distally between the long and medial heads of the triceps muscle.
- Further course: It travels in a posterolateral direction around the humerus within the radial groove between the medial and lateral heads of the triceps toward the flexor side of the arm.
- Branches:
  - The posterior cutaneous nerve of the arm extends toward the axillary fold and innervates the skin of the posterior upper arm down to the olecranon.
  - The posterior cutaneous nerve of the forearm leaves the radial nerve within the radial groove and supplies the skin of the posterior side of the forearm.
- It innervates the triceps, anconeus, and brachioradialis muscles and the extensor muscles of the hand and fingers.

### Pathology

Damage to the posterior cutaneous nerve of the arm can occur in the axilla, with a corresponding loss of sensation. Damage to the radial nerve may cause paresis of the triceps muscle, which is the first muscle it supplies. The most common causes are trauma and the use of crutches.
Paresis from pressure on the nerve in the upper arm can occur as a complication of a fracture of the shaft of the humerus, or can be caused, e.g., by laying the arm on the back of a park bench for a long time. The most proximal paresis occurs in the brachioradialis muscle. *Wrist drop* demonstrates the paresis of the hand extensors.

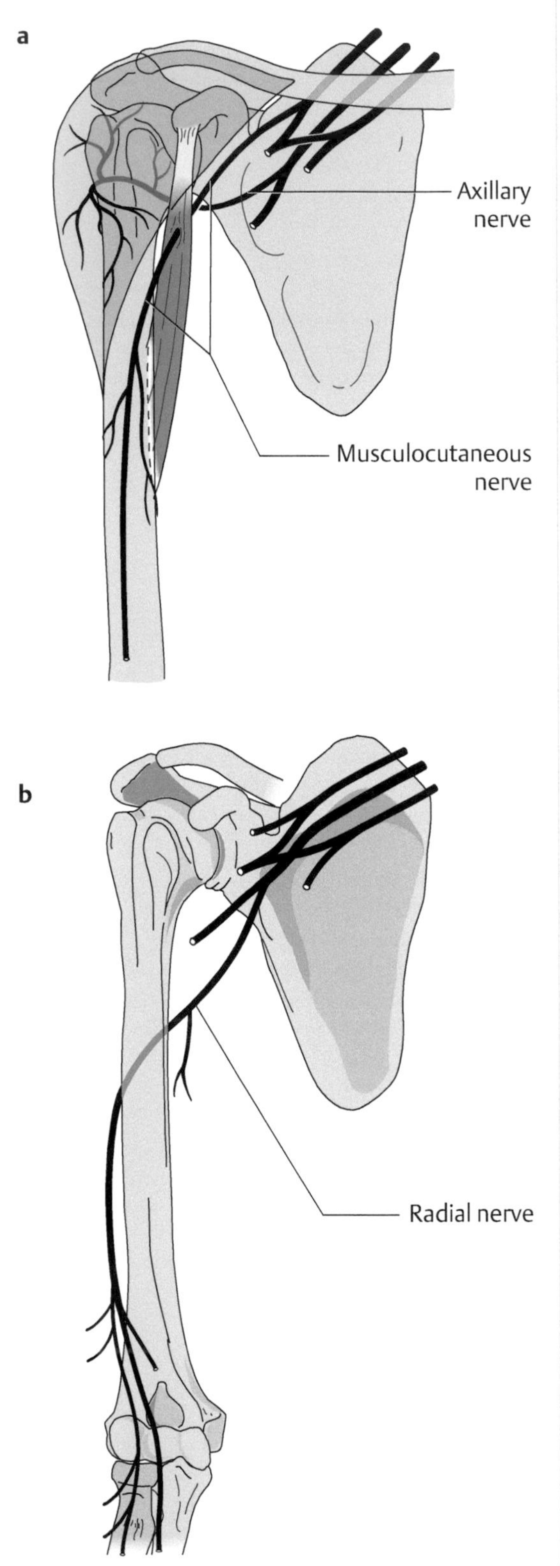


**Fig. 4.98 (a)** Musculocutaneous nerve. **(b)** Radial nerve.

## Median Nerve (C5–T1) (Fig. 4.99)

- This emerges from the lateral and medial cords, running anterior to the axillary artery and distally on the volar side of the upper arm.
- It innervates most of the thenar muscles and the muscles that have their origin on the medial epicondyle, except for the flexor carpi ulnaris muscle.

**Pathology**

A pressure lesion from the head of a sleeping partner on the upper arm ("honeymoon palsy") can lead to distal motor and sensory deficits. When attempting to close the fist, the characteristic *hand of benediction* deformity occurs.

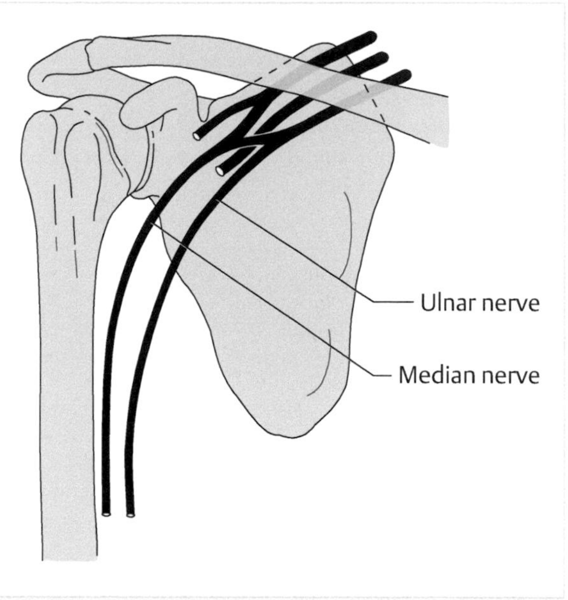


**Fig. 4.99** Median nerve, ulnar nerve.

## Ulnar Nerve (C8–T1) (Fig. 4.99)

- This arises from the middle cord and runs medial to the axillary artery. In the mid-upper arm, it extends toward elbow on the extensor side.
- It innervates the hypothenar muscles, the interosseous and lumbrical muscles, and the flexor carpi ulnaris muscle, as well as parts of the flexor digitorum profundus, flexor pollicis brevis, and adductor pollicis muscles.

**Pathology**

A *claw hand* deformity (extension in the metacarpophalangeal joints and flexion in the interphalangeal joints) develops when there is damage to the ulnar nerve.

Pathology

**Compression Syndrome in the Shoulder Region (Fig. 4.100)**

On its way from the intervertebral foramina to the nerves of the arm, the brachial plexus runs through a few bottlenecks where it can be compressed.

See Chapters 2.1 and 2.3, sections regarding the cervical spine.

There are two of these narrow spots in the shoulder area, where compression is known as *thoracic outlet syndrome*:

- In the **clavicular region**, the costoclavicular space is bounded by the first rib and the clavicle. Here the brachial plexus, together with the subclavian artery and vein, runs toward the axilla. Lowering and retracting the shoulder girdle narrows the space. The causes of narrowing are drooping shoulders, widening of the superior thoracic aperture from chronic emphysema, and deformity of the clavicle after a fracture.

Practical Tip

A provocation test differentiates this complaint from other conditions. Push the shoulder girdle inferiorly and hold this position while checking the radial pulse at the same time. If the space narrows significantly, the pulse feels weak or completely disappears, and patients describe an increase in their symptoms:

- **In the pectoralis minor muscle region**, the distal brachial plexus, along with the subclavian artery and vein, passes into the axilla under the pectoralis minor muscle and its insertion on the coracoid process. With maximal abduction, the plexus cannot avoid the structures here, so it wraps around the terminal tendon of the pectoralis minor muscle and is thereby stretched. Symptoms caused by a bottleneck in this region are therefore known as a *hyperabduction syndrome*. The structures are usually quite distensible, and the symptoms therefore emerge only after holding the abduction position for a long time, as when sleeping.

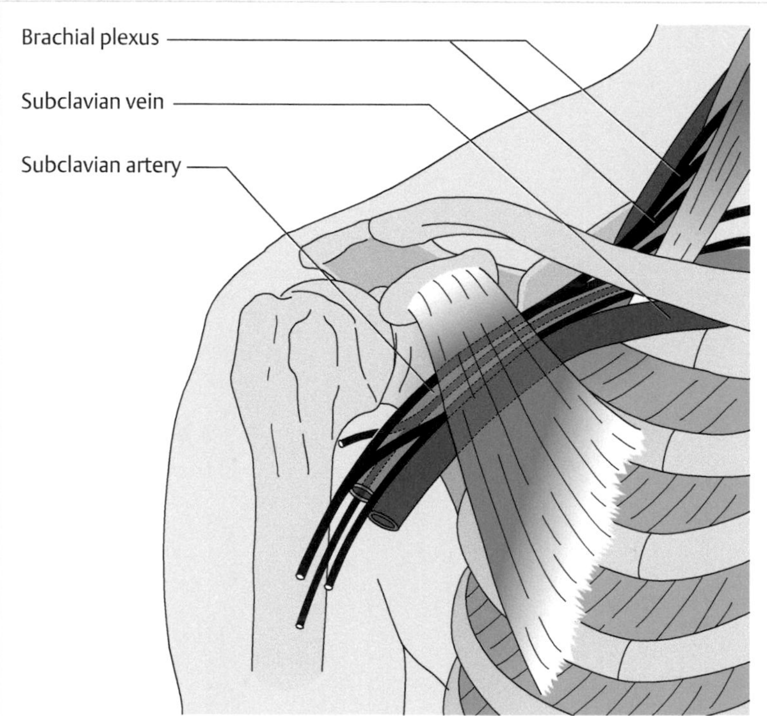


**Fig. 4.100** Compression syndrome in the shoulder area.

# Chapter 5

## Elbow



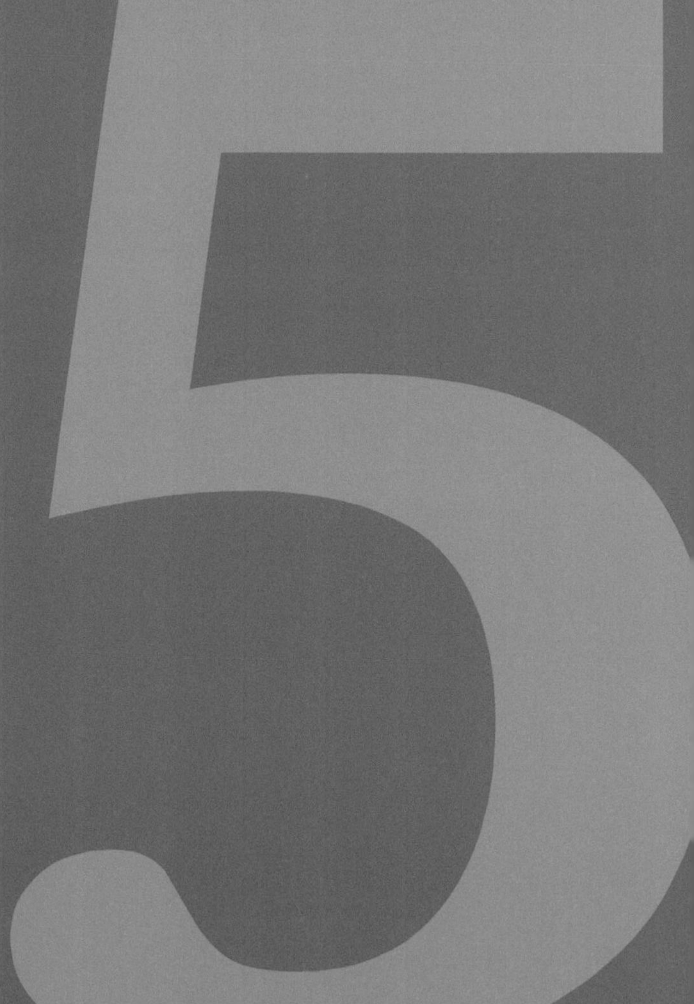

# 5 Elbow

## 5.1 Palpation of Landmarks in the Elbow Region

### Lateral Epicondyle of the Humerus (Fig. 5.1)

This can be identified as an easily palpable, projecting structure on the distal, lateral humerus. The tip is free from any muscle insertion sites.

A small flat area is sited just distal to the tip of the epicondyle and about a fingerbreadth toward the cubital fossa. Several wrist and finger extensors arise from this point. These can be differentiated from each other by palpation only with difficulty because they lie very close together. From proximal to distal, they are as follows:

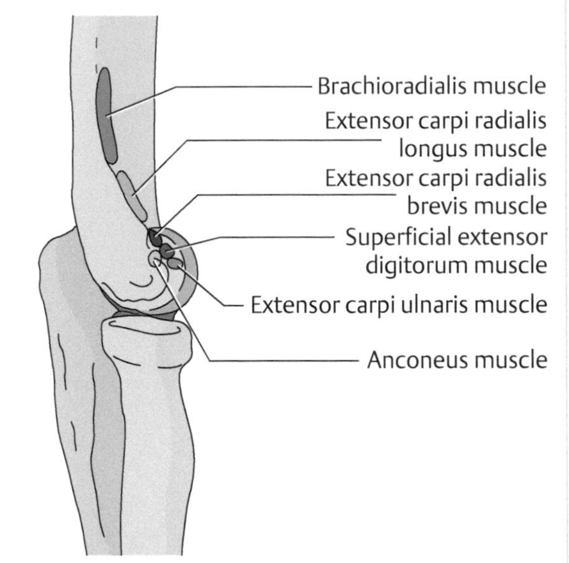


**Fig. 5.1** Palpation of the muscle origins on the lateral epicondyle.

### Extensor Carpi Radialis Brevis Muscle (Fig. 5.2)

This extends to the base of the third metacarpal. It is easier to palpate by tensing the muscle as if extending the wrist with the fingers flexed.

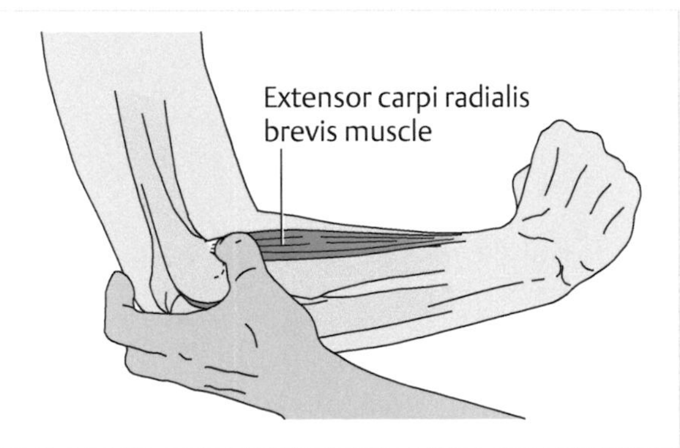


**Fig. 5.2** Palpation of the extensor carpi radialis brevis muscle.

### Extensor Digitorum Muscle (Fig. 5.3)

This extends into the dorsal aponeurosis of the second to fourth fingers and to the base of the middle and distal phalanges. The area of origin can be more exactly localized if the patient flexes and extends the fingers while the hand is stabilized in dorsiflexion.

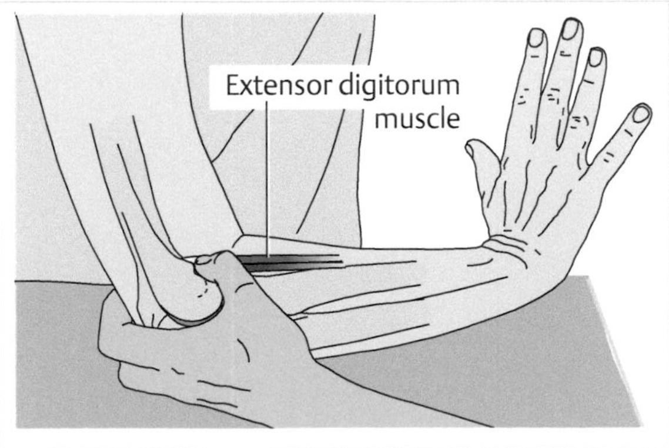


**Fig. 5.3** Palpation of the extensor digitorum muscle.

### Extensor Digiti Minimi Muscle

This muscle runs just to the ulnar side of the extensor digitorum muscle and extends into the dorsal aponeurosis of the fifth finger. Extending the little finger makes localization more obvious.

### Extensor Carpi Ulnaris Muscle

This extends to the base of the fifth metacarpal. The muscle is tensed by extension and ulnar abduction.

**Practical Tip**

Lateral epicondylitis, also known as *tennis elbow*, involves most of the area of origin of the extensor carpi radialis brevis muscle. Find the exact location by palpation and provocation testing by means of extending and contracting the muscle.

## Anconeus Muscle (Fig. 5.4)

This muscle can be palpated between the lateral epicondyle and the olecranon as a small, triangular cushion of muscle.

## Lateral Margin of the Humerus

This bony ridge runs proximally from the lateral epicondyle and is the site of origin for two muscles:

## Brachioradialis Muscle (Fig. 5.5)

This extends from the lateral supracondylar ridge about one handbreadth above the tip of the epicondyle to the radial styloid process. Its origin is about three fingerbreadths wide.

Palpation is easier when flexing the elbow against resistance with the forearm midway between supination and pronation.

## Extensor Carpi Radialis Longus Muscle (Fig. 5.5)

This muscle arises directly inferior to the brachioradialis muscle with a breadth of 1 to 2 fingerbreadths and extends to the base of the second metacarpal.

It is easier to palpate by tensing the muscle as if extending and radially abducting the wrist.

## Radial Collateral Ligament (Fig. 5.6)

This ligament spreads out like a fan, extending from the lateral epicondyle toward the head of the radius into the annular ligament of the radius and to the posterior ulna. It is very easy to palpate between the lateral epicondyle and the olecranon. Further distally, this becomes more difficult because of the overlying extensors.

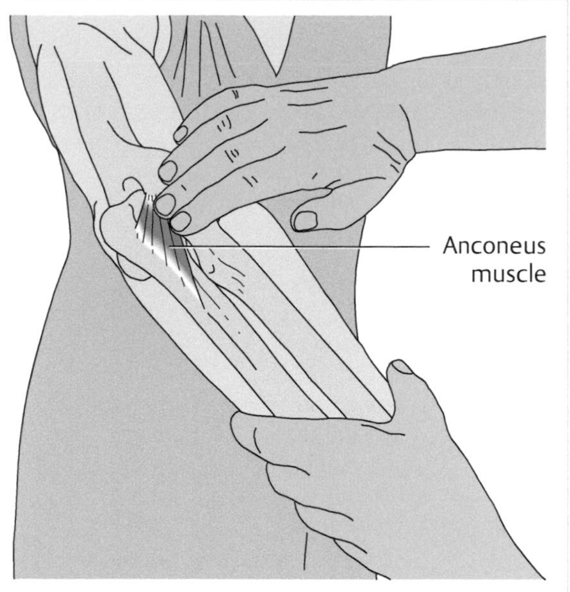


**Fig. 5.4** Palpation of the anconeus muscle.

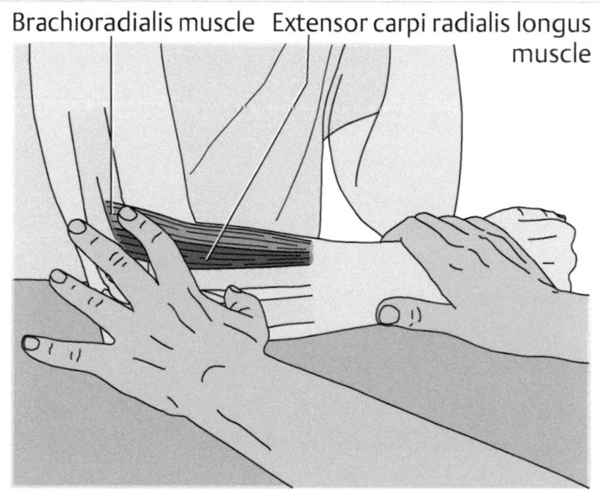


**Fig. 5.5** Palpation of the brachioradialis and extensor carpi radialis longus muscles.

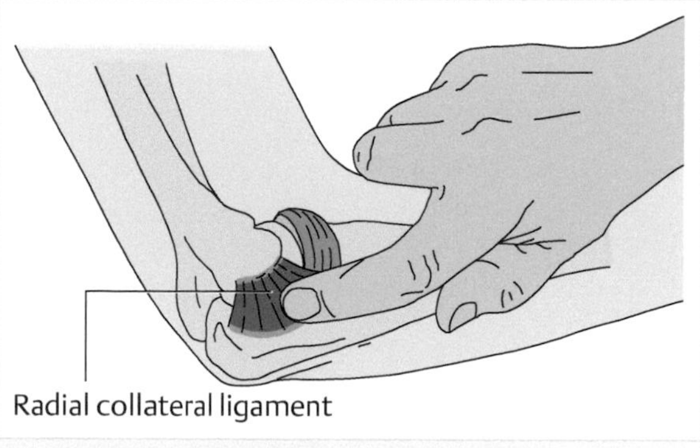


**Fig. 5.6** Palpation of the radial collateral ligament.

## Head of the Radius

The head of the radius lies 2.5 cm distal to the lateral epicondyle. It turns back and forth under the palpating finger when pronating and supinating the forearm.

The **annular ligament of the radius** (**Fig. 5.7**) extends around the radial head and can be palpated between the ulna and radial head as a firm strand.

While palpating the **joint space** (**Fig. 5.8**) of the humeroradial joint bilaterally, carry out a direct side-to-side examination of the position of the radial head in relation to the humerus.

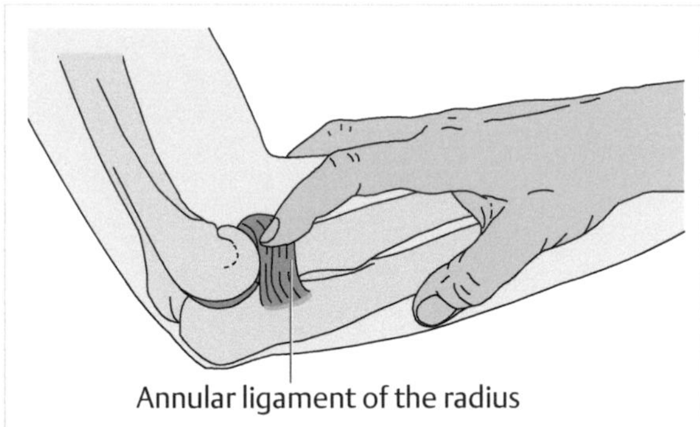


**Fig. 5.7** Palpation of the annular ligament of the radial head.

### Practical Tip

Carry out the evaluation of the position of the radial head in relation to the humerus at rest as well as during movement. To enable a direct comparison, palpate both joint spaces simultaneously using the index fingers while asking the patient to flex and extend the elbow.

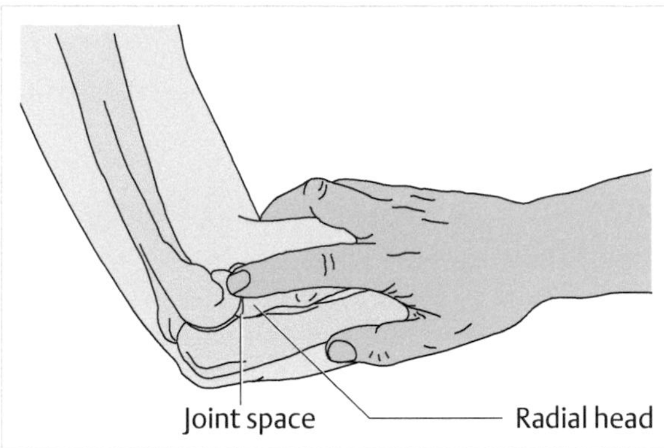


**Fig. 5.8** Palpation of the joint space of the humeroradial joint.

## Medial Epicondyle of the Humerus (Fig. 5.9)

Because the tip of the medial epicondyle is free of muscle insertions, it can be palpated as a distinctly protruding bony structure on the distal medial humerus. The area of origin for the wrist flexors is slightly distal and anterior to the tip of the epicondyle. The origin is a common aponeurosis, so the muscles can only be differentiated during their further course.

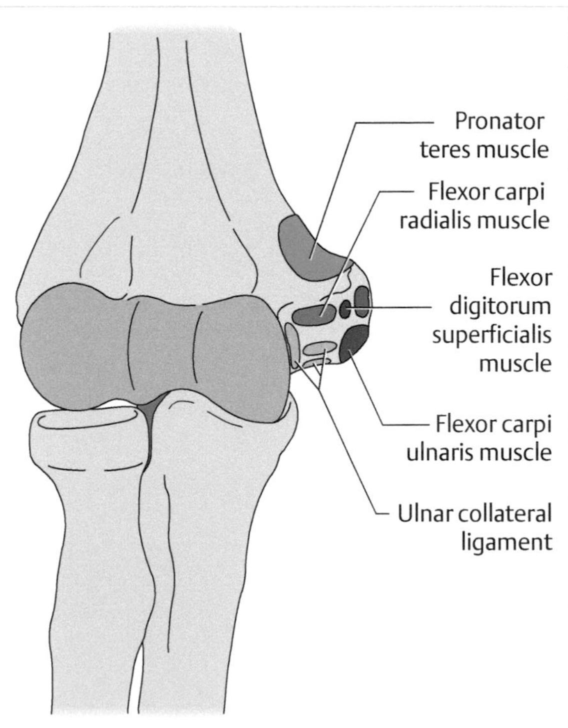


**Fig. 5.9** Palpation of the muscle origins on the medial epicondyle.

The following muscles have a common origin and can therefore be identified in the epicondylar area only with difficulty. As an aid to determining the course of the forearm muscles, place the opposite hand with outstretched fingers and a slightly abducted thumb on the palmar aspect of the forearm with the tubercle of the trapezium of the examiner's hand on the patient's medial epicondyle (**Fig. 5.10**):

- The position of the thumb represents the course of the pronator teres muscle.
- The index finger represents the flexor carpi radialis muscle.
- The middle finger = the palmaris longus muscle.
- The ring finger = the flexor digitorum superficialis muscle.
- The little finger = the flexor carpi ulnaris muscle.

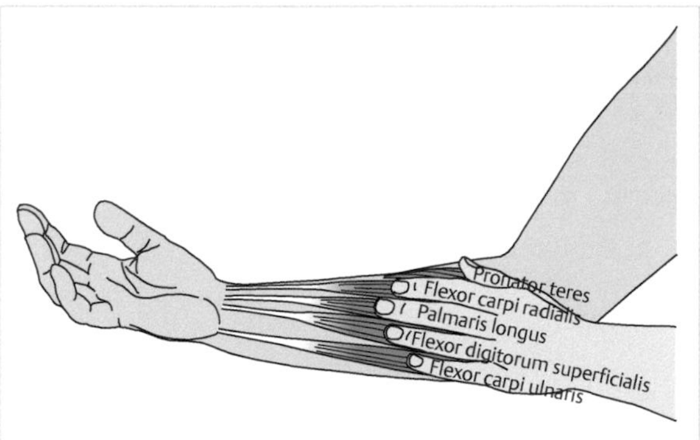


**Fig. 5.10** Palpation of the course of the muscles from the medial epicondyle.

## Flexor Carpi Radialis Muscle

This muscle extends to the base of the second metacarpal. It is easier to palpate when tensing the muscle in palmar flexion and radial abduction. In its further course in the forearm, this muscle is the furthest lateral.

## Flexor Digitorum Superficialis Muscle (Fig. 5.11)

This extends to the middle phalanges. To better palpate it, tense it to flex the wrist and fingers.

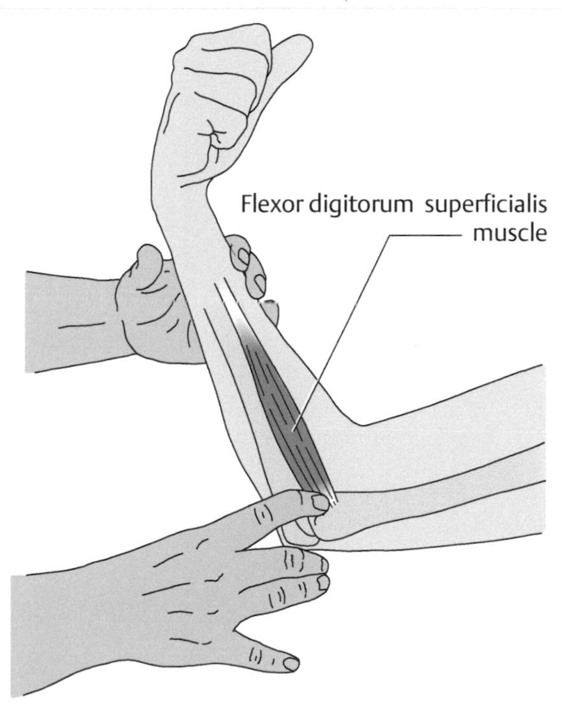


**Fig. 5.11** Palpation of the flexor digitorum superficialis muscle.

## Palmaris Longus Muscle

This extends to the palmar aponeurosis, but it is not always present. Bring the thumb and small finger together and tense the muscle in wrist flexion to help in finding its origin.

## Flexor Carpi Ulnaris Muscle

This extends to the pisiform bone. Tense the muscle in palmar flexion and ulnar abduction.

### Practical Tip

Tendinopathy in the area of the medial epicondyle is known as *golfer's elbow* and encompasses the common flexor origin area. Palpation while simultaneously extending the wrist shows the exact localization of the irritation, as does the wrist flexor resistance test.

## Medial Border of the Humerus

Palpate the medial border as a bony ridge running superiorly from the epicondyle in a straight line.

## Pronator Teres Muscle (Fig. 5.12)

Its origin is the most proximal, and it forms the medial border of the cubital fossa. It can be felt well by tensing the muscle in flexion and pronation.

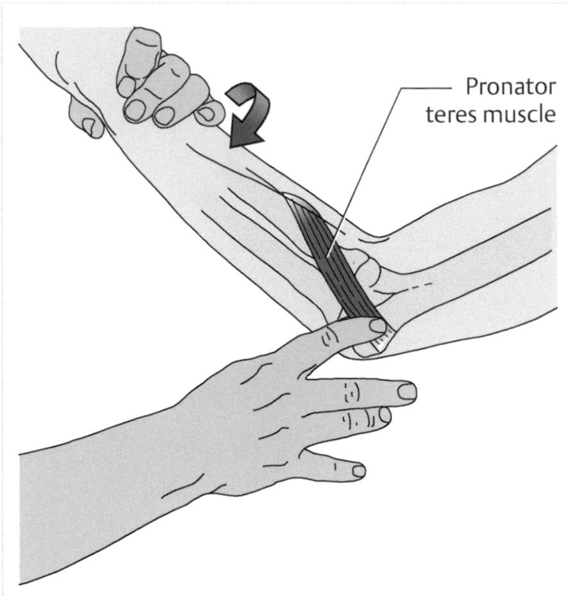


**Fig. 5.12** Palpation of the pronator teres muscle.

## Groove for the Ulnar Nerve (Fig. 5.13)

The groove lies between the medial epicondyle and the olecranon. Within this channel runs the **ulnar nerve**, which can be palpated as a very firm, round strand slightly proximal to the groove. Within the groove, it is protected by ligamentous structures running over it and can therefore only be palpated using considerable pressure. This pressure can trigger a pain like an electric shock that radiates to the side of the little finger.

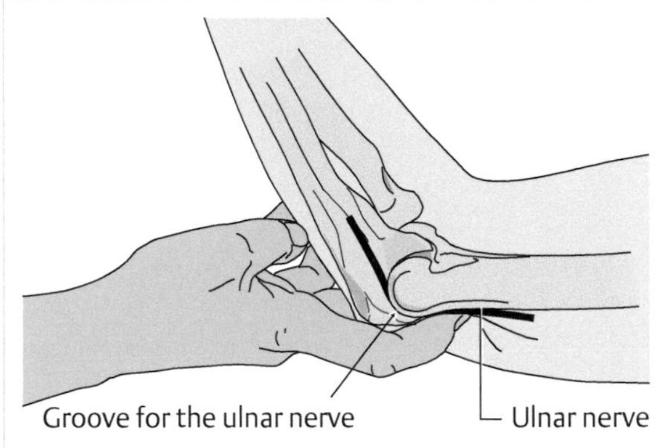


**Fig. 5.13** Palpation of the ulnar nerve; groove for the ulnar nerve.

**Pathology**

Subluxation of the ulnar nerve can occur as a result of a congenital alteration in the anatomy of the groove. When attempting to move, the patient complains of stabbing pain with distal radiation. This occurs during flexion because the medial edge of the triceps brachii muscle can force the nerve out of the groove and push it over the medial epicondyle. This subluxation also occurs in contact sports such as judo and wrestling.

## Ulnar Collateral Ligament (Fig. 5.14)

The ulnar collateral ligament extends like a fan from the epicondyle to the ulna and into the annular ligament of the radius. As on the lateral side, muscles cover a large part of the ligament. The part that extends toward the olecranon is easier to find.

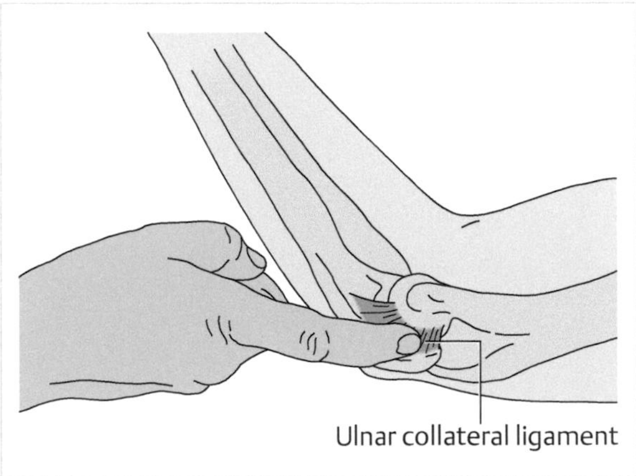


**Fig. 5.14** Palpation of the ulnar collateral ligament.

## Olecranon (Fig. 5.15)

With flexion, the olecranon emerges from the olecranon fossa and thereby becomes accessible to palpation. The triceps muscle inserts on the tip of the olecranon.

The olecranon bursa lies directly on the olecranon and can only be felt clearly if it is swollen.

### Olecranon Fossa

The olecranon fossa can be felt only with slight elbow flexion and some pressure because it must be palpated through the stretched triceps tendon. The olecranon occupies the space when the elbow is extended.

## Borders of the Cubital Fossa (Fig. 5.16)

The cubital fossa is bordered laterally by the brachioradialis muscle and medially by the pronator teres muscle. From lateral to medial, the following structures extend through the cubital fossa:

### Biceps Brachii Tendon (Fig. 5.16)

This is the tendon in the cubital fossa that stands out most clearly. It extends toward the inner margin of the radius.

Medial to this, the continuation of the tendon, the **bicipital aponeurosis** (**Fig. 5.17**), can be palpated as a flat structure with a firm proximal margin as it runs to the ulna and antebrachial fascia.

**Practical Tip**

A change in the contour of the biceps brachii muscle, such as a small balled-up area a little above the cubital fossa, suggests rupture of the tendon, usually of the long head of the biceps in the area of the bicipital groove.

▷ See Chapter 4, Shoulder

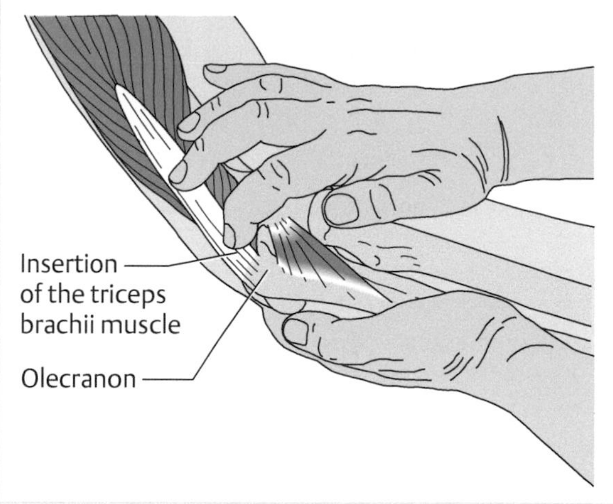


**Fig. 5.15** Palpation of the olecranon; insertion of the triceps brachii muscle.

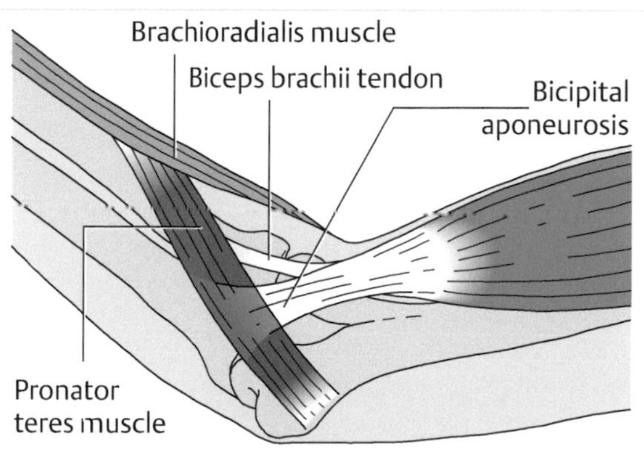


**Fig. 5.16** Palpation of the borders of the cubital fossa.

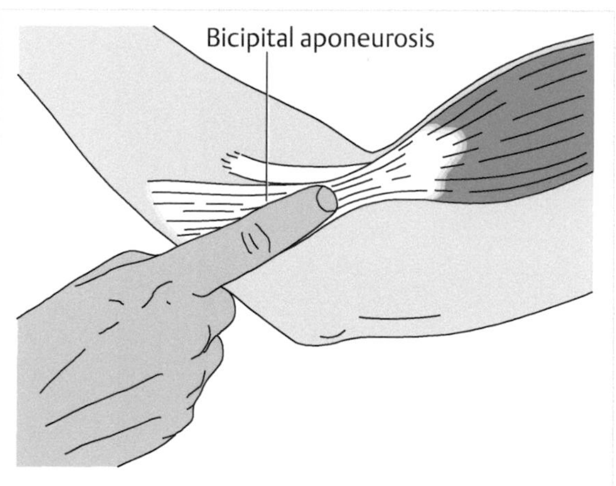


**Fig. 5.17** Palpation of the bicipital aponeurosis.

## Radial Tuberosity (Fig. 5.18)

The insertion of the biceps on the radial tuberosity lies at a very deep level, and it is only accessible to palpation in the following way. With maximal pronation combined with elbow flexion, the tuberosity turns posteriorly and can then be palpated approximately 2 to 3 cm distal to the head of the radius as an elevated area.

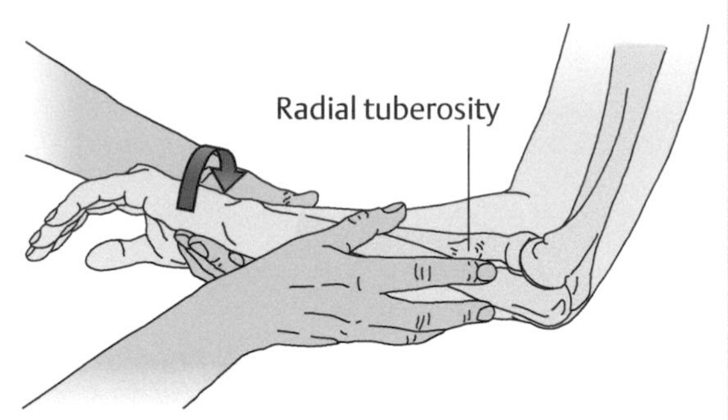


**Fig. 5.18** Palpation of the radial tuberosity.

### Practical Tip

In cases of insertional tendinopathy, a distinct swelling can be felt at the insertion of the biceps brachii tendon. This can become so large that the tuberosity must force itself through the space between the radius and ulna during pronation, which can be very painful.

## Blood Vessels and Nerves

A trough can be palpated between the ulnar margin of the biceps and the pronator teres muscle, with the brachialis muscle forming its floor. Within this trough is found a neurovascular bundle containing the median nerve and brachial vessels.

The lateral border of the biceps muscle and the brachioradialis muscle form another trough, whose floor is again formed by the brachialis muscle. The radial nerve and the radial collateral vessels run deep within this trough. The lateral cutaneous nerve of the forearm runs more superficially.

## Brachial Artery (Fig. 5.19)

The pulse can be felt just medial to the biceps tendon.

## Median Nerve (Fig. 5.19)

This is a tubular structure directly medial to the artery. On its further course distal to the cubital fossa, it travels through the pronator teres muscle.

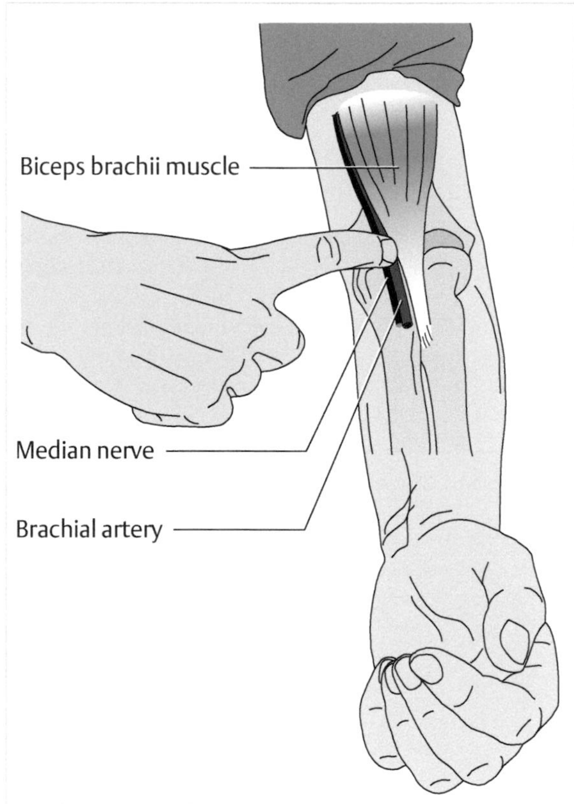


**Fig. 5.19** Palpation of the brachial artery; median nerve.

# 5.2 Functional Anatomy of the Elbow

## 5.2.1 X-Ray Image of the Elbow

### Anteroposterior View (Fig. 5.20)

#### Position: Extension / Supination

- Gap between the capitulum of the humerus and the radius: approximately 3 mm.
- The angle formed by the axis of the humeral shaft and the axis of the ulnar shaft is the axial angle of the elbow. Normal: 170°.

### Lateral View (Fig. 5.21)

#### Position: 90° Elbow Flexion

- Projection of both epicondyles superimposed over each other.
- Joint space of the humero-ulnar joint:
  - Uniform gap between the trochlea and ulna.
  - Smooth, congruent joint surfaces.

**Pathology**

In pathologic conditions, the joint space can narrow because of inflammation or arthritic changes.
An arthritic deformity of the radial head in chronic polyarthritis is just as recognizable as the well-defined findings of diagnostic radiology in trauma medicine, such as dislocation of the radial head or an avulsion fracture of an epicondyle or the olecranon.

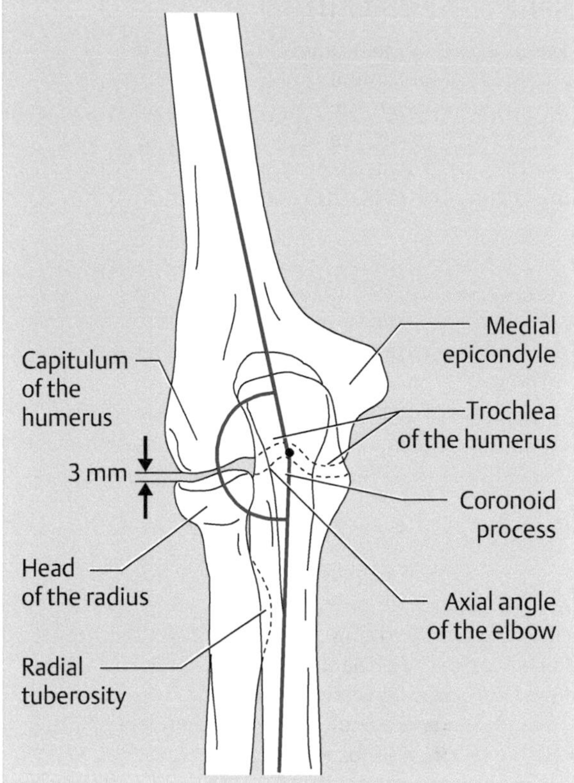


**Fig. 5.20** X-ray image: anteroposterior view.

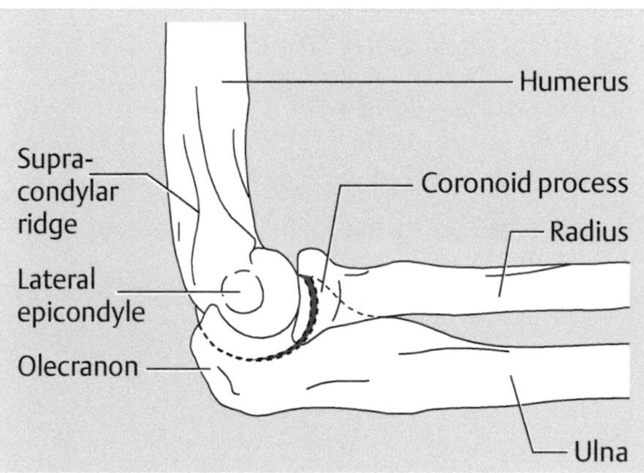


**Fig. 5.21** X-ray image: lateral view.

## 5.2.2 Elbow Joint

Unlike the proximal joint surfaces on the head of the humerus, which are oriented medially, the joint surfaces of the distal humerus are oriented anteriorly. The elbow joint is thereby optimally oriented for its functional use, which is primarily anterior to the body.

The elbow joint is composed of three joints that form a functional unit:

- The **humero-ulnar joint** represents the articulated connection between the humerus and the ulna. Functionally, it is a saddle joint.
- The **humeroradial joint** attaches the humerus to the radius.
- The **proximal radio-ulnar joint** is the joint between the radius and ulna in the proximal area. It is obligatorily linked with the **distal radio-ulnar joint**.

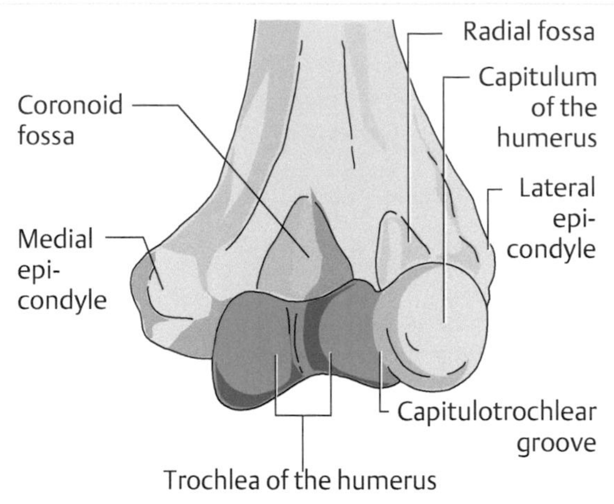


**Fig. 5.22** Trochlea of the humerus.

### Humero-Ulnar Joint

#### Humerus

- The *trochlea of the humerus* (**Fig. 5.22**) is shaped like a champagne cork. The ulnar part is somewhat wider that the radial part, and an hourglass-type constriction divides the two parts. It is oriented slightly medially.
- At the distal end of the humerus, the trochlea and the capitulum are angled approximately 45° anteriorly to the axis of the shaft.
- The *coronoid fossa* (**Fig. 5.22**) is located anteriorly above the trochlea. In flexion, it accommodates the *coronoid process*.
- Posteriorly, the *olecranon fossa* (**Fig. 5.23**) is very deep and filled with some fatty tissue. In extension, it accommodates the olecranon.

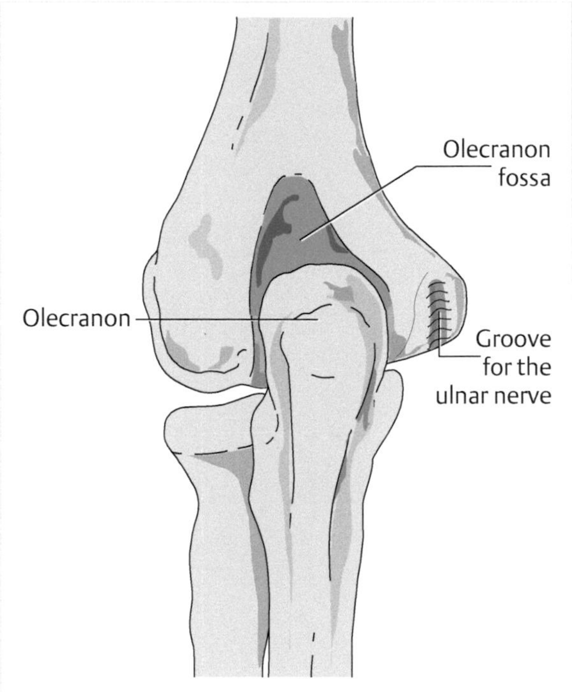


**Fig. 5.23** Olecranon fossa.

## Ulna

- The *trochlear notch* (**Figs. 5.25 and 5.26**) encloses the trochlea like a pipe wrench. It has a ridge that fits into the furrow in the trochlea. The middle portion of the notch is not covered with cartilage.
- Posteriorly, at the end of the notch, is the *olecranon* (**Figs. 5.24–5.26**). This serves as the insertion for the triceps brachii muscle and the origin for the flexor carpi ulnaris muscle.
- At the anterior end is the *coronoid process* (**Figs. 5.24–5.26**). Immediately distal to the coronoid process is the ulnar tuberosity. This is the insertion site for the brachialis muscle and the area of origin of the flexor digitorum superficialis muscle.
- A line running from the olecranon to the coronoid process forms an angle of 45° with the axis of the ulnar shaft. The large range of flexion is due to this orientation and the angularity of the distal humerus.

### Practical Tip

An isolated fracture of the olecranon is treated surgically with osteosynthesis using the tension-band wiring technique, because otherwise the triceps muscle will pull the proximal end of the fracture superiorly. In subsequent therapy, passive muscle stretching and concentric resistive training from the position of maximum flexion must therefore be avoided.
When treating the humero-ulnar joint with traction, the 45° angle formed by the tip of the olecranon and the coronoid process must be taken into consideration. The trochlear notch is the concave joint partner and thereby corresponds to the treatment plane of this angle, which must be considered when changing the position of the ulna. Not accounting for this angle while applying traction in a position of 90° will produce compression in certain parts of the joint.

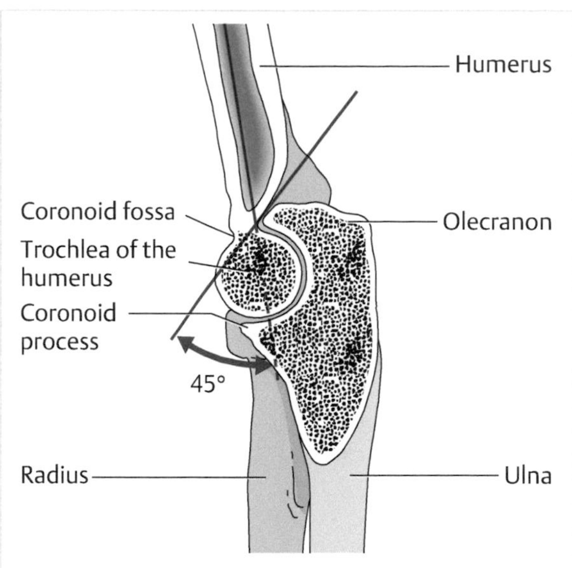


**Fig. 5.24** Position of the trochlea of the humerus.

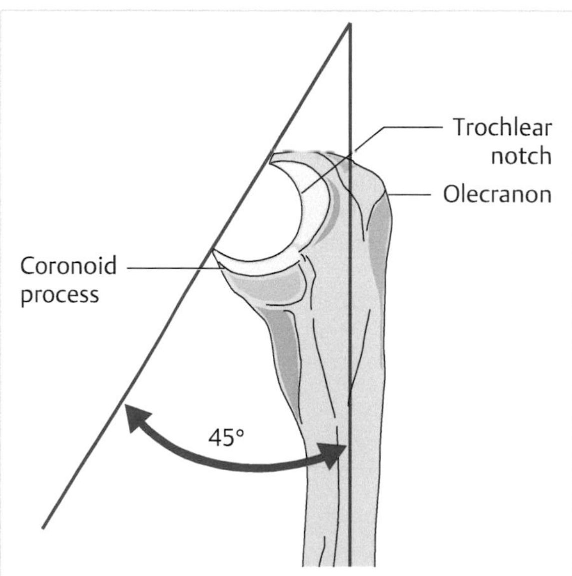


**Fig. 5.25** Trochlear notch of the ulna.

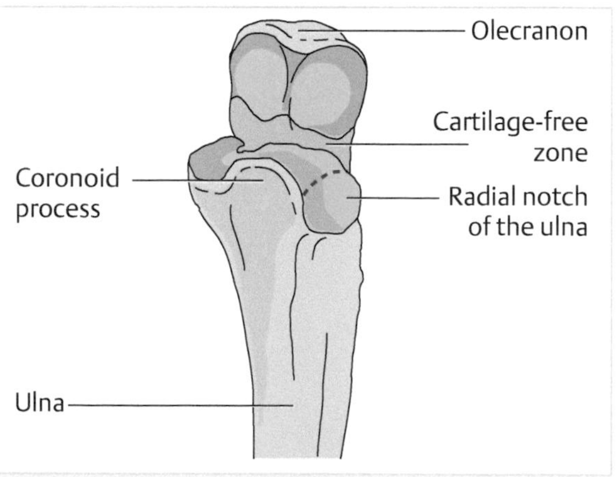


**Fig. 5.26** Position of the trochlear notch.

## Humeroradial Joint

### Humerus (Figs. 5.27 and 5.28)

- The *capitulotrochlear groove* demarcates the *capitulum of the humerus* from the trochlea.
- Above the anterior capitulum is the *radial fossa*, which accommodates the head of the radius at maximal flexion.

### Radius (Fig. 5.29)

- The *articular facet of the radius* is the concave joint surface on the radial head.
- Around the rim of the fovea is a small circular bulge, the *lunula obliqua*. This articulates with the capitulotrochlear groove of the humerus.

The radius is closely coupled to the movements of the ulna through the annular ligament of the radius, so that neither the humero-ulnar joint nor the humeroradial joint can be moved separately, but only together as a unit.

**Practical Tip**

The usual treatment of a fracture of the head of the radius is surgical screw fixation. The follow-up functional therapy should proceed very carefully, avoiding the forbidden positions of pronation and supination. Excess effort and duration in the implementation of physical therapy can lead to calcification and other complications.

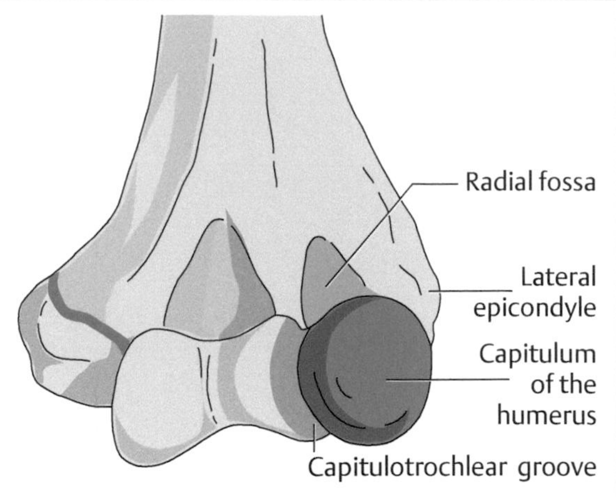


**Fig. 5.27** Capitulum of the humerus.

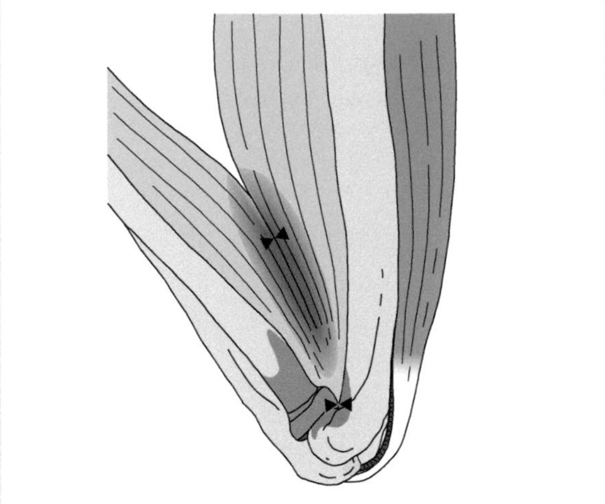

**Fig. 5.28** Position of the radial head in maximal flexion.

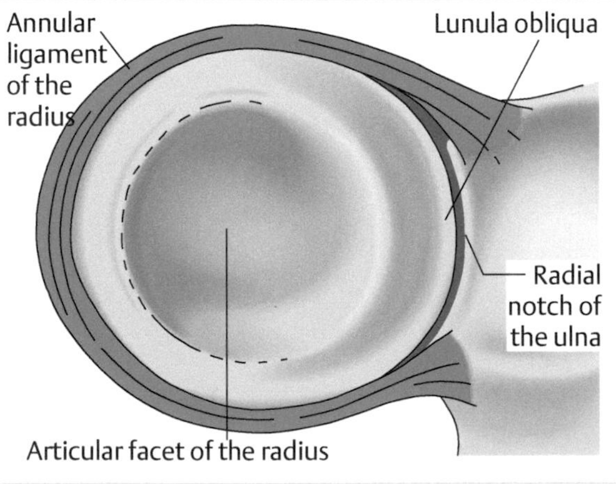


**Fig. 5.29** Articular facet of the radius.

## Proximal Radio-Ulnar Joint (Fig. 5.30)

### Ulna

- The *radial notch of the ulna* is concave and sagittally oriented.
- The *annular ligament of the radius* is approximately 1 cm wide and fixed to the anterior and posterior rim of the notch. It encircles most of the radial head—only the lunula obliqua is uncovered.
- In the area of the radial notch of the ulna, the ligament consists of fibrocartilage, which merges into connective tissue composed of collagen fibers. This inclusion of cartilage cells is indicative of a locally limited transfer of pressure and takes over the important function of centering the head of the radius in the notch, while the other ligaments experience more tensile stress.
- The radial and ulnar collateral ligaments extend into the annular ligament, thereby providing an interrelationship between the humero-ulnar, humeroradial, and radio-ulnar joints.
- A few fibers of the supinator muscle radiate into the ligament.
- The *quadrate ligament* attaches to the inferior aspect of the radial notch of the ulna and extends to the base of the articular circumference of the radius. On the ulna, a few fibers of this ligament extend into the annular ligament of the radius.

### Radius

The ***articular circumference of the radius*** is convex and articulates with the annular ligament of the radius and with the radial notch of the ulna.

**Practical Tip**

The close interconnection between the joints of the elbow demonstrates that a disturbance in one will always also involve the others, which is why all the joints must be examined and treated.

**Pathology**

In chronic polyarthritis of the elbow, arthritic deformity primarily affects the head of the radius. After therapeutic resection of the head of the radius, there is a resultant instability of the elbow, because the bracing from the humeral support is missing. In addition, due to the transection of the annular ligament of the radius, the stabilizing connection to the collateral ligaments is no longer present. Another consequence is that there is a change in the stress placed on the distal radio-ulnar joint.

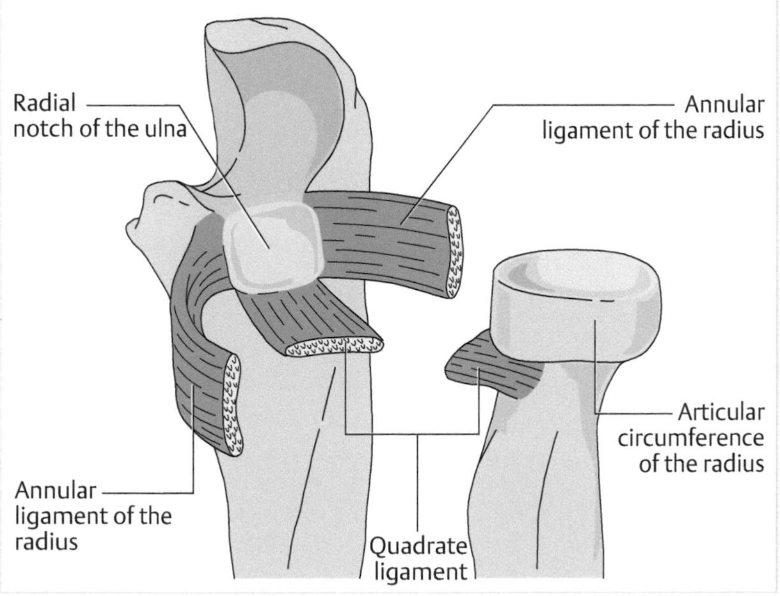


**Fig. 5.30** Proximal radio-ulnar joint.

## Joint Capsule (Figs. 5.31–5.34)

A thin capsule enfolds the three joints. The **insertions on the humerus** enclose the radial, coronoid, and olecranon fossae but omit the epicondyles and the groove for the ulnar nerve.

The capsule forms small recesses anteriorly and posteriorly, which unfold during maximum movements. A few muscle fibers of the brachialis muscle and the anconeus muscle extend anteriorly and posteriorly to the capsule and prevent the folds of the recesses from becoming entrapped. The collateral ligaments reinforce the sides of the capsule, as do bands of muscle fibers from the supinator and extensor carpi radialis brevis muscles.

On the **ulna**, the insertion is located on the bone–cartilage border of the trochlear notch, and in the radial area, it encloses the radial notch of the ulna.

On the radius, the insertion lies somewhat below the bone–cartilage border of the articular circumference.

**Pathology**

Outpouchings of the capsule, which can become fibrosed and thus very firm, lead to recurring episodes of entrapment with movement. They must be removed surgically.

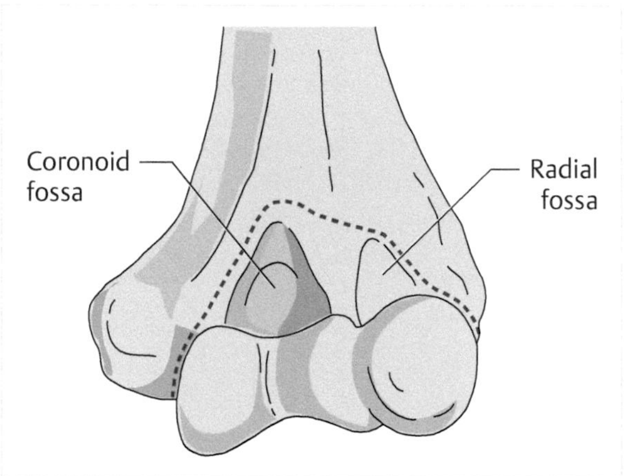


**Fig. 5.31** Capsule insertion on the anterior humerus.

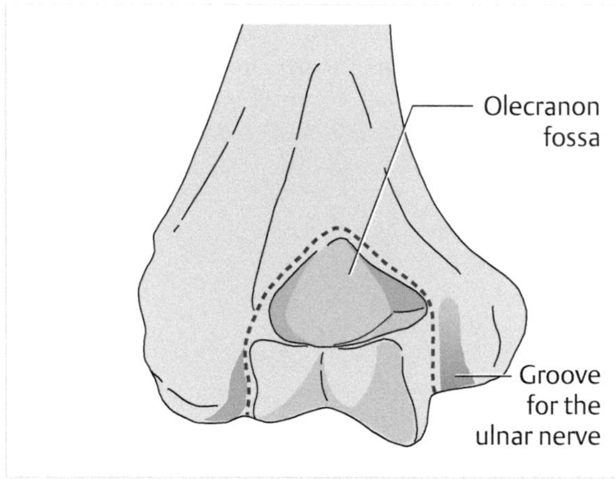


**Fig. 5.32** Capsule insertion on the posterior humerus.

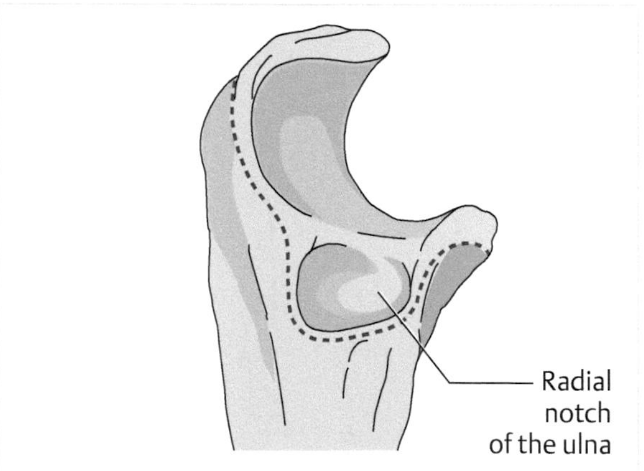


**Fig. 5.33** Capsule insertion on the ulna, radial region.

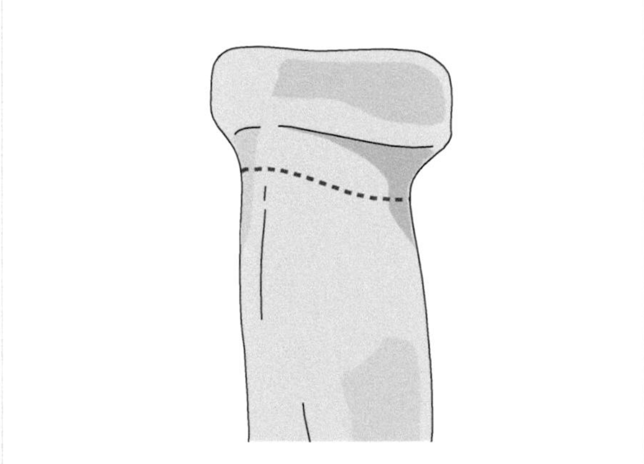

**Fig. 5.34** Capsule insertion on the radius.

## Perfusion (Fig. 5.35)

The terminal arteries form an anastomotic network around the olecranon. The medial collateral artery from the profunda brachii artery, the posterior branch of the ulnar collateral artery from the brachial artery, and the posterior branch of the ulnar recurrent artery from the ulnar artery supply the capsule–ligament apparatus in the lateral, medial, and posterior sections.

The anterior region of the elbow is supplied by the anterior branches of the brachial artery.

These vessels also supply the surrounding muscles.

## Innervation (Figs. 5.36 and 5.37)

The region of the lateral epicondyle is supplied exclusively by branches of the radial nerve.

Branches of the ulnar nerve innervate the posterior area around the medial epicondyle, and branches of the median nerve innervate the anterior area.

The posterior capsule–ligament apparatus receives its innervation from the radial and ulnar nerves, and the anterior area from the radial, musculocutaneous, and median nerves.

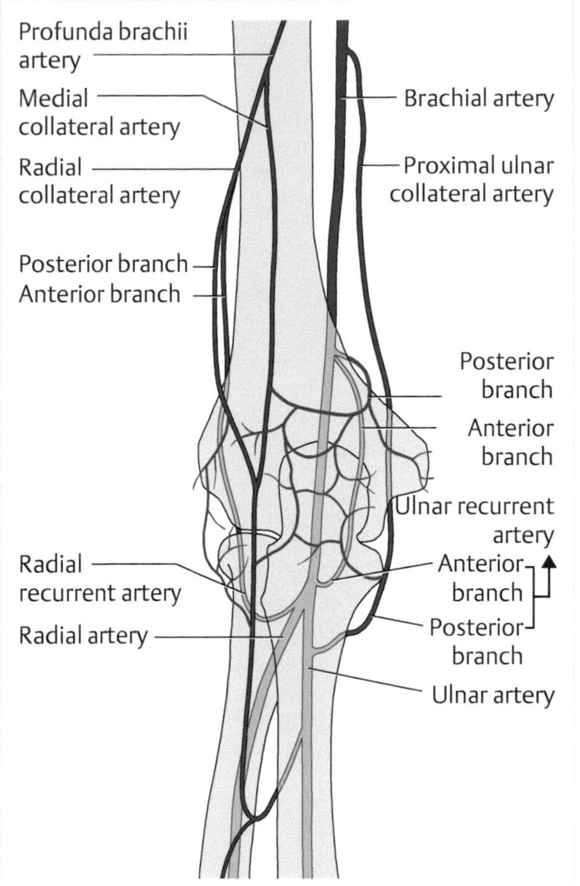


**Fig. 5.35** Arterial supply of the elbow joint.

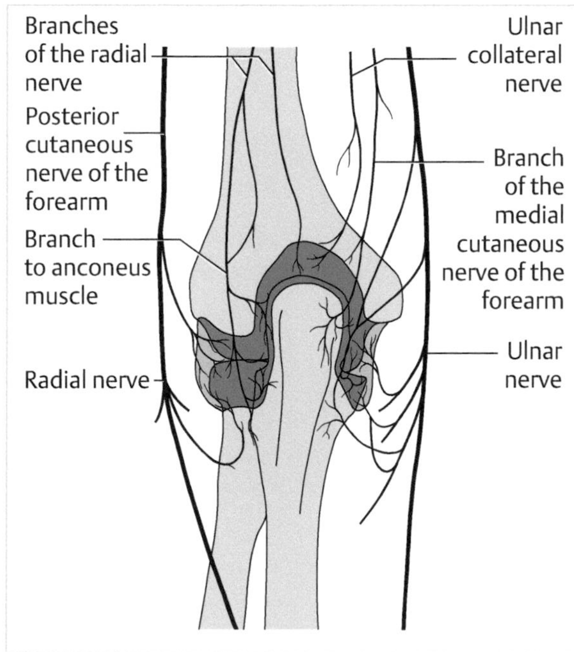


**Fig. 5.36** Innervation of the posterior elbow.

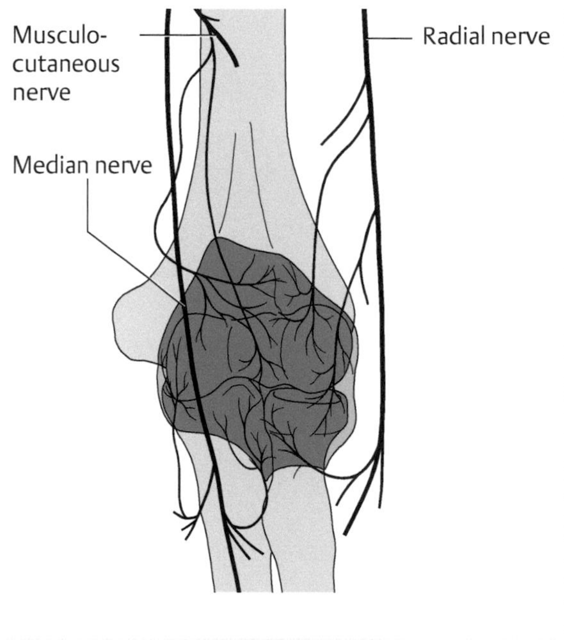


**Fig. 5.37** Innervation of the anterior elbow.

## Distal Radio-Ulnar Joint (Fig. 5.38)

### Ulna

- The *articular circumference of the ulna* on the ulnar head is convex.
- The articular disk (**Fig. 5.39**) lies distal to the ulna. Because of its fixation to the radius, it participates in the movements of pronation and supination.

▷ See Chapter 6, Hand

### Radius

The *ulnar notch of the radius* is concave.

#### Pathology

A fracture of the distal radius occurs through a fall onto the dorsally extended hand. It is the most common of all fractures. When this occurs, the distal fragment shifts dorsally and radially, resulting in the *bayonet* (or *dinner fork*) *deformity*. Proper fracture reduction and follow-up immobilization in a cast is essential to prevent carpal tunnel syndrome and incongruity of the joint surfaces of the distal radio-ulnar joint and proximal wrist joint (radiocarpal joint).

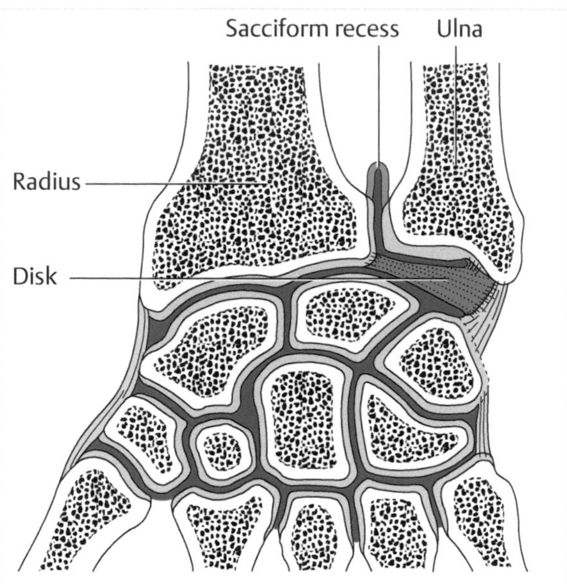


**Fig. 5.38** Distal radio-ulnar joint.

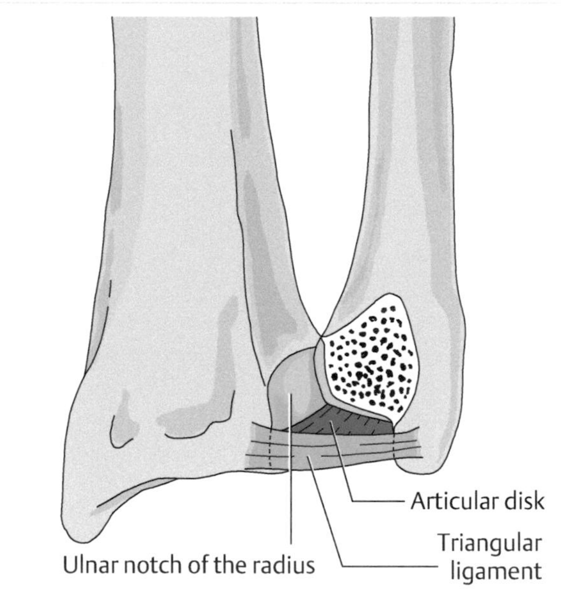


**Fig. 5.39** Articular disk of the radio-ulnar joint.

### Joint Capsule

- The capsule inserts on the bone–cartilage border.
- It has an evagination, the sacciform recess, which is approximately 1 cm long and extends proximally between the radius and ulna.
- The capsule is reinforced by the distal radio-ulnar ligament and a few posterior bands of the interosseous membrane.
- At the borders of the disk, the capsule merges with the capsule of the wrist joint.

#### Pathology

During the movements of pronation and supination, the proximal and distal radio-ulnar joints form a functional unit and must be considered as such in their examination and treatment.

## 5.2.3 Ligaments

### Ulnar Collateral Ligament (Fig. 5.40)

The ulnar collateral ligament consists of three fibrous bands:

- The **anterior part** extends from the anterior aspect of the medial epicondyle to the medial edge of the coronoid process. It radiates into the annular ligament of the radius.
- The **posterior part** extends from the posterior aspect of the epicondyle to the medial border of the olecranon.
- The **intermediate part** is relatively thin and fills the space between the above two parts. A small, transversely running bundle—Cooper's ligament—splits off and connects the bases of the anterior and posterior parts.

A branch of the ulnar collateral ligament, the **epicondylo–olecranon ligament**, extends from the medial epicondyle to the medial border of the olecranon. Its function is to stabilize the ulnar nerve as it runs distally within the groove for the ulnar nerve.

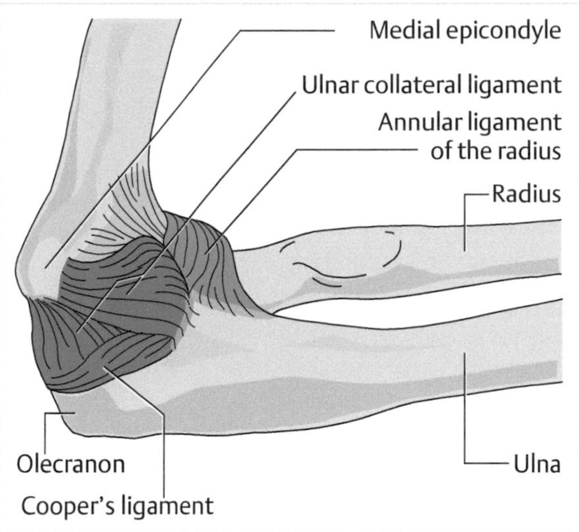


**Fig. 5.40** Ulnar collateral ligament.

#### Pathology

Ligament injuries of the ulnar collateral ligament are seen in conjunction with acute or chronic valgus trauma, such as occurs in throwing sports. The symptoms only occur with clear provocation, such as athletic strain.

### Radial Collateral Ligament (Fig. 5.41)

The radial collateral ligament divides into two divergent sections that extend from the anterior and posterior parts of the lateral epicondyle to the anterior and posterior margin of the radial notch of the ulna. These give off fibers to the annular ligament of the radius and to the tendons of the supinator and extensor carpi radialis brevis muscles.

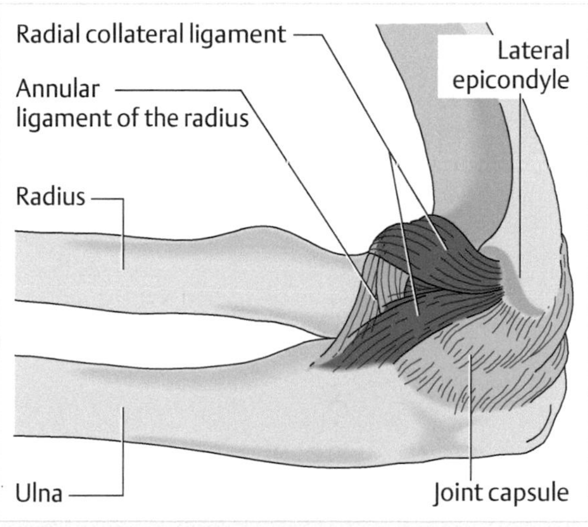


**Fig. 5.41** Radial collateral ligament.

**Function.** Because of their delta-shaped structure, the collateral ligaments are proportionally tight in all positions of the joint.

#### Practical Tip

Test the stability of the ligaments by checking for joint gapping medially and laterally with the elbow extended, because in this position most parts of the ligaments are taut.

**Posterior bands** (**Fig. 5.42**) extend medially and laterally into the collateral ligaments and reinforce the capsule as longitudinally and obliquely running fibrous tracts.

**Anterior bands** (**Fig. 5.43**) reinforce the capsule as diagonal longitudinally and obliquely running fibrous bands. They also radiate into the collateral ligaments and into the annular ligament of the radius.

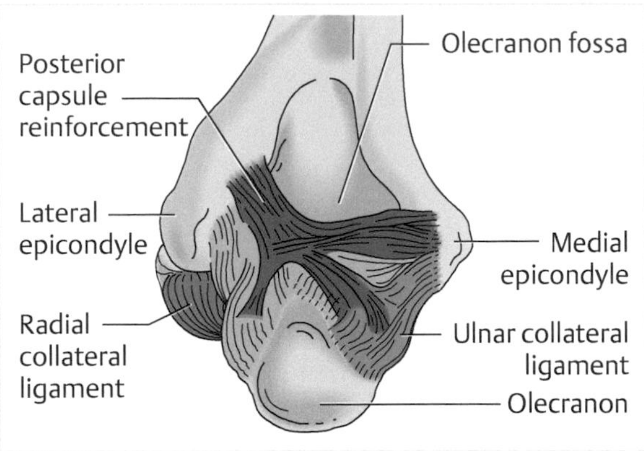


**Fig. 5.42** Posterior capsule–ligament apparatus.

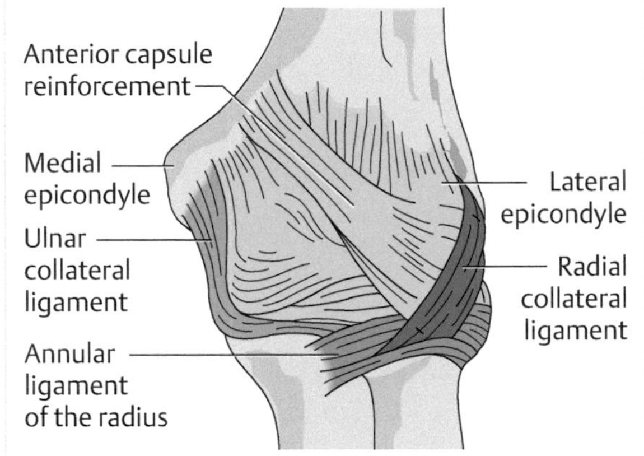


**Fig. 5.43** Anterior capsule–ligament apparatus.

## Interosseous Membrane (Fig. 5.44)

- This begins about two fingerbreadths below the radial tuberosity and ends shortly before the distal radio-ulnar joint, except for a few fibers that extend into the joint capsule there.
- Bundles of fibers run obliquely, crossing over each other, and are particularly strongly pronounced in the middle section of the membrane.
- Between the various parts are openings to allow blood vessels to pass through.
- The membrane serves as the origin for the deep finger flexors and extensors.
- Distally, it prevents the radius from shifting against the ulna.
- Most parts are taut in supination.
- Due to the alignment of the fibrous structure, the membrane can compensate for variously directed tensile strains.

## Oblique Cord

- This is a small ligamentous structure.
- It inserts a little below the radial notch of the ulna and directly below the radial tuberosity.

**Pathology**

In rheumatoid patients who have had the radial head resected, the interosseous membrane is of great importance because it holds the two forearm bones together during pronation and supination.

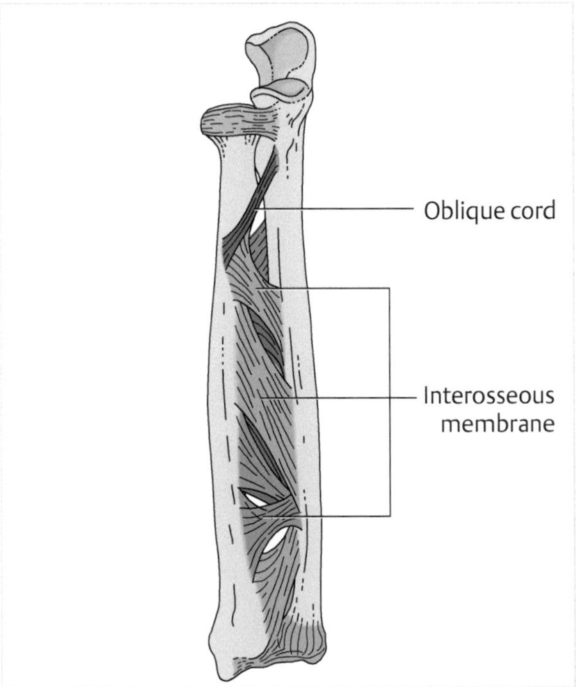


**Fig. 5.44** Interosseous membrane.

## 5.2.4 Axes and Movements

### Flexion/Extension (Fig. 5.45)

The axis runs below the epicondyles through the capitulum of the humerus and the trochlea of the humerus.

### Range of Motion

*Flexion* is possible to a maximum of 130 to 150°. The movement is inhibited either by the soft tissue that lies between the upper arm and the forearm or by the posterior capsule–ligament apparatus.

**Practical Tip**

In individuals with poorly developed soft tissues and an unstable capsule–ligament apparatus, the end-feel for passive flexion can be hard because, in this case, the coronoid process is pressed against the coronoid fossa on the humerus.

*Extension:* approximately 10°. The end-feel here is hard. Due to the tightening of the anterior capsule–ligament apparatus and the collateral ligaments, the notch and the trochlea are pressed together, leading to the firm-elastic end-feel.

### Cubital Angle (Fig. 5.46)

Due to the shape of the trochlea and a small tilt of the ulna in the medial area, there is a valgus position of approximately 10° (cubital angle) at full extension.

The cubital angle is evident primarily with elbow extension with supination, and it disappears in flexion.

**Practical Tip**

Test the tilt of the ulna for medial gapping using a position of slight elbow flexion, because in this position the capsule and ligaments yield to allow gapping at the sides of the joint.
Adhesion in the medial capsule–ligament apparatus can limit extension because it does not yield enough to allow this tilting movement.

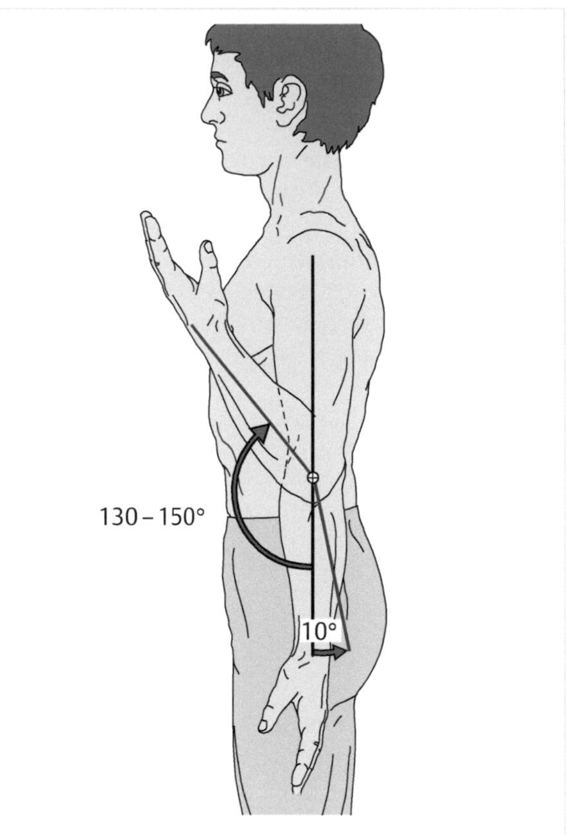


**Fig. 5.45** Range of motion: flexion and extension.

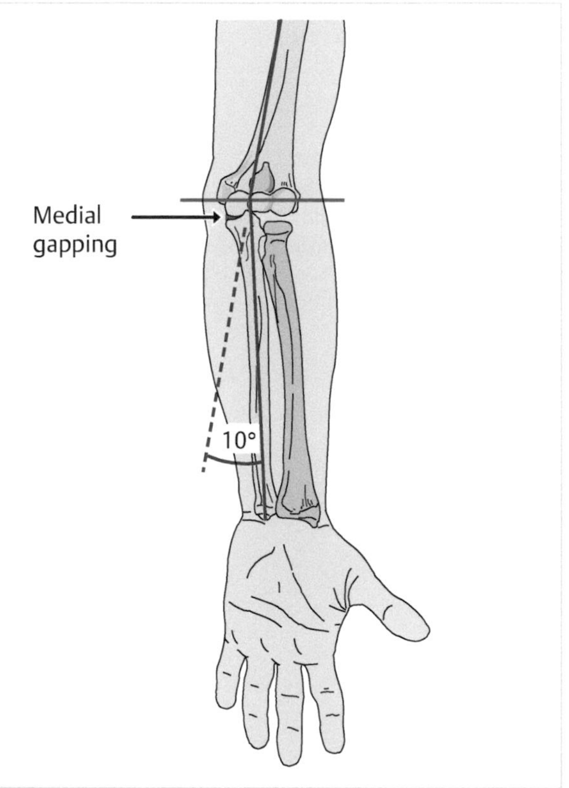


**Fig. 5.46** Axis of motion for flexion/extension and the cubital angle.

## Supination/Pronation (Fig. 5.47)

The **axis for supination/pronation** goes through the capitulum of the humerus, the middle of the radial head, and the ulnar styloid process.

## Range of Motion (Fig. 5.48)

*Supination/pronation:* 80°/90°, respectively, from neutral. The point at which the largest contact area in both radio-ulnar joints occurs is in the midposition between pronation and supination, an area that is used extensively in the movements of everyday life.

The following joint surfaces move against each other (**Fig. 5.49**):

- Proximal radio-ulnar joint: The articular circumference of the radius moves against the radial notch of the ulna and the annular ligament of the radius.
- Humeroradial joint: The articular facet of the radius rotates against the capitulum of the humerus, and the lunula obliqua glides within the capitulotrochlear groove.
- Distal radio-ulnar joint: The ulnar notch of the radius glides against the articular circumference of the ulna.
- The articular disk of the distal radio-ulnar joint, which lies distal to the ulna, shifts during the movements of pronation and supination because of its fixation to the radius.

### Practical Tip

When there is limited movement, these joints must be examined to establish the exact therapy. For example, if pronation is limited, the movement of the radial head gliding dorsally against the ulna must be tested, because the articular circumference on the proximal radius is convex in its apposition to the ulna. Applying traction to the humeroradial joint provides information about possible disturbances in this joint. Because the joint surface of the distal radius is concave, the radius must be tested as it glides in a palmar direction. In addition, the flexibility of the disk against the ulna should be examined.

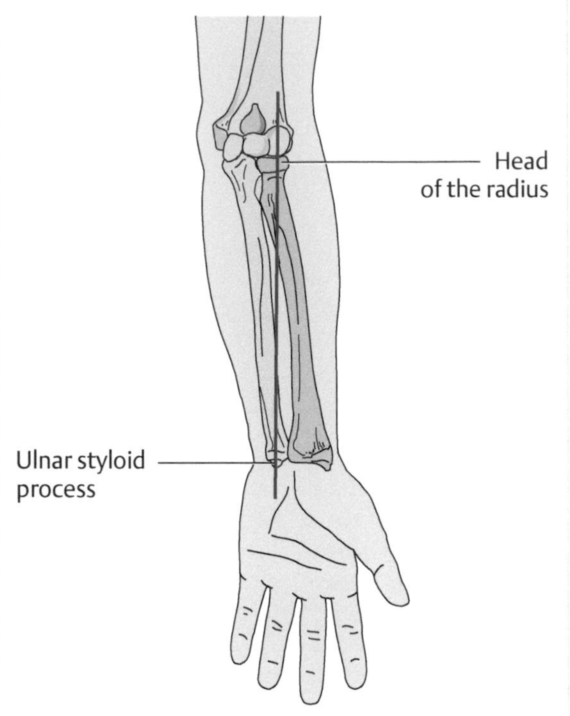


**Fig. 5.47** Pronation and supination axes.

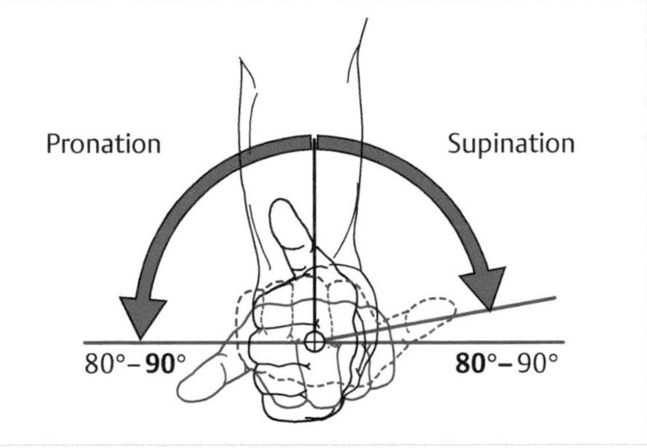


**Fig. 5.48** Range of motion: pronation and supination.

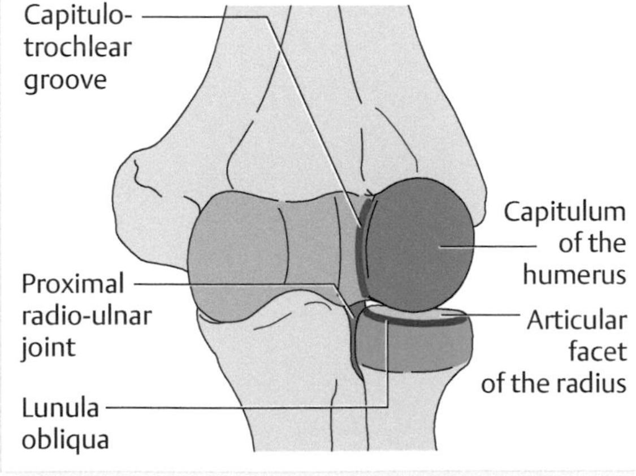


**Fig. 5.49** Joint surface contact in pronation and supination.

## Pronation Position (Figs. 5.50 and 5.51)

In the pronated position, the *radius* lies obliquely over the ulna. Due to this movement, the articular facet of the radius tilts about 5° distally.

The *ulna* also performs a tilting movement. The distal part shifts laterally, resulting in gapping of the medial joint space of the humero-ulnar joint. It is comparable to the tilting that occurs with elbow extension.

Pronation is limited by the capsule–ligament apparatus. In addition, soft tissue, especially the flexor digitorum profundus and flexor pollicis longus muscles, becomes sandwiched between the bones as they cross.

In the pronated position, the greater diameter of the oval radial head lies obliquely, resulting in more room for the radial tuberosity, which turns towards the ulna with increasing pronation. At maximal pronation, it has turned so far that it can be palpated on the posterior side about 2 to 3 fingerbreadths distal to the radial head.

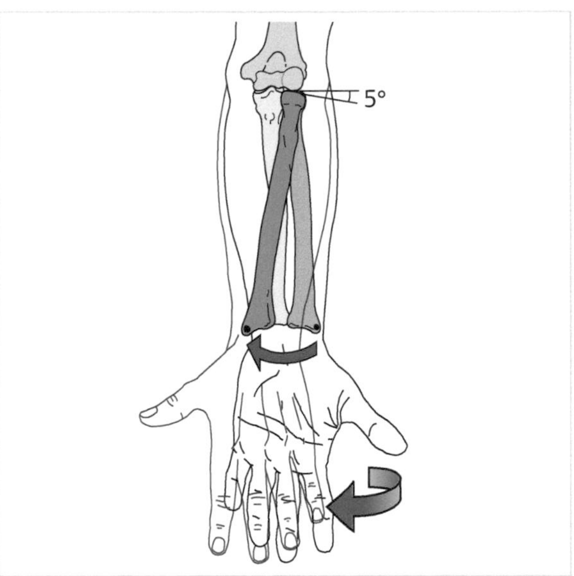


**Fig. 5.50** Tilting and turning of the radius during pronation.

### Practical Tip

In the evaluation of limited pronation, medial gapping must be examined in addition to the translatory joint tests described, because the capsule–ligament apparatus must give way on the medial side to accommodate for the shift of the distal ulna laterally.

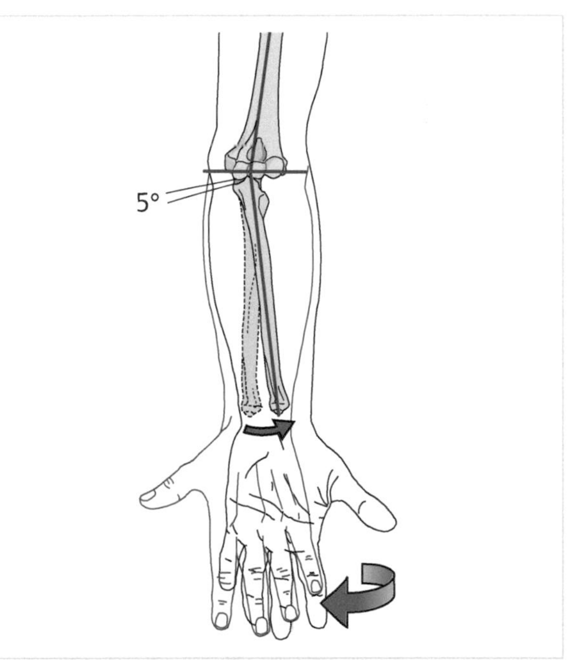


**Fig. 5.51** Tilting and displacement of the ulna during pronation.

## Supination Position (Fig. 5.52)

In the supinated position, the radius and ulna are parallel. The movement is inhibited by the tension of the capsule–ligament apparatus, the quadrate ligament, and in part the interosseous membrane.

During supination, the distal ulna simultaneously shifts minimally to the medial side.

The greater diameter of the oval radial head lies parallel to the radial notch of the ulna, and the radial tuberosity points in a anteromedial direction.

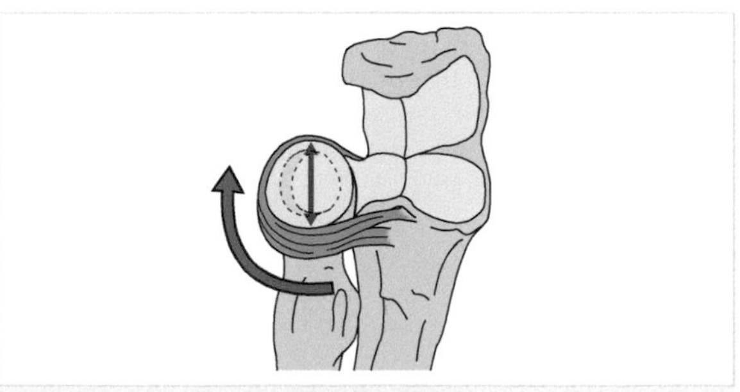

**Fig. 5.52** Supination.

## 5.2.5 Muscles: Flexors

### Biceps Brachii Muscle (Fig. 5.53)

- The round tendon of this muscle extends to the radial tuberosity.
- A flat part of the tendon, the **bicipital aponeurosis**, extends medially toward the ulna and into the antebrachial fascia.

**Function.** Elbow flexion/supination.

In terms of flexion, the maximum degree of efficiency is attained at 90° of flexion and in the supinated position.

### Third-Class Lever (Fig. 5.54a)

| | |
|---|---|
| Fulcrum: | Elbow joint. |
| Force: | Biceps brachii muscle. |
| Effort arm: | Distance from the fulcrum to the insertion, approximately 5 cm. |
| Load: | Forearm + weight = 20 N. |
| Load arm: | Distance from the fulcrum to the point of the impact of the weight, approximately 35 cm. |

The impact point of the force is between the fulcrum and the load; therefore this is a third-class lever.

### Mechanics of the Work of the Biceps Brachii Muscle (Fig. 5.54b)

The ulna is well stabilized on the humerus due to its special form. The radius, on the other hand, is not, so it depends on other structures to stabilize it, with the biceps muscle playing a major role. With diminished force from the biceps in the extended position, the longitudinal force component (Ft) approximates the longitudinal course of the radius and humerus and passes through the fulcrum. When the biceps muscle contracts, it causes compression of the articular facet of the radius against the capitulum of the humerus, stabilizing the humeroradial joint.

At a position of 45° of flexion (**Fig. 5.54b**), the alignment of the vector (Ft) is no longer longitudinal to the humerus, so that the compression in the humeroradial joint decreases and the rotatory component (Fr) ensures that the radius glides anteriorly in relation to the humerus. With increasing flexion, the vector (Ft) becomes ever smaller, while the vector (Fr) becomes ever larger. That means that the anterior gliding is even more pronounced. At this moment, the stabilization function of the annular ligament of the radius is called upon to hold the radius to the ulna, which is itself stable because of the shape of its notch articulating with the trochlea of the humerus, thus preventing subluxation.

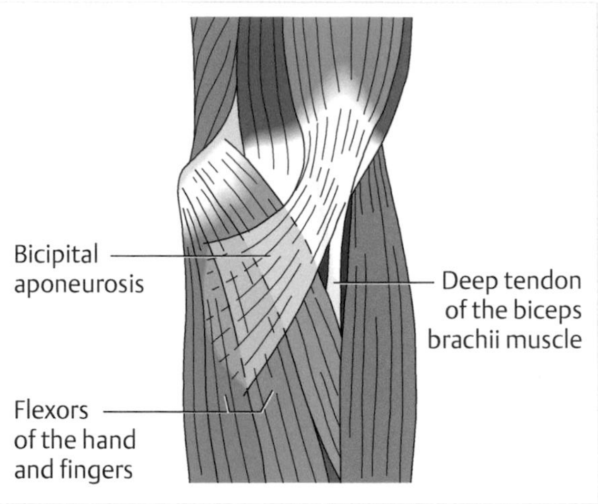


**Fig. 5.53** Biceps tendon and bicipital aponeurosis.

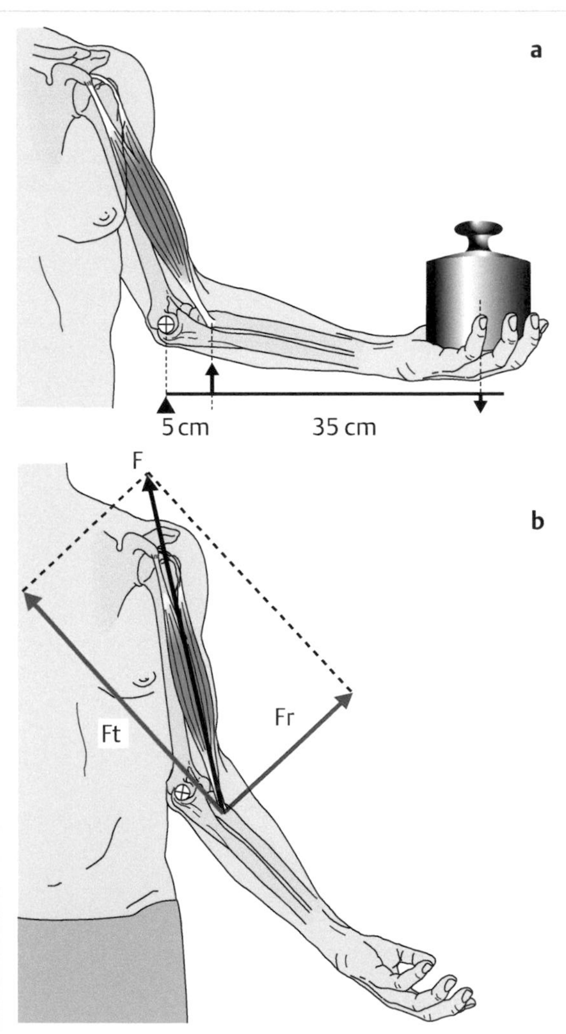


**Fig. 5.54 (a)** Biceps brachii muscle as a third-class lever. **(b)** Mechanics of the work of the biceps brachii muscle in the 45° flexed position. Ft, tendon force; Fr, rotatory vector; F, resultant force.

## Brachialis Muscle (Fig. 5.55)

- Together with the brachioradialis muscle, it forms a tunnel through which the radial nerve runs.
- The biceps muscle lies directly over the brachialis muscle.

**Function.** It is an important flexor as it can fulfill its function in both supination and pronation.

## Brachioradialis Muscle (Fig. 5.56)

**Functions:**
- Flexion: Brachoradialis has its best flexor effect in the midposition between pronation and supination.
- From maximal supination, it produces pronation up until the midposition, and from maximum pronation, it produces supination.

With increasing flexion, it loses the supinator effect. In maximal flexion, it exclusively pronates.

The following muscles help with flexion of the elbow:
- Pronator teres muscle (**Fig. 5.56**).
- Extensor carpi radialis longus muscle (**Fig. 5.57**).
- Flexor carpi ulnaris and flexor carpi radialis muscles (only minimally).

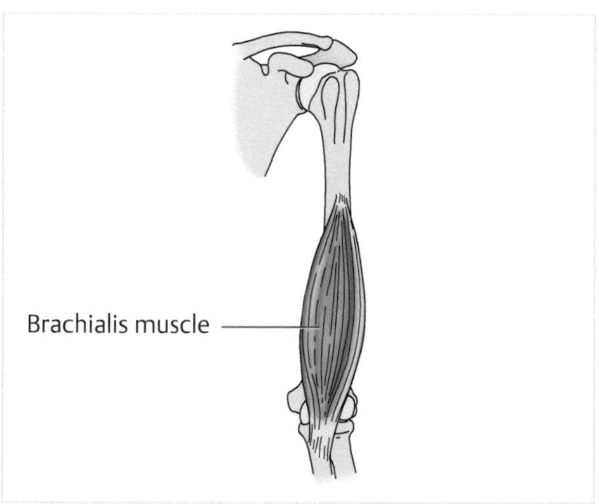


**Fig. 5.55** Brachialis muscle.

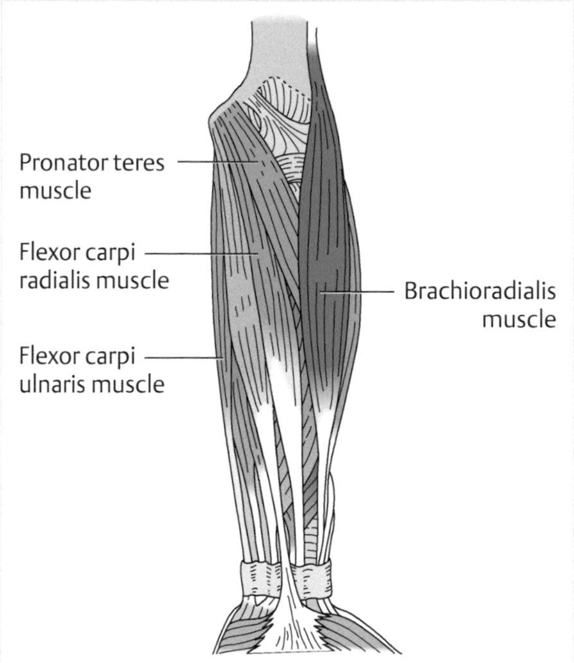


**Fig. 5.56** Flexors of the elbow: the brachioradialis, pronator teres, flexor carpi ulnaris, and radialis muscles.

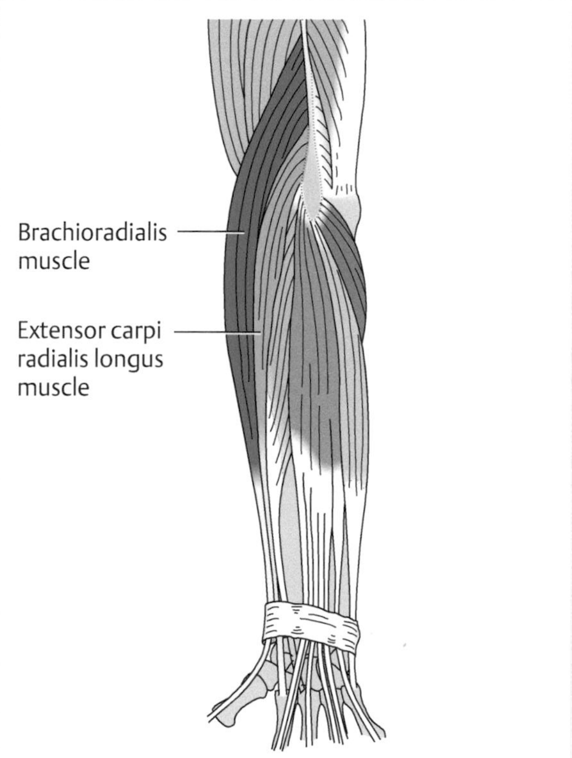


**Fig. 5.57** Flexors of the elbow: extensor carpi radialis longus muscle.

## 5.2.6 Muscles: Extensors (Fig. 5.58)

### Triceps Brachii Muscle

- The medial and lateral heads, together with the radial groove, form the radial canal, in which the radial nerve and accompanying blood vessels run.
- Many of the fibers of the triceps muscle extend into the antebrachial fascia, thereby merging directly into the extensor carpi radialis brevis muscle. Training the triceps muscle can therefore strengthen the latter as well.

**Function.** Extension of the elbow; the medial head is the strongest part.

### Anconeus Muscle

This runs immediately distal to the lateral head of the triceps muscle and is considered to be a continuation of it.

**Function.** Due to its origin on the capsule, it influences the state of tension of the joint capsule and prevents the posterior parts of the capsule from shifting into the joint during extension.

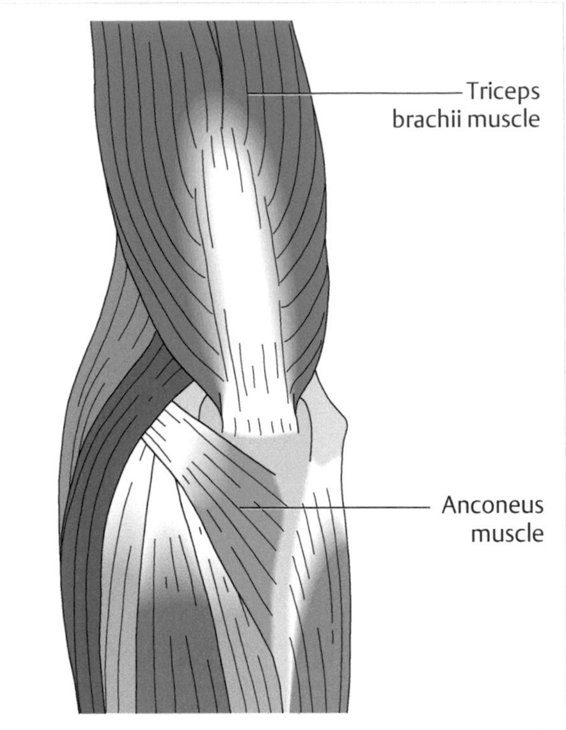


**Fig. 5.58** Extensor muscles of the elbow: triceps brachii and anconeus muscles.

## 5.2.7 Muscles: Pronators (Fig. 5.59)

### Pronator Teres Muscle

The humeral and ulnar heads form the pronator canal, in which the median nerve runs.

**Function.** Pronation, especially with the elbow flexed (it lessens in extension); elbow flexion.

### Pronator Quadratus Muscle

- This flat muscle runs transversely between the palmar aspects of the distal radius and ulna.
- It runs deeply, directly over the interosseous membrane. Deeper lying parts extend into the membrane and to the joint capsule of the distal radio-ulnar joint.

**Function.** Pronation, independent of the flexion or extension position of the elbow. It tenses the capsule of the distal radio-ulnar joint.

*Synergists:* Brachioradialis muscle (especially in elbow flexion and from maximal supination), extensor carpi radialis longus muscle and flexor carpi radialis muscle.

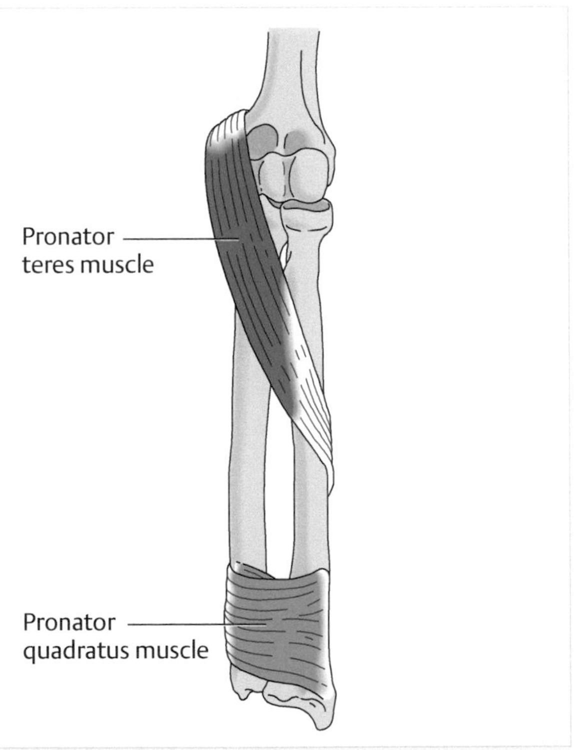


**Fig. 5.59** Pronators of the elbow: pronator teres and pronator quadratus muscles.

## 5.2.8 Muscles: Supinators

### Supinator Muscle (Fig. 5.60)

- This muscle connects to the annular ligament of the radius and to the joint capsule, from there it connects to the radial collateral ligament as well.
- It consists of superficial and deep parts.
- The upper border of the superficial part is strengthened by tendons and forms an arch, the *arcade of Frohse* (supinator arch). Here the radial nerve tracks through the supinator canal between the two parts of the muscle.

**Function.** Supination in both flexion and extension of the elbow. It initiates supination, and only thereafter is it supported by the biceps muscle. In addition, it stabilizes the lateral elbow region through its connection to the capsule and the collateral ligament.

### Further Supinators

- The biceps brachii muscle is the strongest supinator, with two to four times the power delivery.
- The brachioradialis muscle in also involved, but only from the position of maximal pronation to the mid-position.
- The following finger muscles, which run obliquely from ulnar to radial on the posterior side, also help (**Fig. 5.61**):
  - Extensor pollicis muscles.
  - Abductor pollicis longus muscle.
  - Extensor indicis muscle.

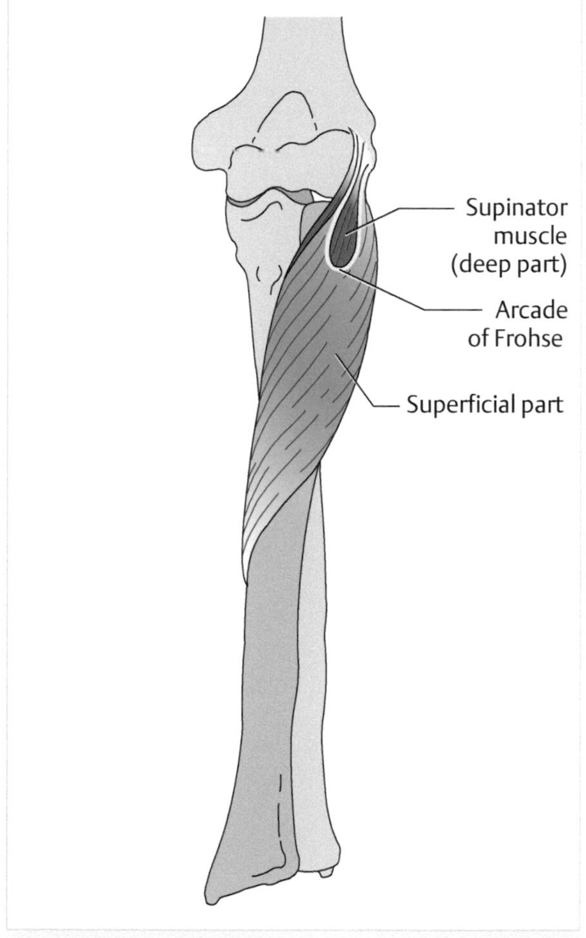


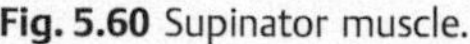
**Fig. 5.60** Supinator muscle.

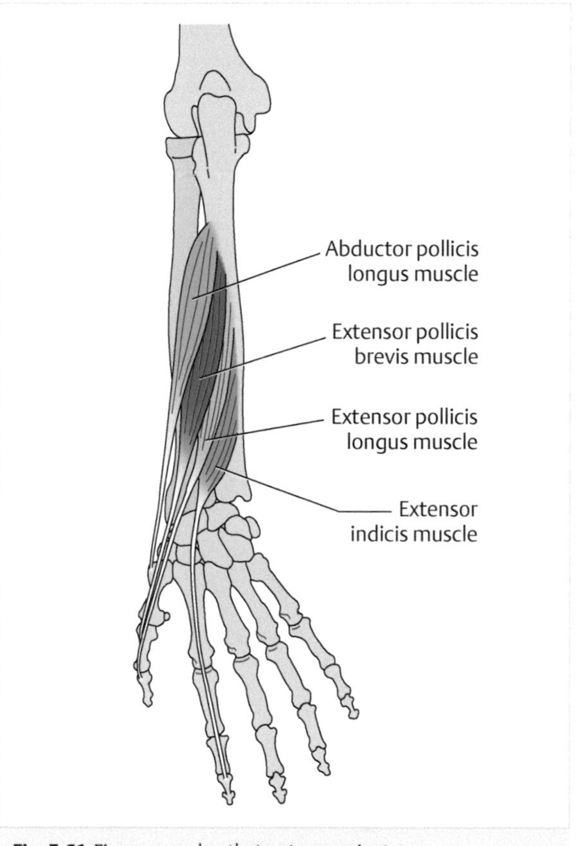


**Fig. 5.61** Finger muscles that act as supinators.

# 5.3 Course of Nerves in the Elbow Region

## Radial Nerve (Fig. 5.62)

The radial nerve runs within the *radial groove* between the medial and lateral heads of the triceps muscle. After leaving the canal, it pierces the lateral intermuscular septum of the arm. There it enters the anterior compartment, so that it lies within the gap between the brachialis and brachioradialis muscles and anterior to the lateral epicondyle. The two muscles, together with the lateral intermuscular septum of the arm, form the radial tunnel for the nerve. Just proximal to this (but sometimes not until the level of the elbow joint), the radial nerve divides into its superficial and deep branches.

The **deep branch of the radial nerve** is a motor branch that extends under the extensor carpi radialis muscle and then through the fibrous arch of the supinator muscle, the *arcade of Frohse*. In its further course, it lies between the two parts of this muscle, which form a canal, the supinator canal. It pierces the muscle in its distal region, runs on the dorsal side of the forearm, and here becomes the **posterior interosseous nerve**, which runs to the proximal wrist joint.

Before reaching the supinator compartment, the deep branch gives off branches to innervate the brachioradialis muscle and the radial wrist extensors, and, within the supinator canal, to the supinator muscle. Distal to the canal, it gives off branches to the finger and thumb extensors and to the abductor pollicis longus muscle.

The **superficial branch of the radial nerve** is a sensory branch that runs lateral to the radial artery under the anterior border of the brachioradialis muscle. At the level of the distal forearm, it extends onto the extensor side and divides into the dorsal digital nerves to supply the skin of the thumb, index finger, and half of the middle finger.

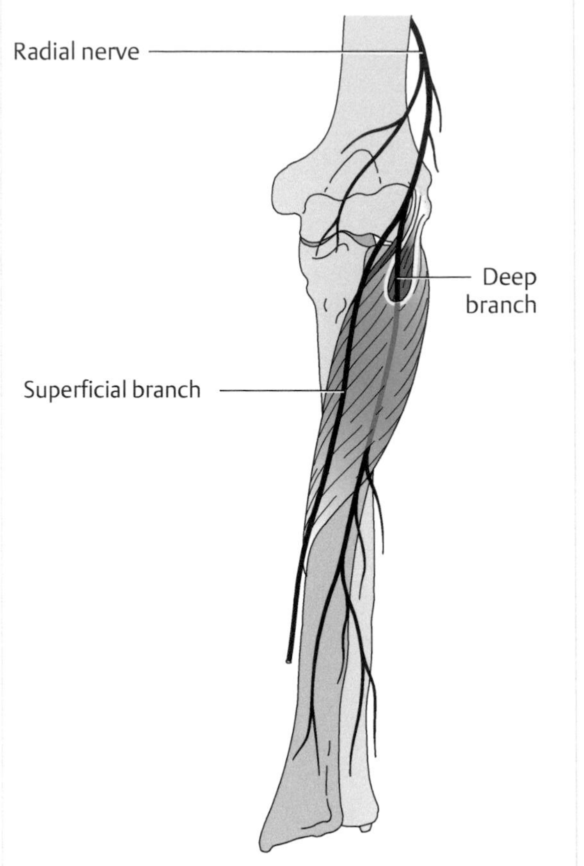


**Fig. 5.62** Course of the radial nerve in the supinator muscle region.

**Pathology**

Radial nerve lesion: The typical site for a compression injury to the radial nerve is in the area of the arcade or in the supinator canal. Because the sensory branch, having exited the radial stem earlier, is not affected in this case, this injury causes purely motor symptoms—wrist drop.

## Median Nerve (Fig. 5.63)

This nerve runs on the medial side of the brachial artery toward the cubital fossa under the bicipital aponeurosis. Further distally, it lies between the two heads of the pronator teres muscle, pierces it, and runs down between the flexor digitorum profundus and superficialis muscles toward the hand.

*Branches*

- Under the bicipital aponeurosis, it gives off branches to the pronator teres, flexor carpi radialis, palmaris longus, and flexor digitorum superficialis muscles.
- Distal to the pronator teres muscle, the anterior interosseous nerve branches off, extends to the pronator quadratus muscle, and innervates it and the flexors of the thumb and second and third fingers.

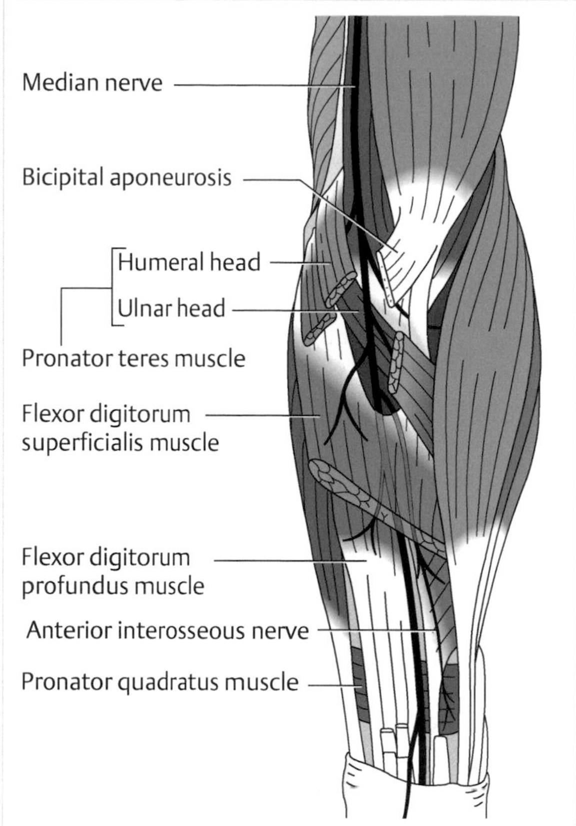


**Fig. 5.63** Course of the median nerve in the elbow region.

**Pathology**

If the pronator teres muscle becomes hypertonic through frequently repeated pronation movements, it can compress the median nerve. The same applies to the bicipital aponeurosis.

**Practical Tip**

Provocation testing of the injured median nerve within the pronator bottleneck is performed through maximal supination and extension or through pronation against resistance.

## Ulnar Nerve (Fig. 5.64)

The ulnar nerve runs down the extensor side of the distal humerus and further distally through the groove for the ulnar nerve. It reaches the flexor side of the forearm between the two heads of the flexor carpi ulnaris muscle and extends between the flexor carpi ulnaris and the flexor digitorum profundus muscles to the wrist joint.

*Branches*

- Immediately distal to the elbow joint, branches are given off to the flexor carpi ulnaris and the ulnar part of the flexor digitorum profundus muscles.
- In the final third of the forearm, it divides into its two terminal branches, the dorsal and palmar branches. The dorsal branch extends to the extensor side and the palmar branch extends on the flexor side toward the hypothenar region.

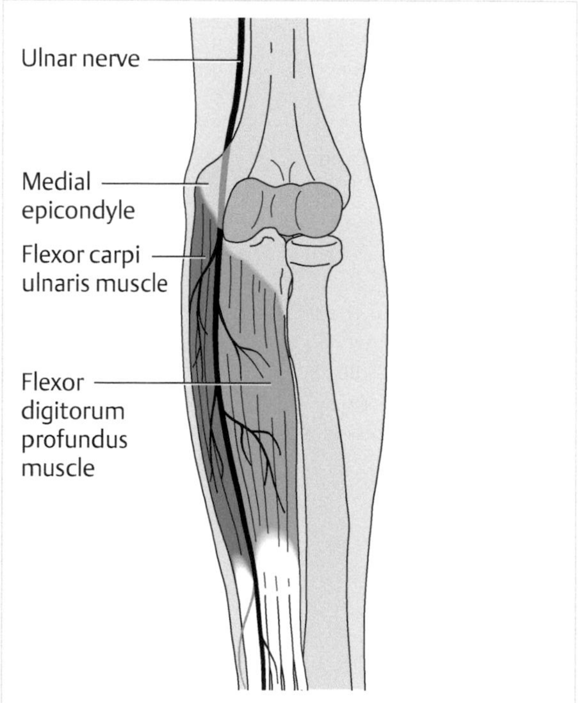


**Fig. 5.64** Course of the ulnar nerve in the elbow region.

**Pathology**

Ulnar nerve injury may occur due to compression within the groove from trauma or by propping oneself up on the elbows for a prolonged time.

# Chapter 6

## Hand and Wrist

# 6 Hand and Wrist

## 6.1 Palpation of Structures in the Hand and Wrist

### 6.1.1 Radial Side of the Hand and Wrist

#### Radial Styloid Process (Fig. 6.1)

Palpate this as a round process on the distal lateral end of the radius.

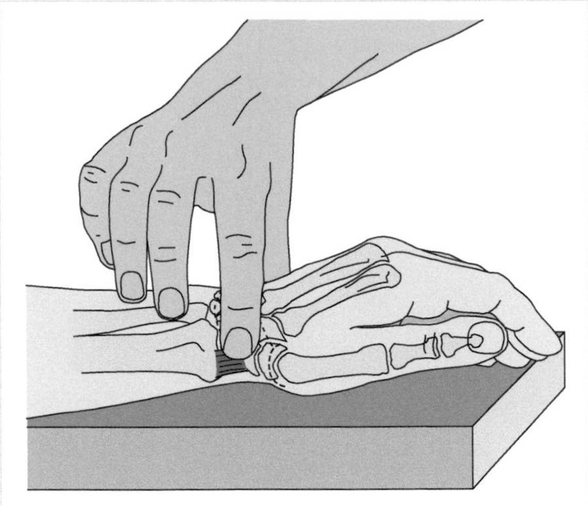

**Fig. 6.1** Palpation of the radial styloid process with the radial collateral ligament.

#### Radial Artery

Palpate the radial artery pulse on the palmar side of the styloid process, slightly proximal to it.

#### Radial Collateral Ligament (Fig. 6.1)

This extends from the radial styloid process to the scaphoid bone and is easier to palpate when it is tensed by ulnar abduction.

#### Scaphoid Bone (Fig. 6.2)

This bone lies directly distal to the radial styloid process. During ulnar abduction, it presses up against the palpating finger.

The **tubercle of the scaphoid bone** can be felt as an elevation on the palmar side at the level of the distal wrist crease under the tendon of the flexor carpi radialis muscle.

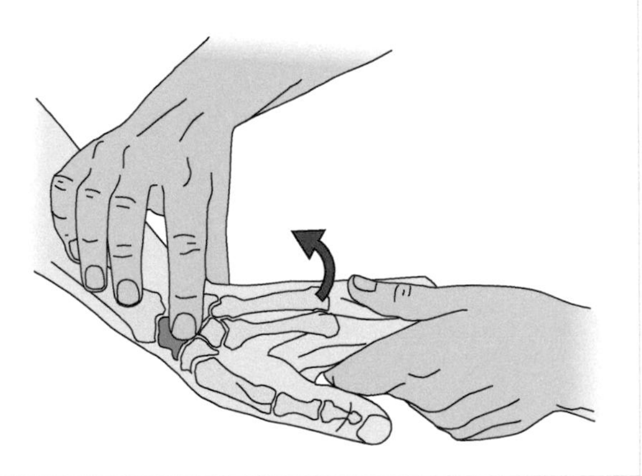

**Fig. 6.2** Palpation of the scaphoid bone.

#### Trapezium (Fig. 6.3)

The trapezium lies distal to the scaphoid bone. Palpate it by finding its prominence, the **tubercle of the trapezium**, directly proximal to the base of the first metacarpal on the palmar side.

#### Base of the First Metacarpal

This distinct, round proximal part of the first metacarpal can be palpated from both the radial and palmar sides. Passive circumduction of the thumb facilitates palpation.

#### Anatomical Snuffbox (Fig. 6.3)

This distinct hollow is recognizable by maximally extending the thumb.

The scaphoid and trapezium lie here deep within the depression. Its borders are as follows—proximal: styloid process of the radius; distal: base of the first metacarpal; radial: tendons of the abductor pollicis longus and extensor pollicis brevis muscles; dorsal: extensor pollicis longus tendon.

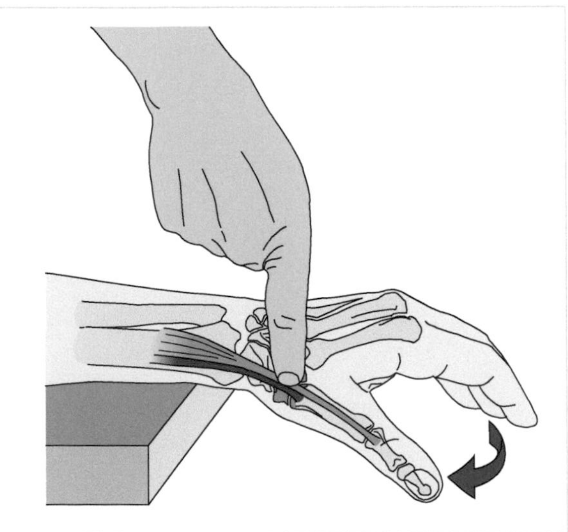

**Fig. 6.3** Palpation of the trapezium in the anatomical snuffbox.

## 6.1.2 Dorsum of the Hand and Wrist

### Capitate (Fig. 6.4)

This is located proximal to the base of the third metacarpal in a depression that is easily palpable on passive dorsiflexion.

### Trapezoid

This bone lies at the level of the capitate on the radial side and proximal to the base of the second metacarpal.

### Lunate

This lies to the ulnar side and proximal to the capitate bone. Its articulation with the scaphoid is located under the tendon of the extensor carpi radialis brevis muscle.

### Triquetrum

This is the first bony structure palpable distal to the ulnar styloid process. It shifts toward the ulnar side with radial abduction.

The pisiform bone, overlying it on the palmar side, helps with orientation.

### Hamate

This lies proximal to the bases of the fourth and fifth metacarpal bones.

**Pathology**

Hard, protruding structures called ganglia are often palpable in the area of the carpal bones. These can emanate from the periosteum, the capsule, or tendon sheaths. The presence of a ganglion indicates a dysfunction of one of these structures and will only resolve if the disturbance is eliminated. This is why they invariably disappear and reappear.

### Dorsal Tendon Compartments

### First Tendon Compartment (Fig. 6.5)

- Abductor pollicis longus muscle.
- Extensor pollicis brevis muscle.

Both these muscles border the anatomical snuffbox on the radial side. They lie close together. Tensing the thumb in extension alternating with abduction elucidates the course of each tendon. The extensor tendon runs dorsally and extends to the base of the proximal phalanx. That of the abductor lies on the palmar side and extends to the base of the first metacarpal.

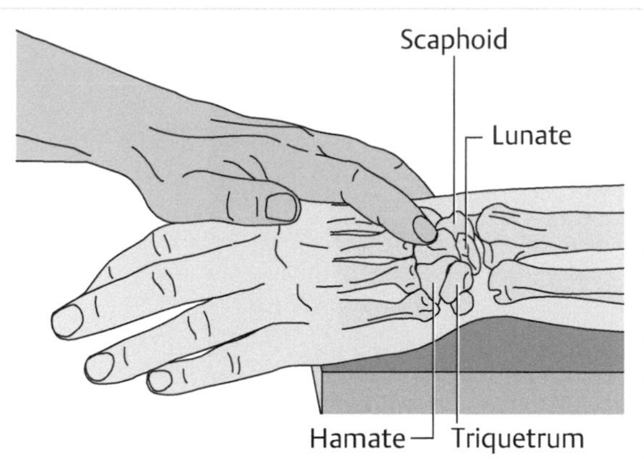


**Fig. 6.4** Palpation of the carpal bones; here, the capitate bone.

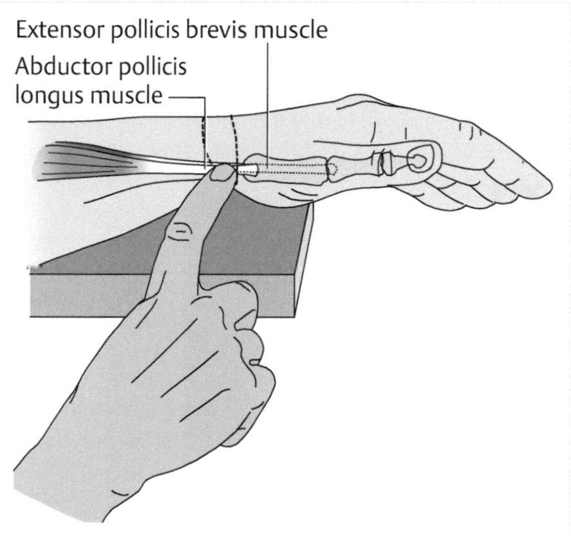


**Fig. 6.5** Palpation of the first tendon compartment.

**Pathology**

When de Quervain's tenosynovitis is suspected, one can test both tendons with provocation with direct pressure as well as with resistance and stretch testing.

## Second Tendon Compartment (Fig. 6.6)

- Extensor carpi radialis longus muscle.
- Extensor carpi radialis brevis muscle.

The tendons can be palpated as thick, round cords proximal to the bases of the second and third metacarpals. The tendon of the extensor carpi radialis brevis muscle extends to the base of the third metacarpal. This can be found easily and followed proximally by balling the hand into a loose fist and tensing in dorsiflexion.

Tensing the wrist in dorsiflexion and radial abduction aids in finding the tendon of the extensor carpi radialis longus muscle proximal to the base of the second metacarpal. The tendons can be palpated over the scaphoid bone as they separate in a V-shape.

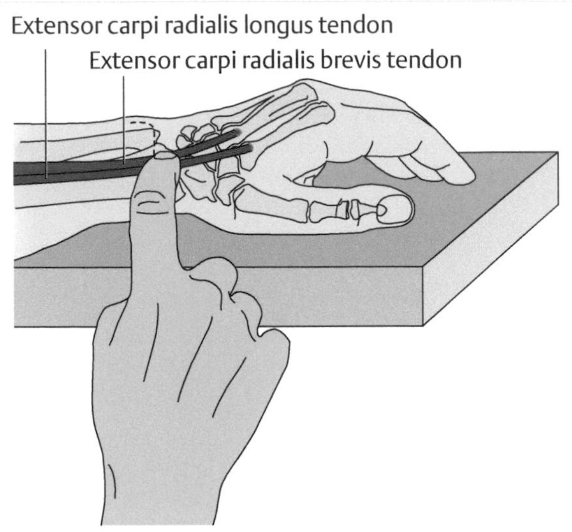


**Fig. 6.6** Palpation of the second tendon compartment.

## Third Tendon Compartment (Fig. 6.7)

- Extensor pollicis longus muscle.

Because the tendon uses Lister's tubercle (dorsal tubercle of the radius) as a hypomochlion, this can be used to follow its further course. The tubercle is located as a protruding point on the ulnar third of the radius in line with the proximal projection of the third metacarpal. From here, the tendon runs obliquely to the radial side to the base of the distal phalanx of the thumb. It borders the anatomical snuffbox dorsally and stands out clearly when extending the thumb.

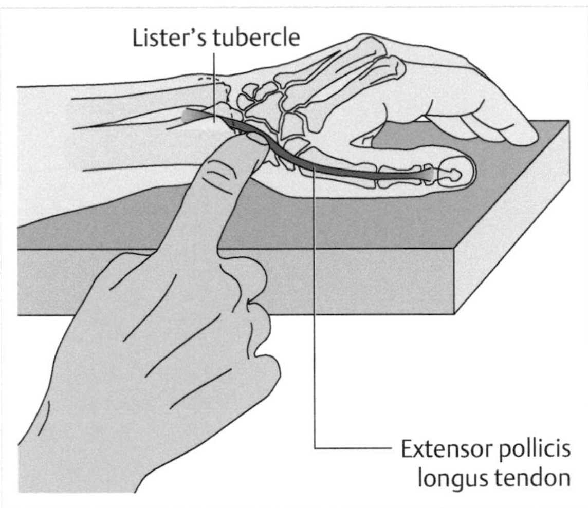


**Fig. 6.7** Palpation of the third tendon compartment.

## Fourth Tendon Compartment (Fig. 6.8)

- Extensor digitorum muscle.
- Extensor indicis muscle.

The tendon of the extensor digitorum muscle runs in the middle of the wrist and divides at the level of the proximal row of carpal bones into the four tendons that proceed to the bases of the terminal phalanges. The tendons stand out clearly on alternating flexion and extension movements of the fingers.

The tendon of the extensor indicis muscle runs ulnar to the extensor digitorum tendon.

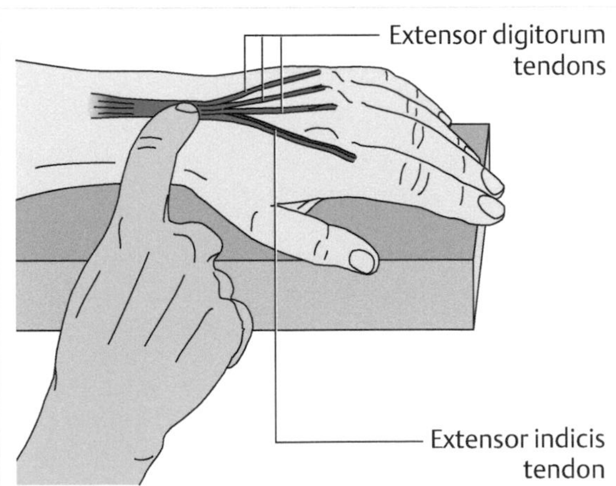


**Fig. 6.8** Palpation of the fourth tendon compartment.

## Fifth Tendon Compartment (Fig. 6.9)

- Extensor digiti minimi muscle.

This runs on the ulnar side of the tendon of the extensor digitorum muscle. It lies over the distal radio-ulnar joint, which is found along a line extending from the fourth metacarpal. To facilitate its palpation, lay the hand flat and extend the little finger.

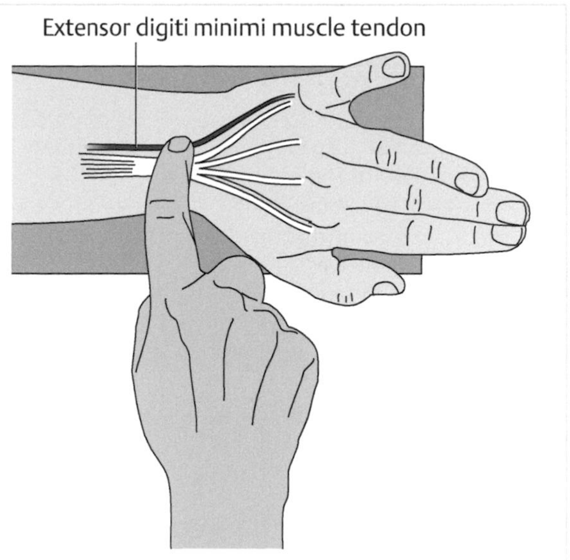


**Fig. 6.9** Palpation of the fifth tendon compartment.

## Sixth Tendon Compartment (Fig. 6.10)

- Extensor carpi ulnaris muscle.

The tendon extends from the ulnar head and the ulnar styloid process to the base of the fifth metacarpal. Tensing toward dorsiflexion and ulnar abduction allows for good palpation of the course of the tendon.

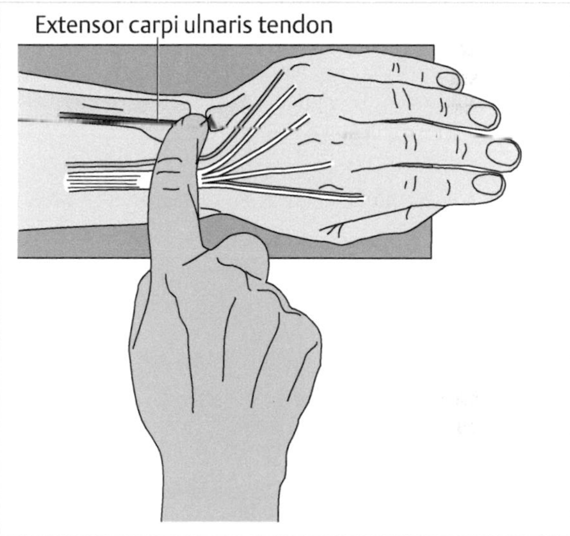


**Fig. 6.10** Palpation of the sixth tendon compartment.

# 6.1.3 Ulnar Side of the Hand and Wrist

## Ulnar Styloid Process (Fig. 6.11)

This can be palpated as a clearly protruding extension ulnar and distal to the ulnar head. It lies further proximally than the radial styloid process.

## Ulnar Collateral Ligament (Fig. 6.11)

This extends from the ulnar styloid process to the triquetrum. Radial abduction causes it to come under tension, making it more distinctly palpable.

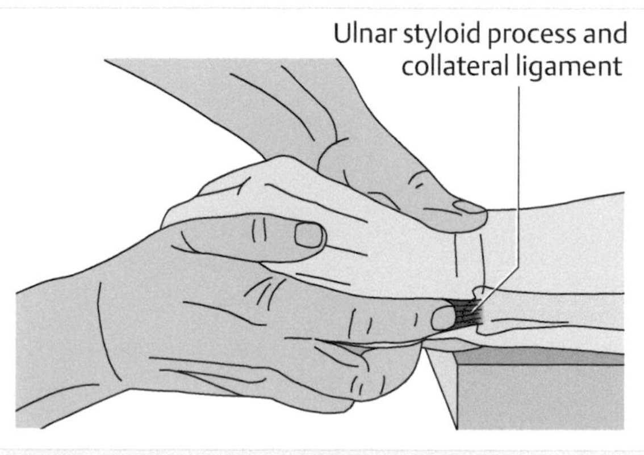


**Fig. 6.11** Palpation of the ulnar collateral ligament.

## 6.1.4 Palmar Region

### Pisiform Bone (Fig. 6.12)

The pisiform bone is found as a distinctly protruding point at the level of the distal wrist crease at its ulnar end. In the position of relaxed palmar flexion, it can be moved over the triquetrum bone from the radial to the ulnar side.

By tensing in palmar flexion and abduction of the little finger, the flexor carpi ulnaris and abductor digiti minimi muscles fixate it in place.

### Ulnar Artery

The artery can be palpated just proximal to the pisiform bone.

### Hook of the Hamate (Fig. 6.13)

This well-padded, protruding bony point is located on the palmar side of the hamate bone. It can be located by placing the interphalangeal joint of the palpating thumb on the patient's pisiform bone and pointing the tip of the thumb obliquely toward the palm. The hook now lies under the tip of the thumb and can be palpated as a round prominence by using firm palpation through the muscles of the hypothenar eminence.

### Guyon's Canal (Ulnar Canal) (Fig. 6.14)

This is located between the pisiform bone and the hook of the hamate. The pisohamate ligament extends over the canal and protects the ulnar nerve, which runs deep within it, from compression.

**Pathology**

Putting pressure on this canal can trigger typical nerve pain, such as an uncomfortable prickling feeling in the area of the little finger. A healthy nerve will perceive these as mildly uncomfortable sensations, whereas the pain reaction is significantly greater when nerve irritation is present.

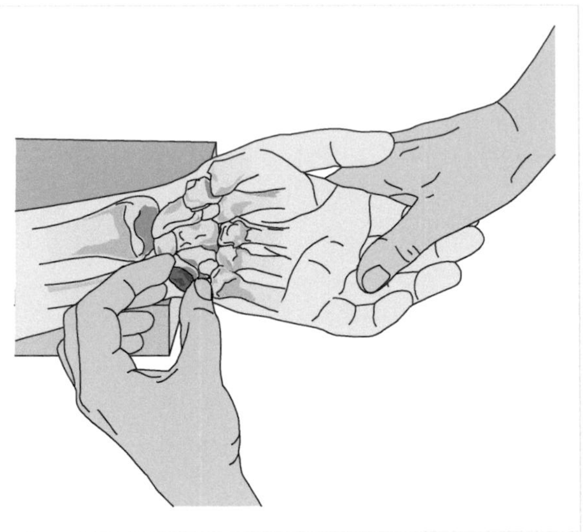

**Fig. 6.12** Palpation of the pisiform bone.

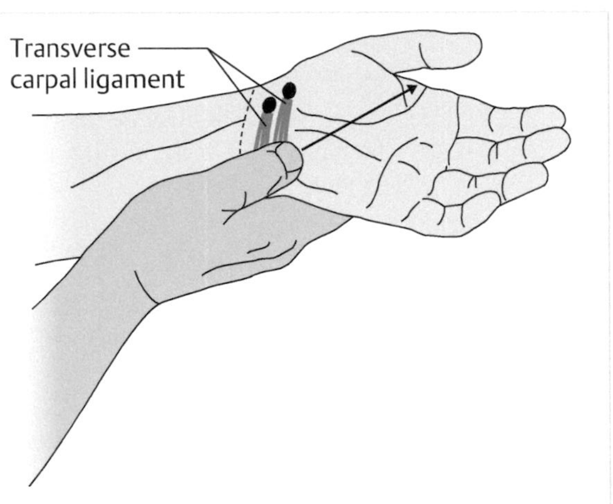


**Fig. 6.13** Palpation of the hook of the hamate.

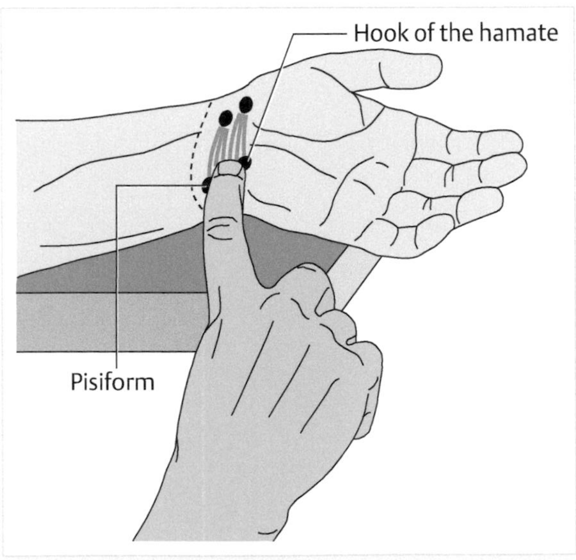


**Fig. 6.14** Palpation of Guyon's canal.

## Transverse Carpal Ligament (Flexor Retinaculum) (Fig. 6.15)

This is a ligamentous structure that extends transversely over the carpal bones. It consists of two main bands:

- The proximal part runs from the pisiform to the tubercle of the scaphoid bone.
- The distal band goes from the hook of the hamate to the tubercle of the trapezium.

A distinctive wrist crease results from the fixation of the transverse carpal ligament to the skin. This is where the ligament begins on the proximal side. About a thumb's breadth distally is the distal border of this transverse connection.

Place the palpating finger between the bony structures described above and move it transversely and longitudinally to the orientation of the fibers.

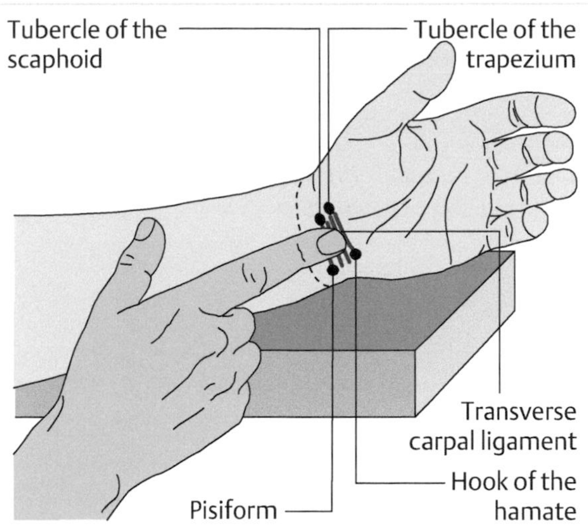


**Fig. 6.15** Palpation of the flexor retinaculum.

> **Practical Tip**
>
> The retinaculum borders the carpal tunnel on the palmar side. Firm pressure on the retinaculum can compress the tendons and the median nerve running under it—a test that is very painful in carpal tunnel syndrome.

## Palmar Tendons

### Flexor Pollicis Longus Muscle (Fig. 6.16)

This tendon can be palpated near the radial pulse between the tendons of the brachioradialis and flexor carpi radialis muscles while tensing the thumb in flexion.

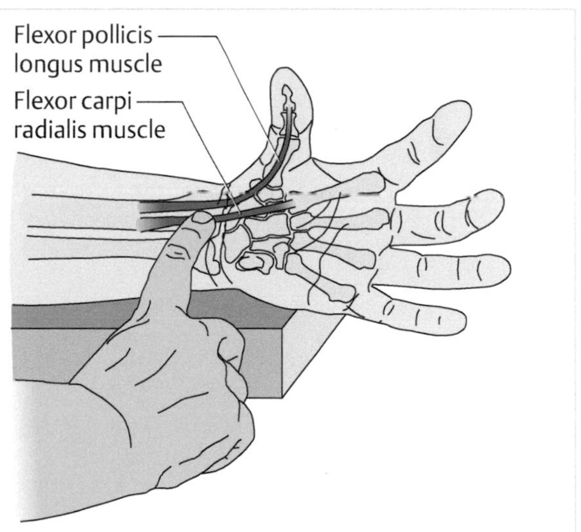


**Fig. 6.16** Palpation of the flexor pollicis longus and flexor carpi radialis muscle tendons.

### Flexor Carpi Radialis Muscle (Fig. 6.16)

This extends to the base of the second metacarpal and crosses the scaphoid bone en route. The tendon can be palpated as a clearly demarcated, round strand running toward the thenar eminence.

Tense the hand in a position with the fingers extended and the wrist in palmar flexion and radial abduction.

### Flexor Digitorum Superficialis Muscle (Fig. 6.17)

Its tendons run immediately ulnar to the flexor carpi radialis muscle. To find the tendons more easily, place the hand with the dorsal side down on the table and then move the fingers in flexion.

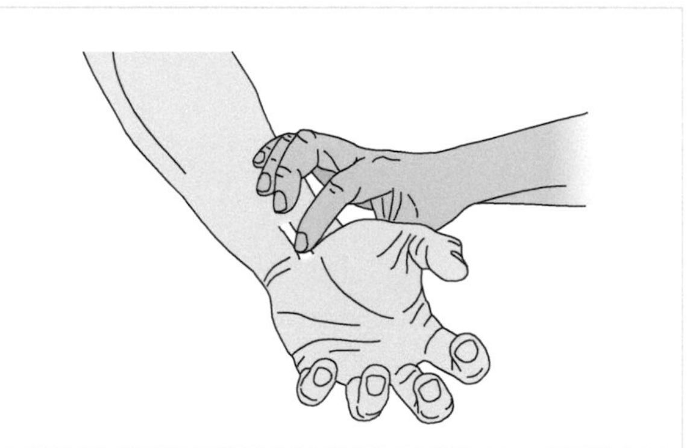

**Fig. 6.17** Palpation of the flexor digitorum superficialis tendon.

## Flexor Digitorum Profundus Muscle

The tendons of the flexor digitorum profundus muscle lie deep under those of the flexor digitorum superficialis and can only be differentiated from them with great difficulty. Because the profundus flexes the distal interphalangeal (DIP) joints while the superficialis flexes the proximal interphalangeal (PIP) joints, it is possible to differentiate them by tensing the distal joints in flexion.

## Palmaris Longus Muscle (Fig. 6.18)

The palmaris longus muscle has the most superficial tendon, which runs in the middle of the wrist joint. It can be palpated by tensing the wrist in palmar flexion with the thumb and little finger opposed.

## Median Nerve

The nerve can be identified as a very firm, round strand directly under and slightly radial to the tendon of the palmaris longus muscle.

## Flexor Carpi Ulnaris Muscle (Fig. 6.19)

The tendon runs into and inserts on the ulnar side of the pisiform bone as a thick, round strand. In addition, offshoots extend toward the hamate bone and the fifth metacarpal. Tensing in palmar flexion and ulnar abduction with the fingers extended facilitates palpation.

## Palmar Aponeurosis (Fig. 6.20)

The aponeurosis is an extension of the palmaris longus muscle. Its exact borders are difficult to locate because of the density of the subcutaneous tissue.

**Pathology**

In Dupuytren's contracture, the aponeurosis contracts, especially in area of the ring finger, and draws the finger into a flexed position.

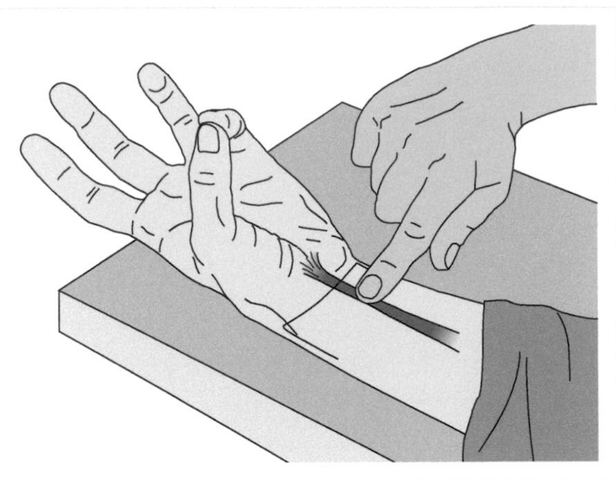

**Fig. 6.18** Palpation of the palmaris longus muscle tendon.

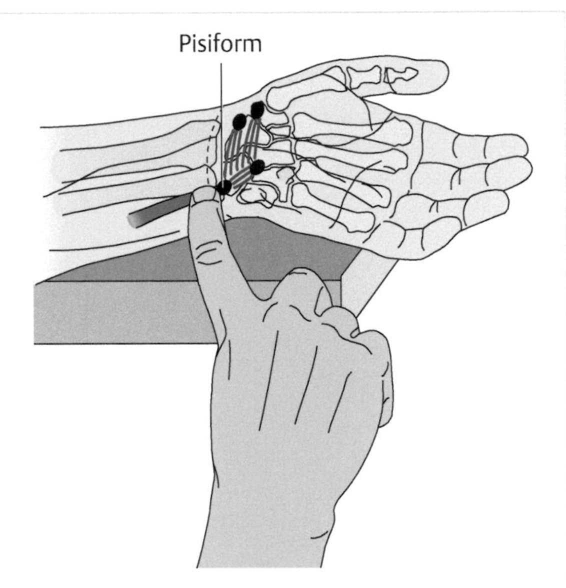


**Fig. 6.19** Palpation of the flexor carpi ulnaris muscle tendon.

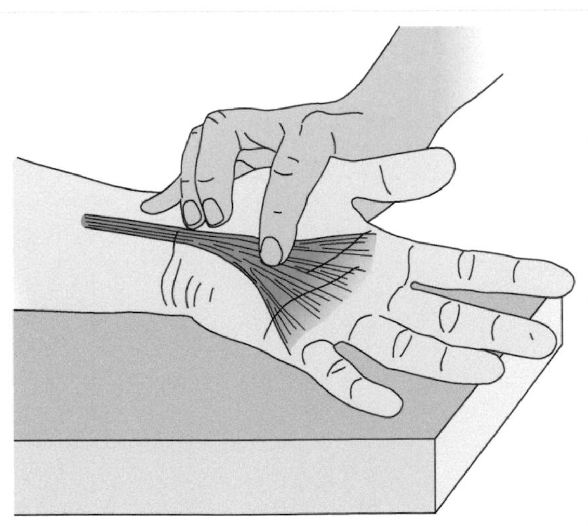

**Fig. 6.20** Palpation of the palmar aponeurosis.

### Thenar Muscles (Fig. 6.21)

From distal to proximal, starting from the area of the proximal transverse palmar crease, from the index finger right up to the radial border of the thumb, the following muscles can be palpated while tensing the appropriate muscle:

- Adductor pollicis muscle.
- Flexor pollicis brevis muscle.
- Abductor pollicis brevis muscle.
- Opponens pollicis muscle.

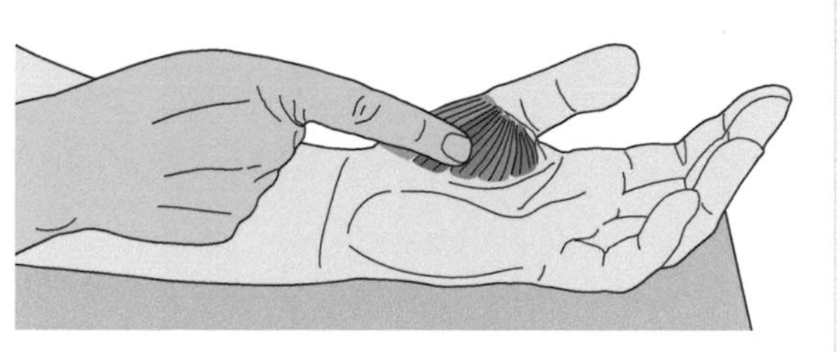

**Fig. 6.21** Palpation of the thenar muscles.

### Hypothenar Muscles (Fig. 6.22)

While the little finger is being abducted, the abductor digiti minimi can be palpated as the muscle furthest to the ulnar side of the hypothenar eminence, as it runs parallel to the first metacarpal bone. Then come the following, moving toward the palm:

- Flexor digiti minimi brevis muscle.
- Opponens digiti minimi muscle.

Tensing the appropriate muscle helps with palpation.

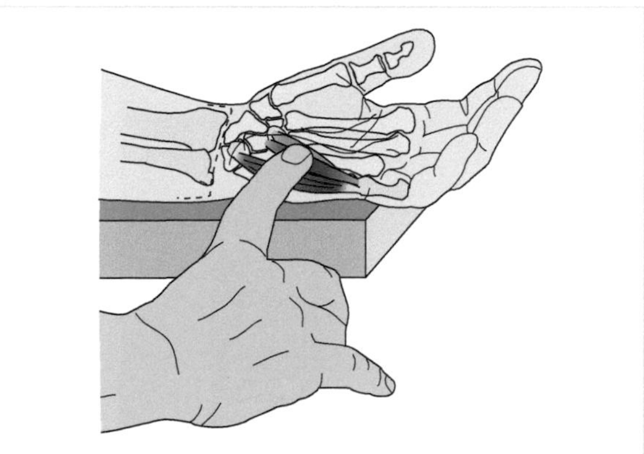

**Fig. 6.22** Palpation of the hypothenar muscles.

## 6.1.5 Phalanges

### Metacarpophalangeal Joints (Fig. 6.23)

While passively moving the finger in flexion, the joint space of each finger can be palpated on both sides of the extensor tendon approximately 1 cm distal to the proximal tip of the phalanx.

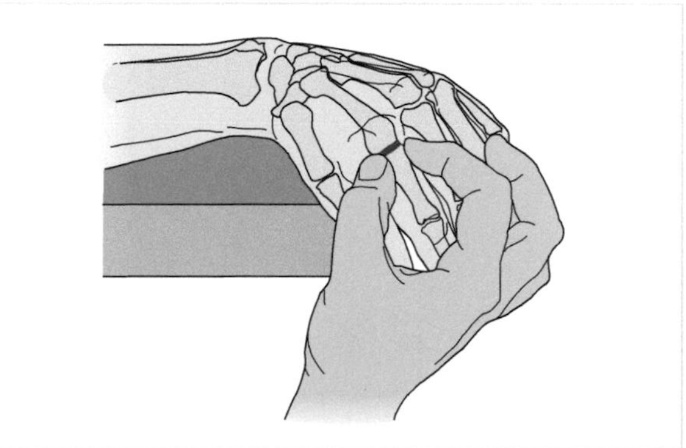

**Fig. 6.23** Palpation of the second metacarpophalangeal joint.

### Interphalangeal Joints (Fig. 6.24)

On the dorsal side, both the proximal (PIP) and the distal (DIP) joints can be palpated immediately next to the extensor tendons while passively flexing and extending the finger.

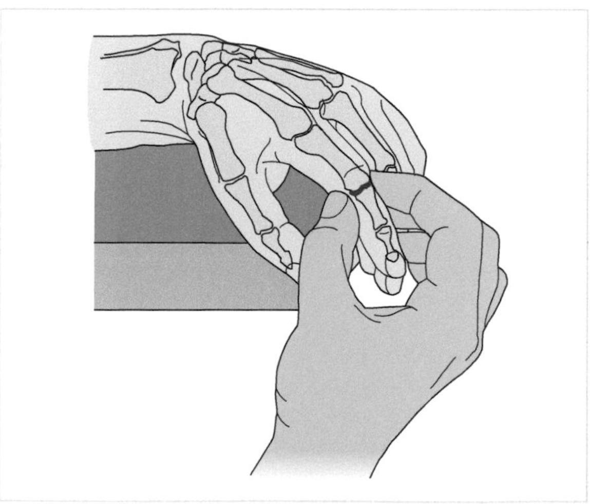

**Fig. 6.24** Palpation of the second proximal interphalangeal ▸ joint.

# 6.2 Functional Anatomy of the Hand and Wrist

## 6.2.1 X-Ray of the Hand and Wrist

### Posteroanterior View of the Wrist (Dorsopalmar View) (Fig. 6.25)

In the neutral position (0°):

- The angle of inclination of the radius in relation to the ulna distally is the base angle; normal: 20°.
- The proximal wrist joint (radiocarpal joint) and a portion of the distal wrist joint (midcarpal joint) form smooth, harmonious arcs running parallel to each other.
- Check the position of the carpal bones to each other and in relation to the radius and ulna and to the bases of the metacarpals.

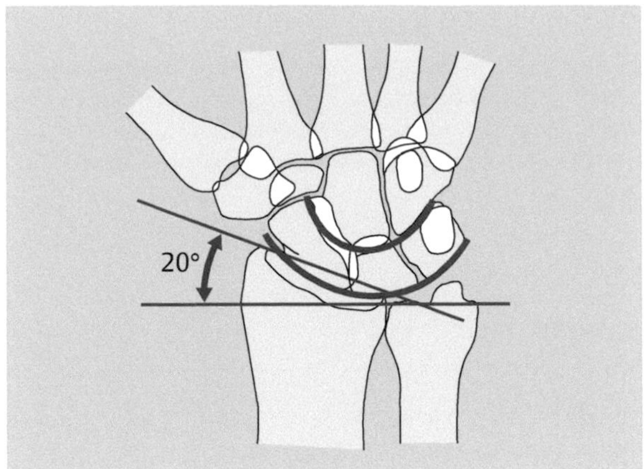


**Fig. 6.25** X-ray of the wrist: posteroanterior view.

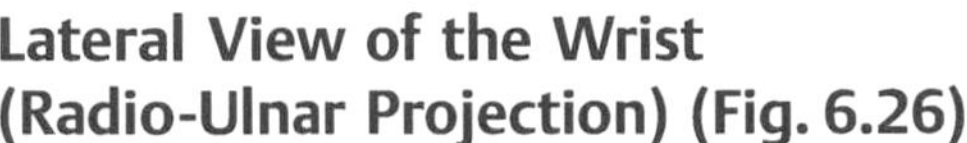

### Lateral View of the Wrist (Radio-Ulnar Projection) (Fig. 6.26)

- Typical shape of the lunate bone.
- Palmar tilt of the radius: 10°.
- Capitolunate angle: 10 to 20°.
- Scaphocapitate angle: 40 to 50°.

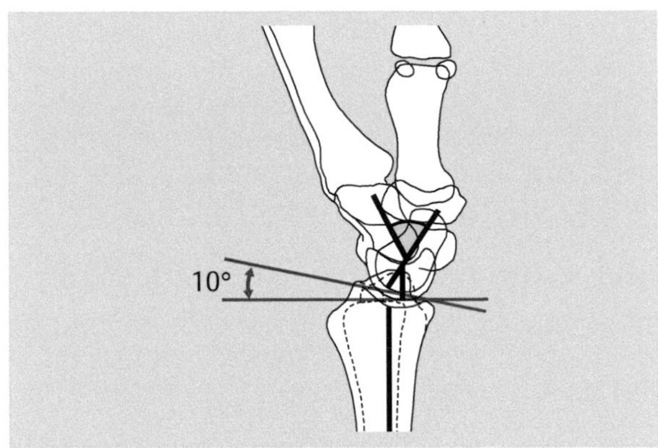


**Fig. 6.26** X-ray of the wrist: lateral view.

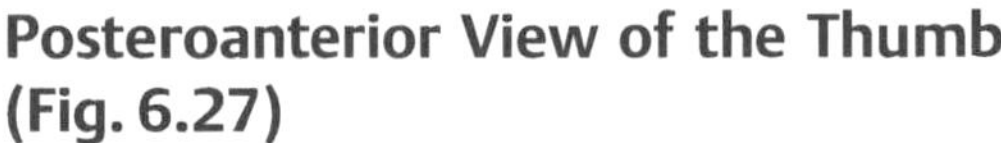

### Posteroanterior View of the Thumb (Fig. 6.27)

- The first carpometacarpal joint is saddle-shaped.
- A sesamoid bone can be seen at the head of the first metacarpal.
- The metacarpophalangeal (MCP) and interphalangeal joint space width: normal: 2 mm.

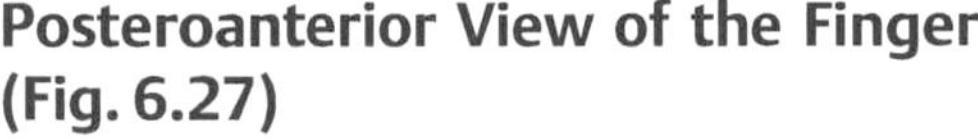

### Posteroanterior View of the Finger (Fig. 6.27)

- Shape of joint surfaces: slightly undulating.
- Normal width of joint spaces:
  - MCP joint: approximately 2 mm.
  - PIP joint: 1.5 mm.
  - DIP joint: 1 mm.

Stress views show the extent of instability in cases of ligament injury.

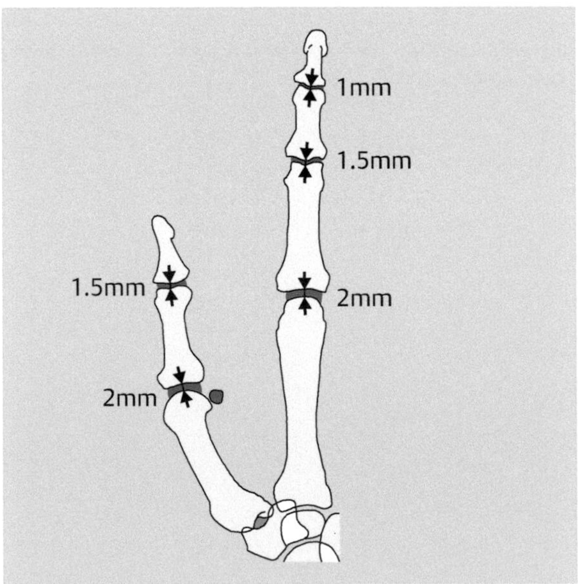


**Fig. 6.27** X-ray of the finger and thumb in the neutral position: posteroanterior view.

**Pathology**

Fractures in the carpal area are often only detectable using tomography or by a fine ossification line that develops after 2 to 3 weeks.

Indications of polyarthritis: Erosions in the joint contours, narrowing of the joint space, thickening of the subchondral spongiosa, small subchondral cysts, and areas of calcification in the joint capsule occur.

Tendinoses and ligamentoses are represented by the ossification of tendon or ligament insertion sites as humped and pin-like shapes or as calcium deposition a few millimeters away from the insertion site.

## 6.2.2 Wrist Joint (Fig. 6.28)

The wrist joint is composed of the **radiocarpal joint** proximally and the **midcarpal joint** distally.

The joint lines are quite varied: that of the radiocarpal joint runs in a harmonious arc, while the midcarpal joint is notched.

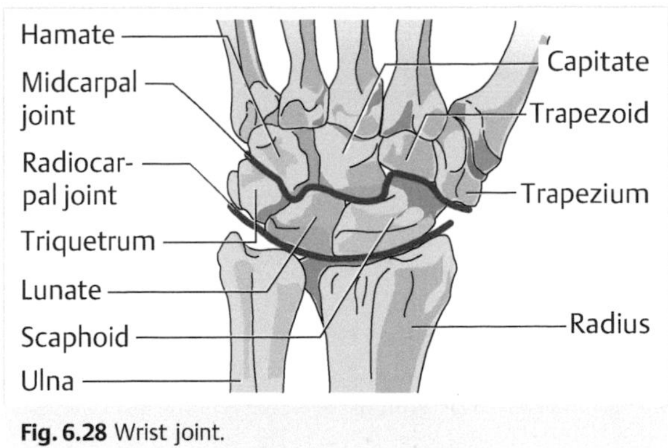


**Fig. 6.28** Wrist joint.

### Radiocarpal Joint

### Joint Surfaces

#### *Proximal Row of Carpal Bones (Fig. 6.29)*

The distal joint partners consist of the scaphoid, lunate, and triquetrum bones.

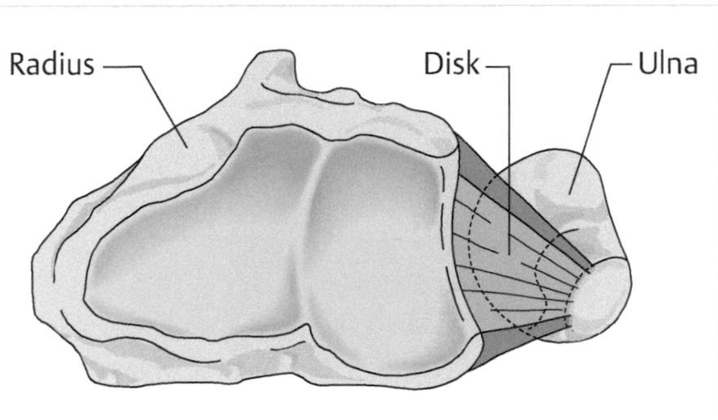


**Fig. 6.29** Proximal joint surfaces of the wrist joint.

#### *Radius*

The distal end of the radius has concave facets: a triangular one for the scaphoid bone and an oval one for the lunate bone. The two joint surfaces are separated by a small elevation.

#### *Radius Joint Surface Angle (Fig. 6.30a)*

This angle is determined from a base line that is 90° from the longitudinal axis of the radius and extends through the ulnar edge of the radius. The second line connects the tip of the radial styloid process with the ulnar edge of the radius. This tangent runs obliquely, resulting in an angle of approximately 20°.

#### *Sagittal Radius Joint Angle (Fig. 6.30b)*

This angle, also called the **radius tilt**, is observed from the side. Of the two lines forming the angle, one is a perpendicular to the longitudinal axis of the radius and the other is a tangent through the dorsal and palmar edge points of the radius. Viewed from the radial side, the dorsal radial edge is further distal than the palmar, so that the joint socket is tilted approximately 10°.

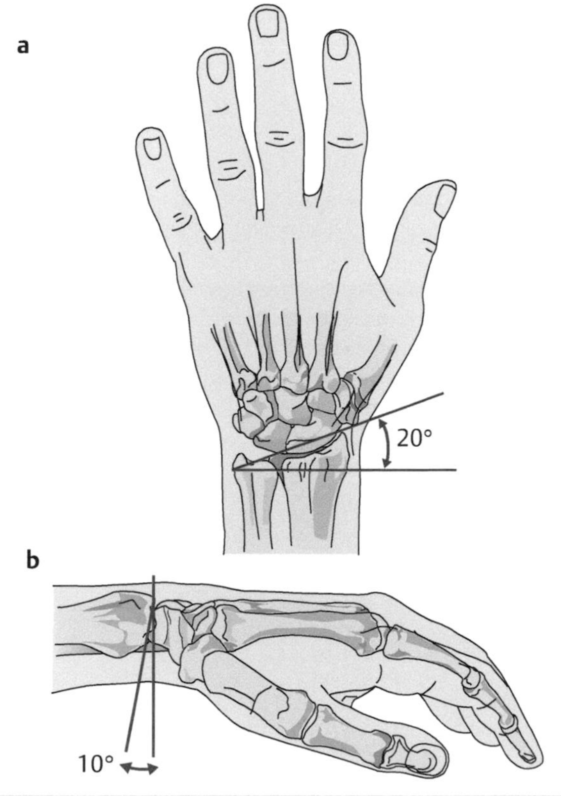


**Figure 6.30** Inclination of the radius. **(a)** Radius joint surface angle. **(b)** Sagittal radius joint angle.

**Practical Tip**

Due to the oblique orientation, the carpal bones on the dorsal side are palpated further distally than on the palmar side.

### *Articular Disk (Fig. 6.31)*

The articular disk lies distal to the ulna and forms the concave joint surface for parts of the lunate and triquetrum bones.

Seen from distally, it has a triangular shape. It is thin in the center, and becomes thicker towards its margins. The base of the disk is attached to the radius distal to the ulnar notch of the radius. Its tip is affixed to the inner side of the ulnar styloid process and to the ulnar collateral ligament of the wrist joint.

The palmar and dorsal borders of the disk merge with the joint capsule as well as with the ligaments that connect the triquetrum bone with the lunate bone. On the radial side, palmar and dorsal bands of fibers of the radio-ulnar ligaments extend into the disk. On the palmar side, it is also strengthened by a few fibrous bands of connective tissue called the **triangular ligament**. A few fibers join with the tendon sheath of the extensor carpi ulnaris muscle.

Appropriate to the tensile forces and compressive load that it has to handle, the disk consists of fibrocartilage with some hyaline cartilage.

Nutrition for the disk is supplied by the dorsal and palmar vascular arches. However, the branches only penetrate into the outer layers; the remaining disk area is avascular.

During the movements of pronation and supination, the radius takes the disk with it, so it has to slide against the ulna.

▷ See Chapter 5, Elbow

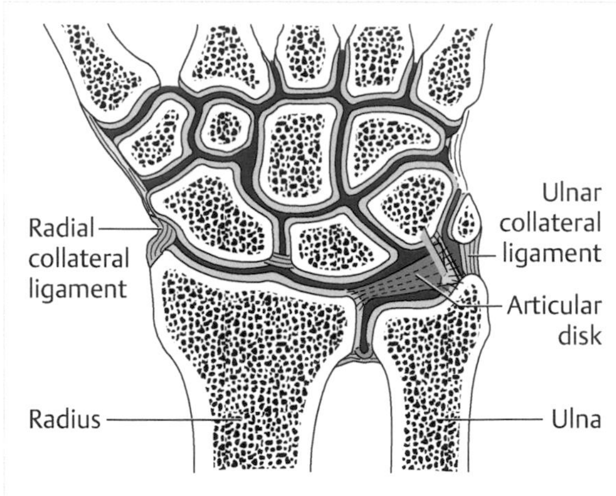


**Fig. 6.31** Articular disk of the distal radio-ulnar joint.

**Pathology**

Perforation of the disk, which is quite common in old age, produces an incongruity between the lunate and head of the ulna, so the loading of the joint cartilage becomes unphysiologic and a defect becomes apparent. In rheumatoid arthritis, disk destruction often occurs very early. This, along with synovial thickening in the distal radio-ulnar joint and in the communicating tendons of the fourth tendon compartment, causes the development of *ulnar head syndrome*. It is characterized by the gradual destruction of the ulnar head. Treatment consists of resection of the head of the ulna. As a result, there is a loss of stabilization of the ulnocarpal area and a change in the way force is transmitted.

## Midcarpal Joint (Fig. 6.32)

### Proximal Row of Carpal Bones

- The *scaphoid bone* has a somewhat pronounced convexity toward the trapezium and a small, concave, more ulnar-positioned facet to the capitate bone. There is a tubercle on the palmar side.
- The *lunate* has a concave facet facing the capitate bone.
- The *triquetrum* has a concave joint surface for its articulation with the hamate bone. On the palmar side, the pisiform bone can be seen as a clearly protruding structure.

### Distal Row of Carpal Bones

- The *trapezium* has a small, concave joint surface to the scaphoid bone. It has a tubercle on the palmar side.
- The *trapezoid* has a concave facet to the scaphoid bone.
- The *capitate bone*'s convex head articulates with the scaphoid bone and the lunate.
- The *hamate* has convex facets for the triquetrum and lunate bones. On the palmar side, there is a clear protuberance, the hook of the hamate.

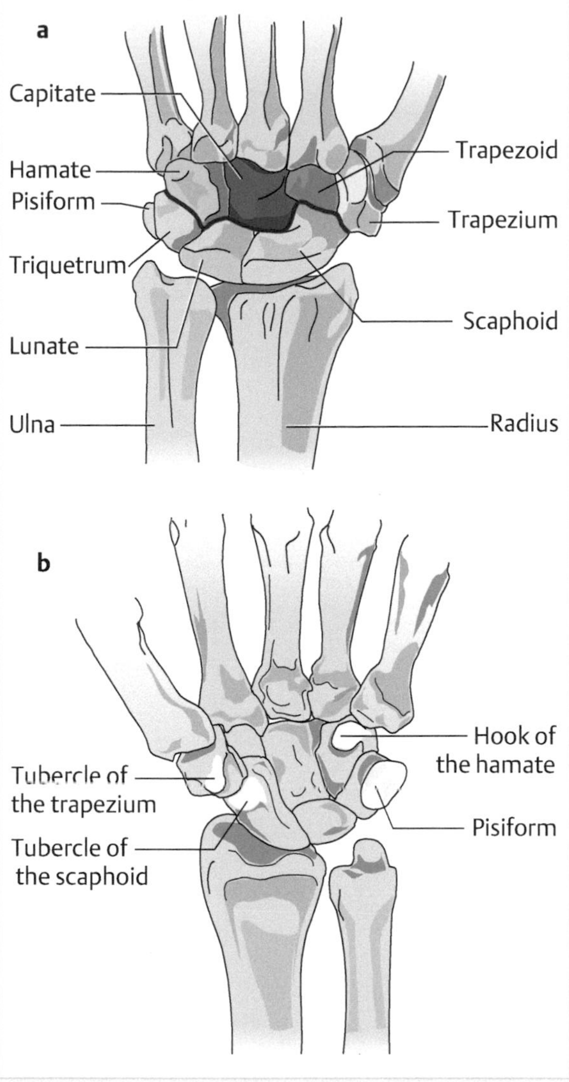


**Fig. 6.32** Midcarpal joint. **(a)** Dorsal view. **(b)** Palmar view.

## 6.2.3 Joint Capsules of the Hand, Wrist, and Finger Joints

### Radiocarpal Joint (Fig. 6.33)

Both layers of the joint capsule have their insertions on the bone–cartilage border of the proximal row of carpal bones and on the radius. In addition, the articular disk of the radio-ulnar joint is embedded in the capsule.

The ulnar recess protrudes from the capsule from radial to palmar toward the ulnar styloid process. It lies between the meniscus and the articular disk of the radio-ulnar joint. There are other small recesses on the radial side, both palmar and dorsal. There is usually no connection with the distal radio-ulnar joint—this would occur if the disk were perforated.

The fibrous layer merges with the palmar and dorsal ligaments. Dorsally, the floors of the tendon sheaths merge with it in most cases.

The joint spaces between the proximal carpal bones are closed by the interosseous ligaments. In approximately 50% of cases, there is a communication with the distal wrist joint (midcarpal joint).

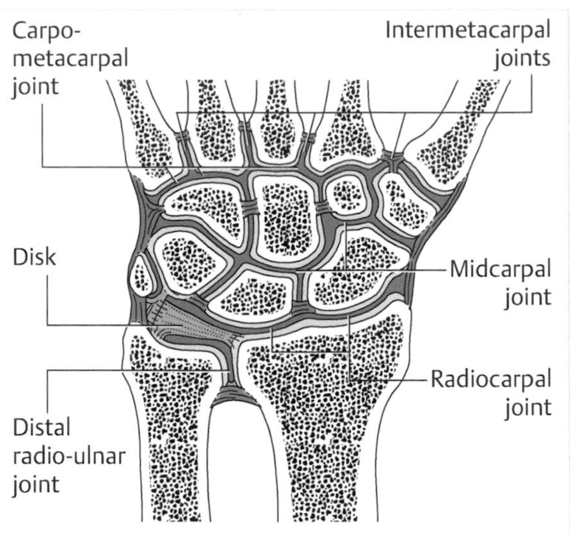


**Fig. 6.33** Joint capsules of the hand and wrist.

### Midcarpal Joint (Fig. 6.33)

The joint capsule of the midcarpal joint inserts at the bone–cartilage border of both rows of carpal bones and forms small recesses dorsally, while the palmar side is taut.

The joint spaces usually communicate with the carpometacarpal joints.

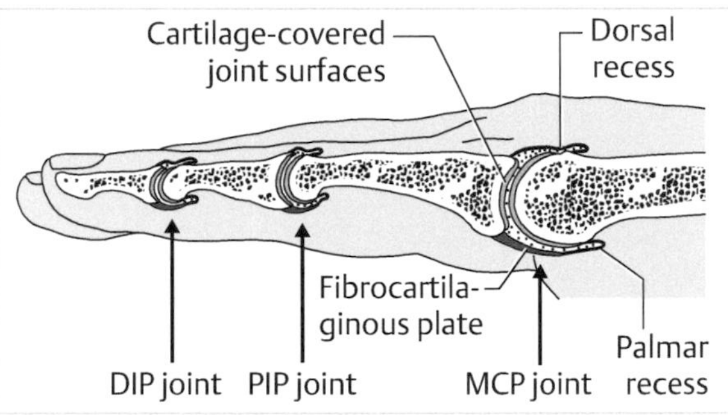


**Fig. 6.34** Joint capsules of the finger joints. DIP, distal interphalangeal; MCP, metacarpophalangeal; PIP, proximal interphalangeal.

### Metacarpophalangeal Joints (Fig. 6.34)

In the MCP joints, the joint capsule forms dorsal and palmar recesses. On the palmar side, the outpouchings are longer because the palmar fibrocartilaginous plate is embedded. Here and at the connection to the base of the phalanx, the capsule has a ligamentous reinforcement, the *palmar ligament*. There are also small outpouchings on the radial and ulnar sides of the joints.

The insertions of the capsule for each joint are at the bone–cartilage border or at the tip of the palmar fibrocartilaginous plate. Dorsally, a few fibers of the dorsal aponeurosis extend into the joint capsule.

### Interphalangeal Joints (Fig. 6.34)

In the PIP joints, the joint capsule forms recesses on both the dorsal and palmar sides, which reach up to 8 mm proximally. In the DIP joints, there is a dorsal recess with an extension of approximately 6 mm, while the palmar recess is only minimally developed. On the palmar side, the palmar fibrocartilaginous plate is embedded in the capsule.

The insertions of the capsule in each of the joints are at the bone–cartilage border or at the tip of the palmar fibrocartilaginous plate.

## 6.2.4 Perfusion (Fig. 6.35)

The dorsal and palmar carpal branches from the ulnar and radial arteries provide the arterial supply for the wrist joint and the carpal bones. These two arteries form the deep and superficial palmar arches to supply the midhand and finger areas. The digital palmar arteries arise from the arches to supply the fingers. The dorsal side of the hand is also supplied by these arteries through individual branches.

**Pathology**

In a third of all people, the blood supply to the scaphoid bone is concentrated at one end of the bone, so that the chances of healing after a fracture that goes through the thinner, middle area are understandably poor. This often results in the formation of a pseudarthrosis.
Reflex sympathetic dystrophy can develop from a cast that is too tight because the deep and superficial palmar arches are compressed.

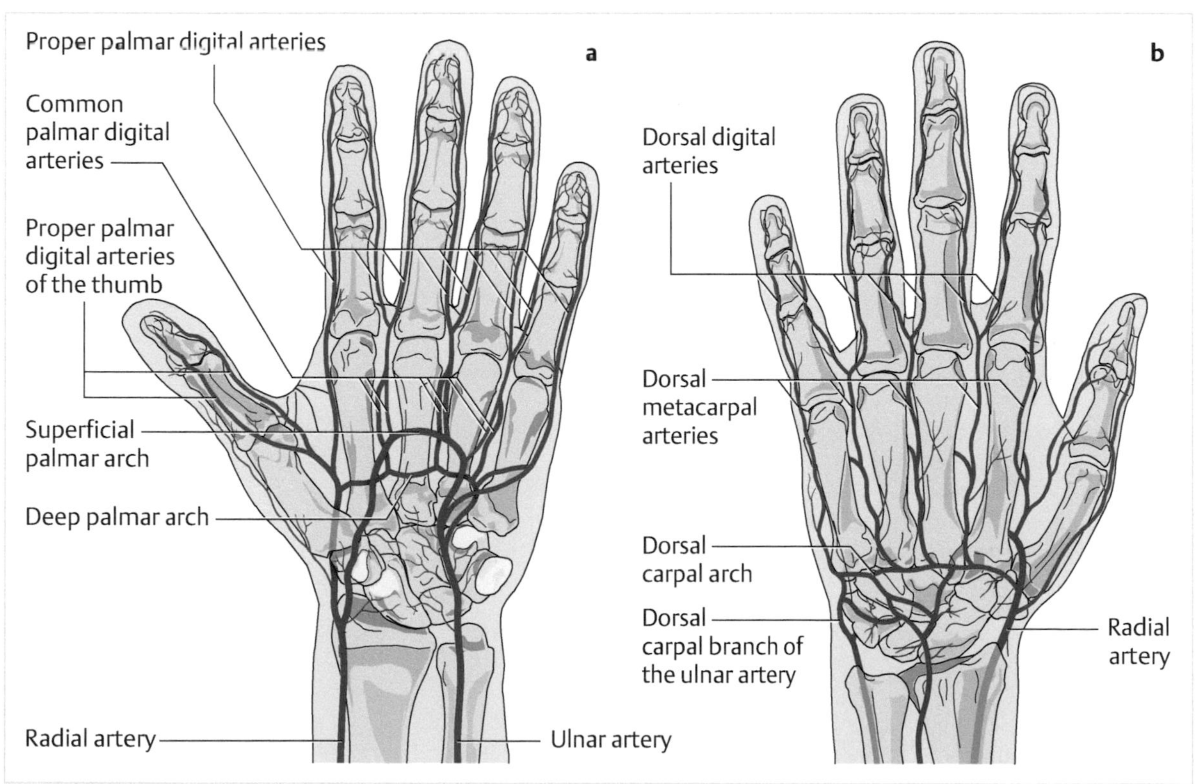


**Fig. 6.35** Perfusion of the hand and wrist. **(a)** Palmar view. **(b)** Dorsal view.

## 6.2.5 Innervation (Fig. 6.36)

### Hand and Wrist

The palmar aspect of the capsule–ligament apparatus of the wrist joint is supplied by the ulnar, anterior interosseous, and median nerves.

The lateral cutaneous nerve of the forearm and the superficial branch of the radial nerve innervate the radial side. The ulnar side is supplied by the dorsal branch of the ulnar nerve.

Dorsally, the innervation occurs through the posterior interosseous nerve and the posterior cutaneous nerve of the forearm.

### Finger

The palmar sections of the capsule–ligament apparatus of the finger are innervated by the articular branches from the deep branch of the ulnar nerve and the proper palmar digital nerves.

The articular branches of the dorsal digital nerves innervate the dorsal aspects. In the MCP joint area, the intermetacarpal branches also contribute.

The distal areas of the finger are supplied by articular branches of the palmar digital nerves.

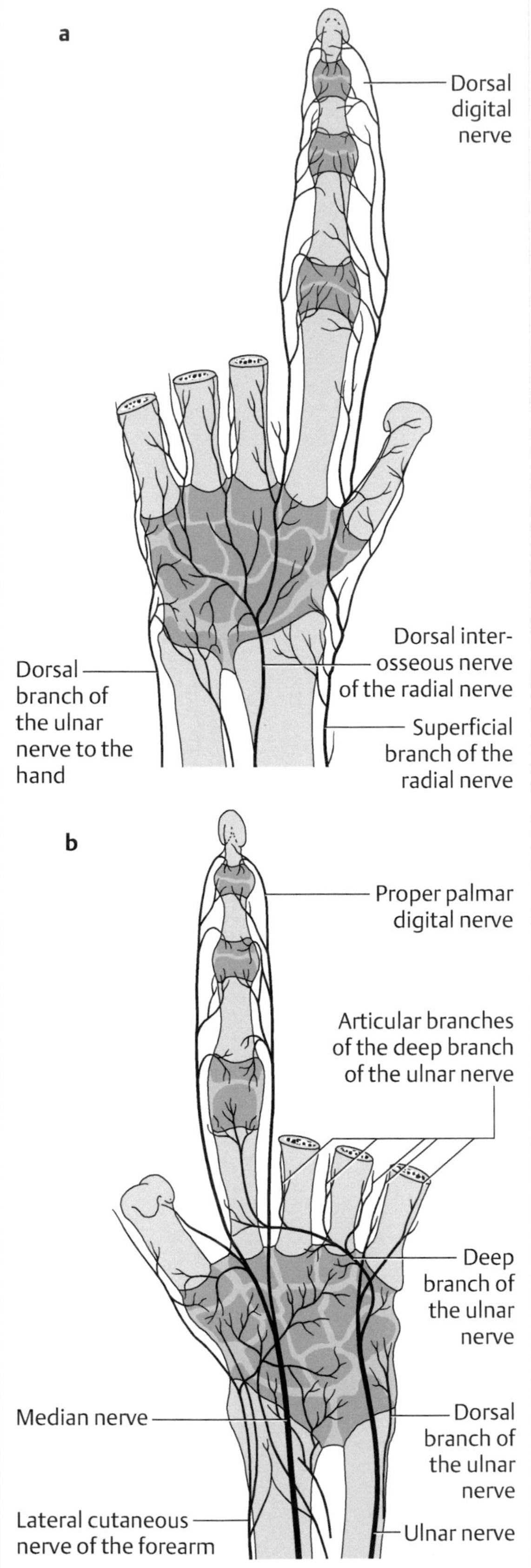


**Fig. 6.36** Innervation of the joint capsules. **(a)** Dorsal view. **(b)** Palmar view.

## 6.2.6 Ligaments

### Collateral Ligaments

#### Radial Collateral Ligament of the Wrist Joint

A dorsal section extends from the radial styloid process to the radial side of the scaphoid bone, and the palmar section to the tubercle of the scaphoid bone. It slows ulnar abduction.

#### Ulnar Collateral Ligament of the Wrist Joint

The ligament is subdivided into the dorsal and palmar bands. The dorsal part extends from the ulnar styloid process and the disk to the triquetrum; the palmar part extends to the pisiform bone. It slows radial abduction.

### Dorsal Ligaments (Fig. 6.37)

#### Dorsal Radiocarpal Ligament

- It has a broad-based origin on the dorsal surface of the radius and the dorsal radio-ulnar ligament.
- It extends with its longest fibers obliquely in an ulnar direction up to the triquetrum bone. Deeper and shorter fibrous bands connect with the lunate bone and the lower border of the scaphoid.
- It is a major stabilizing influence on the radiocarpal joint.

#### Arcuate Ligament of the Wrist

- The proximal band consists of transversely running cords of fibers extending from the scaphoid bone to the triquetrum. From there, there is a connection to the ulnar collateral ligament and the dorsal radiocarpal ligament.
- Distal bands of fibers also run transversely and connect the triquetrum bone with the trapezium.
- These bands provide transverse bracing for the rows of carpal bones.

#### Dorsal Intercarpal Ligaments

- These are included in the intrinsic ligaments of the wrist.
- They are very short ligaments that join adjacent carpal bones in both the transverse and longitudinal directions.

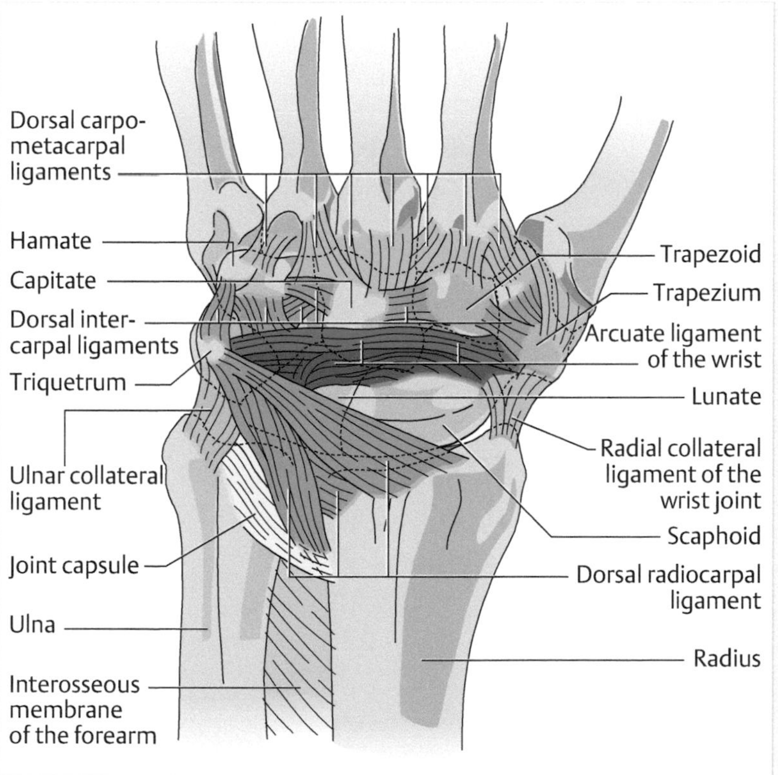


**Fig. 6.37** Dorsal ligaments.

## Palmar Ligaments (Fig. 6.38)

### Radiate Carpal Ligament

- This extends from distal to proximal where it broadens in a fan-like fashion.
- It connects the capitate bone with the hamate, triquetrum, and scaphoid bones and less often with the lunate bone. It also gives off a small band to the trapezoid bone.

### Palmar Radiocarpal Ligament

- The fibers of the superficial layer are thin and connect the radial styloid process with the capitate and triquetrum.
- Deep, strong fibrous bands are shorter and connect the radius with the scaphoid and lunate bones. They merge with the joint capsule.

### Ulnocarpal Ligament

- From the ulnar styloid process and the disk, bands extend to the lunate, triquetrum, and capitate bones.
- Together with the palmar radiocarpal ligament, it forms a **V**-shaped structure.

### Palmar Intercarpal Ligaments

- These join all the carpal bones to each other.
- They rest on the joint capsule and merge with it.
- The **pisohamate ligament** joins the pisiform bone with the hook of the hamate. It closes off a deep gap between the two bones, **Guyon's canal**, on the palmar side.

### Transverse Carpal Ligament (Fig. 6.39)

- This consists of deep, reinforcing bands of the flexor retinaculum, which span over the wrist as a transverse band at the level of the carpal bones.
- It is fixed to the tubercle of the scaphoid and the pisiform bone, and distally to the tubercle of the trapezium and the hook of the hamate.
- The ligament is somewhat narrower on the radial side than on the ulnar side.
- It forms the palmar border of the carpal tunnel and braces the arch of the wrist.

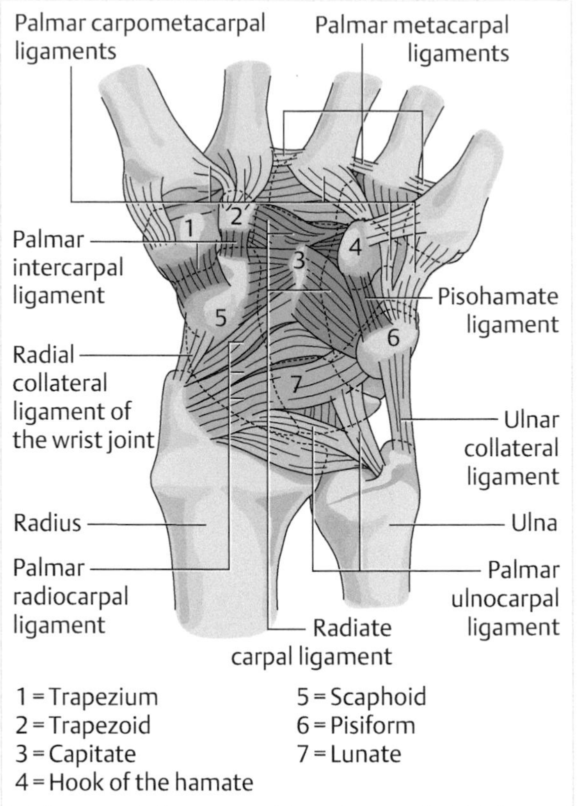


**Fig. 6.38** Palmar ligaments.

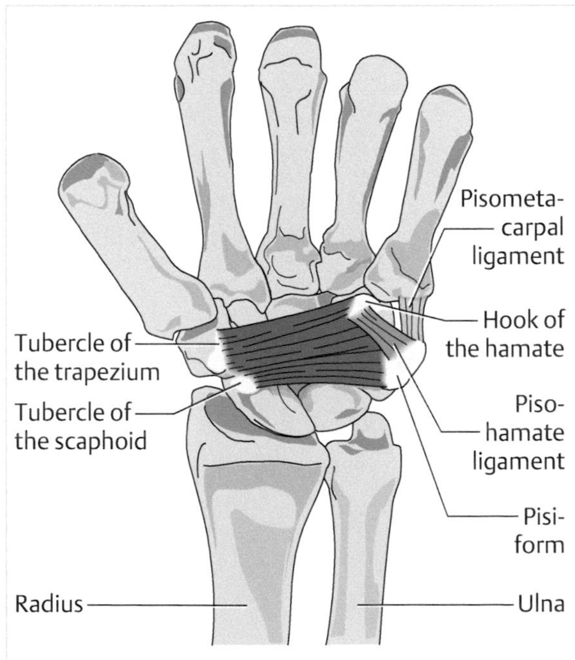


**Fig. 6.39** Transverse carpal ligament.

## Functions of the Ligaments

The wrist joint consists of labile chains of joints, which are stabilized only by the ligaments and by their diverse arrangement. The ligaments play a major role in controlling the position of the carpal bones in relation to each other. They allow movements to occur, but also limit them.

The collateral ligaments primarily stabilize the wrist joint on the sides and thus control the radial and ulnar abduction movements.

The palmar ligaments come under tension during *dorsiflexion*. They also secure the carpal arch. The palmar ligaments between the radius and scaphoid and between the scaphoid and trapezium have a particular role—when they are tensed during dorsiflexion, they clamp the scaphoid bone between the trapezium and the radius.

During *palmar flexion*, it is primarily the dorsally running ligaments that come under tension, thus limiting this movement.

## Longitudinal Column System

The joints of the wrist, hand, and fingers function as a system of three longitudinal movement columns:

### *Lunate Column (Fig. 6.40)*

The central column consists of the radius–lunate–capitate chain and continues on distally to the third metacarpal and the middle finger. It is the most stable of the three columns.

The palmar ligamentous connections between the radius and lunate and between the radius and capitate are tensed during dorsiflexion, producing a centralizing force in a radial direction. A portion of the dorsal radiocarpal ligament between the radius and lunate also comes under tension.

The ligamentous connections between the dorsal radius and lunate provide stability through their increasing tension during palmar flexion.

**Pathology**

Lunatomalacia occurs when the lunate becomes jammed because it does not move sufficiently during dorsiflexion and palmar flexion. This condition develops from repeated minor trauma over a long period of time, gradually leading to osteomalacia. Thus, an important component of the lunate column is missing, causing it to lose its stability.

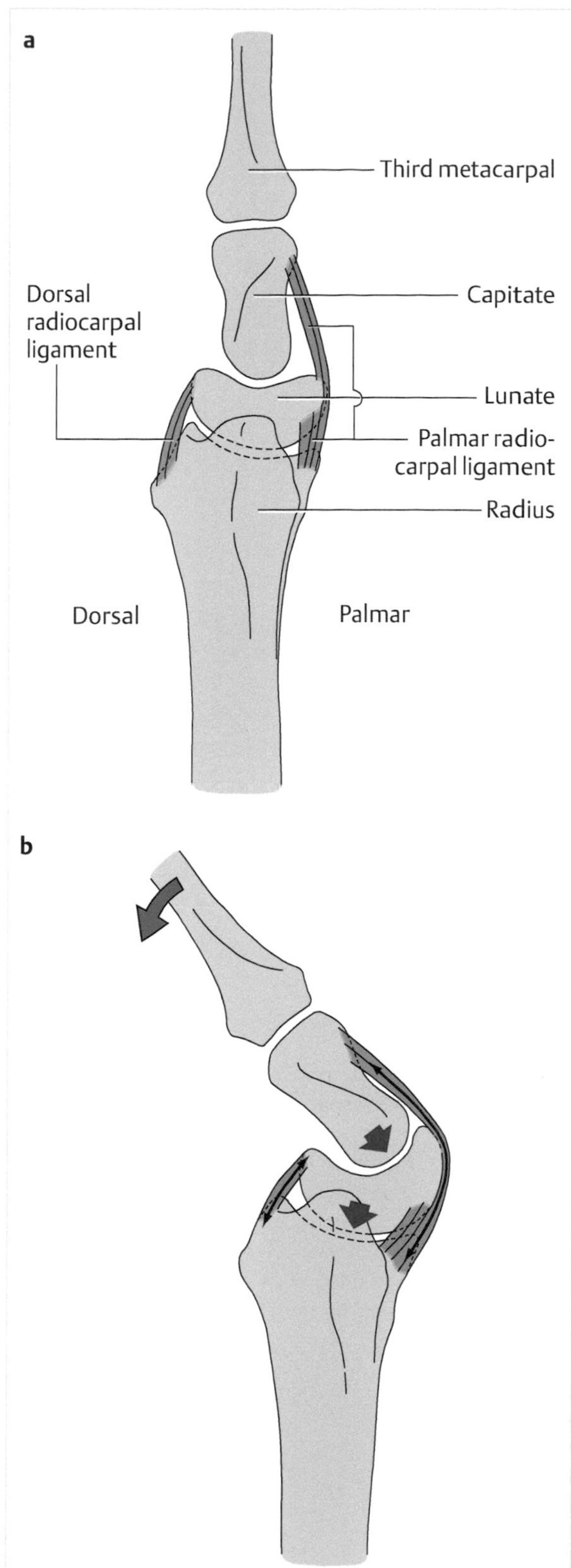


**Fig. 6.40 (a)** Lunate column (left hand, radial view). **(b)** Performance of the lunate column ligaments during dorsiflexion.

### *Scaphoid Column (Fig. 6.41)*

The radial column is composed of the radius–scaphoid–trapezium bone chain. Its distal continuation comprises the first and second metacarpals with the thumb and index finger. During dorsiflexion, the scaphoid bone is clamped between the trapezium and the radius by the tension of the palmar ligaments between the radius and scaphoid and between the scaphoid and trapezium. The dorsal ligamentous connection between the radius and scaphoid, on the other hand, is relaxed.

The thickening of the subchondral bone in the area of the scaphoid facet on the radius suggests that this area handles a large amount of stress. The particular demands are caused by many activities using the thumb and index finger, as well as through muscular forces, which put the scaphoid column under stress.

**Pathology**

#### Fracture of the Scaphoid

In falls onto the dorsiflexed hand, the scaphoid bone is fixed and completely jammed at both ends between the radius and trapezium bones. Therefore it breaks at its thinnest part, known as the waist of the scaphoid.

The capitate is also a long carpal bone, but it is stressed axially rather than transversely during falls onto the dorsiflexed hand, and therefore does not break.

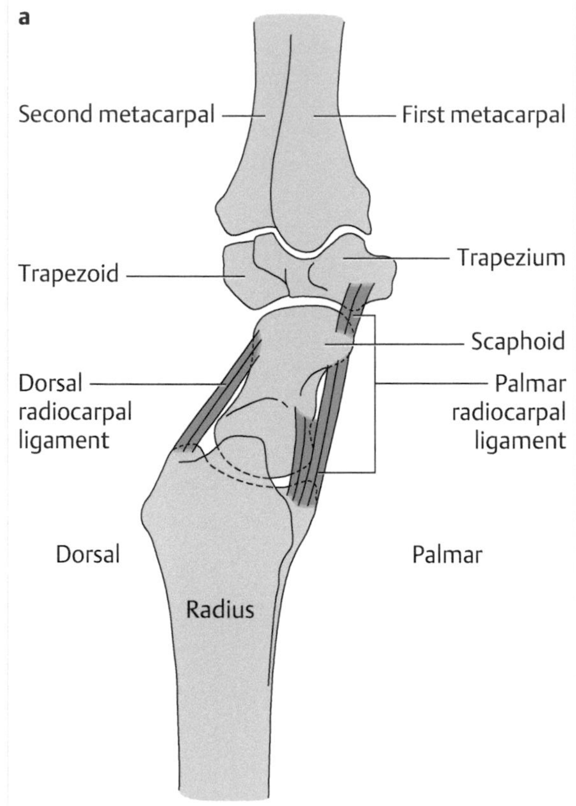


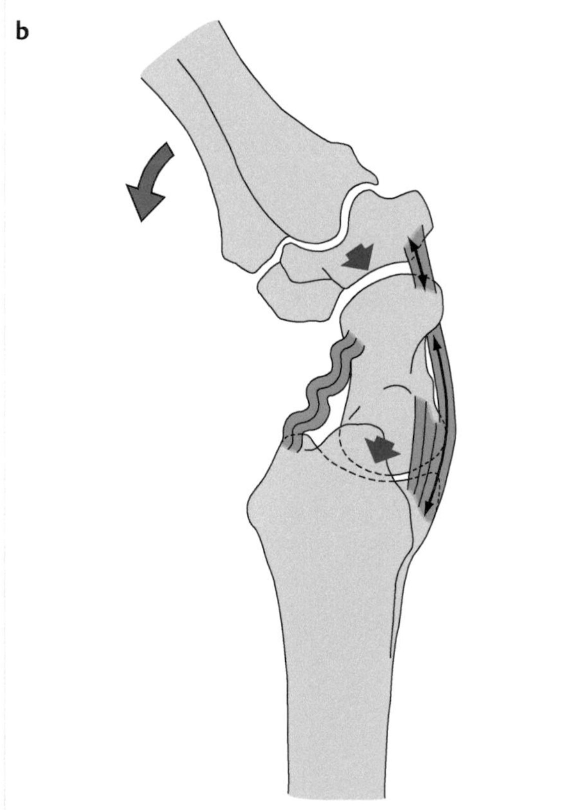


**Fig. 6.41 (a)** Scaphoid column (left hand, radial view). **(b)** Performance of the ligaments of the scaphoid bone during dorsiflexion.

### *Triquetrum Column (Fig. 6.42)*

The ulnar column consists of the bone chain formed of the ulna (with the disk), triquetrum, hamate and fourth and fifth metacarpals, with the ring and little fingers.

In dorsiflexion, the palmar ligaments (radius–triquetrum and pisiform–hamate) come under tension, as do the dorsal ligamentous bands between the hamate and the triquetrum. At the same time, the dorsal connections between the radius/ulna and the triquetrum bone are relaxed.

Because of their course, both the dorsal and palmar bands of the radiocarpal ligament have a centralizing force toward the radius; thus, they act as the "reins of the triquetrum." Contingent on their oblique course, they rein in the ulnar-directed forces that develop from the tilt of the radius. Thus, they function to prevent the translation of the carpus in an ulnar direction.

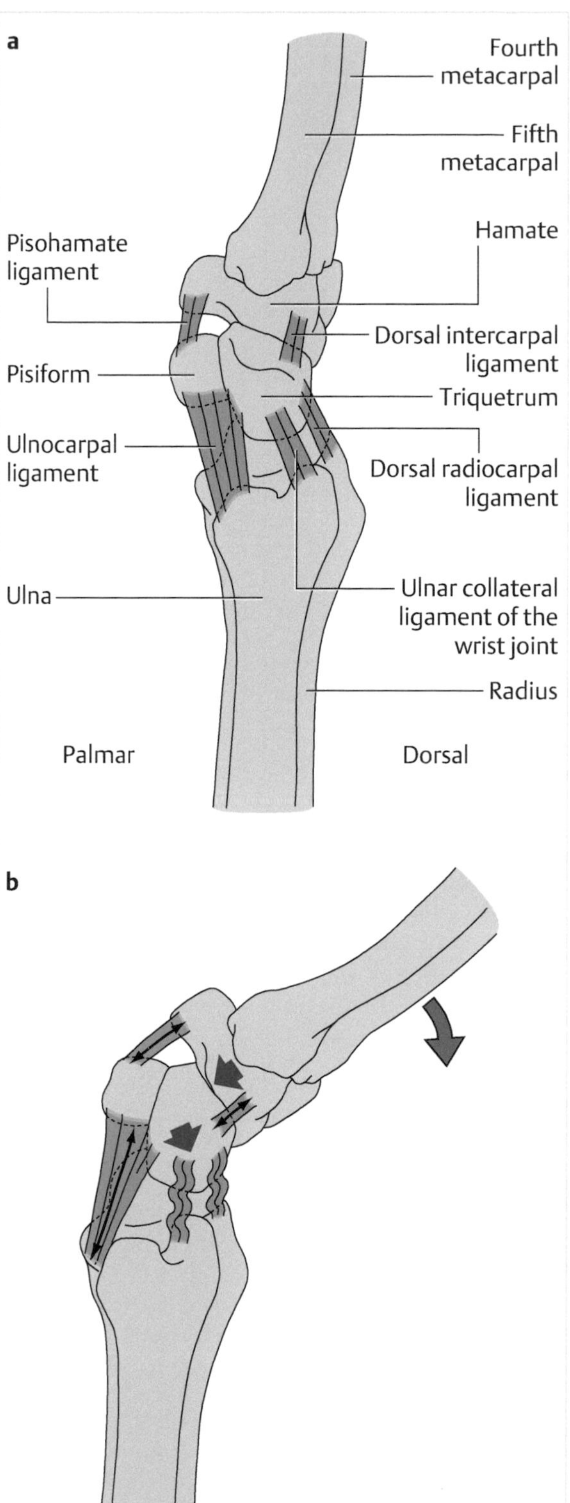


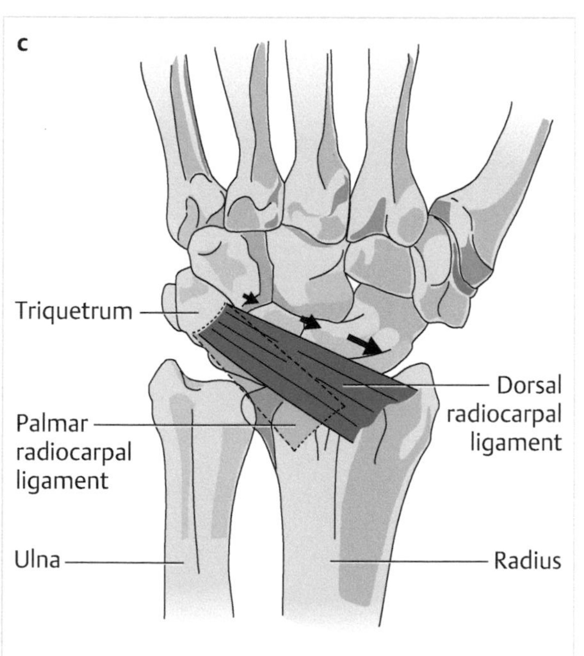


**Fig. 6.42 (a)** The triquetrum column (left hand, ulnar view). **(b)** Performance of the triquetrum column ligaments during dorsiflexion. **(c)** The "reins of the triquetrum" (dorsal view).

## 6.2.7 Carpal Tunnel (Fig. 6.43)

The carpal bones are not arranged in a straight line, but rather form a transverse arc in which the carpal bones at the ends of the arc are aligned toward the palmar side. This bony arch is closed off on the palmar side by the transverse carpal ligament, which results in the formation of a very narrow, osteofibrotic canal.

All the flexor tendons are bundled within this carpal tunnel, after which they spread out like a fan. The *flexor pollicis longus tendon* runs on the radial side. Further in an ulnar direction, the tendons of the *flexor digitorum profundus muscle* run deep within the tunnel and, above them, those of the *flexor digitorum superficialis muscle.* They are enclosed in a common tendon sheath. The *median nerve* is located above these tendons and directly under the ligament, approximately in the center.

The *flexor carpi radialis muscle* runs on the radial side in a small compartment, which is separated from the actual carpal tunnel by bands of connective tissue. It is also covered by the transverse carpal ligament.

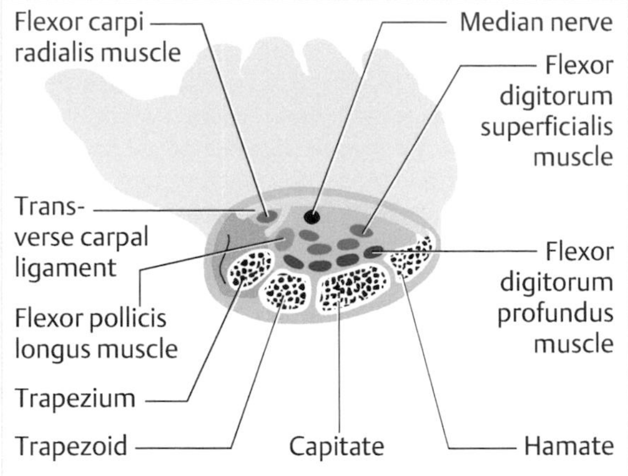


**Fig. 6.43** Carpal tunnel (transverse section at the level of the distal row of carpal bones).

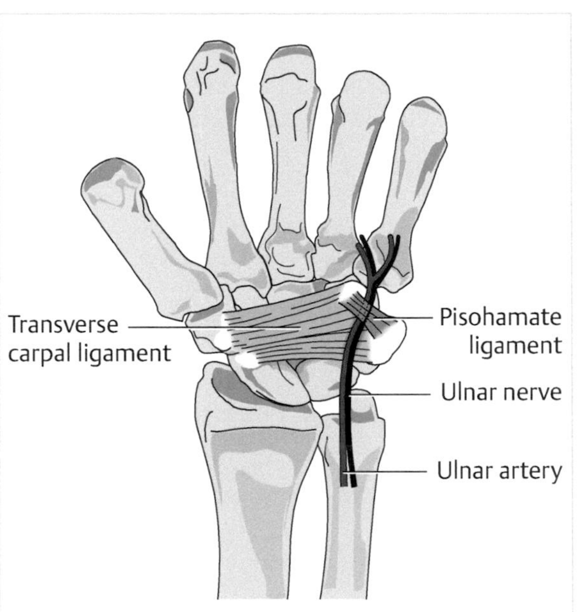


**Fig. 6.44** Guyon's canal.

**Pathology**

*Carpal tunnel syndrome* is a set of symptoms that develop as a result of overstraining the flexor tendons with tenosynovitis and swelling. The result is compression of the median nerve. The patient complains of a feeling of numbness in the supply area, of the hand "going to sleep," and of morning stiffness of the fingers. In terms of motor symptoms, difficulty with grasping can develop because of failure of opposition.
Another cause for the compression syndrome is edema from hormonal changes, such as in pregnancy or menopause.

## 6.2.8 Guyon's Canal (Fig. 6.44)

In the palmar, ulnar area of the wrist is another osteoligamentous canal, *Guyon's canal.* This is formed between the hook of the hamate and the pisiform bone and is bordered on the palmar side by the pisohamate ligament. The ulnar border of the transverse carpal ligament runs somewhat further dorsally. The deep branch of the ulnar nerve and a small branch of the ulnar artery pass distally through this canal.

**Pathology**

**Ulnar neuropathy** (handlebar palsy) is seen in cyclists. Pressure of the dorsiflexed hand on the handlebar narrows the canal, thus compressing the nerve. Cyclists complain of a numb feeling in the area of the little finger and weakness in spreading the fingers.

## 6.2.9 Axes and Movements (Fig. 6.45)

The proximal (radiocarpal) and distal (midcarpal) wrist joints each form an independent joint, but, from a functional point of view, they form a unit.

Because of the complex motion sequences, determining an **axis** is not easy. Each movement segment has its own axis. The closest approximation of the various axes is in the proximal capitate bone, near the capitate–lunate articulation.

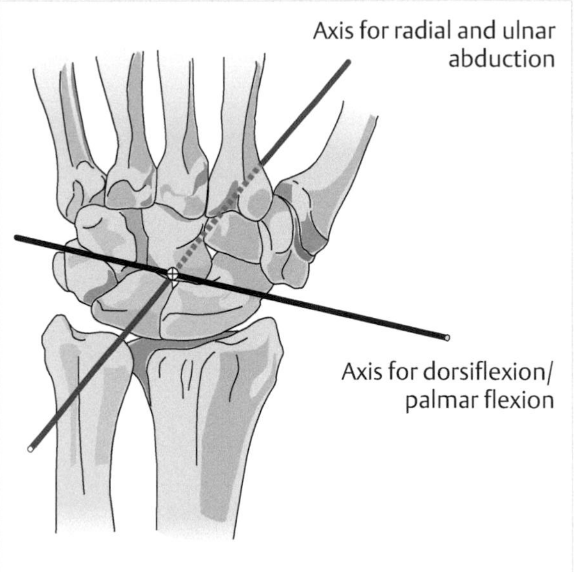


**Fig. 6.45** The axes of the wrist joint (dorsal view).

### Movements

### Dorsiflexion / Palmar Flexion (Fig. 6.46)

Dorsal/palmar: 70°/80° from neutral.

A range of 40° dorsiflexion and 30° palmar flexion is sufficient for the movements of everyday life. This range of movement is divided evenly over the radiocarpal and midcarpal joints. Only at maximum dorsiflexion does the larger proportion of movement takes place in the distal joint—approximately 1.5 times that in the proximal joint. At maximal palmar flexion, the converse is true.

In the first phase of motion, the scaphoid column moves somewhat faster than the lunate column, but it come to a stop sooner because of the jamming of the scaphoid bone. The lunate column moves still further until the palmar ligamentous connections between the radius and lunate bone stop the movement.

**Practical Tip**

Because the columns move against each other to varying degrees, one should examine the mobility of the scaphoid column compared with the lunate column when there are disturbances in the maximum range of motion.

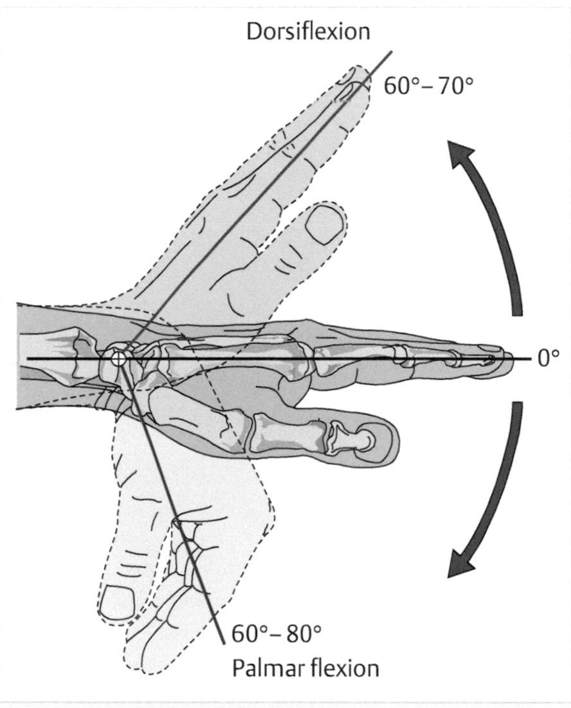


**Fig. 6.46** Dorsiflexion and palmar flexion of the hand.

## Movements of the Carpal Bones (Fig. 6.47)

During dorsiflexion, the scaphoid tilts up as its base glides in a palmar direction, and the trapezium shifts over the scaphoid, gliding dorsally.

The lunate glides in a palmar direction, as does the capitate against the lunate.

The triquetrum glides in a palmar direction, as does the hamate against the triquetrum.

Most of the hand muscles end on the distal carpal bones. Therefore movement begins in the distal row of carpal bones. For instance, when the extensor carpi radialis longus muscle contracts, it pulls the base of the second metacarpal dorsally. Because the mobility in the carpometacarpal joint is quite limited, the trapezoid bone is drawn dorsally as a direct continuation of this movement, and it shifts on the scaphoid bone. The scaphoid, due to its convexity, then glides against the radius in a palmar direction.

In *palmar flexion*, the scaphoid lies transversely, gliding dorsally, and the trapezium glides in a palmar direction. The lunate glides dorsally, putting the thickest part of the lunate between the capitate bone and the radius. The capitate also glides dorsally against the lunate. The triquetrum glides dorsally, as does the hamate bone.

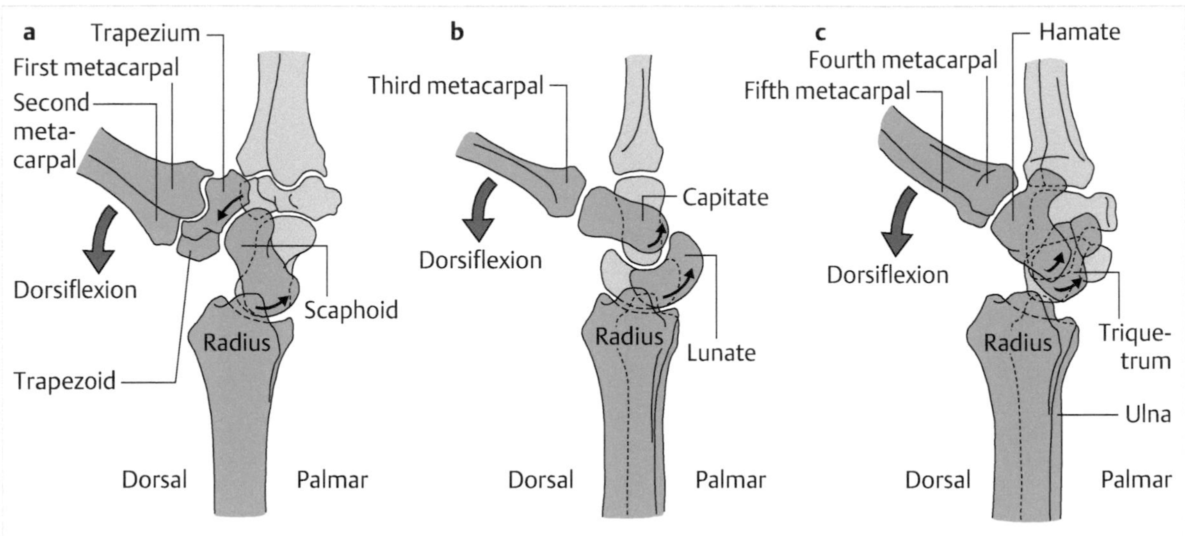


**Fig. 6.47** Performance of the carpal bones in dorsiflexion (radial view of the left hand). **(a)** Scaphoid column. **(b)** Lunate column. **(c)** Triquetrum column.

## Radial and Ulnar Abduction (Fig. 6.48)

Radial/ulnar: 20°/35° from neutral.

These movements take place primarily in the radiocarpal joint because the interdigitation of the distal row of carpal bones permits only limited side-to-side gliding in the midcarpal joint. However, the movements of flexion and extension take place in both the distal and proximal joints.

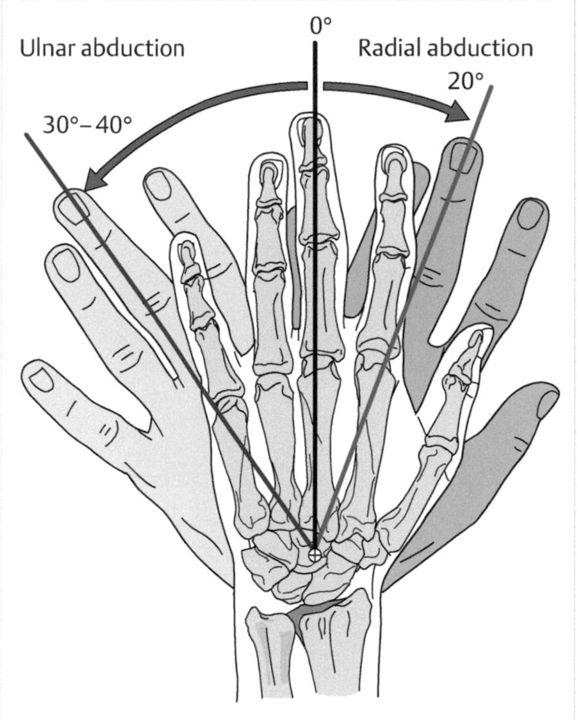


**Fig. 6.48** Radial and ulnar abduction of the hand.

## Movements of the Carpal Bones

*In ulnar abduction* (**Fig. 6.49**):

- The proximal row shifts in a radial direction until the lunate bone is opposite the radius.
- The capitate and hamate glide minimally to the radial side.
- The proximal row of carpal bones performs an extension movement: the scaphoid, lunate, and triquetrum glide against the radius and the disk in a palmar direction.
- A flexion movement takes place in the midcarpal joint: the trapezium glides in a palmar direction, and the capitate and hamate glide dorsally.

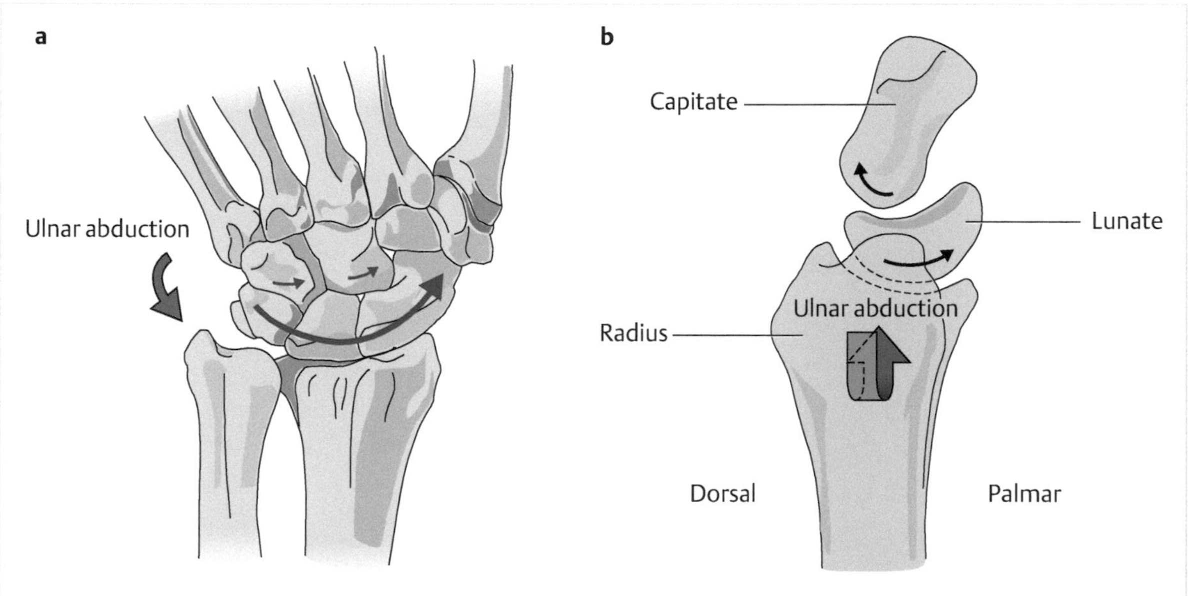


**Fig. 6.49** Performance of the carpal bones in ulnar abduction. **(a)** Dorsal view. **(b)** Radial view of the lunate column by way of example.

*In radial abduction* (**Fig. 6.50**):

- The proximal row shifts to the ulnar side, so that half of the lunate bone is opposite the ulna.
- The capitate bone glides slightly in an ulnar direction.
- A flexion movement takes place in the radiocarpal joint. For example, the lunate bone glides dorsally against the radius.
- In the midcarpal joint, an extension movement takes place. As an example, the capitate bone glides in a palmar direction against the lunate bone.

In everyday life, a predominant movement range of 20 to 30° of ulnar abduction and approximately 10° of radial abduction is sufficient.

## Practical Tip

When dealing with restricted mobility of wrist abduction, either ulnar or radial, one must evaluate the ability of the individual carpal bones to glide in dorsal and palmar directions, among others, because this could be the cause of the restriction.

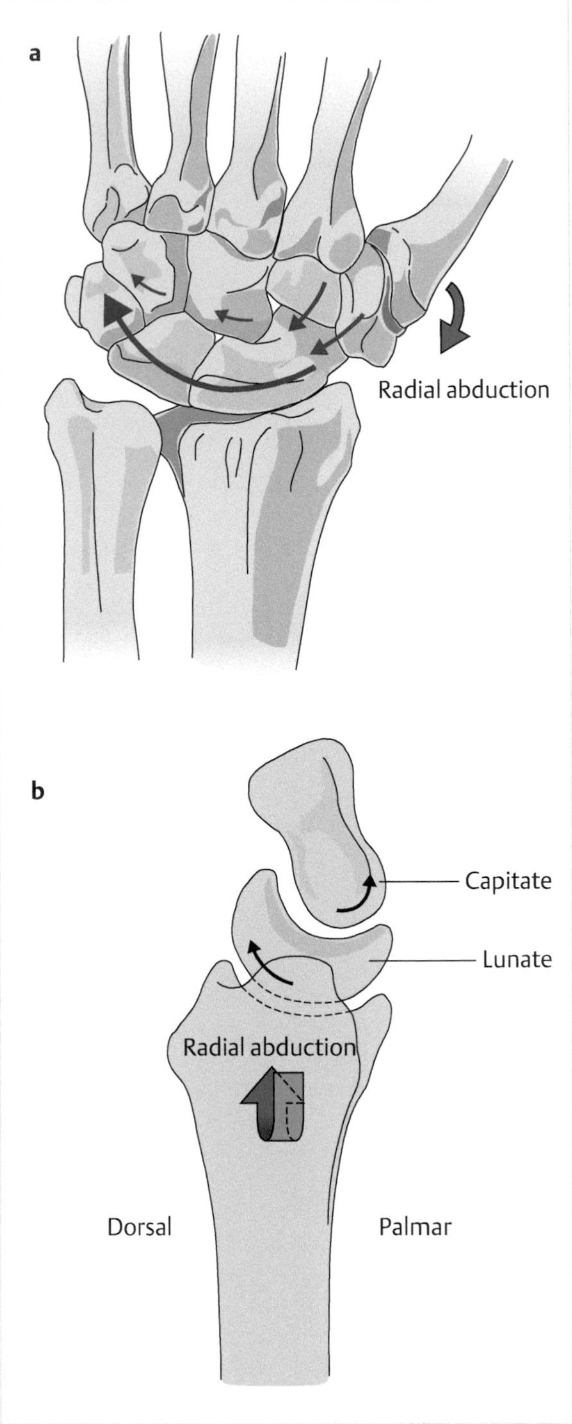


**Fig. 6.50** Performance of the carpal bones in radial abduction. **(a)** Dorsal view. **(b)** Radial view of the lunate column by way of example.

## 6.2.10 Muscles of the Wrist Joint: Extensors (Fig. 6.51)

### Extensor Carpi Radialis Longus Muscle

- This connects the lateral supracondylar ridge of the humerus with the base of the second metacarpal bone.
- In the distal third of the forearm, it is crossed by the abductor pollicis longus and extensor pollicis brevis muscles as they make their way to the radial side of the arm.
- Along with the tendon of the extensor carpi radialis brevis muscle, it extends under the extensor retinaculum through the second tendon compartment.

**Function.** Dorsiflexion and radial abduction at the wrist joint. It also helps with elbow flexion and supination.

### Extensor Carpi Radialis Brevis Muscle

- This connects the lateral epicondyle of the humerus with the base of the third metacarpal.
- It is crossed in the distal third of the forearm by the thumb muscles of the first tendon compartment.
- Along with the tendon of the extensor carpi radialis longus muscle, it extends through the second tendon compartment.

**Function.** Dorsiflexion. It also helps with radial abduction at the wrist joint and produces weak elbow flexion.

### Extensor Carpi Ulnaris Muscle

- This connects the lateral epicondyle of the humerus with the base of the fifth metacarpal.
- Its origin on the epicondyle lies between the origins of the anconeus and extensor digitorum muscles.
- It runs far over to the ulnar side and transitions into its terminal tendon in the distal third of the forearm.
- Its tendon extends through the sixth tendon compartment, which lies in the dorsal-ulnar area.

**Function.** Dorsiflexion and ulnar abduction at the wrist joint; also stabilization of the ulnocarpal area.

The following finger muscles help with dorsiflexion:

- Extensor digitorum muscle.
- Extensor pollicis longus muscle.
- Extensor pollicis brevis muscle.
- Abductor pollicis longus muscle.
- Extensor indicis muscle.
- Extensor digiti minimi muscle.

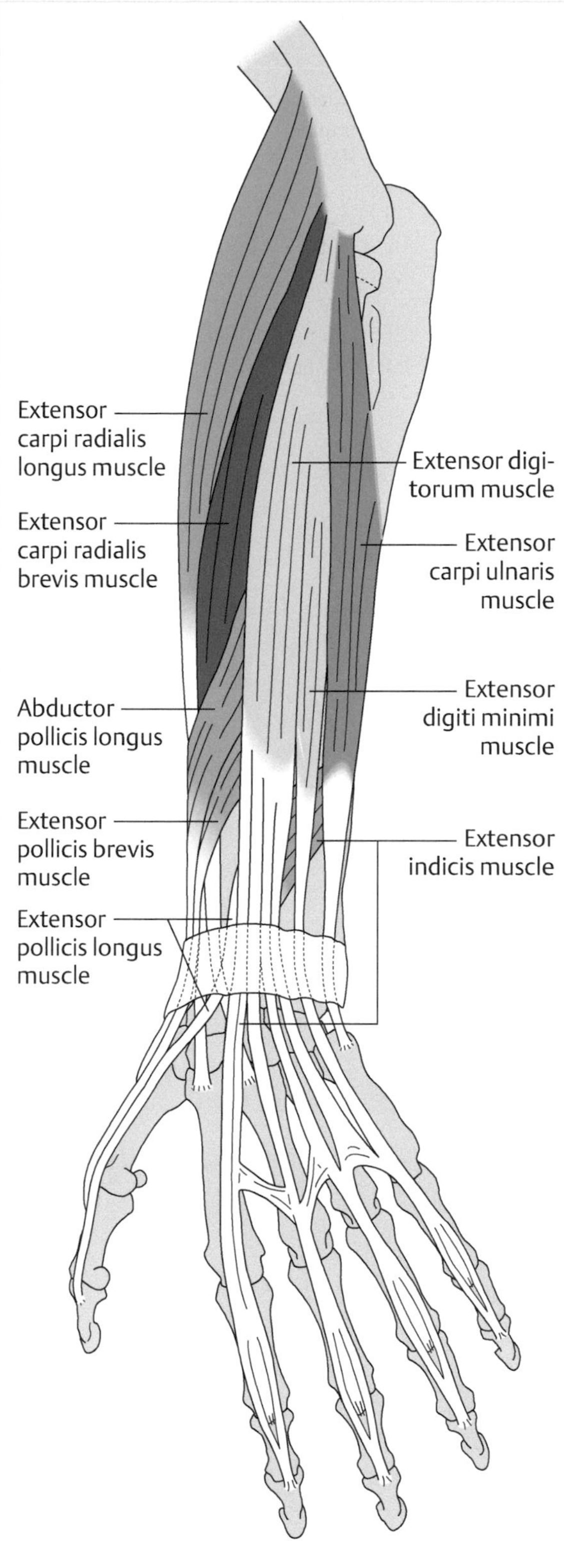


**Fig. 6.51** Extensors of the hand (posterior view).

## 6.2.11 Muscles of the Wrist Joint: Flexors (Fig. 6.52)

### Flexor Carpi Radialis Muscle

- It connects the medial epicondyle with the base of the second metacarpal.
- In the proximal third, its muscle belly is crossed by the bicipital aponeurosis. At this point it runs superficially, centered between the pronator teres and palmaris longus muscles.
- At the beginning of the lower third of the forearm, it transitions into its terminal tendon.
- Its tendon runs under the transverse carpal ligament where it is located within the carpal tunnel, but it is separated from the other tendons by a dividing septum.

**Function.** Palmar flexion and radial abduction at the wrist joint. It also produces weak elbow flexion.

### Flexor Carpi Ulnaris Muscle

- This consists of two heads:
  - The **humeral head** arises from the medial epicondyle of the humerus.
  - The **ulnar head** arises on the medial edge of the olecranon and the posterior border of the ulna. The two heads join and extend to the hook of the hamate and the base of the fifth metacarpal.
- At the area of origin, the two heads form a slit through which the ulnar nerve travels on its way from the posteriorly lying groove for the ulnar nerve to the anterior side of the forearm.
- The pisiform bone is embedded in the tendon as a sesamoid bone.

**Function.** Palmar flexion and ulnar abduction at the wrist; also weak elbow flexion.

The following finger muscles are also involved in flexion:

- Flexor digitorum superficialis muscle.
- Flexor digitorum profundus muscle.
- Palmaris longus muscle.
- Flexor pollicis longus muscle.

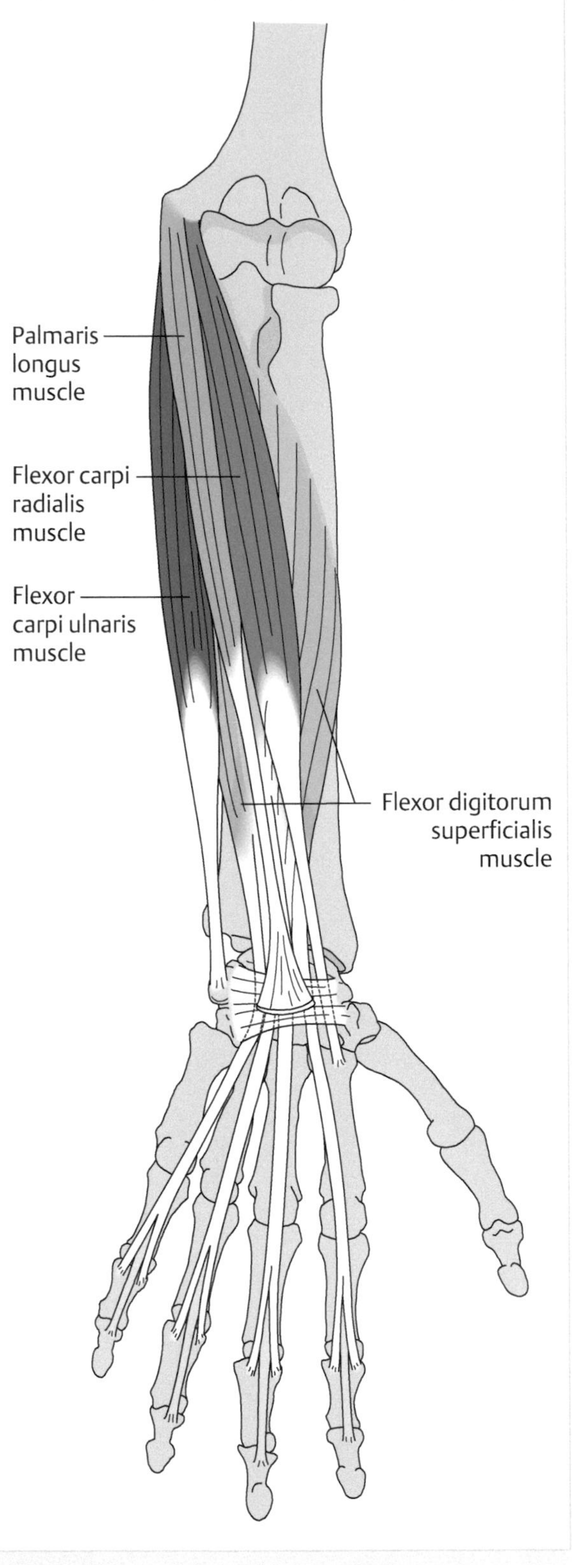


**Fig. 6.52** Flexors of the hand (anterior view).

## 6.2.12 Muscles of the Wrist Joint: Radial Abductors (Fig. 6.53)

Muscles that run radial to the abduction axis perform radial abduction. These are:

- Extensor carpi radialis longus muscle.
- Extensor pollicis longus muscle.
- Extensor pollicis brevis muscle.
- Abductor pollicis longus muscle.
- Extensor indicis muscle.
- Flexor carpi radialis muscle.
- Flexor pollicis longus muscle.

**Pathology**

In rheumatoid arthritis, the radial muscle group predominates due to the very painful, destructive process in the area of the head of the ulna, leading to a restriction of ulnar abduction.

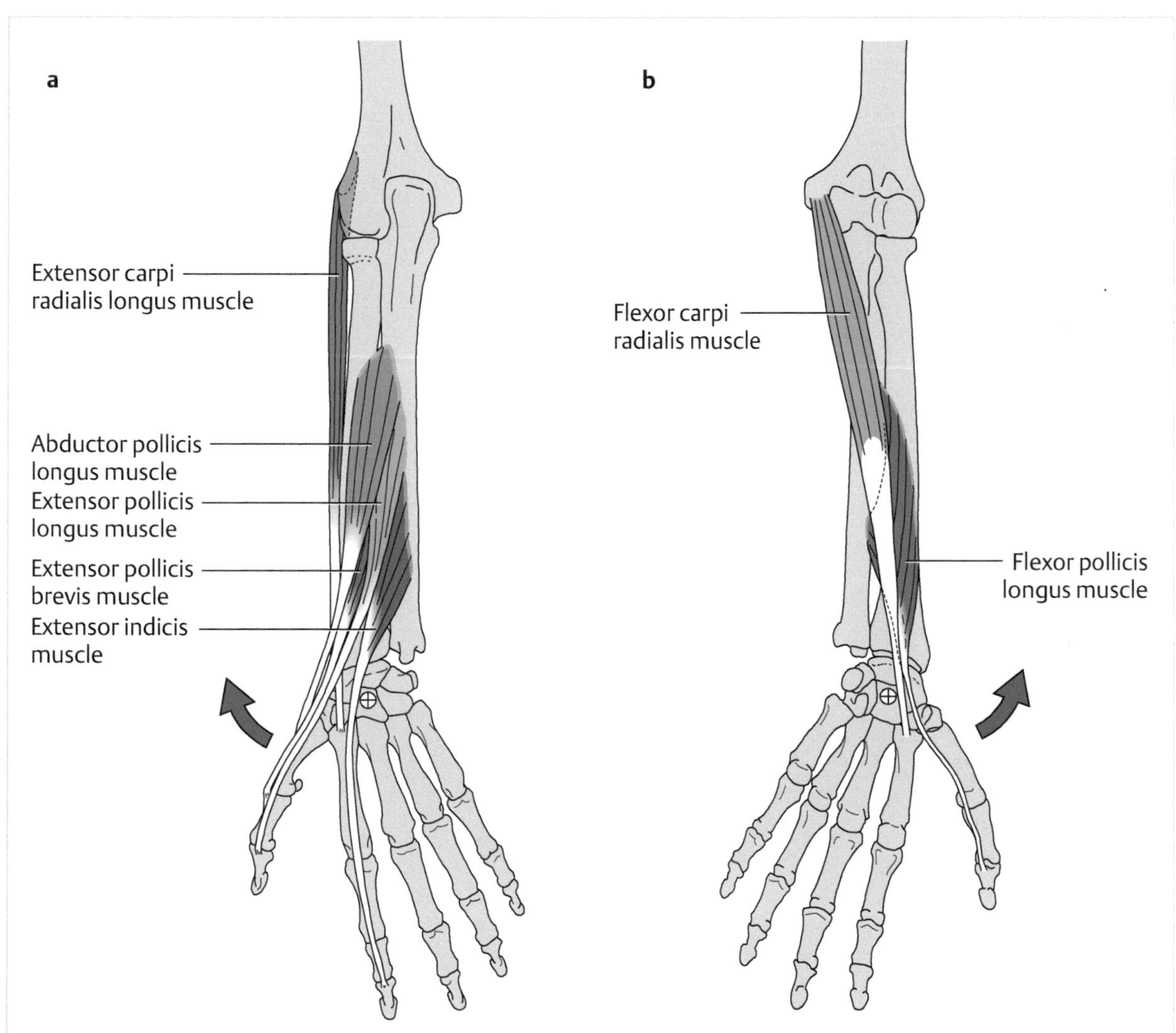


**Fig. 6.53** Radial abductors of the hand. **(a)** Posterior view. **(b)** Anterior view.

## 6.2.13 Muscles of the Wrist Joint: Ulnar Abductors (Fig. 6.54)

All the muscles that run ulnar to the abduction axis produce ulnar abduction. They are:

- Extensor carpi ulnaris muscle.
- Flexor carpi ulnaris muscle.
- Extensor digiti minimi muscle.

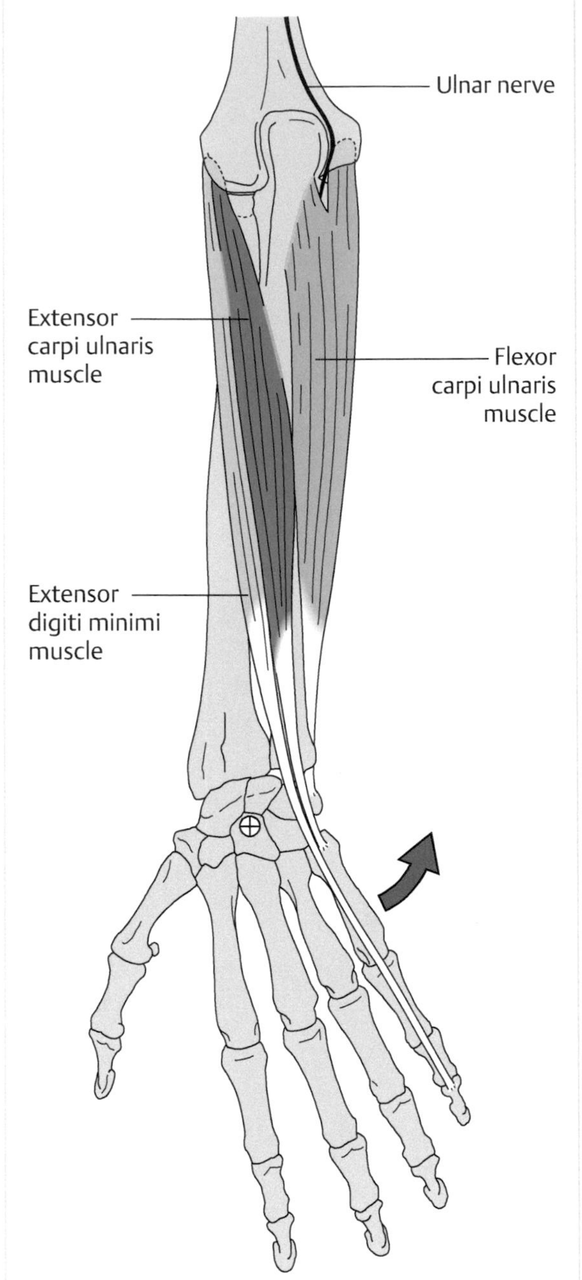


**Fig. 6.54** Ulnar abductors of the hand (posterior view).

## 6.2.14 Joints of the Midhand Region

The movement dynamics of the midhand area are determined by the carpometacarpal and intermetacarpal joints. Good mobility in these joints is a prerequisite for the various forms of grasp.

### Carpometacarpal Joints

- Articulating surfaces: the distal rows of carpal bones and the bases of the metacarpal bones.
- They are amphiarthroses with varying degrees of mobility.
- The bases have special shapes (**Fig. 6.55**):
  - The second metacarpal has a forked shape, giving it a high degree of stability and allowing articulation with the trapezoid and the trapezium.
  - The third metacarpal has a small styloid process that makes contact with the second metacarpal and the capitate bone. This joint is very stable; it is part of the central column of the wrist.
  - The base of the fifth metacarpal is somewhat saddle-shaped—concave in the radio-ulnar direction and convex in the dorsopalmar direction. This joint has the greatest mobility.
- In the fourth and fifth carpometacarpal joints, both flexion and extension movements of approximately 15 to 30° and limited side-to-side and rotatory movements are possible.
- The palmar and dorsal carpometacarpal ligaments provide stability. They connect all the distal carpal bones with the metacarpals.

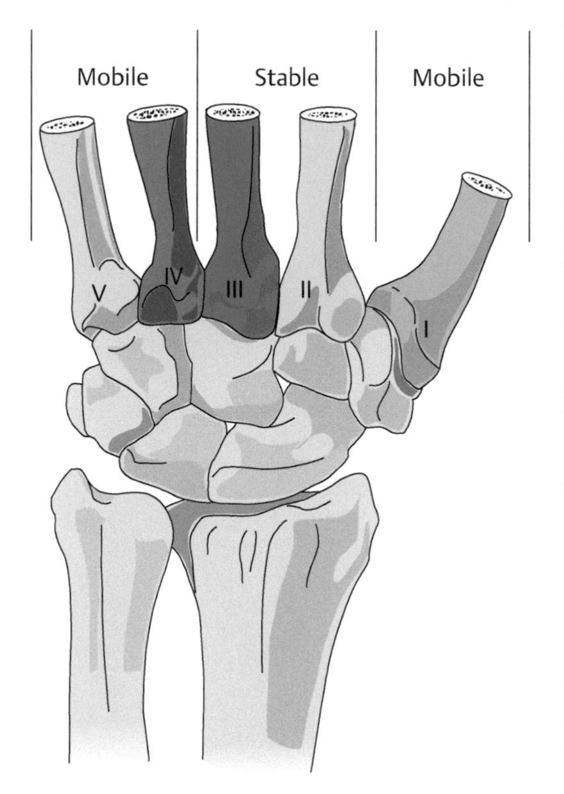


**Fig. 6.55** Shapes of the bases of the metacarpal bones (dorsal view).

## First Carpometacarpal Joint

The carpal bones are organized in an arc—they form a stable, transverse arch with the capitate bone forming the center (**Fig. 6.56**).

The scaphoid bone and the trapezium bones have a distinct radiopalmar orientation. Because of this, the metacarpal of the thumb is not in line with the other fingers but is rotated approximately 60° to the palmar side (**Fig. 6.57**).

This becomes clearly visible when the course of the flexion–extension axis of the other carpometacarpal joints is compared with that of the thumb.

It is only because of this deviation of the thumb that the various forms of grasp are possible (**Fig. 6.58**).

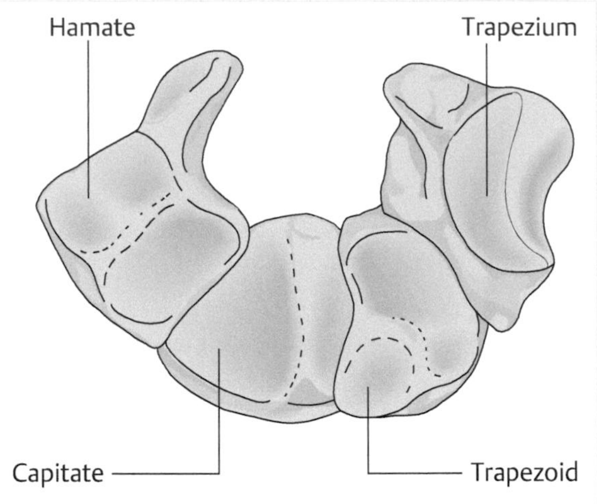


**Fig. 6.56** The carpal arch (distal view of the distal row of carpal bones).

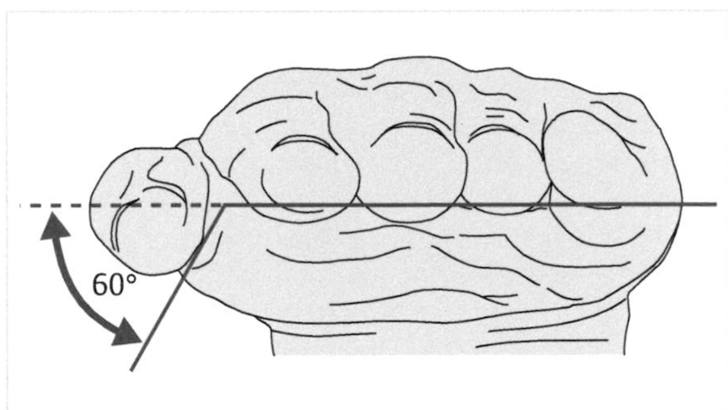


**Fig. 6.57** Position of the thumb in relation to the fingers.

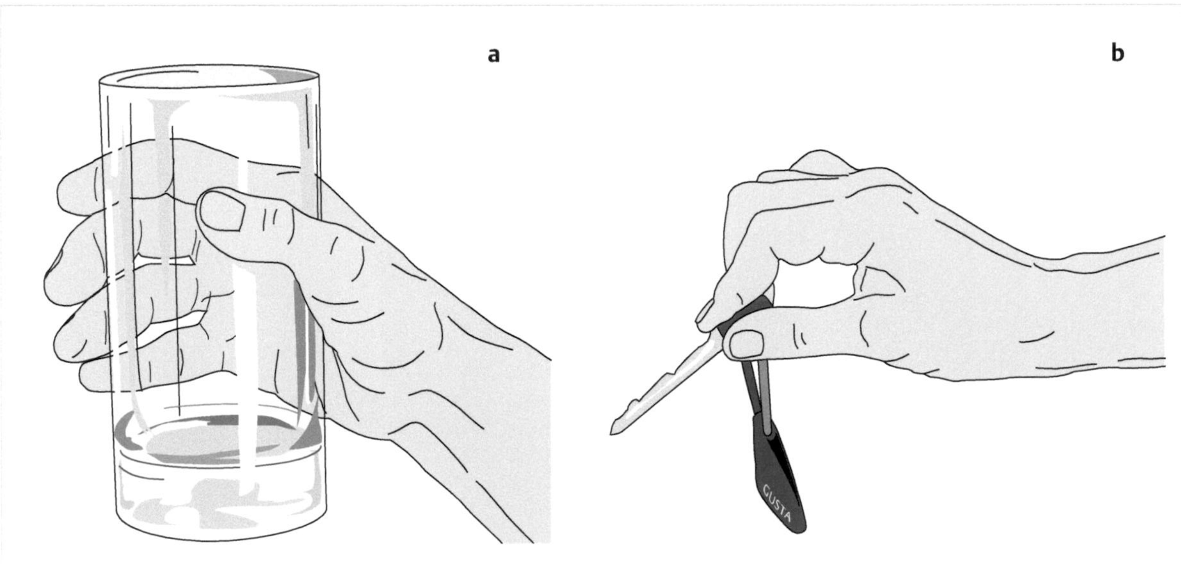


**Fig. 6.58 (a, b)** Types of grasp that require the thumb.

The **first carpometacarpal joint** is a saddle joint (**Fig. 6.59**).

Seen from the radial view, the base of the metacarpal is convex; from the dorsal view, it is concave.

The joint surface on the trapezium bone is inversely curved. From the radial view, it has a concave shape, and in the dorsal view, a convex shape. The joint surfaces are arranged so that they have congruence with each other.

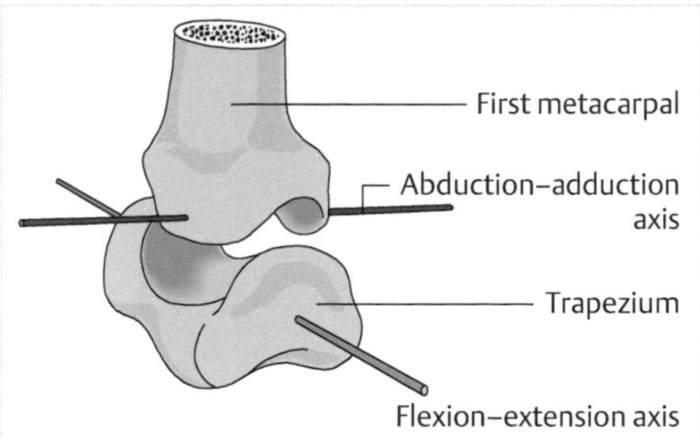


**Fig. 6.59** Thumb saddle joint: movement axes.

**Pathology**

**Rhizarthrosis**

Prolonged instability of this saddle joint of the thumb can lead to dorsal and radial subluxation of the thumb. Destruction of cartilage and pain cause restricted motion in the joint, and pollex adductus ensues. Any demanding movement, but especially opposition, is very painful. A firm grip is scarcely possible. Surgical treatment for severe rhizarthrosis includes inserting a prosthesis or performing an arthrodesis in mild flexion.

## Movements in the Saddle Joint of the Thumb

In spite of the strong congruence of the joint surfaces, the movement possibilities are comparable to those of a ball and socket joint:

### Flexion and Extension (Fig. 6.60)

The axis of movement for flexion and extension runs from radial to ulnar through the distal area of the trapezium bone.

Active *range of motion* for flexion/extension: 20°/45° from neutral; passive: +5°

#### *Joint Mechanics for Flexion*

In flexion, the metacarpal bone moves parallel to the palm. To allow this movement, the joint surface at the base of the first metacarpal is concave, and a concurrent gliding toward the thumb side of the palm takes place.

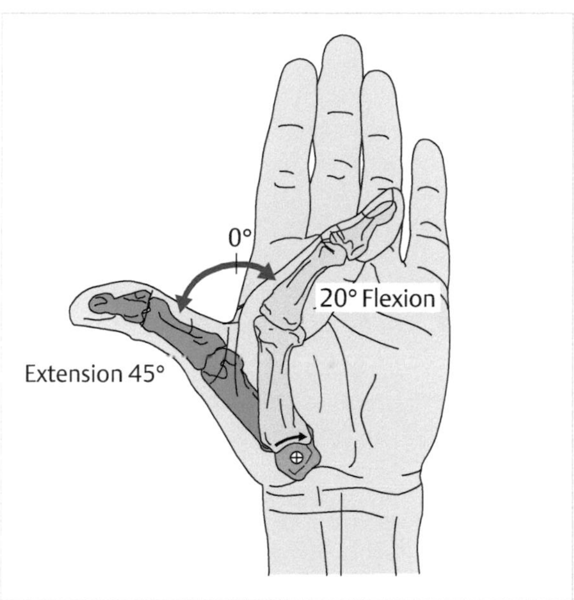


**Fig. 6.60** Flexion and extension in the saddle joint of the thumb; gliding performance in flexion (palmar view).

### Abduction and Adduction (Fig. 6.61)

The axis for abduction–adduction goes through the first metacarpal bone and runs from the palmar to the dorsal surface of the thumb.

Active *range of motion:* 45°/0° from neutral; passive: +5°.

#### *Joint Mechanics during Adduction*

The joint surface on the base of the metacarpal is convex from the radial to the ulnar side of the thumb. Therefore the base glides to the radial side of the thumb during adduction. This equates to a gliding behavior in the opposite direction to the movement of the metacarpal bone.

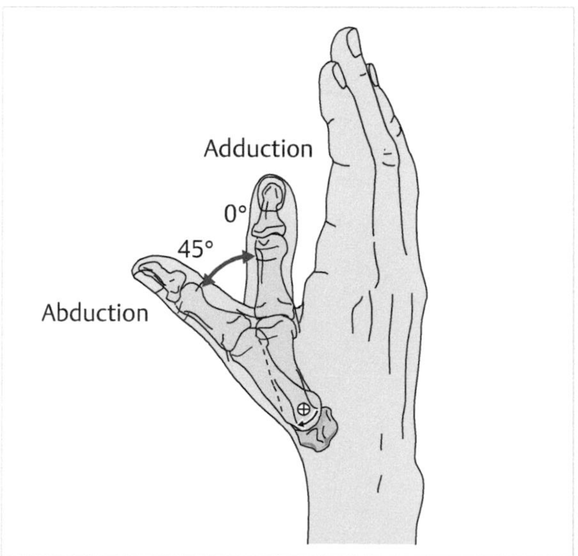


**Fig. 6.61** Abduction and adduction at the saddle joint of the thumb; gliding performance in adduction (radiodorsal view).

### Opposition (Fig. 6.62)

It is not possible to determine an axis of movement for opposition, because it is a mixed movement, consisting of the coupling of flexion and adduction with axial rotation.

During this movement, the metacarpal base rotates approximately 20 to 30° against the trapezium.

This movement is only possible by unlocking the joint, which means that the joint surfaces in this position lose congruence. At the end position, the force-bearing surface is very small, which increases the load many times over.

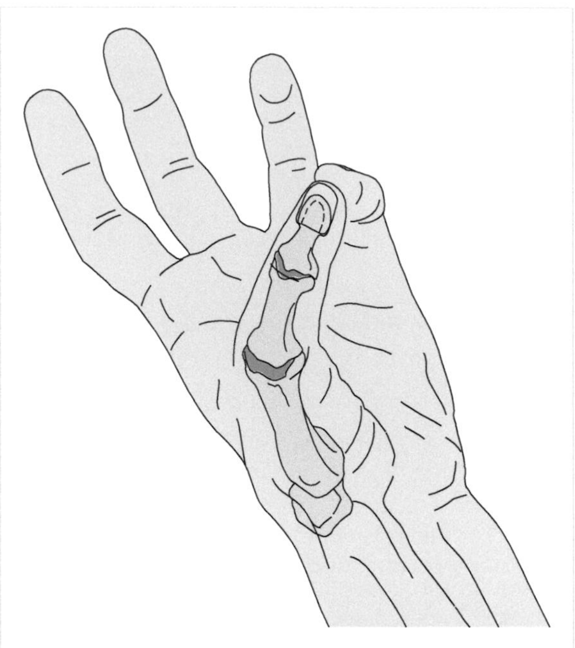

**Fig. 6.62** Opposition movement in the saddle joint of the thumb.

### Reposition

Reposition is the return of the thumb from opposition.

## Capsule and Ligaments

The **capsule** is wide and allows room for larger movements. It forms dorsal and palmar recesses. The insertion of both membranes is on the bone–cartilage border on each of the bones.

The **ligaments** lie directly over the capsule and stabilize the joint. They are so arranged that a portion of the ligaments is tensed in every position of the thumb.

The following ligaments can be differentiated (**Fig. 6.63**):

- An obliquely running ligament extends from the palmar side of the trapezium bone around the base of the first metacarpal and inserts onto the ulnar side of the metacarpal.
- In addition, a straight ligament here runs from the trapezium to the base of the metacarpal.
- On the dorsal side of the thumb, an obliquely running ligament extends around the base and inserts onto the palmar side.

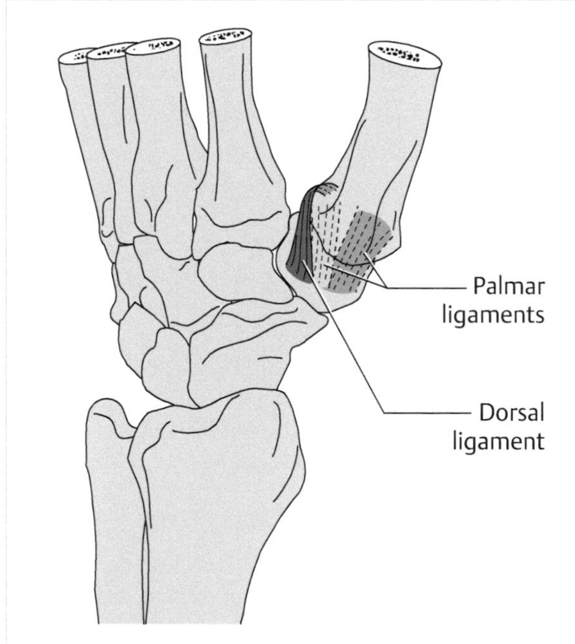


**Fig. 6.63** The ligaments of the saddle joint of the thumb (dorsal view).

## Intermetacarpal Joints (Fig. 6.64)

- The connections between the **metacarpal bases** are amphiarthroses.
- The joint facets on their radial and ulnar sides are cartilage-covered to articulate with each other. They are flat and vary in size.
- The joint capsule is taut, allowing only limited movement, and it usually connects with the carpometacarpal joint.
- The **dorsal and palmar metacarpal interosseous ligaments** are short ligaments that connect the bases of the metacarpal bones to each other. They lie directly distal to the joint capsule on both the dorsal and palmar sides. They perform the task of holding the metacarpal bones together and thus stabilize the movement of spreading the fingers.
- The **distal intermetacarpal connections** consist of obliquely running ligaments and are very mobile. This becomes important during grasping large objects, opposition, and spreading the fingers (**Fig. 6.65**).
- The **deep transverse metacarpal ligament** is a deep palmar ligament that spreads out transversely from radial to ulnar at the level of the metacarpal heads. It is fixed to the sides of the cartilage plates of the MCP joint and to the annular ligament as well. It limits the spreading of the metacarpals and thereby stabilizes the transverse metacarpal arch. Through its connection with the annular ligament and the cartilage plate, it supports the guidance system for the flexor tendons.
- The **superficial transverse metacarpal ligament** is a transverse ligament that runs over the distal metacarpals, almost at the level of the bases of the proximal phalanges. It is a component of the palmar aponeurosis and merges with the tendon sheaths of the flexors.
- As with the carpal bones, there is a transverse arch at the level of the metacarpal heads with its center at the third metacarpal head (**Fig. 6.66**).

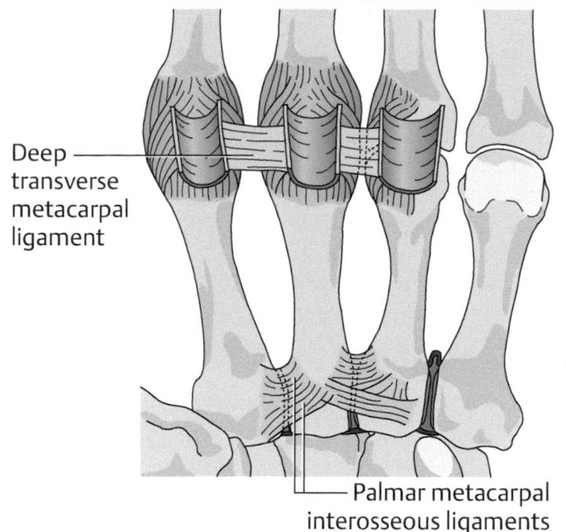


**Fig. 6.64** Intermetacarpal joints (palmar view).

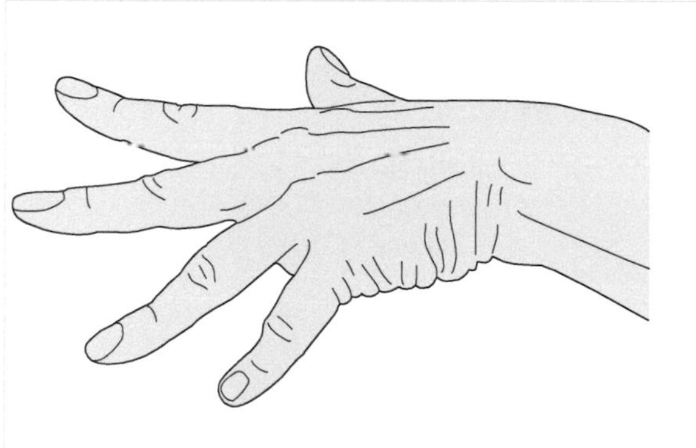

**Fig. 6.65** Mobility of the metacarpal connections during finger spreading.

## Movements

Isolated movements of the intermetacarpal joints are not possible. They are fundamentally combined with the movements of the carpometacarpal joints. The articulations on the radial and ulnar sides are very good, while the central column is the most immobile. It is impossible to determine the axes of movement. The movements that take place are primarily translational. For example, during opposition, the base of the fifth metacarpal glides against the base of the fourth metacarpal in a palmar direction. At the same time, the joint surfaces separate, and the base of the fifth metacarpal rotates as it would in supination.

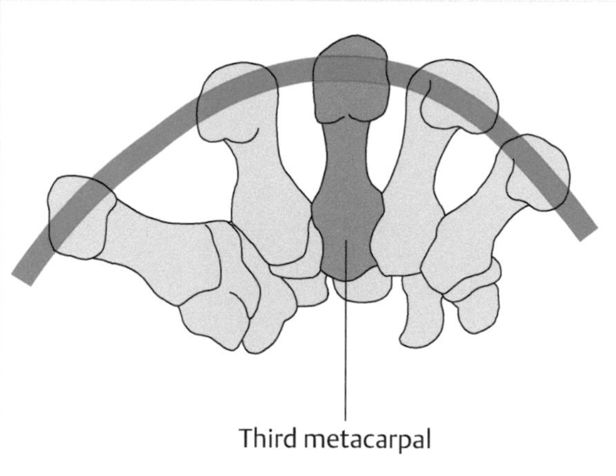


**Fig. 6.66** Transverse arch at the metacarpal head level.

## 6.2.15 Finger Joints

### Metacarpophalangeal Joints (Fig. 6.67)

- The MCPs are ball and socket joints.
- Articulating joint surfaces:
  - The base of the proximal phalanx forms the concave surface of the joint. It is enlarged on the palmar side by a fibrocartilage plate, which merges with the joint capsule. At this location as well as at its connection to the base of the phalanx, the capsule has a ligamentous reinforcement, the *palmar ligament*.
    A connection to the flexor tendon sheaths can be appreciated.
    In the neutral position, the cartilage plate has contact with the head of the metacarpal, but it loses this with increasing flexion as it glides in a palmar direction.
  - The metacarpal head forms the convex surface of the joint.
- The joint capsule is wide, with dorsal and palmar recesses. The insertion follows the bone–cartilage border of the joint surfaces in each of the joints.

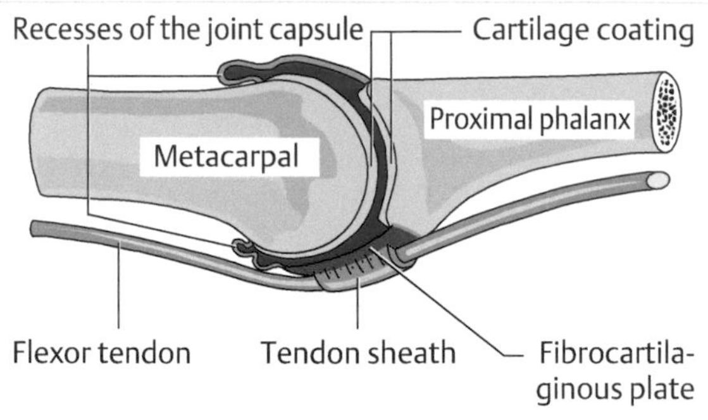


**Fig. 6.67** Metacarpophalangeal joints.

### Collateral Ligaments of the Second to Fifth Metacarpophalangeal Joints (Figs. 6.68 and 6.69)

- The radial and ulnar ligaments are fixed proximally on the metacarpal heads dorsal to the joint axis. The distal insertion is toward the palmar side on the base of the proximal phalanx.
- Because of both the course of the ligaments and also the thicker palmar side of the metacarpal head, the ligaments come under tension during flexion, meaning that side-to-side movements are possible in extension but not when the joint is flexed.
- A few fibers of the dorsal aponeurosis extend into the joint capsule.

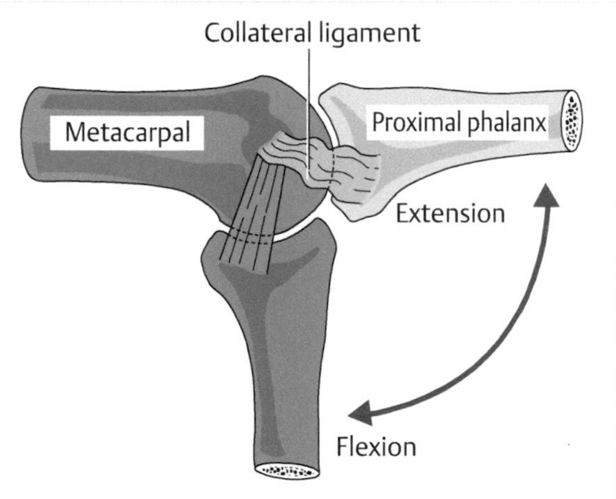


**Fig. 6.68** Collateral ligament of the metacarpophalangeal joints.

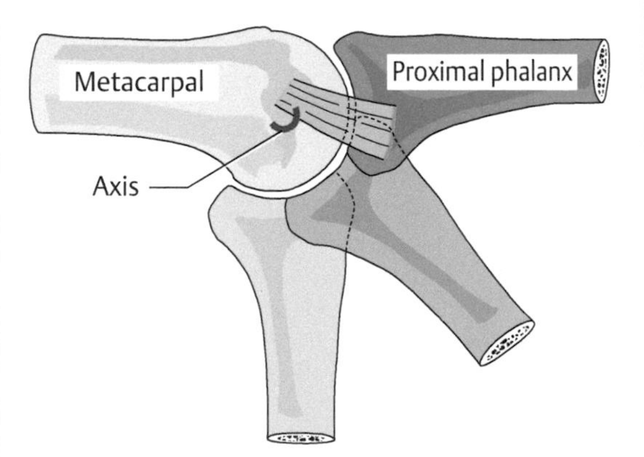


**Fig. 6.69** Metacarpophalangeal axis in relationship to the ligament.

## Radial and Ulnar Collateral Ligaments of the Thumb (Fig. 6.70)

- The radial and ulnar ligaments divide into two fibrous bands. The actual collateral ligament is the *proper collateral ligament*. This is fixed on the metacarpal head and on the base of the proximal phalanx and so runs obliquely from dorsal-proximal to palmar-distal.
- Two fibrous bands, the *accessory collateral ligaments*, one on each side of the metacarpal head, arise slightly to the palmar side and extend in a palmar direction to the respective radial or ulnar sesamoid bone. A few fibers also merge with the palmar cartilage plate.
- *Functions of the collateral ligaments:* Because of the varying courses of the collateral ligaments, there is an increase in tension in both extension and maximal flexion. Because of this, the joint is stable from side to side in both positions. In slight flexion, all the fibrous bands are relaxed, so that lateral and rotatory movements are possible, which is necessary, for example, when grasping objects.
- *Control of the sesamoid bones:* The sesamoid bones are restrained by the accessory collateral ligaments. Small ligaments extending from the sesamoid bones to the palmar metacarpal also contribute to this. Between the two sesamoid bones lies the palmar cartilage plate, with which the outer edges of the accessory ligaments merge. They also merge with the annular ligament. Through this rein-like arrangement, the sesamoid bones offer fixed ends for both heads of the adductor pollicis muscle, which insert onto the ulnar sesamoid bone, and for the flexor pollicis brevis and longus muscles, which extend to the radial sesamoid bone.

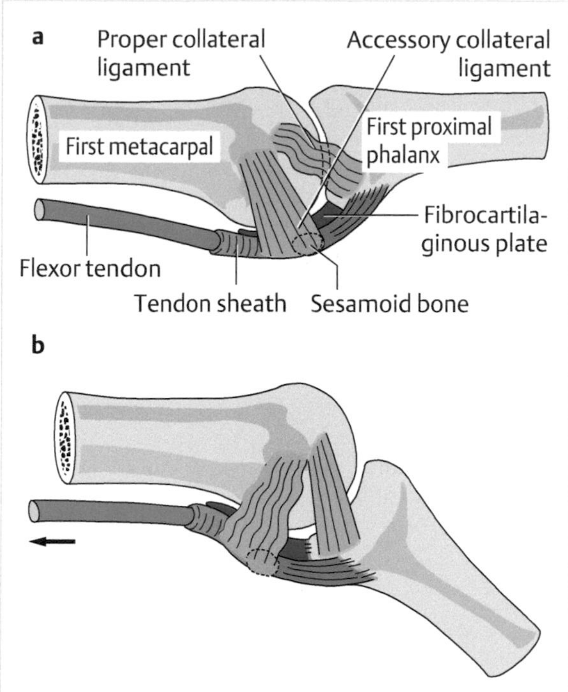


**Fig. 6.70** Collateral ligament of the first metacarpophalangeal joint. **(a)** In the neutral position. **(b)** In flexion.

## Axes and Movements of the Metacarpophalangeal Joints (Figs. 6.71–6.73)

### Horizontal Axis (Figs. 6.69 and 6.71)

The horizontal axis runs from radial to ulnar and lies in the head of the metacarpal. The joint rotates around it in flexion and extension. At the same time, the base of the phalanx adopts a gliding motion in the same direction.

The profile of the metacarpal head does not have a uniformly curved surface but is shaped unevenly in the dorsopalmar direction. Therefore the axis migrates from dorsal to palmar with increasing flexion. If all the axes are lined up next to each other, the result is an elliptical curve.

### Flexion/Extension

- Active *range of motion* of the **second to fourth MCP joints:** 90 to 100°/0 to 40° of flexion/extension from neutral; passive: +10 to +20°

The mobility in the MCP joints improves from the index finger to the little finger. The difference can amount to 20°.

As a result of the differences in the distance that the palmar joint surfaces reach proximally on the heads of the second and third metacarpals, the range of motion of the MCPs is greater on the ulnar side of the hand than on the radial side. Therefore a small accompanying rotation —a pronating twist—takes place during flexion.

- Active *range of motion* of the first MCP joint: 50°/5° of flexion/extension from neutral; passive: +5°.

### Sagittal Axis

The axes for abduction and adduction run from dorsal to palmar and lie in the middle of the head of the metacarpal.

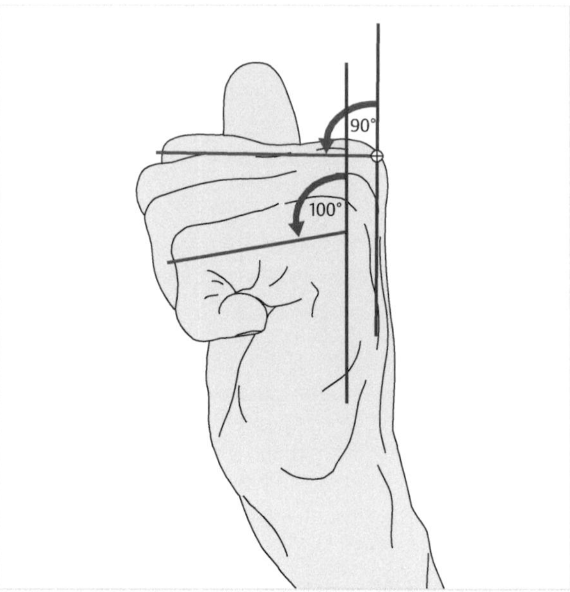


**Fig. 6.71** Active flexion in the metacarpophalangeal joints.

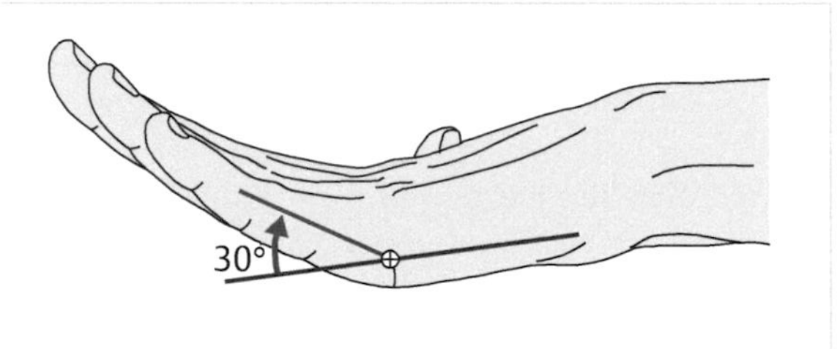


**Fig. 6.72** Active extension in the metacarpophalangeal joints.

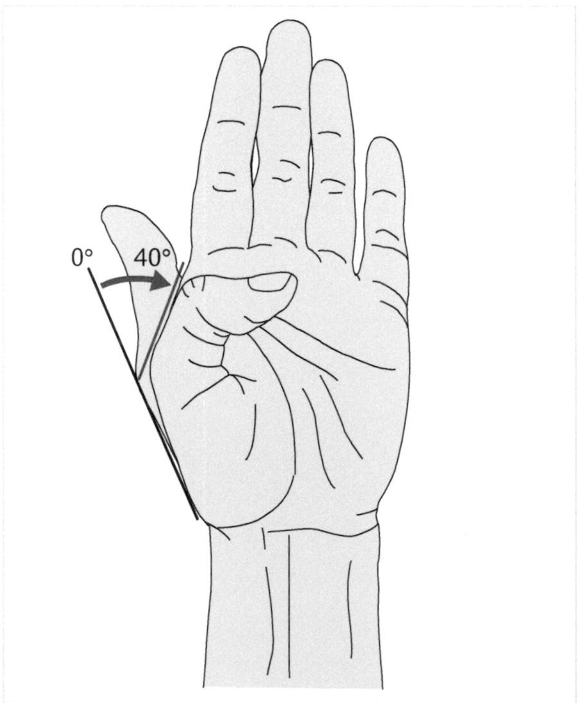


**Fig. 6.73** Flexion and extension in the first metacarpophalangeal joint.

### Abduction/Adduction (Figs. 6.74 and 6.75)

The terminology for movement is based on the middle finger. All movements away from the middle finger are designated "abduction," and all movements towards it "adduction."

- Active *range of motion* of the **second to fourth MCP joints:** 20 to 30°/10 to 20° of abduction/adduction from neutral; passive: +5 to +10°.

The index finger has the greatest side-to-side movement, followed by the little finger.

The combination of all four movements is termed circumduction.

- **First MCP joint:** Movements in this joint are only passive and limited, amounting to only approximately 5 to 10°.

## Longitudinal Axis

The axis for rotation corresponds to the longitudinal axis of the metacarpal bone.

### Rotation

- **Second to fifth MCP joints:** Rotation occurs as a movement accompanying flexion, because the palmar joint surface has an asymmetrical shape. A combination of flexion and rotation takes place, in that there is a pronating twist in the second and third MCP joints, and a supinating twist in the fourth and fifth joints. However, the range of motion is very limited. A purely axial rotation is only possible passively, with approximately 5° possible in each direction.
- **First MCP joint (Fig. 6.76):** In order to grasp with the greatest possible palmar thumb surface, the rotation, which begins in the saddle joint of the thumb, starts in a distal direction. That means that, in opposition, the proximal phalanx turns inward toward the fingers. However, the rotational range of motion is very limited.

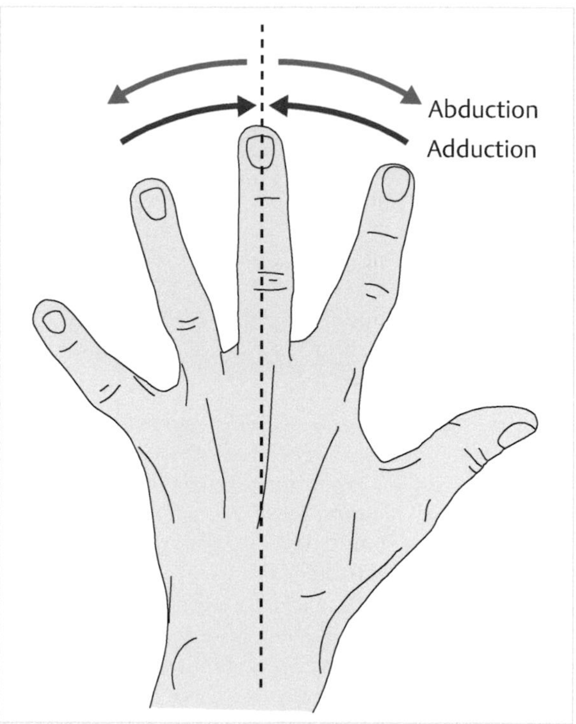


**Fig. 6.74** Movement terminology for abduction and adduction in the metacarpophalangeal joints.

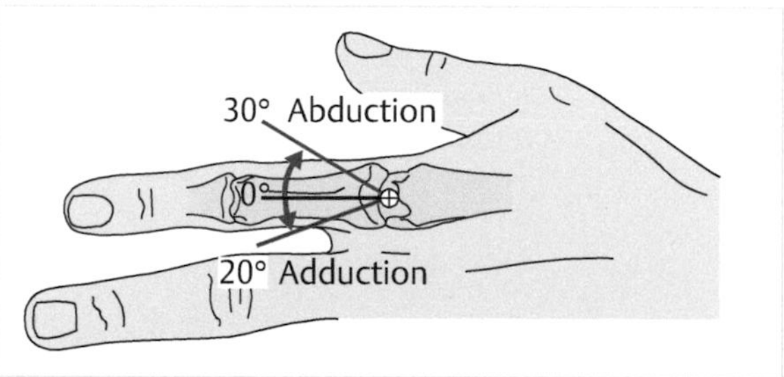


**Fig. 6.75** Abduction and adduction in the second metacarpophalangeal joint.

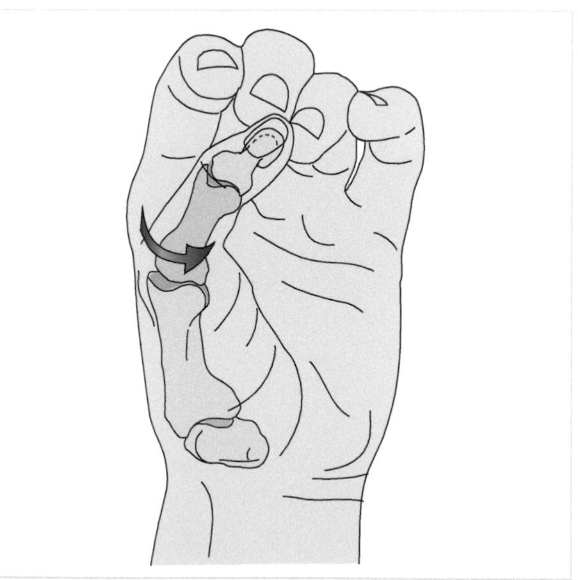

**Fig. 6.76** Rotation in first metacarpophalangeal joint. ▸

## Proximal and Distal Interphalangeal Joints (Fig. 6.77)

- These are hinge joints.
- Joint surfaces:
  - Concave: The base of the middle and distal phalanx of each finger has a small ridge in the middle of the concave joint surface that matches a corresponding furrow in its joint partner—this increases lateral stability. As with the MCPs, the joint surface is enlarged by a small fibrocartilaginous plate.
  - Convex: The heads of the proximal and middle phalanx are convex, with a furrow in the middle.
- The joint capsule is comparable to that of the MCPs.
- The collateral ligaments (**Fig. 6.78**) are tensed both in extension and at maximal flexion throughout their course from the head to the base and from the head to the fibrocartilaginous plate.
- Axis and movements: flexion/extension (**Fig. 6.79**):
  PIP: 110°/0° from neutral.
  DIP: 70–80°/5° from neutral (passive extension: 30°).
- The axis for each joint lies in the proximal joint partner.
- The palmar view of the hand with the MCP and PIP joints of the fingers flexed shows that the fingertips in the little and ring fingers point more or less obliquely in a radial direction. The course of the fingertips points to the scaphoid bone; this relationship plays a role in the movements involved in opposition (**Fig. 6.80**).

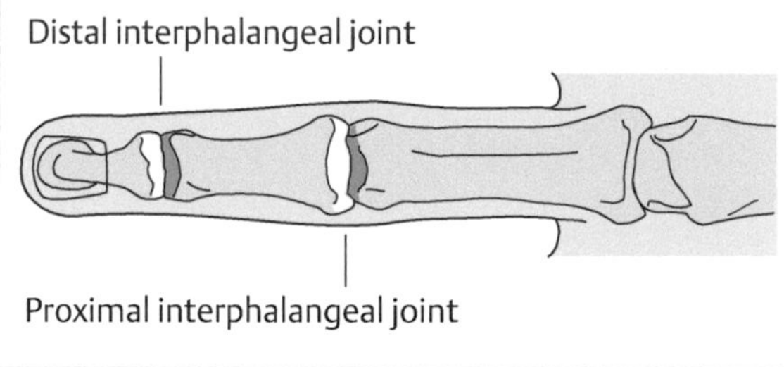


**Fig. 6.77** Interphalangeal joints, proximal and distal.

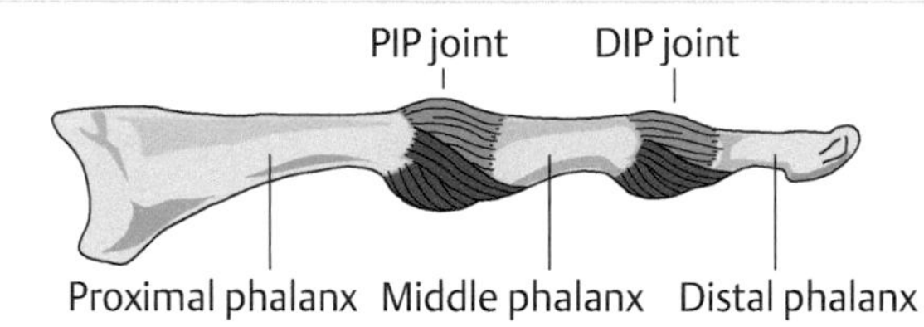


**Fig. 6.78** Ligaments of the proximal interphalangeal joints and dorsal interphalangeal joints. DIP, distal interphalangeal; PIP, proximal interphalangeal.

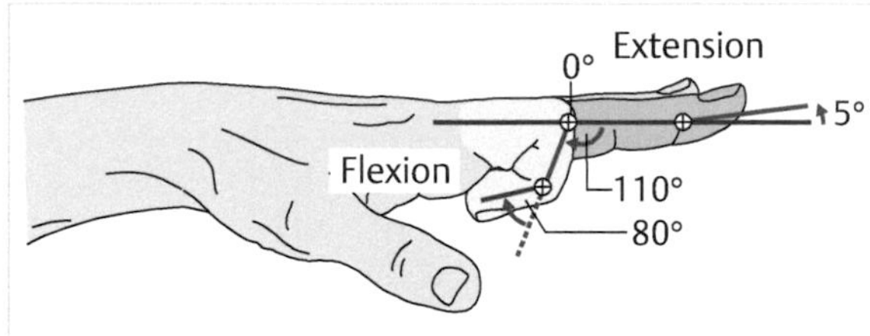


**Fig. 6.79** Active flexion and extension in the proximal interphalangeal joints and dorsal interphalangeal joints.

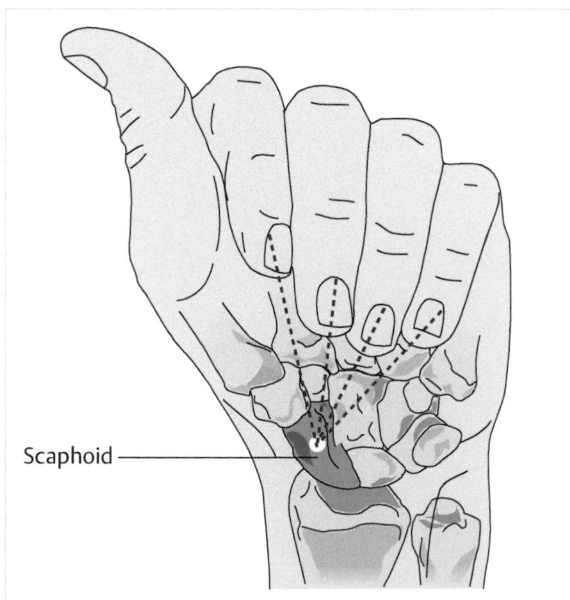


**Fig. 6.80** Orientation of the fingers toward the scaphoid bone during flexion.

## Interphalangeal Joint of the Thumb (Fig. 6.81)

- The capsule and ligaments are comparable to those of the PIP and DIP joints.
- Special characteristics: The end of the proximal phalanx is uneven, with the ulnar part of the condyle being slightly thicker. Because of this, the ulnar collateral ligament comes under tension before the lateral. That means that the movement in the radial part of the joint is greater, leading to a palmar orientation of the inner surface of the thumb. This continues the previously described tendency of the thumb to rotate, further improving the grasping function. (**Fig. 6.82**).
- *Range of motion* (**Fig. 6.83**):
  Flexion/extension: active: 80°/5 to 10° from neutral; passive: 100°/30° from neutral.

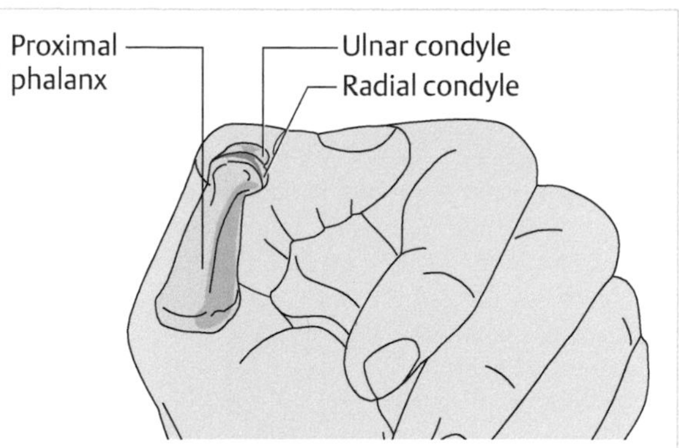


**Fig. 6.81** Distal end of the first proximal phalanx.

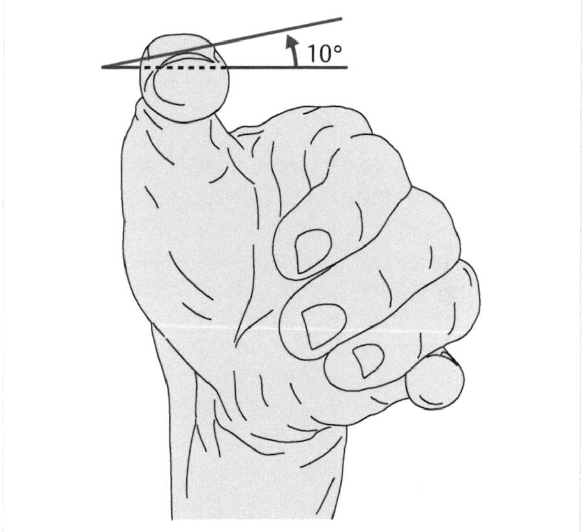


**Fig. 6.82** Tilting of the first distal phalanx in flexion.

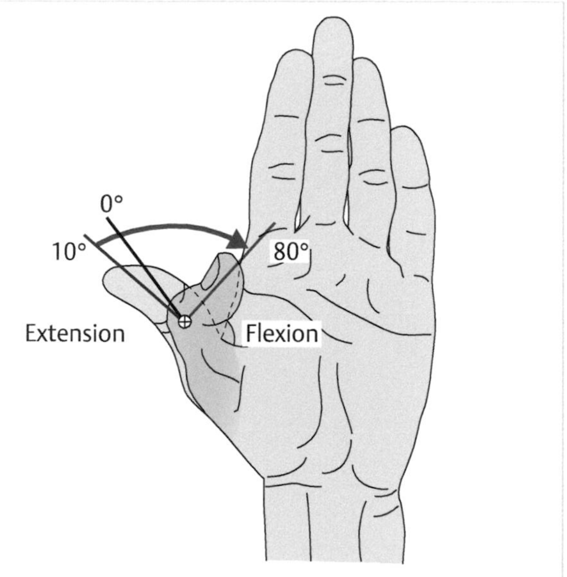


**Fig. 6.83** Active flexion and extension in the first interphalangeal joint.

## 6.2.16 Muscles of the Finger: Extensors (Fig. 6.84)

### Extensor Digitorum Muscle

- It forms four tendons, one to each of the fingers.
- They run through the fourth tendon compartment.
- Proximal to the MCPs, the tendons are connected by transversely extending fibrous bands called **intertendinous connections**—this limits the movements of the individual fingers.
- Each tendon divides distally into three parts: a centrally running band of fibers extends to the base of the middle phalanx. Distal to the MCP joints, two lateral slips branch off. These give off fibers to the collateral ligaments at the level of the PIP joints and insert onto the base of the distal phalanx.
- They form the dorsal aponeurosis, which connects with the capsule of the MCP joints.

**Functions:**

- It extends all the finger joints, with the main effect occurring in the MCP joints through the connection with the dorsal aponeurosis to the capsule and the proximal phalanx. The extensor digitorum muscle pulls the dorsal aponeurosis proximally, thereby allowing the lumbrical and interosseous muscles to extend the fingers. When relaxed, the aponeurosis moves distally, and the intrinsic muscles can flex the MCP joint.
- It produces dorsiflexion of the hand.
- It helps with ulnar abduction.

**Pathology**

In rheumatoid arthritis, collapse of the radial carpal bones can occur, leading to radial deviation of the hand. This causes a change in the course of the extensor tendon in the area of the MCP joint to the ulnar side, which in turn causes *ulnar deviation* of the fingers and the formation of a "zig-zag deformity."

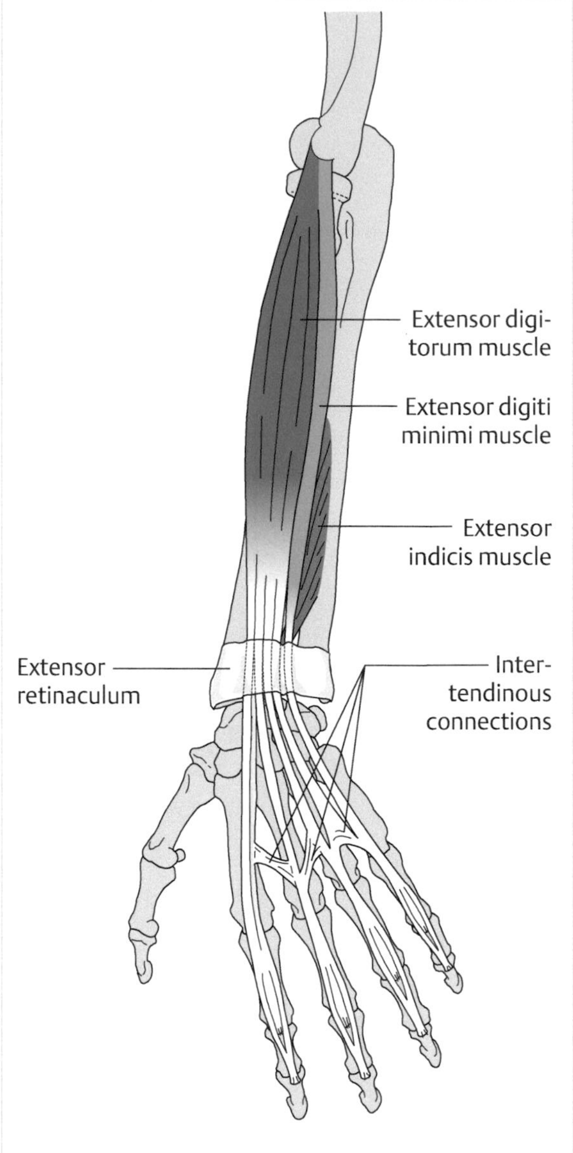


**Fig. 6.84** Extensors of the finger.

### Extensor Indicis Muscle

- This also runs through the fourth tendon compartment.
- At the level of the midmetacarpal, it extends into the dorsal aponeurosis of the index finger from the ulnar side and merges with the tendon of the extensor digitorum muscle.

**Functions:**

- Isolated extension of the index finger.
- Dorsiflexion of the hand.
- Contributes to radial abduction.

### Extensor Digiti Minimi Muscle

- This merges with the extensor digitorum muscle.
- It travels through the fifth tendon compartment.
- Its terminal tendon is involved in the formation of the dorsal aponeurosis, and it runs ulnar to the extensor digitorum muscle.

**Functions:**

- Extension of all the joints of the little finger.
- Abduction of the little finger.
- Dorsiflexion and ulnar abduction of the hand.

## Lumbrical Muscles (Fig. 6.85)

- The first and second lumbrical muscles arise from the radial edge of the tendon of the flexor digitorum profundus muscle. The third and fourth lumbricals are commonly bipennate, arising from both the ulnar and radial edges of the flexor tendons.
- They insert on the radial border of the joint capsule of the MCP joint, and, with a long tendon slip, the *pars obliqua*, to the radial area of the dorsal aponeurosis of each of the four fingers.

**Function.** Because of the connection with the radial bands of the dorsal aponeurosis, their main function is extension of the interphalangeal joints. They also provide a minimal force for flexion of the MCP joints, which they also stabilize.

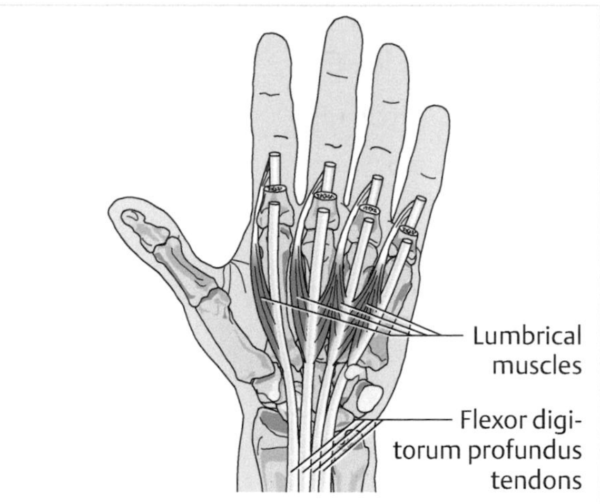


**Fig. 6.85** Lumbrical muscles (palmar view).

## Palmar Interosseous Muscles (Fig. 6.86a)

- The first palmar interosseous muscle arises from the ulnar side of the second metacarpal bone, and the second and third muscles from the radial side of the fourth and fifth metacarpal bones. They extend with long tendons as interosseous slips into the dorsal aponeurosis of the index, middle, and ring fingers. A small offshoot from each interosseous muscle extends to the capsule of the MCP joint and to the base of the proximal phalanx of the same finger.
- The palmar interossei lie between the metacarpal bones at a deep level.

**Function.** Abduction of the finger, flexion of the proximal phalanx, and extension in the interphalangeal joints.

## Dorsal Interosseous Muscles (Fig. 6.86b)

- These consist of four muscles, each with two heads.
- They arise with two heads from facing side surfaces of the metacarpal bones, and extend with long tendon slips into the lateral band of the corresponding dorsal aponeurosis.
- On its way to the palm, the radial artery runs through the gap between the two heads of the first dorsal interosseous muscle.

**Function.** Abduction of the finger. They cause flexion of the proximal phalanx because they run palmar to the flexion axis, and extension at the interphalangeal joints because they merge with the dorsal aponeurosis.

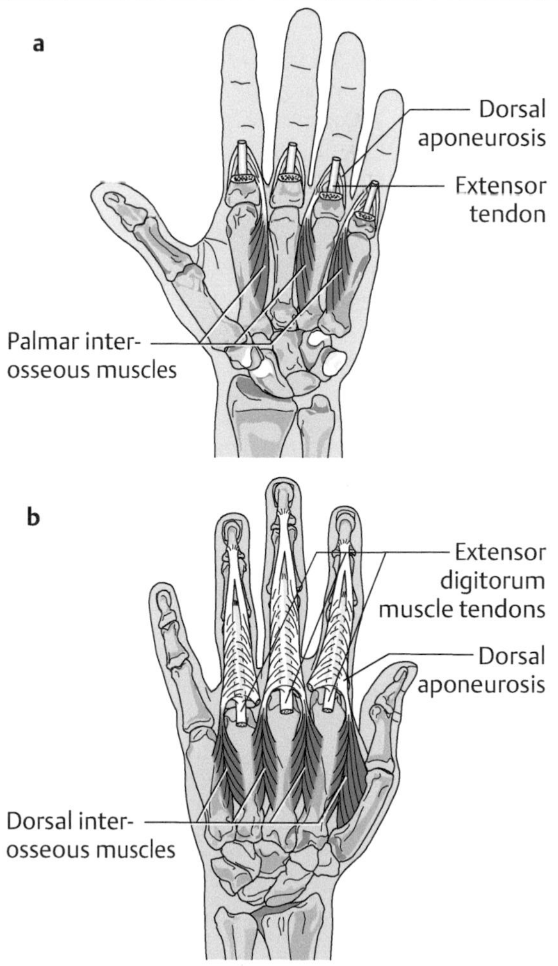


**Fig. 6.86** Interosseous muscles. **(a)** Palmer interosseous muscles (palmar view). **(b)** Dorsal interosseous muscles (dorsal view).

## Dorsal Aponeurosis of the Finger (Fig. 6.87)

The tendons of the extensors digitorum, indices, and digiti minimi and of the interossei and lumbricals extend into the *dorsal aponeurosis*. This is a tendinous sheet or plate (aponeurosis) that consists of interwoven fibrous bands of connective tissue. It starts at the MCP joint and reaches to the base of the distal phalanx. It has a triangular shape, wide proximally and becoming narrow distally.

The central slip is formed by the tendon of the extensor digitorum muscle. Fibrocartilaginous tissue is embedded in the side of the aponeurosis facing the joint over the MCP and PIP joints, which suggests an adaptation to increased compressive forces during extension. The interosseous muscles radiate into the aponeurosis from the side, and the lumbrical muscles from a palmar direction. Obliquely running fibrous bands, the *pars obliqua*, extend dorsally from the lumbrical muscle. The interosseous muscles form transverse bands of fibers, the *pars transversa*. On the palmar side, the interosseous slips join with the palmar fibrocartilaginous plate of the MCP joint and with the deep transverse metacarpal ligament.

The distal part of the aponeurosis consists of the collateral tendon slips of the extensor digitorum muscle, which end on the base of the distal phalanx.

The dorsal aponeurosis represents an important stabilizing mechanism. The connections to the intrinsic muscles and the ligaments on the sides keep the aponeuroses and the extensor tendons centralized. In addition, the connection to the palmar side helps with the lateral stability.

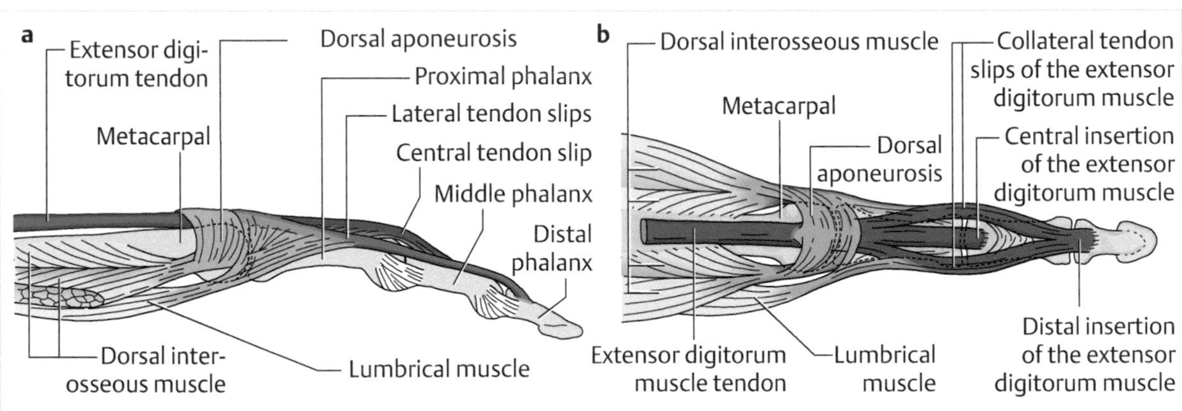


**Fig. 6.87** The dorsal aponeurosis with muscle insertions. **(a)** Radial view. **(b)** Dorsal view.

Pathology

### Deformities in Rheumatoid Arthritis

In rheumatoid arthritis, various deformities of the fingers can develop due to the destruction of joints and ligamentous apparatus.

#### Boutonnière Deformity (Fig. 6.88a)

The boutonnière deformity occurs at the level of the PIP joint because of destruction of the central tendon slip of the dorsal aponeurosis. Both parts of the lateral bands lose their control lines and slide in a palmar direction. In this position, they flex the PIP joints and extend the DIP joints. The head of the proximal phalanx pushes through the gap in the aponeuroses like a button through a buttonhole.

Treatment: Conservative therapy can help if the degree of deformity is minimal. To keep the lateral band in the correct position, flexion in the DIP joint must be exercised consistently with the PIP joint in the extended position. This is supported by wearing a splint at night that fixes the MCP joint in 30° of flexion and the PIP joint in extension, leaving the DIP joint freely mobile.

Surgical treatment involves shortening the intermediate tract and repositioning and fixation of the lateral band.

#### Swan-neck Deformity (Fig. 6.88b)

A swan-neck deformity involves a disturbance of the balance between the flexors and extensors. Due to the collapse of the carpal bones and subluxation of the MCP joint in a palmar direction, the transverse part of the dorsal aponeurosis shifts in the same direction. Because of this, the intrinsic muscles (e.g., the interosseous muscles) come under tension and produce flexion at the MCP joint and hyperextension at the PIP joint. In addition, the collateral bands of the extensor tendon can become inadequate, so that the flexor digitorum profundus muscle predominates, pulling the distal phalanx into flexion.

Surgical therapy is based on the cause. It usually involves reconstruction and refixation of the tendons and parts of the ligamentous structure. In extreme cases, arthrodesis of the DIP joint is considered.

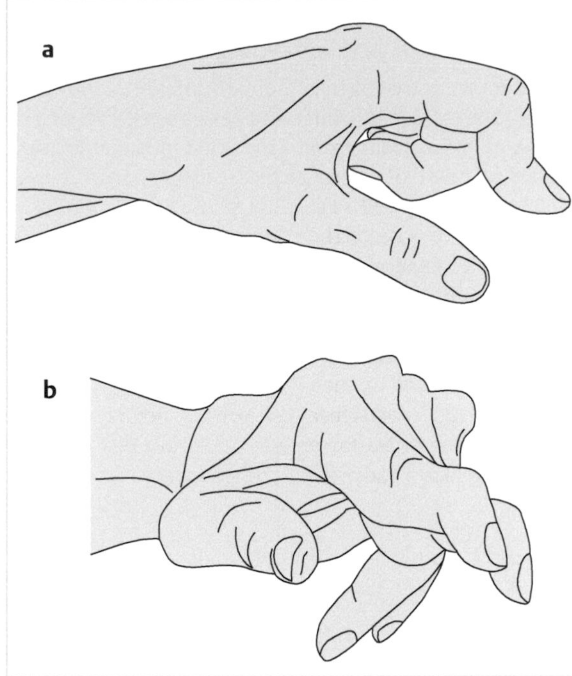


**Fig. 6.88 (a)** Boutonnière deformity. **(b)** Swan-neck deformity.

## Dorsal Tendon Compartments and Tendinous Sheaths (Figs. 6.89 and 6.90)

The extensor muscle retinaculum encompasses the distal dorsal forearm and a portion of the proximal row of carpal bones. It functions to hold the dorsal tendons in place on the forearm. Six vertically placed connective tissue septa extend from the underside of the retinaculum in a palmar direction and attach the radius and ulna.

These form osteofibrotic canals that determine the courses of the tendons. Deep retinacular fibers form the floor of the tendon compartments.

The *first tendon compartment* lies on the lateral aspect of the radius and carries the tendons of the abductor pollicis longus and extensor pollicis brevis muscles. Each tendon is encased in a synovial sheath that is longer for the extensor than it is for the abductor.

In the *second tendon compartment*, the tendon of the extensor carpi radialis longus muscle runs on the radial side, and that of the extensor carpi radialis brevis muscle on the ulnar side. The surrounding tendon sheath is usually arranged so that the fibrous sheath wraps around both tendons while the synovial sheath encloses each tendon individually.

In the *third tendon compartment*, the extensor pollicis longus muscle extends distally. Proximal to the dorsal tubercle of the radius, it runs longitudinally, and then bends radially in an arc around the tubercle, so it lies over the tendons of the second tendon compartment. Its tendon sheath reaches far distally—all the way up to the saddle joint of the thumb.

The *fourth tendon compartment* contains the tendons of the extensor digitorum and extensor indicis muscles. Compared with the other tendons, the extensor indicis muscle runs in a deeper position, on the floor of the compartment. All the tendons in this compartment are enclosed within a common tendon sheath.

The *fifth tendon compartment* crosses over the distal radio-ulnar joint and carries the extensor digiti minimi muscle distally. Its tendon sheath is very long—it can reach up to the middle of the metacarpal bone.

The *sixth tendon compartment* lies on the ulnar side and contains the extensor carpi ulnaris muscle. The enveloping tendon sheath begins proximal to the retinaculum and ends beyond the distal border of the retinaculum.

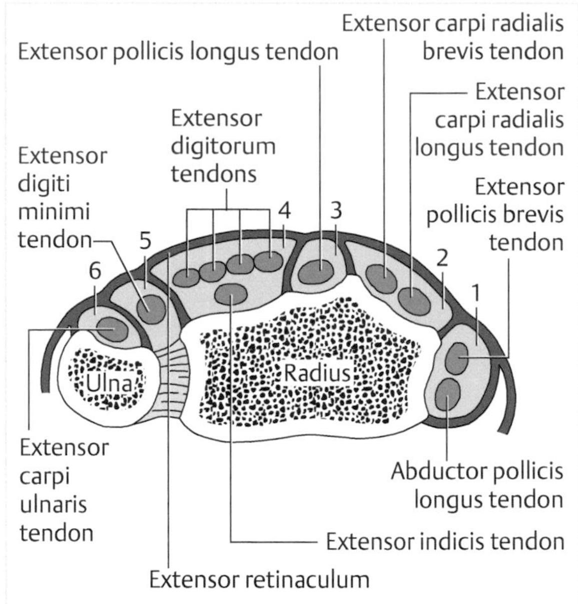


**Fig. 6.89** The dorsal tendon compartments of the hand in transverse section.

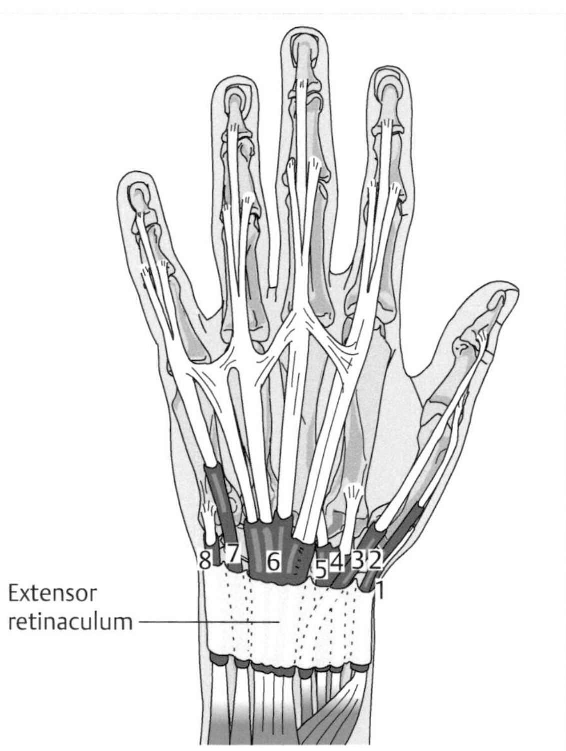


1 = Tendinous sheath, abductor pollicis longus muscle
2 = Tendinous sheath, extensor pollicis brevis muscle
3 = Tendinous sheath, extensor pollicis longus muscle
4 = Tendinous sheath, extensor carpi radialis longus muscle
5 = Tendinous sheath, extensor carpi radialis brevis muscle
6 = Tendinous sheath, extensor digitorum and extensor indicis muscles
7 = Tendinous sheath, extensor digiti minimi muscle
8 = Tendinous sheath, extensor carpi ulnaris muscle

**Fig. 6.90** Dorsal tendinous sheaths of the hand. ▸

## 6.2.17 Muscles of the Finger: Flexors

### Flexor Digitorum Superficialis Muscle (Fig. 6.91)

- This emerges with two heads: the humero-ulnar head and the radial head. The humero-ulnar head arises from the medial epicondyle of the humerus, the ulnar capsule–ligament apparatus, and the medial edge of the ulnar coronoid process. The radial head originates from the radius, distal to the radial tuberosity. It extends to the palmar side of the base of the second to fifth middle phalanges.
- The humero-ulnar and radial heads form an arch, the tendinous arch, through which the median nerve tracks distally.
- The four terminal tendons run within the carpal tunnel.
- Shortly before the PIP joint, each terminal tendon splits into two parts, through which a slit develops (hence the alternate name for the muscle, *flexor digitorum perforatus muscle*). The tendon of the flexor digitorum profundus muscle travels through this opening. After that the two lateral slips join, forming the terminal tendon.

**Function.** Flexion of the MCP and PIP joints, palmar flexion at the wrist joint, and minimal flexion at the elbow joint.

### Flexor Digitorum Profundus Muscle (Fig. 6.92)

- This connects the proximal half of the anterior ulna and the interosseous membrane with the palmar side of the base of the distal phalanges.
- It runs on the ulnar side of the forearm and proximally forms the deepest layer of anterior forearm muscles.
- It extends with its four terminal tendons through the carpal tunnel and lies directly over the capsule–ligament apparatus of the carpal bones.
- At the level of the proximal phalanges, its tendons pierce those of the flexor digitorum superficialis muscle (hence the alternative name of *flexor digitorum perforans muscle*).

**Function.** Flexion at all the finger joints and palmar flexion at the wrist joint. The ulnar part of the tendon causes ulnar abduction.

Flexor digitorum superficialis muscle
Humeral head
Ulnar head
Radial head
Transverse carpal ligament

Fig. 6.91 Flexor digitorum superficialis muscle.

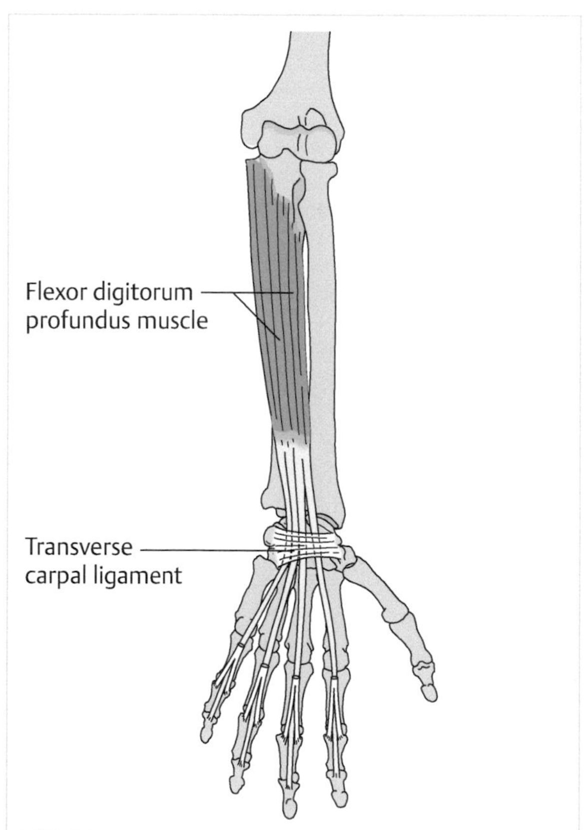


Fig. 6.92 Flexor digitorum profundus muscle.

## Flexor Tendinous Sheaths (Fig. 6.93)

- These enclose the tendons of the finger flexors.
- Along with the bony structures, they form an osteofibrotic canal through which the tendons run. They are reinforced by the palmar ligaments in the joint areas.
- The inner layer is the tenosynovium, which reduces the friction caused by the gliding of the tendon and contributes to the tendon's nutrition.
- The tendon sheaths start somewhat proximal to the MCPs; only the thumb and little finger tendons are almost completely enclosed by tendinous sheaths as far proximally as the carpal tunnel. Distally, they end at the base of the distal phalanx.
- Circularly arranged fibrous bands, the annular part of the fibrous sheath (*annular ligaments of the fingers*), which are connected to the *cruciate ligaments*, provide reinforcement. They ensure that the tendons are guided close to each phalanx.
- In the carpal tunnel, the tendons are also enclosed by tendinous sheaths, which reach proximally up to 3 cm beyond the flexor retinaculum.

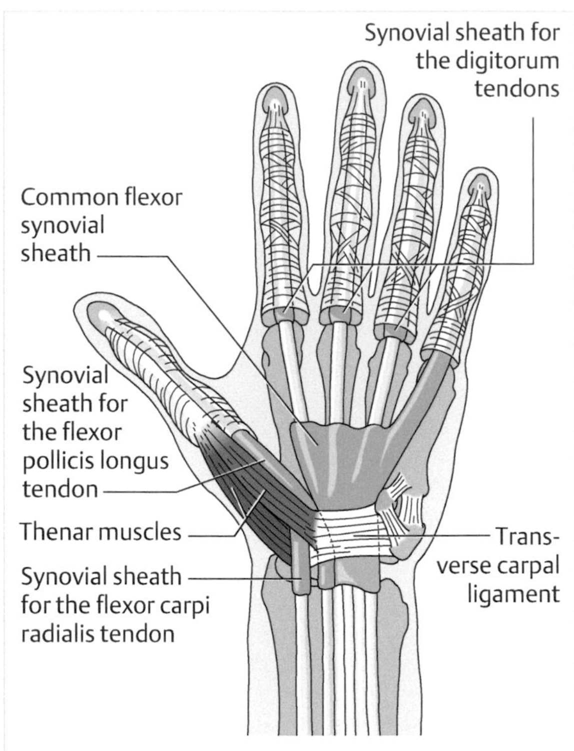


**Fig. 6.93** Palmar tendon sheaths of the hand and wrist.

**Pathology**

*Trigger finger* is a disparity between a thickened tendon and its tendon sheath. Due to the formation of rheumatic nodules, there is little room under the annular ligament. In flexion, the thickened tendon must be forced through the narrow space, which happens in a jerky manner. The treatment is tenosynovectomy and division of the annular ligament.

## Palmar Aponeurosis (Fig. 6.94)

- This is a connective tissue sheet, spread out like a fan in the palm area, that consists of two layers: a deep layer with transversely running bands of fibers, and a superficial layer with longitudinal bands. The transversely running fibrous bands radiate into the fascia of the thenar and hypothenar muscles. The longitudinal bands extend distally into the superficial transverse metacarpal ligament, merge with the most proximal of the annular ligaments and partly insert onto the proximal phalanges.
- Small, strong fiber bundles merge with the subcutaneous tissue, so that only limited skin movement is possible in the palm area. These bundles subdivide the subcutaneous fat tissue into chambers and carry blood vessels to the skin.
- The palmaris longus and brevis muscles extend into the aponeurosis.

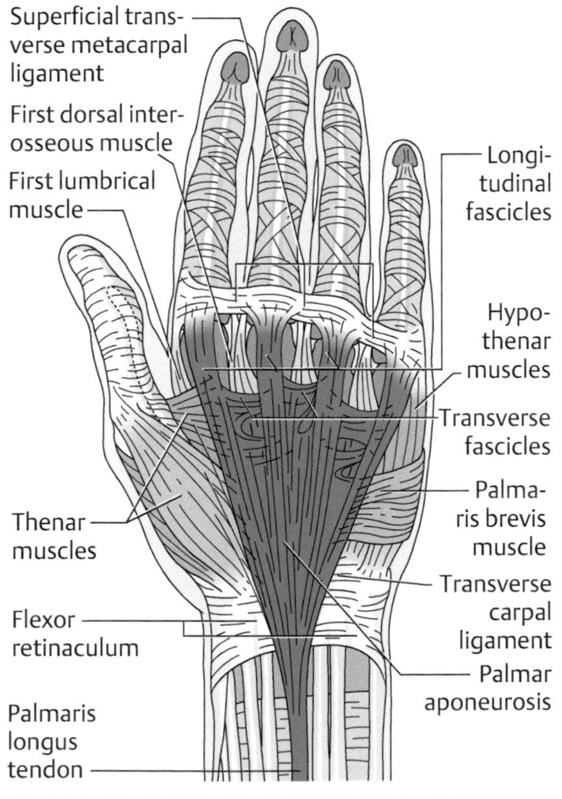


**Fig. 6.94** The palmar aponeurosis.

## 6.2.18 Long Thumb Muscles (Fig. 6.95)

### Extensor Pollicis Longus Muscle

- This extends from the posterior surfaces of the ulna and the interosseous membrane to the dorsal base of the distal phalanx of the thumb.
- It passes through the third tendon compartment under the extensor retinaculum.
- It uses the dorsal tubercle of the radius as a hypomochlion to turn in the direction of the thumb over the dorsum of the wrist. In doing so, its tendons cross the radial extensors of the wrist joint.
- The muscle forms the dorsal border of the anatomical snuffbox.
- It combines with the dorsal aponeurosis, which surrounds the dorsal side of the MCP joint like a cap and has a connection to the sesamoid bone on the palmar side of the thumb by way of the collateral band on the same side.

**Function.** Extension of all the thumb joints, dorsiflexion, and radial abduction at the wrist.

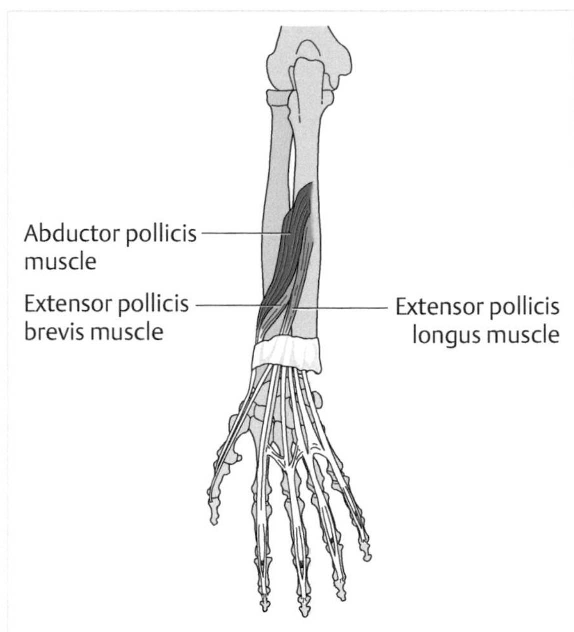


**Fig. 6.95** The long muscles of the thumb.

### Extensor Pollicis Brevis Muscle

- This connects the posterior side of the last third of the radius and the interosseous membrane with the dorsal side of the base of the proximal phalanx of the thumb.
- Its course is oblique in a proximal-ulnar to distal-radial direction.
- Proximal to the retinaculum, it crosses the tendons of the wrist extensors.
- It travels through the first tendon compartment with the abductor pollicis longus muscle.

**Function.** Extension at the saddle joint of the thumb and the MCP joints. It also supports radial abduction of the hand.

### Abductor Pollicis Longus Muscle

- This extends from the posterior surfaces of the ulna and radius in the midforearm and the interosseous membrane to the radial surface of the base of the first metacarpal.
- The muscle fibers have an oblique course from proximal-ulnar to distal-radial.
- Its terminal tendon begins at the level of the distal third of the forearm and runs longitudinally, parallel to the radius.
- It passes under the extensor retinaculum with the extensor pollicis brevis muscle through the first tendon compartment.

**Function.** Abduction and extension at the saddle joint of the thumb, and dorsiflexion and radial abduction at the radiocarpal joint.

### Flexor Pollicis Longus Muscle

- This originates from the anterior surface of the radius distal to the radial tuberosity up to the midradius and the interosseous membrane and extends to the palmar surface of the distal phalanx of the thumb.
- In the forearm, it lies deep within the tissue and radial to the flexor digitorum profundus muscle.
- It runs on the radial side of the carpal tunnel.
- Its tendon sheath begins proximal to the carpal tunnel and ends on the distal phalanx.
- In the thenar area, it runs deeply between the superficial and deep heads of the flexor pollicis brevis muscle.
- Its tendon is held in place next to the bone by proximal and distal annular ligaments at the levels of the MCP and interphalangeal joints, respectively.

**Function.** Flexion of all the thumb joints, and flexion and radial abduction of the wrist joint.

## 6.2.19 Short Thumb Muscles (Thenar Muscles) (Fig. 6.96)

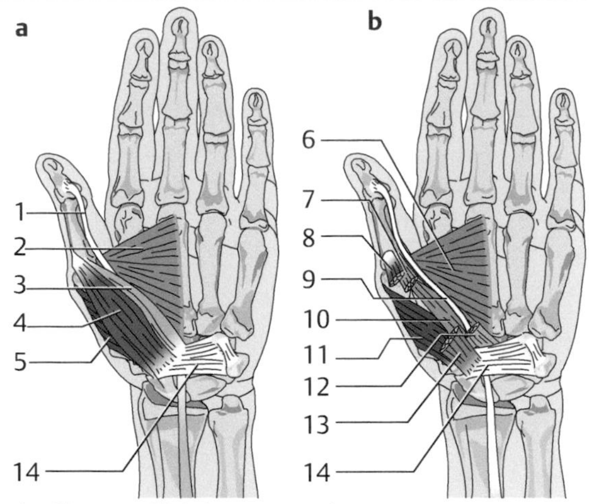


1 = Flexor pollicis longus tendon
2 = Adductor pollicis muscle
3 = Superficial head, flexor pollicis brevis muscle
4 = Abductor pollicis brevis muscle
5 = Opponens pollicis muscle
6 = Adductor pollicis muscle
7 = Superficial head, flexor pollicis brevis muscle
8 = Abductor pollicis brevis muscle
9 = Flexor pollicis longus tendon
10 = Flexor pollicis brevis muscle (deep head)
11 = Opponens muscle
12 = Superficial head, flexor pollicis brevis muscle (cut)
13 = Abductor pollicis brevis muscle (cut)
14 = Transverse carpal ligament

**Fig. 6.96** The thenar muscles. **(a)** Superficial layer. **(b)** Deep layer.

### Flexor Pollicis Brevis Muscle

- This has two heads: the superficial head from the distal radial edge of the transverse carpal ligament, and the deep head from the dorsal surfaces of the trapezium, trapezoid, and capitate bones. It extends to the radial sesamoid, the joint capsule of the MCP joint, and the base of the proximal phalanx.
- The tendon of the flexor pollicis longus muscle runs between the superficial and deep heads and then extends further distally.

**Function.** Flexion at the carpometacarpal and MCP joints of the thumb. It also supports opposition and adduction at the saddle joint of the thumb.

### Abductor Pollicis Brevis Muscle

- The abductor pollicis brevis muscle originates from the tubercles of the scaphoid and trapezium bones and the transverse carpal ligament, and inserts onto the radial sesamoid, the base of the proximal phalanx, and the joint capsule of the MCP joint of the thumb.
- It lies directly under the skin and, along with the opponens pollicis muscle, forms the contour of the thenar eminence.
- At its insertion, it merges with the tendon of the flexor pollicis brevis muscle.

**Function.** Abduction of the thumb at the saddle joint of the thumb. It also supports flexion of the MCP joint of the thumb.

### Opponens Pollicis Muscle

- This extends from the tubercle of the scaphoid bone and the transverse carpal ligament to the radial edge of the diaphysis of the first metacarpal bone.
- It has an oblique course from proximal-ulnar to distal-radial.
- It is overlain by the abductor pollicis brevis muscle.

**Function.** Opposition. It also supports flexion and (minimally) adduction at the saddle joint of the thumb.

### Adductor Pollicis Muscle

- This has two heads: the transverse head arises from the palmar diaphysis of the third metacarpal bone, and the oblique head arises from the bases of the second and third metacarpals, the capitate bone, and the transverse carpal ligament. It extends to the ulnar sesamoid bone, the base of the proximal phalanx, and the joint capsule of the first carpometacarpal joint.
- It is the largest and most powerful thenar muscle.
- In its distal portion, there is a gap between it and the deep head of the flexor pollicis brevis muscle, through which the tendon of the flexor pollicis longus muscle runs.
- A gap forms between the two heads of the muscle, through which the deep palmar arch of the radial artery and the deep branch of the ulnar nerve run.

**Function.** Adduction at the saddle joint of the thumb. It also supports opposition and flexion at the saddle joint of the thumb.

## 6.2.20 Hypothenar Muscles (Fig. 6.97)

### Abductor Digiti Minimi Muscle

- This arises from the pisiform bone, the pisohamate ligament, the transverse carpal ligament, and the tendon of the flexor carpi ulnaris muscle. It extends to the ulnar border of the base of the fifth proximal phalanx.
- It lies directly under the skin on the ulnar side of the hand.

**Function.** Abduction of the little finger. It also supports flexion in the carpometacarpal and MCP joints.

### Flexor Digiti Minimi Brevis Muscle

- This extends from the hook of the hamate and the transverse carpal ligament to the palmar side of the base of the fifth proximal phalanx.
- It borders radially on the abductor digiti minimi muscle.

**Function.** Flexion of the MCP joint of the little finger.

### Opponens Digiti Minimi Muscle

- This arises from the hook of the hamate and the transverse carpal ligament, and connects with the ulnar edge of the diaphysis of the fifth metacarpal.
- Its direction of pull is oblique, from proximal-radial to distal-ulnar.
- It becomes wider towards its insertion.

**Function.** Opposition of the little finger. It also supports flexion at the fifth carpometacarpal joint.

## 6.2.21 Palmaris Brevis Muscle

Its effect on hand movement is negligible. It is fixed to the skin distal to the pisiform bone and extends into the ulnar border of the palmar aponeurosis. It cushions Guyon's canal, tenses the palmar aponeurosis from the little-finger side, and can wrinkle the skin.

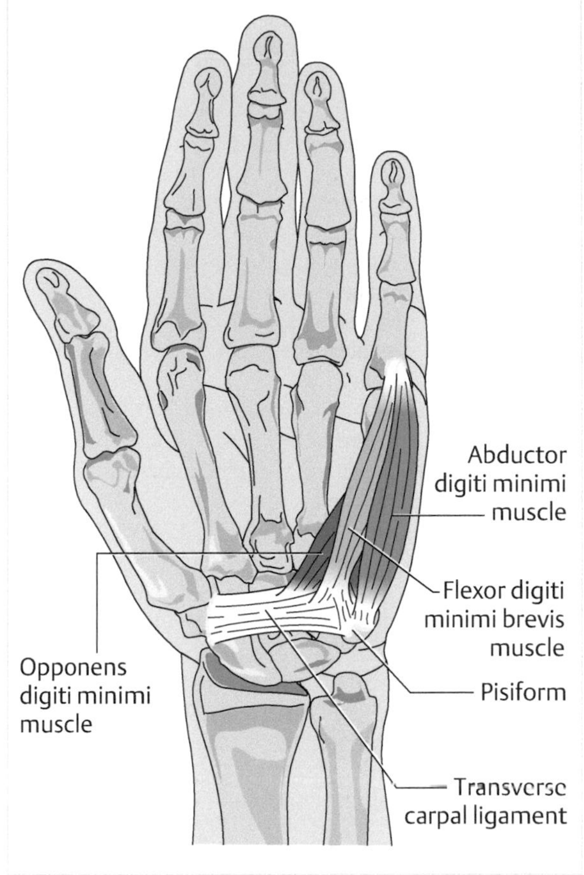


**Fig. 6.97** The hypothenar muscles.

## 6.3 Course of Nerves in the Hand and Wrist Region (Fig. 6.98)

### Median Nerve

Distal to the pronator teres muscle, the median nerve gives off the **anterior interosseous nerve**, which supplies the flexor pollicis longus muscle, the digitorum profundus muscle (excluding the ulnar part), the pronator quadratus muscle, and the wrist joint.

In the carpal tunnel, the median nerve runs ulnar to the tendon of the flexor pollicis longus muscle and palmar to the other tendons that go through the tunnel.

Distal to this, it branches off into muscular branches to the thenar eminence for the abductor pollicis brevis, flexor pollicis brevis, and opponens muscles, and sensory branches, the **proper palmar digital nerves**, which innervate the skin of the thumb, index, and middle fingers, as well as the radial side of the ring finger. The first and second common palmar digital nerves supply the corresponding lumbrical muscles.

The **palmar branch** exits proximal to the wrist joint, supplies the skin in the thenar area, and forms anastomoses with the palmar branch of the ulnar nerve.

▷ See Fig. 6.43, Carpal Tunnel

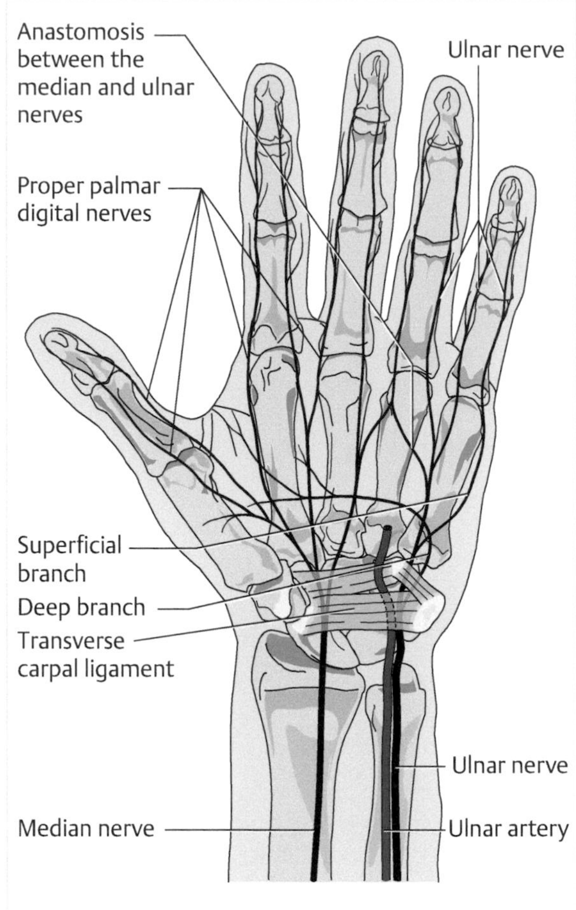


**Fig. 6.98** Course of nerves in the hand and wrist region: median nerve and ulnar nerve.

### Ulnar Nerve

At the wrist level, the ulnar nerve divides into the **dorsal digital nerves** for the skin on the dorsal side of the ring and little fingers and the ulnar side of the middle finger up to the proximal interphalangeal joint.

The sensory **palmar branch of the ulnar nerve** supplies the ulnar part of the palmar side of the wrist joint and the proximal part of the hypothenar eminence.

The main part of the nerve runs on the palmar side and divides into two branches:

The **superficial branch** runs superficially over the pisohamate ligament and extends on the ulnar side to the fingertips of the little and ring fingers. It gives off a motor branch to the palmaris brevis muscle and then divides into the fourth and fifth **common palmar digital nerves**, sensory nerves that supply the little finger and the ulnar side of the ring finger as the proper palmar digital nerves.

The **deep branch** is a purely motor nerve. It extends between the transverse carpal ligament and the pisohamate ligament through Guyon's canal and enters into the deep area between the hypothenar muscles ulnar to the hook of the hamate. Here it gives off muscular branches in an ulnar direction to these muscles.

It then extends in a radial direction as an arch at the level of the proximal third of the metacarpal bone, lying immediately over the metacarpal bones and the interosseous muscles. With further muscular branches arising from the arch, it innervates the ulnar two lumbrical muscles, all the interosseous muscles, and, radially, the adductor pollicis muscle and the deep head of the flexor pollicis brevis muscle.

It connects with the median nerve through an anastomosis.

▷ See Fig. 6.44, Guyon's Canal

## Radial Nerve (Fig. 6.99)

The sensory **superficial branch** extends distally on the dorsal side of the forearm. It runs above the retinaculum and further radially across the anatomical snuffbox before dividing into six branches to the fingers, the **dorsal digital nerves**, which supply the dorsal side of the thumb up to the distal proximal phalanx and the dorsal skin areas of the proximal phalanx of the index and middle fingers. It joins with the ulnar nerve through an anastomosis.

### Pathology

The median nerve is especially vulnerable to injury in the carpal tunnel.
The most common treatment is surgery. The surgeon divides the transverse carpal ligament to decompress the nerve. The ulnar nerve becomes compressed in its course over the transverse carpal ligament or in Guyon's canal.

### Practical Tip

Differential diagnostics are important in this context. Examination of the cervical spine can exclude a problem of the C6–C7 vertebrae as a cause, and provocation testing in the area of the thoracic outlet can eliminate compression from bottlenecks there as a cause.
The level of a nerve injury can be determined by appropriate muscle provocation testing (e.g., of the pronator teres muscle), through medial nerve compression at the elbow, or by manual compression of the carpal tunnel.

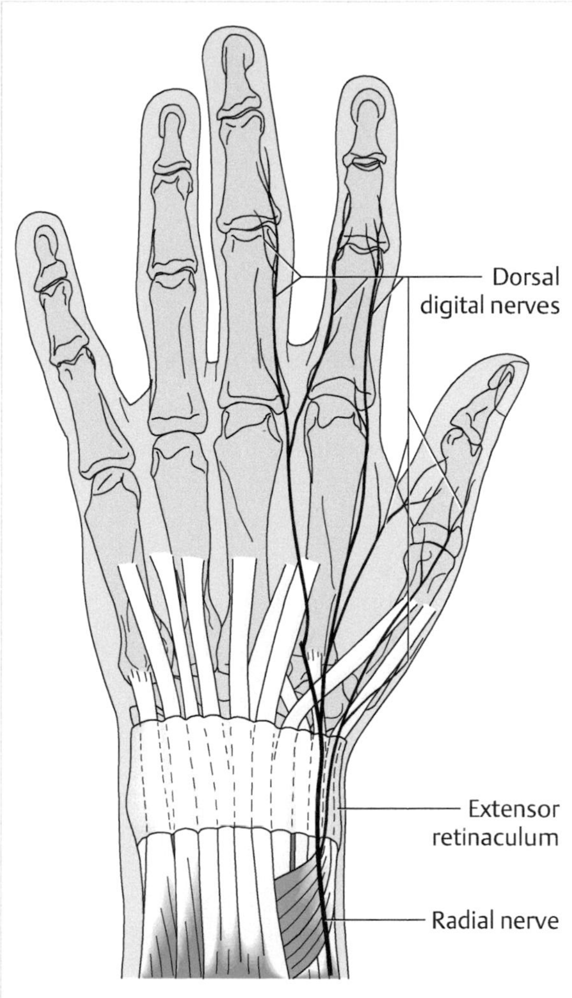


**Fig. 6.99** Course of the radial nerve in the hand and wrist.

# Chapter 7

## Lumbar Spine

# 7 Lumbar Spine

## 7.1 Palpation of Landmarks in the Lumbar Spine and Abdominal Areas

### Bony Landmarks

### Spinous Process

Use the index or middle finger to palpate the superior, inferior, and lateral aspects of the tip of the spinous process. A step-off suggests instability—a segment can shift anteriorly or posteriorly in relation to the next superior or inferior segment. The following muscle insertion sites are palpable from the tip of the spinous process toward the vertebral arch (**Fig. 7.1**):

1 = Latissimus dorsi muscle
2 + 6 = Longissimus thoracis muscle
3 = Long rotator muscle
4 = Multifidus muscle
5 = Interspinalis lumborum muscle

The iliac crest can be used as a guide to determine the level of a spinous process accurately:

- Place the index finger on the iliac crest with the thumb extended over the spine at the same level. The lower edge of the L4 spinous process can be found here (**Fig. 7.2**).
- The projecting median sacral crest of S2 is found at the level of the posterior superior iliac spine (**Fig. 7.3**).

**Pathology**

The most common site for a step-off to occur is the L4–L5 level. A gap can develop between the two articular processes in the L5 segment, which can lead to spondylolisthesis—the slippage of the vertebral body of L5 along with the overlying spinal column, while the L5 spinous process and the sacrum do not move.

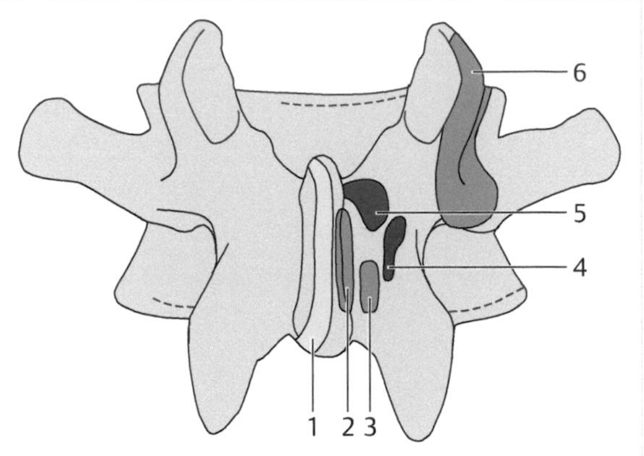


**Fig. 7.1** Palpation points on the spinous process.

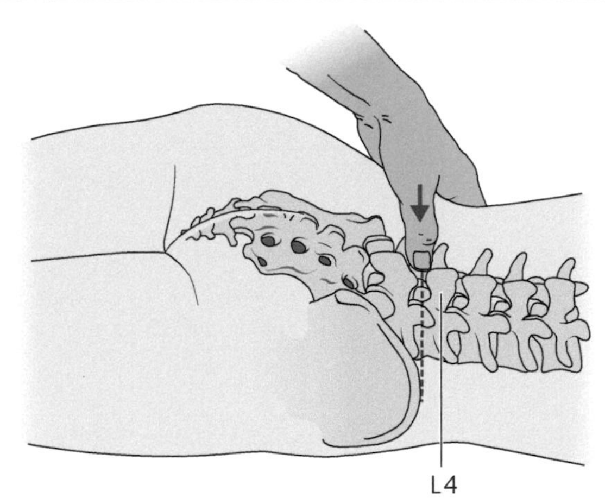


**Fig. 7.2** Palpation: determining the level of L 4.

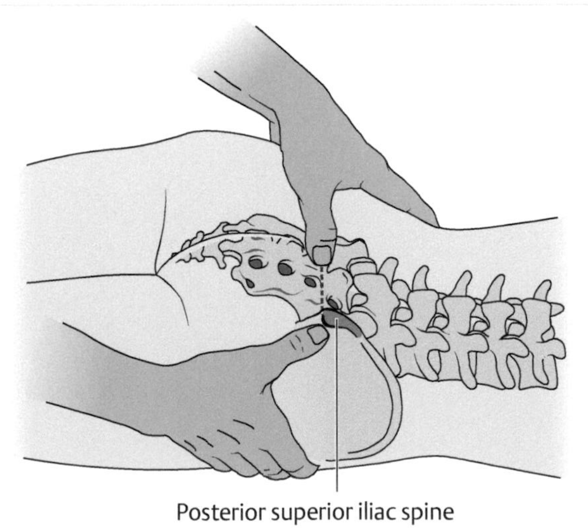


**Fig. 7.3** Palpation: determining the level of S 2.

## Ligaments

### Supraspinous Ligament (Fig. 7.4)

This runs between the spinous processes and is found superficially on the upper and lower margins of the tip of the spinous processes.

### Iliolumbar Ligament (Fig. 7.5)

Palpation of this ligament is possible only using deep palpation at the margin of the iliac crest, which bends inferiorly at this point and then ends at the posterior superior iliac spine.

This is a ligament that is often sprained because every change in pelvic position puts tension on it.

## Musculature

### Erector Spinae Muscle (Fig. 7.6)

The medial border of the erector spinae muscle runs alongside the spinous processes, while the lateral border is about 3 to 4 fingerbreadths further laterally. Furthest medially, and found only in the thoracic and upper lumbar spine, is the spinalis muscle. The iliocostalis lumborum muscle lies furthest laterally, and the longissimus thoracis muscle lies between the two. The courses of muscle layers at a deeper level are noted here but cannot be precisely identified.

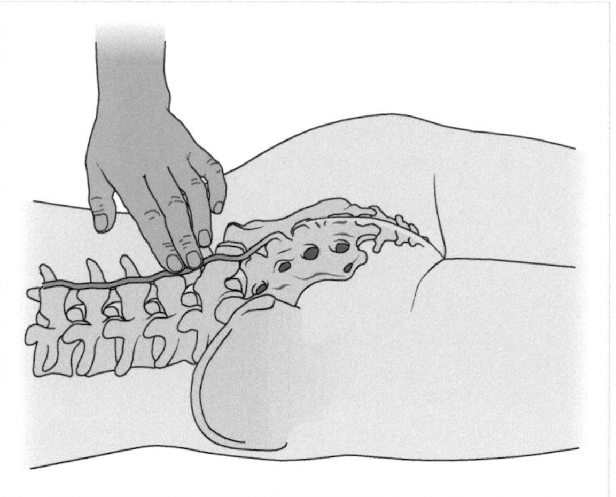

**Fig. 7.4** Palpation of the supraspinous ligament.

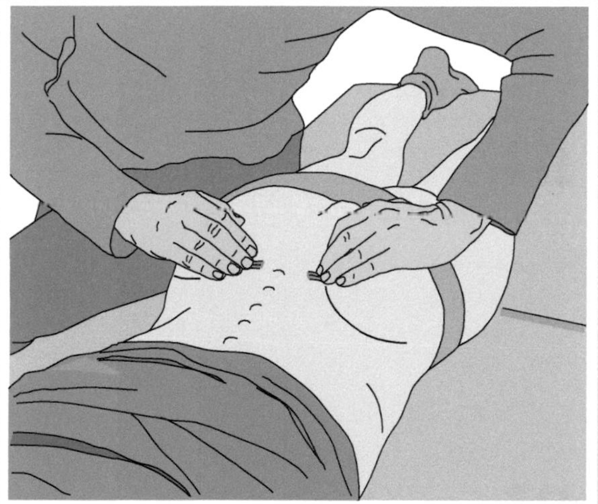

**Fig. 7.5** Palpation of the iliolumbar ligament.

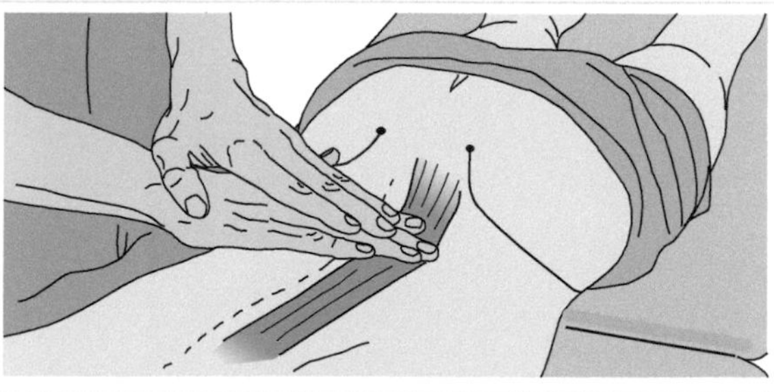

**Fig. 7.6** Palpation of the erector spinae muscle.

## Quadratus Lumborum Muscle (Fig. 7.7)

Its lateral edge can be palpated deeply between the lower rib and the iliac crest immediately next to the outer margin of the erector spinae muscle. Palpation is barely possible at the origin and insertion sites (the 12th rib and iliac crest).

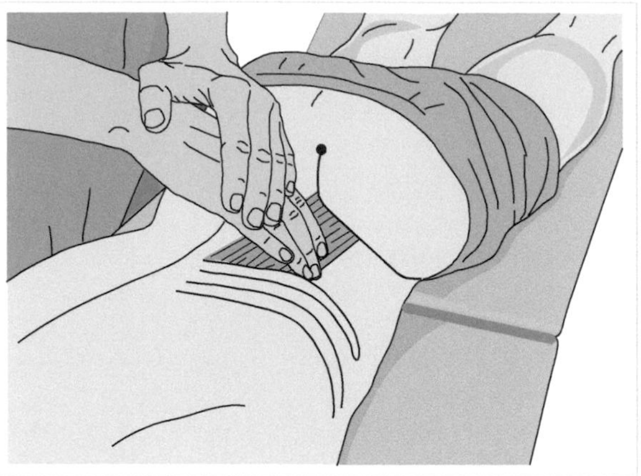

**Fig. 7.7** Palpation of the quadratus lumborum muscle.

## Rectus Abdominis Muscle (Fig. 7.8)

The rectus abdominis muscle can be palpated at the xiphoid process, at the fifth to seventh costal cartilages, as well as in the epigastric angle and at the pubic symphysis. Intermediate tendinous bands, the tendinous intersections, can be recognized as transverse furrows, conditions permitting.

## External Oblique Muscle (Fig. 7.8)

The external oblique abdominal muscle can be palpated on the lateral thorax as its fibers run obliquely over the eight lower ribs from superolateral to inferomedial. Because of its fleshy attachment to the outer margin of the iliac crest, it can be easily identified there. It joins with the inguinal ligament in a broad aponeurosis and can be felt above the ligament.

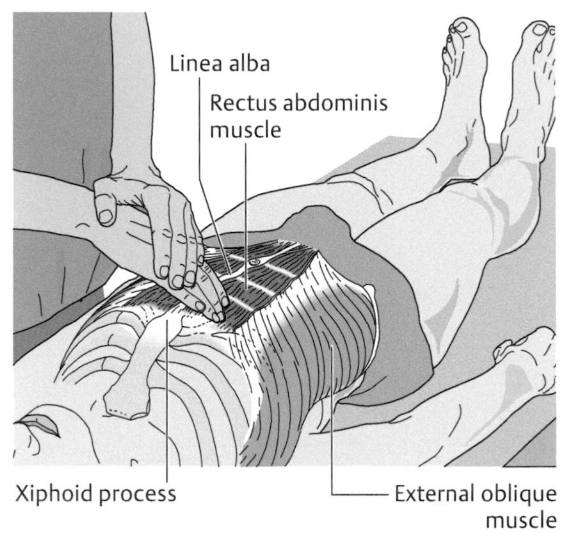


**Fig. 7.8** Palpation of the rectus abdominis muscle.

## Internal Oblique Muscle (Fig. 7.9)

More pressure must be used to palpate this inner, diagonally running abdominal muscle because it lies underneath the external oblique muscle. Its origin is on the lateral aspect of the inguinal ligament and deep on the iliac crest. Its fibers are oriented from inferolateral to superomedial and end with fleshy insertions on the lower three ribs.

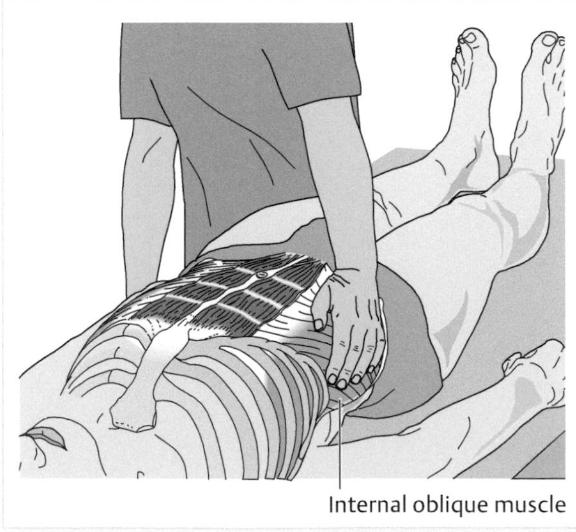


**Fig. 7.9** Palpation of the internal oblique muscle.

## Iliopsoas Muscle (Fig. 7.10a, b)

Starting position: Place the subject in the supine position with hips flexed and the knees up to relax the abdominal wall.

The umbilicus usually lies at the level of the L3–L4 disk space. The *psoas major muscle* can be palpated above and below this point, alongside and anterior to the lumbar vertebrae. Using two to four fingertips, first flat and then with the tips, carefully probe deeply with increasing pressure between the abdominal organs. The muscle can be clearly felt as a round cord.

The *iliacus muscle* cannot be palpated throughout its entire course in the iliac fossa. Carefully palpate downward through the abdominal muscles from the inner brim of the iliac crest to feel the iliacus muscle along the inner wall of the ilium. This is best done using an anterior approach.

See Chapter 8, Pelvis and Hip Joint, for further palpation techniques that are important in relation to lumbar spine problems.

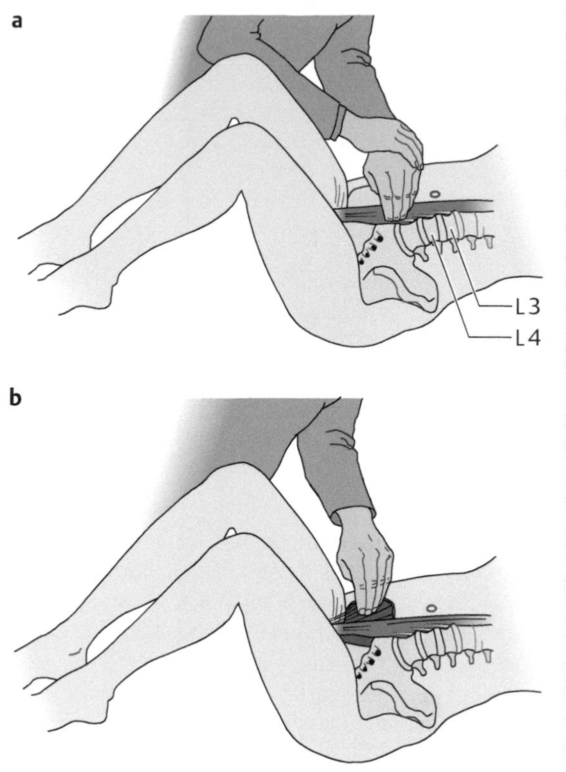

Fig. 7.10 Palpation of the iliopsoas muscle. (a) Psoas major muscle. (b) Iliacus muscle.

## Projection of the Internal Organs

### Liver (Fig. 7.11)

The liver is located under the right dome of the diaphragm and extends to the left into the epigastrium:

- Upper border: approximately 1 cm below the right nipple and 2 cm below the left nipple.
- Lower border: 9th to 10th costal cartilage on the right; 7th to 8th on the left.

### Spleen (Fig. 7.11)

The spleen lies in the left thoracic area. It is approximately 11 cm long, 7 cm wide, and 4 cm thick:

- Superior border: 9th rib.
- Inferior border: 11th rib.

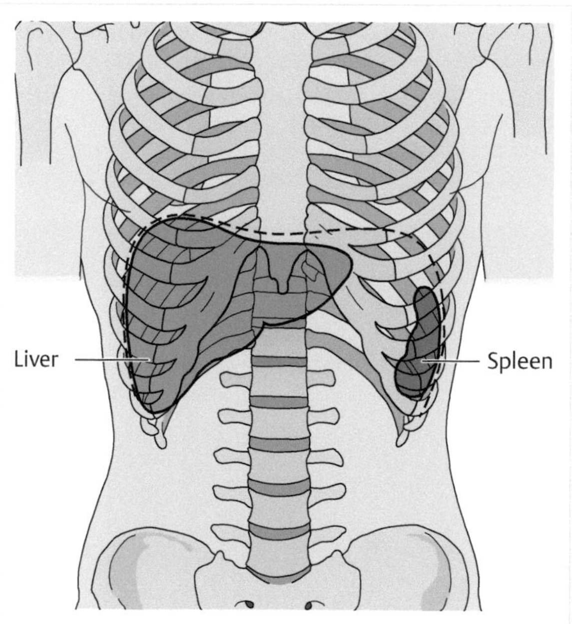

Fig. 7.11 Projection of the internal organs: liver and spleen.

## Stomach (Fig. 7.12)

Most of the stomach lies within the left upper abdominal area. The various areas of the stomach are situated as follows:

- The esophageal junction is approximately at the level of the left seventh costal cartilage.
- The fundus lies under the left dome of the diaphragm.
- The pylorus lies at the level of the first lumbar vertebra and extends inferiorly to the fourth lumbar vertebra.

## Duodenum (Fig. 7.12)

The duodenum is approximately 25 to 30 cm long and lies as a large **C**-shaped loop at the level of L1–L3, i.e., above the umbilicus.

## Jejunum and Ileum

At the level of L2, the duodenum merges into the jejunum, which then soon merges into the ileum. Both of these sections of the intestine consist of multiple loops that are free to move within the abdominal cavity.

## Pancreas (Fig. 7.12)

The pancreas lies retroperitoneally in the upper abdominal area as follows:

- The head of the pancreas lies within the **C**-shaped curve of the duodenum, i.e., between the first and third lumbar vertebrae.
- The body of the pancreas lies transversely in the left upper abdomen.
- The tail of the pancreas lies over the left kidney and ends laterally at the level of 9th to 10th ribs.

The large intestine consists of the caecum, colon, and rectum and has a total length between 1.2 and 1.4 m.

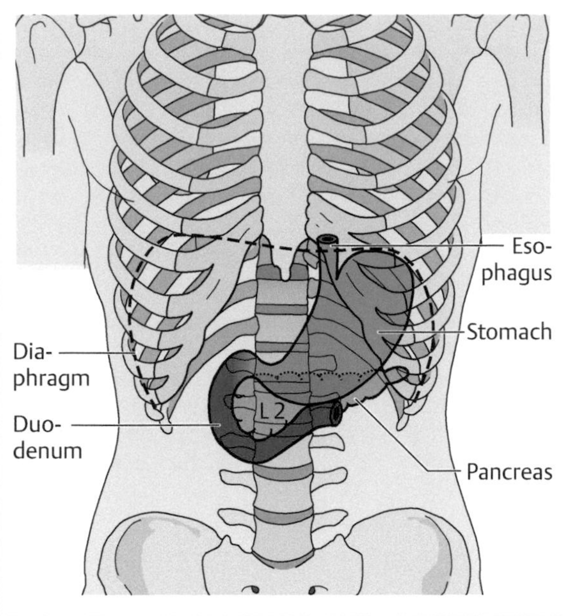


**Fig. 7.12** Projection of the internal organs: stomach, pancreas, and duodenum.

## Caecum (Fig. 7.13)

To identify an irritated appendix, locate McBurney's point, which lies near the middle of a line connecting the navel with the anterior superior iliac spine. The location of the appendix can, however, be quite variable.

## Colon (Fig. 7.13)

The colon surrounds the loops of the small intestine like a picture frame. Its various parts are situated as follows:

- The ascending colon lies in the right lateral abdominal cavity and extends up to the level of the ribs.
- The right colic flexure lies at the level of the T12–L3 vertebrae.
- The transverse colon extends across the posterior abdominal cavity at the level of the lower ribs.
- The left colic flexure lies at the level of the T11–L2 vertebrae.
- The descending colon runs in the left lateral abdominal cavity.

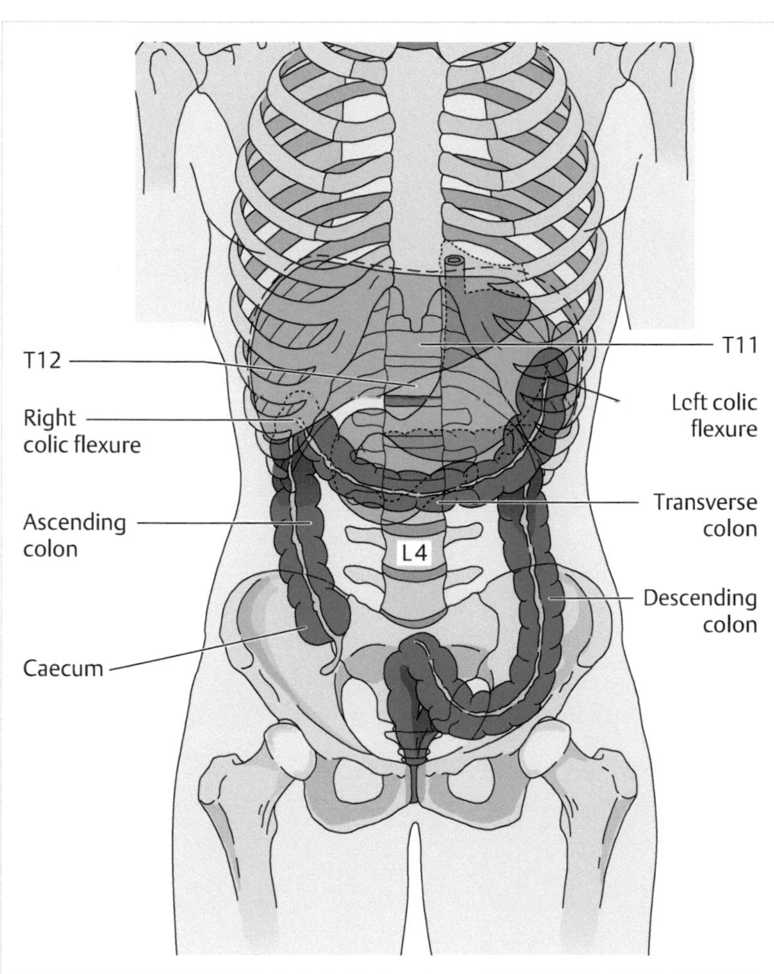


**Fig. 7.13** Projection of the internal organs: colon.

## Kidneys (Fig. 7.14)

The kidneys are approximately 11 to 12 cm long, 5 to 6 cm wide, and 3 to 4 cm thick. The left kidney is slightly larger than the right. They lie partly over the psoas major muscle and partly over the quadratus lumborum muscle.

The upper pole of the kidney is at the level of the 11th thoracic vertebra and is overlain by the pleura and the diaphragm. The lower border is at the level of the third lumbar vertebra.

## Ureter (Fig. 7.14)

The ureter is approximately 25 to 30 cm long. It runs over the psoas major muscle and then passes through the retroperitoneal space distally into the bladder. Its course is represented by the following landmarks:

- The level of the L3 transverse process.
- The middle of the sacro-iliac joint.
- The level of the pubic tubercle.

**Pathology**

Kidney stones can become lodged at various narrow points in the ureter, such as the ureteropelvic junction and the ureterovesical junction. They cause severe pain in a segmental distribution, such as paravertebral pain in the lumbar spine with radiation to the groin.

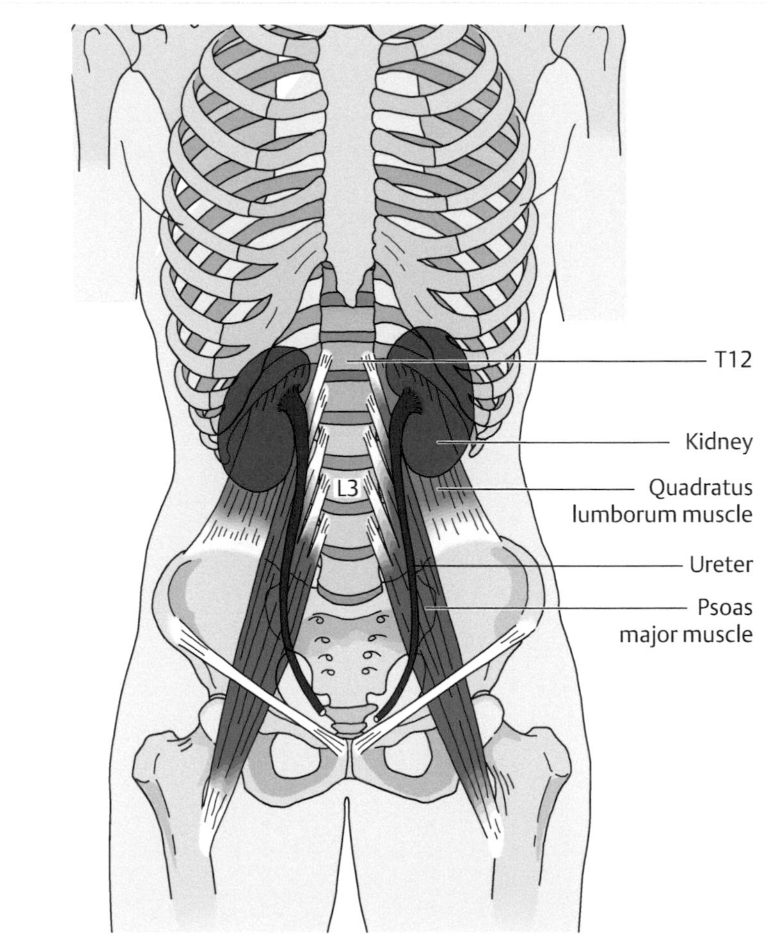


**Fig. 7.14** Projection of the internal organs: kidney and ureter.

# 7.2 X-Ray Image of the Lumbar Spine, Pelvis, and Hips

## Anterior-Posterior View in the Standing Position (Fig. 7.15)

Note the *perpendicular arrangement* of the row of vertebral bodies:

- Pedicles of the vertebral arches: oval, paired, symmetrical, and one above the other.
- Spinous processes: midline, one above the other, with no contact.
- Inferior and superior end plates: parallel.
- Intervertebral disk space: the height increases as one moves inferiorly: L1 < L2 < L3 < L4 < L5.

Note the *width of the spinal canal* (measured as the distance between the pedicles), which is wide enough that two pedicles could be placed next to each other.

Note the course of the *plumb line*: pubic symphysis → median sacral crest → row of spinous processes → middle of the vertebral bodies.

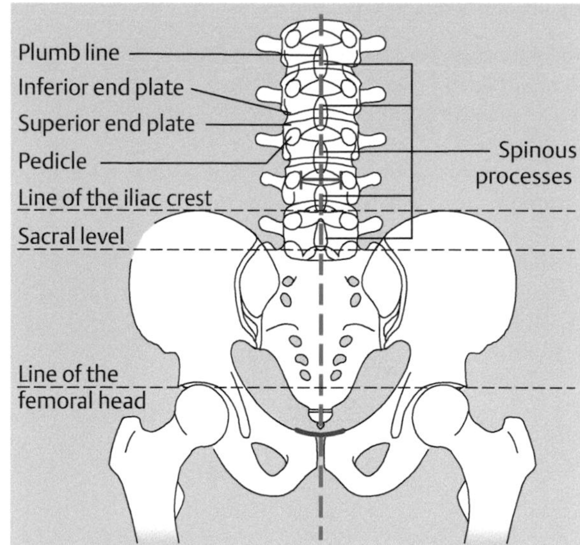


**Fig. 7.15** X-ray image: anteroposterior view of the lumbar spine, pelvis, and hips.

### Pathology

The X-ray image can demonstrate the following changes (**Fig. 7.16**):

- The pedicles of the vertebral arches are shifted to the right or left. For example, if one pedicle is half visible and the other is shifted toward the midline, this indicates a rotational deformity such as scoliosis.
- Osteophyte formation in the vertebral body (*spondylosis*) due to intervertebral disk degeneration in the marginal ridge area; this is usually associated with narrowing of the disk space and *spondylophytes* of the zygapophysial joints.
- Lumbosacral assimilation disturbance, e.g., *sacralization*, in which the transverse process of L5 merges with the base of the sacrum. In *lumbarization*, S1 has the form of a lumbar vertebra.

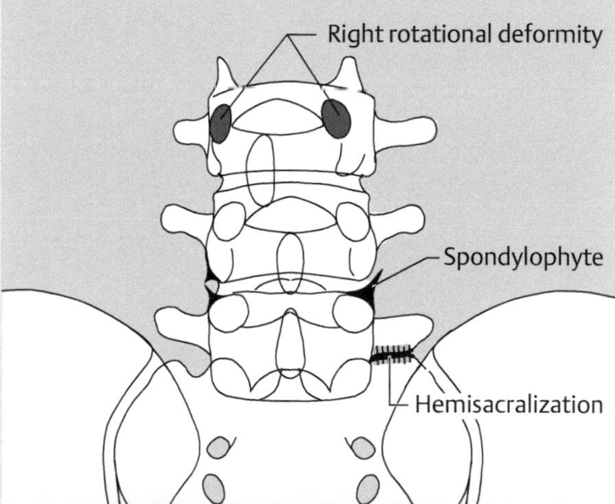


**Fig. 7.16** X-ray image: pathologic changes in anteroposterior view.

## Lateral View (Fig. 7.17)

- The *contours* of the anterior and posterior *vertebral bodies* form harmonious arcs.
- The *intervertebral disk spaces*, particularly L5–S1, are increasingly wedge-shaped.
- The *vertebral bodies* are tapered and box-shaped with uniform contours and no spurs.
- The spinous processes show a small gap between the tips.
- Normally formed *lordosis*: lordotic angle—supine, 50°; standing, 70°. If a line is drawn from the superior end plate of L1 and another from the base of the sacrum, the angle that these form is the lordotic angle.
- The *static axis* is determined by dropping a perpendicular inferiorly from the center of the third vertebral body to the front edge of the superior end plate of the sacrum.
- *Lumbosacral angle*: This is formed by the longitudinal axis of the fifth lumbar vertebra and that of the sacrum, and is usually 130 to 150°.

### Pathology

- *Spondylolisthesis*: There is a significant step-off between L5 and S1 due to an anteroinferior displacement of L5 (**Fig. 7.18**).
- *Retrolisthesis*: Due to the instability of a motion segment, a vertebra is displaced in a posterior direction in relation to the next lower vertebra. This is recognized by a step-off.
- *Baastrup's disease*: The tips of the spinous processes come into contact (kissing spines) as the result of an extreme lordosis.
- *Osteoporosis*: Vertebral body variations occur, such as wedge-shaped vertebrae and butterfly vertebrae.

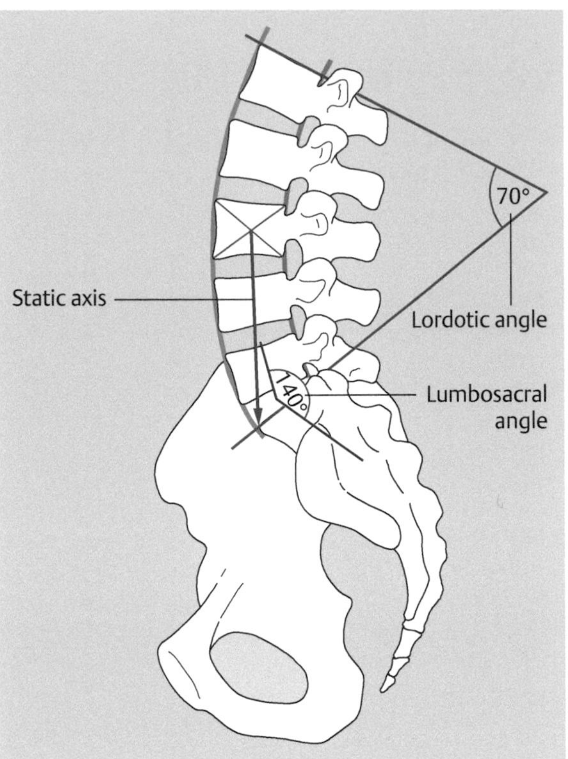


**Fig. 7.17** X-ray image: lateral view of the lumbar spine, pelvis, and hips.

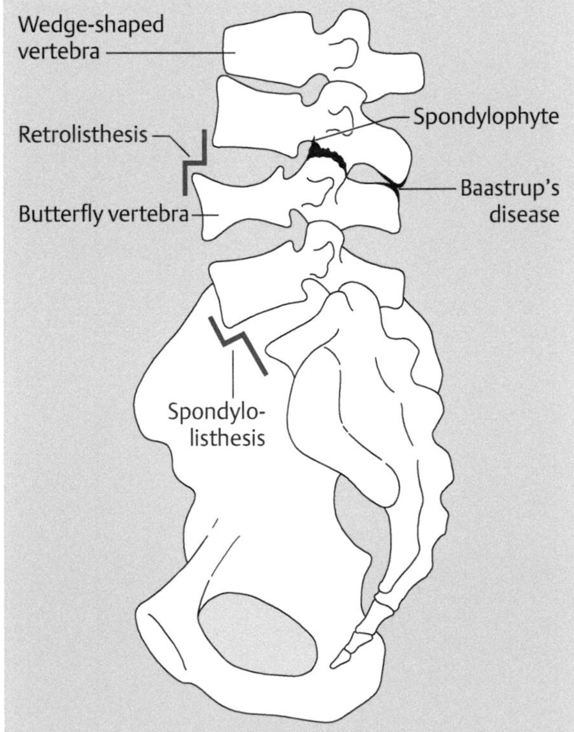


**Fig. 7.18** X-ray image: pathologic changes in the lateral view.

## Oblique (45°) View (Fig. 7.19)

Critical evaluation of the configuration of *pars interarticularis:* The contours can be visualized as a "Scotty dog":

- Snout = transverse process.
- Ear = superior articular process.
- Forepaw = inferior articular process.
- Neck = pars interarticularis.
- Body = vertebral arch.
- Hindquarters = vertebral arch with the articular processes of the contralateral side.

## Zygapophysial Joints

- Joint space width: 1.5 to 2 mm.
- Articulating joint surfaces: smooth and sharply defined.

### Pathology

*Spondylolysis* (**Fig. 7.19**): If a gap develops between the superior and inferior articular processes of a vertebra, the Scotty dog appears to be wearing a collar.

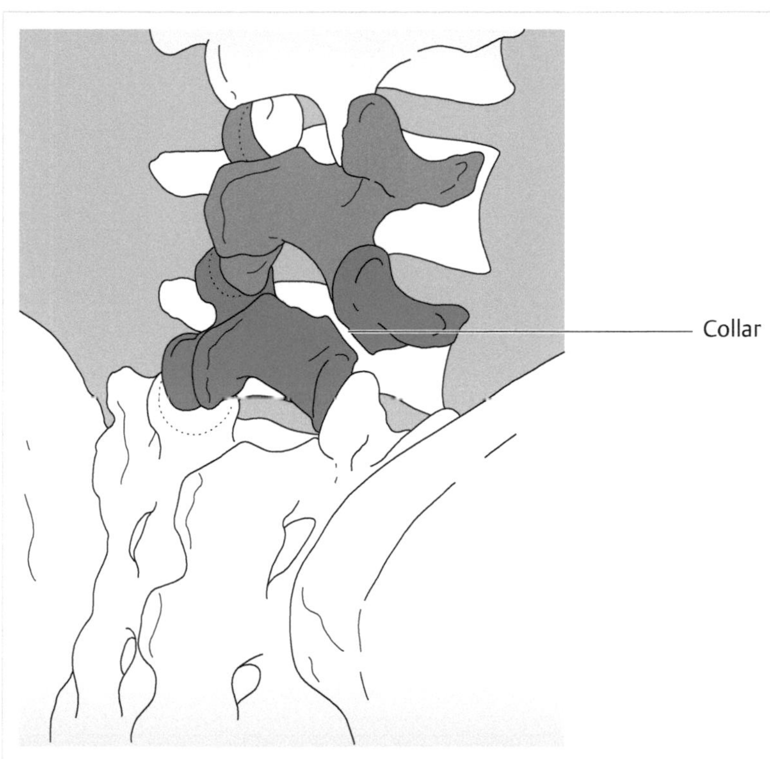


**Fig. 7.19** X-ray image: lumbar spine in oblique (45°) view. Gray: normal vertebra. Red: spondylolysis.

# 7.3 Lumbar Vertebrae

## Vertebral Body (Fig. 7.20a, b)

- The transverse axis is longer than the anteroposterior axis, producing a slightly oval shape.
- They become increasingly wedge-shaped moving inferiorly, so that the body of the fifth lumbar vertebral is 3 to 5 mm thicker anteriorly than posteriorly.

## Transverse Process (Fig. 7.20a, b)

- This is formed by the fusion of a large rib rudiment (*costal process*) with the primordial small transverse process (*accessory process*).
- The costal process is very long and horizontally oriented, except at L5, where it is aligned more anteriorly.
- The accessory process arises at the base of costal process.

## Spinous Process (Fig. 7.20a, b)

The spinous processes extend horizontally and are very strong.

## Articular Processes (Fig. 7.20a, b)

They are designed to be very strong.

- The *superior articular process* has a small protuberance, the *mammillary process*. The articular surface faces posteromedially.
- The *inferior articular process* is located more medially, and its articular surface faces anterolaterally.

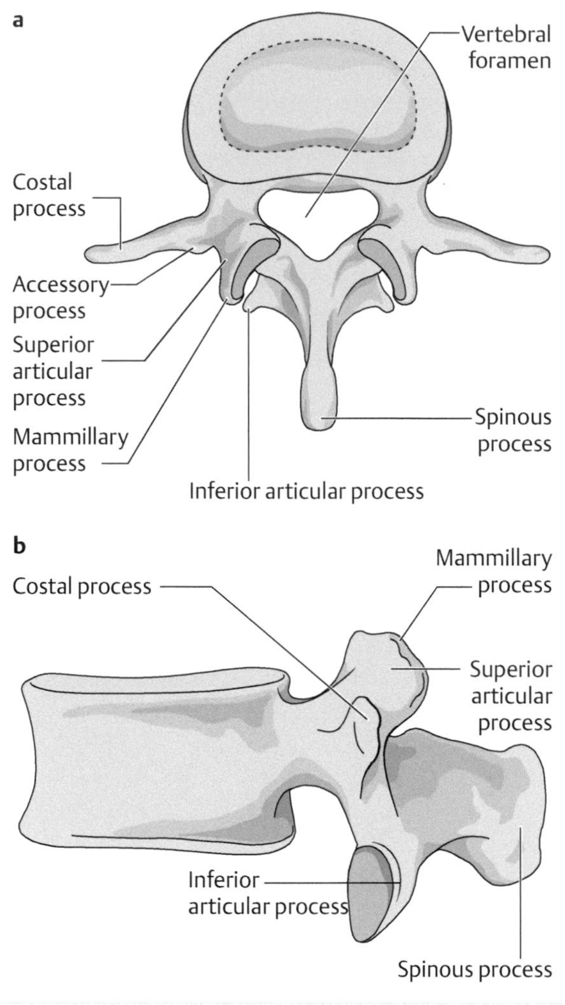


**Fig. 7.20** Lumbar vertebra. **(a)** Superior view. **(b)** Lateral view.

## Orientation of the Zygapophysial Joints

The facets form a 90° angle from the horizontal plane, allowing for very little rotation.

Up to an angle of 45°, a good ability to rotate would be expected. The closer the angle moves to 90°, the less rotation is possible (**Fig. 7.21**).

At the L1 level, the facets form an angle of 15° to the sagittal plane (**Fig. 7.22a**).

Moving inferiorly, they orient themselves increasingly in the direction of the frontal plane and are also positioned far apart.

The orientation of the articular surfaces in the frontal plane is the most favorable for lateral flexion (**Fig. 7.22b**).

The articular facets are slightly curved so that the anterior part lies nearly in the frontal plane, while the posterior part of the facet is in the sagittal plane.

The facet of the inferior articular process is convex, while that of superior articular process is concave.

## Absorption of Force

The estimated force absorption of the joint facets is approximately 18 to 20% of the total load on a motion segment. The remainder acts on the intervertebral disk. If the disk has degenerated, the load that the zygapophysial joint facets must absorb increases to as much as twice the normal load.

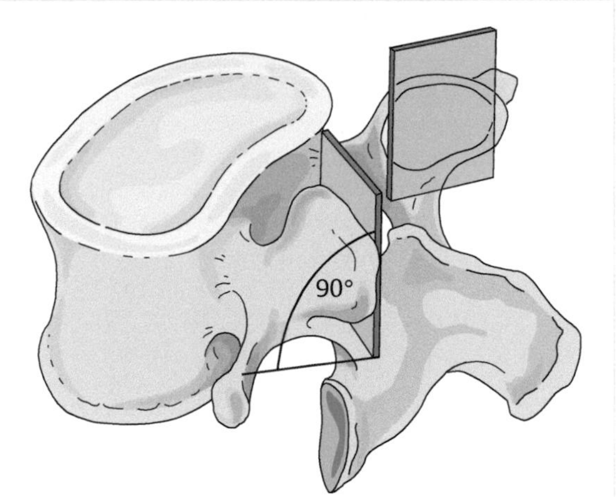


**Fig. 7.21** Position of the joint facets relative to the horizontal.

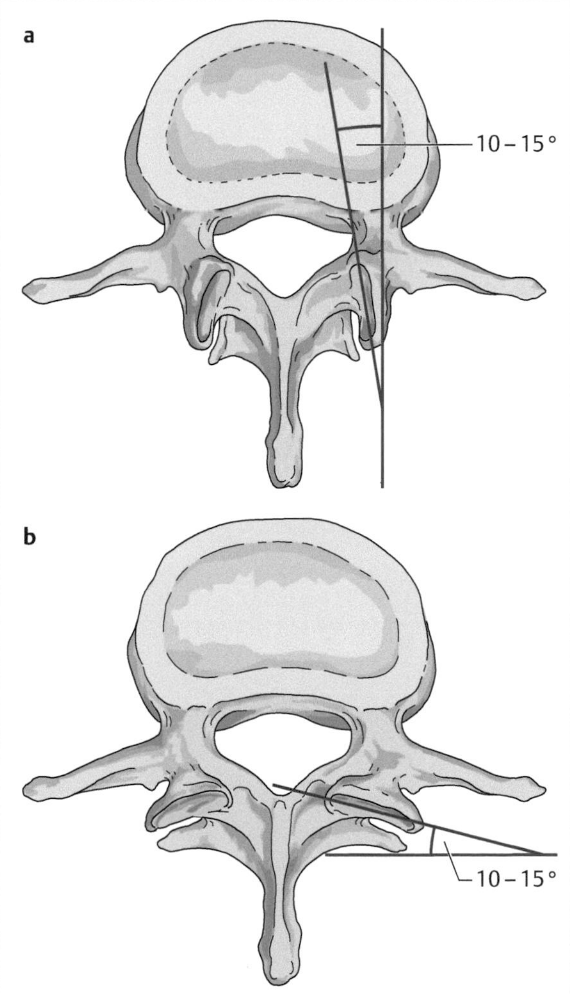


**Fig. 7.22** Position of the joint facets. **(a)** Upper lumbar spine with sagittal orientation. **(b)** Lower lumbar spine with frontal orientation.

## Joint Capsule (Fig. 7.23)

The *synovial membrane* has meniscus-like eversions, the synovial folds, which can extend up to 0.5 cm into the joint. These folds are smoothed out and tensed by the divergent movements of the joint surfaces. With convergence movements (telescoping the joint surfaces), they can become entrapped in the joint space, thus inhibiting movement.

The fibers of the *fibrous layer* run in part diagonally from superomedial to inferolateral and in part horizontally.

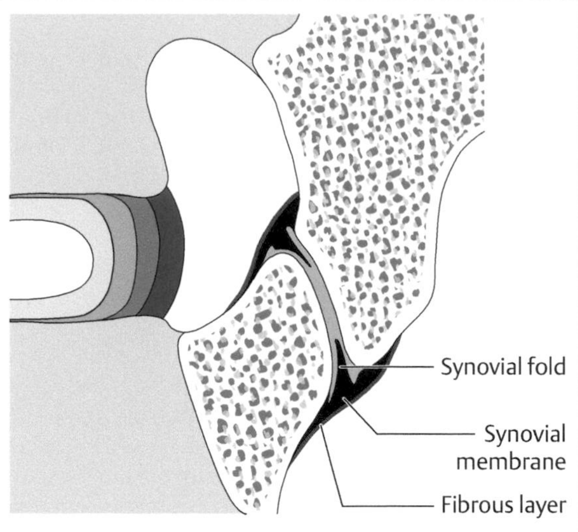


**Fig. 7.23** Joint capsule.

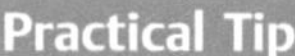

**Pathology**

The increased pressure load on the zygapophysial joints and the resultant reduction in stress on the ligamentous and capsular structures can lead to a displacement of portions of the capsule into the joint, thus inhibiting movement.

**Practical Tip**

If the joint facets lose optimal contact, the use of intensive traction can take the pressure off the joint and free up the jammed capsule recesses.
It can also be effective, as with a jammed door, to mobilize the blocked facet first in the direction in which it is jammed before moving it in the direction in which movement is limited.

## Vertebral Foramen (Fig. 7.24)

In transverse section, the vertebral foramen appears triangular, almost cloverleaf, in shape. The anterolateral portion of the triangle is called the *lateral recess*.

The foramen is bordered anteriorly by the posterior vertebral body and the disk, anterolaterally by the pedicle, laterally by the vertebral arch and zygapophysial joints, and posteriorly by the ligamentum flavum.

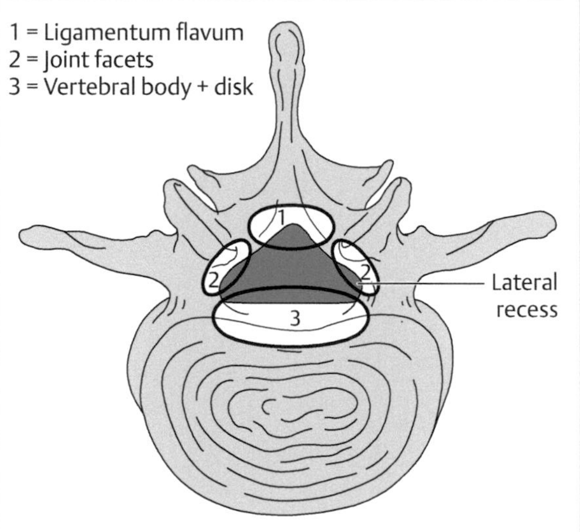


**Fig. 7.24** Borders of the vertebral foramen.

## Vertebral Canal (Fig. 7.25)

The vertebral foramina, stacked one on top of the other, form the spinal canal. The spinal cord (or the cauda equina, depending on the level) lies centrally in the canal. The laterally located recesses form a channel through which the nerve roots run, surrounded by the spinal dura mater, after they branch off from the dural sac and before they reach the intervertebral foramen.

In addition to the nerve roots, epidural fatty tissue is also found in this channel, protecting the root sleeve from the bony walls. A vascular plexus and meningeal branches of the spinal nerve are located in this fatty tissue.

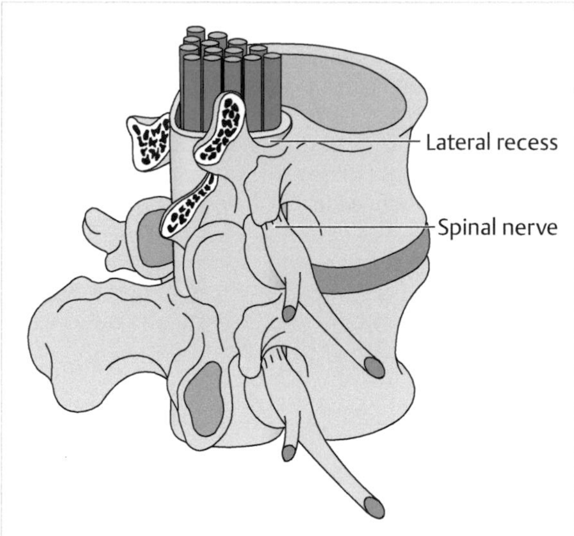


**Fig. 7.25** Vertebral canal.

### Variations in Length

The spinal canal undergoes extreme variations in length:

- In flexion, the posterior region of the spinal canal elongates by 30%, but the anterior region by only 13%. In extension, the anterior portion is slightly longer than the posterior part.
- In lateral flexion, the contralateral side elongates by approximately 15%.

**Pathology**

*Spinal stenosis*: In lumbar spinal stenosis, there is a bony narrowing of the spinal canal that can lead to compression of the nerve root or cauda equina. It can develop from degenerative disk disease with subsequent overloading of the zygapophysial joints due to the formation of osteophytes that constrict the lateral recess.
Retrolisthesis, which develops as a result of instability, can also constrict the spinal canal and the intervertebral foramen. The symptoms usually occur unilaterally and in a monoradicular pattern as intermittent claudication.
Congenital narrowing of the spinal canal represents an unfavorable anatomical variation, although the structures involved are able to adapt to this. Symptoms are only triggered if, for example, segmental instability supervenes.
Treatment: surgical decompression by thinning the inner rim of the arch and removing the osteophytes. If there is instability, spinal fusion of the segment is also carried out.

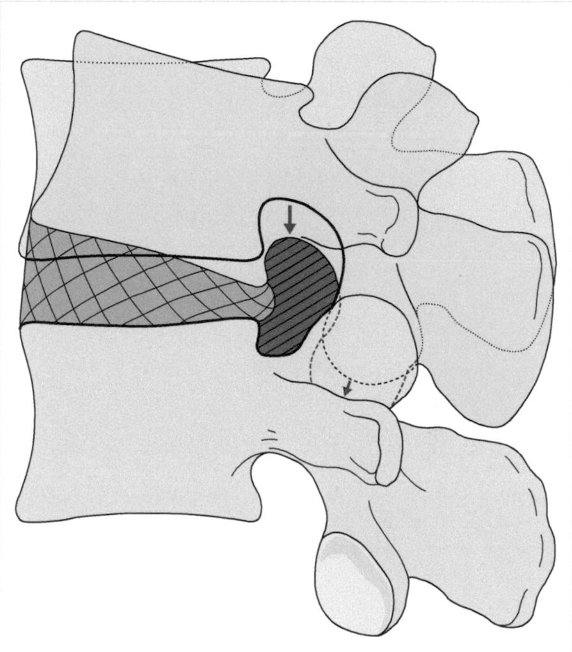

**Fig. 7.26** Changes in the lumen of the intervertebral foramen during extension = hatched area.

## Intervertebral Foramen (Fig. 7.26)

The foramina are located at the level of the intervertebral disk spaces and look like an external ear when viewed laterally. The nerve root passes through the upper part of the foramen and occupies about a quarter of the space.

During lateral flexion, the foramen narrows on the concave side and widens on the convex side. Flexion widens the foramen by approximately 30%. Extension narrows it as much as 20%. Rotational movements result in only minimal changes.

## Lumbosacral Junction (Fig. 7.27)

This junction is an important interface because here forces are transferred from the spine to the lower extremities and vice versa.

Because of the inclination of the sacral base, the fifth lumbar vertebra has a tendency to slip in an anteroinferior direction. The extent of the anterior thrust component depends on the degree of inclination of the sacral base. This tendency to slip is counteracted by the ligaments and muscles of the back as well as by the apposition of the facets with the superior articular processes of the first sacral vertebra.

### Pathology

*Instability* of the lumbar spine is most common at the lumbosacral junction, occurring in 56 % of cases, while instability at L4–L5 follows with 44 % and at L3–L4 with only 2 %. The body can potentially compensate for this for 20 years or more. Symptoms occur only if another factor is added.

*Spondylolysis* is a gap in the vertebral arch area between the upper and lower articular processes, usually at L5. It can occur as a growth disorder or due to long-standing hyperlordosis. If this gap formation occurs bilaterally, slippage in an anteroinferior direction can occur due to the oblique position of the fifth lumbar vertebra in relation to the sacral base—*spondylolisthesis* (**Fig. 7.28**).

*Overload of the pars interarticularis* (**Fig. 7.29**): During excessive extension, the inferior rims of the lower facets (of L4 in this example) compress the L5 lamina. The pivot point for further extension shifts from the posterior disk space to the pars interarticularis. This means that the anterior parts of the disks are overstretched, and the axial transmission of pressure through the disk is no longer possible. The total transmission of axial forces takes place between the facet of the inferior articular process of L4 and the pars interarticularis of L5. Frequent extension, even at low loads, may lead to a fatigue fracture of the pars interarticularis.

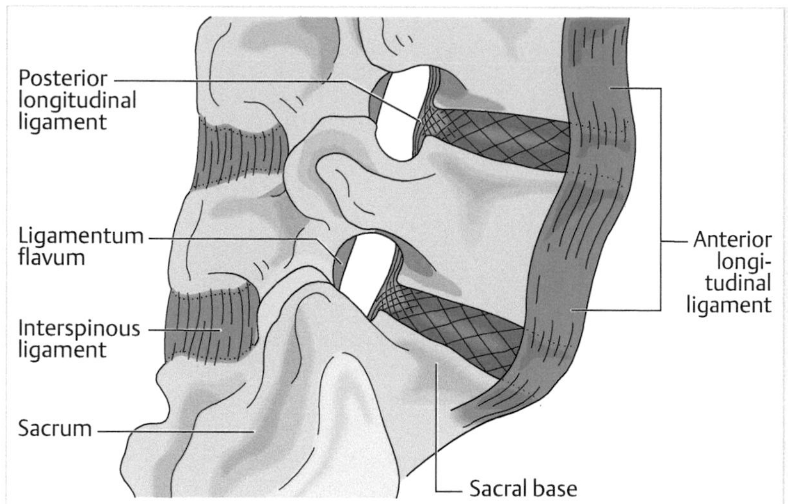


**Fig. 7.27** Lumbosacral junction.

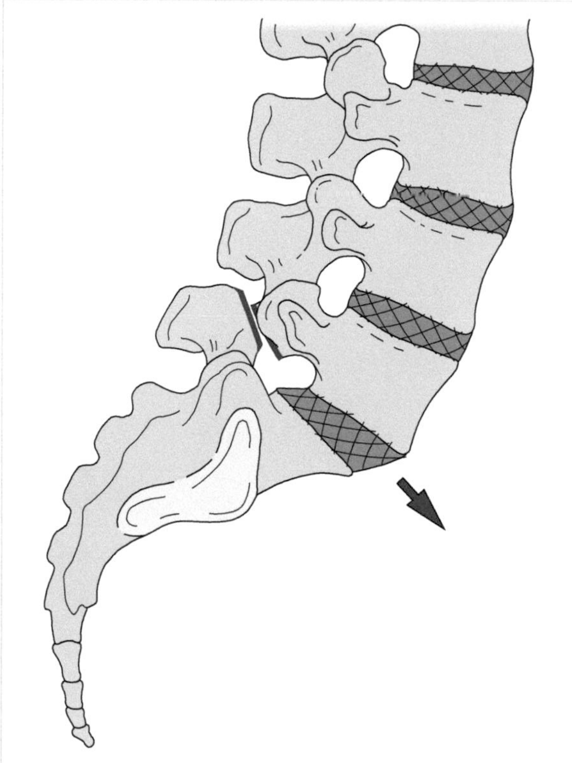

**Fig. 7.28** Inferior slippage of the fifth lumbar vertebra due to spondylolisthesis.

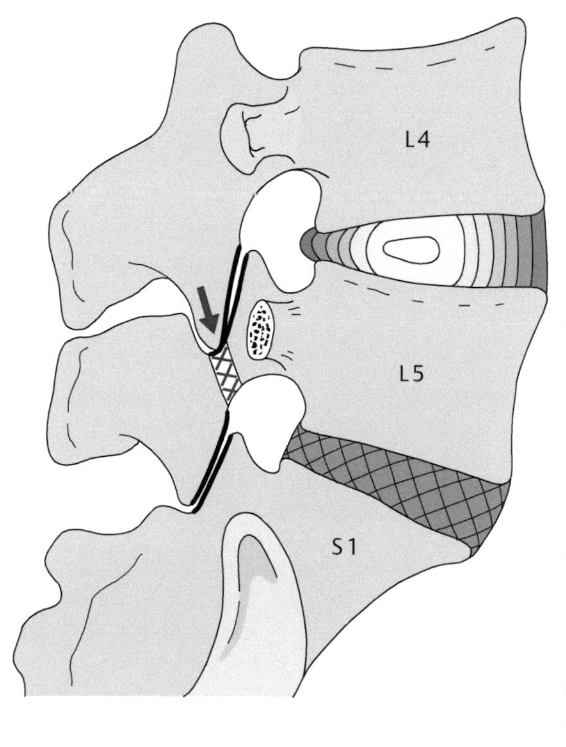


**Fig. 7.29** Overload of the pars interarticularis due to hyperextension.

## 7.4 Ligaments of the Lumbar Spine

The lumbar area is surrounded by a complex of ligamentous structures that pull in different directions, thus stabilizing the lumbar spine from every side.

### Posterior Longitudinal Ligament (Fig. 7.30)

- This ligament contains many elastic components.
- It is a deep layer with short fibers that track from segment to segment. It is approximately 1 cm wide as it passes the vertebral bodies but then widens outward towards the intervertebral disks.
- A thicker, superficial layer with long fibers ends at the level of the L3–L4 motion segment, continuing as a very thin fiber bundle down to the sacrum.
- The posterior longitudinal ligament does not cover the posterolateral region of the intervertebral disk.
- It stabilizes the posterior disk space, especially during flexion.

### Anterior Longitudinal Ligament (Fig. 7.31)

- This tracks as a deep layer from vertebral body to vertebral body and connects with the intervertebral disk by a few thin fibers.
- A superficial layer consists of long fibers that skip several segments.
- The ligament is stretched by extension.

### Ligamentum Flavum (Fig. 7.31)

- The ligamentum flavum contains a large amount of elastic fibers.
- For most of its course, it is 3 to 10 mm thick, but between L5 and S1, it is significantly narrower and thinner.
- It stretches out between the laminae and forms the posterior wall of the spinal canal and the posterior part of the intervertebral foramen.
- In its midsection, it interconnects with the interspinous ligament.
- In its lateral aspect, it merges with the joint capsule of the zygapophysial joint.
- It has a protective function in that it completes the spinal canal posteriorly, limits flexion, and, by its lateral parts, limits lateral flexion on the contralateral side.

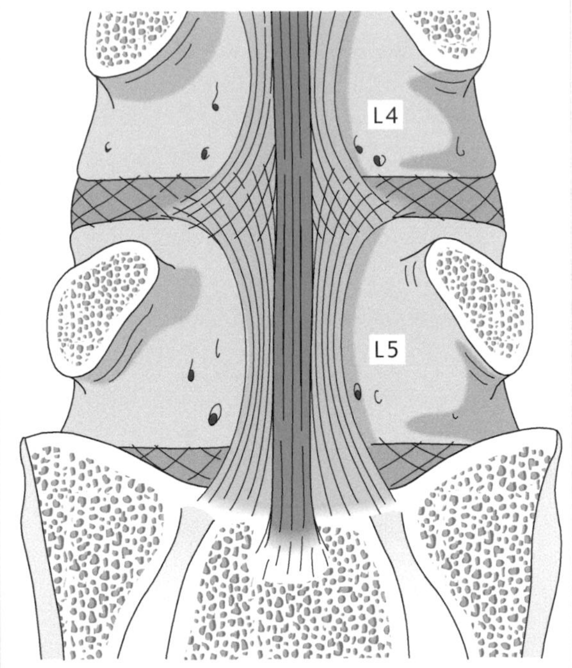


**Fig. 7.30** Posterior longitudinal ligament.

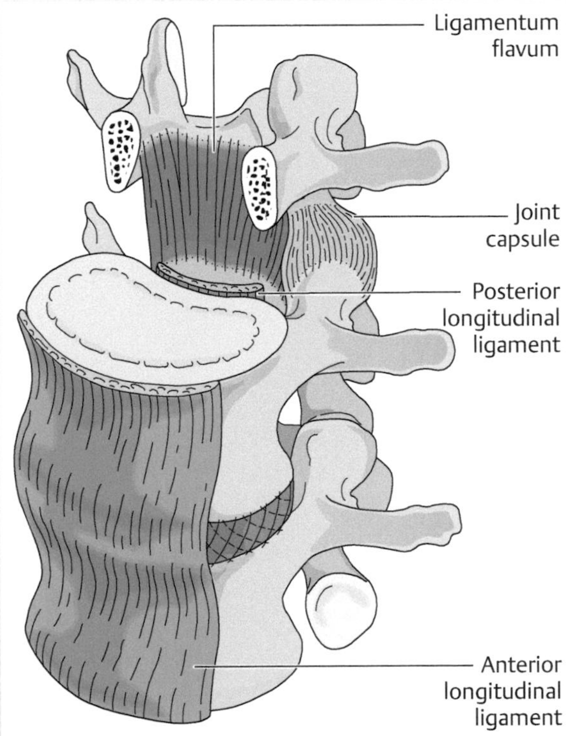


**Fig. 7.31** Ligaments of the lumbar spine (anterolateral view).

## Supraspinous Ligament (Fig. 7.32)

- This ligament stretches out superficially between the tips of the spinous process and ends at L5.
- It continues into the thoracolumbar fascia.
- It inhibits flexion and rotation.

## Interspinous Ligament (Fig. 7.32)

- This ligament runs between the spinous processes at a deep level.
- The deepest portion tracks into the ligamentum flavum, while the superficial part intertwines with the supraspinous ligament.
- It inhibits flexion.

## Intertransverse Ligament (Fig. 7.32)

- The intertransverse ligament connects the transverse processes of one vertebra to the one below.
- It is relatively thin and wide.
- A few of its fibres track into the lateral joint capsule, and it is replaced by the iliolumbar ligament at the lumbosacral junction.
- It inhibits rotation and lateral flexion to the contralateral side.

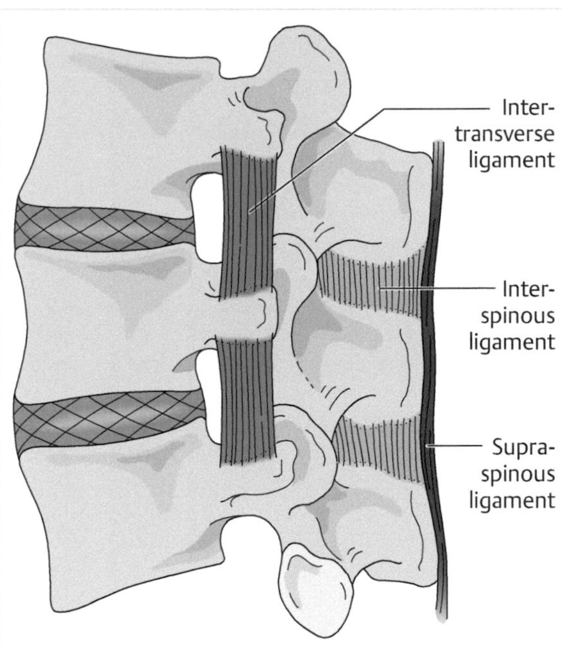


**Fig. 7.32** Ligaments of the lumbar spine (lateral view).

## Iliolumbar Ligament (Fig. 7.33)

- The *superior part of the iliolumbar ligament* connects the iliac crest with the costal process of L4 and the anterolateral vertebral body.
- The *inferior part of the iliolumbar ligament* (lumbosacral ligament) originates from the costal process and the anterolateral vertebral body of L5, and extends in a **V**-shape, the upper part running to the iliac crest and the lower part, in an anteroinferior direction, to the base of the sacrum, where it radiates into the anterior sacro-iliac ligaments.
- The obturator nerve runs between the two parts of the ligament.
- There is a fibrotic transformation of the quadratus lumborum muscle, which gives off fibers to the ligament.
- The ligament is significant for lumbosacral stability in that it prevents L5 from slipping in an anteroinferior direction and inhibits lateral flexion and rotation, while allowing flexion and extension.

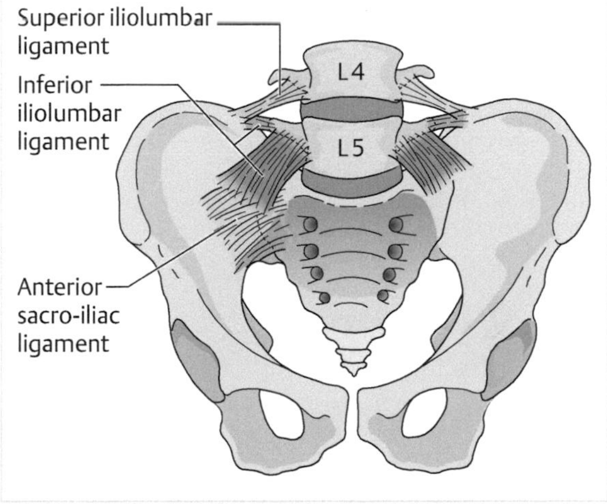


**Fig. 7.33** Ligaments of the lumbar spine: iliolumbar ligament.

# 7.5 Circulation and Innervation

## Arterial Supply (Fig. 7.34)

- The *lumbar arteries* exit the aorta at the segmental levels.
- As they course posterolaterally, they give off branches to the iliopsoas muscle and the peritoneum.
- They form anastomoses with the arteries of the levels above and below.
- The last branching of lumbar arteries from the aorta is at the L4 level.
- Every third lumbar artery divides in close proximity to the intervertebral foramen into:
  - The *spinal branch*, which subdivides into (1) branches to supply the vertebral body and the dura mater, and (2) the *segmental medullary arteries*, which enter the dural sac with the spinal nerve, and supply this as well as the cauda equina by way of the anterior spinal artery and the right and left posterior spinal arteries. The anterior and posterior segmental medullary arteries divide into ascending and descending branches and thus combine with the arteries of the next segments, forming the arterial spinal trunks (anterior and posterior spinal arteries).
  - The *dorsal branch*, which supplies the skin, muscles, and other structures as it courses posteriorly.
- At the L4 level, the aorta divides into the right and left *common iliac arteries*, which in turn divide into the external and internal iliac arteries at the L5–S1 level.
- The internal iliac artery divides into anterior and posterior branches; the anterior branch supplies primarily the surrounding organs, and the posterior branch supplies the L5–S1 segment by way of the iliolumbar artery.
- The external iliac artery becomes the femoral artery, which travels under the inguinal ligament and further distally.

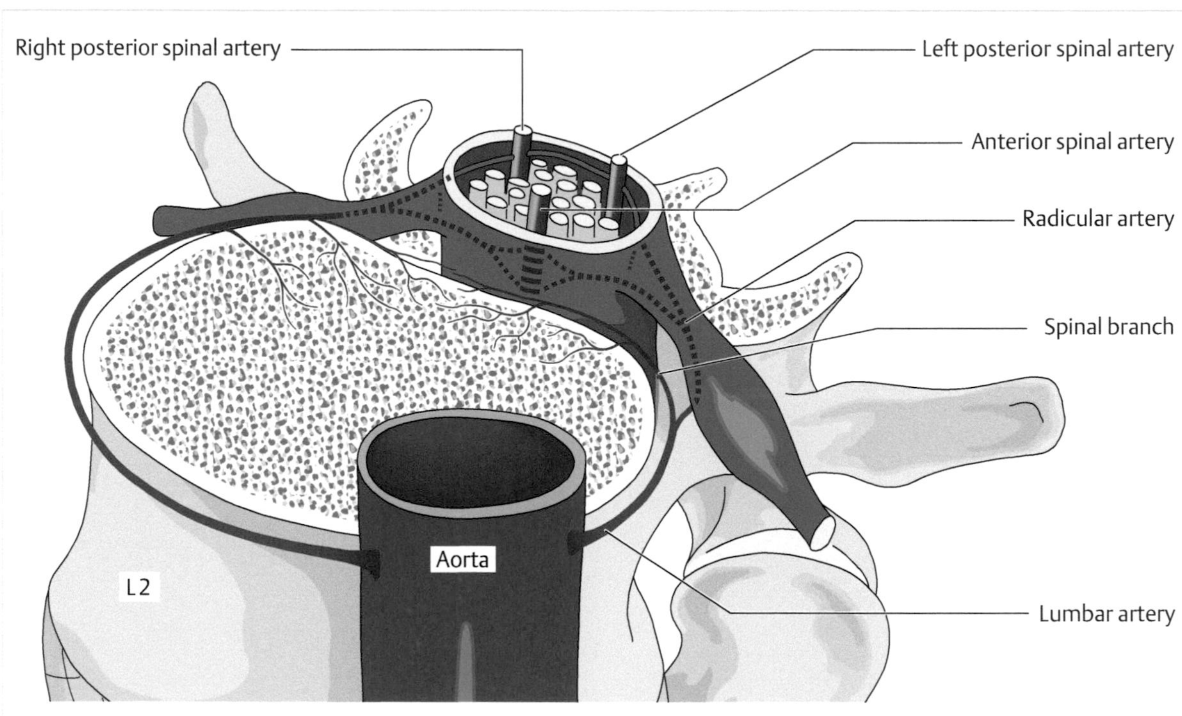


**Fig. 7.34** Arterial supply in the lumbar spine area.

## Venous Return (Fig. 7.35)

- The veins run parallel to the lumbar arteries.
- The *intradural venous system* drains blood from the spinal cord via the longitudinal veins and joins the internal vertebral venous plexus.
- The *extradural system* consists of the external and internal vertebral venous plexuses:
  - The *external vertebral venous plexus* is formed by the veins that run between the spinous process and the laminae to the intervertebral foramen. They empty into the inferior and superior vena cavae.
  - The *anterior internal vertebral venous plexus* consists of two large longitudinal veins that extend immediately lateral to the posterior longitudinal ligament and are interconnected by many transverse anastomoses. They give off the basivertebral vein into the vertebral body. In the area of the intervertebral foramen, they connect to the external vertebral venous plexus (**Fig. 7.35**).
  - The *posterior internal vertebral venous plexus* is located, along with many smaller vessels, in the posterior aspect of the spinal canal and also connects via the intervertebral foramen with the external venous plexus and the segmental veins, which are branches of the ascending lumbar veins and the internal iliac veins.

Extending the dura and the spinal cord through movement influences the tension in the surrounding tissue, and thus also affects perfusion and drainage. An unimpeded blood flow into and out of the lumbosacral region is essential for normal functioning of the nerve root.

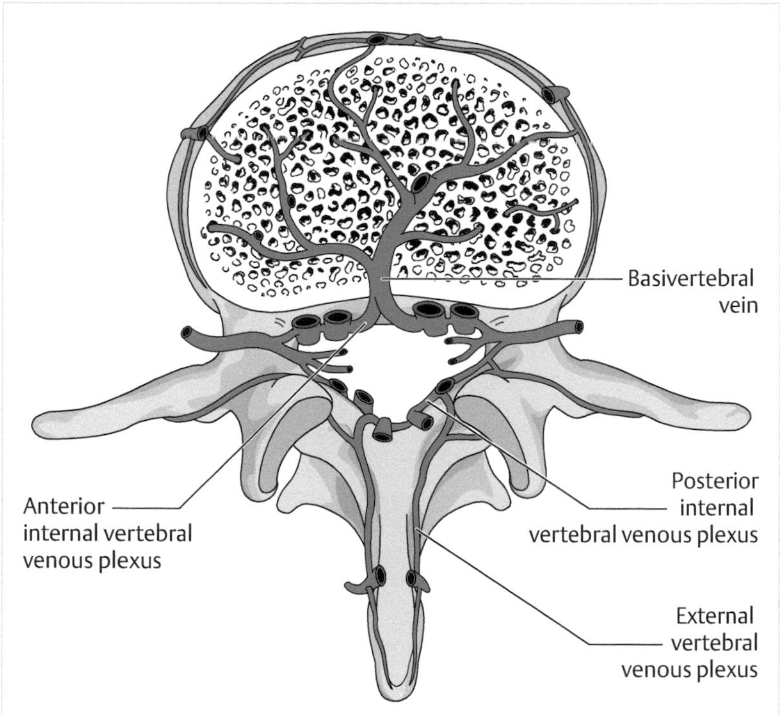


**Fig. 7.35** Venous network in the motion segment.

## Innervation of the Lumbar Region (Fig. 7.36)

The anterior and posterior nerve roots unite to form the spinal nerves. Shortly after exiting the intervertebral foramen, the meningeal branch of the spinal nerve (or recurrent branch) goes back through the foramen and supplies all the structures within the spinal canal.

The posterior ramus supplies the posteriorly lying parts of the motion segment, the muscles, and the skin. The anterior ramus forms the lumbar and sacral plexuses.

▷ See Chapter 1, Fundamentals of the Spinal Column

### Practical Tip

**Injections**

To break the vicious cycle of nerve irritation → faulty posture → muscle tension → neurogenic pain, a mixture of anti-inflammatory drugs and anesthetics can be injected at various sites, with the aim of desensitizing the nerve and the surrounding area, and reducing edema:

- Epidural injection through the interlaminar window into the epidural space.
- Facet infiltration in which receptors in the joint capsule are "turned off."
- Intrathecal injection directly into the subarachnoid space.
- Nerve root block, in which the spinal nerve is desensitized immediately after it exits the intervertebral foramen.
- Paravertebral injection, e.g., injection at myotendinous or ligamentous insertion sites.
- Intradermal injections.

**Therapeutic Approach (Fig. 7.37)**

Keep the following in mind when considering the causes of discomfort in the lumbar region:

- Could disk degeneration and its consequences be responsible for the discomfort?
- Is there a problem with regulation of the muscles and ligaments due to a faulty posture?
- Could it involve cystic hypertrophy of the ligamentum flavum or transformation of the ligament to adipose tissue with resultant irritation of the segment?
- Is there a drainage problem? Could venous congestion be causing the complaints?
- Could the cause lie internally? For example, the kidneys operate in close proximity to the lumbar spine and become less functional in the elderly.
- Could it be resulting from postpartum loosening of the ligaments, which can occur in women 40 to 50 years of age?

This approach can lead to the implementation of appropriate therapy in many areas. However, it should consist not only of mobilizing blocked segments and relieving muscular imbalance, but also of taking care of other structures.

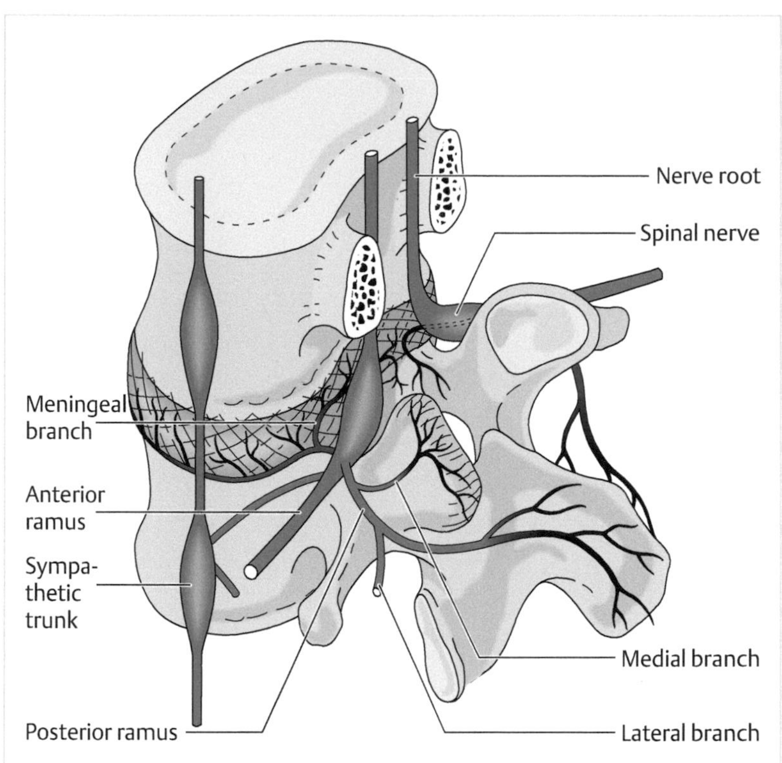


**Fig. 7.36** Innervation of the lumbar region.

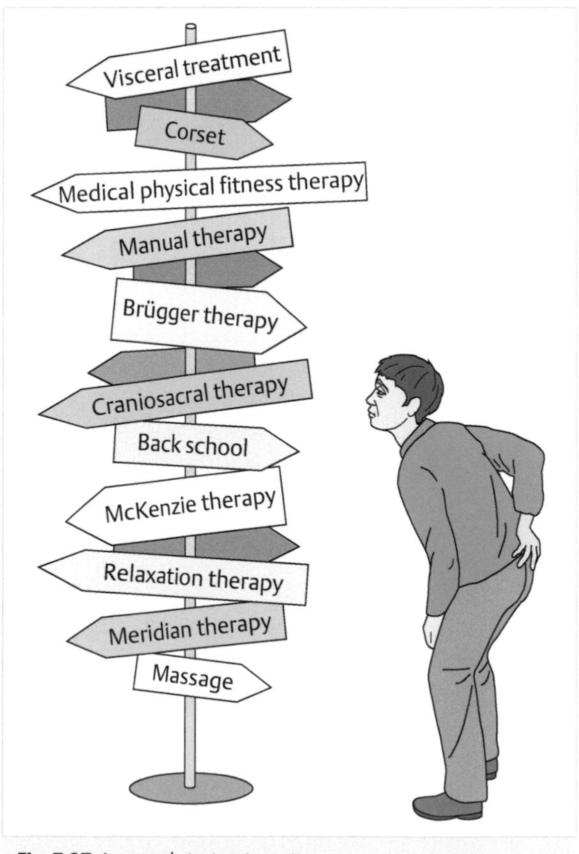


**Fig. 7.37** Approach to treatment.

# 7.6 Lumbar Spine Movements

## Flexion (Fig. 7.38)

In the initial phase of flexion, the posteroinferior portion of the joint loses contact, and there is an increase in the compressive load on the anterior, more frontally configured part of the joint. This movement apart is termed *divergence*.

**Mobility:**
- There is good mobility from the thoracolumbar junction to L2, and at the lumbosacral junction.
- Mobility is less favorable between L2 and L5.
- Total mobility: 40–45° (**Fig. 7.40**).

The *extent of movement is limited* by the increase in resistance from the ligamentum flavum, supraspinous ligament, and posterior longitudinal ligament, as well as from the capsule and its reinforcing bands and the posterior fibers of the anulus fibrosus. The end-feel is firm-elastic.

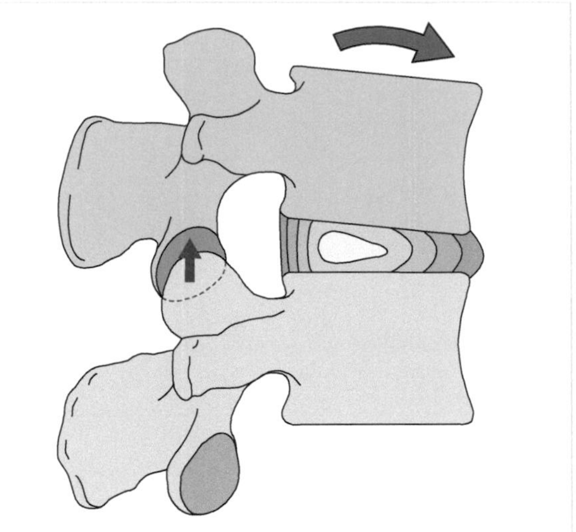

**Fig. 7.38** Flexion of the lumbar spine.

## Extension (Fig. 7.39)

At maximum extension, contact of the articular surface is lost, as shown here in midsagittal section. The ends of the inferior articular processes are pressed into the recesses and impinge on the pars interarticularis. The telescoping of the articular surfaces (convergence) can be severe at times and is referred to as facet closure.

**Mobility:**
- The mobility is good in all segments.
- There is very good mobility at the lumbosacral junction, which accounts for one-quarter of the total extension.
- Total extension: approximately 40° (**Fig. 7.40**).

The *extent of the movement is limited* by anterior portions of the anulus fibrosus and the anterior longitudinal ligament, as well as bony inhibition during end-range motion as a result of facet contact. The end-feel is firm-elastic due to facet closure.

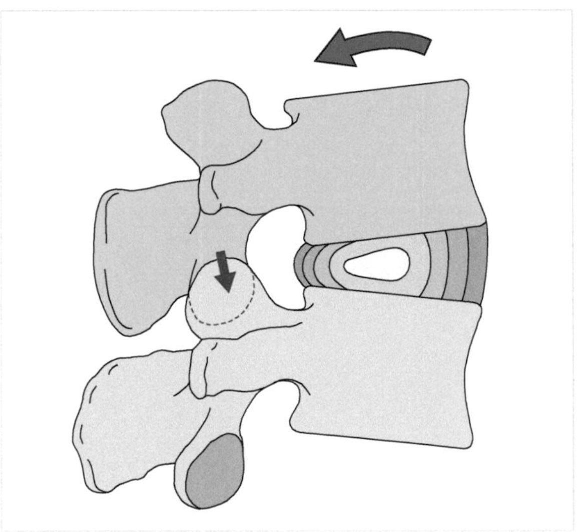

**Fig. 7.39** Extension of the lumbar spine.

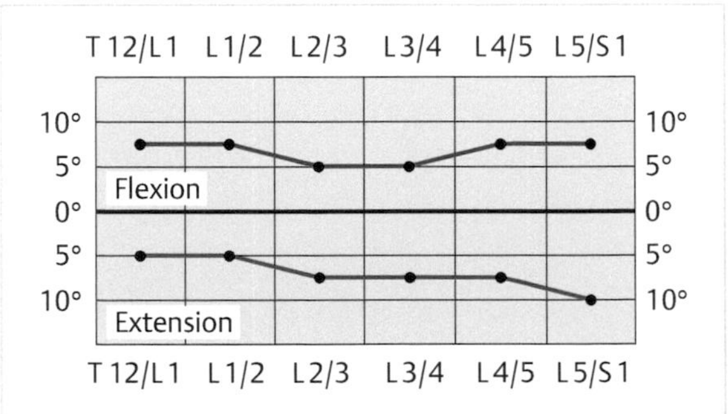


**Fig. 7.40** Movement diagram: flexion/extension.

## Lateral Flexion (Fig. 7.41)

During lateral flexion, there is also a wedge-shaped widening of the zygapophyseal joint space. There is divergence on the contralateral side and convergence on the ipsilateral side. At the same time, there is inevitably a contralateral rotation.

Lateral flexion is generally more feasible in a flexed position than in the neutral position.

**Mobility:**
- Mobility is good in the thoracolumbar section.
- It is not as good in the middle section but improves further inferiorly.
- In the final segment, little movement is possible because it is prevented by the iliolumbar ligament.
- Total mobility on either side: approximately 30° (**Fig. 7.43**).

The *extent of the movement is limited* by the convex lateral portions of the anulus fibrosus, the ligamentum flavum, parts of the capsule, and the intertransverse ligaments. Furthermore, there is compression of the joint surfaces on the concave side due to convergence gliding. The end-feel is firm-elastic.

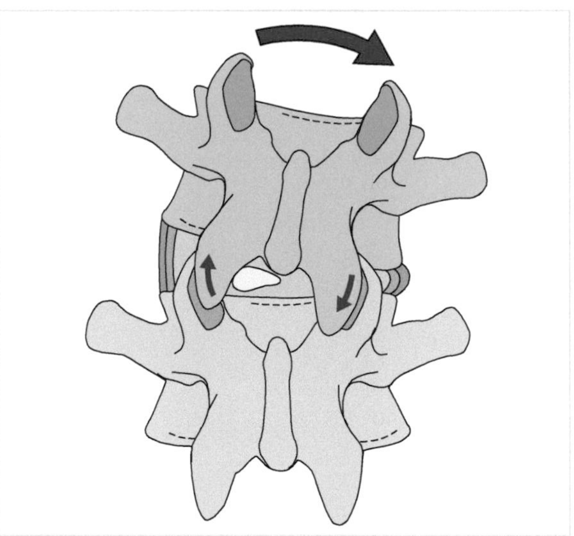

**Fig. 7.41** Lateral flexion of the lumbar spine to the right.

## Rotation (Fig. 7.42)

Rotation is only possible in combination with lateral flexion. In extension, only very small rotational movements can be made. In flexion, by contrast, there is a slight widening of the joint space and thus an improved ability to rotate.

**Mobility:**
*Range of motion*: A total of 3 to 4° of rotation occurs in each segment (**Fig. 7.43**).

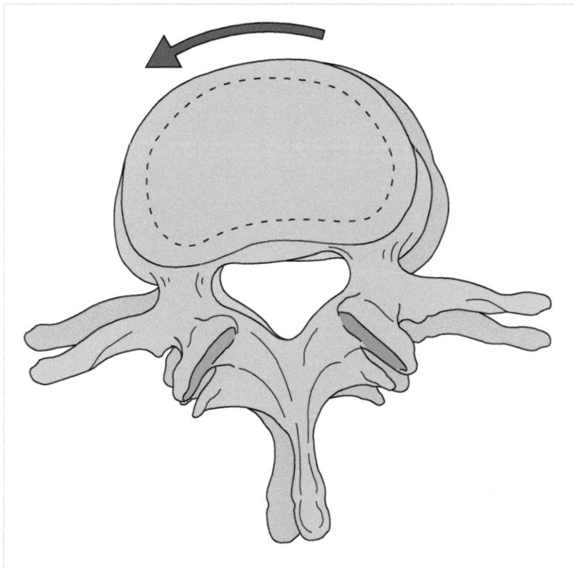

**Fig. 7.42** Rotation of the lumbar spine to the left.

**Practical Tip**

As a result of narrowing of the disk space after intense strain on a segment, the facets may slip into convergence. To center the joint surfaces, the upper joint facet should be mobilized tangentially in a superior direction, and the lower facet in an inferior direction.
Loosening the joint surfaces by applying posterior glide mobilization on the convex side can relieve the pressure. Delivering opposing rotary thrust impulses to the spinous processes of two adjacent vertebrae causes joint compression on one side and traction on the other.

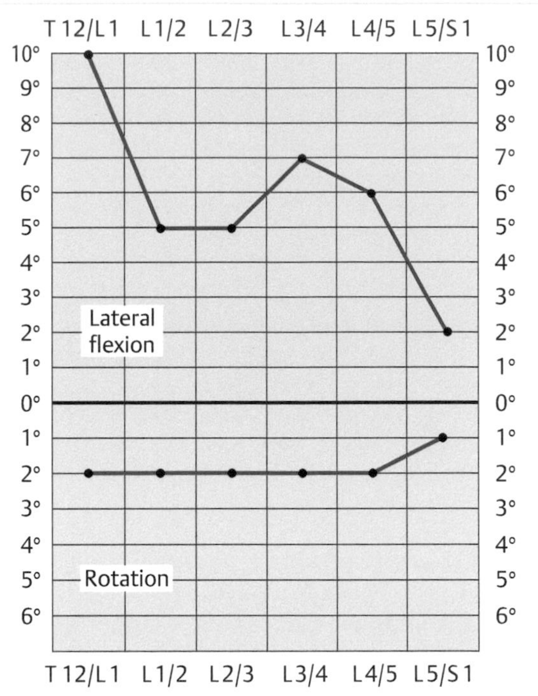


Fig. 7.43 Movement diagram: lateral flexion/rotation.

## Kinematic Coupling of Movements (Fig. 7.44)

Various factors play a role in motion coupling, including the position of the zygapophysial joints and the fiber orientation of the capsular and ligamentous structures.

Computer modeling was used to represent the particular positions of the lumbar joints while exerting a lateral torque of 10 N on the upper vertebra of the segment. This demonstrated a coupling of lateral flexion with axial rotation, the rotation being very limited.

White and Panjabi (1990) also examined movement coupling. With flexion/extension in the neutral position, he found that, between L1 and L4 (as shown in **Fig. 7.44**), right lateral flexion was coupled with rotation to the left, while between L4 and S1 it was coupled with rotation to the right. In addition, in the flexed position, there is a tendency toward extension, and in the extended position a tendency toward flexion.

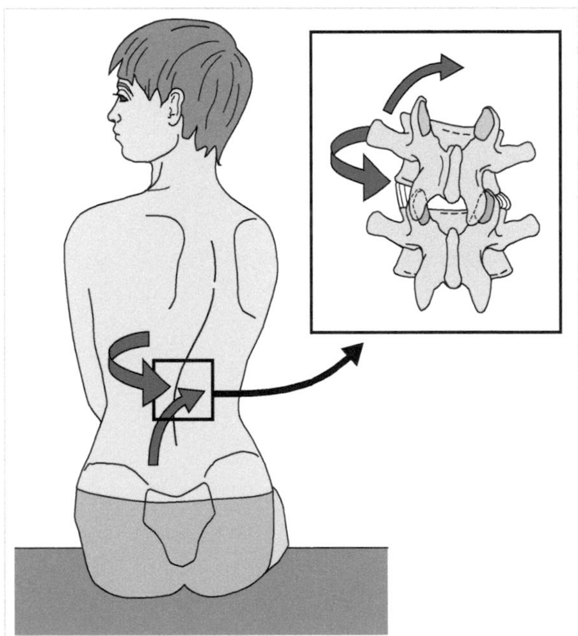

Fig. 7.44 Motion coupling: right lateral flexion with rotation to the left.

## Measurement of Mobility (Fig. 7.45)

It is not possible to measure mobility using a goniometer. Therefore, testing is carried out based on estimates. For example, in a subject with normal mobility, the spine forms a harmonic arc during flexion and lateral flexion. Plateau formation suggests hypomobility, whereas kinks in the arc suggest hypermobility. To assess segmental motion, the therapist needs to know the expected range of motion and be able to assess the extent of restriction.

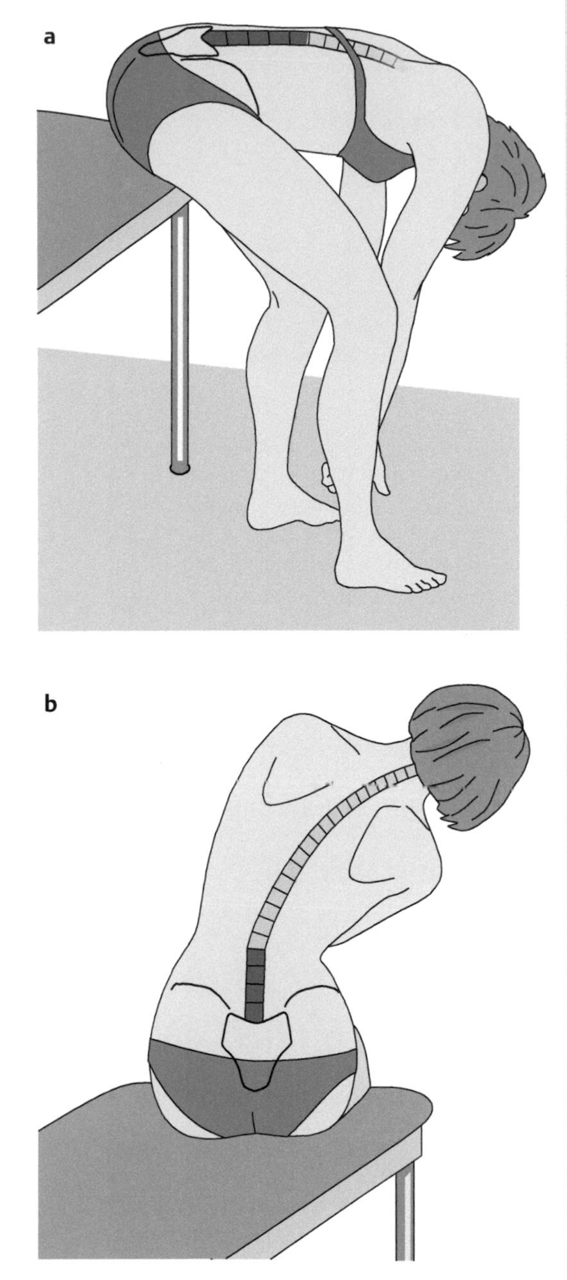


**Fig. 7.45** Measurement of mobility. **(a)** Hypomobility of the lumbar spine in flexion. **(b)** Hypermobility at L1–L2 during right lateral flexion.

# 7.7 Muscles of the Lumbar Spine Region

## Abdominal Muscles

### Rectus Abdominis Muscle (Fig. 7.46)

- This muscle connects the fifth to seventh costal cartilages with the pubic tubercle.
- Three transverse, narrow intermediate tendinous bands (tendinous intersections) divide the muscle into three approximately equal sections above the navel and a larger one below. These intermediate bands are located only in the superficial layer—they are lacking in the deep layer.
- The aponeuroses of the other abdominal muscles run toward the linea alba, partly anterior to the rectus abdominis muscle and partly posterior to it, thus forming the rectus sheath.
- The *linea alba* is a tendinous strip that runs from the xiphoid process to the pubic symphysis and is approximately 10 to 25 mm wide, being narrower toward the inferior end. It arises from intersecting connections of the aponeuroses of the oblique and transverse abdominal muscles and separates the right rectus abdominis muscle from the left.

*Innervation*: 5th to 12th intercostal nerves.

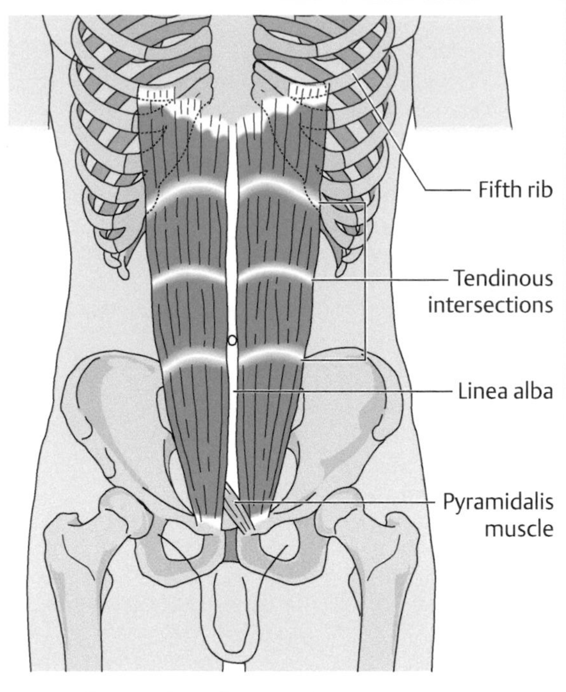


**Fig. 7.46** Abdominal muscles: rectus abdominis muscle.

### Pyramidalis Muscle (Fig. 7.46)

- This lies anteroinferior to the rectus abdominis muscle and runs from the symphysis pubis to the linea alba.
- It runs within the aponeurosis of the oblique abdominal muscles.
- It acts to tense the linea alba.

### Transversus Abdominis Muscle (Fig. 7.47)

- This connects the lower six ribs and thoracolumbar fascia to the rectus sheath and the pubic symphysis.
- The upper section is oriented in a horizontal direction; the lower portions form a slightly curved arch running anterior-medial-inferior.
- Below the navel, the fibers track into the anterior leaf of the rectus sheath; above the navel, the run into the posterior leaf.

*Innervation:* 7th to 12th intercostal nerves, iliohypogastric nerve, and ilio-inguinal nerve.

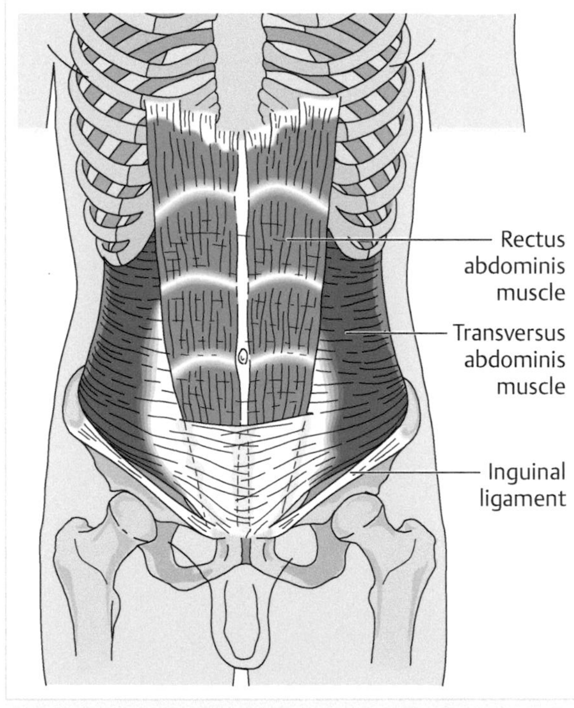


**Fig. 7.47** Abdominal muscles: transversus abdominis muscle.

## Internal Oblique Muscle (Fig. 7.48)

- This connects the iliac crest, the anterior superior iliac spine, and the lateral parts of the inguinal ligament with the lower three ribs.
- The orientation of muscle fibers is from inferolateral to superomedial.
- It participates in the formation of the rectus sheath and belongs to the middle layer of the abdominal muscles.
- Posteriorly, it intertwines with the thoracolumbar fascia.
- The cremaster muscle splits off from the internal oblique to track through the inguinal canal with the spermatic cord.

*Innervation:* 5th to 12th thoracic intercostal nerves, iliohypogastric nerve, and ilio-inguinal nerve.

## External Oblique Muscle (Fig. 7.48)

- This connects the lower ribs to the rectus sheath, the inguinal ligament, and the iliac crest.
- The orientation of the muscle fibers is from superolateral to inferomedial; the lower portions run vertically from the navel.
- Superiorly, its serrations interdigitate with those of the serratus anterior muscle.
- It intertwines with the contralateral internal oblique muscle.
- It represents the superficial layer of abdominal muscles and tenses the linea alba through a broad aponeurosis.

*Innervation:* 5th to 12th thoracic intercostal nerves, iliohypogastric nerve, and ilio-inguinal nerve.

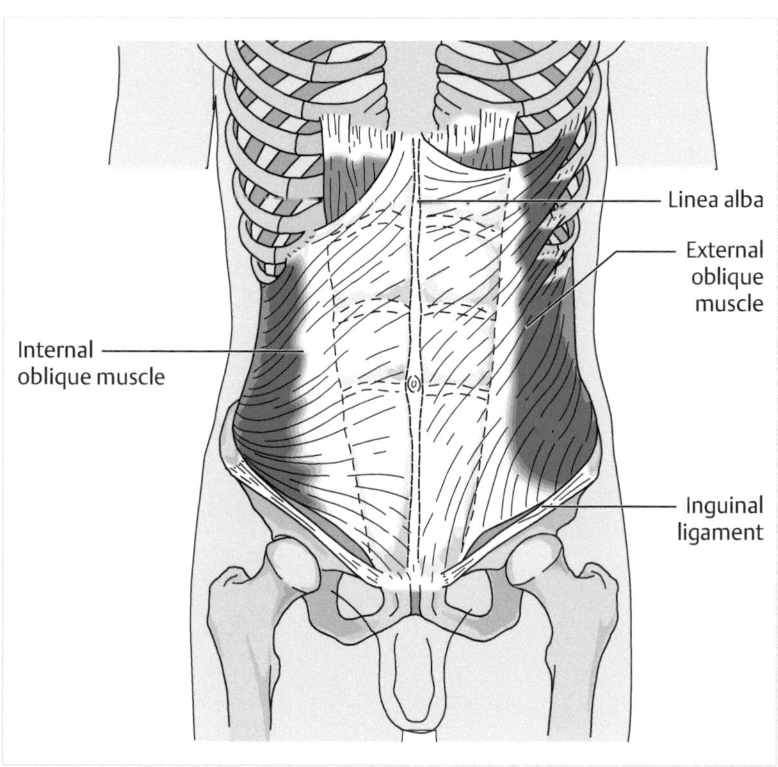


**Fig. 7.48** Abdominal muscles: oblique abdominal muscles.

## Quadratus Lumborum Muscle (Fig. 7.49)

- *Iliocostal part:* The fibers run vertically between the last rib and the iliac crest, and are situated the furthest posteriorly.
- *Costovertebral part:* The fibers run obliquely from the last rib to the costal processes of the lumbar vertebrae, and are located the furthest anteriorly.
- *Ilio-vertebral part:* The fibers run obliquely from the costal process to the iliac crest and lie between the costovertebral and iliocostal parts.

**Function.** By pulling on the 12th rib, this muscle pulls the thorax posteriorly, thus helping with expiration. Conversely, it can also play a role in inspiration because it fixes the ribs posteriorly, serving as a fixed end for the diaphragm.

With a fixed end at the pelvis, it causes extension of the lumbar spine, and, with unilateral contraction, lateral flexion. If its fixed end is reversed, the muscle lifts the pelvis on the ipsilateral side.

*Innervation:* the muscular branches of the lumbar plexus and the 12th intercostal nerve.

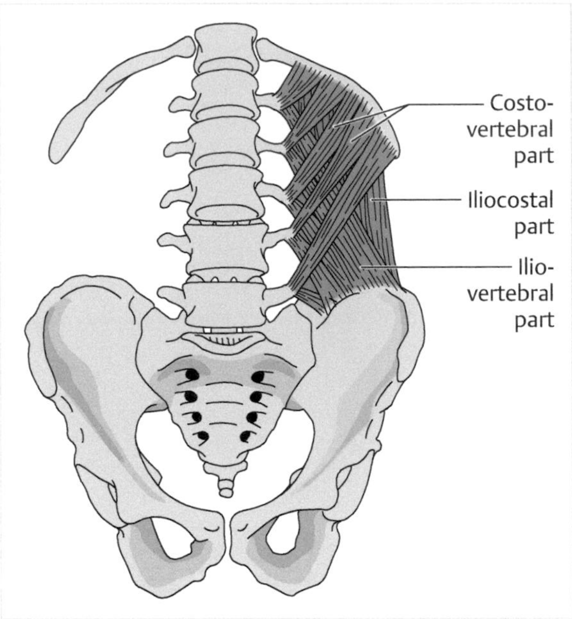


**Fig. 7.49** Abdominal muscles: quadratus lumborum muscle.

## Rectus Sheath

This consists of the following three layers:

- Posterior fascial layer = posterior layer.
- Muscle layer.
- Anterior fascial layer = anterior layer.

### Posterior Layer (Fig. 7.50a)

- In the superior region, the rectus sheath is formed from the posterior leaf of the internal oblique aponeurosis, the transversus abdominis aponeurosis, and the transversalis fascia.
- The posterior aponeurosis of the rectus abdominis muscle is not fused with the posterior layer but glides over it.
- The posterior layer ends approximately 5 cm below the navel in the arched arcuate line, because the aponeuroses tracks into the anterior layer beyond this point.
- Inferior to the arcuate line, the rectus sheath consists only of the transversalis fascia and the peritoneum.
- It continues into the inguinal ligament and the femoral fascia.

### Anterior Layer (Fig. 7.50b)

- This extends over the anterior part of the rectus abdominis muscle.
- Above the arcuate line, the aponeurosis of the external oblique muscle and the anterior leaf of the aponeurosis of the internal oblique muscle participate in forming the anterior layer.
- Below the arcuate line, this layer is composed of the aponeuroses of the oblique and transverse muscles.
- Medially and at the tendinous intersections, the rectus abdominis muscle fuses with the anterior and posterior layers.

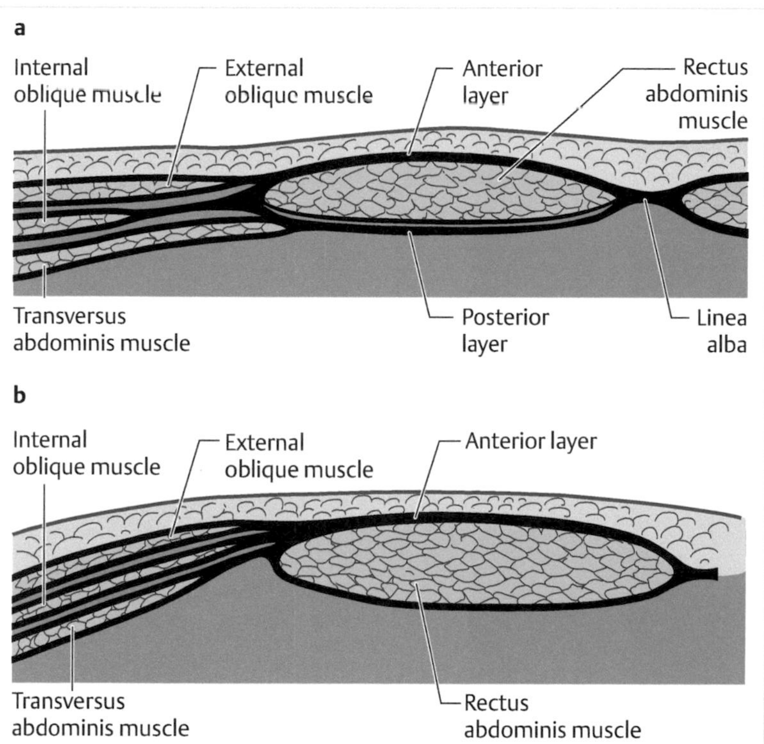


**Fig. 7.50** Rectus sheath. (a) Superior to the arcuate line. (b) Inferior to the arcuate line.

## Function of the Abdominal Muscles

### Flexion (Fig. 7.51)

With the pelvis fixed, the rectus abdominis muscles are the most powerful flexors of the torso. They are supported by the oblique abdominal muscles. With their fixed end on the thorax, they can pull the anterior pelvis superiorly, which corresponds to extension of the pelvis and leads further to flexion of the lumbar spine.

Through the tendinous intersections and their attachment to the anterior leaf of the rectus sheath, individual sections can function independently.

### Abdominal Press

Simultaneous contraction of the transverse abdominal muscles and the diaphragm exerts pressure on the intestines and the muscles of the pelvic floor (*abdominal press*). This passively stretches the pelvic and urogenital diaphragms.

The abdominal press stabilizes the trunk when lifting heavy loads. The erector spinae muscle and the pelvic floor muscles support this feature.

If flexion is prevented by tension caused by the erector spinae muscle, the abdominal muscles will pull the lower ribs inferiorly, thus supporting expiration.

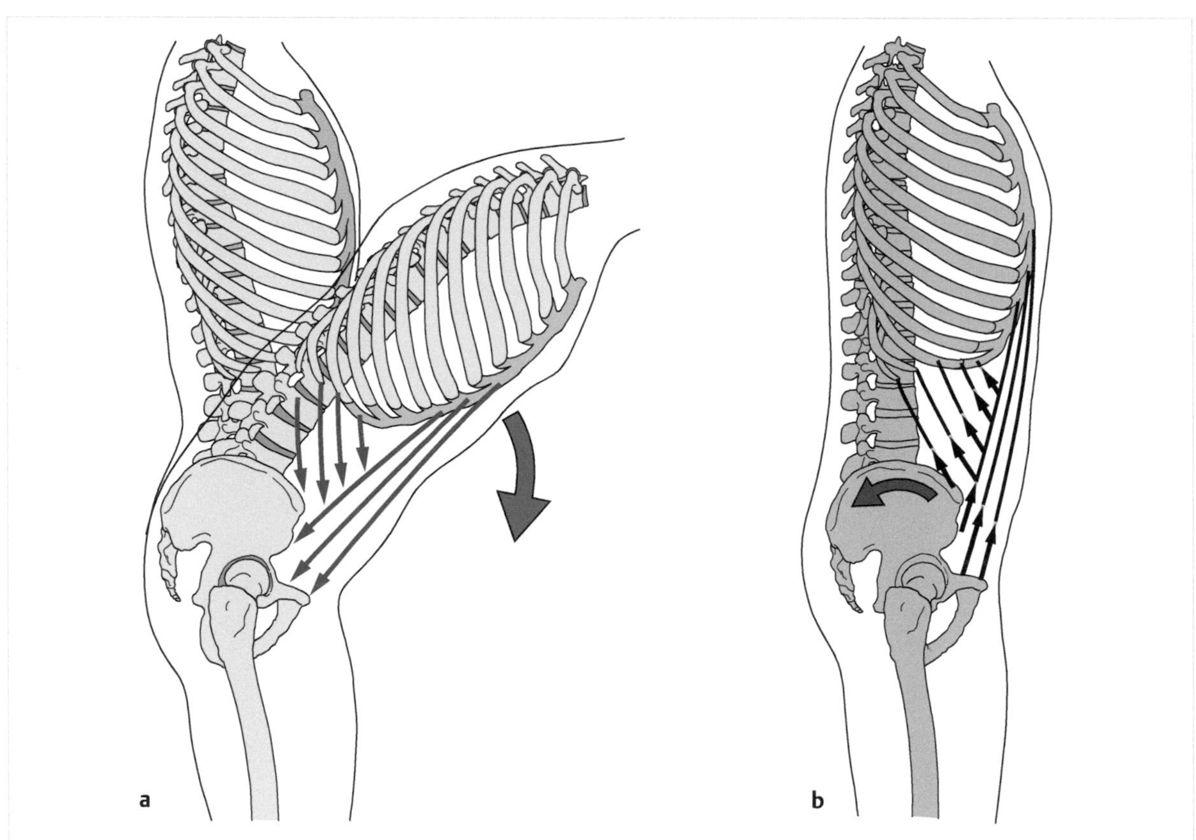


**Fig. 7.51** Function of the abdominal muscles. **(a)** Flexion of the torso. **(b)** Pelvic extension.

## Rotation (Fig. 7.52)

When a diagonal muscle, such as the left external oblique or the right internal oblique, contracts, the torso rotates to the right.

## Lateral Flexion (Fig. 7.53)

Lateral flexion is produced by contraction of the ipsilateral internal and external oblique muscles and the quadratus lumborum muscle. The ipsilateral rectus abdominis muscle supports the movement.

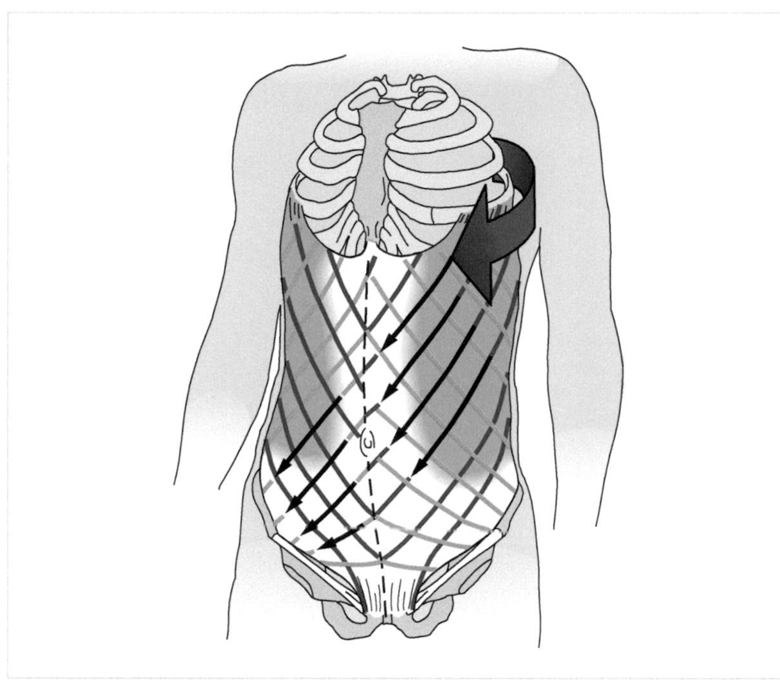

**Fig. 7.52** Function of the abdominal muscles: rotation.

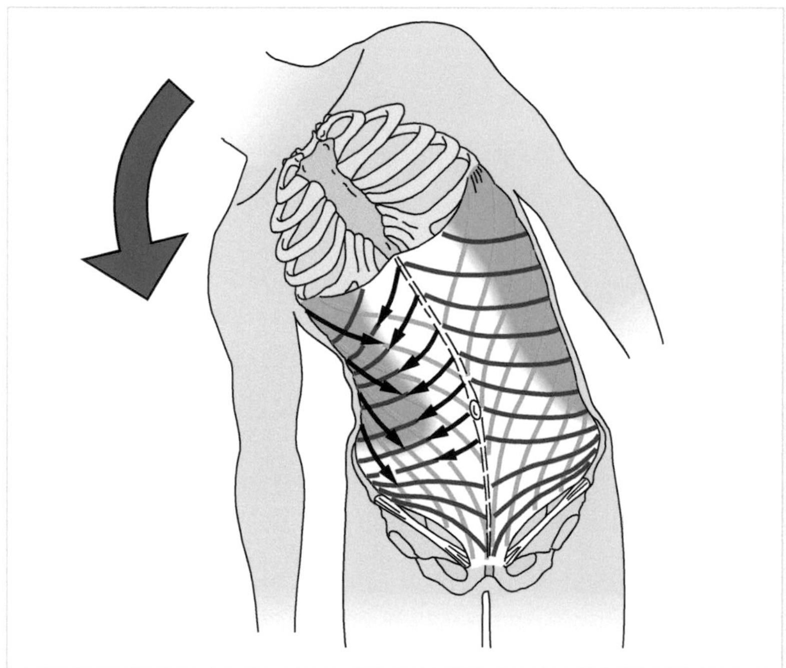

**Fig. 7.53** Function of the abdominal muscles: lateral flexion.

## Abdominal Bracing System

- Among the various directions in which the abdominal muscles pull, the rectus abdominis muscle, the rectus sheath, the linea alba, and the lower fibers of the external oblique aponeurosis present a *vertical orientation.*
- *Diagonal bracing* is provided by the external oblique muscles, which intertwine with the contralateral internal oblique muscles. The linea alba and the two rectus sheaths serve as the interface.
- The transverse abdominis muscle and the horizontally running fibers of the oblique muscles provide *horizontal bracing.* The superior fibers of the transverse abdominal muscle narrow the epigastric angle and thus support forced exhalation.

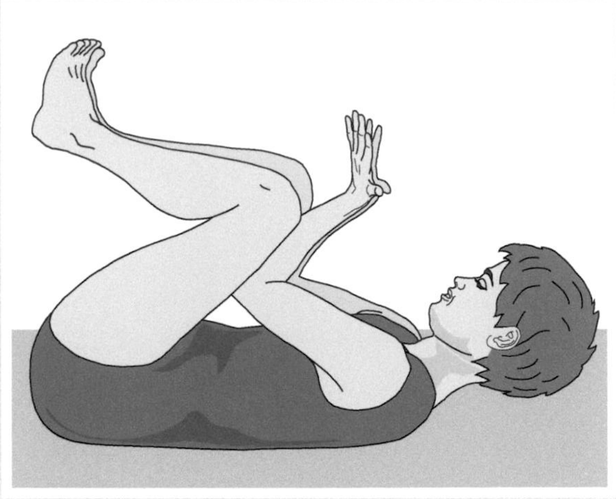

**Fig. 7.54** Functional abdominal training: the "frog."

**Practical Tip**

*Diastasis recti* is a sign of continuing inadequacy of the oblique muscles, which is why a training program for these muscles is so important. To be effective, *abdominal muscle training* should be oriented to the anatomical conditions encountered. The selection of training exercises requires recognition that the abdominal muscles stretch between the pelvis and thorax. Thus, isometric exercises involving tension between points on the thorax and pelvis are optimal, as conceived by Klein-Vogelbach (1991) with her functional abdominal muscle training program. Exercises such as the "frog" (**Fig. 7.54**), involving the legs and arms, are also effective because the limbs act as lever arms attaching to the pelvis and thorax, thereby increasing the expenditure of force.

### Change in Muscle Tension due to Faulty Posture (Fig. 7.55)

Knowing the course of the muscles, the practitioner can deduce which muscles are shortened and which are stretched due to faulty posture. For example, lateral, transverse displacement of the thorax on the pelvis, called a *lateral shift to the right,* shows the following effects on the abdominal muscles:

- The left external oblique muscle and the right internal oblique muscle converge.
- The right external oblique muscle, the left internal oblique muscle, both quadratus lumborum muscles, and the rectus abdominis muscle are under constant tension.

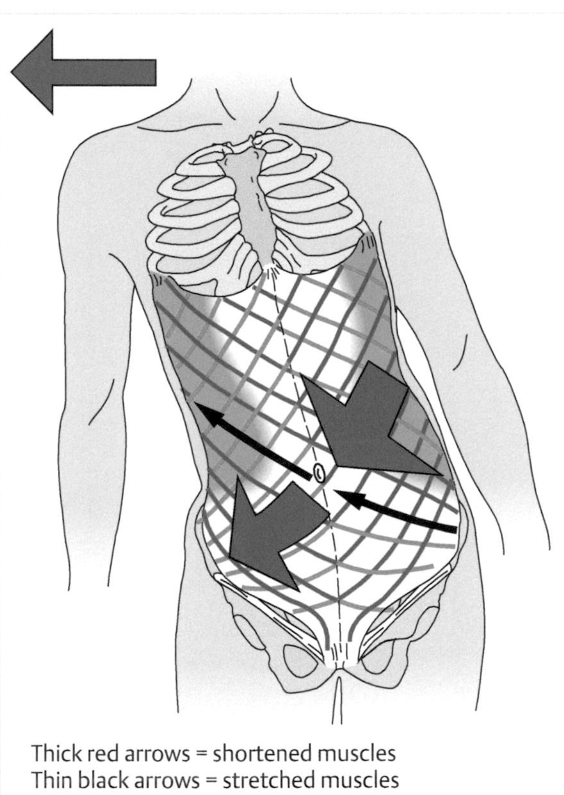


**Fig. 7.55** Change in muscle tension due to faulty posture.

## Superficial Muscles of the Back

### Latissimus Dorsi Muscle (Fig. 7.56)

- Each of its four parts is named according to the region of origin: the *scapular part* from the inferior angle of the scapula; the *vertebral part* over the thoracolumbar fascia from the spinous processes of the lower six thoracic vertebrae and all the lumbar vertebrae; the *costal part* from the lower three ribs; and the *iliac part* from the posterior part of the iliac crest.
- It forms the posterior axillary fold and makes a rotation of 180° shortly before its insertion on the humerus, so that the iliac part inserts the furthest anteriorly and superiorly on the crest of the lesser tubercle of the humerus.

**Functions:**
- If performs adduction, extension, and internal rotation of the arm.
- With the humerus as the fixed end, the scapular part of the muscle causes external rotation of the scapula, and the costal part helps with inspiration.
- During coughing, the ribs are fixed, forming the fixed end for the diaphragm.

*Innervation:* the thoracodorsal nerve.

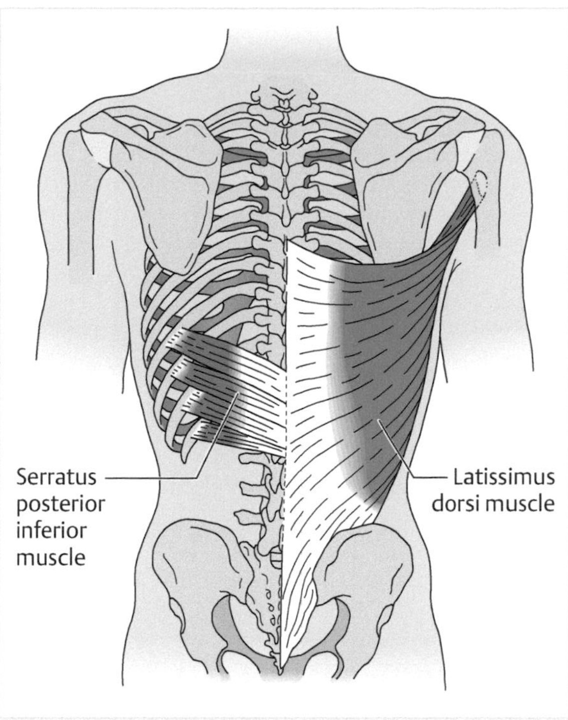


**Fig. 7.56** Back muscles: latissimus dorsi and serratus posterior inferior muscles.

### Serratus Posterior Inferior Muscle (Fig. 7.56)

- This muscle passes over the thoracolumbar fascia as an aponeurosis from the spinous processes of the 12th thoracic vertebra and the first three lumbar vertebrae.
- Its insertion is on the inferior margins of the lower four ribs.

**Function:**
- It pulls the lower ribs inferiorly;
- By fixing the ribs, it offers a fixed end for the diaphragm.

*Innervation:* 9th to 12th intercostal nerves.

## Autochthonous Back Muscles

The term *autochthonous* relates to the embryonic development of these "true" or "intrinsic" back muscles as they take their places at the very beginning of muscle development. They consist of muscle fiber tracts of various lengths: the short ones bridge only one or two motion segments, while the longest tracts bridge up to 10. However, there are none that reach from the pelvis to the occiput. They are innervated by the posterior branches of the spinal nerves.

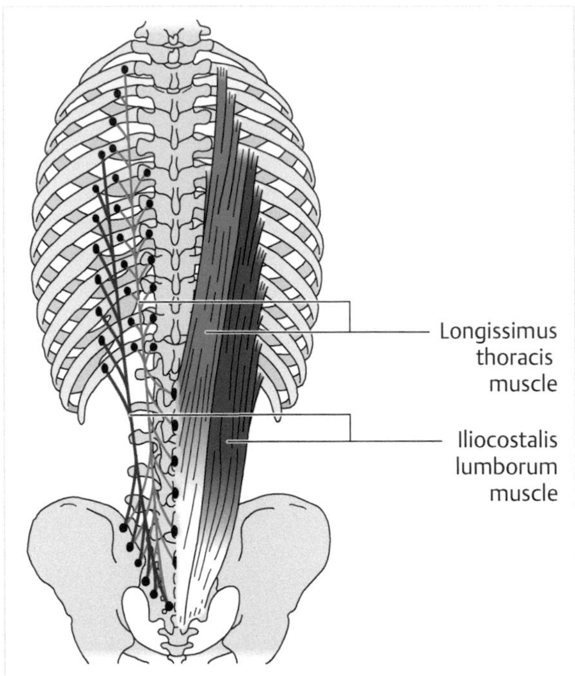


**Fig. 7.57** Back muscles: iliocostalis lumborum and longissimus thoracis muscles.

## 1. Muscles of the Lateral Tract

a) The erector spinae muscle group:

### Iliocostalis Lumborum Muscle (Fig. 7.57)

- This connects the posterior iliac crest and sacrum with the angles of the six to nine lower ribs.
- It is located the furthest laterally.

### Longissimus Thoracis Muscle (Fig. 7.57)

- Its diverse muscle fiber bands extend from the sacrum, the posterior superior iliac spine, the spinous processes of the lower six to seven thoracic vertebrae, and the first and second lumbar vertebra to the transverse processes of all the lumbar and thoracic vertebrae and the angles of the 2nd to 12th ribs.
- It forms the longest system of the erector spinae muscles.
- It has a strong aponeurosis that stretches inferiorly between the two ilia and forms an important part of the lumbar fascia.

*Innervation:* the lateral branches of the spinal nerves at the same segment level.

b) The intertransversarii muscle group:

### Lateral Lumbar Intertransversarii Muscles (Fig. 7.58)

- These run between the ends of costal processes.

*Innervation:* branches of the anterior rami of the lumbar plexus at the same segment level.

### Medial Lumbar Intertransversarii Muscles (Fig. 7.58)

- They connect the mammillary processes with each other.

*Innervation:* medial branches of the spinal nerves at the same segment level.

## 2. Muscles of the Medial Tract

a) The spinal muscle group:

### Interspinales Lumborum Muscles (Fig. 7.58)

- These connect adjacent spinous processes to each other as far as the sacrum.

*Innervation:* the medial branch of the spinal nerve of the same segment.

b) The transversospinales muscle group:

### Multifidus Muscles (Fig. 7.59)

- These join laterally to the interspinales muscles.
- They extend from inferolateral to superomedial from the sacrum and the mammillary processes to the spinous processes, skipping over three or four segments.
- Some fibers track into the aponeurosis of the erector spinae muscle.
- In the sacral area, there is a link to the posterior sacroiliac ligaments.
- They are designated as the key muscles for segmental stabilization of the lumbar spine.

*Innervation:* the posterior branches of the spinal nerves at the same segmental level.

### Long Rotator Muscles (Fig. 7.59)

- These track from the costal processes to the base of the spinous processes on the vertebral arch, passing over two motion segments.
- They are not always present in the lumbar spine.

*Innervation:* the posterior branches of the spinal nerves at the same segmental level.

**Pathology**

In a *hemilaminectomy* (removal of half a vertebral arch), the insertion site of the long rotator muscle of a motion segment is destroyed.

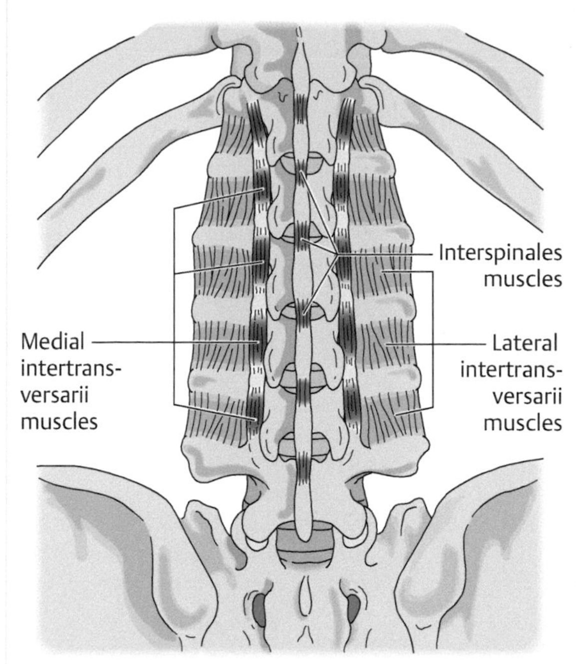


**Fig. 7.58** Back muscles: intertransversarii and interspinales muscles.

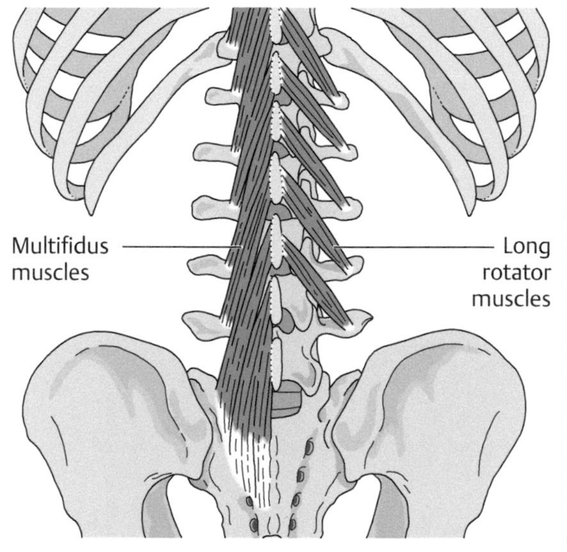


**Fig. 7.59** Back muscles: multifidus and long rotator muscles.

## Function of the Back Muscles

### Extension

Since the muscle groups lie posterior to the axis of movement, they all cause extension. The sacrospinales group is the strongest in this regard. They stabilize end-range extension, i.e., they hold the arc of the extended vertebrae in place.

When straightening up after bending forward, the hamstrings and gluteal muscles take part by bringing the pelvis into extension. The back muscles only become active in straightening up beyond this point.

### Lateral Flexion

By contracting unilaterally, all parts of the erector spinae muscle group participate in this movement. Of the erector spinae muscles, the iliocostalis muscle develops the greatest force because it inserts into the ribs far laterally. Muscles that are located medially, such as the spinalis and interspinous muscles, are only slightly involved.

### Rotation

All obliquely running muscle fiber bands, especially the transversospinales group, have a rotational function.

The *transversospinales group* is an important integral part of the support system of the spine. Due to the varying lengths of its muscle fibers and its course, which is partly horizontal and partly oblique, it can not only optimally stabilize the segments and accentuate facet closure, but also implement movements in any direction.

Another important function of the short muscles is their involvement in spinal proprioception. They provide sensory feedback for position control and the coordination of spinal movement, which is carried out centrally.

**Practical Tip**

The proportion of joint disorders that are muscle-related is very high, showing how important a functioning muscular system is for joint equilibrium.
Treatment should be structured with the goals, first and foremost, of restoring joint harmony and, secondarily, of providing proprioceptive rehabilitation. For example, specialized segmental training with stabilizing and rotational stimuli for the transversospinales group can be utilized to achieve these goals.

# 7.8 Fascial Structures of the Torso

## Thoracolumbar Fascia

This represents a type of retinaculum for the deep muscles of the back and is divided into superficial and deep leaves:

- The superficial leaf stretches medially to the spinous processes of the thoracic and lumbar spines and the sacrum, and laterally to the iliac crest. Inferiorly, this fascia has a sinewy nature and serves as the origin for the latissimus dorsi and serratus posterior inferior muscles.
- The deep leaf connects the posterior ribs, the costal processes, and the iliac crest to each other and separates the quadratus lumborum muscle from the erector spinae muscle. This part of the fascia serves as the origin for a portion of the autochthonous back muscles and the internal oblique and transverse abdominal muscles.
- In the pelvic area, the posterior sacro-iliac ligaments form reinforcing bands in the fascia with a continuation into the sacrotuberous ligament and to the hamstring muscles.

## Abdominal Fascia

- The superficial abdominal fascia covers the anterior abdominal wall superficially and connects superolaterally to the axillary fascia.
- The transversalis fascia is the inner abdominal fascia. It runs on the posterior wall of the rectus abdominis muscle, extending over the quadratus lumborum muscle and, superiorly, over the abdominal surface of the diaphragm as a thin layer. It connects to the parietal peritoneum and, in the region of the iliac crest, with the iliac fascia that surrounds the iliopsoas muscle.

## 7.9 Cauda Equina (Fig. 7.60)

- The end of the spinal cord, the *conus medullaris*, is located at the level of the second lumbar vertebra. Within the spinal canal below that point are found the dural sac, the nerve roots, and the peridural tissue, which consists of a vascular plexus and adipose tissue. **Fig. 7.60** is a section showing the nerve roots, here called the *cauda equina*, and the *filum terminale*, surrounded by the dural sac.
- The *spinal dura mater* forms the dural sac, which extends to the second sacral vertebra and continues on in a fan shape as the dural part of the filum terminale into the periosteum of the sacrum.

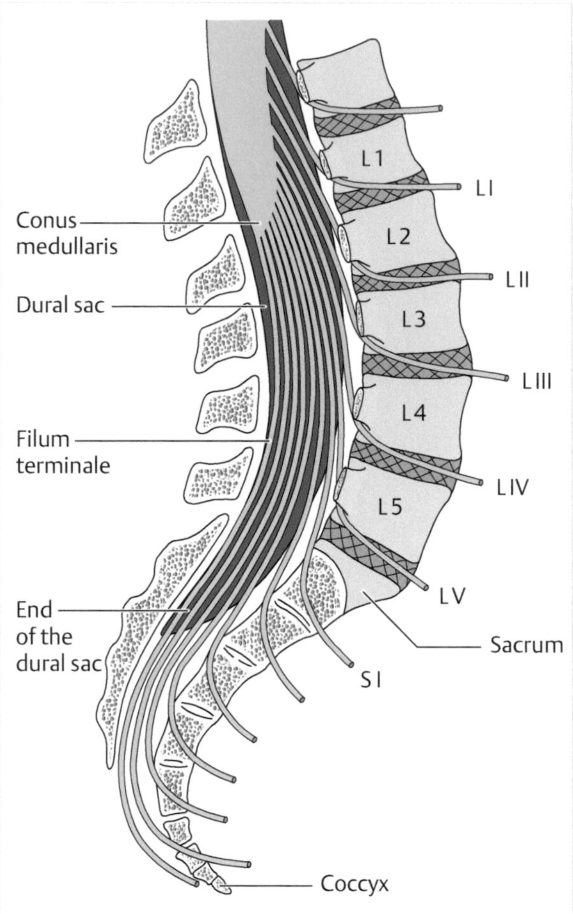


**Fig. 7.60** Cauda equina.

## Course of the Nerve Roots

- In the area of the nerve root outlets, bulges called *root sleeves* form in the dural sac. Within these run the sensory root (posterior root) and the thinner motor root (anterior root). Each root is surrounded by the spinal arachnoid mater, pia mater, and dura mater. The root sleeve is loosely fixed in two places: at the dural hiatus (the exit point from the dural sac) and at the outer boundary of the intervertebral foramen.
- The nerve roots extend steeply downward to a variable degree through the spinal canal. In the upper lumbar spine, the nerve root forms an angle of approximately 80° at the dural hiatus, becomes almost horizontal through the intervertebral foramen, and has a very short path within the spinal canal. The lower nerve roots exit the dural sac with a very acute angle of approximately 10 to 20° and travel a longer distance within the lateral recess (**Fig. 7.61**).
- The nerve roots exit the spinal canal in pairs through the intervertebral foramina.
- In the sacral area, they leave the canal through the anterior sacral foramina.

### Practical Tip

The spinal canal extends when traction is applied. However, the root itself is not affected by the increased tension on the dural sleeve because it has a certain amount of reserve length in the dural sac, within which it glides. Due to the change in tension in the dural membrane, patients may at times develop a headache, because the spinal dura mater merges into the cranial dura mater at the foramen magnum.

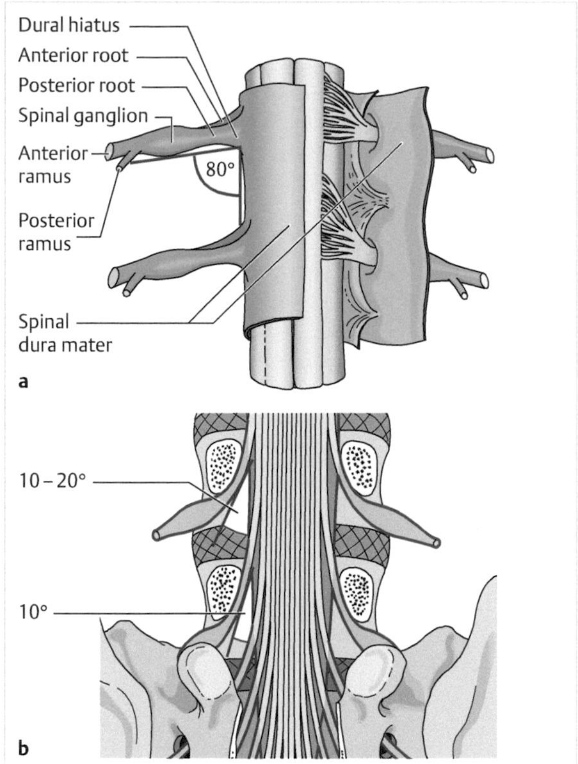


**Fig. 7.61** Nerve roots exiting the spinal cord. **(a)** In the thoracic spine and upper lumbar spine. **(b)** In the lower lumbar spine.

## Nerve Roots and Their Relationship to the Intervertebral Disk (Fig. 7.62)

The L5 nerve root runs from the dural hiatus at the level of superior intervertebral disk (L4–L5) in the lateral recess and then laterally from under L5 into the intervertebral foramen. At the point that it bends, the root lies directly above the L5–S1 disk. This means that it runs very close to two intervertebral disks.

In the event of a prolapsed disk at L5–S1, both the L5 and S1 roots can be affected, depending on the direction of the prolapse.

### Pathology

In the rare case of medial disk prolapse—usually at L3–L4 or L4–L5—the cauda equina can be compressed, in which case all the nerve roots in the lumbar spinal canal are pressed together.

*Symptoms:* There is sphincter insufficiency of the bladder and bowels, saddle anesthesia, and loss of the Achilles reflex. Immediate surgery is required because irreversible damage can occur within a few hours.

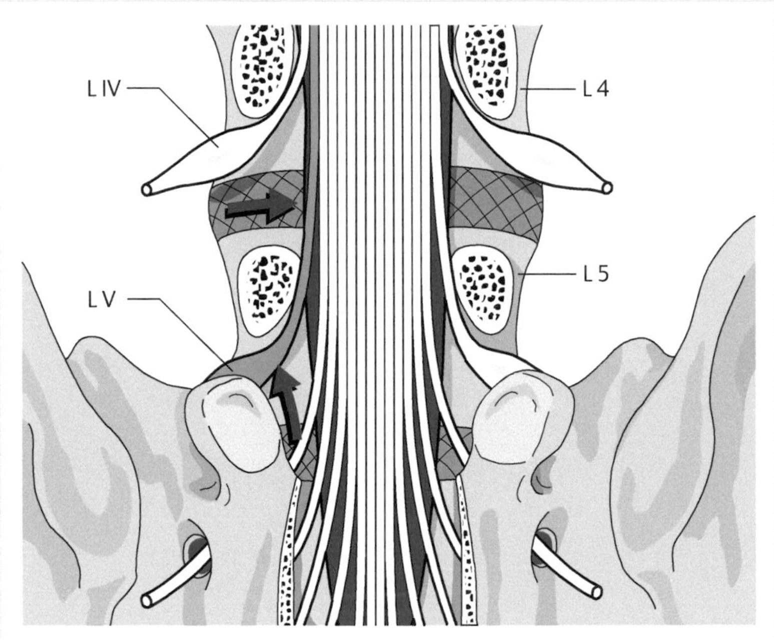


**Fig. 7.62** Course of the nerve roots in the lower segments.

# 7.10 Lumbar Plexus (Fig. 7.63)

- This arises with four anterior rami from the L1–L5 levels and possibly a small branch from T12.
- The anterior rami intertwine with each other; only after this are the muscular branches given off.
- The lumbar plexus passes in front of the costal processes between the fibers of the psoas major muscle.
- The *anterior ramus of L1*, with anastomoses to the 12th intercostal nerve and the anterior ramus of L2, branches more distally into the iliohypogastric nerve (T12–L1) and the ilio-inguinal nerve (L1–L2).
- The genitofemoral nerve arises from the union of the branches of L1 and L2.
- The lateral cutaneous nerve of the thigh develops from the anastomoses of L2–L3.
- The femoral and obturator nerves are formed from the integration of the anastomoses of L2–L4.

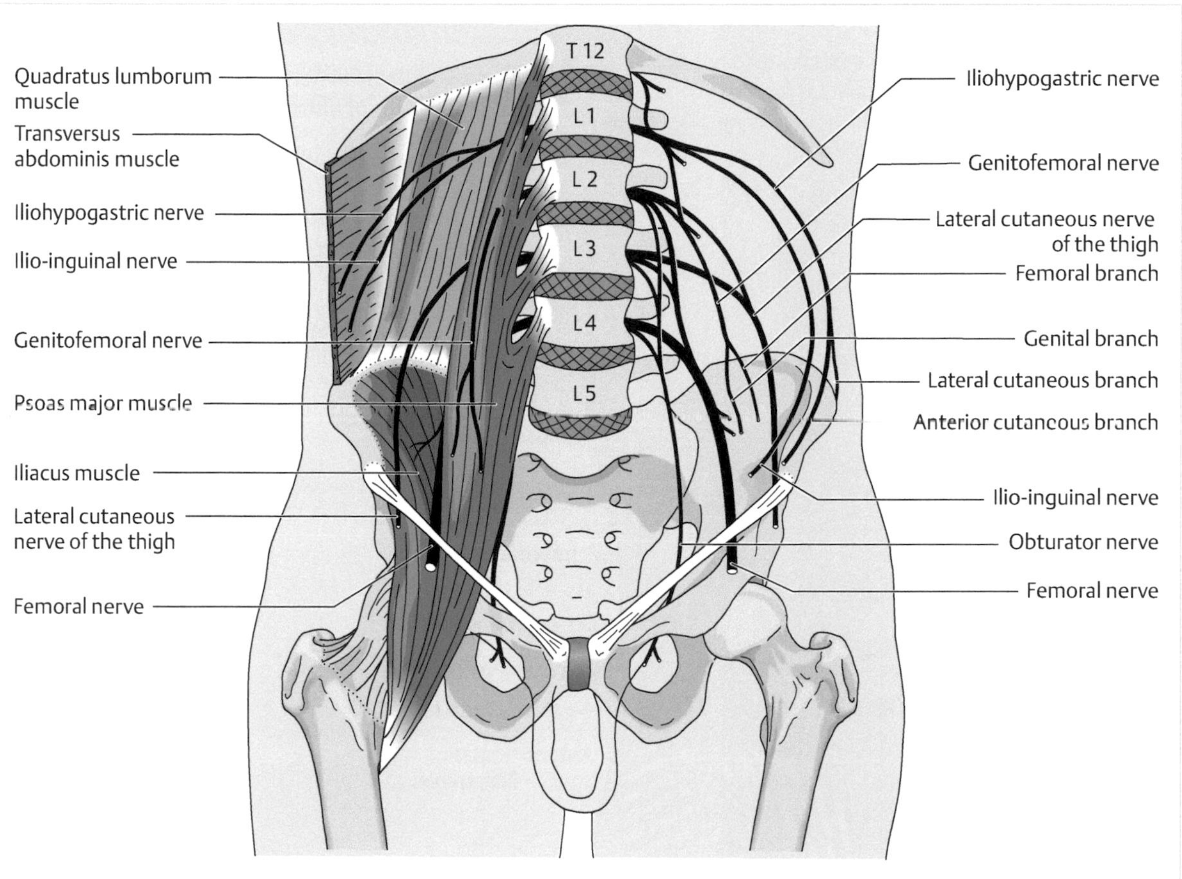


**Fig. 7.63** Lumbar plexus.

## Femoral Nerve—L1–L4 (Fig. 7.66)

- This passes posterior to the lateral border of the psoas major muscle in an inferior direction.
- There it is covered with the psoas fascia between the psoas and iliacus muscles.
- Proximal to the inguinal ligament, it gives off the muscular branches for the *iliopsoas muscle*; another muscular branch passes under the femoral vessels to the *pectineus muscle.*
- The femoral nerve then runs through the muscular space with the iliopsoas muscle.
- Inferior to the inguinal ligament, it divides into a lateral, a medial, and a deep group of terminal branches, each of which has motor and sensory fibers.
- Motor branches track laterally to the *sartorius muscle.* The *anterior cutaneous branches* pierce the sartorius muscle and travel to the great saphenous vein.
- Branches track to the *pectineus* and *adductor longus muscles*, and sensory branches track to the *skin of the medial thigh.* The deep group consists of many motor branches of various lengths to supply of the *quadriceps femoris muscle.* In addition, the saphenous nerve belongs to this group.

## Saphenous Nerve (Fig. 7.66)

- This is the longest branch of the femoral nerve.
- It travels through the adductor canal with the femoral artery and then follows the posterior edge of the sartorius muscle.
- Proximal to the medial condyle of the femur, it gives off the *infrapatellar branch* for the knee joint and for the *area of skin over the medial knee* to below the *tibial tuberosity.*
- On the *medial surface of the lower leg*, anterior and posterior branches go to the skin and track down to the *medial border of the foot.*

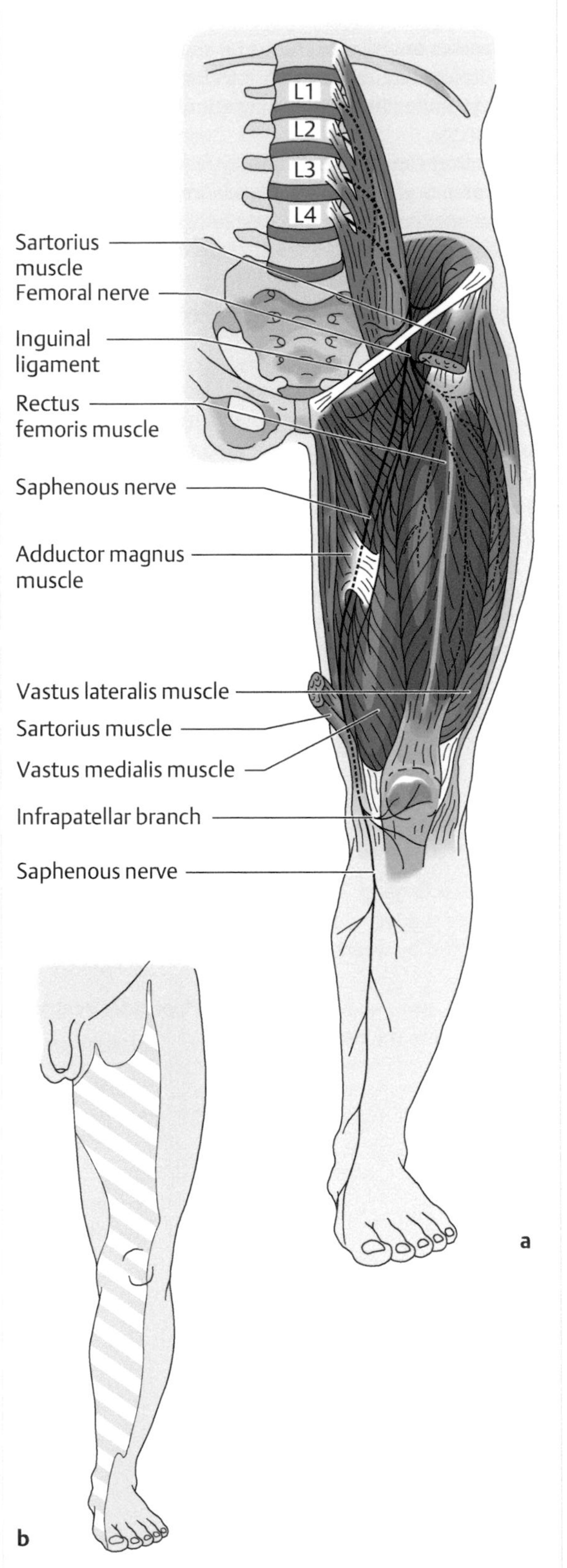


**Fig. 7.66** Femoral and saphenous nerves. **(a)** Course of the nerves. **(b)** Innervated areas of skin.

## Obturator Nerve—L2–L4 (Fig. 7.67)

- This tracks in an inferior direction along the medial border of the psoas major muscle.
- It travels over the sacroiliac joint into the true pelvis to the obturator canal. The nerve, the artery, and the vein run within the canal.
- Within the canal, it divides into the anterior and posterior branches:
  - The **posterior branch** runs between the adductor brevis and magnus muscles and gives off motor branches for the *obturator externus* and the *adductor magnus muscles.*
  - The **anterior branch** runs along the anterior side of the adductor brevis muscle and innervates the *pectineus, adductor longus, adductor brevis,* and *gracilis muscles.* It ends with the sensory cutaneous branch, which supplies the ***skin in the distal and medial areas of the thigh.***

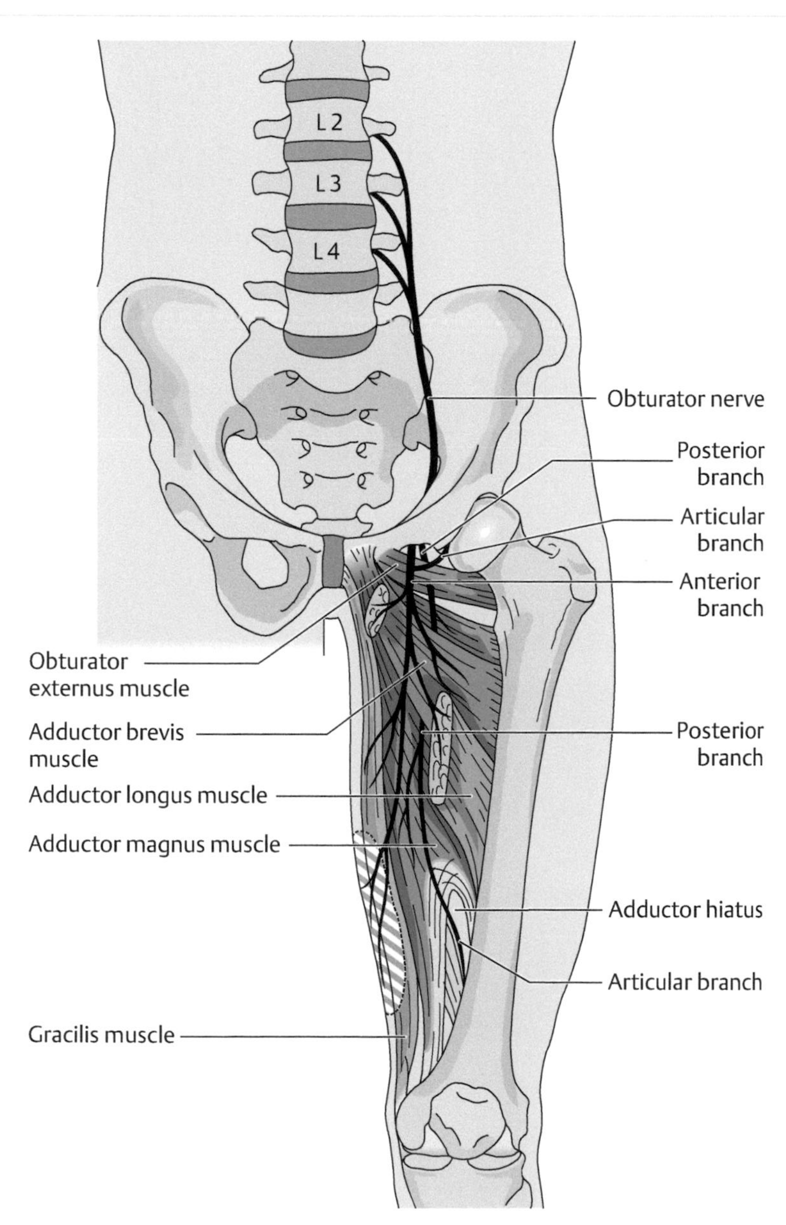


**Fig. 7.67** Course of the obturator nerve. Hatched areas = innervated skin areas.

# Chapter 8

## Pelvis and Hip Joint



8

# 8 Pelvis and Hip Joint

## 8.1 Palpation of Landmarks in the Pelvic and Hip Region

### 8.1.1 Palpation in the Posterior Pelvic Area

#### Iliac Crest (Fig. 8.1)

The iliac crest can be palpated as the broad, upper rim of the pelvis using the radial side of the index finger or the tips of the three long fingers. Posteriorly, it bends downward and ends there as the posterior superior iliac spine (PSIS).

The following muscle insertion sites can be palpated on the iliac crest, moving medially from the lateral rim (**Fig. 8.2**):

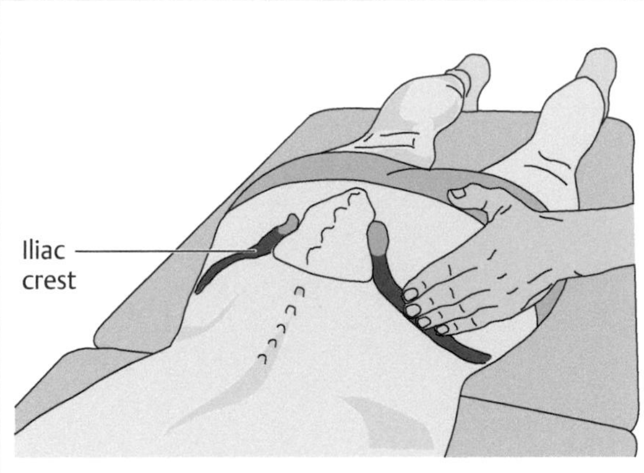


**Fig. 8.1** Palpation of the iliac crest.

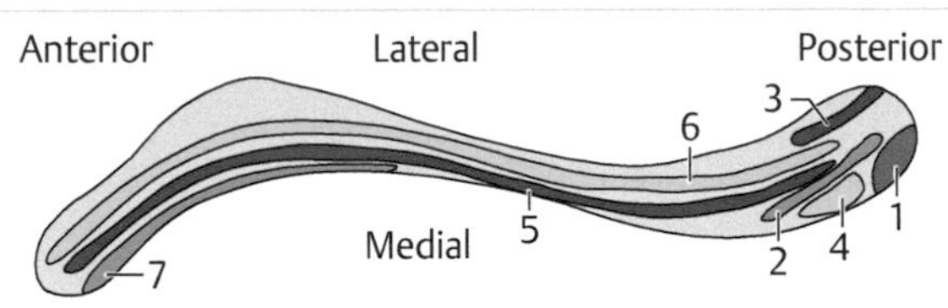


**Fig. 8.2** Palpation of the muscle insertions on the iliac crest.

##### External Oblique Abdominal Muscle

This can be palpated directly on the iliac crest.

##### Internal Oblique Abdominal Muscle

This is located at the posterior end of the iliac crest between the lateral edge of the latissimus dorsi muscle and the posterior edge of the external oblique abdominal muscle. The triangle formed in this way is called the inferior lumbar triangle.

#### Posterior Superior Iliac Spine (Fig. 8.3)

This is located on the posterior end of the iliac crest and is broad and roughened. Place a thumb on the inferior aspect of the tip of each of the spines to determine any difference in their levels.

If pelvic dimples are present, the spines are usually located somewhat inferior to the dimples. To find the PSIS quickly, place the fingertips on the iliac crest laterally and splay the thumbs out as far down as possible. The spines then lie in the immediate area surrounding the thumbs.

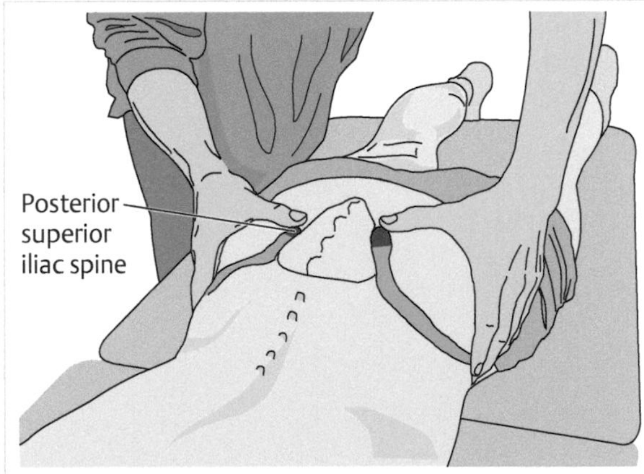


**Fig. 8.3** Palpation of the posterior superior iliac spine.

**Practical Tip**

Small, freely mobile areas of thickening within the subcutaneous fat around the spines and the iliac crest are fibrous, fatty nodules in the subcutaneous fat that can at times be painful.

## Sacral Sulcus (Fig. 8.4)

The sulcus lies just superior and medial to the PSIS. The short interosseous sacro-iliac ligaments pass over it; the sacro-iliac joint (SIJ) lies deep to this area and cannot be palpated.

Palpate across the fiber orientation to gauge the tautness of these ligaments. The sacral mobilization test can be used to check whether your fingers are in fact in the sulcus. Place your fingertips in the sulcus in such a way that the fingertips are touching the rim of the ilium. With your other hand on the ipsilateral anterior superior iliac spine (ASIS), push with a light, springy impulse posteriorly so that the ilium is shifted against the sacrum—this can be detected by the fingertips (**Fig. 8.5**).

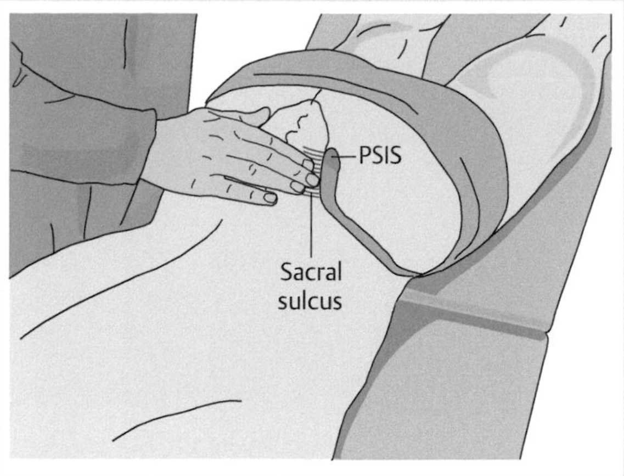


**Fig. 8.4** Palpation of the sacral sulcus.

### Practical Tip

A comparison of the sulcal depths and the differential state of tension of the ligaments in a direct right–left comparison can lead to conclusions on whether there is a malposition of the SIJ. Likewise, if the displacement of the ilium during the sacral mobilization test is either absent or, on the other hand, too great, this might suggest a functional disturbance that can be confirmed through further testing.

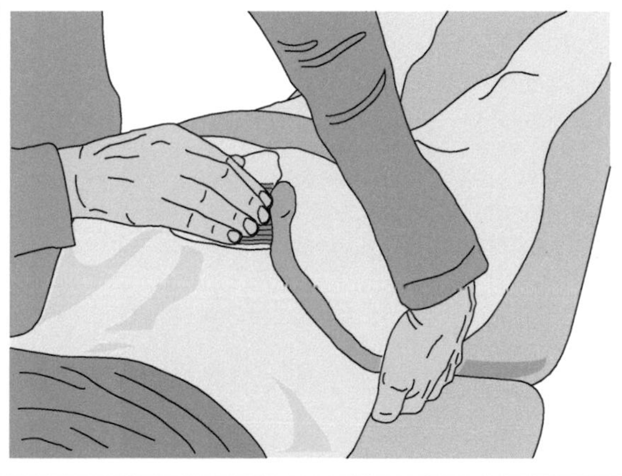

**Fig. 8.5** Sacral mobilization test.

## Inferior Lateral Angle of the Sacrum (Fig. 8.6)

At the level of the upper end of the intergluteal cleft, spread the middle and index fingers out slightly and place them approximately 1.5 cm inferior and lateral to the intergluteal cleft, one on each side. The lateral angle of the sacrum can be found in the area immediately below the fingers. Using this, differing levels of the angle and the tilt of the sacrum can be evaluated.

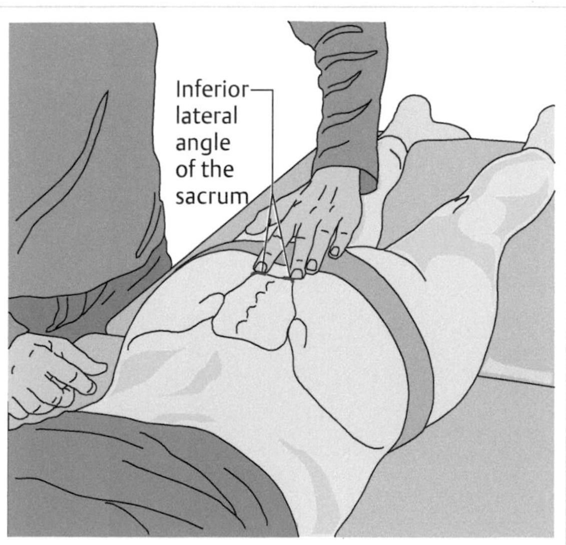


**Fig. 8.6** Palpation of the inferior lateral angle of the sacrum.

## Coccyx (Fig. 8.7)

From the superior end, place the index finger along the intergluteal cleft to palpate the curve of the coccyx. It may be necessary to palpate it per rectum.

**Practical Tip**

Anterior angulation of the coccyx caused by a fall on the buttocks can be palpated by examination of the intergluteal cleft area. Examination per rectum confirms the diagnosis.

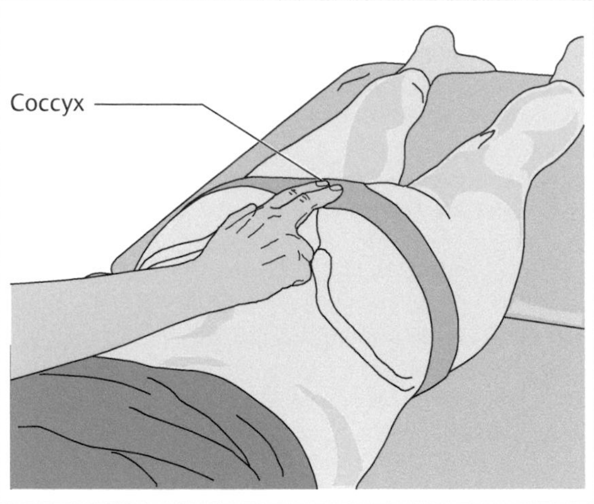


**Fig. 8.7** Palpation of the coccyx.

## Ischial Tuberosity

Palpate deeply in the medial third of the gluteal fold to identify the tuberosity as a broad bulge.

### Sacrotuberous Ligament (Fig. 8.8)

This ligament runs from the tuberosity in a superior and medial direction. It is very firm and broad. By palpating both right and left simultaneously, one can evaluate differences in tension and provoke pain to help diagnose a difficult case. A clear increase in tension in the ligament can be palpated during nutation of the sacrum.

▷ See Chapter 8.4.7, Involving the Sacrum Movements

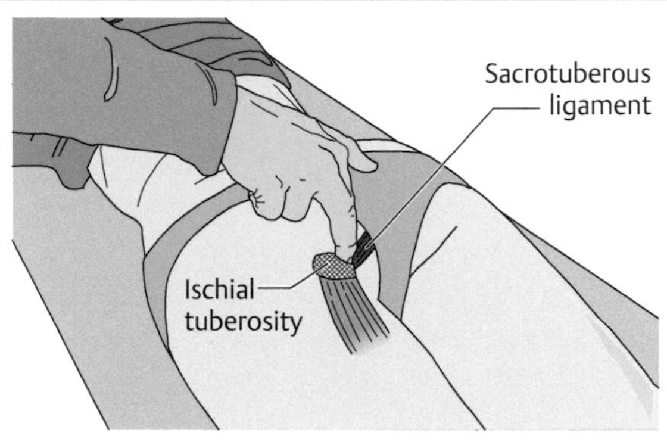


**Fig. 8.8** Palpation of the sacrotuberous ligament.

## Hamstring Muscles (Fig. 8.9)

The common origin of the hamstring muscles can be palpated on the inferior aspect of the tuberosity. The *long head of the biceps femoris muscle* has its origin superficially, covers the other muscles, and tracks laterally. Then it follows the *semitendinosus muscle*, and, deep to this, the *semimembranosus muscle*, both of which track medially. These can be very well palpated when flexing the knee against resistance.

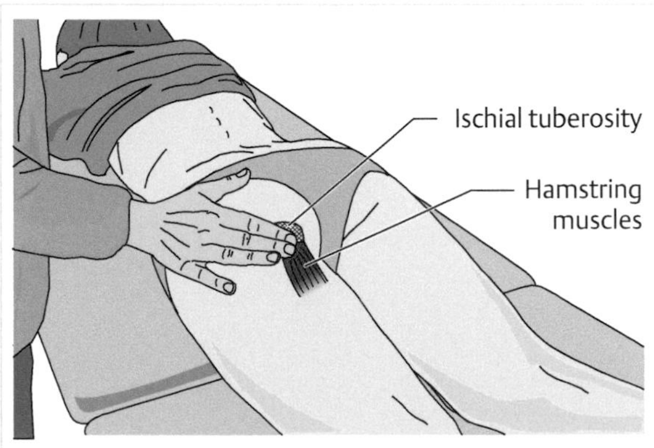


**Fig. 8.9** Palpation of the hamstring muscles.

## Gluteus Maximus Muscle (Fig. 8.10)

To locate the upper margin of the muscle, use a point that lies about two fingerbreadths above the PSIS and identify a line connecting this to the greater trochanter. Isometrically tensing the muscle as if extending the hip confirms the direction of the muscle fibers to be obliquely inferolateral as they track to the gluteal tuberosity on the femur.

The inferior margin of the gluteus maximus crosses the gluteal fold in an obliquely inferolateral direction. The gluteal fold is not the lower margin of the gluteus maximus, but corresponds instead to a reinforced fibrous band that spans from the iliotibial tract to the ischial tuberosity and is fixed to the skin.

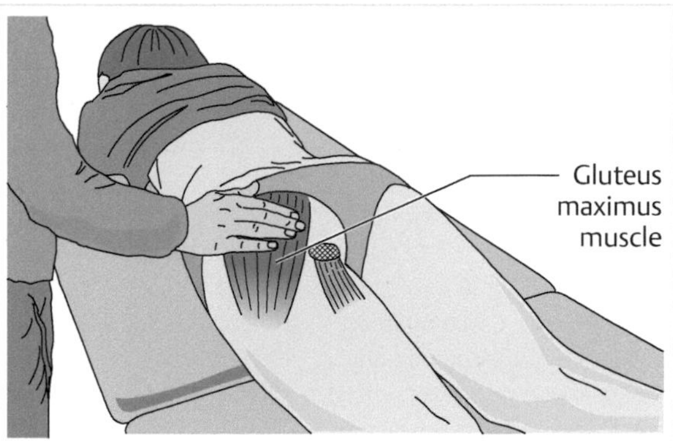


**Fig. 8.10** Palpation of the gluteus maximus muscle.

## Piriformis Muscle (Fig. 8.11a)

The piriformis can be located with the help of two lines, one from the ASIS to the inferior lateral angle of the sacrum, and the other from the PSIS to the upper edge of the greater trochanter. A firm structure can be palpated near the intersection of these lines. The muscle-tendon junction lies here; about one-third of the muscle consists of tendon, which can be traced to its insertion site on the posteromedial aspect of the tip of the trochanter.

## Suprapiriform Foramen (Fig. 8.11b)

Construct a line from the PSIS to the tip of the greater trochanter. Superior to this line, between the median and the medial third, lies the suprapiriform foramen. The superior gluteal nerve and vessels travel through this notch.

## Infrapiriform Foramen (Fig. 8.11b)

The inferior infrapiriform foramen is found lateral to the midpoint of a line between the PSIS and the ischial tuberosity. The inferior gluteal vessels, the pudendal and inferior gluteal nerves, as well as the sciatic nerve travel through this portion of the foramen.

## Sciatic Nerve (Fig. 8.12)

The sciatic nerve crosses the tendon of the internal obturator muscle and both gemellus muscles and, at the transition to the thigh, the quadratus femoris muscle.

At this point, it lies approximately in the middle of a line connecting the ischial tuberosity with the greater trochanter and can be palpated here as a cord that is the same width as a finger. It is, of course, covered here by the gluteus maximus muscle.

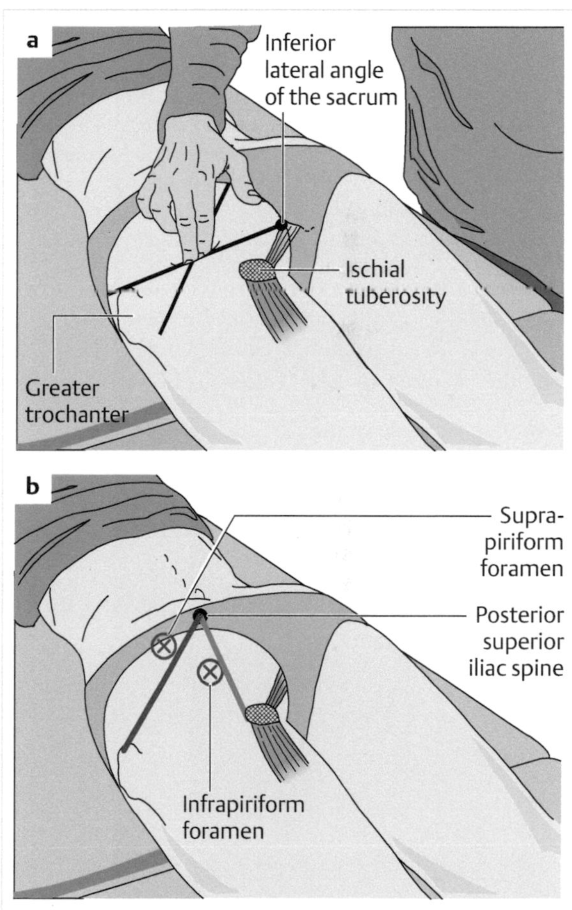


**Fig. 8.11** Palpation. **(a)** Piriformis muscle. **(b)** Suprapiriform and infrapiriform foramen.

## 8.1.2 Palpation in the Lateral Pelvic Area

### Greater Trochanter

Place your thumbs on the ASIS and spread your fingers out in a posteroinferior direction. Feel in the immediate area of the greater trochanter. For purposes of the examination, ask the patient to rotate the leg several times, allowing the trochanter to glide back and forth under your palpating fingers.

The following insertion sites can be palpated on the trochanter.

#### Gluteus Medius Muscle (Fig. 8.13)

Especially when aided by isometric tension toward hip abduction, the posterior margin can be well palpated and traced to its insertion on the greater trochanter. The insertion site is located laterally on the tip of the trochanter and is about 2 to 3 fingerbreadths wide.

The anterior belly of the muscle borders on the tensor fasciae latae muscle. The gluteus medius spreads out and flattens superiorly, so that its posterior border corresponds with the line connecting the PSIS to the tip of the trochanter:

#### Gluteus Minimus Muscle (Fig. 8.13)

Its origin is about one handbreadth posterior to the iliac crest and its insertion is under the gluteus medius on the tip of the trochanter.

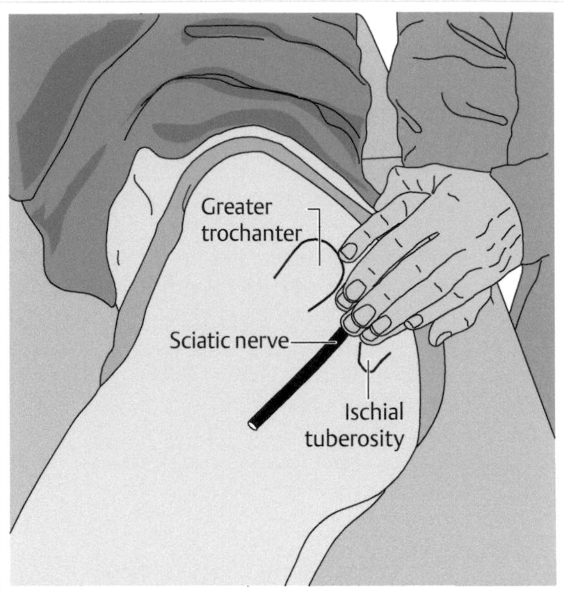


**Fig. 8.12** Palpation of the sciatic nerve.

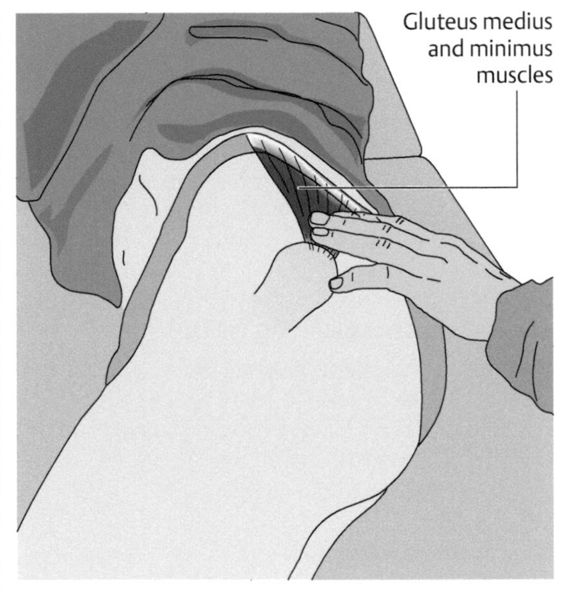


**Fig. 8.13** Palpation of the gluteus medius and minimus muscles.

### Piriformis Muscle (Fig. 8.14)

Its insertion can be palpated on the posterior aspect of the tip of the trochanter. Its tendon is very firm, allowing easy reproduction of the approximately horizontal orientation of its fibers.

### Pelvitrochanteric Muscles (Fig. 8.15)

Directly posterior to the piriformis muscle, the pelvitrochanteric muscles insert onto the intertrochanteric crest.

Moving out from the tip of the greater trochanter, place your fingertips on the posterior edge of the trochanter. Palpate transversely to the fiber orientation, in a superior to inferior direction.

The following muscles cannot be identified individually, because they are bound closely together near the insertions and have the same functions:

- Obturator internus muscle.
- Obturator externus muscle.
- Gemellus muscles.
- Quadratus femoris muscle.

## 8.1.3 Palpation in the Anterior Pelvic Area

### Anterior Superior Iliac Spine (Fig. 8.16a)

Place the fingertips of both hands on the iliac crests with the thumbs spread out widely anteriorly on the crest. The upper anterior spines are found at approximately this level as bulging ends of the crests.

To evaluate the leg lengths, start in the standing position. Then place your thumbs on the spines from below to check for a difference in level, making sure that the malleoli and knee joints are at the same level.

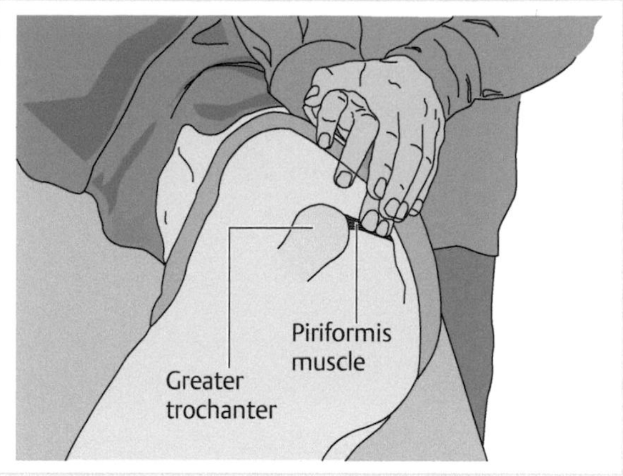


Fig. 8.14 Palpation of the insertion site of the piriformis muscle.

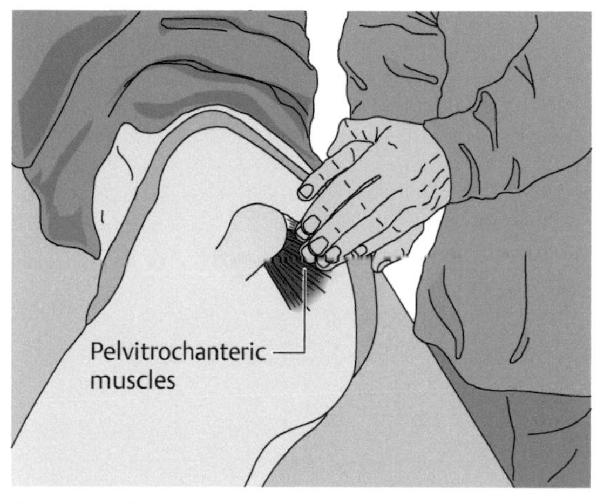


Fig. 8.15 Palpation of the pelvitrochanteric muscles.

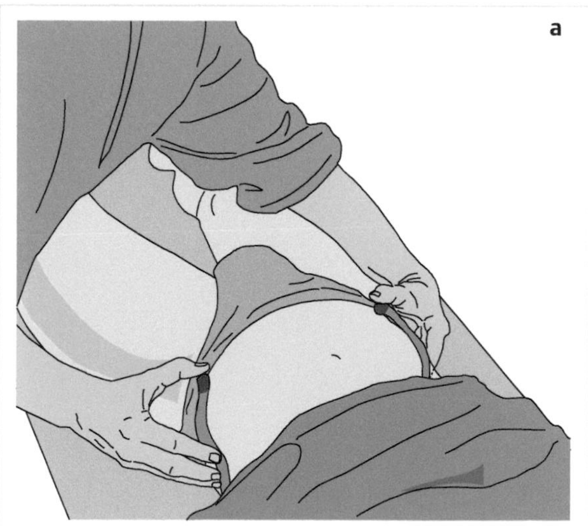


Fig. 8.16 Palpation. (a) Anterior superior iliac spine.

Continued ►

**Practical Tip**

**Differentiation between Leg Lengths and Functional Disturbances in the Sacro-Iliac Joint (Fig. 8.16b, c)**

Evaluation of the PSIS and the ASIS in terms of their height difference is an important examination for differentiating differences in leg length and functional disturbance in the SIJ. Carry out the evaluation in the standing position.

For instance, if both the PSIS and the ASIS on the left side are elevated to the same degree, the difference is caused by a longer leg.

On the other hand, if the right PSIS is lower than the left, and the right ASIS is higher than the left, there is a dysfunction of the SIJ.

Determinations of leg lengths in which only the ASIS or the iliac crest is considered are therefore inexact.

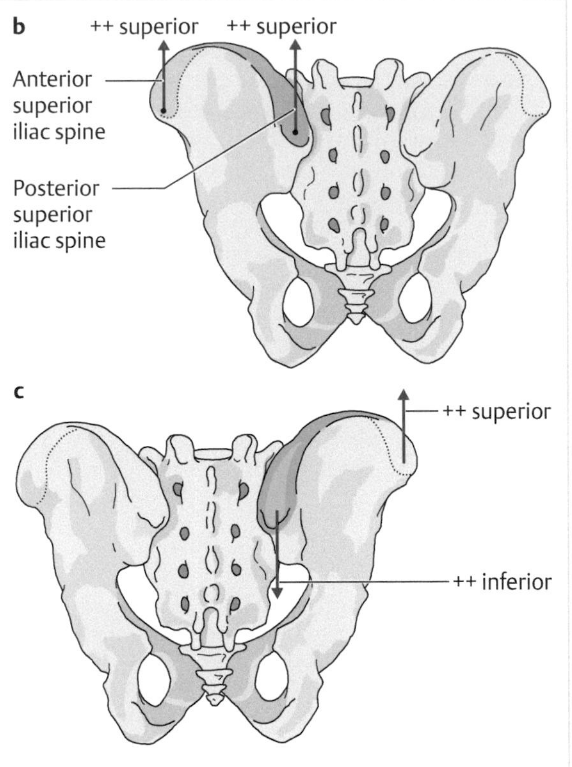


Fig. 8.16 Continued. (b) Difference in leg lengths. (c) Pelvic torsion.

The *ASIS* is the origin for:

## Sartorius Muscle (Fig. 8.17)

This exits right from the tip of the spine in an inferomedial direction and can be well palpated even in the relaxed condition. Tense the muscle in hip flexion if necessary.

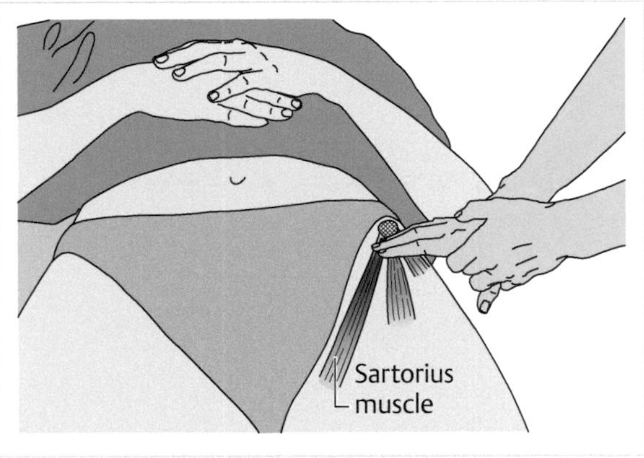


Fig. 8.17 Palpation of the sartorius muscle.

## Tensor Fasciae Latae Muscle (Fig. 8.18)

This lies lateral to the spine and is significantly thicker than the sartorius muscle, but is also easy to find in the relaxed condition. Tensing the muscle in the direction of abduction further improves the presentation.

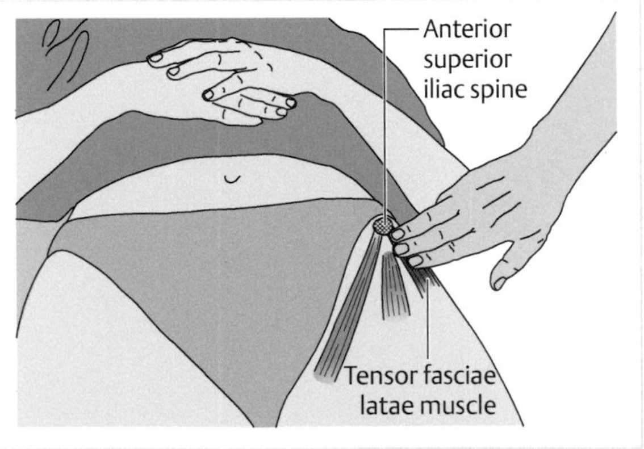


Fig. 8.18 Palpation of the tensor fasciae latae muscle.

## Lateral Triangle of the Thigh

The sartorius and tensor fasciae latae muscles form an upside-down "V" with the tensor muscle as the lateral limb and the sartorius as the medial limb. This area is called the lateral triangle of the thigh. The deep artery and vein of the thigh run through this area at a deep level. The rectus femoris muscle can be palpated here.

### Inguinal Ligament (Fig. 8.19)

The inguinal ligament runs from the medial side of the tip of the ASIS to the pubic tubercle.

Palpate across the orientation of the fibers. The ligament cannot be palpated as a homogeneous cord; rather, there are numerous fibrous components to palpate that are bound together by small connective tissue bridges. These arise from the consolidation of the abdominal muscle aponeuroses that intertwine with the ligament from above and the fascia of the thigh from below.

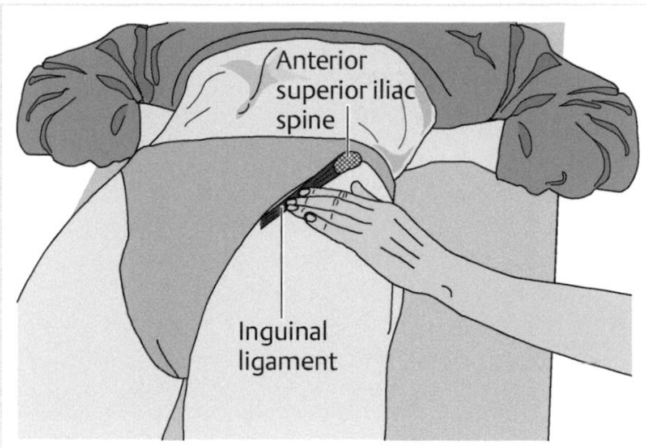


**Fig. 8.19** Palpation of the inguinal ligament.

**Pathology**

Abdominal obesity can exert pressure on the inguinal ligament as the panniculus hangs over it. Nerves that run in the immediate area can be compromised.

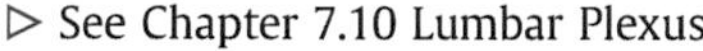
▷ See Chapter 7.10 Lumbar Plexus

**Practical Tip**

Take care when palpating toward the pubic tubercle because of the proximity to the spermatic cord.

## Pubic Tubercle (Fig. 8.20)

Approach the upper margin of the pubic symphysis from the superior side. Palpate with the following in mind:

- Difference in height: Lay the fingers on both sides of the symphysis from above. Both pubic tubercles are at the same height.
- Symmetrical mobility: From the superior side, put the index and middle fingers on the right and left sides of the pubis. Ask the patient to push the outstretched legs downward from the hip, alternating the right and left leg. In this way, the symmetrical mobility can be evaluated. A unilateral blockage can eliminate the symmetry.
- Possible pain at the insertion of the rectus abdominis muscle: Palpate across the orientation of the muscle fibers and continue further toward the inguinal ligament.

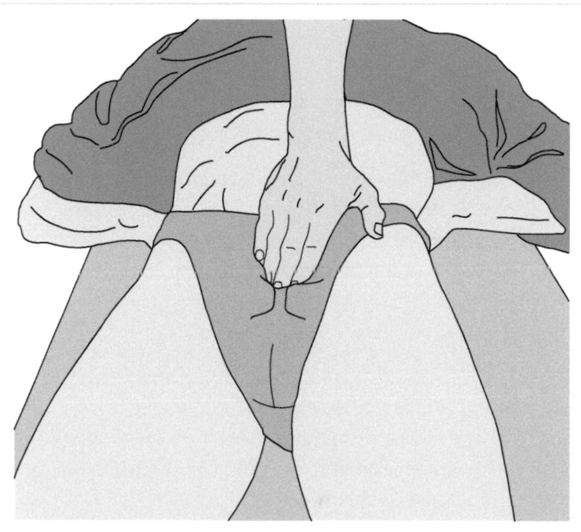

**Fig. 8.20** Palpation of the pubic tubercle.

The origins of the following muscles can be palpated as they leave the pubis:

### Adductor Longus Muscle (Fig. 8.21)

The patient draws the foot up and leans the side of the knee against the therapist. When the leg is tensed in adduction, the muscle can be seen and palpated as a round, protruding cord in the medial thigh area. It can be traced to the superior pubic ramus.

### Gracilis Muscle (Fig. 8.22)

This arises directly posterior and inferior to the adductor longus muscle and tracks as the only adductor over the knee joint. Therefore it can be differentiated from the other adductors by flexing the knee against resistance.

### Adductor Brevis Muscle (Fig. 8.22)

This muscle arises posterior and inferior to the gracilis muscle.

### Adductor Magnus Muscle (Fig. 8.22)

This is barely perceptible on palpation because it is broad and flat as it emerges from the inferior pubic ramus and the ischial tuberosity. It can sometimes be palpated posteromedially next to the hamstring muscles.

### Medial Femoral Triangle (Fig. 8.23)

The sartorius and adductor longus muscles form the medial femoral triangle. The tip of the triangle points inferiorly, and the femoral artery bisects the triangle. Superficially, the great saphenous vein and lymph nodes pass through it. Deep to this lies the iliopectineal bursa.

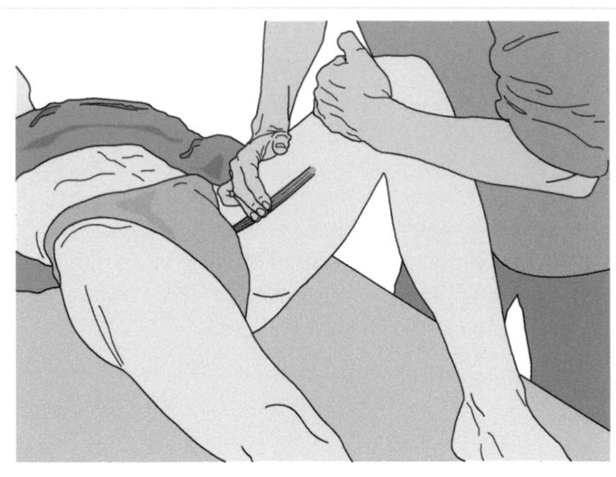

**Fig. 8.21** Palpation of the adductor longus muscle.

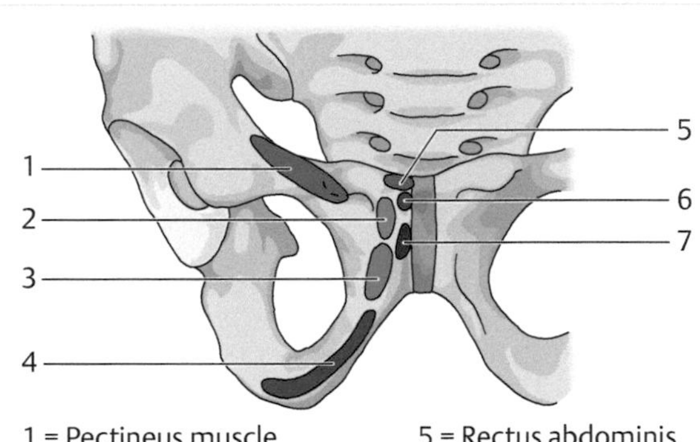


**Fig. 8.22** Palpation of the muscle origins on the pubis.

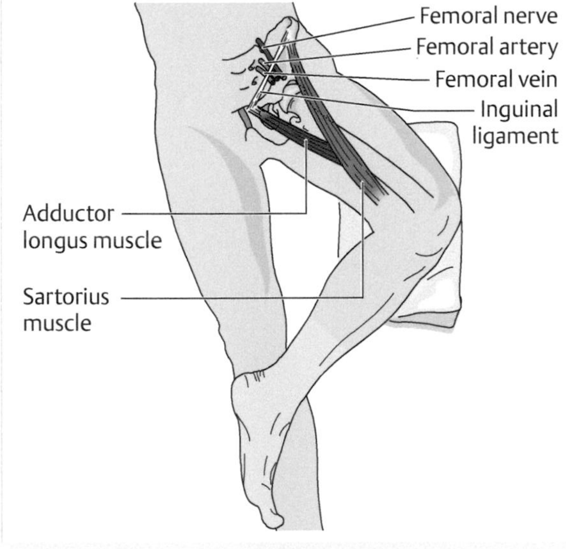


**Fig. 8.23** Palpation of the medial femoral triangle.

## Lesser Trochanter (Fig. 8.24)

To enable palpation, the knee must be significantly flexed and externally rotated, and fully tensed. The insertion of the iliopsoas muscle on the lesser trochanter can be identified using four fingers with flat palpation deeply in the direction of the femur a handbreadth inferior to the medial groin. Feel the trochanter as an elevation that becomes evident by tensing the muscle.

In larger individuals, this palpation can be quite painful and therefore of questionable value. It is preferable to palpate the muscles in the groin area.

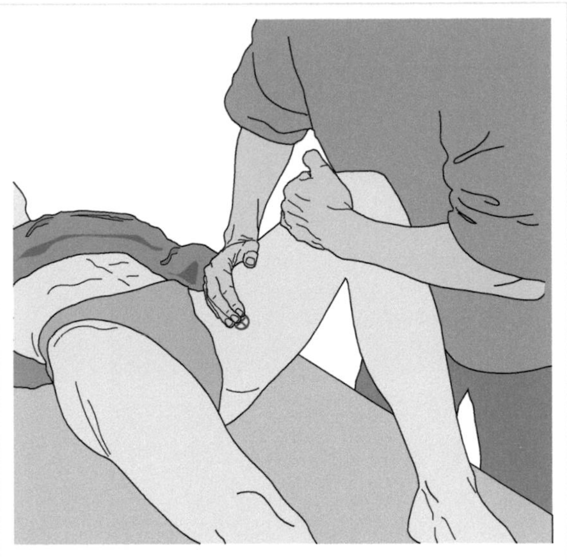

Fig. 8.24 Palpation of the lesser trochanter.

## Rectus Femoris Muscle (Fig. 8.25)

The hip should be flexed to relax the fascia of the thigh by using a thick roll to support the knee. The tensor fasciae latae and sartorius muscles can help with orientation. The rectus femoris muscle can be palpated in the depths between these two muscles and about 2 to 3 fingerbreadths inferior to the ASIS. For confirmation, the rectus femoris should be tensed by extending the knee, because hip flexion will tense all the muscles in the area, making palpation difficult.

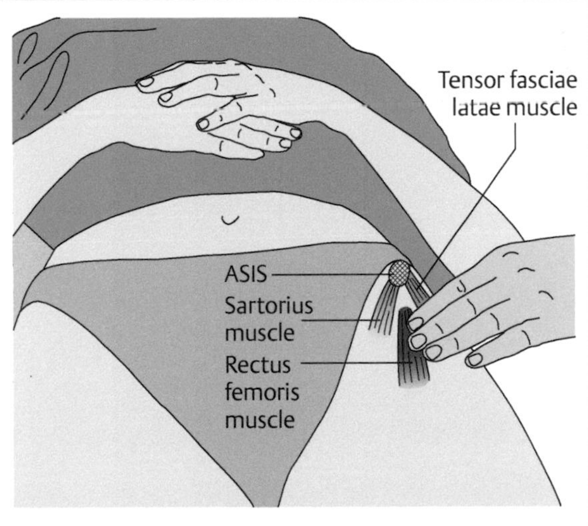


Fig. 8.25 Palpation of the rectus femoris muscle.

### Practical Tip

The lateral cutaneous nerve of the thigh runs through the **V**-shaped space formed by the sartorius and tensor fasciae latae muscles. It is a sensory branch, and if palpation is too strong, this can result in a burning pain in the lateral thigh down to the knee.

## Femoral Artery (Fig. 8.26)

The femoral artery crosses under the inguinal ligament approximately at its midpoint. Placing the leg in mild external rotation makes palpation easier. Palpate deeply with the middle and ring fingers.

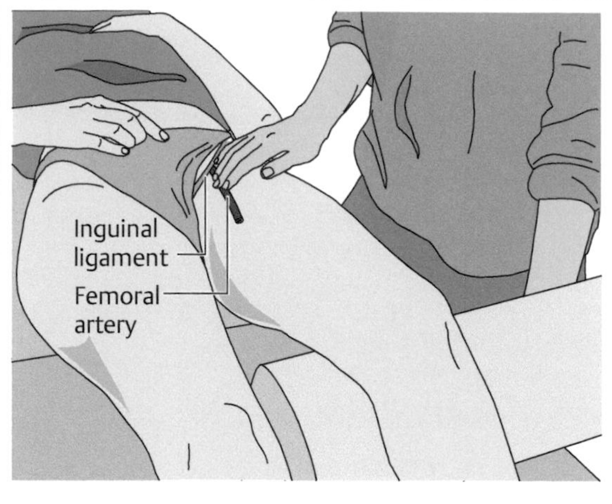


**Fig. 8.26** Palpation of the femoral artery.

## Pectineus Muscle (Fig. 8.27)

This lies medial to the femoral artery. Its very broad origin spreads from the pectineal line to the pubic tubercle. It can be palpated at a deep level immediately posterior to the inguinal ligament, aided by adduction against resistance.

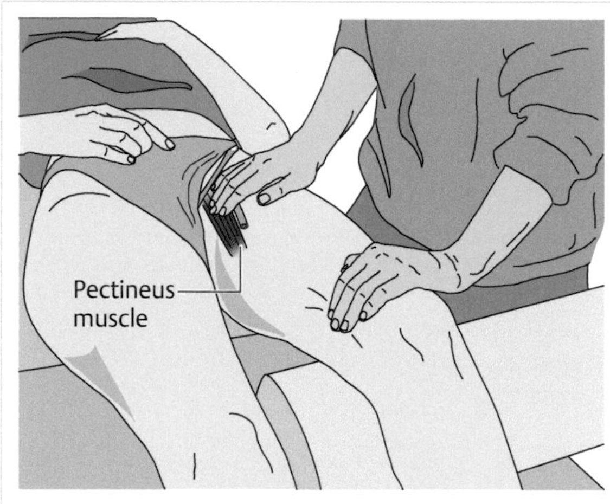


**Fig. 8.27** Palpation of the pectineus muscle.

## Iliopsoas Muscle (Fig. 8.28)

The iliopsoas muscle runs in the muscular space under the inguinal ligament lateral to the femoral artery. Aided by hip flexion against resistance, it can be palpated clearly on deep palpation.

▷ See Chapter 7.1, Palpation of Landmarks in the Lumbar Spine and Abdominal Areas

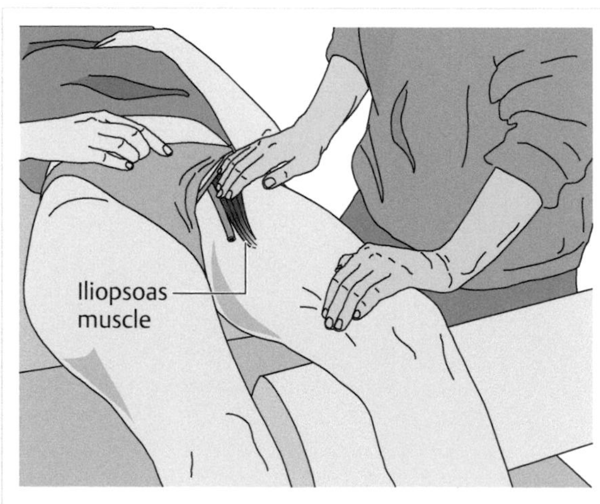


**Fig. 8.28** Palpation of the iliopsoas muscle.

## Femoral Vein (Fig. 8.29)

This is located medial to the femoral artery.

## Hip Joint (Fig. 8.29)

The femoral head is located under the femoral artery. Because of this, palpation of the pulse here is a good aid to orientation. Extension of the leg can help with locating the femoral head more easily because with this movement, the head of the femur turns anteriorly against the palpating finger in the groin.

## Lymph Nodes (Fig. 8.29)

The superficial lymph nodes are located medially in the groin in the subcutaneous fat tissue. Because of their size, they can be felt as small nontender, superficial thickenings that can be moved back and forth.

**Pathology**

### Pain in the Groin

Pain in the groin region has many potential causes:

Enlarged lymph nodes can point to inflammation in the lower extremities or urogenital tract.

Referred pain: Organs in the urogenital tract often cause pain in the groin. Pain of gynecologic origin is usually related to the menstrual cycle, whereas other organs are more likely to cause a colicky discomfort.

Both inguinal and femoral hernias can be linked to pain in the groin. They are reducible swellings that develop either above or below the inguinal ligament and enlarge on coughing.

Compression of single nerve branches may be caused by to a hematoma. It is possible for an obese belly to hang over the inguinal ligament and compromise nerves. This can also occur after various types of surgery in the kidney, groin, or hip areas.

Irritation of the nerves of the lumbar plexus should also be considered as a cause. The dermatome is supplied by T12–L1.

Pains caused by blood vessels are stress-dependent (intermittent claudication).

Possible causes of pain that radiate toward the pubic tubercle are extended standing on one leg, frequent microtrauma, imbalance of the abdominal, pelvic, or leg muscles, and altered body statics.

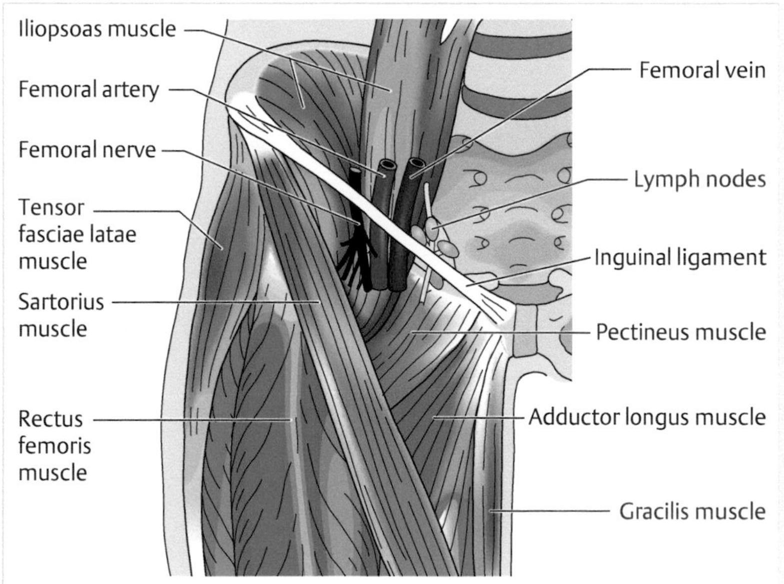


**Fig. 8.29** Palpation of structures in the groin area.

# 8.2 X-Ray and CT Scan

## 8.2.1 Pelvis–Leg Overview (Anteroposterior View in the Standing Position) (Fig. 8.30)

The following reference lines can be used to help determine difference in leg length and pelvic tilt. They should run horizontal or parallel to each other:

- *Femoral head reference line:* through the upper border of the two femoral heads.
- *Intercristal line:* through the highest point of the two iliac crests and through the body of the fourth lumbar vertebra.
- *Sacral level:* the horizontal line through the upper border of the sacrum.
- *Median:* the vertical line through the middle of the sacrum and the pubic symphysis.

- *Pubic symphysis:*
  - No step-off or marginal spurs.
  - Symphysis width: normal up to 6 mm.
  - Joint space: smooth borders.
- *Sacrum:* four foraminal borders: smooth and bilaterally symmetrical.
- *Ilium:* the symmetrical alae of the ilium.
- *Femur:* the ball-shaped head of the femur.
- *Hip joint:* a joint space of 4 to 5 mm with smooth joint surfaces.
- *Obturator foramen:* a symmetrical, slightly oval shape.

### Sacro-Iliac Joint

The complicated shape of this joint makes evaluation difficult. An anteroposterior view can only show a small part of the total picture. The posterior parts of the joints are better appreciated in a lateral view, which shows joint spaces of approximately 3 mm with smooth joint contours. The middle and inferior parts are better viewed with an oblique projection of approximately 30°. Computed tomography (CT) and magnetic resonance imaging (MRI) deliver a clearer picture of the SIJ.

Starting position: standing with approximately 20° internal rotation to compensate for the femoral antetorsion.

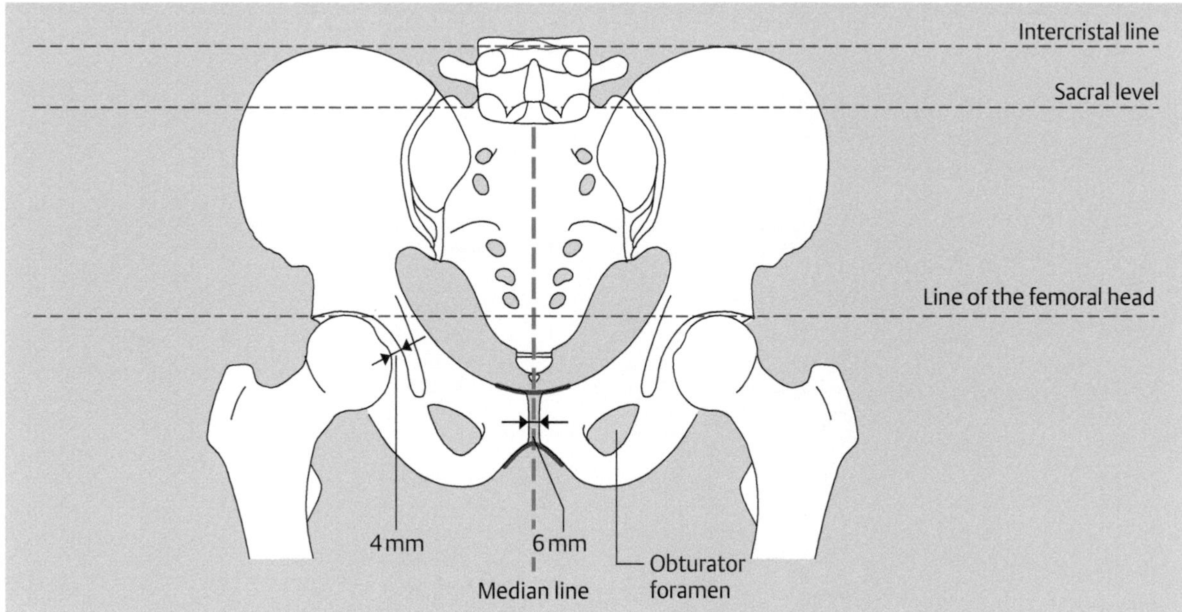


**Fig. 8.30** Pelvis–leg overview in the anteroposterior view.

## Femoral Neck Axis

The femoral neck axis runs through the midpoint of the femoral head and stays at approximately the same distance from the overlying contour of the femoral neck.

## Femoral Shaft Axis

The axis of the shaft of the femur runs in the medullary cavity of the body of the femur.

## Femoral Neck Angle (CCD Angle; Fig. 8.31)

The caput–collum–diaphyseal (CCD) angle is the angle formed by the femoral neck axis and the femoral shaft axis. In infants, it is 150°. The normal value for adults is 125–130°. It decreases with increasing age (50–60 years).

▷ See Chapter 8.7.6, Angles in the Femoral Region

## Acetabular Inlet Plane (Fig. 8.31)

From the bony superior margin of the acetabular roof, draw a line to the inferior margin of the acetabulum. This line represents the acetabular inlet plane and it forms the transverse angle with a line drawn horizontally. This angle is 60° in newborns, approximately 45 to 50° in 10-year-olds, and about 40° in adults.

This measured angle is not always exact, because alterations in the pelvic position, such as pelvic rotation, can have an influence on its magnitude. Further projections such as the faux profile, the Lauenstein projection, and the obturator projection can give a better representation of various parts of the joint if there is a suspicion of dislocation or dysplastic changes.

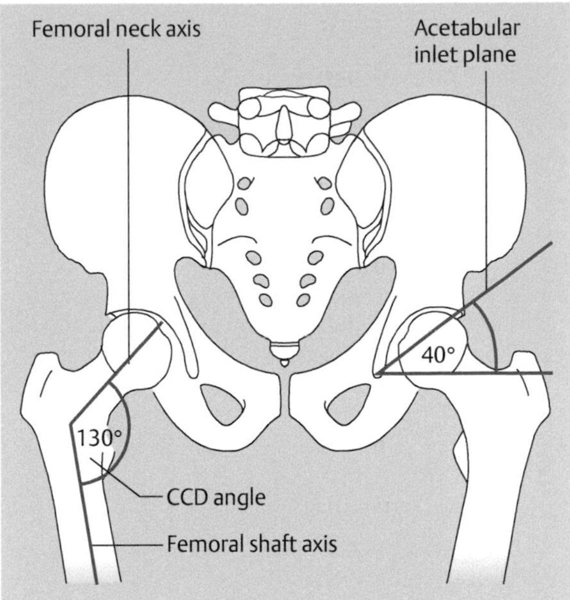


**Fig. 8.31** Acetabular inlet plane and caput–collum–diaphyseal (CCD) angle.

## Pathology

### Degenerative Osteoarthritis of the Hip Joint (Fig. 8.32)

Narrowing of the joint space due shrinkage of the cartilage.

Osteophytes on the acetabular margin.

Loss of congruence of the head of the femur, possibly leading to collapse of the femoral head.

Subchondral zones of sclerosis with cystic lucency and subchondral cysts.

### Slipped Capital Femoral Epiphysis (Fig. 8.33a)

Widening of the epiphysial plate.

Step-off of the head of the femur in relation to the femoral neck.

### Legg–Calvé–Perthes' Disease (Fig. 8.33b)

Apparent widening of the joint space through lateralization of the femoral head.

A foreshortened femoral neck.

Late stage: a mushroom-shaped femoral head.

### Changes in the Femoral Neck Angle (CCD Angle) (Fig. 8.34)

Coxa valga: CCD angle greater than 135°:

- The trabecular orientation changes: there is an increase in the longitudinally oriented compression trabeculae and a decrease in the horizontally oriented traction trabeculae.

Coxa vera: CCD angle less than 120°:

- The spongiosa features highly developed traction trabeculae and compression trabeculae. The compression trabeculae run very near the medial femoral neck.

### Fractures

Medial femoral neck fracture: the fracture gap is intracapsular.

Lateral femoral neck fracture: the fracture line is extracapsular and close to the greater trochanter.

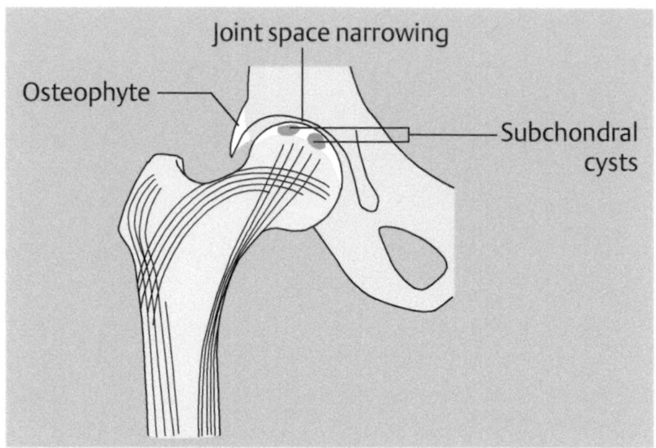


**Fig. 8.32** Degenerative osteoarthritis of the hip joints.

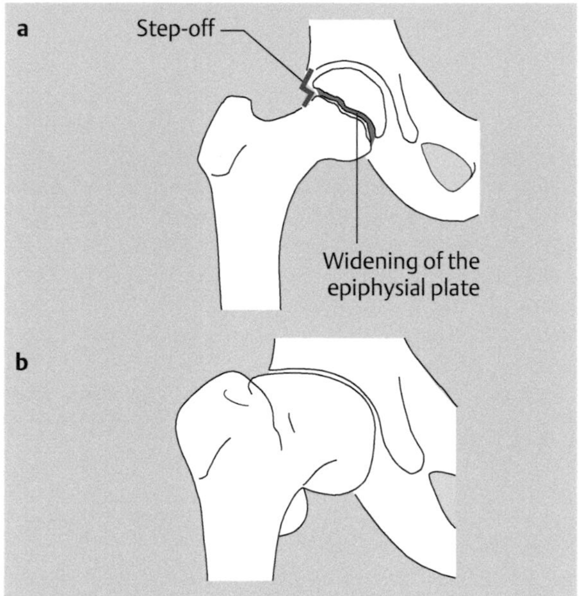


**Fig. 8.33 (a)** Slipped capital femoral epiphysis. **(b)** Late-stage Legg–Calvé–Perthes' disease.

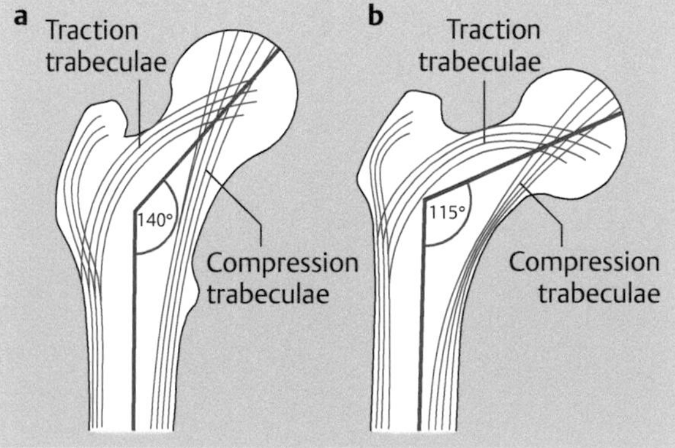


**Fig. 8.34 (a)** Coxa valga. **(b)** Coxa vara.

## 8.2.2 Pelvis–Leg Overview (Lateral View in the Standing Position)

Normal values (**Fig. 8.35**):

- L5 is trapezoid-shaped and is lower posteriorly.
- The sacral base angle is the angle between the line that lies on the sacral base and the horizontal. Normal: 45°.
- The main loading effect occurs in the posterior part of the sacral base.
- The transverse axis of the hip joint is located anterior to the sacral promontory.
- The right and left ASISs and the upper margin of the pubic symphysis lie in the same frontal plane.
- Sacral-coccygeal angle: approximately 10 to 30°.
- The angle of pelvic inclination is the angle that the plane of the pelvic inlet makes with the horizontal. Normal: 50 to 60°.

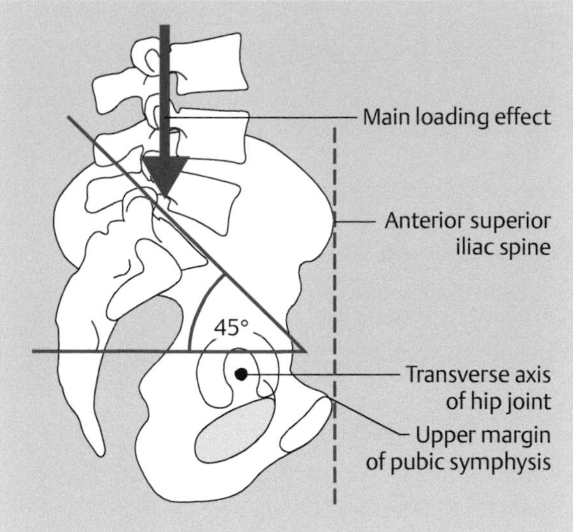


**Fig. 8.35** Pelvis in the lateral view.

**Pathology**

### Steep Pelvis (Fig. 8.36a)

This type of pelvis favors wear and tear on the fifth lumbar intervertebral disk.

The promontory is high between the iliac crests.

The sacral base angle is less than 45° because the sacrum is steeply oriented.

There is a decreased lumbar lordosis.

The main loading effect occurs in the middle of the L5–S1 disk.

The transverse axis of the hip joint is clearly anterior to the promontory.

Both ASISs are further posterior in relation to the superior margin of the pubic symphysis.

### Horizontal Pelvis (Fig. 8.36b)

The hip joints are severely affected because of the unfavorable loading effect, leading to a propensity for degenerative osteoarthritis of the hip joints.

The promontory is deep in the pelvis.

The fifth lumbar vertebra and disk are significantly wedge-shaped.

Increased lumbar lordosis is seen.

The sacral base angle is greater than 45° because the sacrum is almost horizontal.

The main loading effect occurs over the L5–S1 zygapophysial joints, the SIJ, and the hip joints.

The ASIS is clearly anterior in relation to the superior margin of the pubic symphysis.

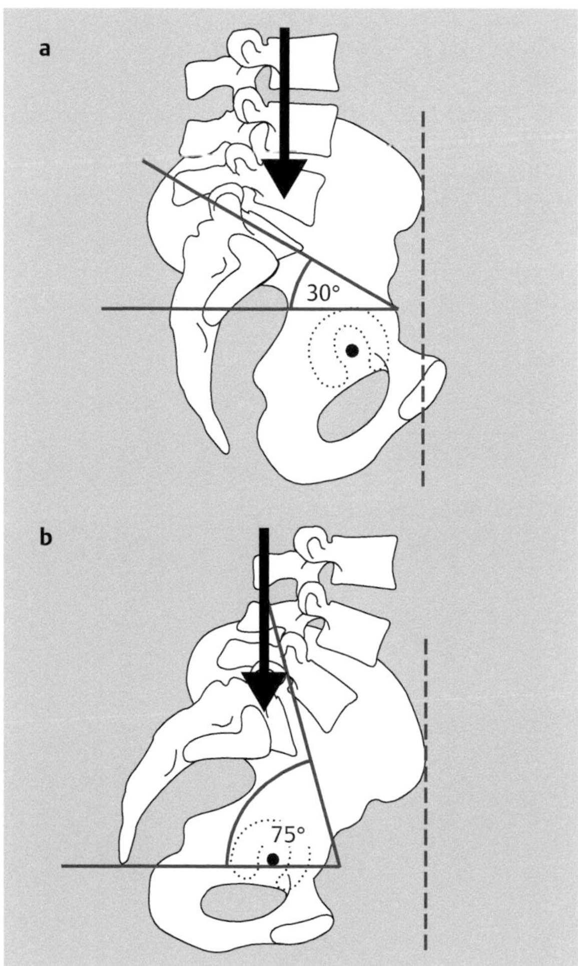


**Fig. 8.36 (a)** Steep pelvis. **(b)** Horizontal pelvis.

## 8.2.3 Lines and Angles to Determine Hip Dysplasia and Dislocation

Ultrasound has become the accepted method for detecting variations in the pelvic region in an infant. X-rays can be used after the third month of life because at this point ossification is sufficient to help with diagnosis.

### Center–Edge Angle (Fig. 8.37a)

The acetabular roof over the head of the femur can be assessed with the help of the center–edge angle, which is formed by a vertical line through the center of the head of the femur and the line from the femoral head center to the lateral acetabular margin.

Normal: 4 to 13 years, 20°; over 14 years, 25°. The vertical line should always be medial to the other line. If the angle is smaller than normal, this should arouse suspicion of hip dysplasia.

### Acetabular Angle (Fig. 8.37a)

The acetabular angle can help to determine if the acetabular roof over the head of the femur is lacking. The angle is made up of a line connecting the superior aspect of both triradiate cartilages of the acetabula with a line that extends from the triradiate cartilage along the acetabular roof.

Normal: newborn, 29°; 3 to 4 years, 15°; 15 years and above, less than 10°.

### Ombrédanne's Cross (Fig. 8.37b)

- *Hilgenreiner's line:* the line connecting the superior aspects of the two triradiate cartilages. It is the horizontal line of the cross.
- *Perkin's line:* a vertical line through the lateral aspect of the acetabular roof bilaterally.

These lines result in a cross delineating four quadrants on each side. To establish whether subluxation has occurred, the quadrant where the femoral head ossification centers lie should be determined.

Normal: The ossification center is found in the inner lower quadrant. The hip is subluxed if the center is in the outer lower quadrant, and dislocated if it is in the upper outer quadrant.

### Ménard–Shenton's Line (Fig. 8.37b)

This line should be a harmonious arc made up of the medial contour of the femoral neck and the obturator crest of the pubic bone. If the femoral head is dislocated or the CCD angle has altered, the arc has step-offs or gaps in its course.

**Pathology**

**Hip Dysplasia**

In hip dysplasia, the acetabulum is defective. The acetabular angle is larger than normal, and the femoral head is less covered. The head can be dislocated superiorly, laterally, or posteriorly.

This change is very commonly found in combination with anteversion of the femoral neck.

▷ See Chapter 8.2.4, Rippstein II View

**Practical Tip**

The following findings on physical examination suggest hip dysplasia:

An inability to make pedaling motions with the affected leg; foreshortening of the affected leg.

Asymmetry of the thigh and gluteal folds.

Limited abduction.

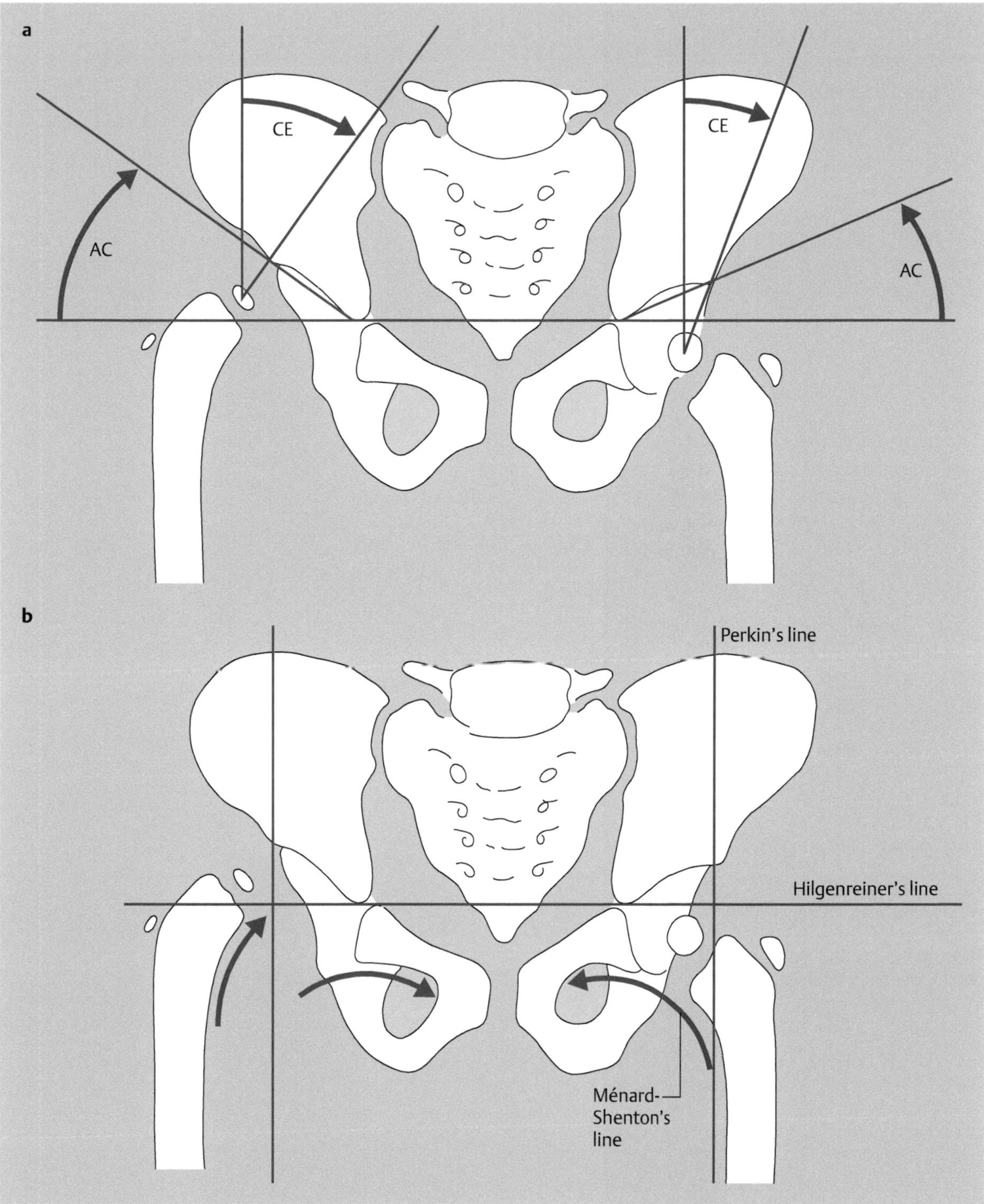


**Fig. 8.37 (a)** Center–edge (CE) and acetabular (AC) angles. Left hip: normal; right hip: dysplasia. **(b)** Ombrédanne's cross and Ménard-Shenton's line. Left hip: normal; right hip: dislocation.

## 8.2.4 Rippstein II View (Fig. 8.38a)

### Anteversion Angle of the Femur (Fig. 8.38b)

Projected onto a horizontal plane, the axis of the femoral neck forms an angle with the transverse axis of the femoral condyles. In newborns, this angle amounts to approximately 30 to 40°, and it declines with growth, so that it is about 25° at age 10 years and 12° in adults.

To represent the anteversion angle (AV angle) of the femur, the technician must position the patient in a particular way: 90° of hip flexion and 20° of hip abduction to delineate the projected anteversion angle.

To determine the actual angle, a conversion table must be consulted.

**Pathology**

**Anteversion of the Femoral Neck**

If the anteversion is too great, for example if growth stops with an anteversion angle of 25°, the head of the femur is too far anterior in relation to the acetabulum, and this is primarily associated with external rotation. To counter this, internal rotation centers the head. This compensation is quite noticeable as a marked internal rotation during walking.

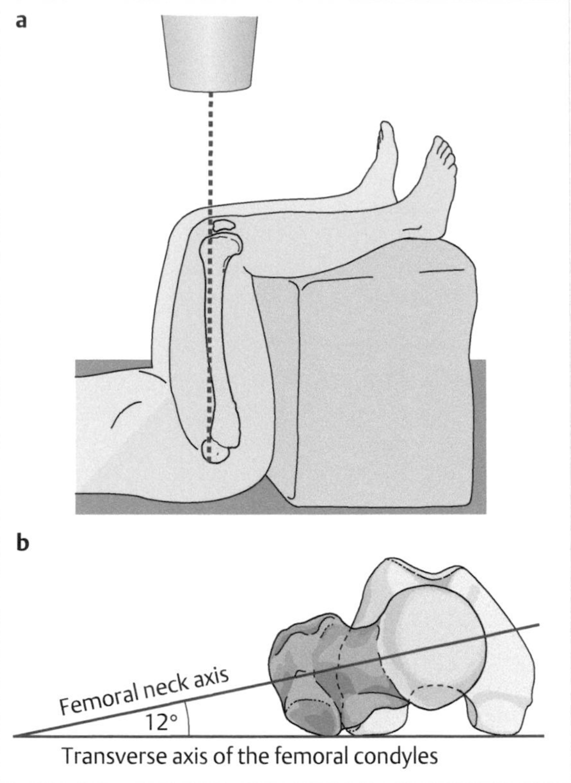


**Fig. 8.38 (a)** Rippstein view. **(b)** Anteversion angle.

## 8.2.5 Computed Tomography

CT scanning makes it possible to show images of transverse sections. Using different density settings, both soft tissue and bones can be accentuated.

### Anteversion Angle (Fig. 8.39)

In cross-section, the anteversion angle of the acetabulum (the anterior acetabular opening angle) can be demonstrated. It provides information concerning the anterior covering of the femoral head. It consists of the angle between the tangent of the anterior and posterior acetabular margins and a sagittal axis generated from the posterior acetabular margin.

Normal: 10 to 15°. Thus the tangent of the acetabulum should always be medial to the sagittal axis.

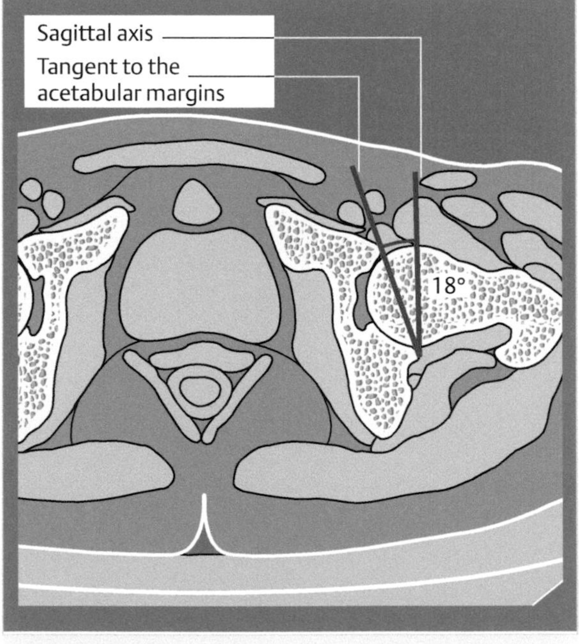


**Fig. 8.39** Anteversion angle.

# 8.3 Pelvic Ring

## 8.3.1 Bony Structure of the Pelvis

The pelvic ring is a ring of bone that operates between the vertebral column, which it supports, and the lower extremities, on which it rests.

The pelvis consists of two hip bones and the sacrum. Each hip bone in turn consists of the ilium, ischium, and pubis. These come together at the triradiate cartilage, a Y-shaped cartilage that fills the gap between the three bones within the concave joint socket of the hip joint. The triradiate cartilage usually ossifies by the 16th year of life.

The pelvis is divided into the greater pelvis and lesser pelvis. The linea terminalis, running from the promontory of the sacrum to the upper margin of the pubic symphysis, represents the border between the two.

### Ilium (Figs. 8.40–8.42)

This is composed of the iliac wing (the ala of the ilium) and the body of the ilium.

#### Ala of the Ilium

*Gluteal Surface*

- This is the outer surface of the ilium.
- It has several ridges that serve as origins for the gluteal muscles:
  - Inferior gluteal line: above the acetabulum.
  - Anterior gluteal line: in the middle area.
  - Posterior gluteal line: in the posterior region of the gluteal surface.

*Iliac Crest*

- This forms the border of the ilium as an arc bowing superiorly.
- There are three ridges on the superior aspect of the crest:
  - The *outer lip:* the origin for the latissimus dorsi and gluteus medius muscle, and the insertion for the external oblique muscle.
  - The *intermediate zone:* the origin for the internal oblique muscle.
  - *Inner lip:* the origin for the inferior part of the transverse abdominis muscle, and the insertion for the quadratus lumborum.

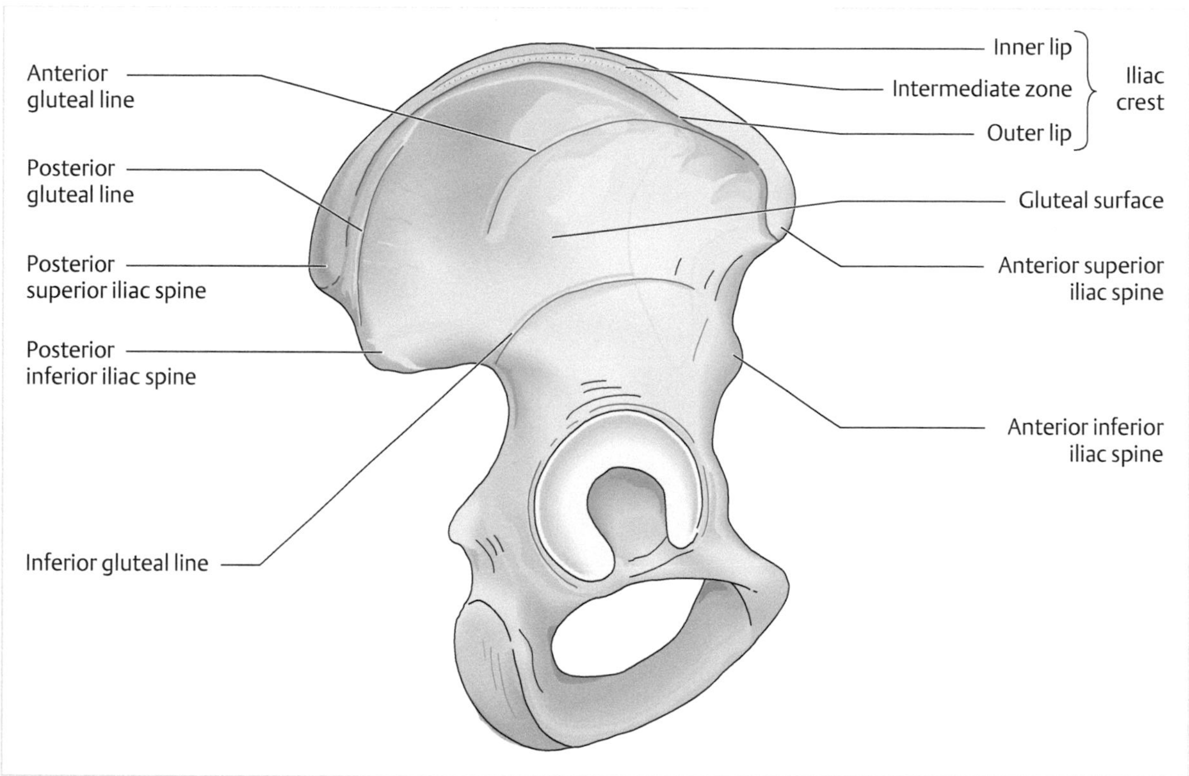


**Fig. 8.40** Ilium (lateral view).

- *ASIS:* This is the anterior end of the iliac crest and is the site of origin for several structures: from here, the sartorius muscle tracks inferiorly; the tensor fasciae latae muscle arises somewhat lateral to the spine; and from the tip, the inguinal ligament runs medially.
- *Inguinal ligament:* This runs in the direction of the pubic tubercle and in part to the pubic ramus, where it is slightly wider. It passes over the retroinguinal space. The abdominal muscles track into the inguinal ligament from superior and lateral directions, and the fascia of the thigh tracks into it from below.
- *Anterior inferior iliac spine:* This lies approximately 2 cm inferior to the ASIS. The rectus femoris muscle arises here.
- *Muscular space:* The anterior side of the ilium along with the inguinal ligament and the superior pubic ramus form a tunnel, which is divided into two spaces by a band of fascia, the iliopectineal arch. The following structures pass through the lateral, muscular space: the iliopsoas muscle and lateral cutaneous nerve of the thigh in the superolateral region, and the femoral nerve in the medial aspect. The iliopectineal bursa lies in the inferior section of the muscular space (**Fig. 8.41**).
- *Vascular space:* The femoral artery and vein as well as the lymphatic vessels pass through this space. The *lacunar ligament*, which is formed from fibers that fan out from the inguinal ligament, forms the medial border, and the iliopectineal arch forms the lateral border (**Fig. 8.41**).
- *Inguinal canal:* This is formed anteriorly by the aponeuroses of the external oblique muscle, and superiorly by the transverse abdominis muscle. It is approximately 5 cm long. Within it runs the spermatic cord or the round ligament of the uterus.
- Posterior end of the iliac crest: the PSIS (**Fig. 8.42**).
- The *posterior inferior iliac spine* lies three fingerbreadths inferior to this.

### *Internal Iliac Fossa*

- This is an indentation on the medial side of the ilium that serves as the origin for the iliacus muscle.
- The *auricular surface* for the SIJ is located posteroinferiorly.

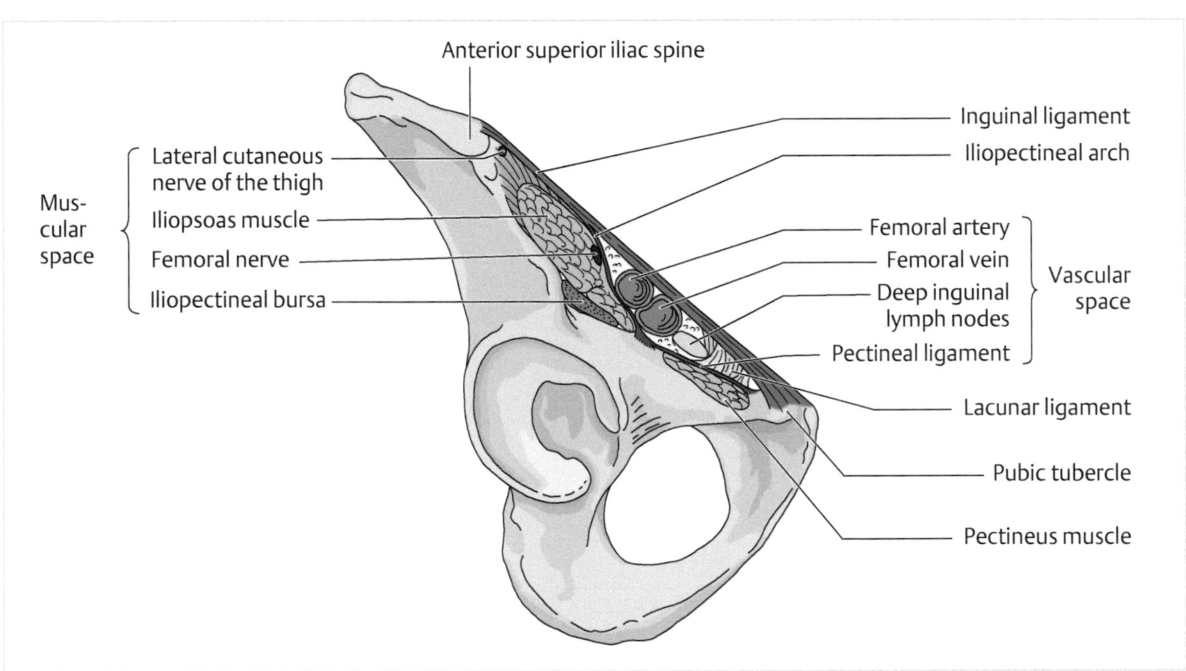


**Fig. 8.41** Ilium with muscular and vascular spaces (anterior view).

- *Iliac tuberosity:* This lies superior and posterior to the auricular surface for the insertion of the short posterior ligaments.

### Body of the Ilium (Fig. 8.42)

- This forms the roof of the acetabulum.
- The arcuate line forms the border between the body and the ala; it corresponds to the linea terminalis, which divides the greater pelvis from the lesser pelvis.

## Ischium (Fig. 8.43)

### Body of the Ischium

- This forms the posterior part of the acetabulum.
- It is the posterior border of the obturator foramen.

#### *Ischial Spine*

- This is located posteriorly on the body and serves as the origin for the gemellus superior muscle and the sacrospinous ligament.
- The *lesser sciatic notch* lies inferior to the ischial spine and has a cartilage-covered surface as it serves as a hypomochlion for the obturator internus.
- The *greater sciatic notch* is located superior to the ischial spine.

#### *Ischial Tuberosity*

- Located inferiorly, this is the origin of the hamstring muscles and the adductor magnus.
- From here, the sacrotuberous ligament tracks in a superomedial direction toward the sacrum.

### Ramus of the Ischium

This forms the inferior boundary of the obturator foramen.

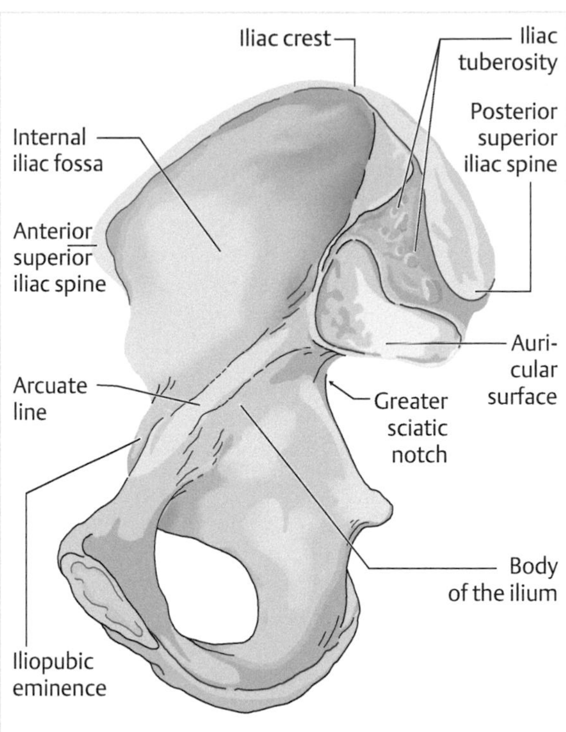


**Fig. 8.42** Ilium (medial view).

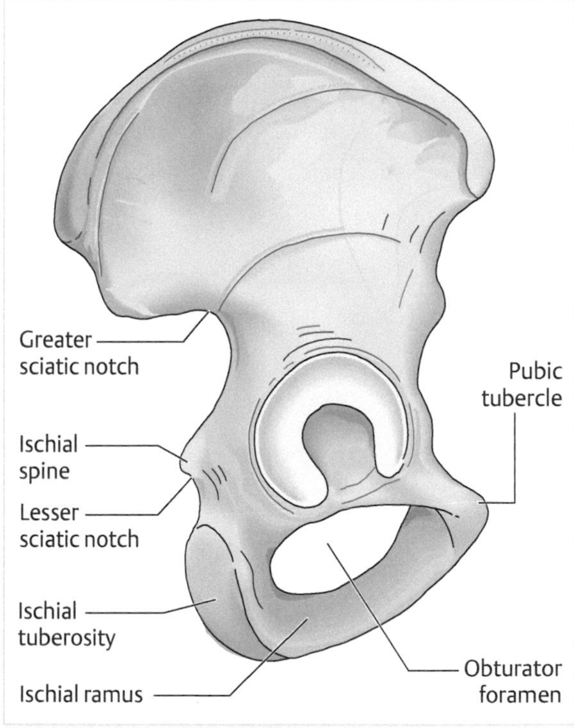


**Fig. 8.43** Ischium (lateral view).

## Pubis (Fig. 8.44)

### Body of the Pubis

- The body of the pubis forms the anterior part in the acetabulum.
- It forms the pubic tubercle.
- It enters the superior pubic ramus at the iliopubic eminence.

### Superior Pubic Ramus

- This forms the superior boundary of the obturator foramen.
- The superior edge protrudes as the pecten pubis; this is the origin of the pectineus muscle.
- Superiorly, the ramus merges into the arcuate line.

#### *Obturator Crest*

This is the bony ridge that runs from the pubic tubercle to the anterior edge of the acetabular notch.

#### *Obturator Groove*

- This is the groove below the obturator crest.
- It forms the superior boundary of the obturator canal.
- *Obturator canal:* This is approximately 3 cm long and runs from posterior to superolateral. The obturator nerve and obturator blood vessels pass through it, and the fat body of the obturator canal forms a cushion of connective tissue and fat.

### Inferior Pubic Ramus

- Medially, this forms the symphysial surface.
- It represents the inferior border of the obturator foramen and connects with the ramus of the ischium there.

### Pubic Arch/Subpubic Angle

In women, both inferior rami and the symphysis form an arc, the arcus pubis, with an angle of approximately 90 to 100°; in men, the subpubic angle is formed, which measures about 70°.

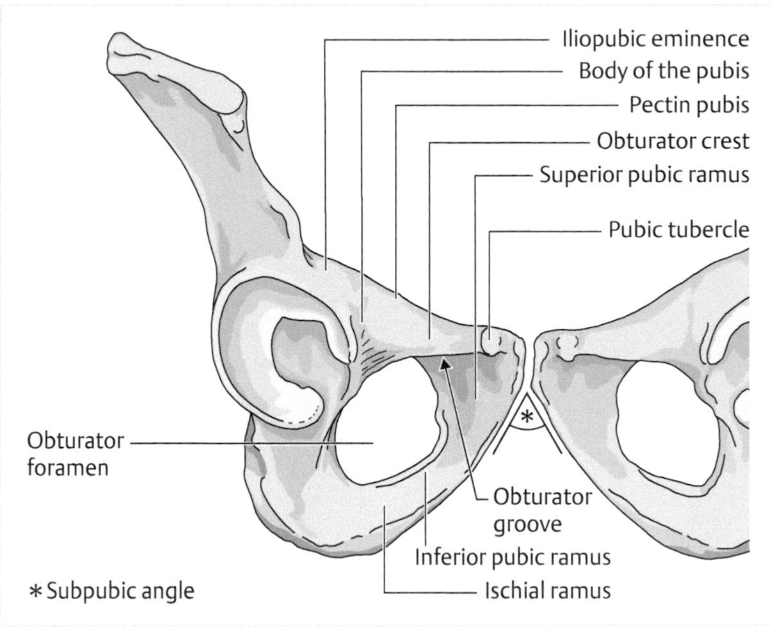


**Fig. 8.44** Pubis (anterior view).

## Obturator Membrane (Fig. 8.45)

- This covers the obturator foramen.
- It consists of tight connective tissue fibers that are woven together into varying layers and orientations.
- It is perforated by some gaps for vessels and nerves.
- It serves as the insertion for the muscles of the pelvic floor, and as origin for the obturator muscles.

## Sacrum (Figs. 8.46–8.49)

- During human evolution five vertebrae fused together into one bone.
- The sacrum is wedge-shaped, being thick and wide at the superior end, and thin and narrow at the inferior end.
- It has a convex outward curve, with the apex of curvature at the S3 vertebral level.

### Base of the Sacrum (Fig. 8.46)

- This is the superior end of the sacrum; the anterior portion projects outward to form the promontory.
- It is connected to the fifth lumbar vertebra by means of the last intervertebral disk.
- The pair of superior articular processes extend in a superior direction, representing the articular connection to the fifth lumbar vertebra.

### Apex of the Sacrum (Fig. 8.46)

- This is the pointed inferior end of the sacrum.
- It connects to the coccyx by way of a narrow disk.

### External Surface of the Sacrum (Fig. 8.47)

- *Outer surface of the sacrum with ridges that are longitudinally arranged:*
  - Median sacral crest: corresponds to the spinous processes.
  - Two intermediate sacral crests: arise from the fusion of the articular processes.
  - Two lateral sacral crests: represent the accessory processes.

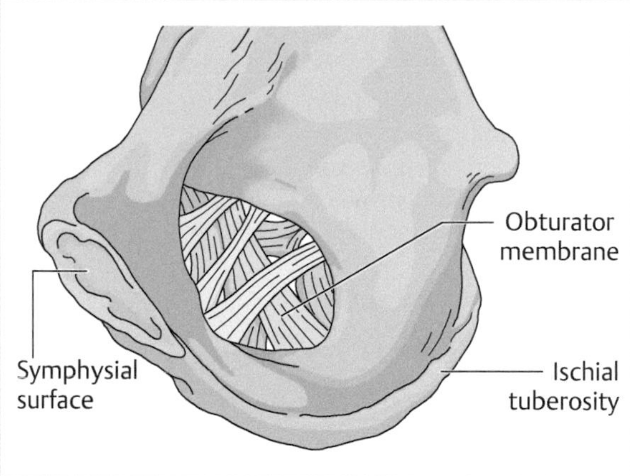


**Fig. 8.45** Obturator membrane (medial view).

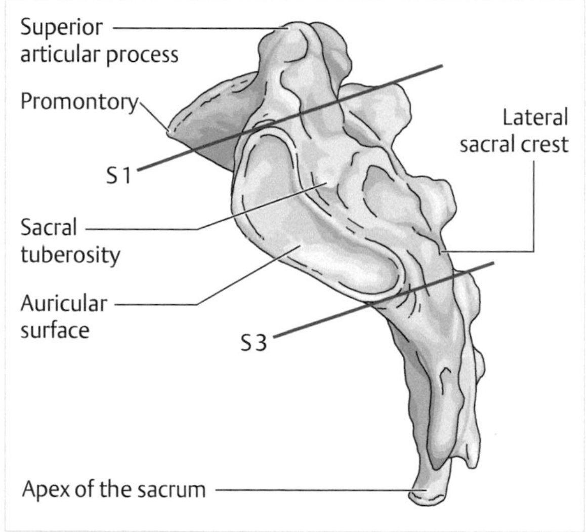


**Fig. 8.46** Sacrum (lateral view).

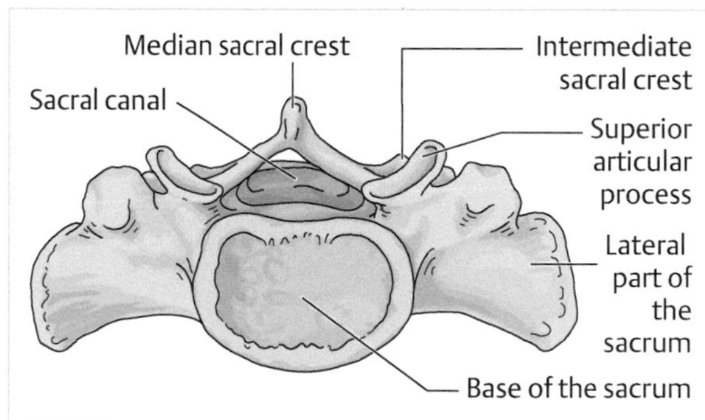


**Fig. 8.47** Sacrum (superior view).

- *Sacral horns* (**Fig. 8.48**):
  - These protrude outward and form the posterolateral end of the sacral canal.
  - They are the vestiges of the articular processes of the fifth sacral vertebra.
- *Sacral canal* (**Figs. 8.47 and 8.48**):
  - This is the caudal continuation of the spinal canal.
  - It ends at the *sacral hiatus*, which is located below the fourth sacral vertebra.
- *Posterior sacral foramina:*
  - These are eight outlet openings for the posterior nerves.
- *Lateral part of the sacrum:*
  - This arises from the fusion of the costal processes.
  - The articular surface of the SIJ—the *auricular surface* —is located in the superior region and extends down to the third sacral vertebra.
- *Sacral tuberosity:*
  - This serves as insertion for the posterior sacro-iliac ligaments.
  - It is located posteriorly at the level of the auricular surface.

### Pelvic Surface (Fig. 8.49)

- Four transverse lines, the *transverse ridges*, are visible in place of the intervertebral disks.
- There are eight laterally located *anterior sacral foramina* through which the nerves forming the sacral plexus pass.

## Coccyx (Fig. 8.50)

- This consists of three or four vertebral vestiges that have fused.
- The first vertebra has short transverse processes and *coccygeal cornua*, representing the remnants of the articular processes. However, they do not articulate directly with the sacrum, but are instead connected to it via a ligament.
- The superior surface of the coccyx, the *articular surface*, is connected to the apex of the sacrum at the *sacrococcygeal joint*.

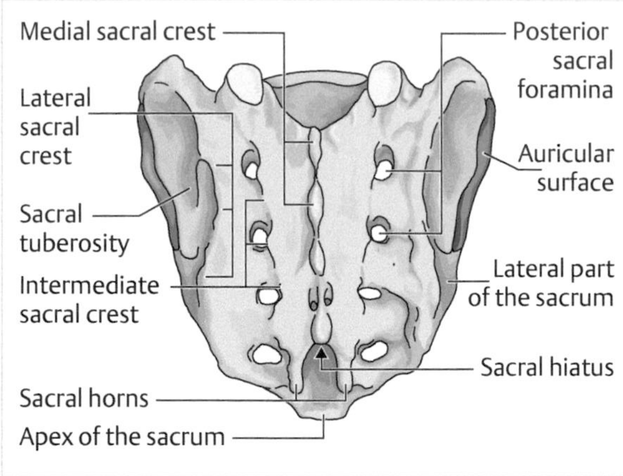


**Fig. 8.48** Sacrum (posterior view).

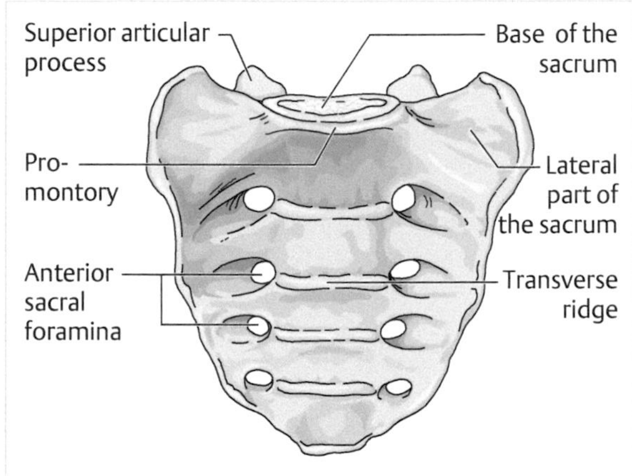


**Fig. 8.49** Sacrum (anterior view).

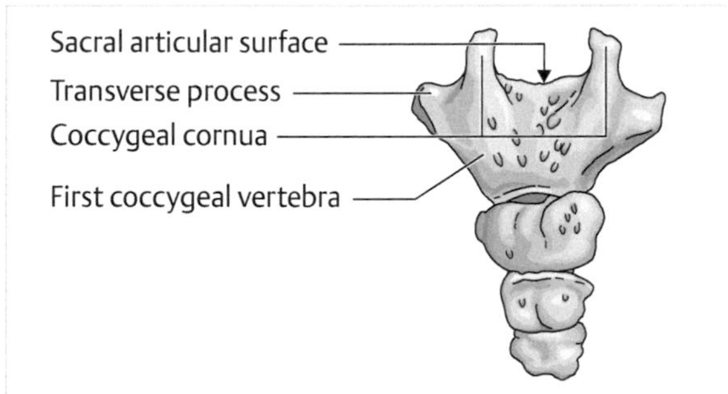


**Fig. 8.50** Coccyx (posterior view).

## 8.3.2 Pelvic Dimensions

### Gender Differences in the Pelvis

#### Female Pelvis (Fig. 8.51a)

- Transverse–oval pelvic inlet area.
- Pelvic outlet wide.
- Alae of the ilia large and extended laterally.
- Obturator foramen triangular.
- Pubic symphysis wide and low.
- Pubic arch of approximately 100°.

#### Male Pelvis (Fig. 8.51b)

- Heart-shaped opening.
- Diameters of the lesser pelvis are smaller than in the female.
- Alae of the ilia steep.
- Obturator foramen oval.
- Pubic symphysis tall and narrow.
- Pubic angle approximately 70 to 80°.

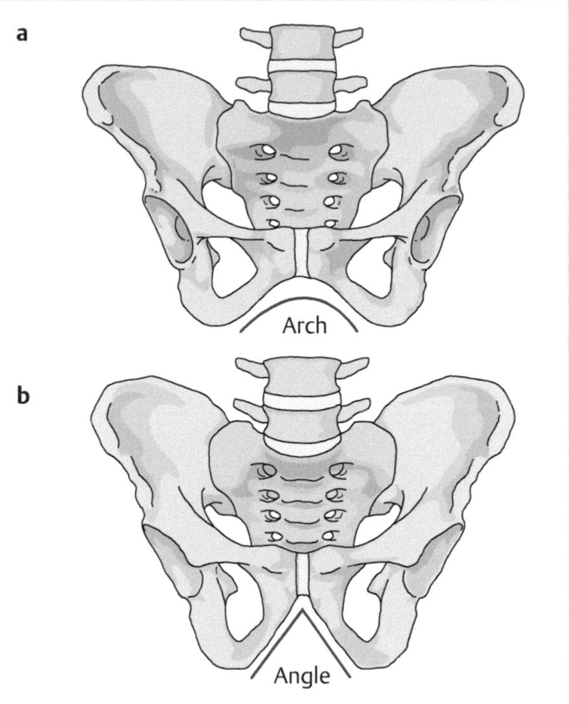


**Fig. 8.51** Gender differences in the pelvis. **(a)** Female pelvis. **(b)** Male pelvis.

### External Pelvic Dimensions

These measurements allow conclusions to be drawn as to the size and shape of the lesser pelvis.

The following dimensions can be determined with regard to the pelvic circle:

- *Intertrochanteric distance* (**Fig. 8.52a**): the distance between the most laterally lying points on the greater trochanter. Normal: approximately 31 to 32 cm. This measurement does not really belong to direct pelvic dimensions, but does allow an inference to be made about the shape of the pelvis.
- *Interspinous distance* (**Fig. 8.52a**): the distance between the two ASISs. Normal: approximately 25 cm.
- *Intercristal distance* (**Fig. 8.52a**): the distance between the most lateral points on the iliac crests in the frontal plane. Normal: approximately 28 cm.

These measurements usually fall within 3 cm of those given here. If they are significantly lower, it suggests a contracted pelvis, which could affect the birth process.

- *External conjugate* (**Fig. 8.52b**): the distance between the upper margin of the pubic symphysis and the L5 spinous process. Normal: approximately 20 cm.

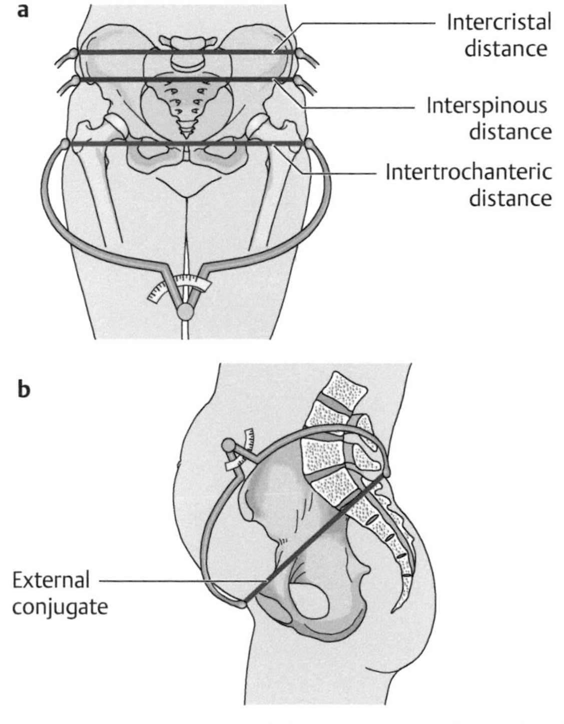


**Fig. 8.52** External pelvic dimensions. **(a)** Intertrochanteric, interspinous, and intercristal distances. **(b)** External conjugate.

## Internal Pelvic Dimensions (Fig. 8.53)

The internal pelvic dimensions can be determined using ultrasound examination. These provide evidence on the bony confines of the pelvis.

The *pelvic inlet* is the narrowest part of the birth canal; it becomes larger when the legs are extended:

- *True conjugate:* the distance between the promontory and the upper inner surface of the pubic symphysis. Normal: approximately 11 cm.
- *Diagonal conjugate:* the distance between the promontory and the lower margin of the pubic symphysis. Normal: approximately 13 cm.
- *Oblique diameter:* the diagonal diameter of the pelvis, measured by the distance between the SIJ and the iliopubic eminence on the opposite side.
- *Transverse diameter:* the distance between the lineae terminales. Normal: 13 cm.

The *pelvic outlet* is enlarged by flexing the legs, which is important for the second stage of labor. For this reason, many people around the world give birth in a squatting position:

- *Conjugates:* the direct diameter of the pelvic outlet, which measure approximately 9 cm; due to the flexibility of the coccyx, the diameter can be increased to 11 cm.
- *Transverse diameter:* the distance between the ischial tuberosities, which measures approximately 11 cm.

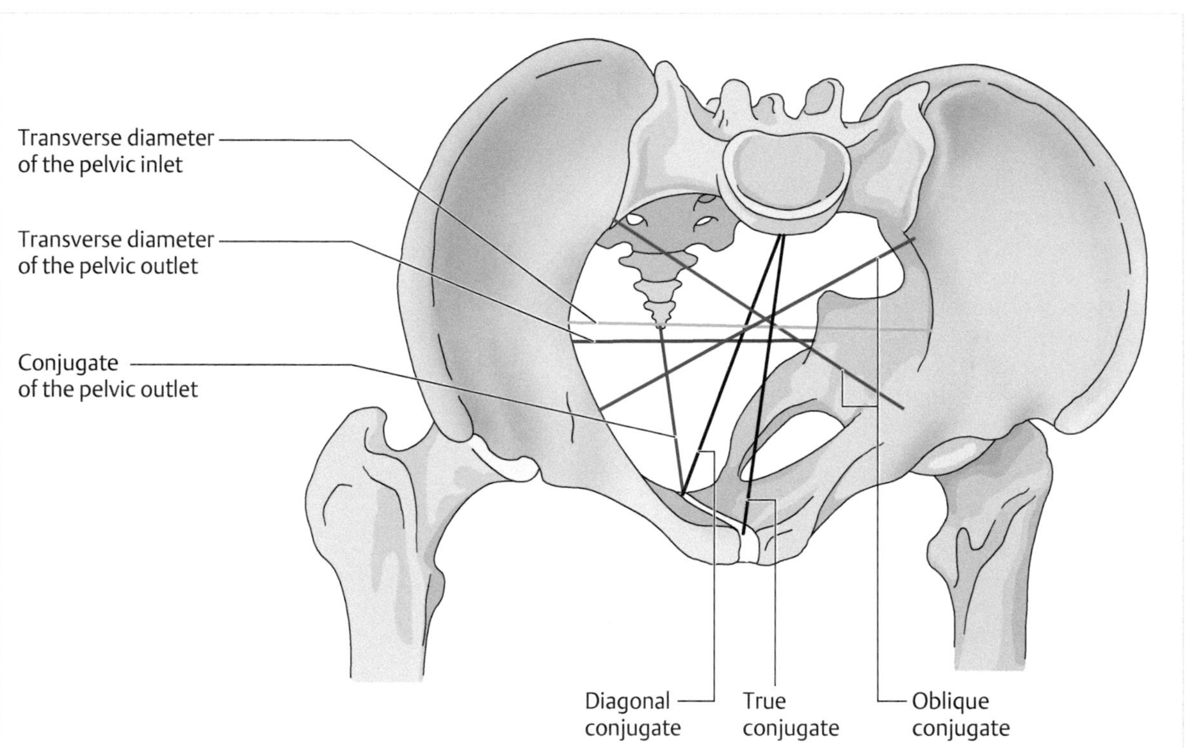


**Fig. 8.53** Internal pelvic dimensions.

## 8.3.3 Distribution of Forces

The pelvic ring has an important mechanical function in that it distributes the forces acting from above and below.

## Effect of Force

### Pressure Load in the Standing Position (Fig. 8.54)

The body weight is applied onto the promontory. The force is transferred over the SIJs and on to the acetabula. When the forces are distributed in the hip joint, one can detect a larger force that is directed inferiorly (**a** in **Fig. 8.54**), and a small component of force that is directed laterally (**b** in **Fig. 8.54**). The inferiorly directed force puts the hip joint under compressive load, whereas the lateral force places the pubic symphysis under tensile stress.

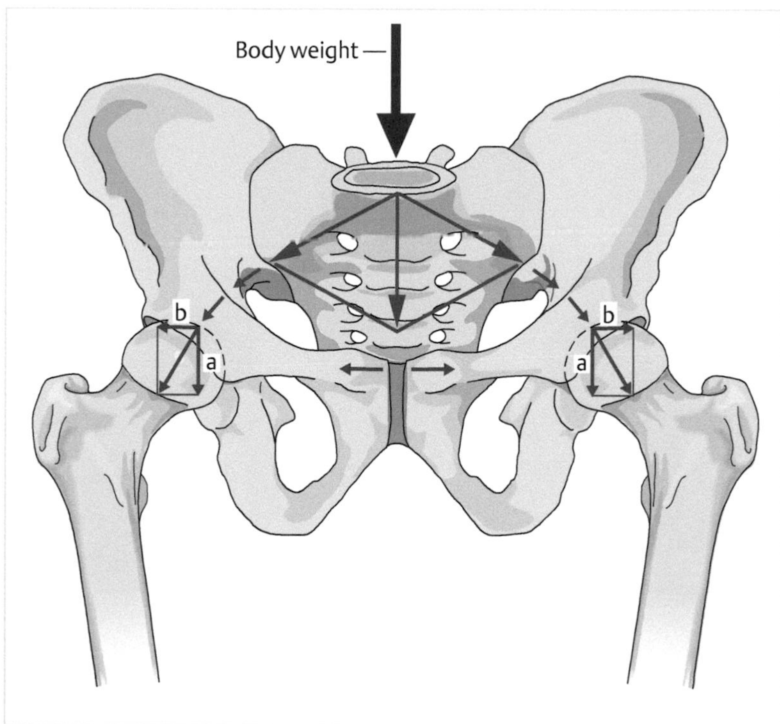


**Fig. 8.54** Pressure load in the standing position.

## Pressure Distribution in the Sitting Position (Fig. 8.55)

In the sitting position, the body weight also rests on the promontory and is propagated over the SIJs. Here, however, it is directed not toward the acetabulum, but toward the ischial tuberosity. In the distribution of the forces, a horizontal and a vertical direction of force can be identified. The vertical component submits the tuberosity to pressure, while the horizontal component puts the symphysis under pressure.

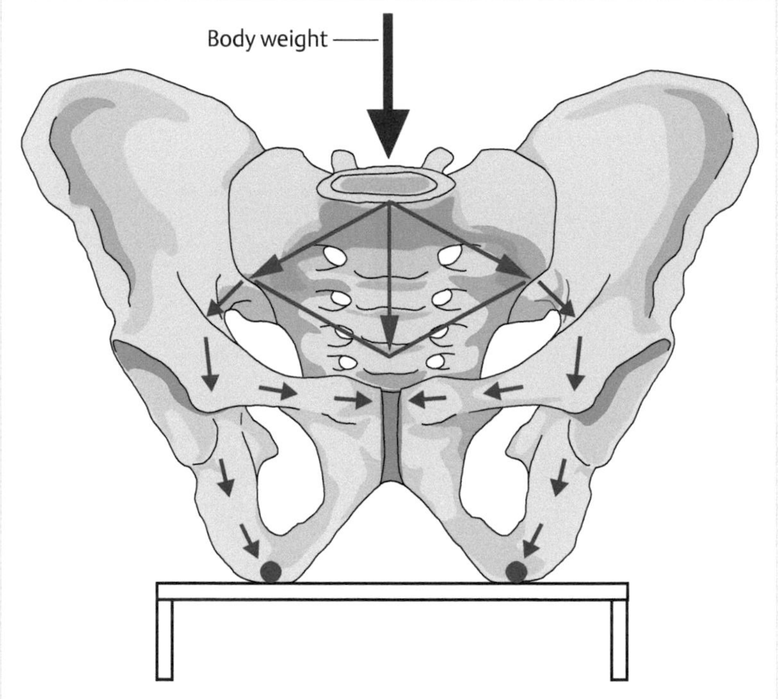


**Fig. 8.55** Pressure load in the sitting position.

## Trabecular (Cancellous) Structure

The distribution of the forces affects the arrangement and density of the trabecular structure.

### Trajectories in the Pelvic Ring (Fig. 8.56)

From the superior region of the auricular surface, the forces pass outward to the posterior margin of the greater sciatic notch and in a line to the ischium and further laterally to the posterior acetabulum. From the auricular surface on the medial side, the density of the arcuate line indicates the magnitude of force that it transfers.

Moving outward from the inferior region of the auricular surface, the trajectories diverge at the level of the superior gluteal line and form the arcuate line. They extend further to the superior region of the acetabulum.

Bundles of trabeculae track inferiorly to the ischium, some toward the ischial tuberosity and others anteriorly toward the pubic ramus.

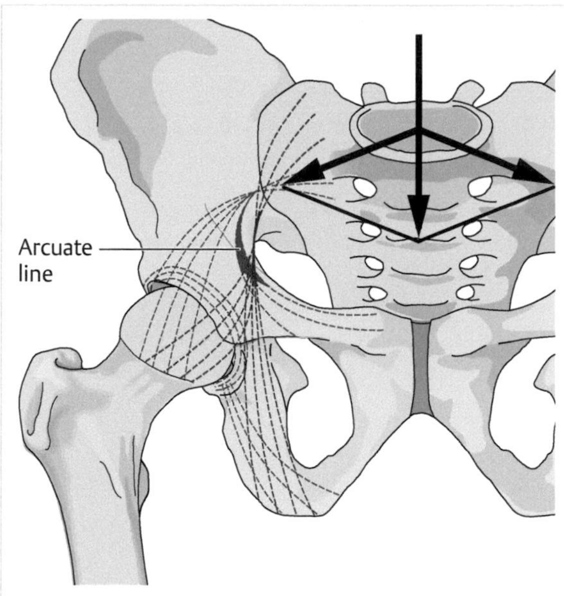


**Fig. 8.56** Course of the trabeculae in the pelvic area.

### Distribution of Trabeculae at the Proximal End of the Femur (Fig. 8.57)

The pressure trajectories meet perpendicular to the articular surface of the femoral head and extend further within the medial aspect of the femoral neck and shaft area (Adams's arch).

Traction trabeculae arising from the medial femoral head cross the compression trabeculae in the proximal region and pass superiorly in an arc before running along the femoral neck in an inferolateral direction. They are crossed by other traction trabeculae that run from the greater trochanter parallel to the intertrochanteric line to the lesser trochanter.

On X-ray, an area of reduced density, called *Ward's triangle*, can be seen between these systems.

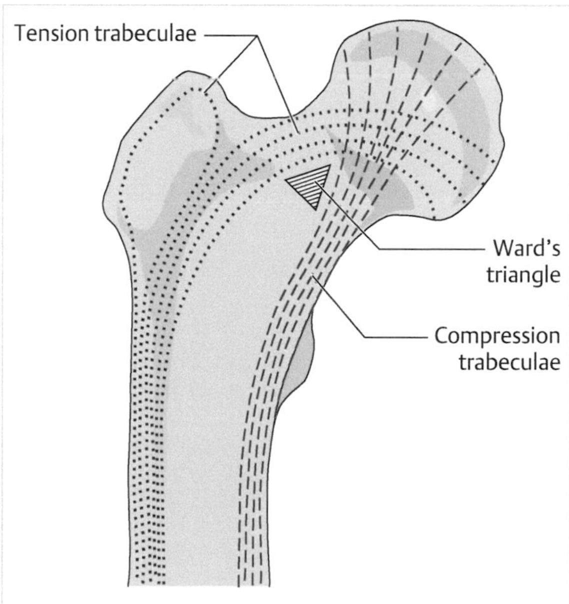


**Fig. 8.57** Distribution of trabeculae in the proximal femur.

**Pathology**

**Coxa Vara**

Since the bending stress of the femoral neck is very large, the densely arranged traction trabeculae run distally in a pronounced arc. The compressive trabeculae, however, run very steeply in an inferior direction. See **Fig. 8.34.**

**Coxa Valga**

In the proximal femoral neck area, there are pronounced compression trabeculae that run steeply inferiorly, while the traction trabeculae are significantly reduced.

## The Sacrum as a Wedge (Figs. 8.58 and 8.59)

The pelvic girdle must be stable to successfully transmit the body weight to the lower extremities. The ligamentous connections, the muscles, and the sacral wedge ensure this stability.

In the frontal view, the sacrum presents as a wedge that narrows at the inferior end and is wedged between the two hip bones.

In the transverse plane, the sacrum is wedged into the pelvic girdle. The strong posterior ligaments that overlay the SIJ and the ligamentous connections of the pubic symphysis stabilize the sacrum.

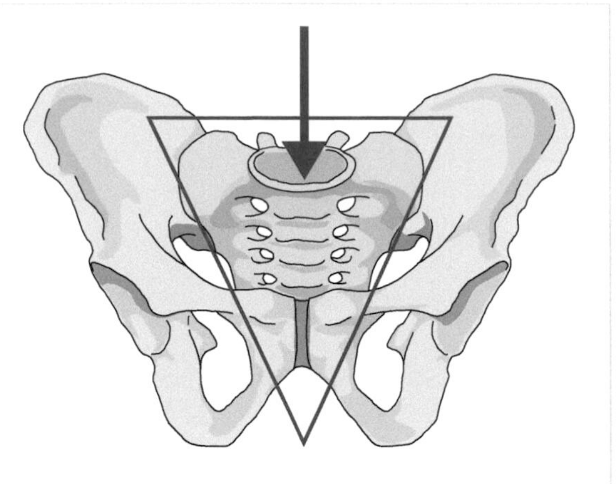

Fig. 8.58 The sacrum as a wedge: frontal plane.

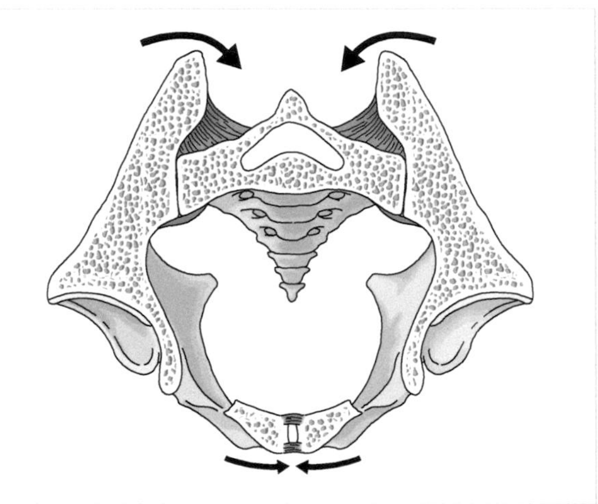

Fig. 8.59 The sacrum as a wedge: the transverse plane.

### Pathology

#### Instability

If the ligaments lose stability at a particular point, the strength of the entire pelvic ring is impaired. During pregnancy, the release of hormones causes loosening of the ligaments of the pelvic girdle, making it more flexible to allow for the birth process. This loosening must normalize after birth; otherwise instability remains.

#### Disruption of the Pubic Symphysis (Fig. 8.60)

During the birth process, disruption of the symphysis can occur. X-ray and palpation can demonstrate dehiscence of the symphysis in which the pubic bones may drift up to 5 cm apart.

Therapy: application of a firm trochanteric belt.

#### Trauma

During a fall on both tuberosities, the ilia wedge the sacrum as they are pushed superiorly.

In pelvic fractures, the ability of the pelvis to bear weight may be lost, with a resultant loss of stability.

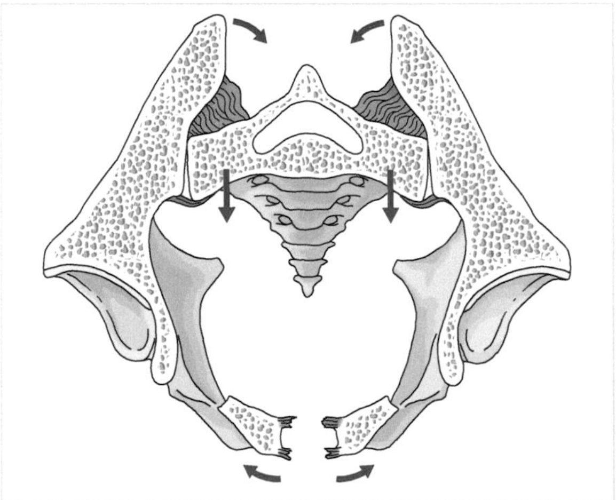

Fig. 8.60 Consequences of disruption of the pubic symphysis.

# 8.4 Sacro-Iliac Joint

## 8.4.1 Articular Surfaces

### Localization (Fig. 8.61)

The *auricular surfaces* of the sacrum and ilium are congruent articular surfaces shaped like a "C" or a boomerang. The inferior part is about one-third longer than the superior part. The ends of the joints are called "poles."

In adults, the articular surfaces extend from the first to third sacral vertebrae. The transition, i.e., the kink between the upper and lower poles, lies approximately at the level of the second sacral vertebra. Overall, the joint surfaces are 6 to 8 cm long and 2 to 3 cm wide.

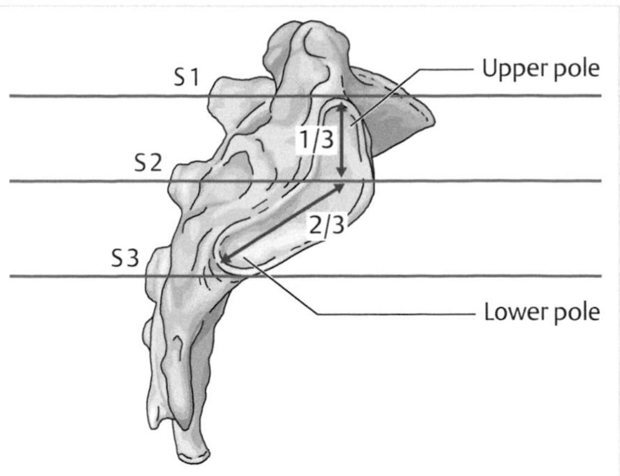


Fig. 8.61 Auricular surface of the sacrum.

### Position

The upper and lower poles meet at an angle of 100–120°. The joint is tilted such that the upper pole points superiorly and the lower posteriorly. Kapandji (2008) describes correlations between shape of the spine and the shape of the auricular surface. A person with a flat back has a less pronounced curvature, whereas when there is significant spinal column curvature, the angle may be 90°.

### Shape (Fig. 8.62)

The joint surfaces are uneven with many furrows and bumps that are quite variable in their characteristics. In transverse section, the articular surfaces of the sacrum exhibit an elevation in the superior region, a change between depression and elevation in the middle section, and a depression in the middle of the inferior section.

The hyaline cartilage layer is thicker on the sacral side than the ilial side.

The joint becomes fixed and acquires its actual shape only after 12 to 13 years of age. Prior to that, the joint surface is flat.

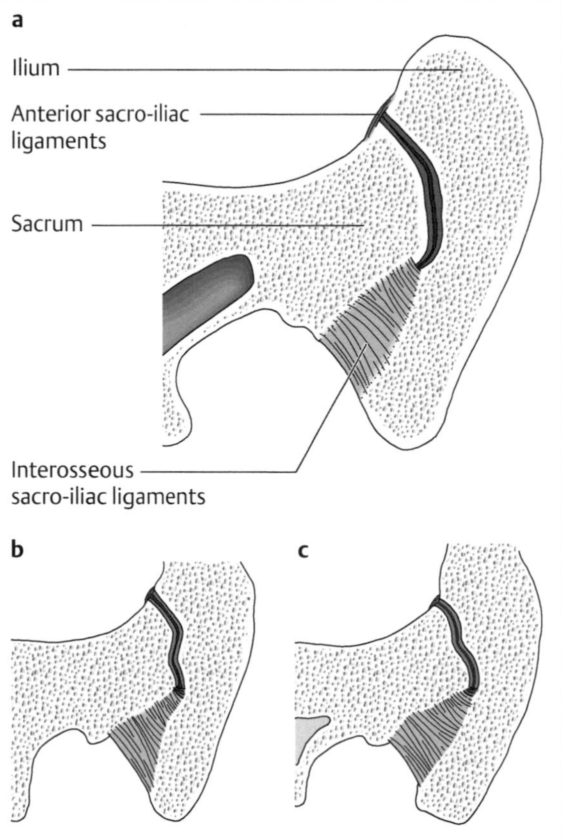


Fig. 8.62 Joint surfaces in transverse section. (a) Superior portion. (b) Middle portion. (c) Inferior portion.

## Differences in the Joint Surfaces in Men and Women

In men, there are numerous distinct grooves and bulges. This means that a large amount of force is needed to move the joint surfaces against each other. Thus, the joint is very stable and has little mobility. This type of joint closure is called *form closure* (**Fig. 8.63**).

In women, there are fewer distinct bulges and furrows. Here the wedging of the sacrum into the pelvic ring and the ligamentous and muscular apparatus play a role in stabilizing the joint. This type of joint closure is called *force closure*. Mobility of the joint is good.

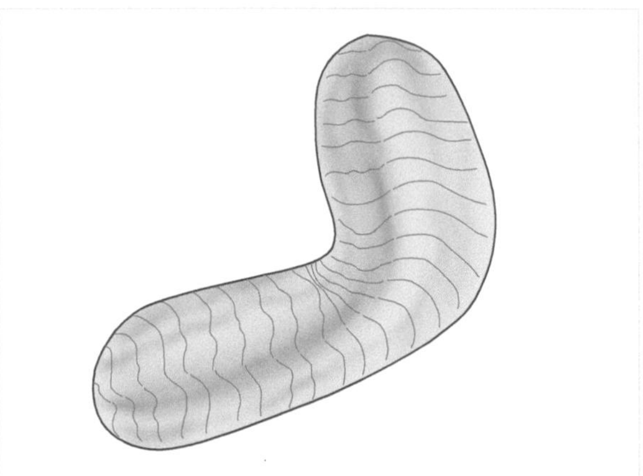

**Fig. 8.63** Articular surface in men.

### Practical Tip

**Provocation of the Joint (Fig. 8.64a)**

Pain provocation tests play a highly significant role in diagnosis. To place pressure evenly on the joint, place the patient in the supine position and apply and maintain uniform pressure on the ASISs with the palms using crossed arms. Reproduction of the pain described by the patient indicates a disorder of the SIJ, which should be confirmed by further provocation tests.

**Releasing the Joint (Fig. 8.64b)**

To achieve a symmetrical release of all parts of the joint, place one hand anteriorly on the ASIS and the fingers of the other hand in the sacral sulcus. Maintain a slight pressure laterally until the joint can be felt to give, i.e., there is a lateral shift.

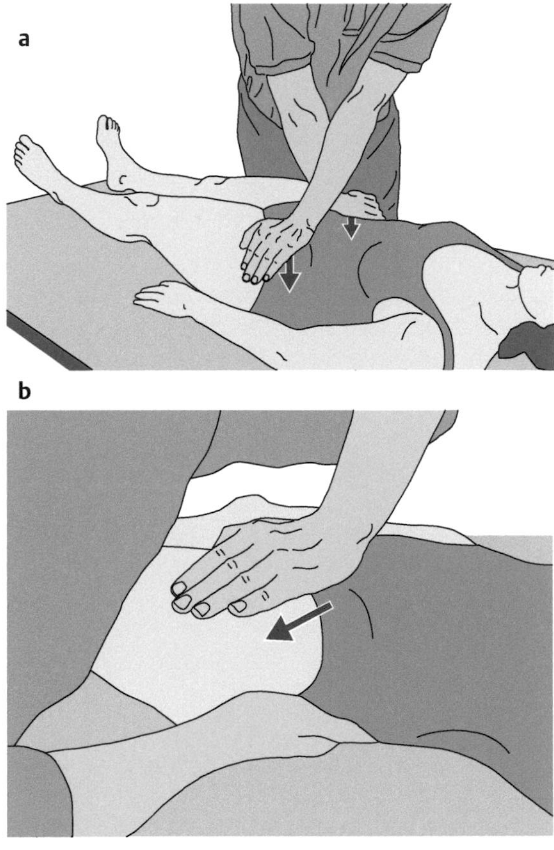


**Fig. 8.64 (a)** Provocation of the sacro-iliac joint. **(b)** Release of the sacro-iliac joint.

## 8.4.2 Joint Capsule

The joint capsule attaches to the bone–cartilage interface with no significant recess being formed. The anterior and interosseous sacro-iliac ligaments are fused with the fibrous layer.

## 8.4.3 Ligaments

In addition to the factors previously mentioned, the sacral wedging and the special construction of the joint interface, an extensive ligament system guarantees the stability of the joint.

### Posterior Sacro-Iliac Ligaments (Fig. 8.65)

Fibrous bands, partly short and thick and partly long, connect the ilium to the sacrum. Among these, various oblique fiber bundles can be distinguished. The longest fibers reaching inferiorly are the *long posterior sacro-iliac ligaments.* These pass into the sacrotuberous ligament and into the ligamentous system of the coccyx.

### Interosseous Sacro-Iliac Ligaments (Fig. 8.65)

These ligaments consist of short fiber tracts that are connected to the joint capsule of the SIJ and fill the sacral sulcus. They are particularly dense in the upper part of the joint.

### Anterior Sacro-Iliac Ligaments (Fig. 8.66)

The anterior ligaments are very thin and intertwine with the capsule. They run at the level of the first to third anterior sacral foramina from the sacropelvic surface of the ilium to the sacrum. The fibers track in two different directions: anterosuperiorly and anteroinferiorly. In the superior region, they intertwine with the iliolumbar ligament.

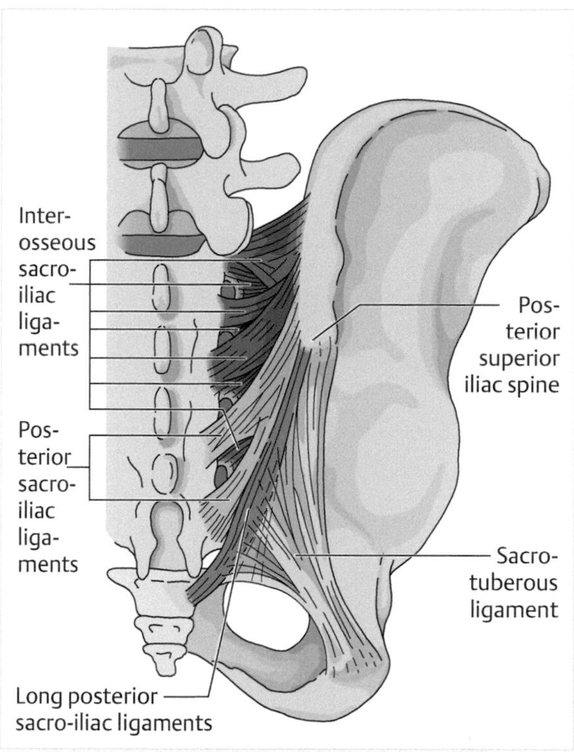


**Fig. 8.65** Posterior and interosseous sacro-iliac ligaments.

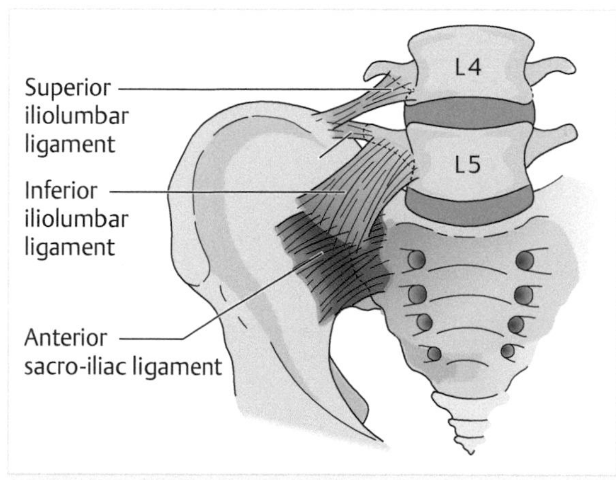


**Fig. 8.66** Anterior sacro-iliac ligaments.

### Sacrospinous Ligament (Fig. 8.67)

This originates on the inferolateral aspect of the pelvic surface of the sacrum and the base of the coccyx, and inserts onto the ischial spine. It crosses over the sacrotuberous ligament in the superior region and interconnects with it at this point.

The sacrospinous ligament forms the greater sciatic foramen from the greater sciatic notch. The lesser sciatic foramen, through which the pudendal nerve and the tendon of the obturator internus pass, lies further inferiorly.

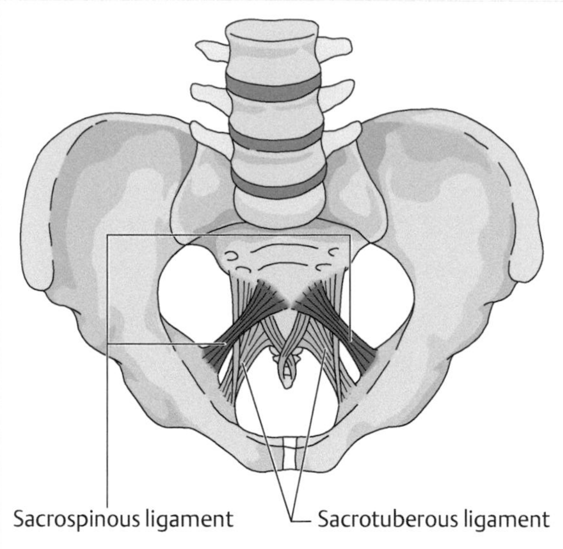


**Fig. 8.67** Sacrospinous and sacrotuberous ligaments (viewed from anterosuperiorly).

### Sacrotuberous Ligament (Fig. 8.68)

This ligament has a triangular shape. It contains long fibers that intertwine with the long posterior sacro-iliac ligament and thus form a connection from the PSIS to the ischial tuberosity and the posterior apex of the sacrum. Shorter fibers run from the posterior apex of the sacrum, the lateral sacrum, and the coccyx to the ischial tuberosity and the ramus of the ischium. In this way, the ligament rotates on its own axis. The right and left ligament enclose the coccyx like a neck tie.

The ligament forms the lesser sciatic foramen and crosses under the sacrospinous ligament. Some fibers of the biceps femoris muscle flow into this ligament from inferiorly. The aponeurosis of the piriformis muscle also intertwines with the superior parts of the ligament. The ligament plays an important role in the stabilization and mobility of the SIJ.

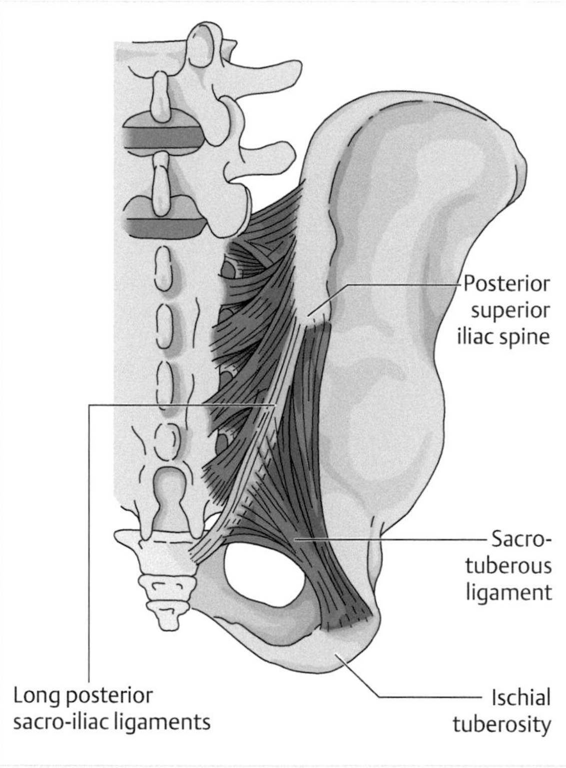


**Fig. 8.68** Sacrotuberous ligament.

### Iliolumbar Ligament

This is the continuation of the anterior sacro-iliac ligaments superiorly and fixes the fifth lumbar vertebra to the ilium.

▷ See Chapter 7.4, Ligaments of the Lumbar Spine and Fig. 7.33

## Function of the Ligaments

They stabilize the SIJ and slow down its movements. For example, the sacrotuberous and sacrospinous ligaments are important in slowing nutation.

▷ See Chapter 8.4.6, Axes of Motion

### Pathology

Malposition of the ilium or sacrum places a long-term burden on the ligamentous structures by bringing them under tension. For example, if the sacrotuberous ligament is very tight, this affects the mobility in the SIJ. There can be a reduction of motion on the affected side of up to 40 %.

### Practical Tip

**Ligament Provocation Tests (Fig. 8.69)**

To provoke the ligaments, place the patient in the supine position. With the patient's leg bent, place stress on the ligaments by using thrusts along the longitudinal axis of the thigh in various positions of the hip joint as follows:

The knee toward the opposite hip joint: iliolumbar ligament.

The knee to the ipsilateral shoulder: sacrotuberous ligament.

The knee to the contralateral shoulder: posterior sacroiliac and sacrospinous ligaments.

It is recommended that the stretch position should be held for about 5 to 10 seconds and that the ligaments should be palpated simultaneously.

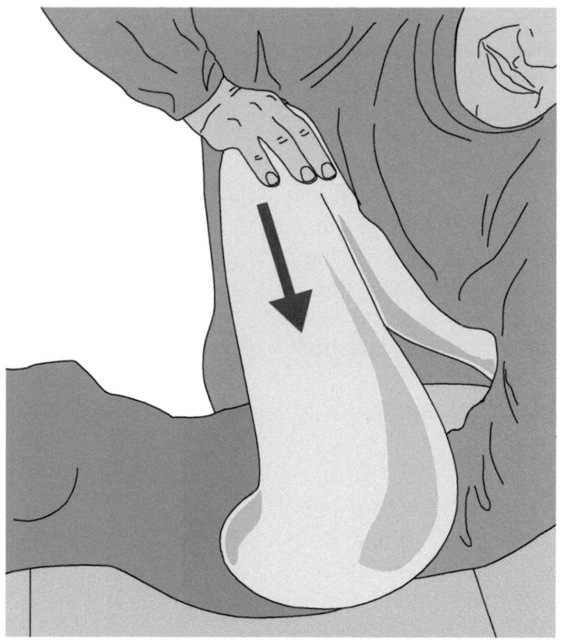

**Fig. 8.69** Provocation test for the iliolumbar ligament.

## 8.4.4 Vascular Supply

### Arterial Supply (Fig. 8.70)

The SIJ is supplied by various arteries. These all form anastomoses, which is why there are very few end-arteries.

#### *Internal Iliac Artery*

- This arises from the common iliac artery at the S1–S2 level.
- It gives off branches to the SIJ, especially to the middle portion of the joint.
- It passes into the lesser pelvis and divides into branches for the organs and other structures.

#### *Iliolumbar Artery*

- This arises from the internal iliac artery.
- It tracks posteriorly to the psoas major muscle and supplies it and other muscles in the area.
- It supplies the last motion segment (L5/S1) through the *lumbar branch* and thus gives off branches to the anterosuperior part of the SIJ.
- The *iliacus branch* supplies the iliacus and gluteal muscles.

#### *Superior Gluteal Artery*

- This is an end-artery of the internal iliac artery.
- It supplies the posterolateral and anteroinferior parts of the SIJ with a few branches.
- It runs through the suprapiriform foramen.
- The artery divides into branches for the gluteal muscles.

#### *Lateral Sacral Artery*

- This arises from the internal iliac artery.
- It supplies the middle and inferior parts of the SIJ.
- It forms anastomoses with the median sacral artery, which arises directly from the aorta at the L4 level.
- It runs through the anterior sacral foramina, supplying it and the sacral canal.

### Venous System

The arteries are accompanied by the veins with the same name. The venous system drains the sacral canal, the organs in the lesser pelvis, the SIJ, and other structures that are in the immediate vicinity. Some veins in the pelvic area do not have valves.

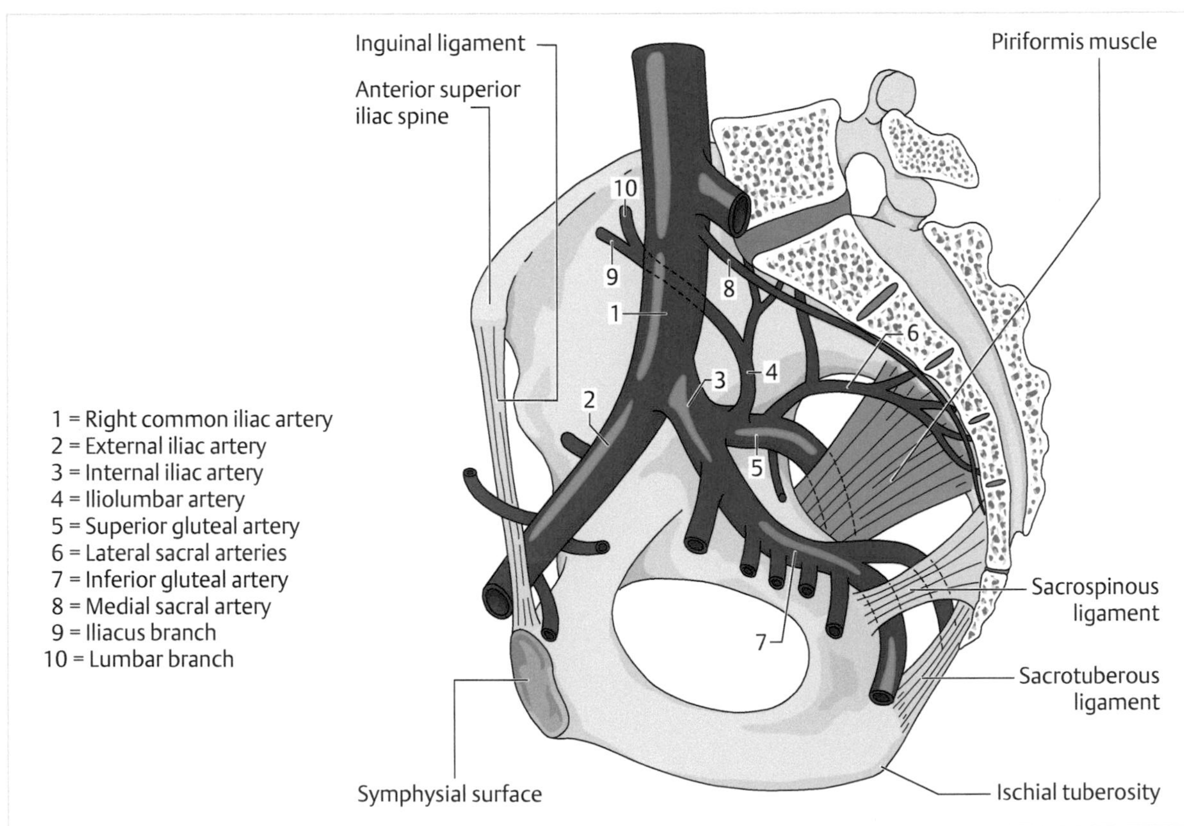


**Fig. 8.70** Arterial supply of the pelvis.

## 8.4.5 Innervation

The joint receives its innervation primarily from the S1 nerve root and possibly also from S2. In addition, the superior gluteal nerve (L4–L5) provides some branches to the joint.

The posterior branches of S2 and S3 give off branches to the posterior sacro-iliac ligaments. Some branches track to the origin of the gluteus maximus muscle. The S3–S4 segments supply the sacrotuberous and sacrospinous ligaments. Fortin et al (1999) describe many thick, myelinated fibers, implying an intensive density of receptors in the capsule–ligament apparatus.

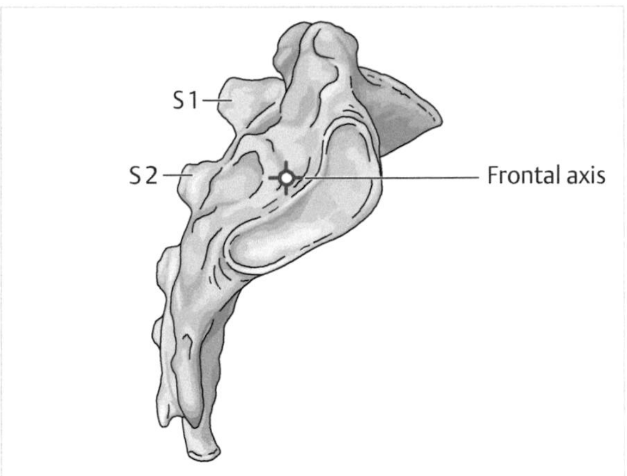


Fig. 8.71 Frontal axis of motion.

## 8.4.6 Axes of Motion

There are many different assertions about the location of the axes of motion. Most authors describe the intersection point of all the axes as being the S2 level in the area of the interosseous sacro-iliac ligament, or immediately posterior to the bend in the joint poles bilaterally.

### Frontal Axis (Frontotransverse Axis; Fig. 8.71)

This axis runs horizontally in the at the S2 level. Nutation and counternutation, also referred to as flexion and extension, occur around this axis.

### Longitudinal Axes (Fig. 8.72)

During walking, the sacrum rotates around this axis, which extends vertically in the standing position and divides the sacrum into right and left halves. A rotation movement occurs, although this is only minimal.

Two other longitudinal axes go through the SIJs.

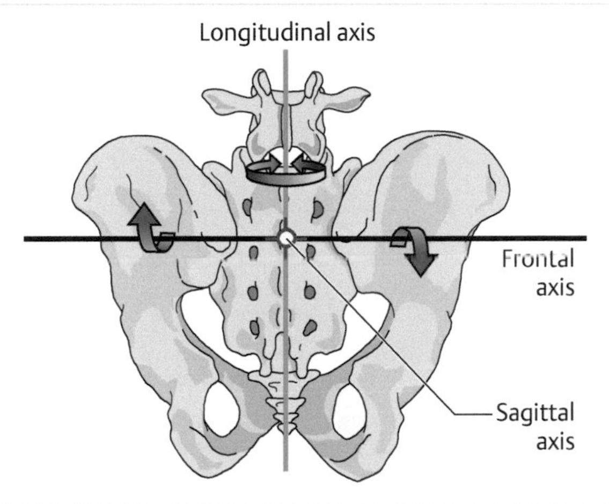


Fig. 8.72 Longitudinal, frontal, and sagittal axes.

## Diagonal Axes (Fig. 8.73)

Greenman (2004) describes, in addition to the horizontal axes, two diagonal axes extending through the sacrum, which are also known as axes of torsion. The right axis runs from the upper right pole to the lower left pole, i.e., from right superior and anterior to left inferior and posterior. The left axis goes from the left upper pole to the right lower pole. The torsion movement that occurs during walking takes place around these axes.

## Sagittal Axis (Sagittotransverse Axis; Fig. 8.73)

This extends from anterior to posterior through S2 and is the point of intersection of most of the axes. The sacrum is balanced around this axis. It is an axis about which lateral deflective deviations can occur. In this way, for example, the right side of the sacral base can be higher posteriorly as opposed to the left.

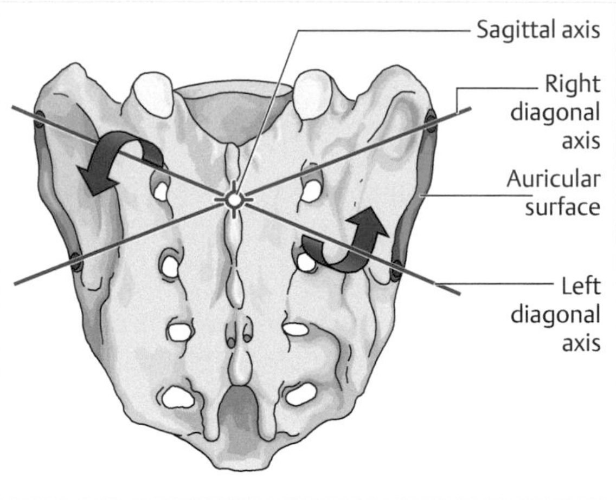


**Fig. 8.73** Diagonal and sagittal axes.

# 8.4.7 Movements

## Nutation

### Movements Involving the Sacrum (Fig. 8.74)

The promontory shifts anteriorly and inferiorly, and the apex of the sacrum in a posterior and superior direction. In the SIJ, a slightly curved slipping motion takes place in an inferior and posterior direction.

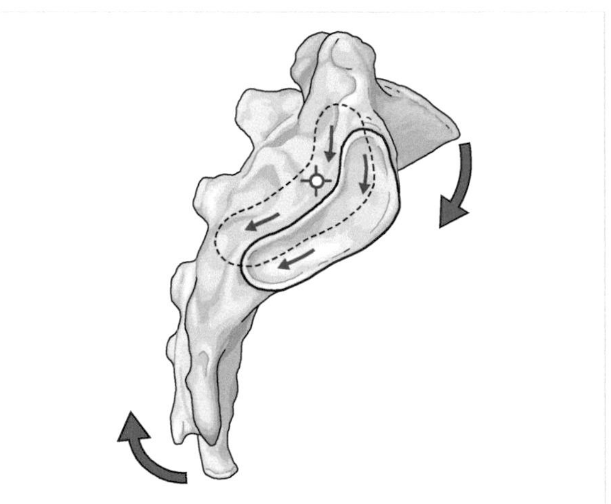

**Fig. 8.74** Nutation of the sacrum.

#### *Ongoing Movements*

The following movements take place continuously:

- Due to the increased tension in the superior posterior ligaments, the alae of the ilia converge, causing the ischial tuberosities to diverge = *inflare movement* (**Fig. 8.75**).
- This results in hyperlordosis of the lumbar spine.

#### *Factors that Limit the Nutation Movement*

Nutation is limited by the tension of sacrospinous and sacrotuberous ligaments and parts of the dorsal and ventral sacro-iliac ligaments. The inflare movement is restricted by the gluteus medius and minimus muscles and the medially running hamstring muscles.

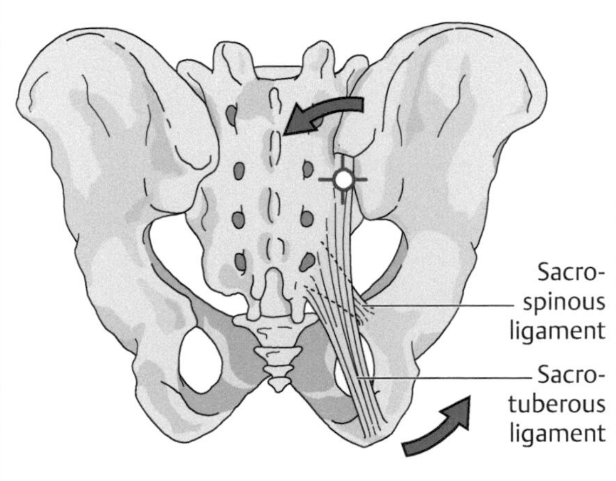


**Fig. 8.75** Inflare of the ilium.

### Movements Involving the Ilium (Fig. 8.76)

The movement of the ilium corresponds to an extension of the pelvis at the hip joints. In relation to the sacrum, the ilium moves in a posteroinferior direction, which is posterior rotation. In the SIJ, the ilium slides anterosuperiorly in relation to the sacrum.

**Practical Tip**

**Palpation of the Movements**

The movements of the ilium posteriorly can be easily palpated using the superior spines. The inflare movements can be felt at the tuberosities, which diverge, and on the upper edge of the crests, which converge.

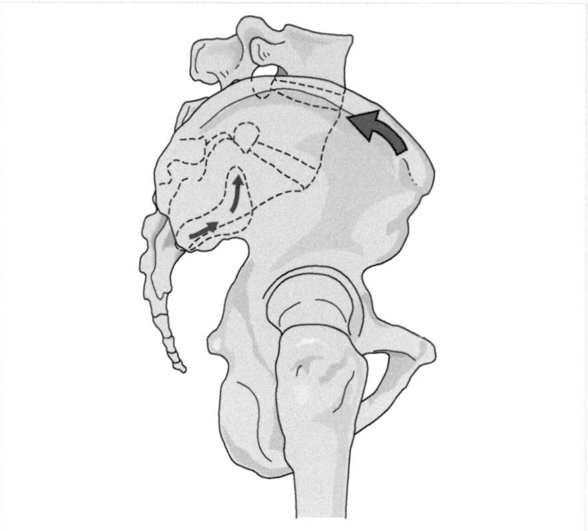

Fig. 8.76 Nutation of the ilium.

## Counternutation (Antinutation)

### Movements Involving the Sacrum (Fig. 8.77)

The promontory shifts posteriorly and superiorly, and the apex of the sacrum in an anterior and inferior direction. In the SIJ, a slipping motion takes place in an anterior and superior direction.

#### *Ongoing Movements*

- The alae of the ilia diverge while the ischial tuberosities converge = *outflare movement* (**Fig. 8.78**).
- Lordosis in the lumbar spine is decreased.

#### *Factors that Limit the Counternutation Movement*

Inferior portions of the posterior sacro-iliac ligaments and superior portions of the anterior sacro-iliac ligaments limit this movement.

The outflare movement is inhibited by the iliolumbar ligament, the upper adductors, the external rotators, and the quadratus lumborum muscle.

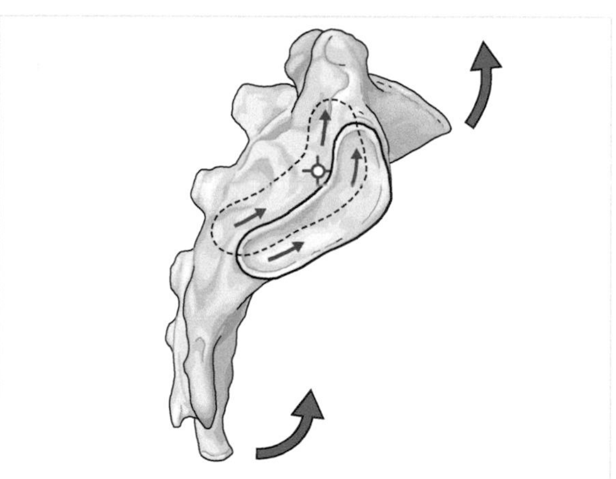

Fig. 8.77 Counternutation of the sacrum.

### Movements Involving the Ilium

The movement of the ilium corresponds to flexion of the pelvis at the hip joints. In relation to the sacrum, the ilium moves in an anteroinferior direction, which is anterior rotation. At the SIJ, the ilium slides inferior and posterior in relation to the sacrum.

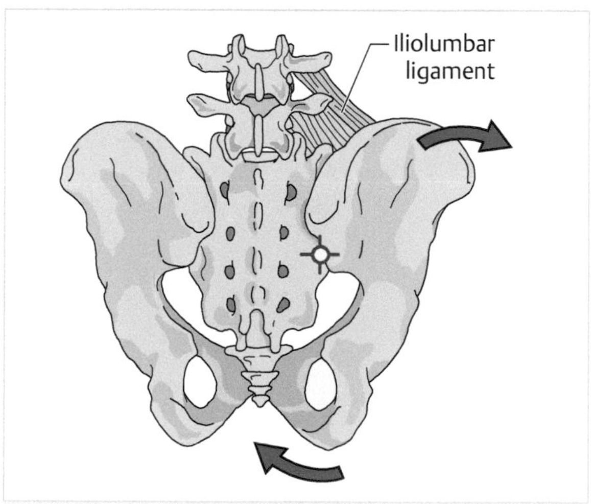


Fig. 8.78 Outflare of the ilium.

## Torsion (Combined Rotation–Lateral Flexion) (Fig. 8.79)

The movement of torsion is carried out primarily when walking. During the gait phase of *left heel strike*, the movement takes place around the right torsional axis, with the left hip bone rotating in a posterior direction, and the right anteriorly.

The sacral base simultaneously tilts to the right, which corresponds to a combined lateral flexion–rotation movement (torsion).

## Range of Motion

The extent of the movement is very small, and there are great individual differences. It is extremely difficult to make an accurate measurement of this complex mixture of movements.

However, the movements are palpable, so a movement around each axis of approximately 2° may be presumed. Active motion is not possible in this joint. Information about the SIJ can be gathered in terms of ongoing movement either from the posterior by way of pelvic and leg movements, or superiorly through the spinal column.

**Pathology**

### Blockage

Blockages in the SIJ can have various causes, such as static disorders during pregnancy and childbirth, reflexive projection of the internal organs, or the foot's suddenly encountering an unexpected step.

**Practical Tip**

### Examination of the SIJ

In the examination of SIJs in terms of a right–left comparison, it is important to remember that asymmetrical joint conditions, and thus differences in amount of joint play, are relatively common. Therefore the following criteria are important in the examination: asymmetrical anatomical landmarks, a significantly different end-feel, changes in the consistency of the tissues, and pain during provocation tests.

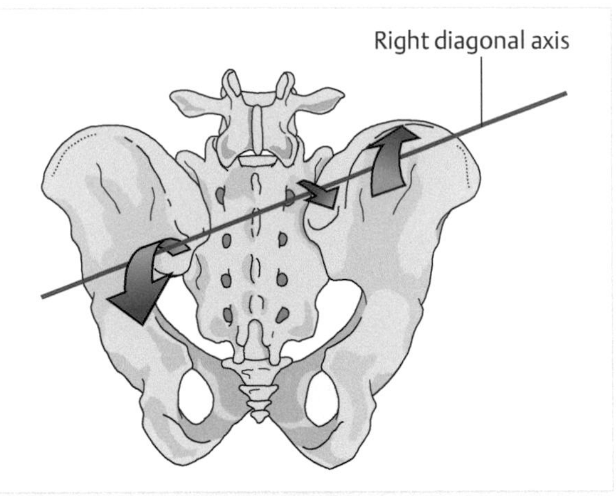


**Fig. 8.79** Movements around the right diagonal axis.

## Movement Tendencies in the Standing Position

### Weight on Both Legs (Fig. 8.80)

When standing on both legs, the tendency toward nutation is accentuated by the force effects from superiorly and posteriorly. The impact of the body weight is located in the anterior region of the base of the sacrum and pushes the promontory posteriorly, corresponding to a nutation motion.

The force that acts from posteriorly presses the pelvis over the femoral heads into an extension position. The axis of motion of the hip joint lies significantly anterior to the axis of the SIJ and pushes the ilium into a posterior position, which is equivalent to a nutation position in the SIJ.

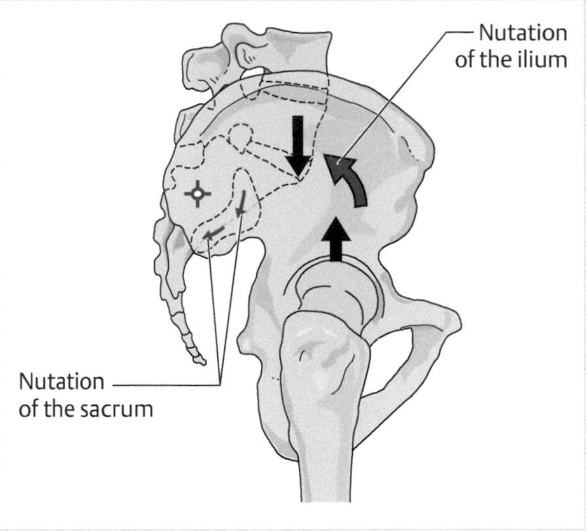


**Fig. 8.80** Tendency toward nutation in the standing position.

### Single-leg Stance (Fig. 8.81)

In the single-leg stance, there is an inflare of the ilium on the side of the supporting leg through the shift in center of gravity toward the supporting leg and a posterior rotation. In addition, the sacrum moves in the direction of nutation because of the body weight. On the side of the free leg, however, the ilium is in anterior rotation and sinks inferiorly.

The impact of the ground reaction force on the supporting leg side leads to a thrust of the ilium in a superior direction.

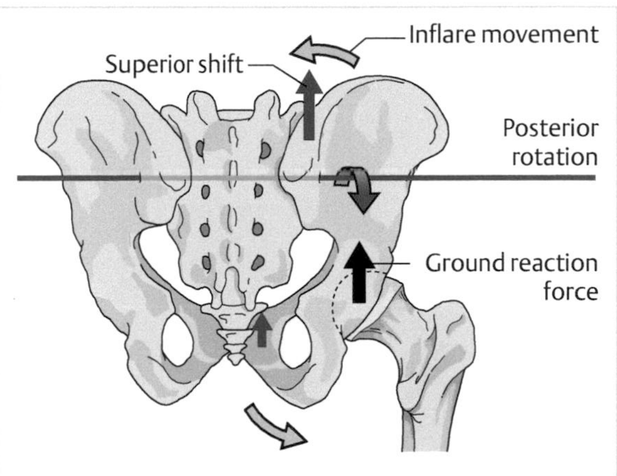


**Fig. 8.81** Movements with weight transfer to the right.

### Movements during Walking (Fig. 8.82)

While walking, minimal, constantly changing movements occur in the SIJs. In *stepping with the right leg*, the following successive movements take place (Greenman 1990):

- The right ilium moves posteriorly and rotates around the longitudinal axis to the left, and the left ilium moves anteriorly. In addition, there is a torsional motion around the left torsion axis, with inclination of the sacral base to the left.
- From the midstance phase, the right hip bone moves in an anterior direction, and the left hip bone in a posterior direction. The sacrum rotates to the right, and the base descends somewhat on this side.

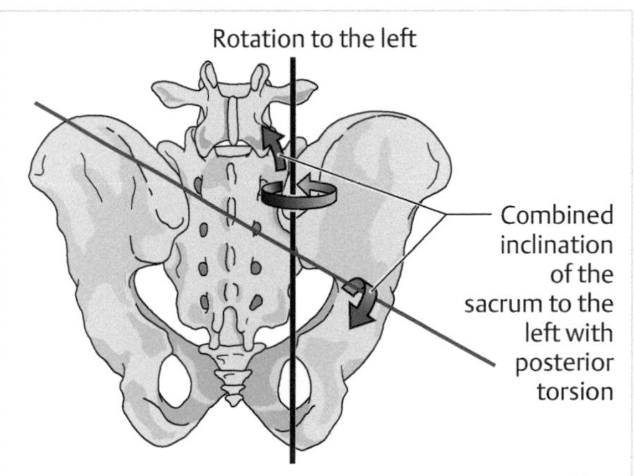


**Fig. 8.82** Movements of the pelvis when stepping out with the right leg.

## Muscles that Move the SIJ

### 1. Nutation

#### Erector Spinae Muscle

Its distal fibers run over and above S2 and thus cause an anterior movement of the sacral base.

#### Hamstring and Adductor Magnus Muscles (Fig. 8.83)

These draw the tuberosity inferiorly. This produces a posterior movement of the ilium relative to the sacrum.

#### Rectus Abdominis Muscle (Fig. 8.83)

This pulls the pubis superiorly and thereby produces a posterior movement of the ilium relative to the sacrum.

### 2. Inflare Movement

#### Quadratus Lumborum Muscle

This draws the ala of the ilium medially, which corresponds to an inflare movement.

#### Pectineus, Adductor Brevis and Adductor Longus Muscles

The sites of origin of these muscles lie below the pivot point; thus, they pull the pubis laterally.

#### Pelvitrochanteric Muscles

The external rotators pull the posterior section of the pelvis laterally.

### 3. Counternutation

#### Latissimus Dorsi Muscle (Fig. 8.84)

Its fibers at the origin, which pull the ilium, can move it anteriorly.

#### Sartorius, Tensor Fasciae Latae and Rectus Femoris Muscles, and the Adductor Muscles (Fig. 8.84)

These pull the pelvis anteriorly and inferiorly.

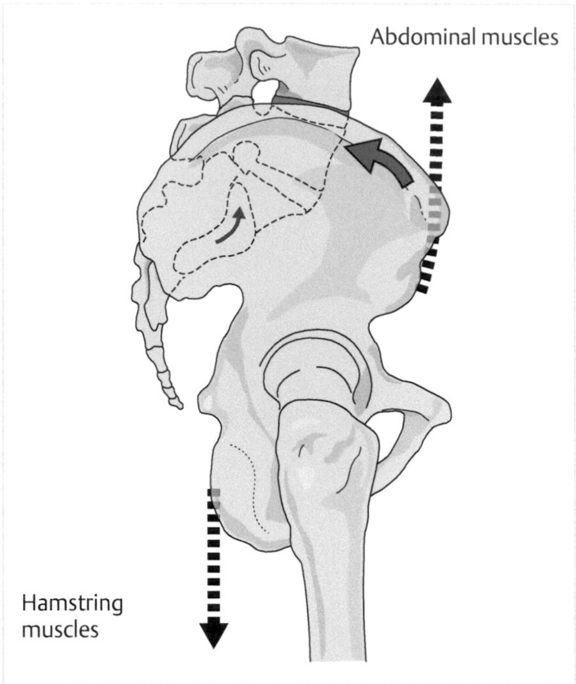


**Fig. 8.83** Nutation by muscle traction.

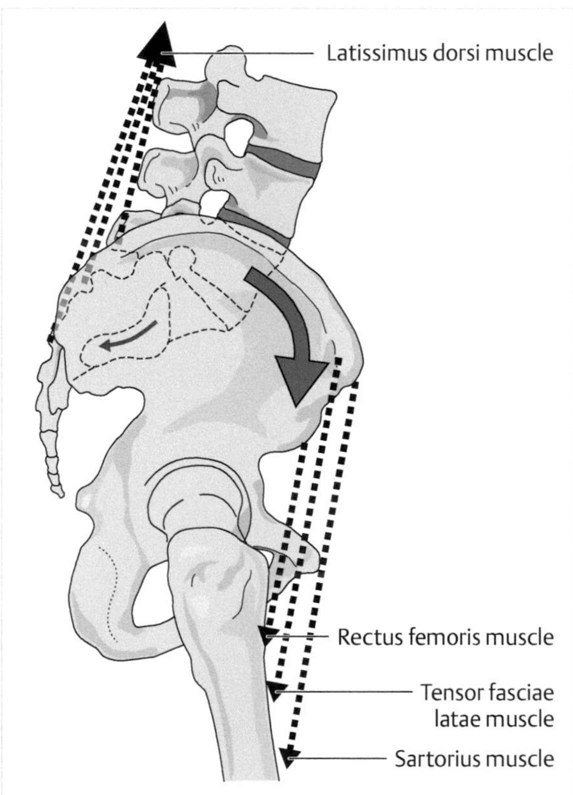


**Fig. 8.84** Counternutation by muscle traction.

## 4. Outflare Movement

### Gluteus Medius and Minimus Muscles and Superior Fibers of the Gluteus Maximus Muscle

These pull the ala of the ilium laterally.

### Semimembranosus and Semitendinosus Muscles

These pull the tuberosity medially.

▷ See Chapter 7.3, Lumbar Vertebrae, and Chapter 8.8, Muscles of the Pelvic and Hip Regions

**Practical Tip**

**Cause and Effect Chain**

1. A sudden application of force, such as in a badly executed jump, can cause the sacrum to become wedged in a position of nutation, causing a blockage to occur. Due to the pressure from posterior, the ilium gets into a *posterior position*. That means that the muscles lying anteriorly come under stress, which can lead to irritation at the insertion sites.

The following areas are predisposed to this:

- Tensor fasciae latae muscle at Gerdy's tubercle.
- Sartorius muscle at the pes anserinus.
- Rectus femoris muscle:
  - At the tibial tuberosity.
  - In patellar apex syndrome from an elevated level of the patella.
  - In chondromalacia patellae, caused by increased pressure in the femoropatellar joint and thereby recurrent joint effusions.

The effects can also be shown in the joints as follows:

- Hip joint: the acetabulum is proximal, and the leg becomes shorter. External rotation is produced by tension on the posterior fibers of the gluteal muscles.
- Knee joint: There is a tendency toward varus caused by compression in the medial aspect of the joint and overextension in the lateral aspect.
- Foot: The tibia is posterior, which means a limited dorsiflexion, a forefoot that is positioned in adduction/pronation, and a medial high arch.

However, this chain of cause and effect also shows that the cause of dysfunction in the SIJ can lie with each of these joints; for example, inversion trauma causes the fibula to be more proximal, which in turn stresses the biceps femoris muscle, causing the ilium to be posterior.

2. If the ilium is in an *anterior position*, it means that there is a strong pull on the hamstring muscles, which can lead to irritation, resulting in functional consequences at the following sites:

- Semimembranosus muscle at the medial meniscus (a tendency toward recurrent effusions).
- Sartorius muscle at the pes anserinus (pes anserine bursitis).
- Biceps femoris muscle:
  - This draws the fibula proximally, which causes tension in the fibularis longus muscle, which in turn rotates the cuboid medially.
  - The interosseous membrane is put under tension; the gaps for the vessels, such as the fibular and tibial arteries, are narrowed, causing a disturbance of blood circulation.

The consequences for the joints:

- Hip joint: The acetabulum becomes situated distally, which lengthens the leg. Tension is placed on the anterior fibers of the gluteal muscles, so that the hip goes into internal rotation.
- Knee joint: There is a tendency toward valgus, compression of the lateral joint space, and overstretching of the structures lying medially.
- Foot: The tibia is turned anteriorly, causing a limitation of plantar flexion. The forefoot is positioned in abduction and supination, and there is flattening of the medial arch of the foot.

## 8.4.8 Stabilizing Structures

### Fasciae (Fig. 8.85)

Because of its course over a joint, a fascia can help with stabilization. In the area around the SIJ, this occurs by interweaving the fibers coming from superior and posterior, which cross the SIJ diagonally and connect with each other.

### Thoracolumbar Fascia

This fascia has a thin fibrous structure in which longitudinally and transversely running fibers intertwine with each other. It consists of three layers:

- *Posterior layer:* This inserts on the spinous processes of the lumbar and sacral vertebrae and their supraspinous ligaments. It continues into the aponeuroses of the latissimus dorsi and serratus posterior inferior muscles, and tracks to the outer lip of the iliac crest and toward the sacrum.
- *Middle layer:* This tracks to the tips of the transverse processes of the lumbar vertebrae and their intertransverse ligaments. It is attached to the last rib and the iliac crest.
- *Anterior layer:* This inserts on the bases of the transverse processes of the lumbar vertebrae, the iliolumbar ligament, and the iliac crest. The erector spinae muscle tracks into the fascia from above and the abdominal muscles from laterally.

### Gluteal Fascia

This inserts on the iliac crest and crosses over the gluteus medius. Fascial fibers move into the muscle fiber bundles in the area of the gluteus maximus muscle. At the insertion site on the sacrum, the fibers intertwine with those of the thoracolumbar fascia.

### Fascia Lata

Portions of the fibers of this tract also pass over the gluteal fascia in the direction of the SIJ. This means that the thoracolumbar fascia uses the greater trochanter as a hypomochlion and arranges itself longitudinally in the lateral thigh area as part of the iliotibial tract.

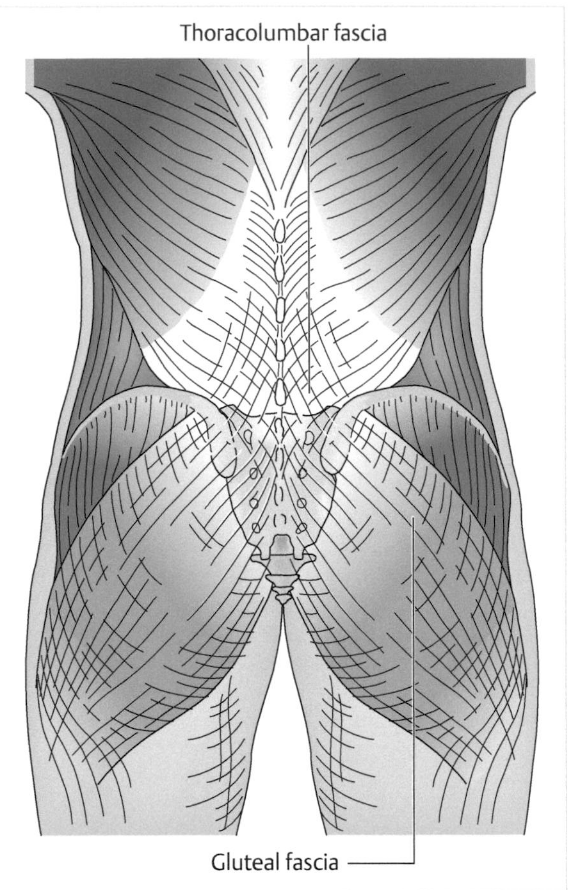


**Fig. 8.85** Stabilizing fasciae: thoracolumbar and gluteal fasciae.

## Ligaments

### Interosseous Sacro-Iliac Ligaments (Fig. 8.86a)

These have a very important stabilizing function because they lie directly posterior to the capsule and fill the entire sacral sulcus as a compact mass. These are short fibers, a portion of which is always tensed in all the different movements.

### Sacrotuberous and Sacrospinous Ligaments (Fig. 8.86b)

In the SIJ, the movement trends toward nutation. Therefore the strongest ligaments serve to stabilize the direction of this motion.

### Iliolumbar Ligaments

These stabilize the anterior SIJ area through their connection to the anterior sacro-iliac ligaments. With the help of the fibers that track to the ilium, they impede shifts to the posteroinferior.

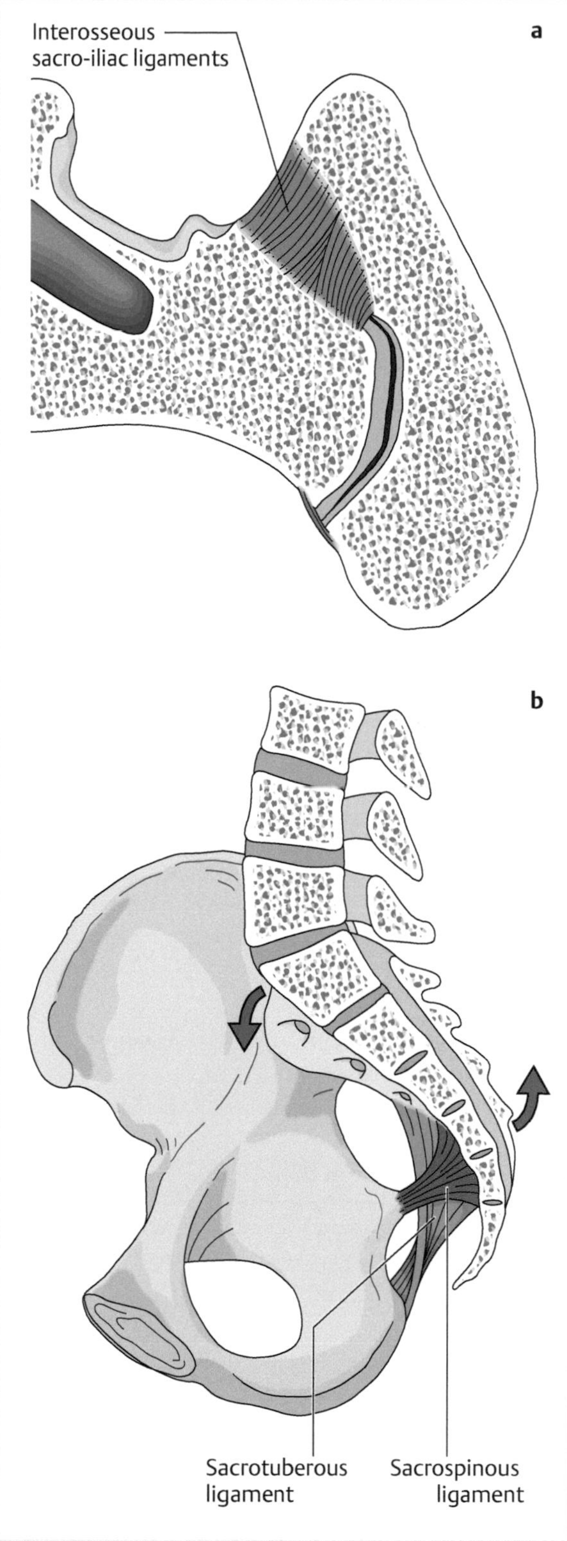


**Fig. 8.86** Stabilizing ligaments. **(a)** Interosseous sacro-iliac ligaments. **(b)** Nutation inhibitors: sacrotuberous and sacrospinal ligaments.

## Muscles

### Gluteus Maximus Muscle (Fig. 8.87)

This is the only muscle that passes posteriorly directly over the SIJ and thus helps to stabilize the joint. The fibers extend at approximately a right angle to the joint line, thus exerting a compressive force on the joint.

Through its connections superiorly to the thoracolumbar fascia, the ilium, the sacrum, the coccyx, and the sacrotuberous ligament, this muscle has a major influence on the pelvic ring.

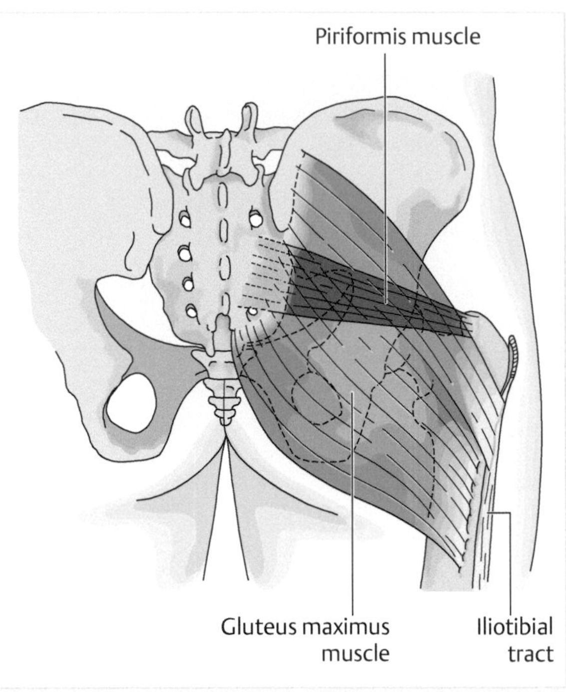


**Fig. 8.87** Stabilizing muscles: gluteus maximus and piriformis.

### Piriformis Muscle (Fig. 8.87)

Through its almost horizontal course, it pulls on the posterior portion of the joint and causes compression in the joint as it draws the sacrum toward the ilium.

### Erector Spinae Muscle

Most of the tendon fibers of the erector spinae muscles end at the level of the middle of the sacral sulcus; only a few longer fibers extend to the apex of the sacrum. These intertwine with the sacrotuberous ligament.

**Practical Tip**

**Examination of Joint Play and Muscles**

Several factors can influence the mobility of the SIJ. Various tests should be performed to assess whether the malfunction lies in the joint play or in the muscles. To check for joint play, the joint's ability to slide is evaluated by fixing one joint partner and mobilizing the other. The affected muscles are examined in terms of elasticity and strength.

**Muscle Training in Terms of SIJ Instability**

When the SIJ is unstable, the gluteus maximus, erector spinae, and piriformis muscles need to be rehabilitated. Since strength training of these muscles often involves repetitive movement of the SIJ, which is contraindicated, the pelvic ring must be passively stabilized. A pelvic-support belt, worn at the level of the greater trochanter, fulfills this function, after which the training program can be safely carried out.

## 8.4.9 Connection between the Sacrum and Cranium (Fig. 8.88)

The sacrum and coccyx represent the inferior end of the craniosacral system. The dura mater is attached circumferentially to the foramen magnum, and the anterior spinal dura mater is attached at the level of C2 and C3. An anterior dural attachment is found again only at the level of S2 and posteriorly at the coccyx.

The spinal dura is at least partially elastic, so positional changes in the pelvic region have consequences for the cranium, and conversely changes in the cranium influence the pelvic region.

### Pathology

Dysfunctions, triggered by birth or trauma, can influence the inferior portion of the spine via the cranial region and vice versa. For example, if an occipital condyle shifts anteriorly and superiorly, the sacrum will shift posteriorly and superiorly on the same side and anteriorly and inferiorly on the contralateral side.

### Practical Tip

**Approach to Treatment**

In handling a functional disturbance in the SIJ, the upper cervical spine and the skull should always be examined and treated, because only then can a balance of activity between the skull and the pelvis be provided.

In addition, it is important to harmonize all the diaphragms lying between the skull and pelvis—the floor of the mouth with the suprahyoid muscles, the cervicothoracic diaphragm (thoracic inlet) at the level of the first rib, the thoracolumbar diaphragm, and the pelvic diaphragm.

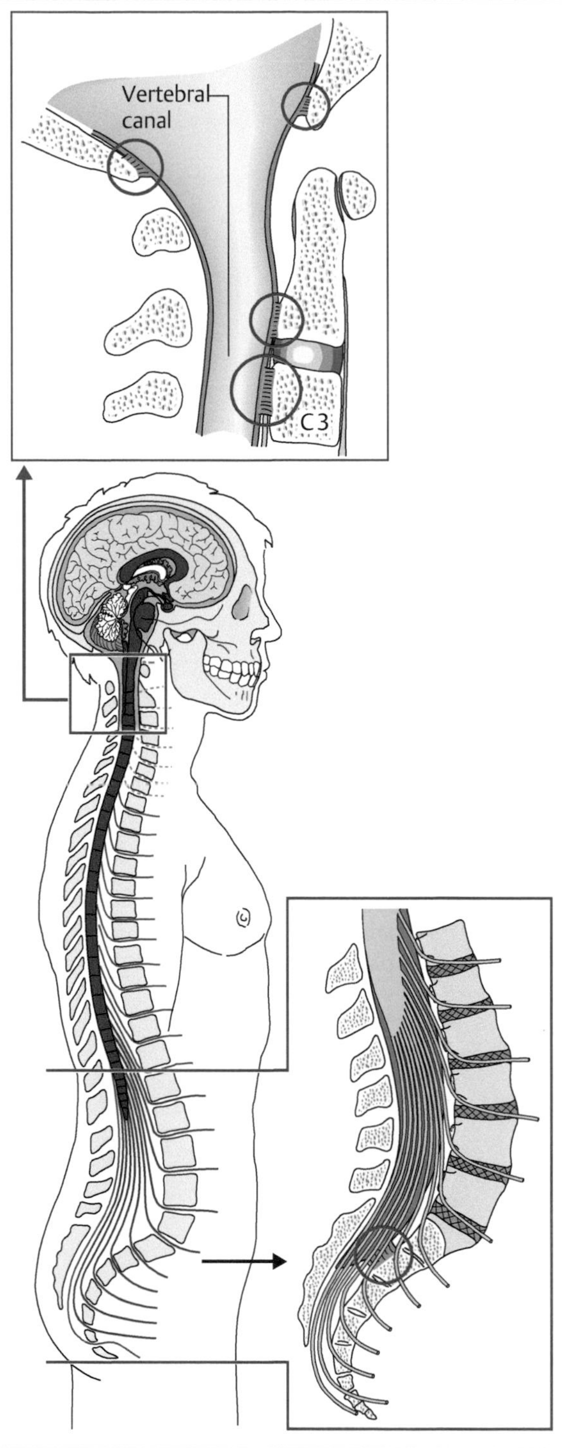


**Fig. 8.88** Connection from sacrum to cranium.

# 8.5 Pubic Symphysis (Fig. 8.89)

## 8.5.1 Articular Surfaces

The articular surfaces of the pubis are flat and oval-shaped with a very thin hyaline cartilage layer.

The *interpubic disk*, composed of fibrocartilage, is adherent to the cartilage-covered articular surface. A longitudinal cleft in the middle forms the *articular cavity*, a synovial fluid-filled space. The disk is wider anteriorly than posteriorly, and it adjusts to the variable pressure and tensile loads by the orientation of its collagen fibers.

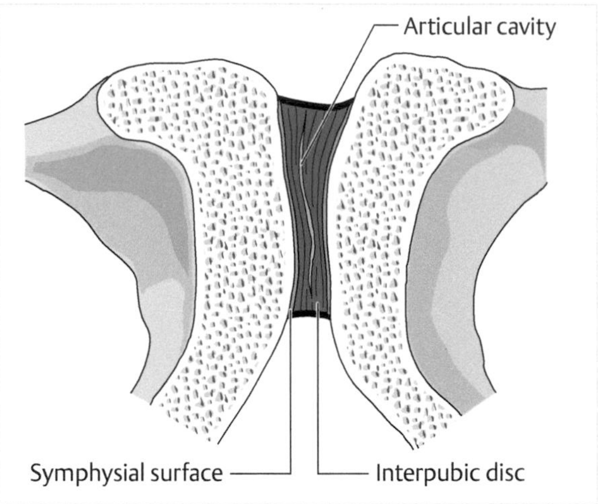


**Fig. 8.89** Pubic symphysis (frontal section, anterior view).

## 8.5.2 Axes of Motion and Movements

The symphysis is part of the articular movement chain of the pelvis. That means that movements of the pelvis always affect the pubic symphysis and vice versa.

### Axes (Fig. 8.90)

There are three axes around which the movements take place:

- Sagittal axis.
- Frontal axis.
- Longitudinal axis.

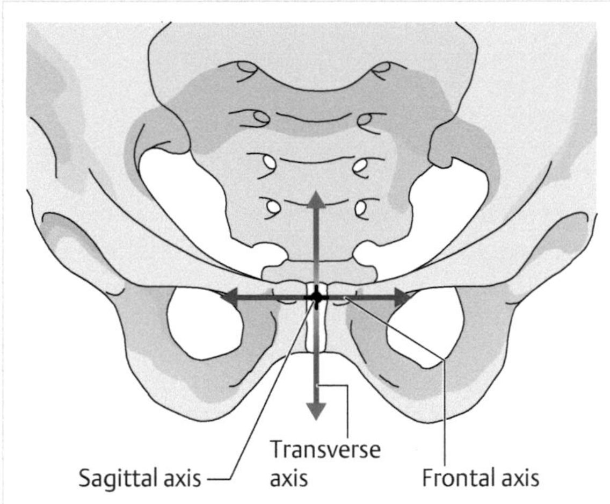


**Fig. 8.90** Axes of the pubic symphysis.

### Directions and Extent of Movement

The pubic symphysis is an amphiarthrosis. During walking, thrust and rotational movements occur. On the side of the supporting leg, the symphysis moves superiorly by approximately 1 to 2 mm and follows the movement of the ilium in posterior rotation. This rotation is 2 mm in women but much less in men. On the swing leg side, the pubis sinks.

## 8.5.3 Ligaments

The ligaments are fused with the disk.

### Anterior Pubic Ligament (Fig. 8.91 a)

This ligament lies anteriorly and consists of transverse fiber tracts that are strengthened by superficial oblique and longitudinal fibers. These fibers are formed from the aponeuroses of the external oblique, rectus abdominis, and pyramidalis muscles, and from the adductor longus and gracilis muscles.

### Posterior Pubic Ligament (Fig. 8.91 a)

This is a thin, wide ligament in the posterior region.

### Superior Pubic Ligament (Fig. 8.91 b)

This extends from one pubic tubercle to the other and combines with fibers of the inguinal ligament.

### Inferior Pubic Ligament (Fig. 8.91 b)

The ligament runs in the pubic arch inferior to the joint.

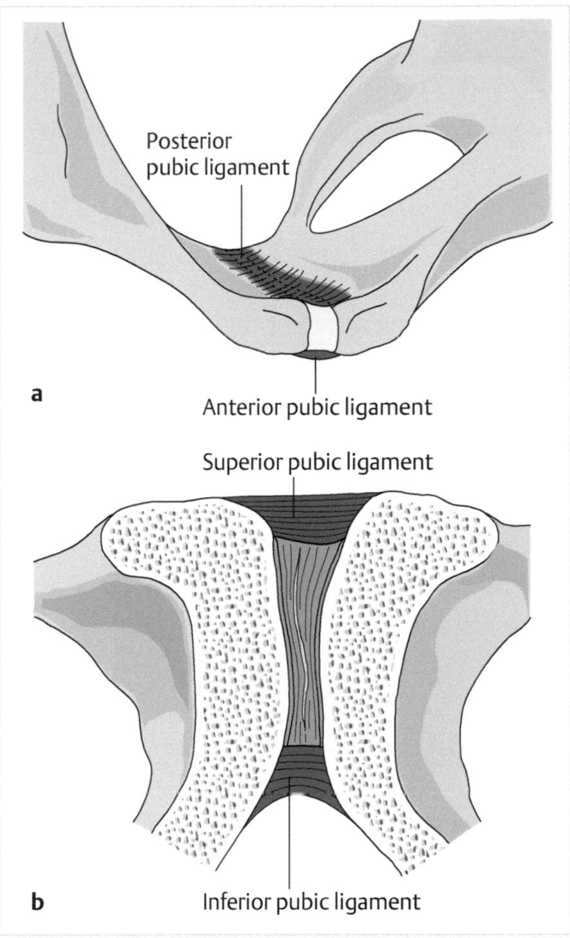


**Fig. 8.91** Ligaments of the pubic symphysis. **(a)** Posterior and anterior pubic ligaments. **(b)** Superior and inferior pubic ligaments.

## 8.5.4 Stabilizing Muscles

### Abdominal Muscles

The external oblique, rectus abdominis, and pyramidalis muscles track into the ligaments from above.

### Adductors

The pectineus and adductor longus muscles enter into a connection with the anterior ligament.

**Practical Tip**

**Examination**

When there is dysfunction in the pubic area, the following evaluation should be performed:

- Palpation of the abdominal muscles and the adductors with regard to their state of tension and trigger points.
- Palpation of the inguinal ligament with regard to pain and changes in tension.
- Examination to see if one pubis is higher than the other.
- An assessment of movement symmetry while the patient pushes the legs outward and during movements of the hip joint.

**Loosening of the Pubic Symphysis (Pubic Symphysis Diastasis)**

Typical symptoms of pubic symphysis diastasis include painful hypermobility during hip movements, especially with abduction, and pain in the area of the symphysis when walking that radiates toward the groin and lumbar region. Intensive strengthening of the surrounding muscles and the use of external stabilization in the form of a pelvic support belt can make the patient symptom-free.

# 8.6 Sacrococcygeal Joint

## 8.6.1 Articular Surfaces

The articular surfaces are flat with an embedded disk.

## 8.6.2 Ligaments

### Posterior Sacrococcygeal Ligament (Fig. 8.92)

The deep and superficial parts of the ligament are superficial structures running along the median sacral crest on the posterior side.

### Interarticular Sacrococcygeal Ligament (Fig. 8.92)

This ligament has short fiber tracts that extend posteriorly over the joint.

### Lateral Sacrococcygeal Ligament (Fig. 8.92)

This connects the transverse processes with the inferior angle of the sacrum. The coccygeal nerve runs between this ligament and the bone.

### Anterior Sacrococcygeal Ligament (Fig. 8.93)

This ligament is virtually the continuation of the anterior longitudinal ligament, but split into two parts. The fibers cross each other at the level of the third to fourth coccygeal vertebrae.

### Intercoccygeal Ligament (Fig. 8.93)

This ligament connects the inferior part of the coccyx with the lateral process.

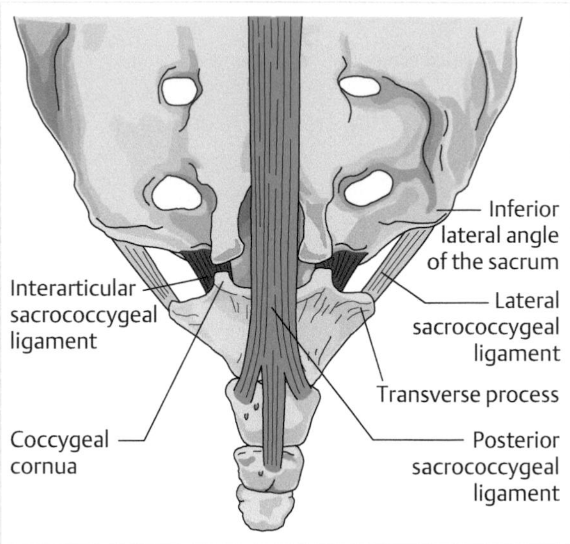


**Fig. 8.92** Posterior ligaments of the sacrococcygeal joint.

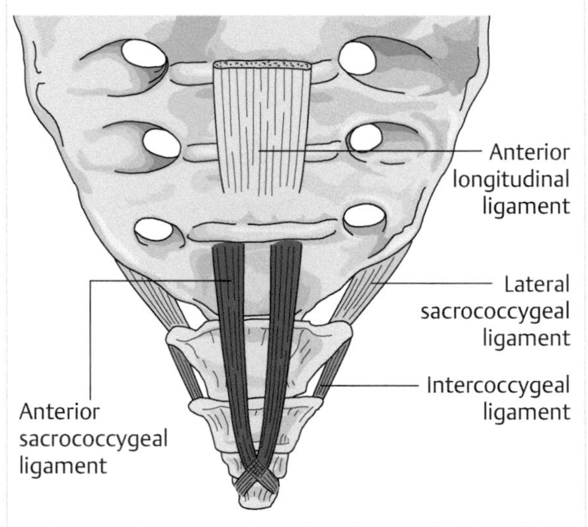


**Fig. 8.93** Anterior ligaments of the sacrococcygeal joint.

### 8.6.3 Axes of Motion and Movements

Flexion and extension occur around the horizontal axis. As a synchondrosis, only limited movements are possible. The coccyx follows the movements of the sacrum.

### 8.6.4 Stabilizing Muscles

The following muscles play a role in stabilizing the joint:
- Levator ani muscle.
- Ischiococcygeus muscle.
- Gluteus maximus muscle.

**Pathology**

Dysfunction of the coccyx almost always occurs in an anterior direction; the following are possible causes:
- Birth trauma.
- Dysfunction of the spinal column.
- A fall on the coccyx.
- Head trauma.

**Practical Tip**

**Treatment after Trauma**

When a fall occurs causing injury to the coccyx, this bends anteriorly and causes pain in the posterior gluteal region, which is aggravated by prolonged sitting or bearing down (e.g., during defecation). The point at which the coccyx is bent can be palpated when examining the anal fold area. Treatment per rectum is required, with relaxation of the ischiococcygeus muscle and the ligaments, followed by decompression of the sacrococcygeal joint and repositioning of the coccyx back into place.

# 8.7 Hip Joint

## 8.7.1 Articular Surfaces

### Acetabulum (Fig. 8.94)

The acetabulum is made up of the three parts of the hip bone:

- Superior: ilium.
- Anterior: pubis.
- Inferior: ischium.

The triradiate cartilage closes between the 14th and 16th year of life and forms the concave joint socket. The outer bony rim is called the *acetabular margin*. It is oriented in an anterior-lateral-inferior direction. This orientation can be seen in the frontal section on the basis of the acetabular inlet plane of 40°, and in the transverse section by means of the anteversion angle of 10 to 15°. It does not completely enclose the head of the femur.

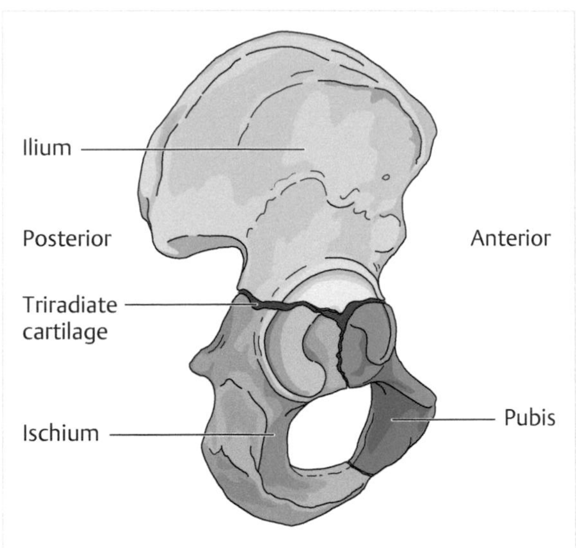


**Fig. 8.94** Acetabulum: triradiate cartilage.

### Acetabular Labrum (Fig. 8.95)

The labrum is a triangularly shaped structure composed of firm connective tissue and fibrocartilage. It encircles the acetabulum like a ring and is fixed to the base of the margin, while the tip extends into the joint. Superiorly and posteriorly, it is approximately 1 cm wide; anteriorly and inferiorly, it is 0.5 cm. It serves to increase the size of joint socket and can deform during movement.

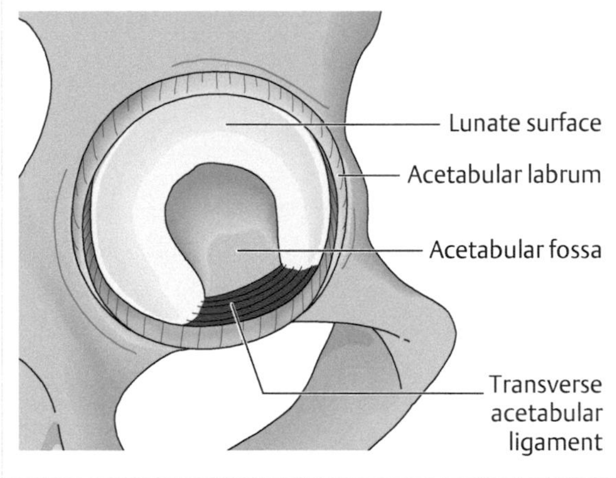


**Fig. 8.95** Acetabular labrum.

### Acetabular Notch (Fig. 8.96)

The notch is a distinct indentation in the lower acetabular margin and represents the interface between the pubis and ischium. The *transverse acetabular ligament* passes over it.

### Lunate Surface (Fig. 8.96)

This crescent-shaped articular surface of the acetabulum is covered with cartilage. It runs posteriorly and anteriorly, and has a horn at each end. The cartilage is thicker in the middle section, especially on the anterolateral acetabular roof, where it is approximately 3 mm thick, than it is on the anterior and posterior horns.

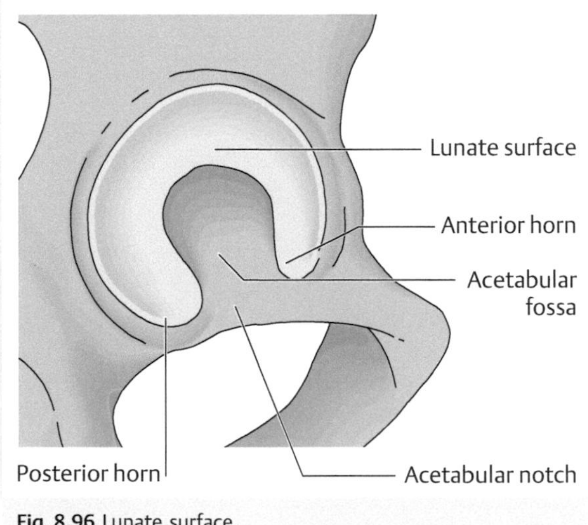


**Fig. 8.96** Lunate surface.

### Acetabular Fossa (Fig. 8.97)

The fossa is a depression of 3 to 4 mm at the medial edge of the lunate surface. It is filled with loose, fatty connective tissue, the *acetabular fat pad*, and the *ligament of the head of the femur*. This fat pad compensates for the difference in level from the surrounding cartilage-covered surface. The cavity provides a small amount of vacuum, which contributes to stability of the joint. The transverse acetabular ligament closes the space on the inferior side.

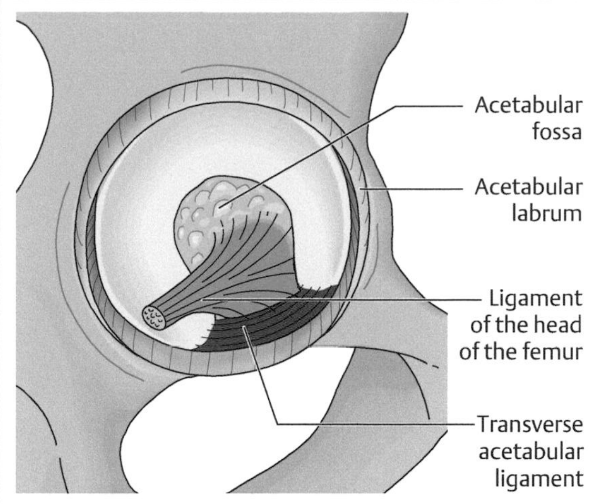


**Fig. 8.97** Acetabular fossa.

## Head of the Femur (Fig. 8.98)

The head is spherical and forms the articulating joint surfaces of the femur.

### Fovea for the Ligament of the Head of the Femur

The fovea is a depression in the posterior-inferior quadrant. It is not covered with cartilage and forms the insertion area for the ligament of the head of the femur.

### Cartilage-Covered Surfaces

With a thickness of 4 mm, the strongest cartilage layer lies superior to the fovea. It is significantly thinner inferomedially, where the surface is narrower and forms an uneven border with the femoral neck. The surface is divided into four quadrants.

The area of contact with the lunate surface changes depending on the position of the joint. Only a portion of the cartilage-covered surface of the femoral head has contact with the entire lunate surface. In adduction, for example, the contact point shifts so far medially that the inner rim of the lunate surface reaches the cartilaginous rim of the fovea.

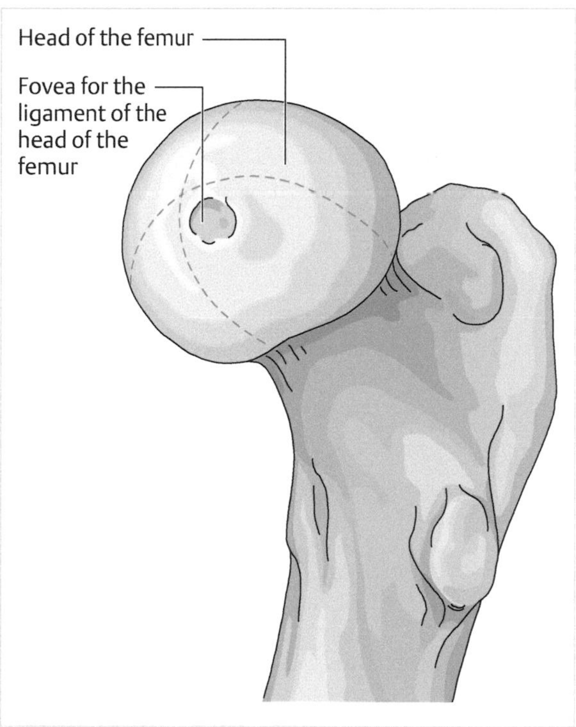


**Fig. 8.98** Head of the femur (posteromedial view).

**Pathology**

**Cartilage Preservation Zones**

The articular cartilage is preserved only where it undergoes repeated elastic compressive stresses through intermittent compressive forces, which must lie within a certain range of physiologic magnitude. In the long run, this means that the articular cartilage remains only in those surface areas in which the transmission of forces takes place within certain tolerance limits.

**Practical Tip**

In the early stages of osteoarthritis, an important goal of treatment is to promote nutrition of the cartilage and joint through graded functional training involving positions that load and unload the joint utilizing the entire range of motion.

## Femoral Structures Near the Joint (Figs. 8.99 and 8.100)

### *Neck of the Femur*

- This connects the head to the shaft.
- It merges into the intertrochanteric line anteriorly and distally, and into the intertrochanteric crest posteriorly.

### *Greater Trochanter*

- It is an apophysis.
- It acts as the insertion site for muscles.
- The trochanteric fossa lies medial to it.

### *Lesser Trochanter*

- This lies medial to the intertrochanteric line.
- It is the insertion site for the iliopsoas muscle.

### *Intertrochanteric Line*

This is an anterior line running from one trochanter to the other.

### Intertrochanteric Crest

This ridge connects the two trochanters posteriorly.

### Trochanteric Fossa

The fossa is a depression located posteromedial to the greater trochanter.

### *Linea Aspera*

- This is a longitudinally oriented ridge on the posterior aspect of the femoral shaft.
- It serves as the insertion for many muscles.

### *Gluteal Tuberosity*

- The gluteal tuberosity acts as the insertion site for the gluteus maximus muscle.
- It lies as a superior extension of the linea aspera.

### *Pectineal Line*

- This is the insertion site for the pectineus muscle.
- It is an anterior extension of the linea aspera toward the lesser trochanter.

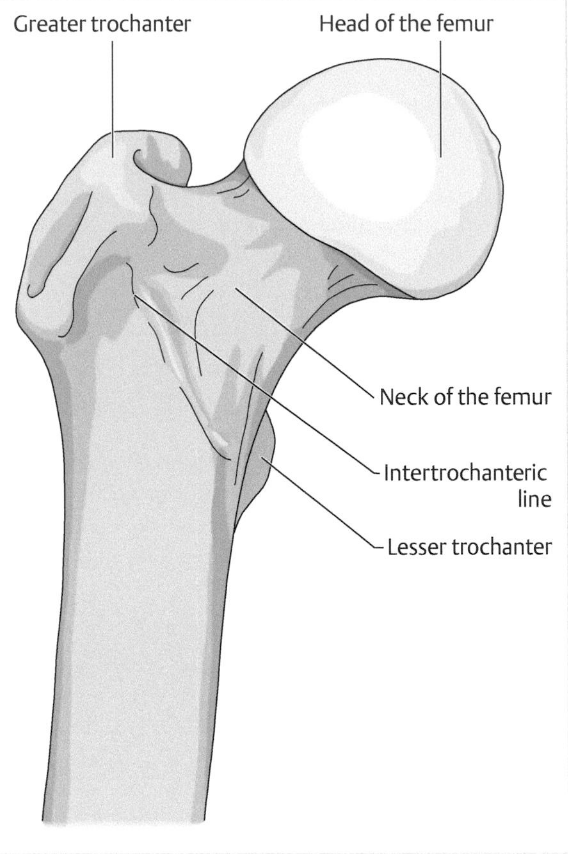


**Fig. 8.99** Proximal femur (anterior view).

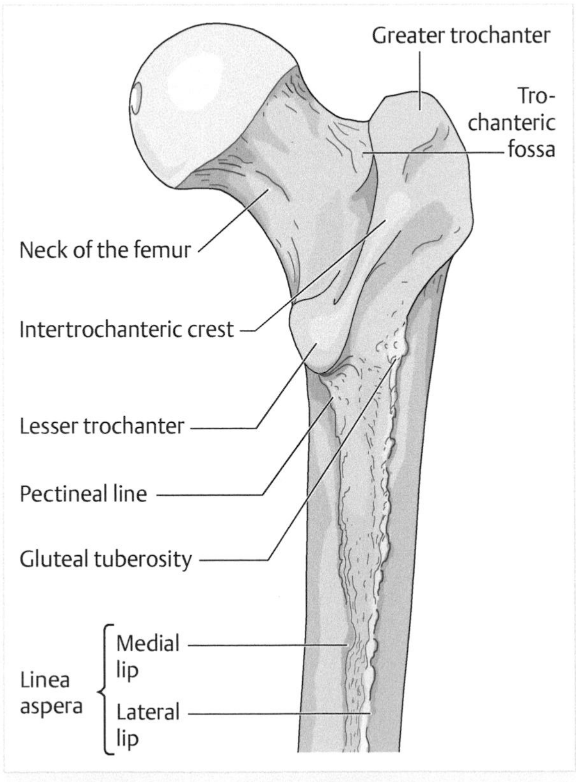


**Fig. 8.100** Proximal femur (posterior view).

## 8.7.2 Joint Capsule

### Fibrous Layer (Figs. 8.101 and 8.102)

The fibrous layer is a firm, thick-walled membrane. It consists of fibril bundles oriented in various directions, running, for example, longitudinally and diagonally. The firm, collagenous fiber content makes up approximately 70 to 80% of this, and the elastic component approximately 5%.

It inserts on the bony rim of the acetabulum, the transverse acetabular ligament, and anteriorly on the femur along the intertrochanteric line. Posteriorly, it attaches to the femoral neck approximately 1 cm medial to the intertrochanteric crest, which, along with the trochanteric fossa, remains outside the joint.

The fibrous layer has many receptors that provide the central nervous system with information on positions, movements, and deviations.

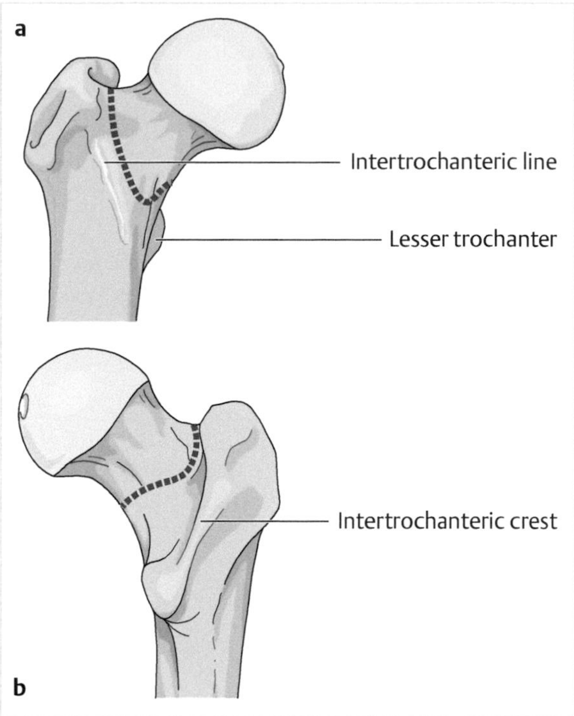


**Fig. 8.101** Insertion of the fibrous layer. **(a)** On the anterior femur. **(b)** On the posterior femur.

## Synovial Membrane (Fig. 8.102)

The synovial membrane inserts on the outer edge of the base of the acetabular labrum and leaves the tapered edge of the labrum to protrude into the joint space. This creates a small annular recess between the capsule and labrum, the *perilimbic recess*. Only inferiorly does the synovial membrane arise from the tip of the labrum.

The synovial membrane inserts anteriorly on the femur at the bone–cartilage junction, forming small outpouchings. Posteriorly it inserts 1.5 cm proximal to the intertrochanteric crest. Around the neck of the femur, especially laterally, medially, and anteriorly, it forms synovial folds, the *frenula capsulae*. These run from the insertion on the femoral neck to the bone–cartilage junction of the femoral head, and direct vessels toward the head of the femur; en route, these vessels supply the femoral neck with blood. The membrane forms a tube that enfolds the ligament of the head of the femur. It originates at the base of the acetabulum, thus closing the joint at the acetabular notch and fossa (**Fig. 8.103**).

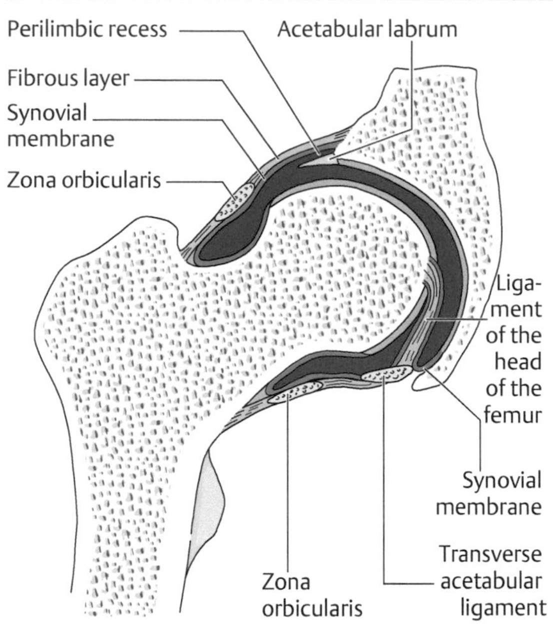


**Fig. 8.102** Synovial membrane (the femoral head has been extracted from the acetabulum for better representation).

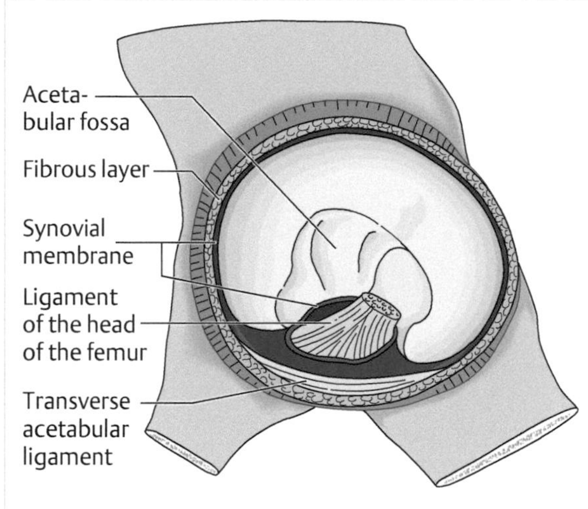


**Fig. 8.103** Synovial membrane on the ligament of the head of the femur.

### Pathology

#### Capsule Patterns

If the entire capsule is irritated, as in osteoarthritis, each joint has its own characteristic pattern of movement limitations that affects the sequence of movements and the degree to which they can be performed. For the hip joint, the capsule pattern is internal rotation/extension → abduction → flexion.

#### Total Hip Replacement

In a total hip replacement, part of the capsule–ligament apparatus is removed. This means that an important part of the regulatory mechanism for static and dynamic functions is missing.

## 8.7.3 Ligaments

A distinction is made between intra-articular and extra-articular ligaments.

### Intra-Articular Ligaments (Fig. 8.104)

#### Ligament of the Head of the Femur

The ligament of the head of the femur is also known as the round ligament of the femur (ligamentum teres femoris). It is approximately 3 cm long and 1 cm wide, lies within the capsule with a flat profile, and is enfolded by a synovial membrane.

Fiber bundles track from the anterior and posterior horns of the lunate surface and the upper margin of the transverse acetabular ligament to the acetabular fossa. The ligament carries the acetabular branch of the obturator artery and provides the blood supply to the head of the femur (see **Fig. 8.112**).

It is tensed by flexion/adduction/external rotation.

#### Transverse Acetabular Ligament

This ligament bridges the acetabular notch and thus supports the femoral head from the inferior side. Its outer layer connects the ends of the labra, and the inner layer connects the horns of the lunate surface. It is approximately 1 cm wide.

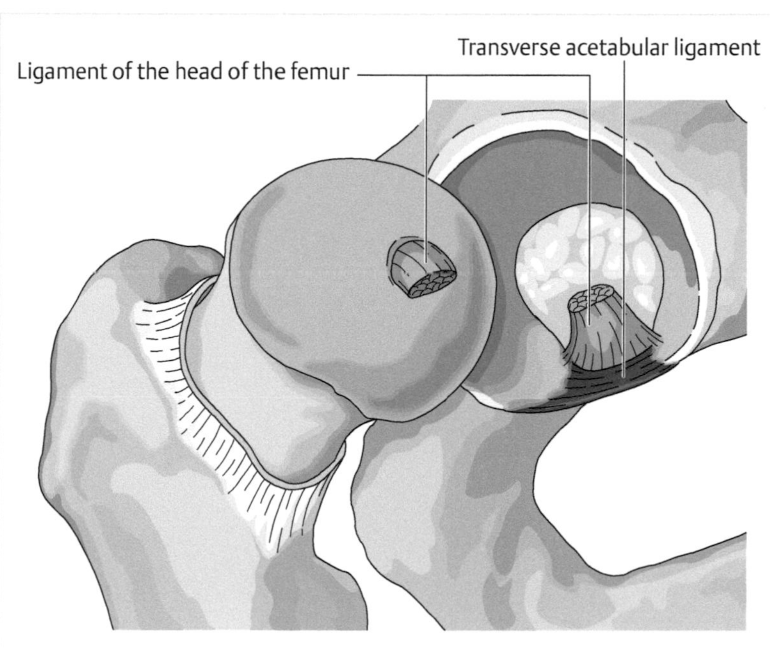


**Fig. 8.104** Intra-articular ligaments: ligament of the head of the femur and transverse acetabular ligament.

## Extra-Articular Ligaments (Fig. 8.105)

### Iliofemoral Ligament

The iliofemoral ligament is a V-shaped ligament. The tip of the **V** lies below the anterior inferior iliac spine, where it merges with the rectus femoris muscle. The insertion is along the intertrochanteric line:

- *Transverse part:* The upper band (Bertini's ligament) runs transversely and is the strongest ligament in the human body. It is up to 1 cm thick. Its tensile strength is 350 kg.
- *Descending part:* The lower, thin band, tracks to the lower half of the intertrochanteric line. The fibers run helically. On the right hip, they turn to the left, and on the left hop, they turn to the right. During external rotation, this part of the ligament untwists and thus relaxes.

### Pubofemoral Ligament

The pubofemoral ligament runs from the iliopubic eminence and the obturator crest, where it intertwines with the tendon of the pectineus muscle, to the inferior part of the intertrochanteric line. Here it intertwines with the iliofemoral ligament. It has a connection to the joint capsule and the zona orbicularis.

On the anterior side, the iliofemoral and pubofemoral ligaments form the *Welcker-Z*, with the following components:

- The transverse part of the iliofemoral ligament.
- The descending part of the iliofemoral ligament.
- The pubofemoral ligament.

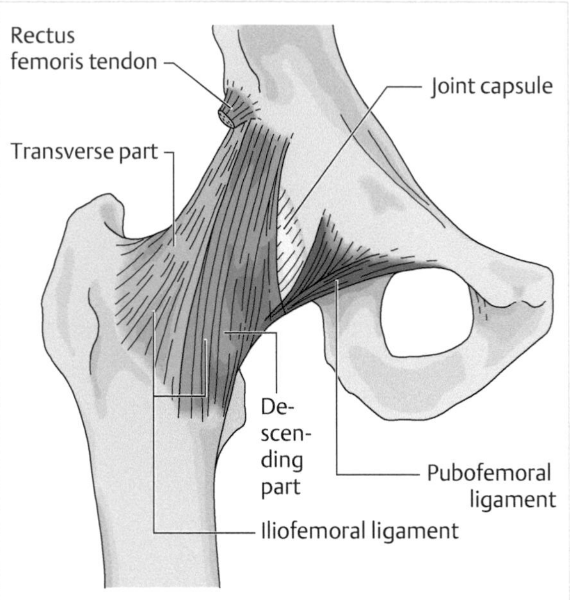


**Fig. 8.105** Anterior extra-articular ligaments: iliofemoral and pubofemoral ligaments.

### Iliopectineal Bursa (Fig. 8.106)

Between the iliofemoral and pubofemoral ligaments, the capsule wall is thin; this is where the iliopectineal bursa lies over the capsule. It communicates with the joint cavity in 10 to 15% of cases. It is oblong and can reach as far as the lesser trochanter. The tendons of the iliopsoas muscle run over it.

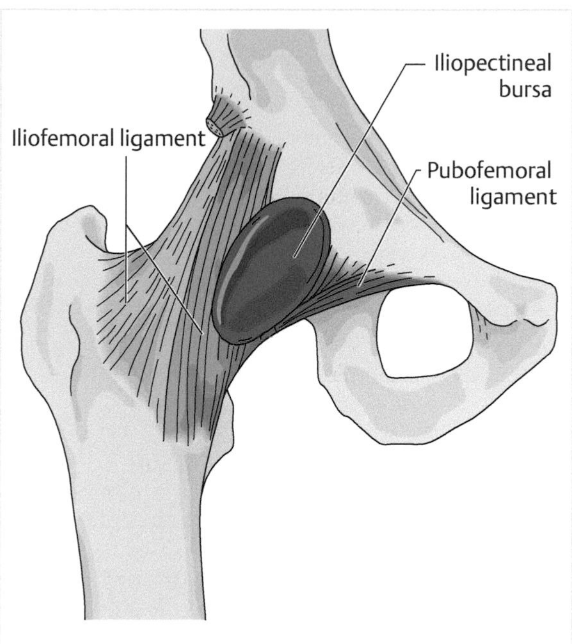


Fig. 8.106 Iliopectineal bursa.

**Pathology**

As the result of inflammation (purulent bursitis) from an underlying infection, the bursa can cause pain on movement, especially when the iliopsoas muscle is contracted.
Changes in static body posture can also cause bursitis, which can sometimes become chronic because it relates to recurrent irritation.

### Ischiofemoral Ligament (Fig. 8.107)

The ischiofemoral ligament has its origin on the posterior, inferior margin of the acetabulum and the superior margin of the ischial tuberosity. It runs as a spiral in a superolateral direction. Its insertion is on the medial side of the greater trochanter and the zona orbicularis. This is also the insertion point for the obturator externus muscle, for which there is a small groove in the ligament.

The ligament intertwines with the lateral part of the iliofemoral ligament.

### Zona Orbicularis (Fig. 8.107)

The zona orbicularis is a ligamentous loop that contains fibers from all three extra-articular ligaments. It is adherent to the joint capsule and wraps closely around the neck of the femur. It exerts pressure on the joint through its connection with the extra-capsular ligaments.

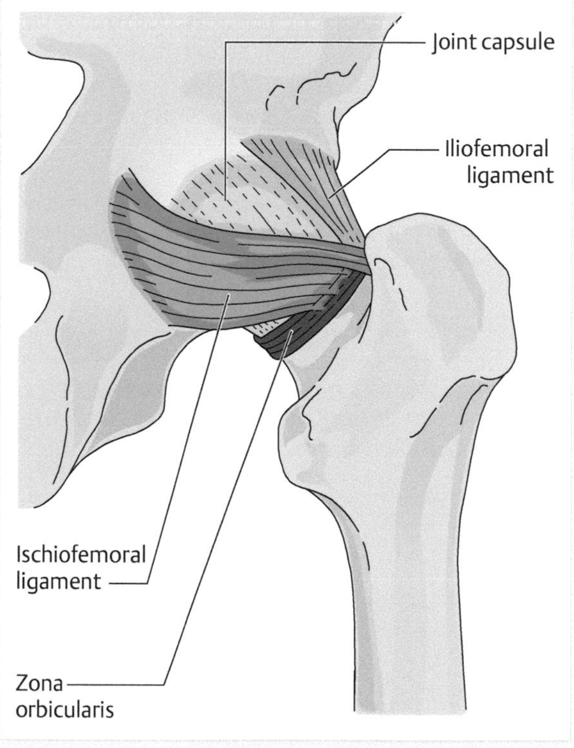


Fig. 8.107 Ischiofemoral ligament.

## Functions of the Ligaments (Figs. 8.108 and 8.109)

These serve both to carry out and to limit the movements of the joint, thereby stabilizing it:

- *Extension:* With extension, the ligaments twist and bring about a joint closure, which limits extension to approximately 10 to 15°.
- *Flexion:* In a mildly flexed position, all the ligamentous structures are relaxed. Not until there is significant flexion does the transverse part of the iliofemoral ligament come under tension.
- *Rotation:* In external rotation, the transverse part of the iliofemoral ligament and the pubofemoral ligament come under tension; in internal rotation, the ischiofemoral ligament and the descending part of the iliofemoral ligament become tensed. If the ligaments are relaxed in flexion, a significantly greater external rotation is possible.
- *Abduction:* In abduction, portions of the descending part of the iliofemoral ligament and the pubofemoral ligament as well as the inferior parts of the ischiofemoral ligament are tensed.
- *Adduction:* In adduction, the transverse part of the iliofemoral ligament prevents large movement deflections.

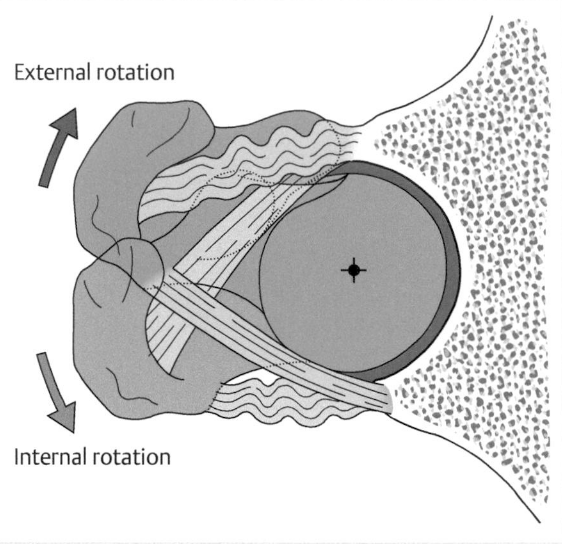

**Fig. 8.108** Ligament tension in external and internal rotation (transverse view).

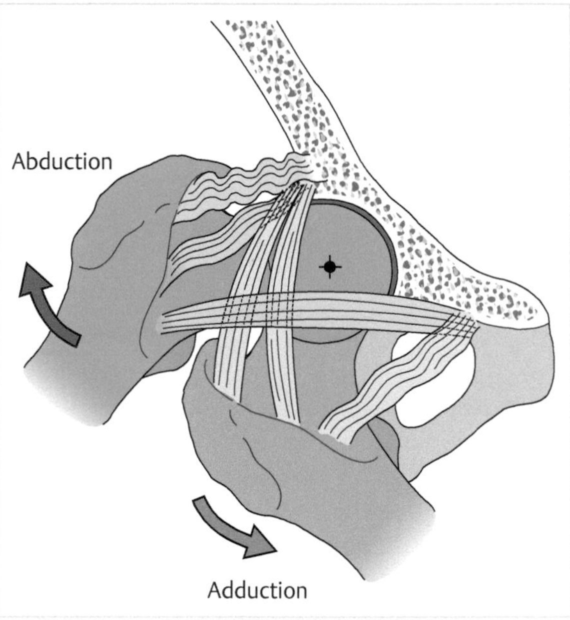

**Fig. 8.109** Ligament tension in abduction and adduction (anterior view).

### *Resting Position*

In the resting position, the capsule–ligament apparatus is relaxed, and the synovial fluid can be optimally distributed. This is the position of comfort, which patients automatically assume when in pain.

In the hip joint, the resting position is at approximately 30° of flexion, 15 to 20° of abduction, and 5 to 10° of external rotation.

### *Locked Position*

In the locked position, the capsule–ligament apparatus is maximally taut, and no joint play is possible. In the hip joint, this occurs at maximal extension with internal rotation combined with either abduction or adduction.

Pathology

### Weak Points

Weak points in terms of stability of the hip joint are the areas in which the various ligamentous structures intertwine. These occur especially between the iliofemoral ligament and the pubofemoral ligament, i.e., in the anterior region.

### Acquired Dislocation of the Hip

A large amount of force is required to dislocate the hip joint. For example, in the case of anterior dislocation of the pubic type, where there is extreme external rotation and the acetabular margin and labrum are used as the hypomochlion, the head of the femur is leveraged out of the joint in an anterior direction. The leg is fixed in the forced position of external rotation and cannot bear weight.

Practical Tip

### Treatment of the Capsule–Ligament Apparatus

#### Alleviation of Pain (Figs. 8.110 and 8.111)

To alleviate pain, treatment involves the application of traction in the patient's current position of rest. The traction should just tighten the capsule, because a stretch impulse can cause discomfort. Search for the current position of rest at approximately 30° of flexion, slight external rotation, and abduction. When this position is found, an elastic "give" can be felt when applying traction.

#### Increasing Movement

In contrast to the method used for pain relief, stretching various parts of the capsule requires intense traction treatment to be carried out at the end-motion position. This begins with minimal traction, is built up gradually, and is carried out intermittently.

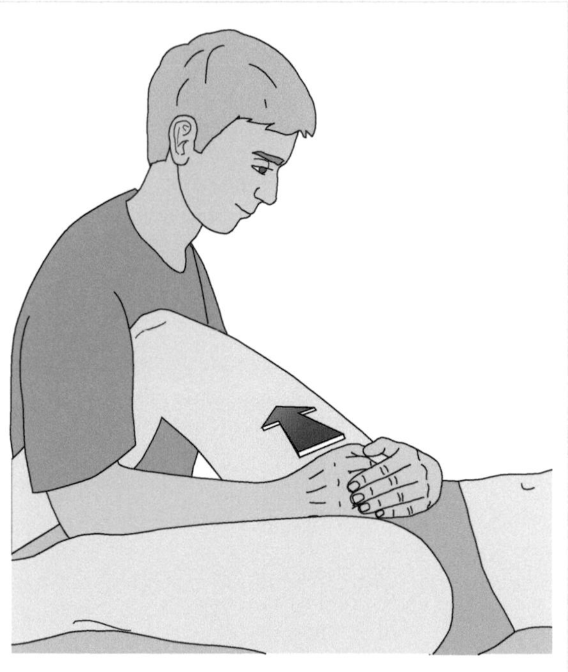

**Fig. 8.110** Traction in the current rest position.

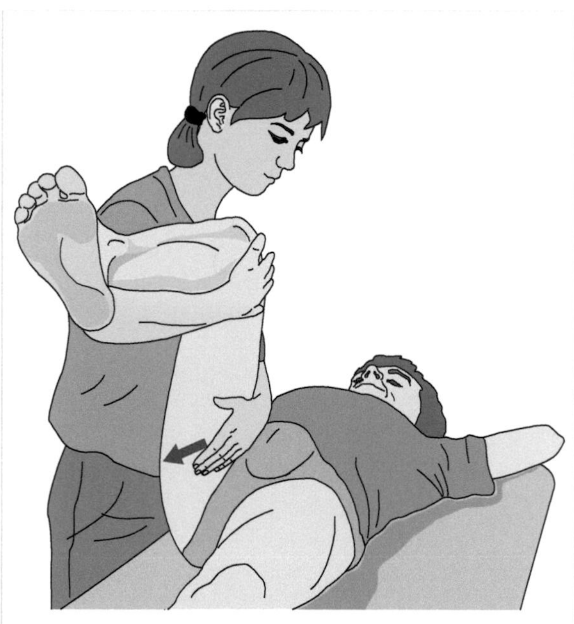

**Fig. 8.111** Traction therapy in the end-motion position. Example: flexion.

## 8.7.4 Arterial Supply (Fig. 8.112)

### *Femoral Artery*

- This is a continuation of the external iliac artery.
- It begins within the vascular space and extends laterally within the space.
- About three fingerbreadths inferior to the inguinal ligament, the *femoral artery* gives off the *deep artery of the thigh* in a posterolateral direction. The lateral circumflex femoral artery branches off this soon after.

### *Lateral Circumflex Femoral Artery*

- The *ascending branch* runs superolaterally along the intertrochanteric line and gives off several branches in the direction of the femoral neck; these run under the synovium and penetrate the femoral head near the bone–cartilage interface.
- The *transverse branch* supplies the area of the greater trochanter.
- The *descending branch* extends distally along the shaft to the knee joint.

The remaining portion of the femoral artery, also called the *superficial femoral artery*, does not give off any major branches into the surrounding area and runs distally into the adductor canal.

### *Medial Circumflex Femoral Artery*

- This arises from the deep artery of the thigh at the same level as the lateral circumflex femoral artery.
- It runs medial to the neck of the femur and bends around the tendon of the iliopsoas muscle in a posterior direction.
- The *deep branch* tracks superiorly and gives off branches to the greater trochanter and femoral neck.
- The *acetabular branch* tracks inferior to the neck, anastomoses with the obturator artery and sends off branches to the anterior acetabulum.

### *Superior and Inferior Gluteal Arteries*

- These arise from the internal iliac artery.
- They supply the posterosuperior and inferior acetabulum.

### *Obturator Artery*

- The acetabular branch passes over the acetabular notch into the interior of the joint.
- It runs further within the ligament of the head of the femur.
- The artery supplies the joint socket, the fat pad, and the femoral head.

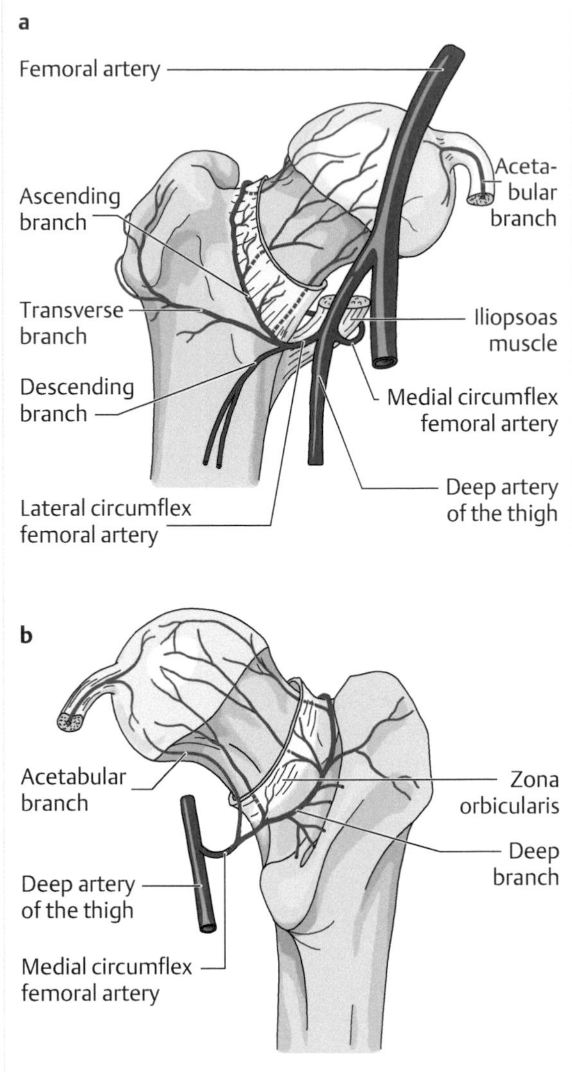


**Fig. 8.112** Arterial supply of the hip joint. **(a)** Anterior. **(b)** Posterior.

**Pathology**

In a fracture of the femoral neck, the blood supply to the femoral head may be interrupted if the fracture line is intracapsular. Nutrition is only guaranteed through the ligament of the head of the femur. Since this can atrophy in old age, necrosis due to a lack of nutrition can develop. In these cases, an endoprosthesis is inserted. If the fracture line is extracapsular, the nutritional conditions are more favorable.

## 8.7.5 Innervation (Fig. 8.113)

### *Femoral Nerve*

Distal to the lateral circumflex femoral artery, the femoral nerve gives off a branch to the anterior joint region.

### *Obturator Nerve*

- The accessory obturator nerve from the L3–L4 nerve roots tracks to the inferior hip joint.
- Further branches extend to the knee joint.

### *Sciatic Nerve*

- The articular branch to the hip branches off just before the infrapiriform foramen.
- It supplies the posterior hip region.

### *Superior Gluteal Nerve*

This sends a small branch to the joint from a superolateral direction.

### *Nerve to the Quadratus Femoris*

- This runs through the greater sciatic foramen.
- It gives off branches to the quadratus femoris muscle and the posteroinferior hip joint.

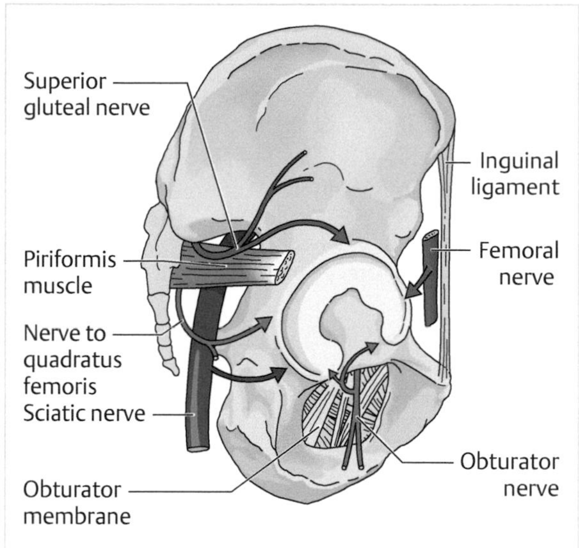


**Fig. 8.113** Innervation of the hip joint.

## 8.7.6 Angles in the Femoral Region

### CCD Angle (Fig. 8.114)

The CCD angle is the angle formed by the femoral neck axis and the femoral shaft axis:

- The *femoral neck axis* runs through the midpoint of the head of the femur and stays at approximately the same distance from the contours of the femoral neck.
- The *femoral shaft axis* runs roughly in the medullary canal of the femoral shaft.

In the newborn, the angle is 150°; after the age of 2, it becomes smaller. Toward the end of the growth it reaches 125 to 130°, and with increasing age, it may continue to decline.

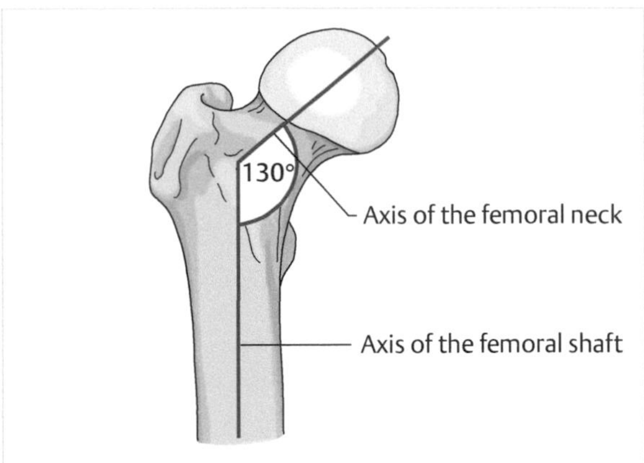


**Fig. 8.114** The caput–collum–diaphyseal angle.

#### *Factors that Impact Angle Changes*

- *Forces that reduce the angle (toward varus)* are the body weight, the abductors, the rectus femoris muscle, the hamstring muscles, the long adductors, and the ground reaction force coming from inferiorly (**Fig. 8.115**).
- *Forces that increase the angle (toward valgus)* are the transversely running adductors, the two muscles that extend into the iliotibial tract (the gluteus maximus and tensor fasciae latae), the pelvitrochanteric muscles, and the transverse fibers of the iliopsoas muscle.

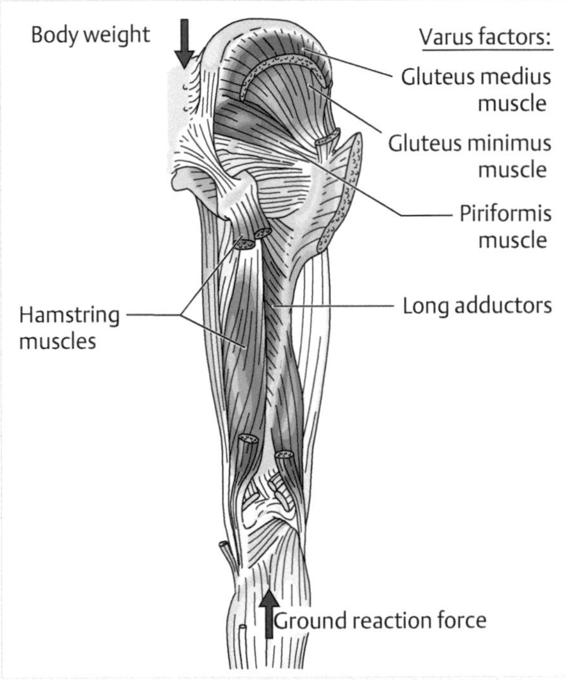


**Fig. 8.115** Forces that reduce the caput–collum–diaphyseal angle.

**Pathology**

**Changes in the Angle (Fig. 8.116)**

- Coxa valga: angle greater than 135°.
- Coxa vara: angle less than 120°.

▷ See Chapter 8.7.8, Biomechanics

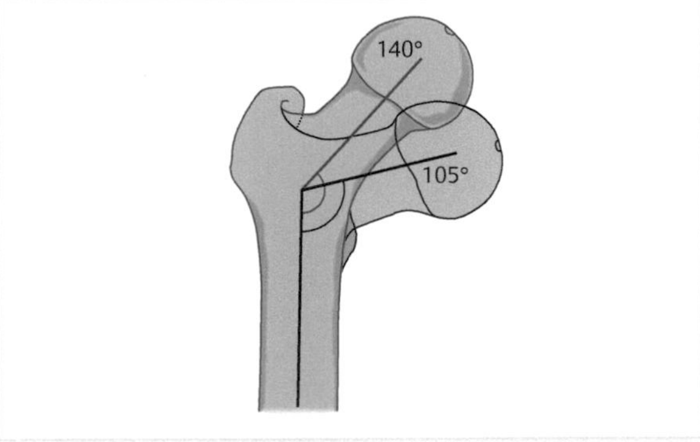


**Fig. 8.116** Coxa valga and coxa vara.

## Angle of Anteversion (Fig. 8.117)

The femoral neck axis forms an angle with the transverse axis of the femoral condyles, which is open anteriorly.

### *Development of Femoral Version*

In newborns, the angle of anteversion is 30 to 40°. After birth, there is regression of anteversion, so that the angle drops to 18° between the 10th and 14th years of life. The normal value for adults is 12°.

## Changes in the Angle and their Consequences (Fig. 8.118)

If the angle of anteversion is greater than the normal values, this leads to increased internal rotation of the leg. Conversely, retroversion causes increased external rotation.

Compensation can be achieved proximally in the area of the acetabulum or distally, with tibial torsion.

> **Practical Tip**
>
> **Observable Rotation Position (Fig. 8.119)**
>
> If the ability to externally rotate is significantly limited, it should be assumed that a femoral torsion error, such as increased antetorsion, is present, because the center point of the rotation has shifted. Inspection of the entire leg shows that the patella and longitudinal axis of the foot are medially directed.
>
> If the foot is medially rotated, the reason is not always increased antetorsion. If the patella points straight forward but there is a clear deviation of the longitudinal axis of the foot medially, the cause could be internal tibial torsion. The evaluation is made on the basis of the position of the malleoli in relation to the proximal transverse axis of the tibia. The angle formed in this way should be 30°, and it should open medially.

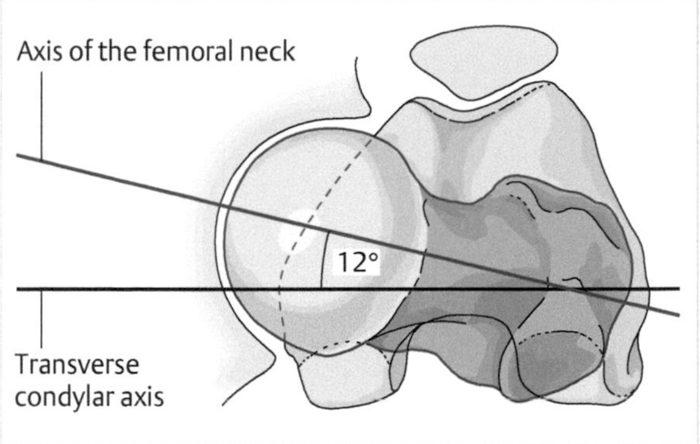


**Fig. 8.117** Angle of anteversion.

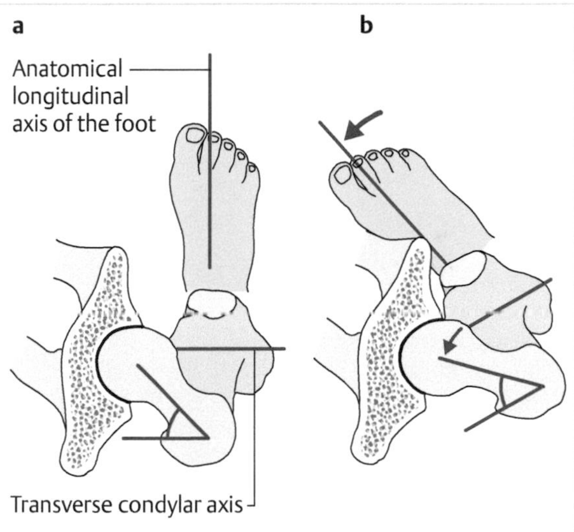


**Fig. 8.118** Increased antetorsion. **(a)** Femoral head in the anterior position. **(b)** Femoral head centered.

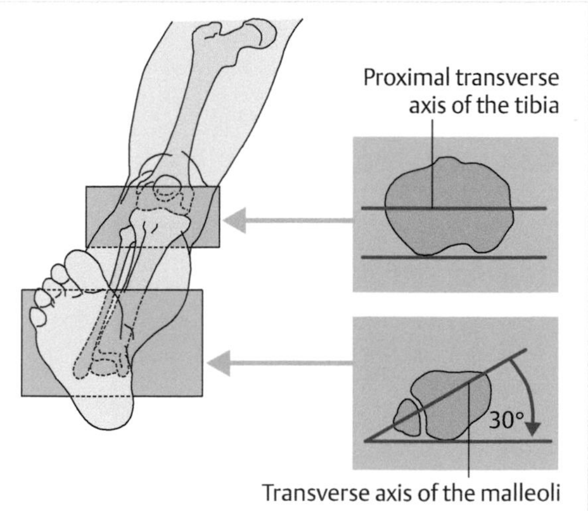


**Fig. 8.119** Determination of tibial torsion.

## 8.7.7 Movements and Axes of Motion

### Axes of Motion (Fig. 8.120)

The hip joint is a ball and socket joint with three axes of motion. All the axes meet at right angles at the pivot point of the hip joint, which is located in the center of the femoral head:

- *Frontal axis:* for flexion and extension.
- *Sagittal axis:* for abduction and adduction.
- *Longitudinal axis:* for rotation; note that the axis of rotation does not correspond to the axis of the shaft but runs medial to it.

In everyday activities, movements are rarely performed around only one axis. Usually, there are combined movements around an infinite number of instantaneous axes of rotation.

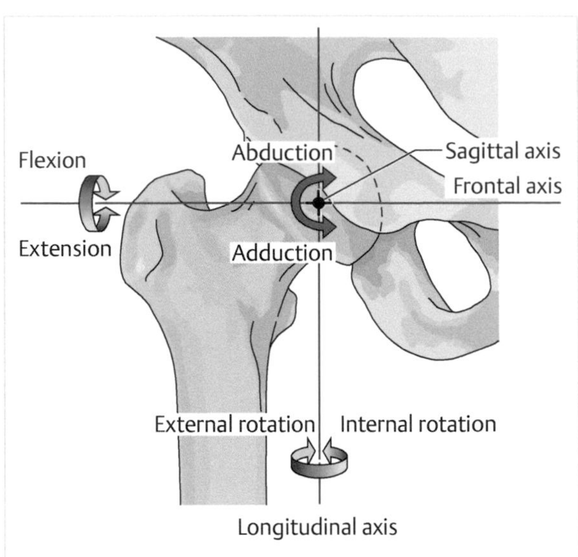


**Fig. 8.120** Axes of motion of the hip joint.

### Movement—Direction and Extent

#### *Flexion/Extension (Fig. 8.121)*

- Active: 130 to 140°/10 to 15°, respectively, from neutral.
- Passive: 150°/15°, respectively, from neutral.

Extension is usually evaluated with the patient in the supine position using Thomas's test. The knee of the opposite side is bent until the pelvic tilt of 12° is reversed. If the thigh stays flat on the table, an extension of 10° has been attained.

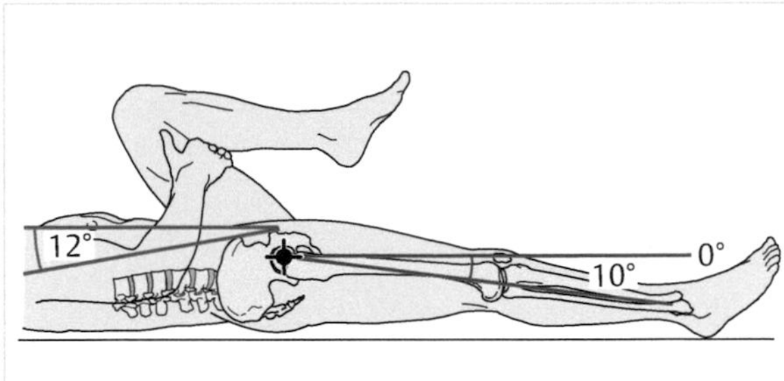


**Fig. 8.121** Thomas's test to determine hip extension.

#### *Physiologic Difference between Hip Movements with the Knee Flexed Versus Extended*

With the knee flexed, the hip can flex to its maximum of approximately 130°, but the ability to extend the hip is significantly reduced. With the knee in extension, hip flexion of approximately 90° is to be expected, while the hip can be extended to its maximum of about 15°. This relates to the reduced elasticity of the hamstring muscles during knee flexion and the rectus femoris muscle during knee extension, due to, in each case, stretching of the component of the respective muscle at the knee.

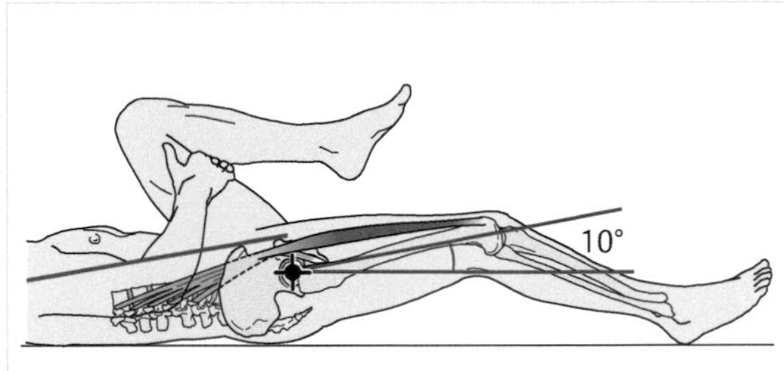


**Fig. 8.122** Flexion contracture.

**Pathology**

**Flexion Contracture (Fig. 8.122)**

In Thomas's test, if the leg being tested for extension gives way in the direction of flexion and cannot be passively extended, a flexion contracture exists.

### *Abduction/Adduction (Fig. 8.123)*

- Active: 30 to 40°/20 to 30°, respectively, from neutral.
- Passive: 10° more in each direction.

Abduction is inhibited by the increasing tension of the anterior ligaments and the adductors.

The ability to adduct is better with the hip flexed because the ligaments are relaxed.

### *External Rotation/Internal Rotation (Fig. 8.124)*

- Active: 40 to 50°/30 to 40°, respectively, from neutral.
- Passive: 10° more in each direction.

Rotation is difficult to assess in the supine position and in the neutral position. Therefore the measurement is performed at 90° of hip and knee flexion, and the lower leg is observed as the indicator. In this position, the ligaments are relaxed and have good motility.

*Alternative method:* Place the patient in a prone position with 90° flexion in the knee joints. Here too, the lower legs are used as the indicator. In this position, less movement is possible due to ligament tension.

### *Prerequisite for Normal Mobility*

The prerequisites for harmonious and maximal movement of the hip are a capsule–ligament apparatus with good elasticity, a femoral head centered in the joint socket, and good coordination of the surrounding muscles.

## Pathology

**Osteoarthritis**

In osteoarthritis, contractures in the positions of flexion, external rotation, and adduction can develop. The result is a functional shortening of the leg, which can be compensated for by changes in the SIJ and lumbar region such as pelvic rotation, hyperlordosis, and lateral flexion. Because of the change in the stride length and the weakening of the abductors, a limping mechanism develops, and the efficiency of ambulation is reduced.

In stage 3 osteoarthritis, a significant restriction of movement is to be expected. Because of decreased mobility due to pain, the cartilage on the joint surfaces changes, and therefore the joint's nutritional status will also change. In this way, a vicious cycle is set up.

Patients rarely sense the limited hip extension as disturbing, but instead feel the resultant compensation and the pain in the lumbar spine and SIJ. In contrast, in terms of everyday movements that occur with worsening osteoarthritis, such as sitting in deep chairs or putting on stockings, they perceive the restricted hip flexion as being very debilitating.

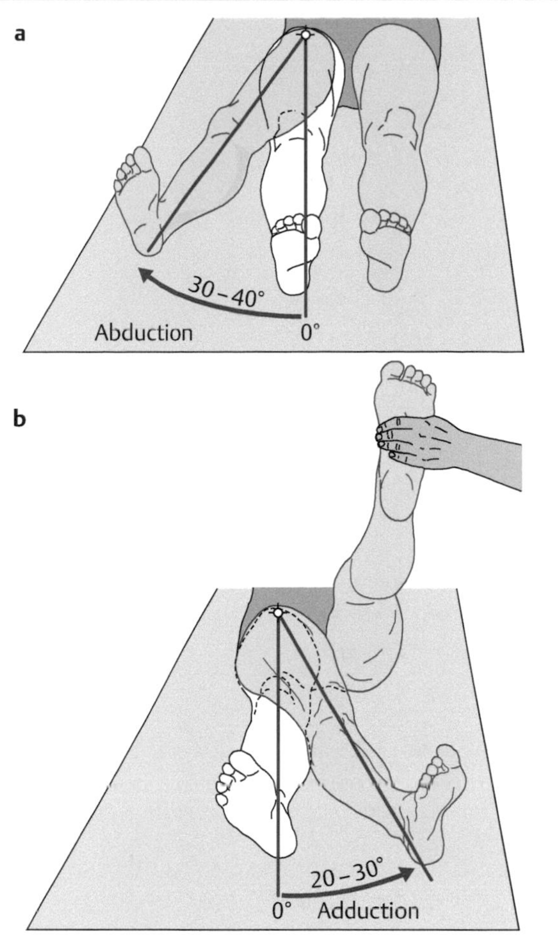


**Fig. 8.123** Movements of the hip joint. **(a)** Abduction. **(b)** Adduction.

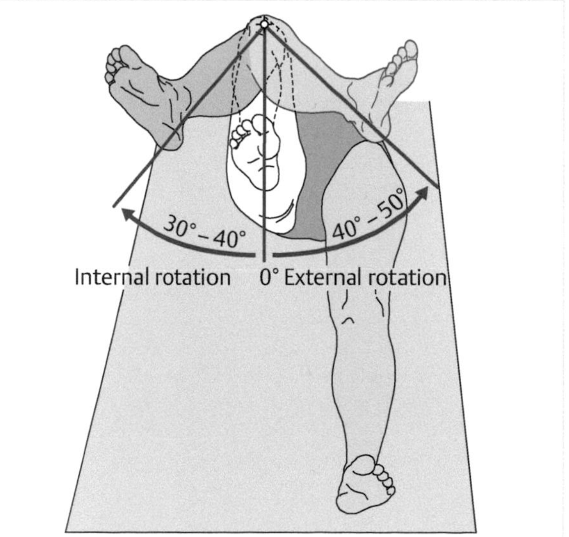


**Fig. 8.124** Movements in the hip joint: external and internal rotation.

## Practical Tip

### Treatment of Movement Restrictions (Figs. 8.125 and 8.126)

The cause (e.g., articular or muscular) of the reduced mobility must be found in order to start therapy at the right place.

The capsule–ligament apparatus is examined in terms of its extensibility and painfulness, and the centering of the femoral head is also assessed. Internal rotation will be limited, for example, if the femoral head is located too far anteriorly, because the pivot point also shifts anteriorly, and thus the posterior capsule–ligament apparatus comes under tension too early in the movement. That means it is necessary to center the femoral head in order to improve mobility. This centering is performed by a thrust posteriorly over the knee with the knee and hip flexed to 90°, combined with decompression of the acetabular roof inferiorly.

The muscles need to be evaluated in terms of their elasticity and of the endurance and coordination of the force components.

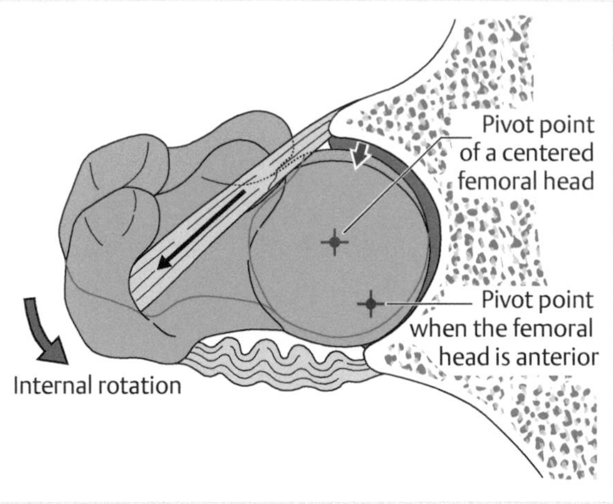


**Fig. 8.125** Shift of the longitudinal axis by an anteriorly positioned femoral head.

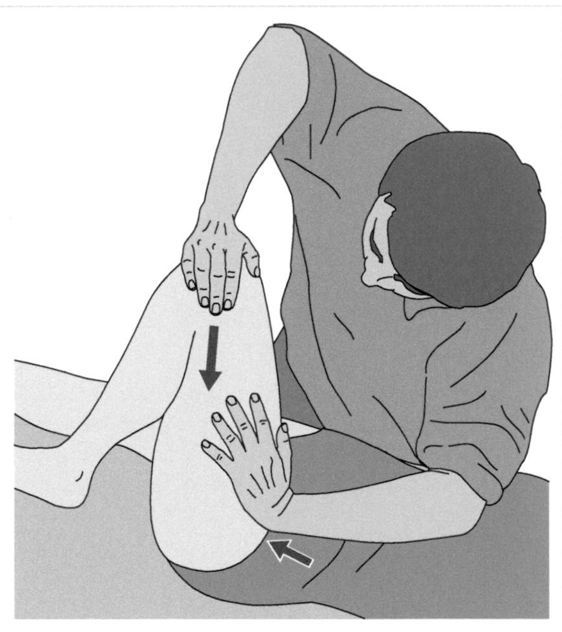

**Fig. 8.126** Centering the femoral head when it is positioned anteriorly.

## 8.7.8 Biomechanics

### Calculation of the Balance of Forces as per Pauwels

The determination of the balance of forces was described by Pauwels (1973). Among other things, he determined the balance of forces on the basis of a two-dimensional static model of the patient standing on one leg. Today, the three-dimensional approach is biomechanically relevant. Since the ball and socket joint has three axes, three moments must be calculated with respect to the state of equilibrium, and the direction and magnitude of the joint's resultant forces must be changed depending on the position and load status.

### Joint Mechanics during Single-Leg Stance (Fig. 8.127)

Assessing the hip joint in the frontal plane according to the law of levers, a first-class lever is involved, i.e., the fulcrum is between the load and force:

- *Fulcrum:* hip joint.
- *Load:* body weight; the center of gravity is shifted slightly to the side of the free leg, trying to pull the pelvis down.
- *Force:* abductors on the side of the standing leg must hold the pelvis in balance.
- *Load arm:* the direct connection from the fulcrum to the action line of the load.
- *Force arm:* the direct connection from the fulcrum to the application of the force.

Since the force arm is much shorter than the load arm, the force must be greater to produce an equilibrium of moments, i.e., to stabilize the joint in this plane. The law of levers states that: force × force arm = load × load arm.

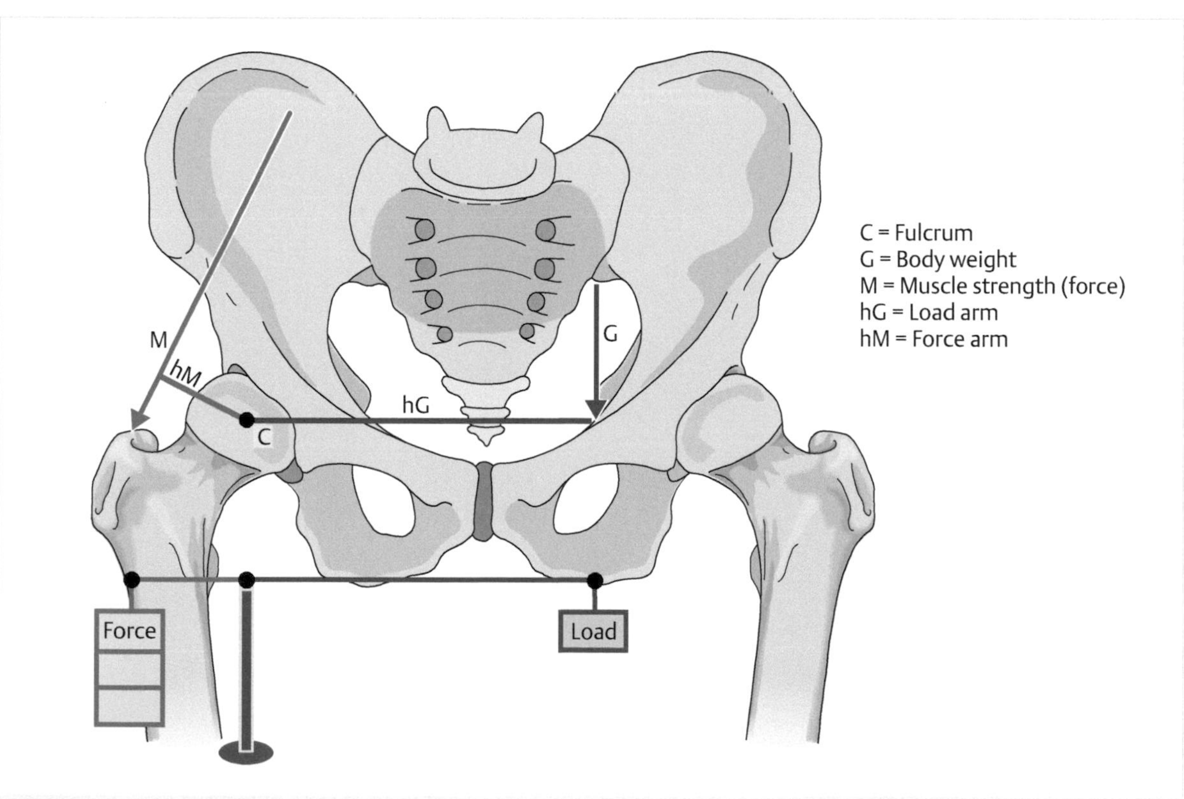


**Fig. 8.127** Joint mechanics during single-leg stance.

## Calculation of the Joint Load (Fig. 8.128)

The actual load on a joint is the resultant of the forces acting on the joint. To calculate the magnitude and direction of the forces, the geometric sum of muscle strength and body weight is determined using a parallelogram of forces.

Body weight is the first vector. The magnitude of this is known and is shown by the corresponding arrow length. It is moved along its line of action until it meets the line of action of the force.

The force is the second vector. Its magnitude is derived from the law of lever. With the two vectors emanating from the reference point, a force parallelogram is formed and the diagonal is drawn, which represents the resultant force, the magnitude of which corresponds to the length of the arrow. The line of action always runs through the pivot point.

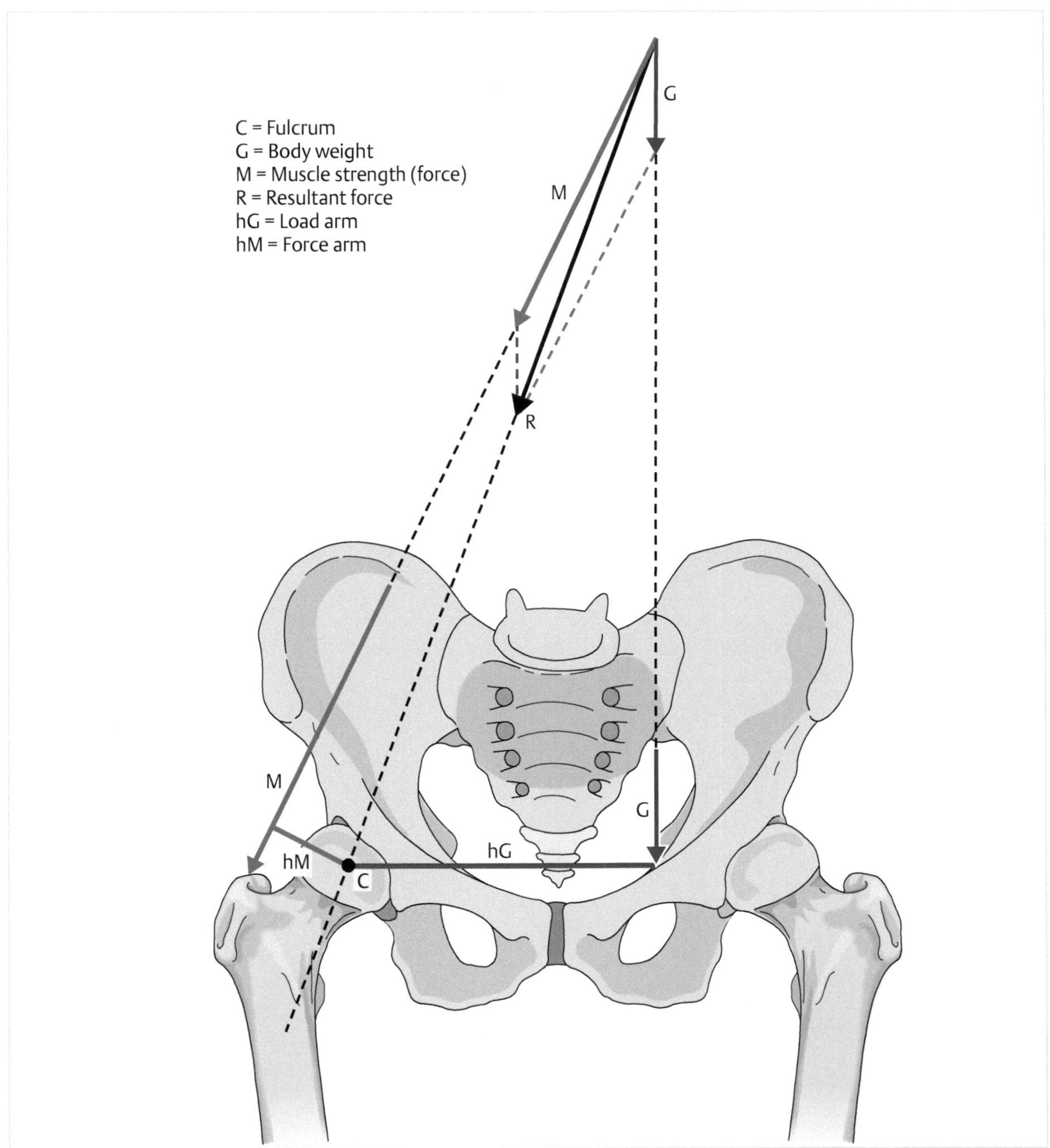


**Fig. 8.128** Calculation of joint load during single-leg stance.

## In Vivo Measurements of Hip Joint Load

Bergmann (1993) developed and implanted an instrumented endoprosthesis at the Freie Universität Berlin. He installed three strain gauges and a mini transmitter in its neck to measure the acting three-dimensional forces.

### Raising and Lowering the Extended Leg (Fig. 8.129a)

While raising the patient's outstretched leg, Bergmann (1993) measured a force of 160% BW (body weight) in the hip joint. When lowering the leg, and while pressing the outstretched leg strongly into the pad, the forces even reached 250% BW.

### Exercises against Resistance (Fig. 8.129a)

During abduction against resistance, forces of up to three times body weight occurred; with internal rotation, the forces were up to double the body weight.

### Assisted Movements (Fig. 8.129a)

Assisted movements put the least strain on the joint at 50% BW.

### Symmetrical Standing on Both Legs (Fig. 8.129a)

While standing symmetrically on both legs, forces between 80% and 100% BW were measured.

### Walking with Support/Walking Stick (Fig. 8.129a)

Walking with support does not significantly unload the joint. In this case, measurements of 180% BW were obtained; only after repeated explicit requests to take the weight off the leg were they reduced. Walking barefoot was only slightly less stressful than walking with shoes.

Using a walking stick on the contralateral side compared with walking without support reduced the load by approximately 20 to 25%.

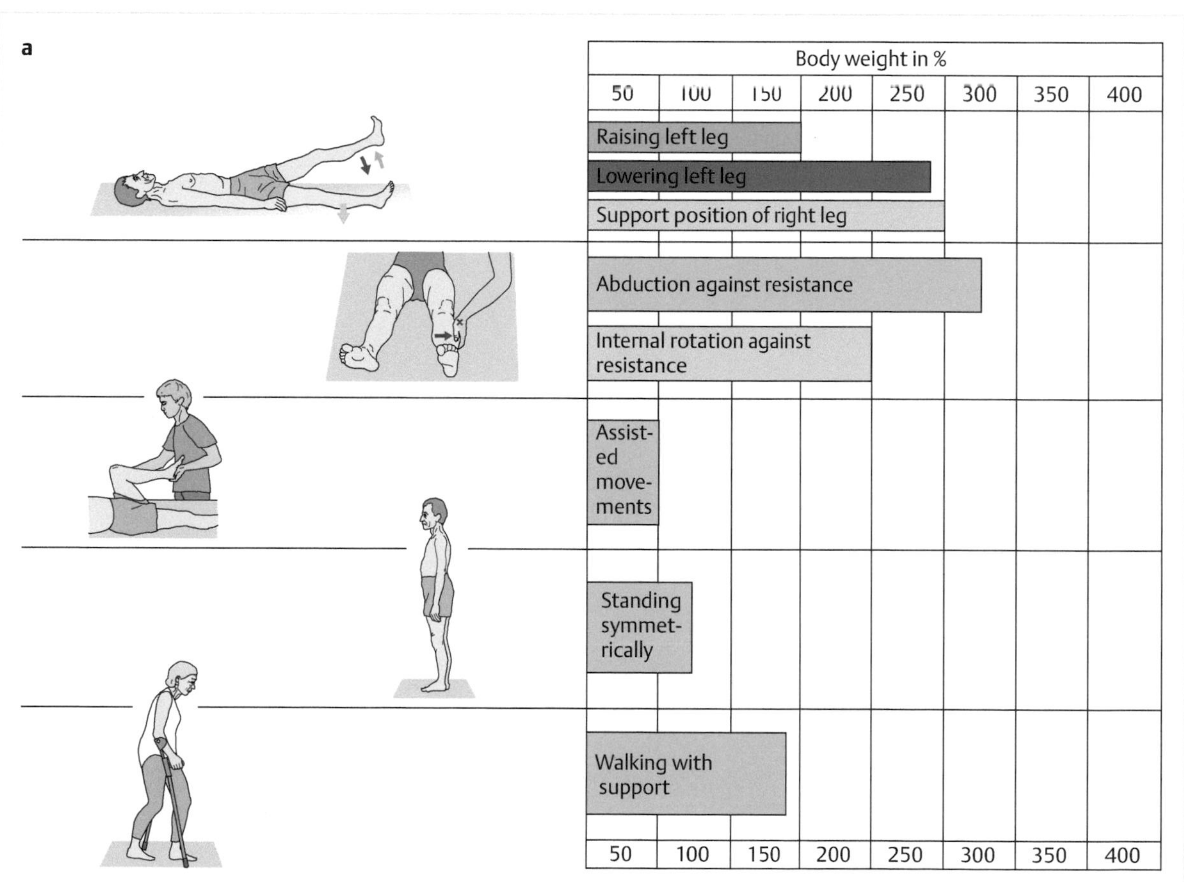


**Fig. 8.129 (a)** Measurements of joint loading during various activities.

Continued ►

## Measurement of Hip Joint Loading (Fig. 8.129b)

- *Sitting:* 30% BW.
- *Standing up:* 200 to 300% BW.
- *Climbing stairs:*
  - Up: 350% BW.
  - Down: 400% BW.
- *Jogging:* 400% BW.
- *Cycling* at 90 to 100 W: 75% BW (the problem being getting on and off the cycle).
- *Bridging:* 200 to 300% BW.

**Practical Tip**

**Consequences after Surgery**

The prescription of partial weight-bearing after a total hip replacement is based on the idea that the bone around the prosthesis requires mechanical rest to grow more densely and strongly to the implant. Extremely high joint forces may shear off the bone that is growing into the porous surface of the implant. The loading forces discussed above exert torque primarily in the shaft area, possibly leading to loosening of the prosthesis. Values of two to three times the body weight should therefore be avoided in the postoperative period.

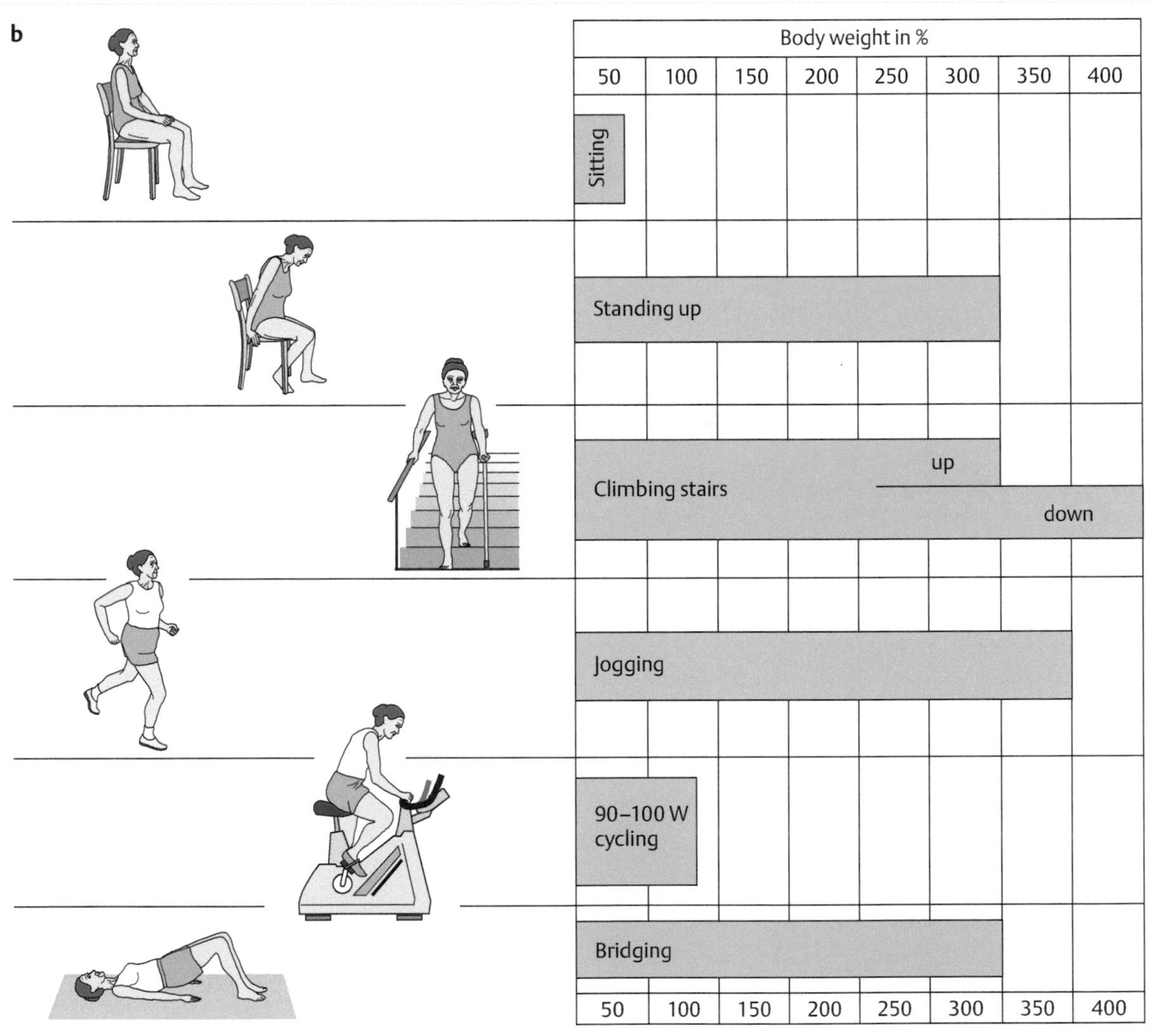


**Fig. 8.129 (b)** Continued.

## Pathology

The CCD angle influences the length of the force arm and its direction of pull, and thereby changes the loading of the joint.

### Coxa Valga

The force arm is shortened, and the load arm is unchanged. To produce a balance between moments, more muscle power must be expended. This means that this vector, and thereby the resultant joint force, increases. The line of action of the abductors is steeper, which is why the direction of the resultant force changes, becoming steeper and approaching the acetabular rim.

The total load on the joint is greater, and in the long run there will be overuse and damage to the cartilage (**Fig. 8.130**).

Compensation occurs through shortening of the load arm in that the point of force is pushed in the direction of the fulcrum. This means that the torso is brought over the standing leg, which corresponds to *Duchenne's limp* (**Fig. 8.131**). The force needed by the abductors to maintain the balance of forces is reduced, and thus the joint load is also reduced.

If not compensated for, and the force of the gluteus medius and minimus muscles is not sufficient to stabilize the pelvis, *Trendelenburg's limp* develops (**Fig. 8.131**). The pelvis lowers on the free leg side with resultant compression in the hip joint, which is very painful.

### Osteoarthritis

The consequence of faulty loading is osteoarthritis. In the long run, *osteophytes* arise in both the stress zones and the nonloaded areas. These are areas of reactive new bone formation in the form of bone spurs. In addition, subchondral cysts develop. These are round cysts in the stress zones that contain a disorderly debris of cancellous bone and have a sclerotic border.

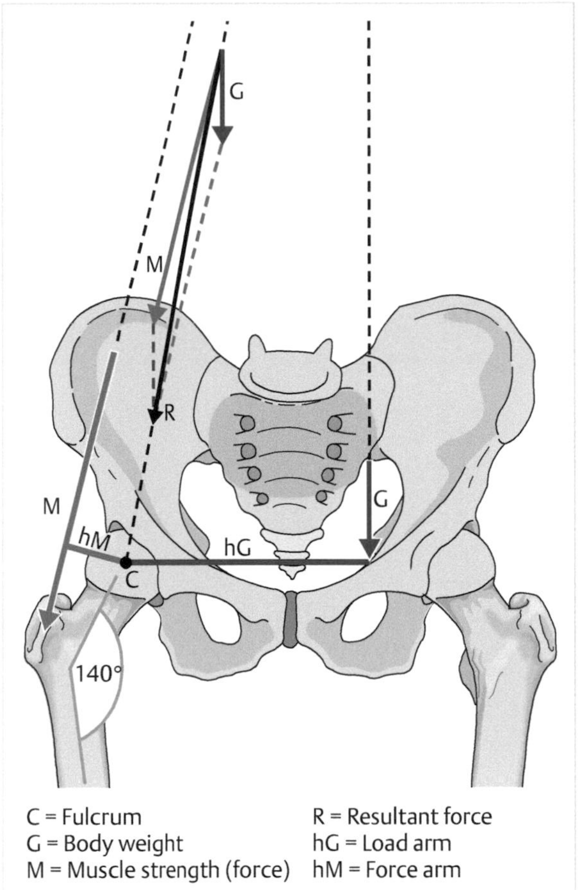


**Fig. 8.130** Joint loading in coxa valga.

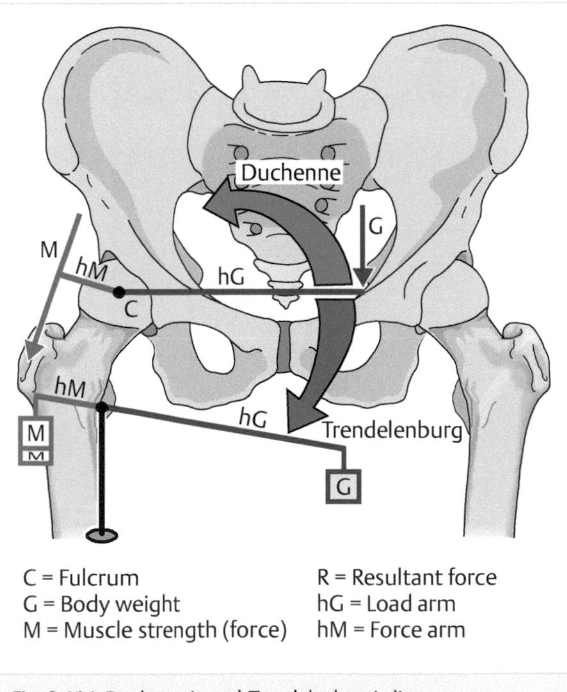


**Fig. 8.131** Duchenne's and Trendelenburg's limps.

### Coxa Vara (Fig. 8.132)

The force arm is lengthened, so the abductors do not have to expend as much force to keep the pelvis in balance. The line of action of the abductors is not as steep.

*Result:* The resultant force on the joint becomes smaller and oriented medially. In due course, this places stress on the medial femoral neck, where increased bending stress develops.

## Practical Tip

### Walking Stick (Fig. 8.133)

To avoid or reduce joint stress factors, the patient should use a cane on the contralateral side. In the stance phase, the distance from the stick to the fulcrum is 40 cm. The load arm is 15 cm, and the force arm 5 cm. The force of the stick is eight times more effective than the force of the abductor muscles. That means that a relatively small force in the direction of the cane causes a significant reduction of the abductor force and thus a relief of the pressure on the joint.

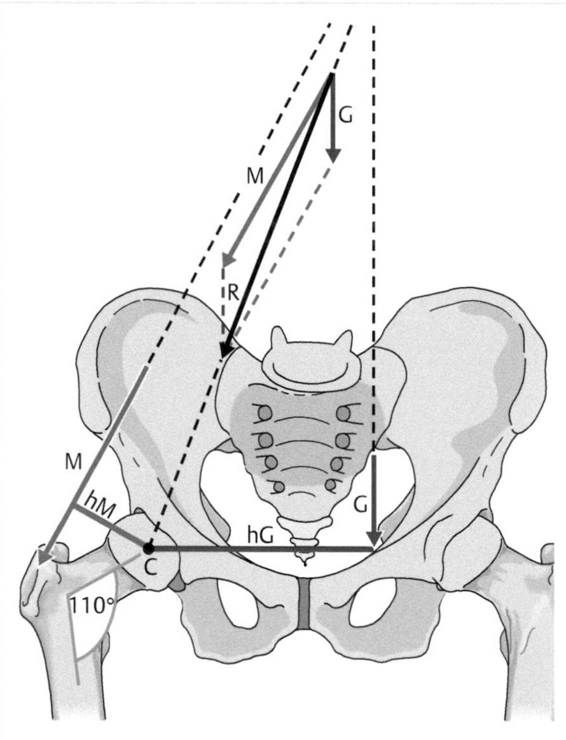


**Fig. 8.132** Joint loading in coxa vara.

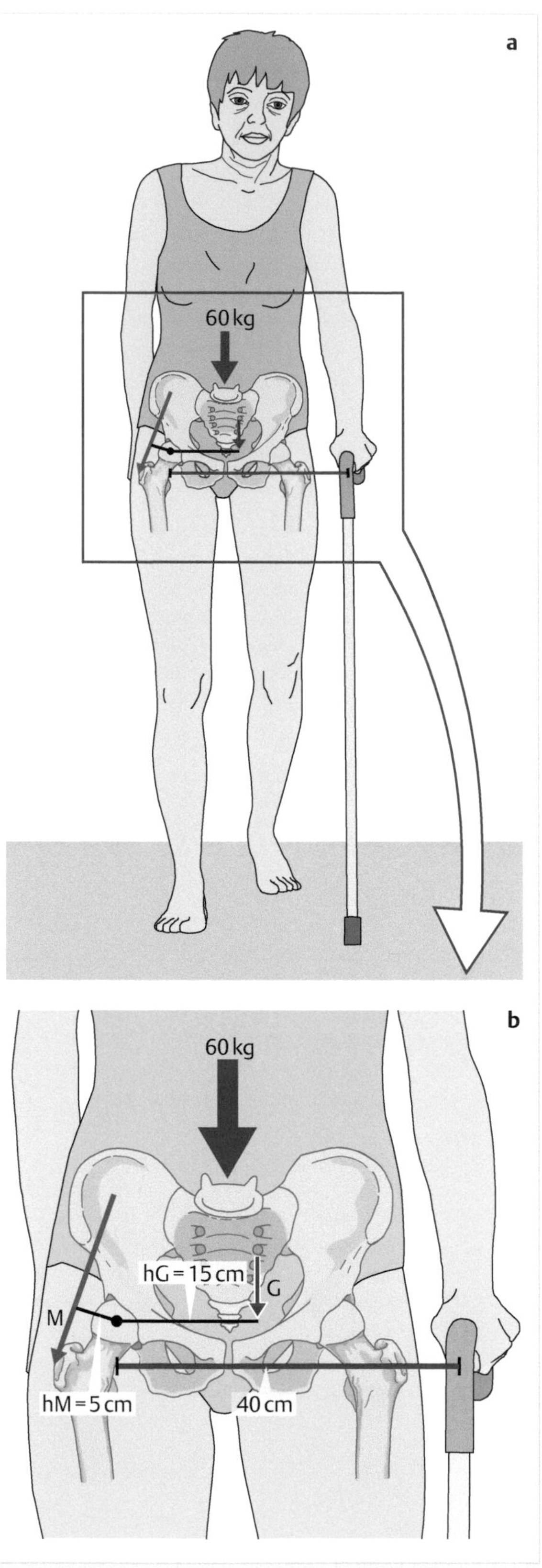


**Fig. 8.133 (a, b)** Load reduction using a walking stick.

## 8.7.9 Stabilization of the Hip Joint

### Surface Covering

In the neutral position, the femoral head is not completely covered by the acetabulum as its cartilage-covered anterosuperior area is uncovered. This is due to the anteversion of the femur and the anteversion of the acetabulum. That means that, in this position, the femoral head is not optimally centered. Three motions are needed to achieve surface coverage: flexion of approximately 70°, slight abduction, and external rotation.

### Enclosing the Joint (Fig. 8.134)

Joint closure is ensured by the following structures.

#### Acetabular Labrum

This compensates for the unevenness of the margin and encloses the femoral head with its tapered ends.

#### Joint Capsule

The capsule is thick and firm, with reinforced fiber tracts in the fibrous layer that run in various directions.

#### Ligaments

All the ligaments described above contribute to stability. In this regard, the zona orbicularis plays an important role through its connection to the joint capsule and the ligaments.

#### Muscles

Muscles whose longitudinal components coincide with the axis of the femoral neck pull the femoral head in a superomedial direction and thereby center it. The muscles that are particularly involved in this are the piriformis, the gluteus medius and minimus, and the obturator externus. Slips of the gluteus maximus and tensor fasciae latae muscles and their connection with the fascia lata also help with this centering function.

The superior portion of the joint is stabilized by the pelvitrochanteric muscles. Anteriorly, the iliopsoas muscle fulfills this function since it runs directly over the femoral head.

Ligaments and muscles are very important for joint closure and complement each other. Anteriorly, the ligaments are very strong, but the muscles are not very numerous; posteriorly, in contrast, the muscles dominate.

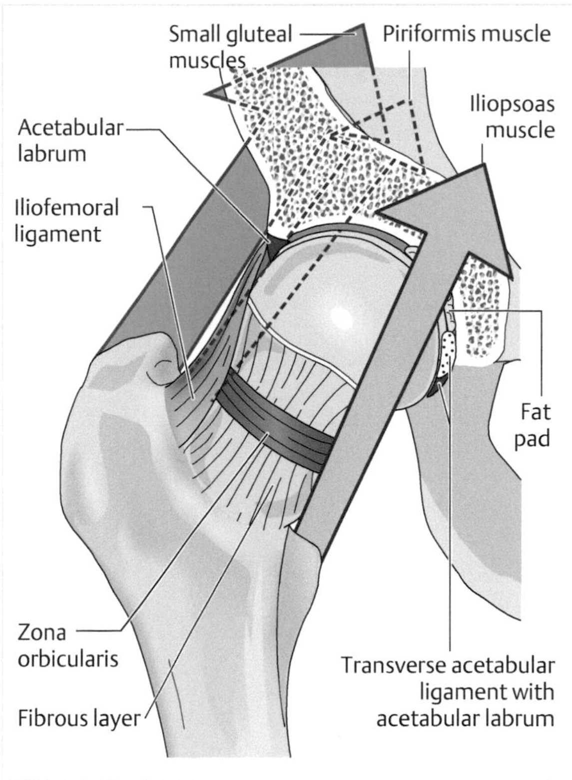


**Fig. 8.134** Stabilization of the hip joint.

# 8.8 Muscles of the Pelvic and Hip Regions

## 8.8.1 Pelvic Diaphragm (Fig. 8.135)

*Levator Ani Muscle*

- This is a broad thin muscle.
- It can be divided into several different, and at times overlapping, parts.
- The *iliococcygeus muscle* connects the tendinous arch with the coccyx.
- The *puborectalis muscle* goes around the rectum and anteriorly to the pubis.
- The *pubococcygeus muscle* consists of long fibers that connect the pubis with the coccyx, running at the edge of the anal and urogenital openings.
- Fibrous bands of the obturator membrane radiate into the muscle.
- The levator ani radiates into the fascia of the prostate and into the vaginal wall, thus affecting their tone.
- The *anal sphincter*, formed from fibers from the levator, wraps around the rectum and has a ligamentous connection to the coccyx, the *anococcygeal ligament*. There is also a connection with the transverse perineal muscles. The muscle has resting tone and basically holds the anus closed.
- *Innervation:* from the third to fourth sacral segments.

*Ischiococcygeus Muscle*

- This connects the ischial spine and the sacrotuberous ligament with the inferior sacrum and the coccyx.
- The lower part is fused with the gluteus maximus muscle.
- It connects to the posterior part of the levator ani muscle.
- Its superior edge, along with the inferior edge of the piriformis muscle, forms a gap through which the sciatic nerve runs.
- It has an influence on the position of the sacrum and causes counternutation.
- *Innervation:* fourth to fifth sacral nerves.

**Practical Tip**

**Consequences of Changing Muscle Tension**

Hypertonus of the ischiococcygeus muscle may hinder nutation of the sacrum. This can result in malfunction of the SIJ, and, as it is transmitted through the dural sac, may result in an unfavorable pulling action on the membrane systems of the cranium.

An altered position of the pubis, or from hypertonus of the abdominal muscles, for example, can affect the tension of the pelvic diaphragm.

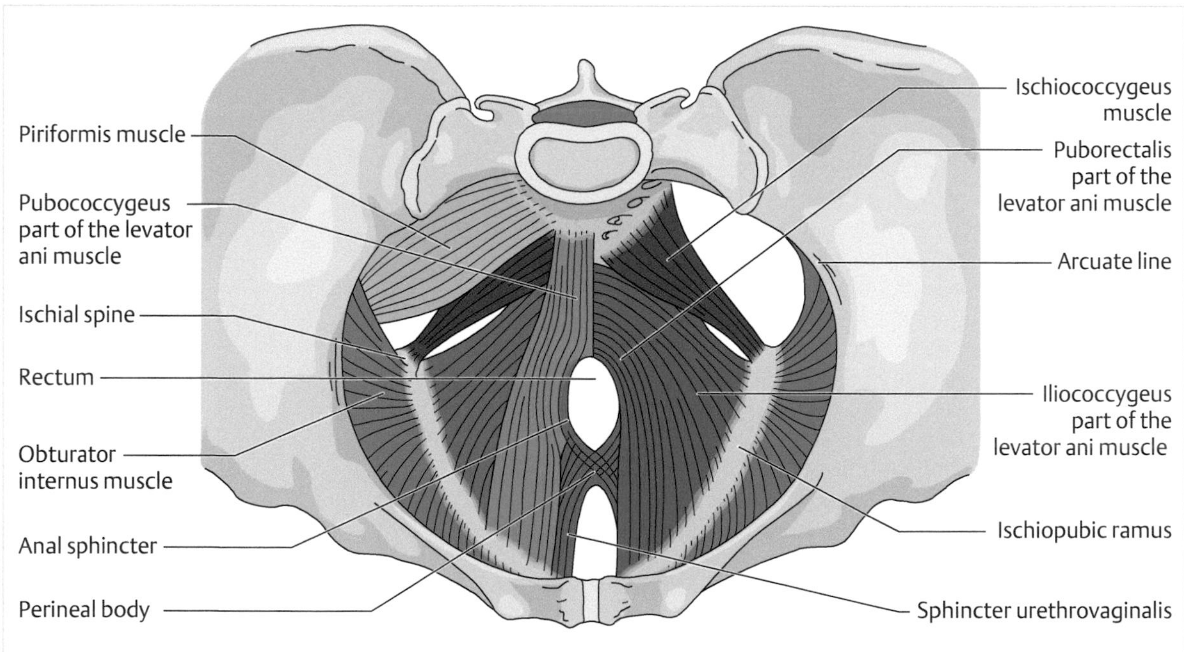


**Fig. 8.135** Female pelvic diaphragm (superior view).

## 8.8.2 Urogenital Diaphragm

The urogenital diaphragm consists of deep and superficial layers that are composed of fascia and muscles. These spread out between the right and left side of the pubis.

*Deep Transverse Perineal Muscle (Fig. 8.136)*

- This runs as a deep layer across the anterior area of the diaphragm.
- It is attached anteriorly to the pubic symphysis and superiorly to the perineal body.
- It leaves passages for the urethra and the vagina and, around this hiatus, connects with the bulbospongiosus, which is the outermost sphincter muscle.
- It acts as a broad, flat support for the bladder.
- The perineal body is the point where the sphincter muscles of the anus and urethra intersect.

*Superficial Transverse Perineal Muscle (Fig. 8.136)*

- This is a narrow muscle that is located at the posterior edge of the deep layer.
- It connects the perineal body to the ischial tuberosity.
- It continues anteriorly, and, along the margin of the ramus of the ischium, forms the *ischiocavernosus muscle.*
- *Innervation:* pudendal nerve.

### Functions of the Diaphragms

- Contraction causes elevation of the pelvic floor.
- Along with the thoracolumbar diaphragm, they take part in abdominal bracing.
- They act as a hammock for the organs of the lesser pelvis, preventing them from descending.
- They also serve as the closure mechanism for the rectum and bladder.
- The diaphragms play a role in reproduction.
- They are also involved in the birth process.
- They play a role in the transmission of forces posteriorly.
- They have an influence on the mobility and position of the sacrum, coccyx, and pubis; therefore changes in the position of these structures can affect the tone of the pelvic floor.

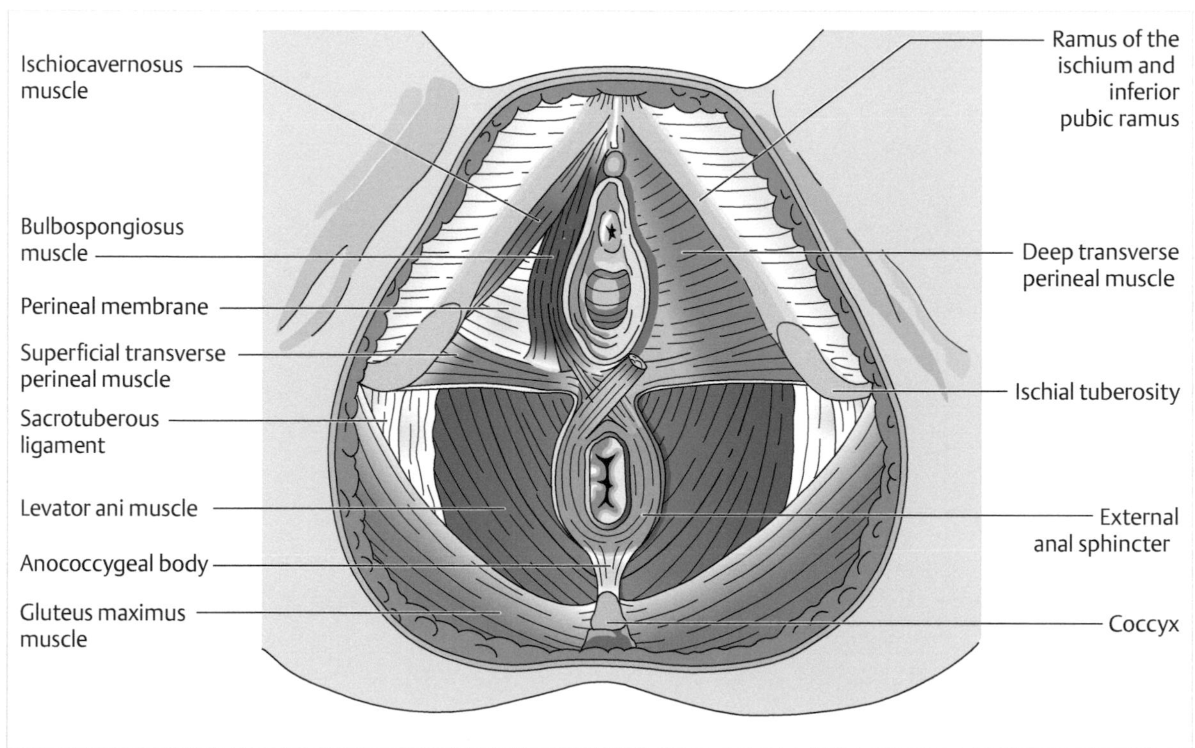


**Fig. 8.136** Female urogenital diaphragm. Left: superficial layer; right: deep layer (inferior view).

**Pathology**

**Pelvic Floor Insufficiency and Urinary Incontinence (Fig. 8.137)**

The bladder, rectum, and female genital organs are suspended by means of ligamentous structures that connect the organs to the inner walls of the sacrum, ilium, and pubis. Relaxation of these ligaments would overburden the pelvic floor muscles over time and allow downward displacement.

By descending vertically, the uterus presses on the bladder and changes the position of the urethra. This disrupts the closure mechanism of the bladder, which can manifest itself in the form of bladder weakness.

Other causes of incontinence include surgery of the urogenital tract because, as a result of reduced venous drainage, any edema is not sufficiently evacuated, thus restricting the closure mechanisms. In addition, the innervation of the pelvic floor muscles is often disturbed due to overstretching.

**Prostatic Hypertrophy (Fig. 8.138)**

Prostatic hypertrophy plays a role in urinary obstruction because the prostate lies immediately inferior to the bladder and, when enlarged, may constrict the urethral orifice.

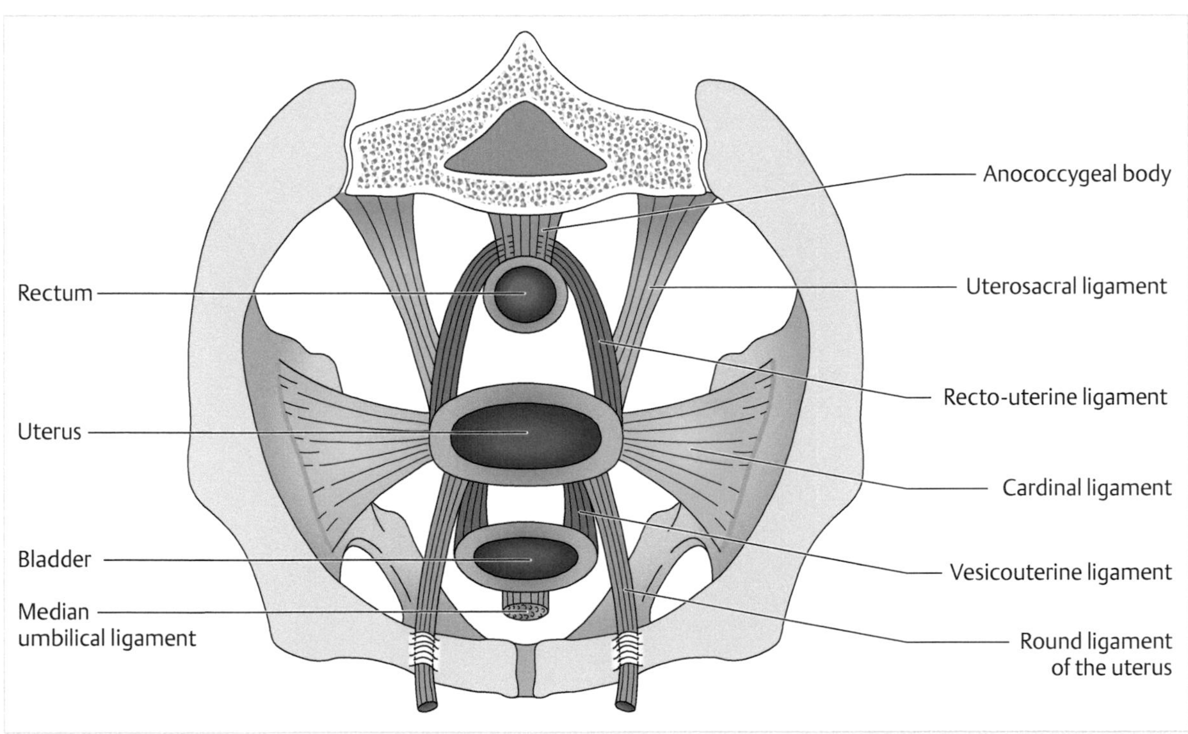


**Fig. 8.137** Suspension of the organs in the female pelvis (superior view).

## Practical Tip

### Pelvic Floor Exercises

After surgery of the urogenital tract, pelvic floor exercises should be started early as prophylaxis for incontinence. They promote blood flow and venous function, involve nerve retraining and may play a role in the position of the urogenital organs. The interval between micturition is extended, the bladder capacity increased, and the strength of the sphincter improved.

However, the exercises should not consist simply of squeezing the buttocks together in various body positions, but rather represent the start of training in the perception of pelvic movements. Examples of the possible exercise options are various activities involving putting pressure on the tuberosity while sitting, practicing cautious constriction of breathing patterns, and the "elevator ride" or the proprioceptive neuromuscular facilitation pattern of anterior elevation/posterior depression.

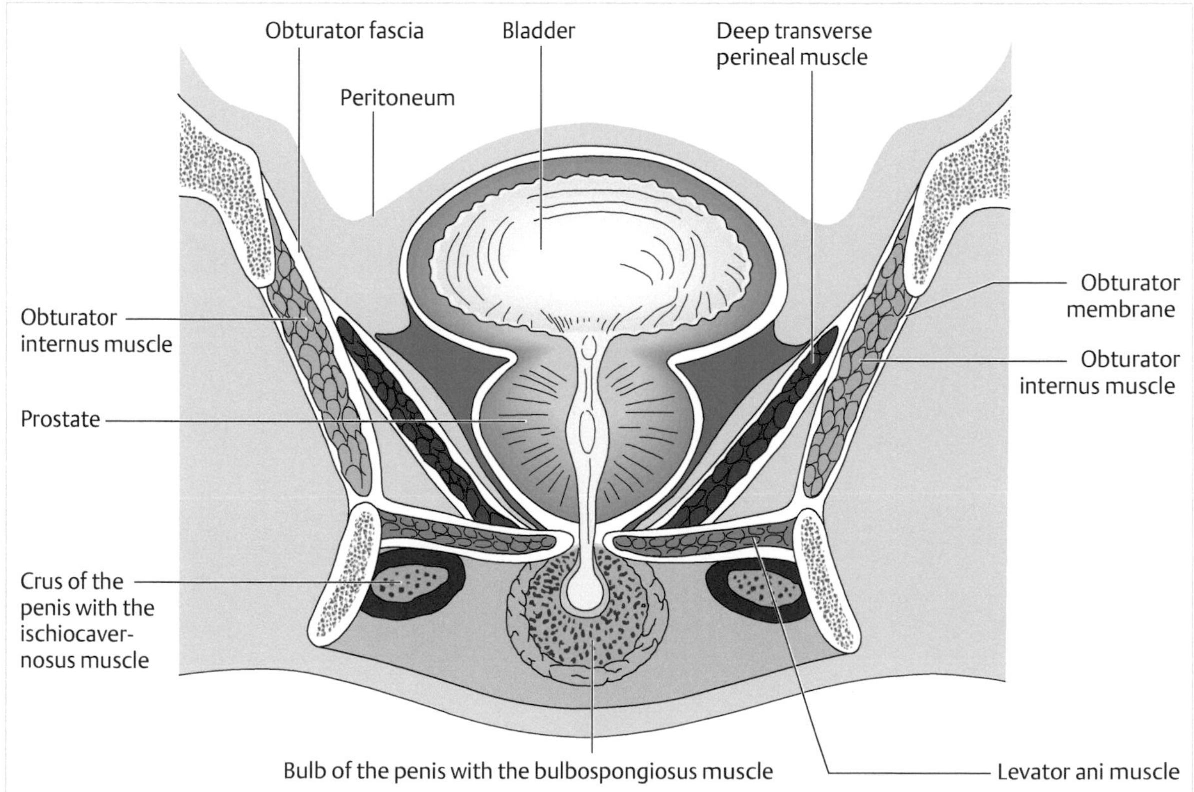


**Fig. 8.138** Male pelvis in frontal section.

## 8.8.3 Flexors of the Hip Joint

### Iliopsoas Muscle (Fig. 8.139)

- This passes under the inguinal ligament anterior to the femoral head.
- It uses the femoral head as a kind of hypomochlion and then moves posteriorly. The muscle possesses a large lifting height.
- It has a large physiologic cross-section and thus is well qualified to be the most powerful hip flexor.
- Rami communicantes of the sympathetic trunk pass under its tendinous arches and connect with the lumbosacral plexus.

#### *Psoas Major Muscle*

- Originating from the first four lumbar and the 12th thoracic vertebrae, the psoas major muscle forms an important functional connection between the spinal column and the lower extremity.
- The superficial layer arises from the lateral surface of the vertebral body, with a few fibers going into the anulus fibrosus.
- The deep layer arises from the costal processes.
- The lumbar plexus lies between the deep and superficial layers.
- A few fibers intertwine with the diaphragm at the median arcuate ligament.

#### *Psoas Minor Muscle*

- This muscle is inconstant.
- It establishes a connection between the vertebral bodies of the 12th thoracic and first lumbar vertebrae and the iliac fascia.

#### *Iliacus Muscle*

- This consists of a thick muscle plate.
- At its insertion site on the lesser trochanter, the fibers of the iliacus muscle arising from the ASIS insert distally on the lesser trochanter and sometimes go as far as the medial lip of the linea aspera.
- *Functions:*
  - Flexion: It is the strongest flexor of the hip joint and exerts its force from the beginning of the movement to the end. It is possible to differentiate its delivery of force from other flexors because it is the only muscle that can flex above 90°.
  - Rotation: Opinions concerning its rotational function are very mixed. However, if the muscle's course is considered in relation to the axis of rotation—it comes from anteromedially and goes in a posterolateral direction—it has to cause external rotation in the neutral position.
  - Extension of the lumbar spine: With the legs as its fixed end, it extends the lumbar spine. However, if the back muscles prevent extension by tensing, then it, along with the abdominal muscles, causes flexion of the torso.
  - Lateral flexion and rotation: In unilateral contraction, it brings about ipsilateral lateral flexion and rotation to the contralateral side.
- *Innervation:* femoral nerve (T12–L3).

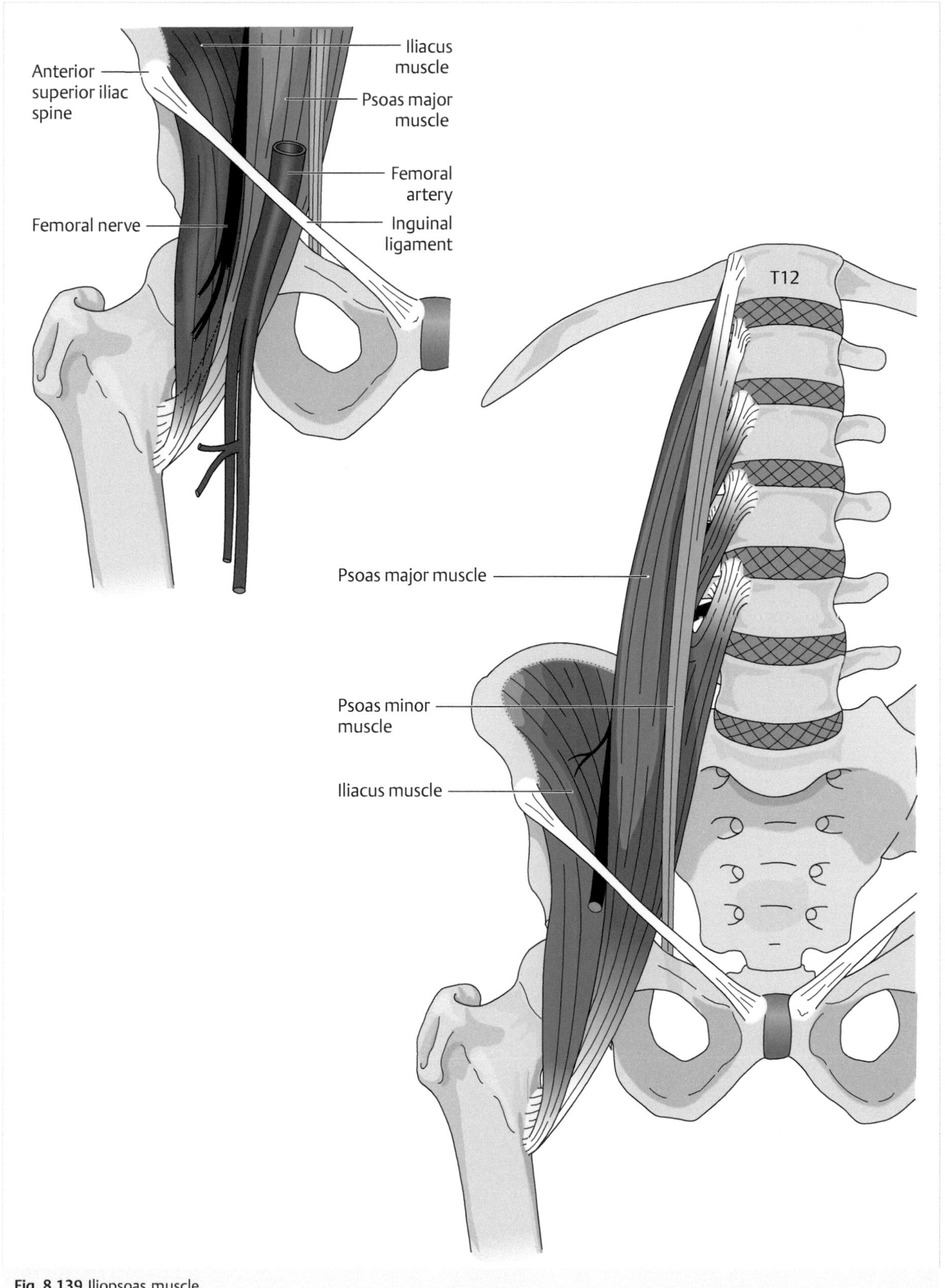


**Fig. 8.139** Iliopsoas muscle.

## Lever Calculation of the Iliopsoas Muscle (Fig. 8.140)

The iliopsoas muscle lies at a distance of 4 cm from the center of the femoral head. The resistance in this calculation is the weight of the leg, whose center of gravity lies approximately 40 cm distal to the hip joint when the knee is extended.

The ratio of the two lever arms means that the muscle force is 10 times the weight of the leg, which is one-sixth of the body weight, or 110 N. Therefore the muscle force is 10 times this (1100 N), which is 1.5 times the body weight.

When the leg is raised further, the lever arm of the leg weight is reduced, thereby improving the efficiency of the iliopsoas muscle. Thus, the forces acting on the hip joint are reduced.

From the small angle of muscle pull, it is also apparent that almost the entire force causes joint compression.

The iliopsoas muscle uses the femoral head as a pulley: it moves from posteriorly, runs anteriorly over the head of the femur, and then runs again posteriorly to the lesser trochanter. In this way, it exerts pressure on the femoral head toward the posterior.

Because of this, there is a small groove in the anterior area of the femoral head in some specimens.

### Practical Tip

The greatest forces are generated in the first phase of raising the leg off the bed. If no weight-bearing on the hip is allowed, this phase is therefore potentially hazardous. To reduce the risk, a short lever arm must be used or the weight of the leg reduced, by using the other leg, for example.

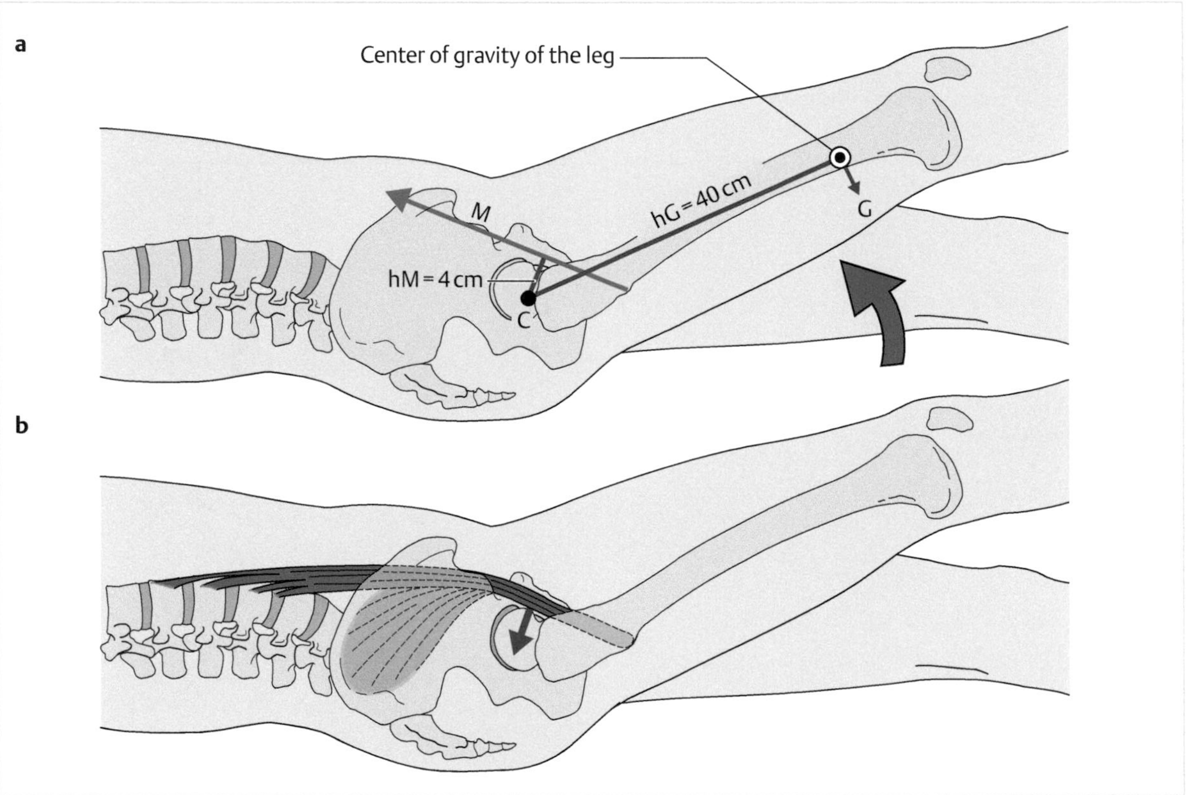


**Fig. 8.140 (a)** Leverage ratios of the iliopsoas muscle. M, muscle force; hM, force arm; hG, load arm; G, body weight. **(b)** Pressure component directed posteriorly.

### Rectus Femoris Muscle (Fig. 8.141)

- The origin is in the vicinity of the hip joint. A broad part arises from the superior rim of the acetabular margin and forms a connection with the fibrous layer of the capsule. A round part of the tendon comes from the anterior inferior iliac spine.
- The tensor fasciae latae and sartorius muscles overlie the area of origin.
- The muscle transitions into the terminal tendon about a handbreadth superior to the patella.
- The continuation of the terminal tendon is the patellar ligament.
- *Functions:*
  - At the hip: flexion is its most important function. The more the muscle is stretched over the knee joint (i.e., set in flexion), the more effective it is. It also supports abduction.
  - At the knee: extension.
- *Innervation:* femoral nerve (L2–L4).

#### Practical Tip

In hip joint surgery, such as total hip replacement, parts of the capsule–ligament apparatus are removed, depending on the size of the acetabulum. That means that some areas of origin of the rectus muscles are cut, and the patient will have difficulty in tensing the quadriceps muscle after surgery.

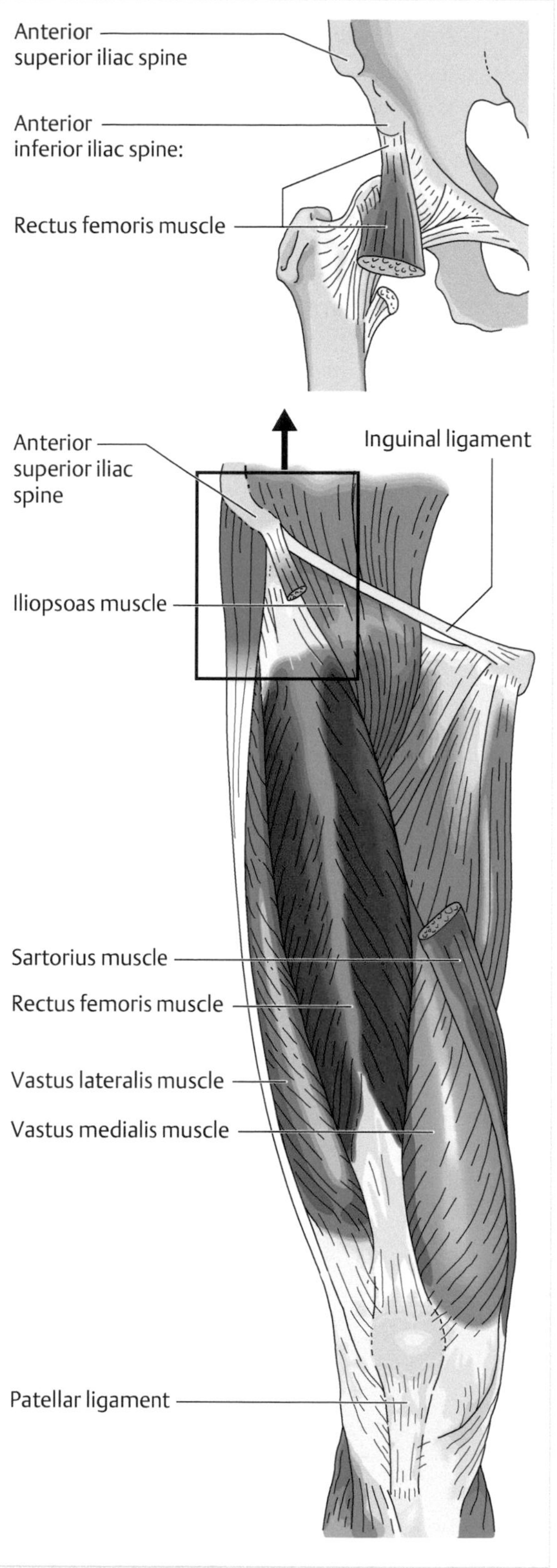


**Fig. 8.141** Rectus femoris muscle.

## Tensor Fasciae Latae Muscle (Fig. 8.142)

- This lies directly anterior to the gluteus medius muscle, from which it derives in evolutionary terms.
- It runs distally in front of the greater trochanter and extends into the iliotibial tract and fascia lata.
- *Functions:*
  - Flexion/abduction/internal rotation.
  - Through its connection to the iliotibial tract, it plays a role in the lateral stabilization of the knee joint.
  - Centering the hip joint, in which it plays a special role. The tensor fasciae latae muscle from the anterior side and the gluteus maximus muscle from the posterior side track into the upper third of the fascia lata, which envelops the entire thigh. They thus form the iliotibial tract, a very firm longitudinal, aponeurotic band that reaches to the tibia. The median fibers of the tract also extend to the iliac crest. Through their connections to the iliotibial tract, these two muscles provide a guiding function for the femoral head, pressing it into the acetabulum (**Fig. 8.143**).
- *Innervation:* superior gluteal nerve (L4/L5).

> **Pathology**
>
> **Snapping Hip Syndrome (Coxa Saltans)**
>
> Too much tension on the entire lateral fascia, especially in the iliotibial tract, can lead to the snapping hip syndrome. During flexion and extension movements, the tract slides over the greater trochanter. The result is a snapping sound, and a painful bursitis may develop.

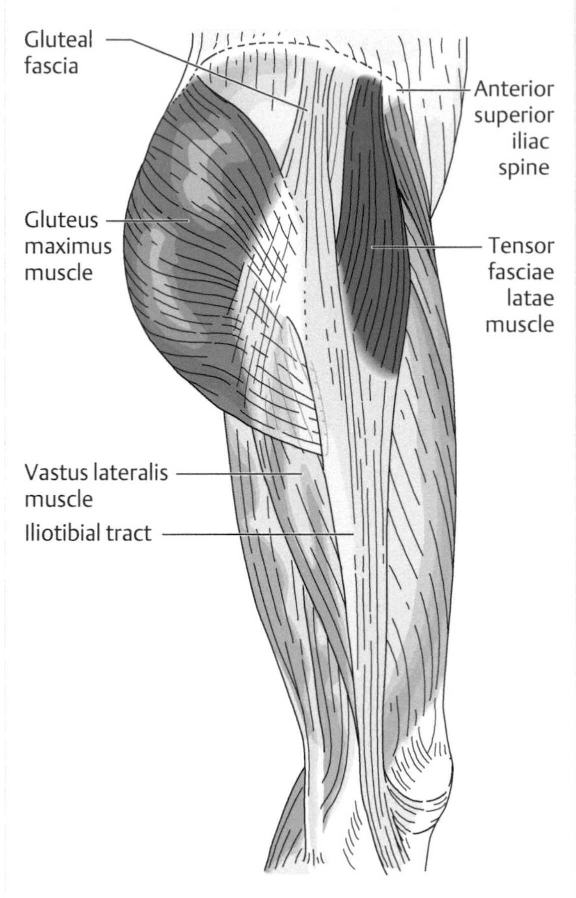


**Fig. 8.142** Tensor fasciae latae muscle.

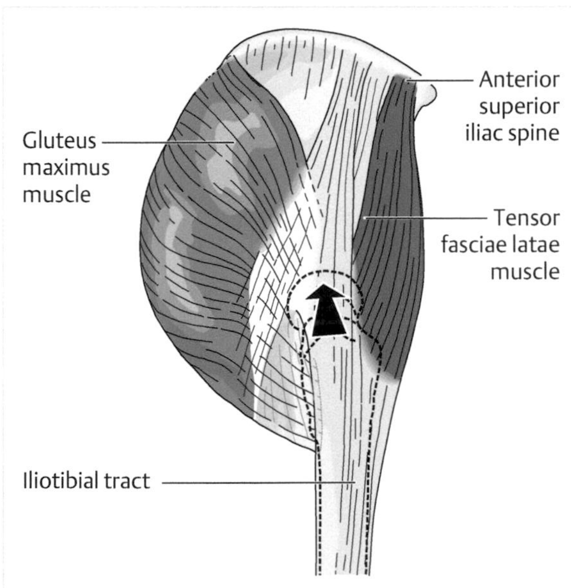


**Fig. 8.143** Tensor fasciae latae and gluteus maximus muscles holding the femoral head in place.

**Practical Tip**

**Flexor Stretch Test (Fig. 8.144)**

The flexors of the hip joint include primarily muscle fibers with type I collagen. These muscles belong to the tonic muscle system and have sustained power, a slower contraction speed, and a good capillary supply. In testing for their elasticity, Thomas's test, with the legs hanging over the end of the table, is used to test the iliopsoas, rectus femoris, and tensor fasciae latae muscles. If shortened, the iliopsoas muscle forces the hip joint to flex, the shortened rectus muscle pulls the knee into extension, and the tensor fasciae latae muscle pulls the leg into abduction.

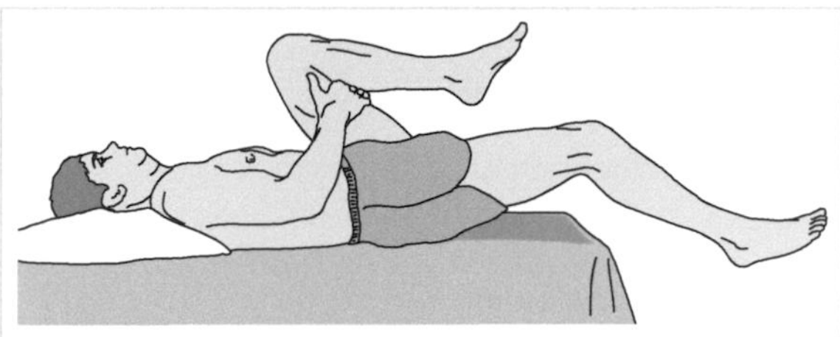

**Fig. 8.144** Flexor stretch test for the flexors of the hip joint showing decreased elasticity of the iliopsoas and rectus femoris muscles.

## Sartorius Muscle (Fig. 8.145)

- This is a muscle crossing two joints.
- The muscle fibers are very long.
- It moves spirally around the anterior thigh from proximal-lateral to distal-medial.
- Its tendon of insertion forms the superficial part of the pes anserinus.
- *Functions:*
  - Flexion/abduction/external rotation.
  - Knee flexion and internal rotation.
- *Innervation:* femoral nerve (L2–L3).

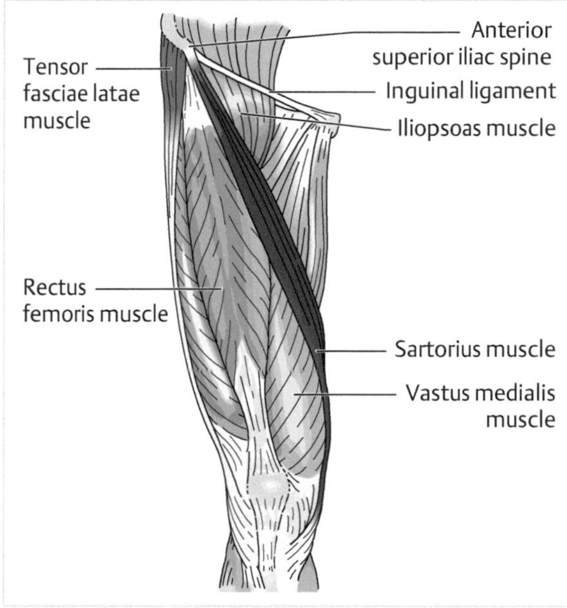


**Fig. 8.145** Sartorius muscle.

## Additional Flexors (Fig. 8.146)

The following muscles assist in flexion and will be described later:

- Pectineus muscle.
- Adductor longus muscle.
- Adductor brevis muscle.
- Gracilis muscle.
- Gluteus medius and minimus muscles.

### *Classification of the Flexor Muscles According to Their Function*

The flexors may be divided into two groups with respect to their other functions:

- *Flexion/abduction/internal rotation:* parts of the gluteus medius and minimus muscles and the tensor fasciae latae muscle.
- *Flexion/adduction/external rotation:* the iliopsoas, pectineus, gracilis, and adductor longus and brevis muscles.

### *Influence on Muscle Force by Altered Pelvic Position*

The position of the pelvis influences the development of power by the flexor muscles. Through a flexed position of the pelvis and increased lordosis of the lumbar spine, the iliopsoas, rectus femoris, and sartorius muscles are in a shortened position and cannot develop their optimal power. Therefore more areas of the gluteus medius and minimus muscles function as flexors, because in the flexed position they clearly lie anterior to the axis of motion.

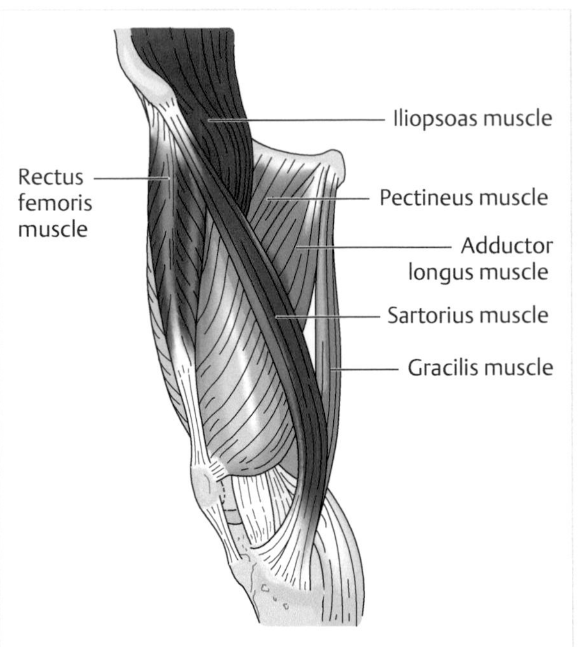


**Fig. 8.146** Flexors of the hip joint (anteromedial view).

## 8.8.4 Extensors of the Hip Joint

### Gluteus Maximus Muscle (Fig. 8.147)

- At its origin, this a continuation of the thoracolumbar fascia.
- A broad superior part merges into the iliotibial tract; a step-off is recognizable at the transition point.
- The posterior part tracks to the gluteal tuberosity and to the linea aspera on the femur.
- There is a connection to the lateral intermuscular septum.
- The muscle continues into the vastus lateralis muscle.
- Connective tissue septa span between the muscle bundles and provide a kind of compartmentalization.
- The fascia lata forms a halter-like support for the inferior edge of the muscle. Fibers running transversely are tensed during sitting and pull the muscle border superiorly and laterally. When sitting, the ischial tuberosity is thus padded by chambered subcutaneous adipose tissue.
- *Functions:*
  - Extension: Significant force—about one to two times body weight—is required to activate the muscle. It is most effective at a hip flexion of approximately 90°. When the fixed end of the muscle is on the femur, it is involved in all extension movements that require power, such as rising from a sitting position, getting up from squatting, and straightening the torso from a flexed position. When the fixed end is on the pelvis, the muscle is involved in activities such as going up steps, mountain climbing, and running quickly.
  - External rotation: The muscle is a powerful external rotator.
  - It is an autoantagonist. Because of its broad course, some of its fiber components are located superior to the sagittal axis and thus perform *abduction*, while others are inferior to it and perform *adduction* (**Fig. 8.148**).
  - Through the connection with the iliotibial tract, it has the effect of *centering the femoral head* (see **Fig. 8.143**) and *stabilizing the knee joint.*
- *Innervation:* inferior gluteal nerve (L4–S1).

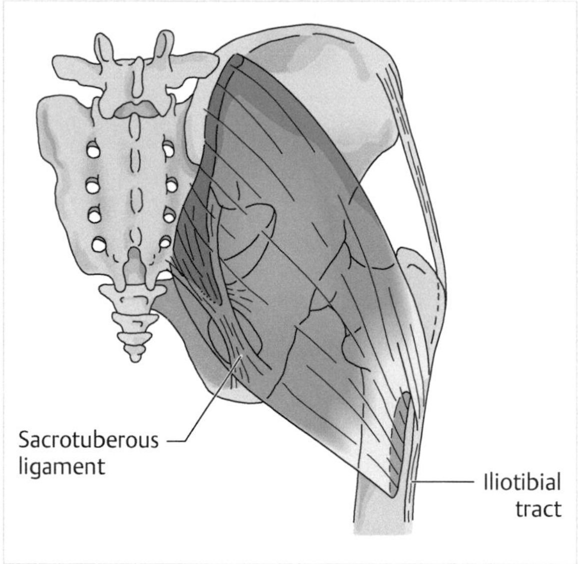


**Fig. 8.147** Gluteus maximus muscle.

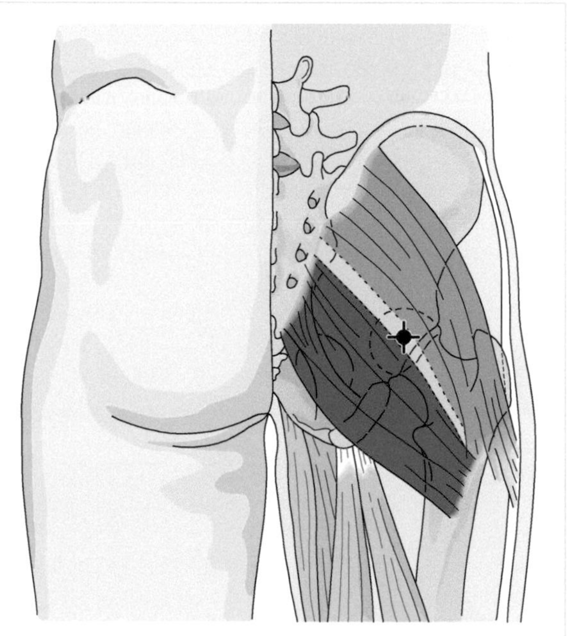

**Fig. 8.148** Autoantagonism: the gluteus maximus muscle with respect to abduction and adduction. Brown part: abduction; red part: adduction.

## Hamstring Muscles

### Biceps Femoris Muscle, Long Head (Fig. 8.149)

- This uses the ischial tuberosity as a pulley because some of the muscle fibers track into the sacrotuberous ligament.
- The origin on the tuberosity is superficial. It forms a common head with the semitendinosus muscle.
- It runs just medial to the vastus lateralis muscle and is separated from it by the lateral intermuscular septum.
- At the knee, it forms the lateral boundary of the popliteal fossa.

### Semitendinosus Muscle (Fig. 8.149)

- This has a connection to the sacrotuberous ligament.
- It lies in a groove formed from the semimembranosus muscle.
- At the beginning of the lower third of the thigh, it transitions into its long terminal tendon.

### Semimembranosus Muscle (Fig. 8.150)

- Inferior to its origin, the muscle widens into an aponeurosis over which the two above-mentioned muscles run.
- Its muscle fibers run from superolateral to inferomedial.
- The medial part of the muscle transitions into its tendon earlier than the lateral part, where muscle fibers continue to run distally.
- At the knee, the insertions spread out in five different directions. See Chapter 9.3.5, Medial Functional Complex, and **Fig. 9.97.**
- It forms the medial border of the popliteal fossa.

### Functions of the Hamstring Muscles

- The work performance of the hamstring muscles corresponds to about two-thirds that of the gluteus maximus.
- All parts of the hamstring muscles contribute to hip *extension.*
- *External rotation* is brought about by the biceps femoris muscle.
- *Internal rotation* is achieved by the semitendinosus and semimembranosus muscles.
- *Flexion of the knee* and *external rotation* of the lower leg are caused by the biceps femoris muscle, and *internal rotation* by the semitendinosus and semimembranosus muscles.

*Innervation:* sciatic nerve (L5–S2).

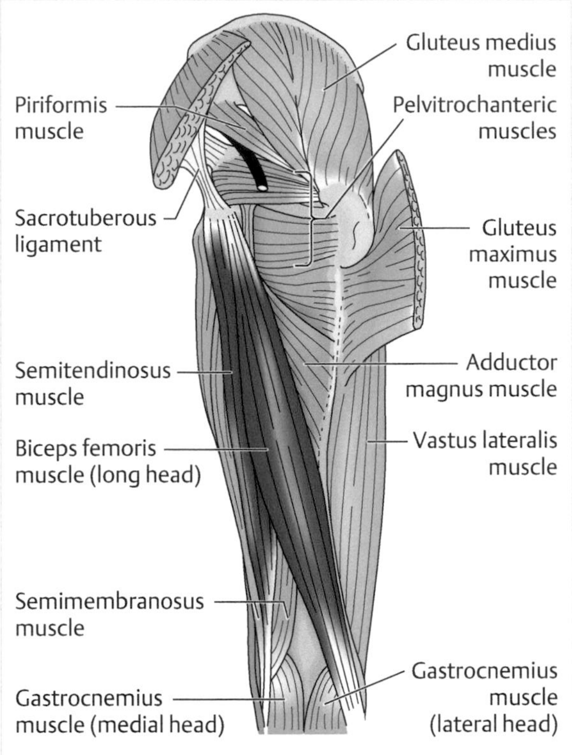


**Fig. 8.149** Hamstring muscles: biceps femoris and semitendinosus muscles.

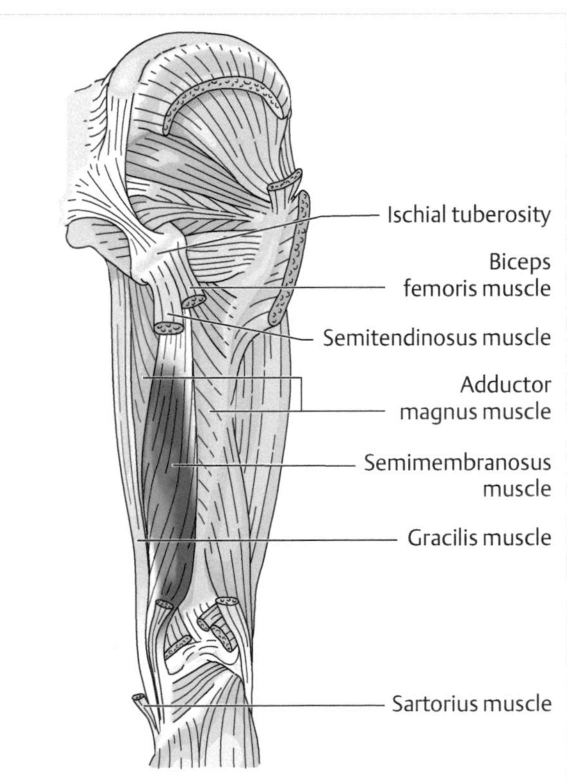


**Fig. 8.150** Hamstring muscles: semimembranosus muscle.

### Stabilization in the Sagittal Plane (Fig. 8.151)

- When the patient is standing in a comfortable position, the center of gravity lies centrally behind the hip joints. The iliofemoral ligament and tensor fasciae latae impede extension beyond this point.
- If the plumb line from the center of gravity passes through the center of the hip joint, both flexors and extensors are relaxed, giving rise to an unstable equilibrium.
- If the pelvis is in a slightly flexed position, the hamstring muscles act to stabilize the pelvis.
- Only with further flexion does the gluteus maximus muscle also become active.

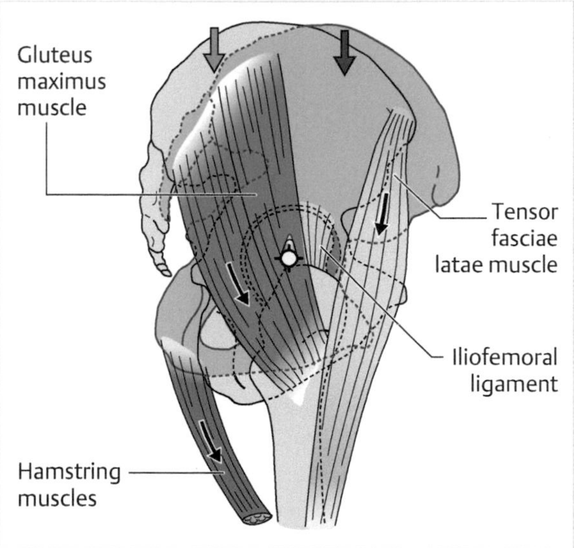


**Fig. 8.151** Stabilization in the sagittal plane. Gray: the center of gravity of the body behind the pivot point. Red: the center of gravity of the body in front of the pivot point.

## Additional Extensors (Fig. 8.152)

The following muscles assist with extension and will be described later:

- Gluteus medius and minimus muscles.
- Adductor magnus muscle.
- Short external rotators (e.g., piriformis and obturator muscles).

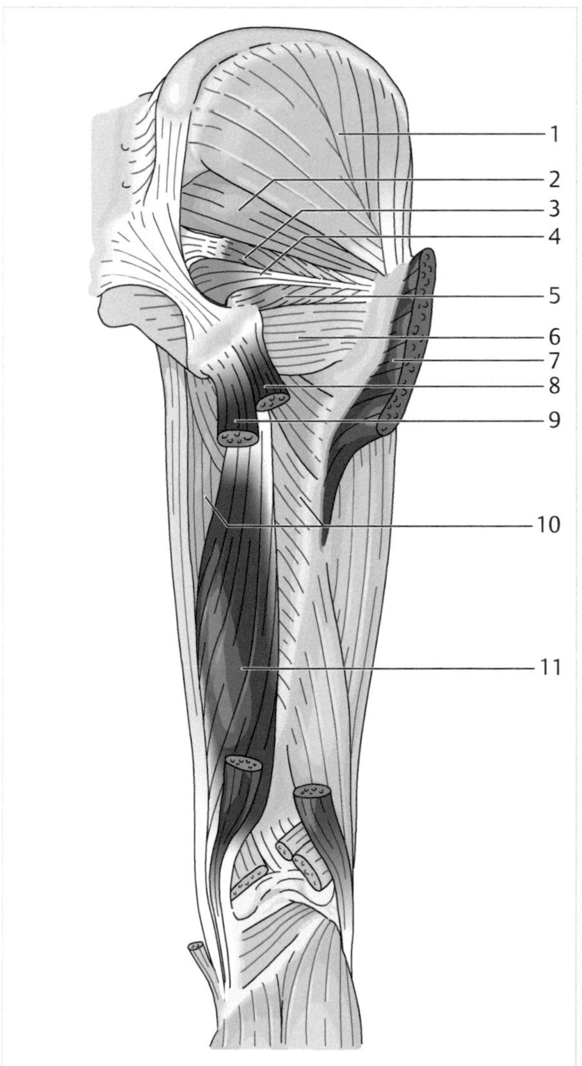


1 = Gluteus medius muscle
2 = Piriformis muscle
3 = Gemellus superior muscle
4 = Obturator internus muscle
5 = Gemellus inferior muscle
6 = Quadratus femoris muscle
7 = Gluteus maximus muscle
8 = Biceps femoris muscle (long head)
9 = Semitendinosus muscle
10 = Adductor magnus muscle
11 = Semimembranosus muscle

**Fig. 8.152** Extensors of the hip joint. ▸

## 8.8.5 Abductors of the Hip Joint

### Gluteus Medius Muscle (Fig. 8.153)

- The anterior fibers run helically in a posterior direction and lie on top of the posterior fibers at the greater trochanter.
- The posterior third is covered by the gluteus maximus muscle.
- The insertion occupies the lateral surface of the greater trochanter.
- The superficial trochanteric bursa of the gluteus medius muscles lies between the tendon and the greater trochanter.

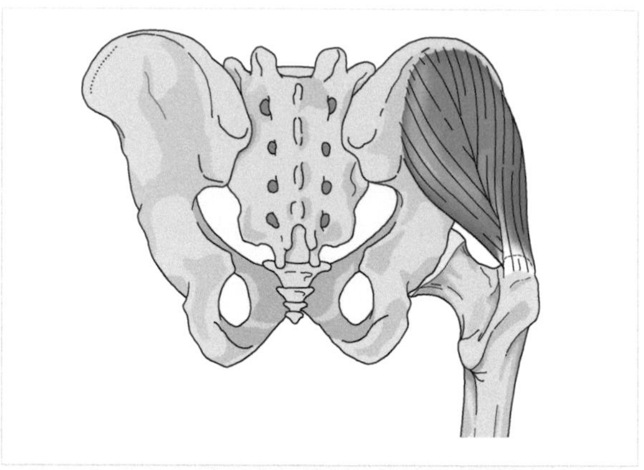

**Fig. 8.153** Gluteus medius muscle.

### Gluteus Minimus Muscle (Fig. 8.154)

- This is covered by the gluteus medius muscle.
- It runs anteriorly to the greater trochanter; the trochanteric bursa of the gluteus minimus muscle lies here between the tendon and bone.
- *Functions:*
  - Abduction: These two abductors play an important role in body balance—with the distal ends fixed in the stance phase, they prevent the pelvis on the free-leg side from dropping. In doing this, they perform eccentric work. With the fixed end at the pelvis, they abduct the leg.
  - Influence on pelvic tilt (**Fig. 8.155**): from a lateral view, one can easily discern the division of the fibrous components and the relationship to the flexion-extension axis. If the fiber orientation is anterior to the axis, there is flexion; if it is posterior, there is extension.
  - Rotation: the anterior fibers cause internal rotation; the posterior fibers cause external rotation.
  - The magnitude of the CCD angle influences the effect of the gluteus medius and minimus muscles:
    - Coxa valga alters the course of the muscle fibers, which becomes steeper and thus less favorable for the functions of abduction and stabilization because the moment of force is very low.
    - In coxa vara, the course of the muscles is almost horizontal. This implies a very good moment of force, but this is nullified because the origin and insertion sites move close to each other due to the lowering of the femoral neck.
- *Innervation*: superior gluteal nerve.

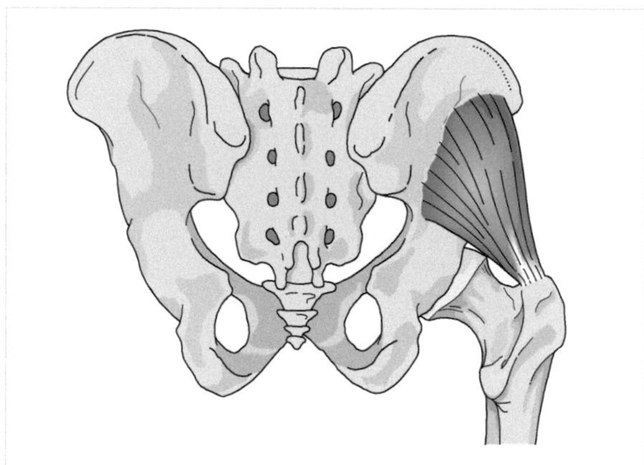

**Fig. 8.154** Gluteus minimus muscle.

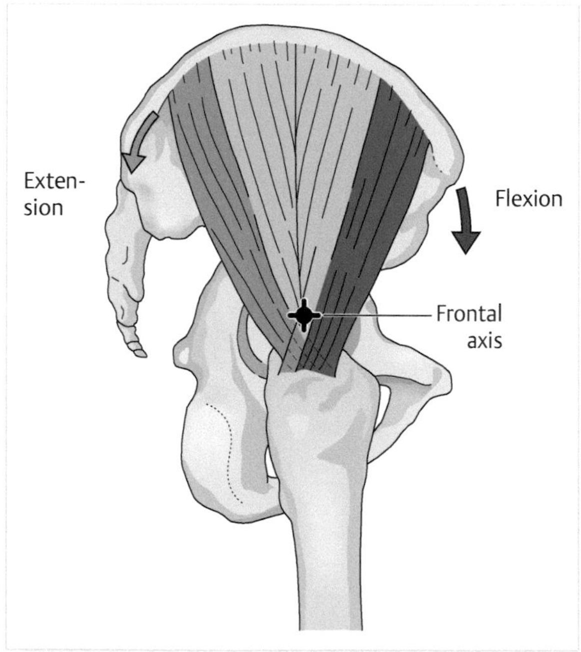


**Fig. 8.155** Influence of the gluteus medius muscle on pelvic tilt.

## Piriformis Muscle (Fig. 8.156)

- This travels in an anteroinferior direction over the SIJ.
- It runs almost horizontally through the greater sciatic foramen, dividing it into the suprapiriform and infrapiriform foramina.
- The *suprapiriform foramen* is a gap through which the superior gluteal artery and vein and the superior gluteal nerve travel, and which is filled with connective tissue.
- The inferior gluteal vessels and the pudendal and the inferior gluteal nerves travel through the *infrapiriform foramen*, with the sciatic nerve also passing through the lateral part of the foramen.
- The piriformis muscle has a connection to the sacrospinous ligament.
- *Functions:*
  - Abduction: in the neutral position, it performs flexion and external rotation.
  - At 60° of hip flexion, a *reversal of function* takes place. The path of the muscle changes in relation to the axis of rotation: in the extended position, the muscle runs posteriorly, which means it produces external rotation. In the flexed position, it runs anteriorly, which means it produces internal rotation. It also changes its course in the frontal axis: at a flexion of approximately 60°, its insertion on the greater trochanter is clearly shifted inferiorly, which is why it acts as an extensor in this position.
  - Stabilization of the SIJ: see Chapter 8.4.8, Stabilizing Structures.
- *Innervation:* sacral plexus (L5–S2).

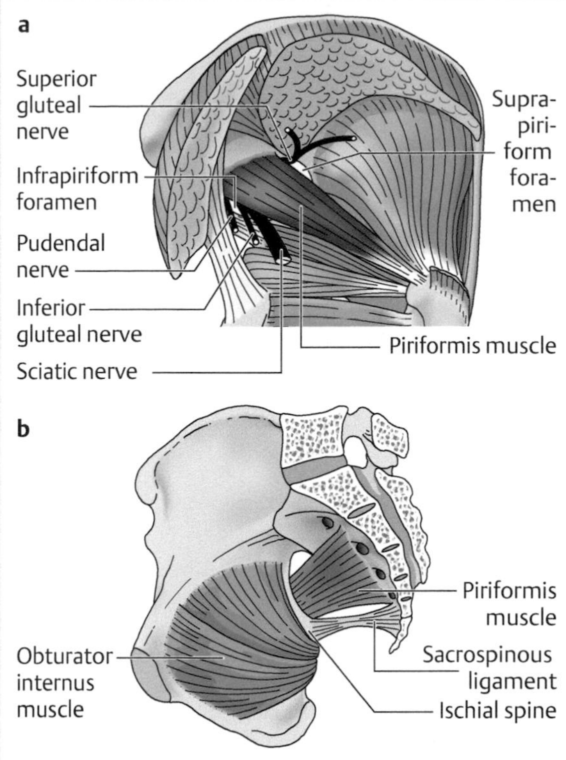


**Fig. 8.156** Piriformis muscle. **(a)** Superior view. **(b)** Medial pelvic view.

Pathology

### Piriformis Syndrome

The piriformis syndrome, in which the sciatic nerve is irritated, can have the following causes:

- Hematoma with consequent swelling of the muscle and surrounding tissue.
- Hypertonicity of the muscle.
- Proliferation of the vessels: The inferior gluteal vein lies below the muscle. It tends to form outpouchings that build up into a large tangled mass that can press on the sciatic nerve. If this goes on for an extended period, a neuroma can develop, which takes a long time to regress.

**Practical Tip**

**Examination and Treatment of the Piriformis Syndrome**

To determine whether the piriformis muscle is responsible for a patient's sciatica, straight leg raising is carefully performed to approximately 70°, even if it causes pain. In this position, the leg is placed in internal rotation and abduction. This allows the piriformis muscle to relax; the pain decreases and flexion can be increased. External rotation/adduction, in contrast, will increase the pain.

To enlarge the space for the sciatic nerve, the tone of the piriformis muscle must be reduced. This can be achieved by longitudinal stretching or cautious inhibitory compression. The subsequent mobilization of the sciatic nerve should not be forgotten.

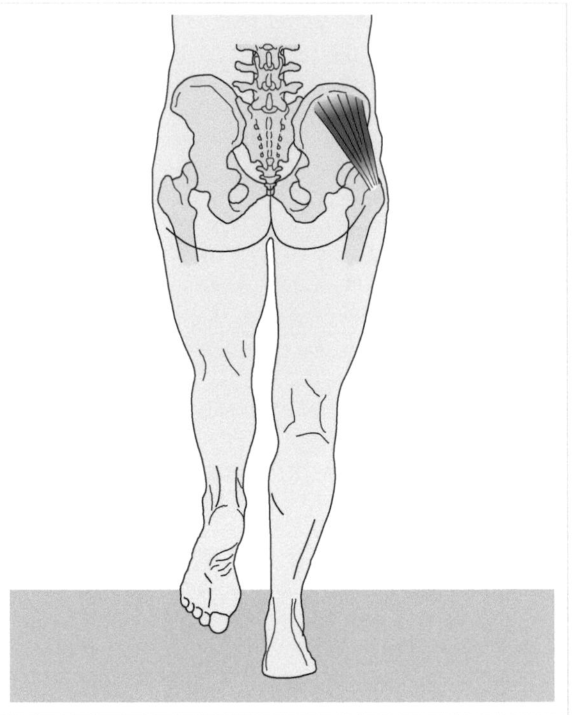

**Fig. 8.157** Stabilization of the pelvis in the neutral position.

## Additional Abductors

- Tensor fasciae latae muscle.
- Gluteus maximus muscle (superior part).

### *Stabilization of the Pelvis in the Frontal Plane (Fig. 8.157)*

In various flexed positions of the hip joint in standing and walking, stabilization in the frontal plane is guaranteed by various abductors. These prevent descent of the pelvis on the free-leg side:

- If the load of the partial body weight falls behind the transverse axis, the pelvis is stabilized by the iliofemoral ligament, the tensor fasciae latae muscle, and the anterior parts of the gluteus medius muscle.
- If the plumb line passes through the rotational center, the gluteus medius and minimus muscles stabilize the pelvis, as they do when the patient's leg is slightly flexed.
- With increasing flexion, the superior portions of the gluteus maximus and the piriformis muscle come into play.

**Pathology**

While walking, a near-neutral position of the pelvis must be maintained to support the body's weight and stabilize the pelvis. Weakening of the gluteus medius and minimus muscles is thus especially noticeable—they can no longer hold the pelvis up, so it drops on the free-leg side—Trendelenburg's sign.

▷ See Chapter 8.7.8, Biomechanics

## 8.8.6 Adductors of the Hip Joint

### Pectineus Muscle (Fig. 8.158)

- Together with the iliopsoas muscle, this forms a V-shaped depression, the iliopectineal fossa, in which the vessels run distally.
- The posterior surface of the muscle comes into contact with the anterior ligaments of the hip joint, the adductor brevis and obturator externus muscles.
- *Functions:* adduction/flexion/external rotation.
- *Innervation:* femoral nerve and possibly the obturator nerve as well.

### Adductor Longus Muscle (Fig. 8.158)

- This borders the entrance of the adductor canal, through which the femoral artery and vein run.
- Together with the sartorius muscle and the inguinal ligament, it forms the *medial femoral triangle*, a V-shaped space through which the femoral artery, veins, and lymphatic vessels run.
- *Functions:*
  - Adduction.
  - Flexion from the neutral position to 70° of flexion; beyond that, extension.
  - External rotation: this function can be explained if one considers the course of the muscle to the linea aspera (from anteromedial to posterolateral) in relation to the axis of rotation (**Fig. 8.159**).
- *Innervation:* anterior branch of the obturator nerve (L2–L4).

### Gracilis Muscle (Fig. 8.158)

- This has a wide area of origin on the inferior pubic ramus and then becomes narrower.
- It crosses two joints because of its insertion on the anteromedial tibia, the superficial pes anserinus.
- *Functions:*
  - Adduction/hip flexion up to flexed position of 50°, and hip extension beyond that.
  - Knee flexion and internal rotation.
- *Innervation:* anterior branch of the obturator nerve (L2–L4).

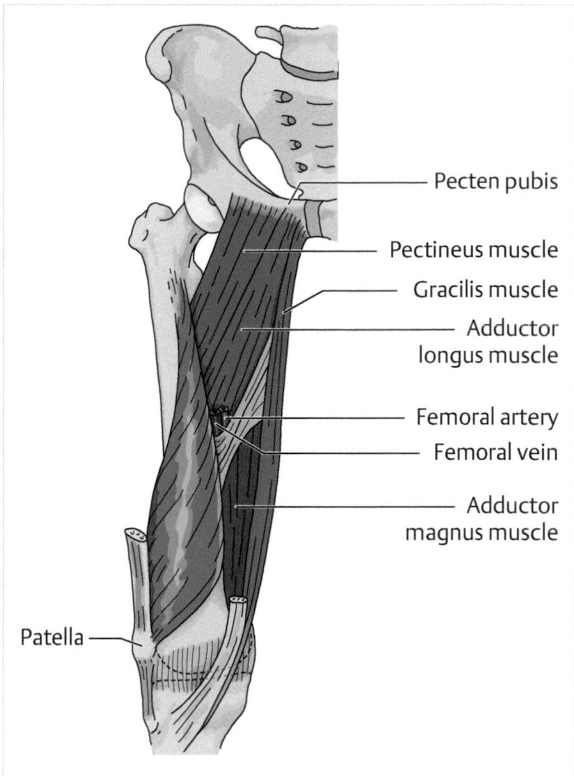


**Fig. 8.158** Adductors of the hip joint: pectineus, adductor longus, and gracilis muscles (anteromedial view).

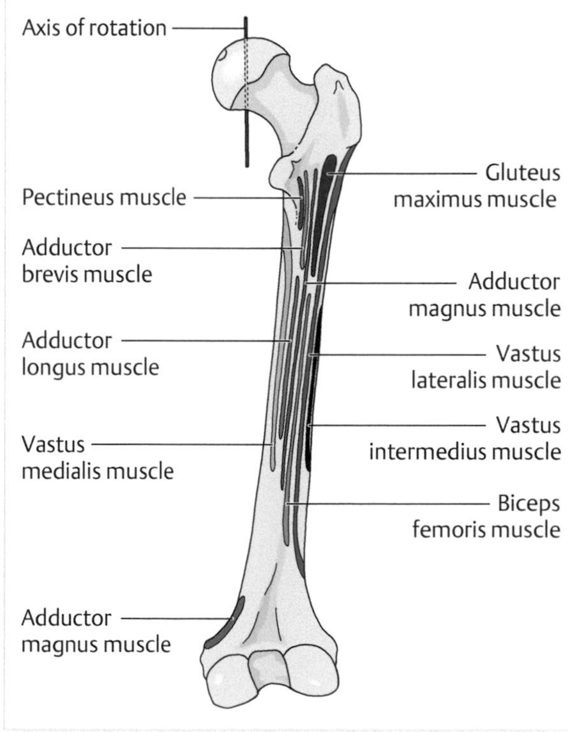


**Fig. 8.159** Insertions of the adductors on the linea aspera.

### Adductor Brevis Muscle (Fig. 8.160)

- Together with the adductor magnus muscle, it forms the deep adductor layer.
- *Functions:* see the adductor longus muscle.
- *Innervation:* see the adductor longus muscle.

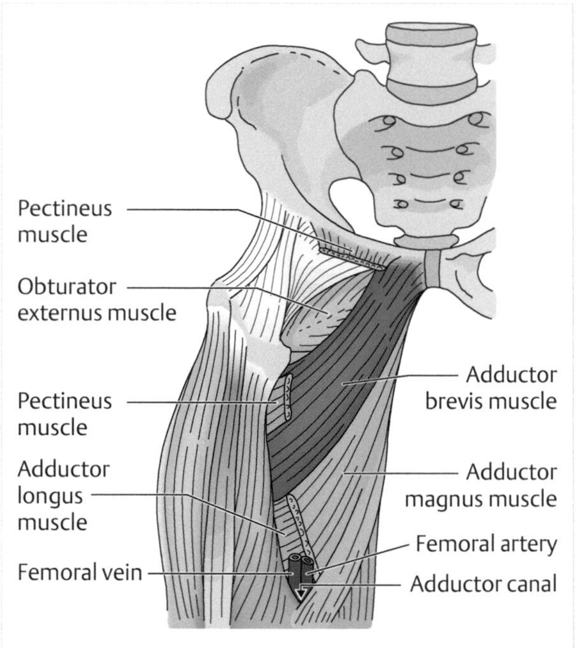


**Fig. 8.160** Adductor brevis muscle.

### Adductor Magnus Muscle (Fig. 8.161)

- This is located the furthest posteriorly; its posterior surface is in contact with the hamstring muscles.
- It is the most powerful adductor.
- The muscle has the shape of an opened fan.
- It is divided into three parts: The *proximal part* extends transversely and is also referred to as the adductor minimus muscle. The *middle part* has the broadest insertion—the entire linea aspera. The *distal portion* tracks to the adductor tubercle, on the medial femoral condyle.
- Together with the vastus medialis muscle, the adductor magnus forms the anteromedial intermuscular septum, a connecting aponeurotic sheet that, along with the muscle insertion at the linea aspera, represents the superior part of the adductor canal. The vessels run distally through this. The canal is bordered distally by a slit-like opening, the adductor hiatus, which is located between the deep and superficial layers of the adductor magnus muscle.
- *Functions:*
  - Adduction/powerful extension over the entire movement sequence, especially the supracondylar part of the muscle; *external rotation* by its proximal parts; *internal rotation* by its distal parts.
  - The interplay between the abductors and adductors is important in the balance of the pelvis because the pelvis can be kept stable only if there is a good balance between the two muscle groups.
- *Innervation:* double innervation: the superior areas by the posterior branch of the obturator nerve (L3–L4), and the inferior areas by the tibial part of the sciatic nerve (L4–L5).

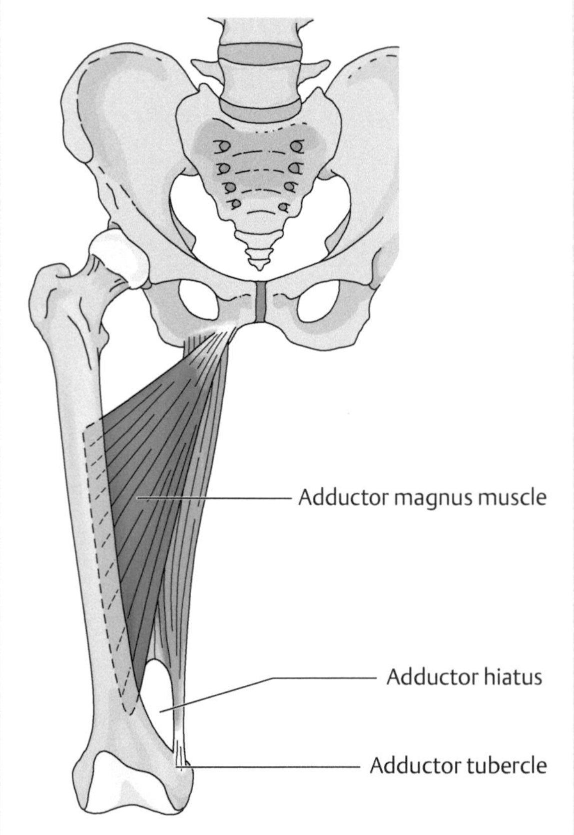


**Fig. 8.161** Adductor magnus muscle (anteromedial view).

## Additional Adductors

- Hamstring muscles.
- Gluteus maximus muscle (inferior fibers).
- Quadratus femoris muscle.

## 8.8.7 External Rotators of the Hip Joint

These muscles are located in the inferior gluteal region and are known as the pelvitrochanteric muscles. They run posterior to the longitudinal axis, which makes them external rotators.

They consist of the following muscles, arranged from superior to inferior:

### Piriformis Muscle (Fig. 8.162)

▷ See Chapter 8.8.5, Abductors of the Hip Joint

### Obturator Internus Muscle (Fig. 8.162)

- This consists of a short, broad, muscular portion and a long terminal tendon.
- The inner side of the obturator membrane serves as its origin.
- It runs in a sharp bend around the lesser sciatic notch, which it uses as a hypomochlion; this is why the surface of this area is covered with cartilage.
- It has a connection to the pelvic diaphragm and the gemellus muscles.
- Together with the bony obturator groove, it forms the obturator canal, which runs from superolateral to inferomedial, through which the obturator nerve and vessels run.
- *Functions:*
  - From the neutral position: external rotation/adduction and extension.
  - From approximately 90° of hip flexion: abduction.
- *Innervation:* variations include the sacral plexus, the gluteal nerve, and possibly the pudendal nerve.

### Gemellus Muscles (Fig. 8.163)

- These originally belonged to the obturator internus muscle, which is why they are known collectively as the triceps coxae muscle.
- They run immediately superior and inferior to the obturator internus muscle; the tendons of both muscles radiate into its terminal tendon.
- *Functions:*
  - From the neutral position: external rotation/adduction and extension.
  - From approximately 90° of hip flexion: abduction.
- *Innervation:* varies between the sacral plexus, the inferior gluteal nerve, and possibly the pudendal nerve.

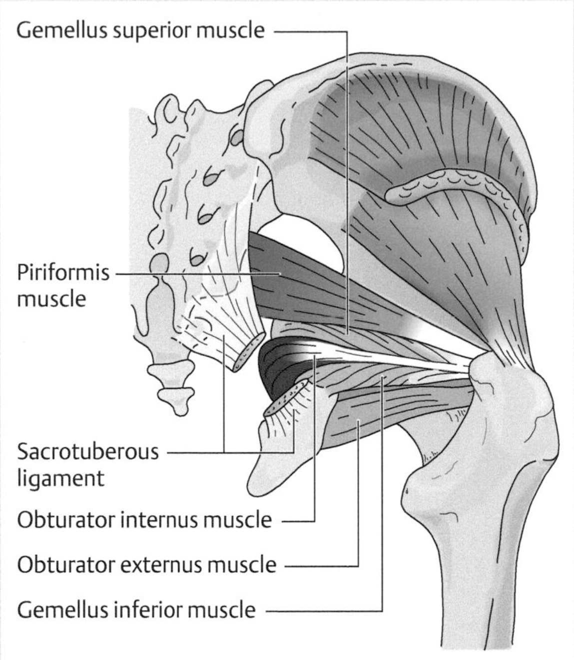


**Fig. 8.162** Piriformis and obturator internus muscles.

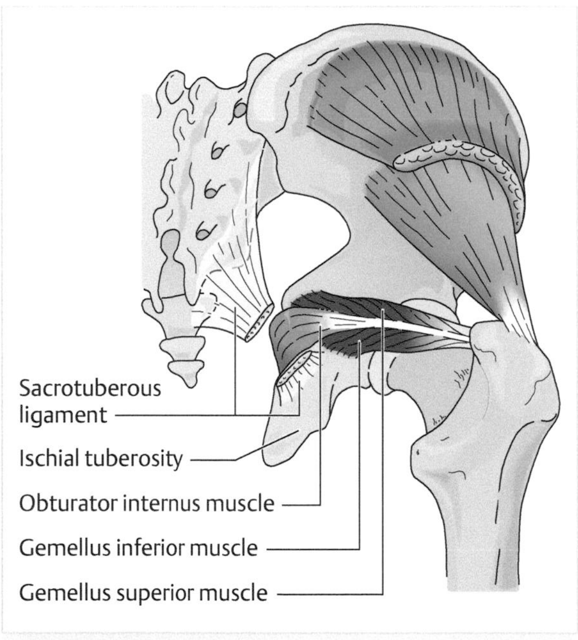


**Fig. 8.163** Gemellus muscles.

### Obturator Externus Muscle (Fig. 8.164)

- This has a connection to the external surface of the obturator membrane.
- It gives off some fibers to the zona orbicularis.
- It forms a spiral arc around the femoral neck, which, together with the ischiofemoral ligament, forms a figure-of-eight that envelops the femoral neck.
- It is covered by the quadratus femoris muscle.
- *Functions:* centering of the femoral head, external rotation/weak adduction.
- *Innervation:* obturator nerve (L3–L4).

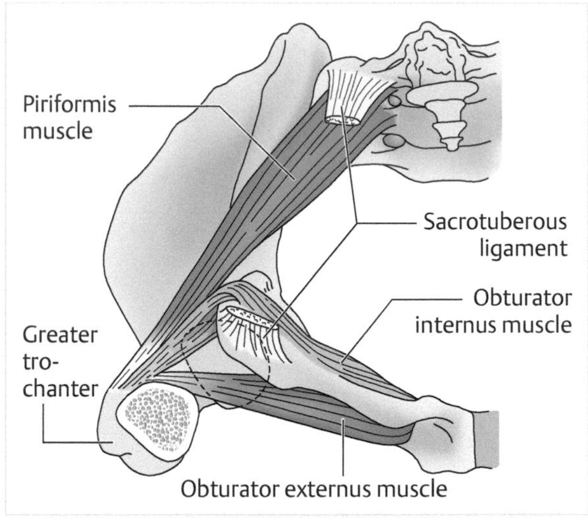


**Fig. 8.164** Obturator externus muscle (posterior view).

### Quadratus Femoris Muscle (Fig. 8.165)

- This lies immediately posterior to the inferior gemellus muscle, to which it may be adherent.
- *Functions:*
  - External rotation/adduction.
  - Can bring the leg from flexion to extension and vice versa.
- *Innervation:* inferior gluteal nerve and tibial portions of the sciatic nerve.

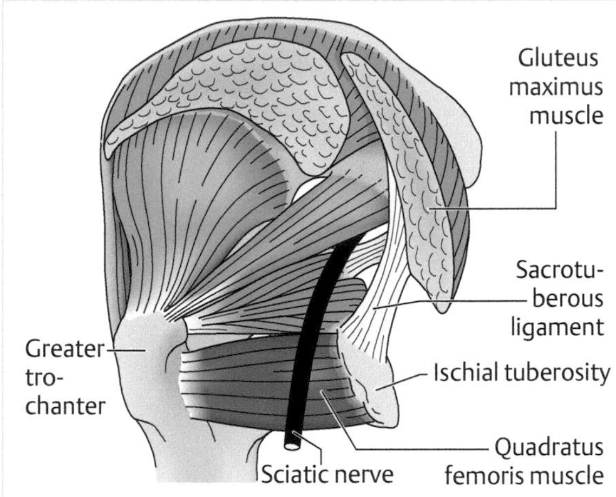


**Fig. 8.165** Quadratus femoris muscle.

## Additional External Rotators

- Gluteus maximus, which is the strongest external rotator; it provides about a third of the total force.
- Gluteus medius and minimus muscles (posterior part).
- Some adductors.
- Sartorius muscle.
- Biceps femoris muscle.
- Iliopsoas muscle.

The largest development of power in the direction of external rotation can be expected at approximately 60° of flexion. If the force components of the external rotators could be disassembled, the following differences would be found (**Fig. 8.166**):

- The piriformis, obturator internus, gluteus maximus, gluteus medius, and gluteus minimus muscles act mainly in the direction of external rotation and have a small joint-centering force.
- In the case of the pectineus, quadratus femoris, and obturator externus muscles, the joint-closure component is the dominant force.

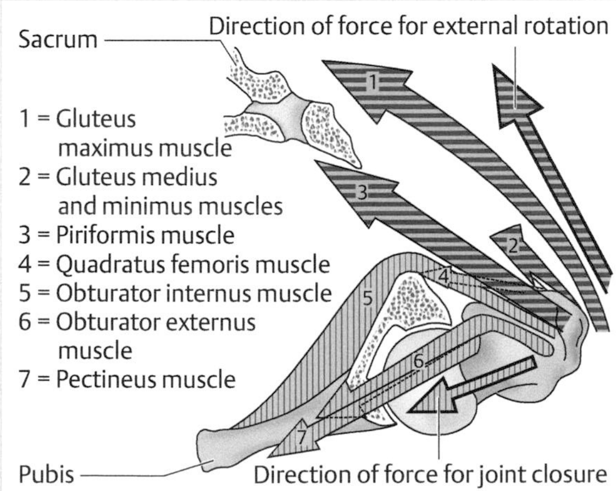


**Fig. 8.166** Force components of the external rotators (superior view).

### Reversal of Muscle Function (Fig. 8.167)

During internal rotation, a reversal of the rotational muscle function can occur. In this position, a portion of the *adductors*, the *obturator externus muscle*, and the *pectineus muscle* can become internal rotators due to the change of their course in relation to the axis of rotation.

## 8.8.8 Internal Rotators of the Hip Joint (Fig. 8.168)

Very few muscles cause internal rotation. Their power delivery is only one-third the power of the external rotators:

- Gluteus medius and minimus muscles (anterior fibers).
- Tensor fasciae latae muscle.
- Adductor magnus muscle (distal fibers).

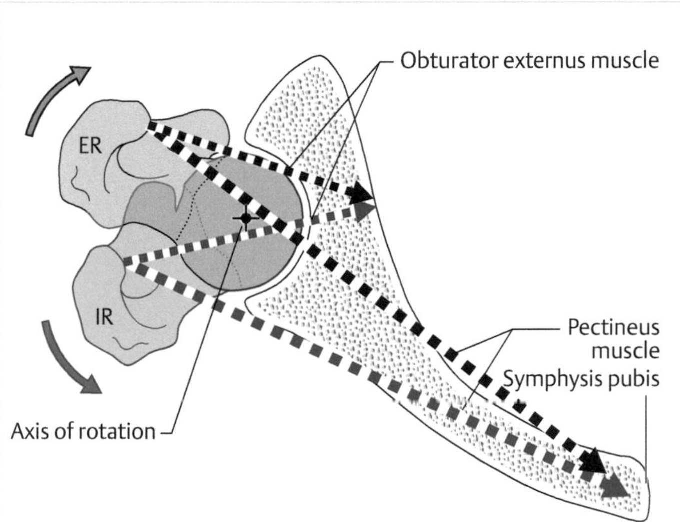


**Fig. 8.167** Muscle function reversal: obturator externus and pectineus muscles. ER = external rotation; IR = internal rotation.

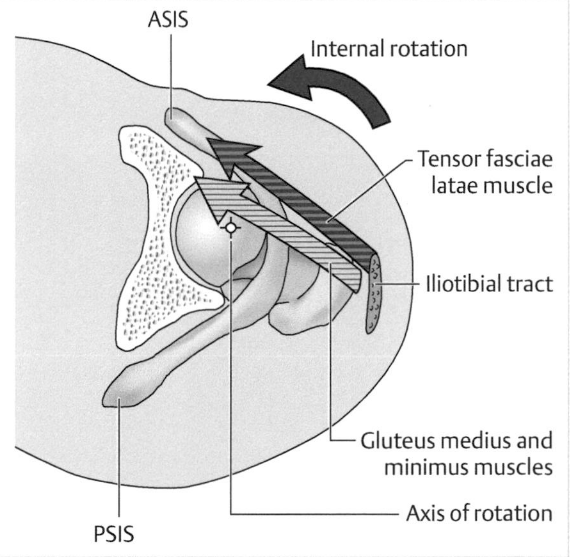


**Fig. 8.168** Gluteus medius and minimus muscles and tensor fasciae latae muscle (transverse view). ASIS, anterior superior iliac spine; PSIS, posterior superior iliac spine.

# 8.9 Neural Structures in the Pelvis–Hip Area

## 8.9.1 Sacral Plexus (Fig. 8.169)

- The sacral plexus can be subdivided into a sciatic plexus (L4–S3) and a pudendal plexus (S2–S4).
- It arises from the anterior rami of the fourth and fifth lumbar and the upper three sacral nerve roots.
- The anterior rami of L4 and L5 form the lumbosacral trunk, which runs into the lesser pelvis.
- The rami divide into a preaxial division, running anteriorly, and a postaxial division, running posteriorly.
- The anterior division forms the tibial part of the sciatic nerve, and the posterior division forms the common fibular part.
- The course of the sacral plexus is located on the anterior side of the piriformis muscle.
- The branches combine shortly before passing through the infrapiriform foramen.

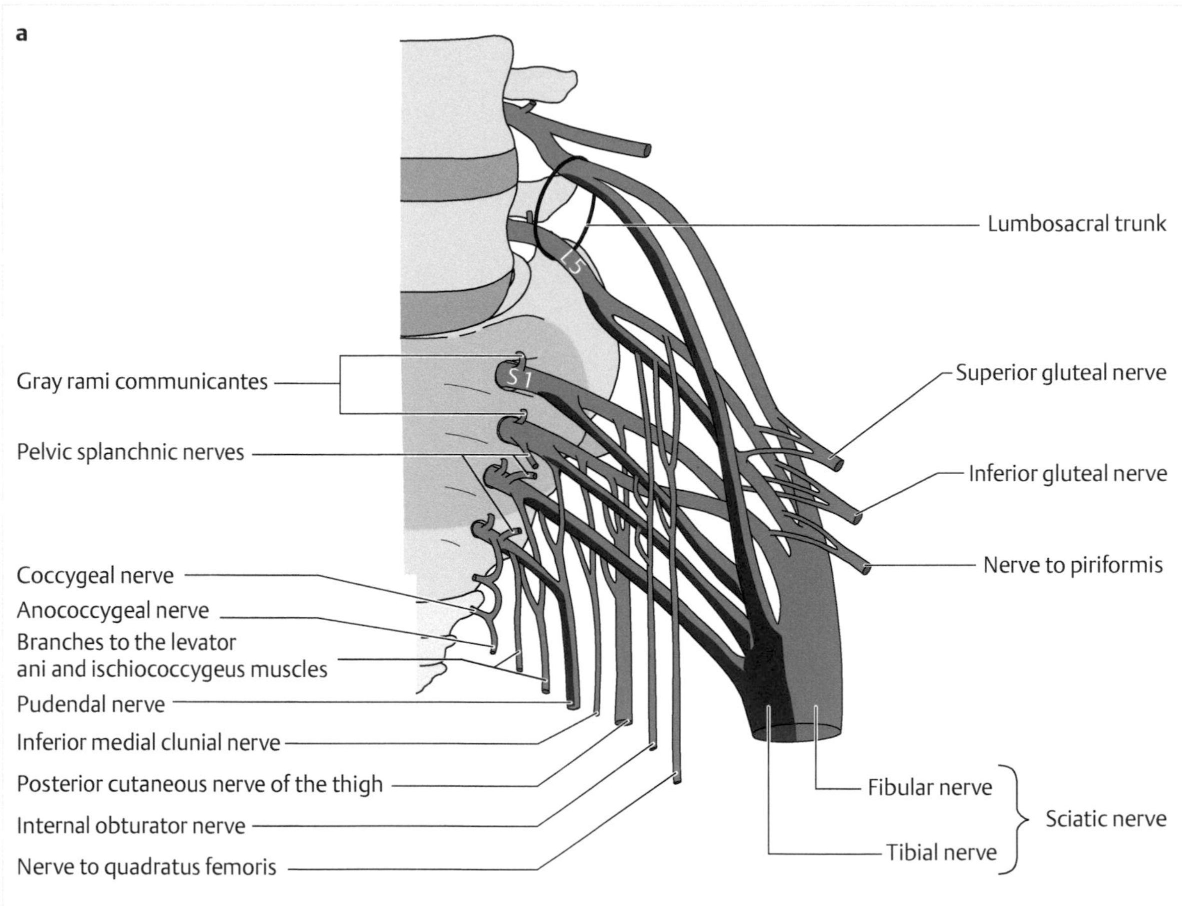


**Fig. 8.169** Sacral plexus. **(a)** Schematic drawing, anterior view.

Continued ►

**Pathology**

### Plexus Palsies

- *Fractures* of the sacrum, especially with involvement of the sacral foramina, can contribute to overstretching and possibly even disruption of parts of the plexus, leading to neurologic deficits.
- *Tumors:* Uterine, prostatic and colorectal tumors can put pressure on the plexus.
- Hip joint *surgery:* In total arthroplasty of the hip, the prosthetic head is leveraged out of the acetabulum with powerful traction and internal rotation. This can lead to overstretching of individual parts of the plexus.
- In *pregnancy*, the baby's head or buttocks may be lying in such an unfavorable position that the plexus is compressed.

**Practical Tip**

To diagnose a plexus lesion, functional tests of the muscles of the foot and lower leg as well as the hip extensors and abductors must be carried out. This is the only way in which a plexus paresis can be distinguished from a sciatic lesion.

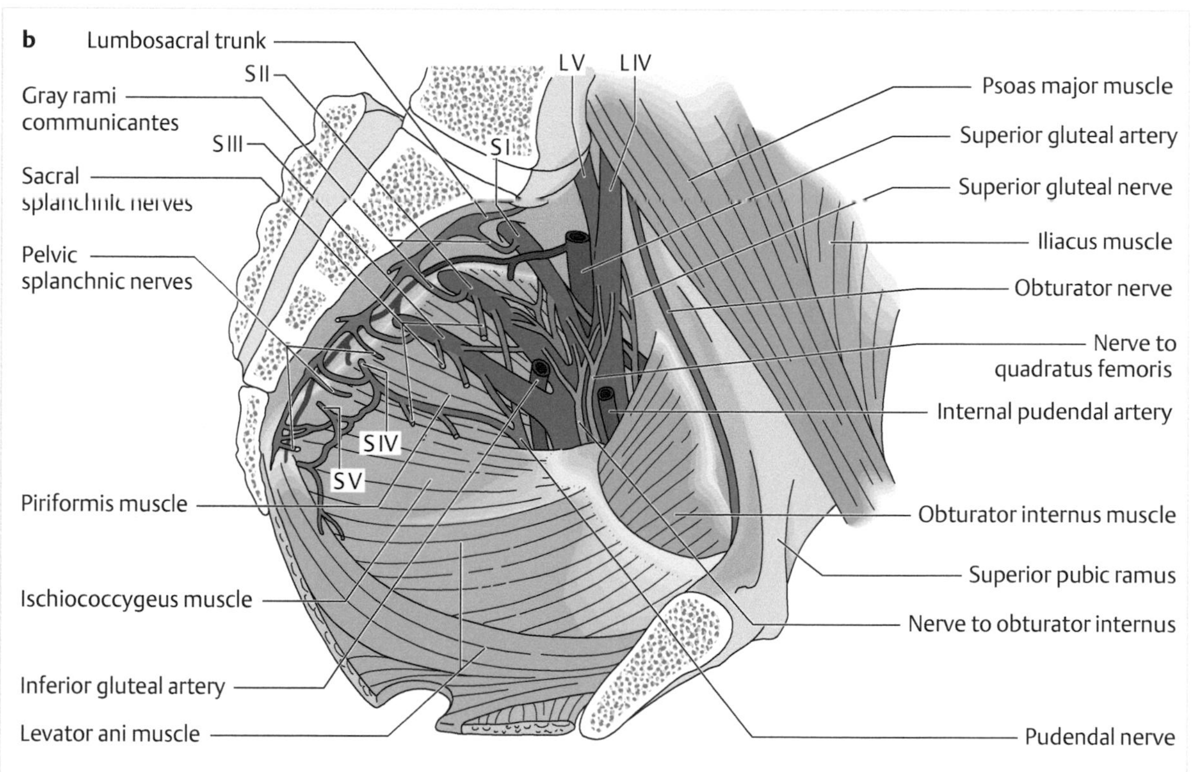


**Fig. 8.169** Continued. **(b)** Medial pelvic view.

## Offshoots of the Sacral Plexus

### Superior Gluteal Nerve (L4–S1; Fig. 8.170)

- This arises from the posterior branches of the anterior rami of L4–S1.
- It runs through the suprapiriform foramen.
- After this, it runs within the *intergluteal space*, the connective tissue between the gluteus medius and minimus muscles.
- It innervates the gluteus medius and minimus muscles, the tensor fasciae latae muscle, and parts of the capsule of the hip joint.

### Inferior Gluteal Nerve (L5–S2; Fig. 8.170)

- This arises from the posterior branches of the anterior rami of L5–S2.
- It leaves the pelvis through the infrapiriform foramen posteromedial to the sciatic nerve.
- Several branches innervate the gluteus maximus muscle, and individual branches go to the capsule of the hip joint.

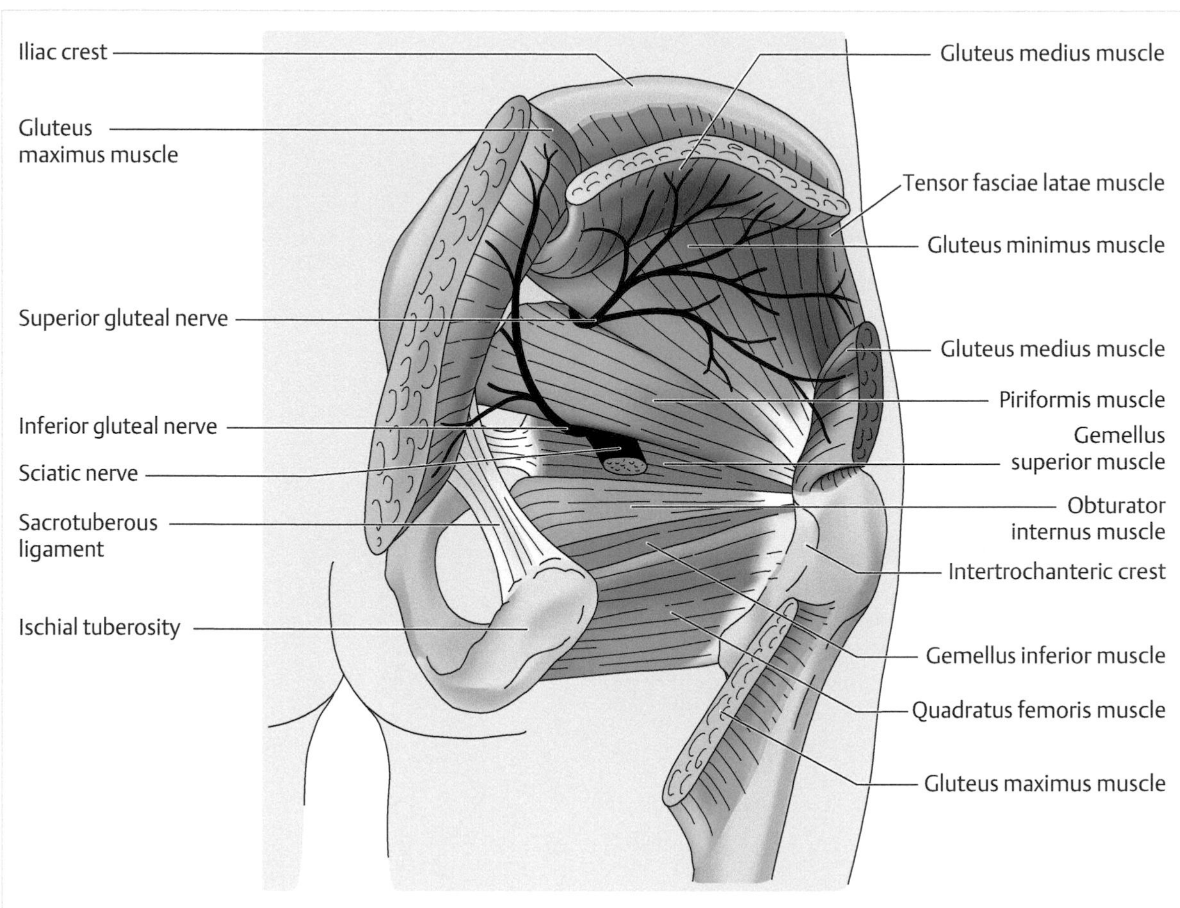


**Fig. 8.170** Superior and inferior gluteal nerves.

### Sciatic Nerve (L4–S3; Fig. 8.171)

- This is the longest and strongest of the peripheral nerves.
- It arises from all parts of the sacral plexus and leaves the pelvis through the infrapiriform foramen.
- It runs laterally and crosses the tendons of the obturator internus, gemellus, and quadratus femoris muscles.
- It then passes under the gluteus maximus muscle in a space filled with adipose tissue and blood vessels—the subgluteal space.
- In the proximal third of the thigh, it runs into the posterior compartment of the thigh.
- At the level of the popliteal fossa—possibly more proximally or more distally—it divides into its two terminal branches, the tibial nerve and the common fibular nerve.
- The sciatic nerve provides motor innervation to the hamstring muscles and all the muscles of the lower leg and foot.

**Pathology**

#### Lesion of the Sciatic Nerve

There can be many causes:

- *Surgery* in the immediate vicinity.
- *Tumors* and *hematomas* after fractures.
- Inflammation spreading through the subgluteal space.
- *Damage from injections:*
  - Nerve compression from direct needle trauma with the subsequent injection of a quantity of liquid. The result is pressure within the neural tissue, which can affect the blood supply to the nerve. Patients note burning, radiating pain immediately at the time of the needlestick event.
  - Nerve compression by a hematoma when the puncture injures the blood vessels in the immediate vicinity of the nerve. The hematoma can compress the nerves. There may be hours or days between the time of injection and the onset of the symptoms.
  - Nerve irritation from toxic damage. The peripheral nerves may show a toxic reaction, with inflammation as a result of analgesics, anti-rheumatic medications, or antibiotics. Patients describe a pain with associated sensorimotor deficits that occur promptly.

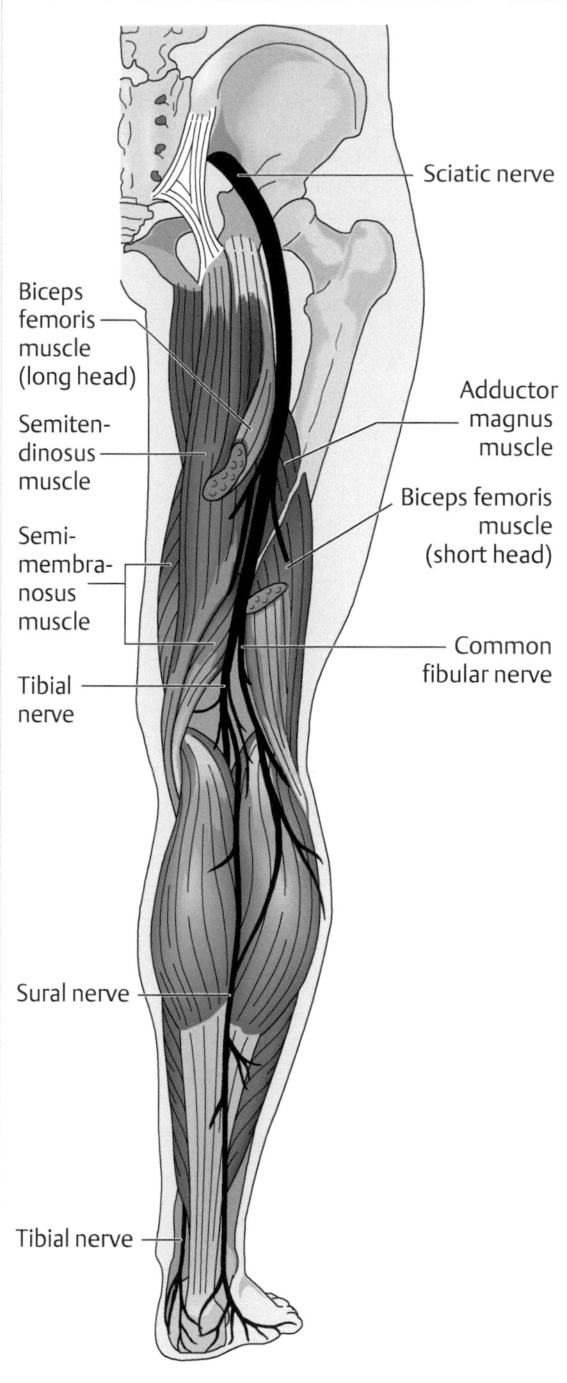


**Fig. 8.171** Sciatic nerve.

**Practical Tip**

**Examination**

With complete failure of the sciatic nerve, the only flexors of the knee joint that remain functional are the muscles innervated by the femoral nerve—the sartorius and gracilis. In gait analysis, the examiner notes a lack of stability of the foot, whereas the hip and knee joints can be stabilized by the gluteal muscles and muscles innervated by the femoral nerve.

## Pudendal Nerve (S1–S4; Fig. 8.172)

- This arises from the anterior rami of S1–S4.
- It carries sympathetic and parasympathetic fibers.
- The nerve passes through the infrapiriform foramen, tracking around the ischial spine into the lesser sciatic foramen and then anteriorly into a duplication of the internal obturator fascia, the pudendal canal.
- It innervates the pelvic and urogenital diaphragms, the ischiococcygeus muscle, and the buttock, anal, and genital regions.

**Pathology**

During biking, medially extending branches of the pudendal nerve can be compressed by the pressure of the seat. The results are temporary sensory disturbances in the affected area and impotence.

## Posterior Cutaneous Nerve of the Thigh (S1–S3; Fig. 8.172)

- This arises from the anterior and posterior rami of S1–S4.
- It runs with the inferior gluteal nerve through the #infrapiriform foramen, and then further posteriorly in the middle of the thigh to the popliteal fossa.
- It gives off branches to the skin in the vicinity of the gluteal fold and supplies the entire posterior thigh region during its further course to the popliteal fossa.

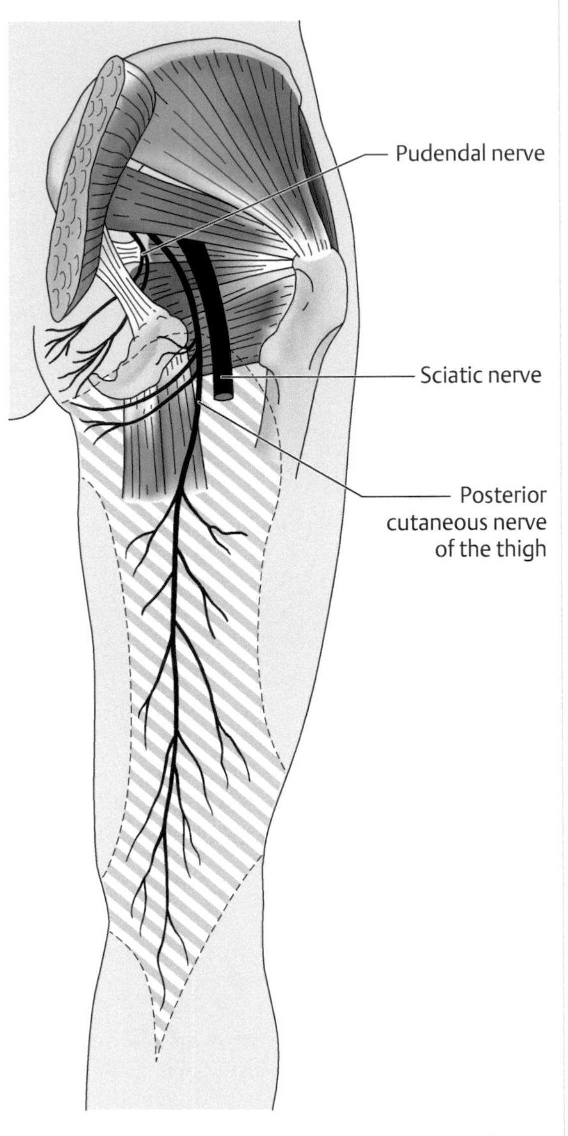


**Fig. 8.172** Pudendal nerve and posterior cutaneous nerve of the thigh. Hatched areas, innervated areas of skin.

# Chapter 9

## Knee



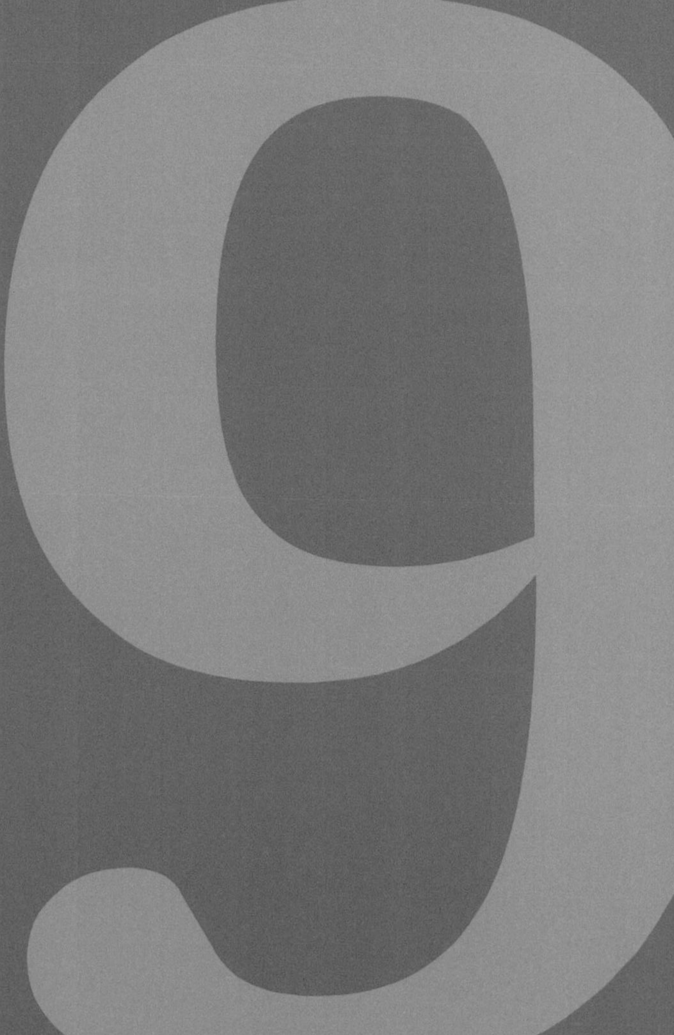

# 9 Knee

## 9.1 Palpation of Knee Structures

Palpation of the knee structures is carried out in various positions. For structures in the anterior and medial regions, use the supine position, with a small roll under the patient's knees. For the lateral area, use the lateral decubitus position, and for the posterior area, the prone position.

### 9.1.1 Palpation of Anterior Knee Structures

#### Patella (Figs. 9.1 and 9.2)

Check the surface of the patella with your hand; some fibers of the rectus femoris muscle run distally over it, and the small bursa lying there can sometimes swell.

Many structures run at the margins of the patella, all of which should be carefully palpated.

The tendon of the rectus femoris muscle tracks broadly to the entire base of the patella. To help with palpation, press the apex of the patella toward the patellar surface so that the base rises and the tendons are put under more tension. At the upper edge of the patella, palpate across the fiber orientation.

The tendons of the vastus medialis and lateralis muscles track to the superomedial and superolateral margins of the patella.

The apex of the patella deserves special attention. By applying pressure to the base of the patella, the apex rises somewhat, the patellar ligament here is tensed, and the insertion area can be palpated.

#### Patellar Ligament (Fig. 9.3)

The ligament can be traced from the apex of the patella inferiorly and somewhat laterally to its insertion. Palpate longitudinally along the medial and lateral borders of the ligament, and transverse to the fiber orientation over its surface.

#### Tibial Tuberosity (Fig. 9.4)

The patellar ligament ends at the tibial tuberosity. This is a clearly palpable, bony elevation on the tibia about 3 to 4 fingerbreadths inferior to the apex of the patella.

**Practical Tip**

Palpate the patella at rest as well as during flexion and extension, to detect abnormal tilts and course deviations, such as lateral deviation of the patella. Crepitus can also be detected here.

**Pathology**

**Patellar Tendinitis (Jumper's Knee)**

In this disorder, the insertion site of the patellar ligament on the apex of the patella is extremely sensitive to pressure, and the pain intensifies with extension against resistance. Some of the many causes are specific to sports, such as sudden deceleration, as well as factors such as the nature and consistency of the playing surface and the footwear. Other factors are constitutional, such as malalignment and muscular imbalances. All these causes produce an unfavorable force impact on the patellar ligament.

**Osgood–Schlatter's Disease**

This is a disturbance of ossification of the tibial tuberosity, which is thick, reddened, and painful to palpation.

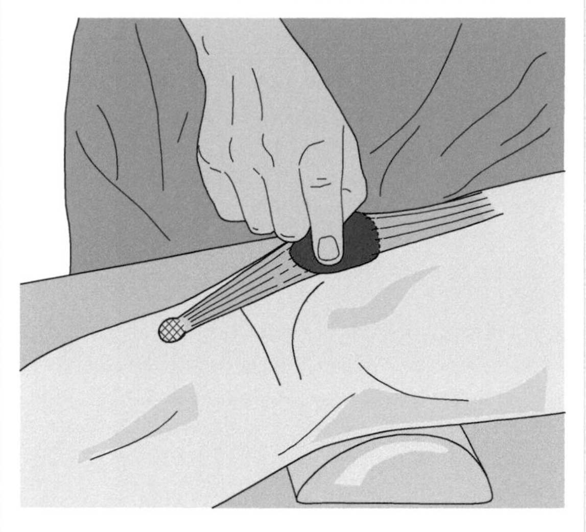

**Fig. 9.1** Palpation of the surface of the patella.

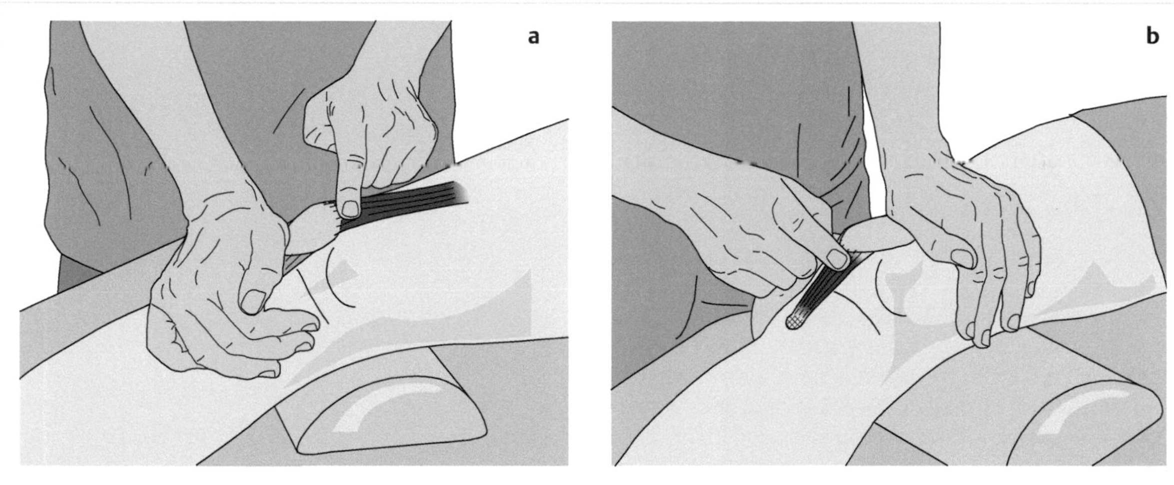


**Fig. 9.2** Palpation. **(a)** Tendon of the rectus femoris muscle at the base of the patella. **(b)** Patellar ligament at the apex of the patella.

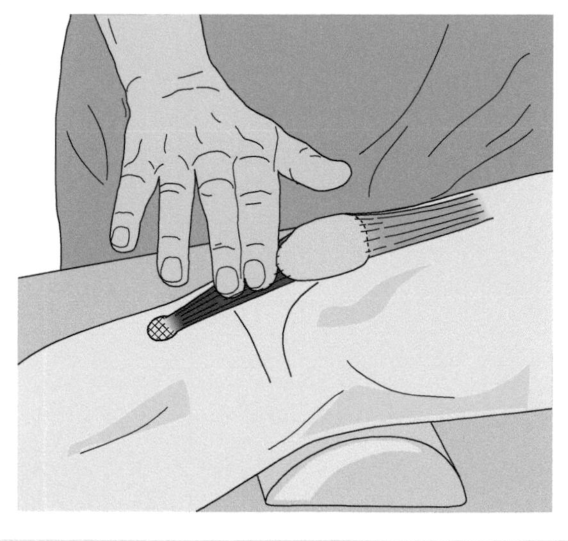

**Fig. 9.3** Palpation of the patellar ligament.

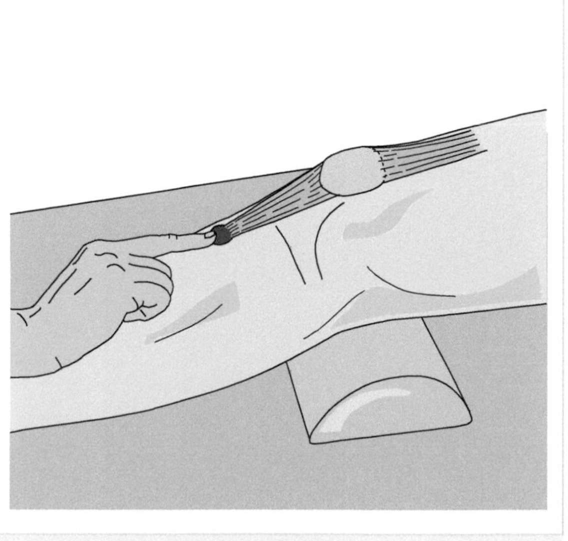

**Fig. 9.4** Palpation of the tibial tuberosity.

## Infrapatellar Fat Pad (Fig. 9.5)

With the knee flexed, one can palpate the fat pad deep under the dimples on either side of the patellar ligament. In extension, firm structures clearly bulge out medially and laterally adjacent to the ligament. This is the fat pad, which is pressed anteriorly in extension because of a lack of space in the joint.

### Practical Tip

**Hypertrophy of the Fat Pad**

Because everyone's fat pad bulges out visibly when the knee is extended, it is very important to compare the right and left sides to assess the degree of swelling. Hypertrophy is a sign of faulty static loading of the knee joint.

## Suprapatellar Bursa (Fig. 9.6)

The reflection of the suprapatellar bursa can be palpated approximately 8 cm superior to the base of the patella by feeling deeply through the tendon of the rectus femoris muscle, where it can be identified as a bulge. The direction of palpation goes from inferior to superior, i.e., transverse to the fold.

## Rectus Femoris Muscle (Fig. 9.7)

This can be palpated in the mid-thigh area as a significant muscle mass while tensing it as if to extend the knee. The muscle–tendon transition occurs about 1 to 1½ handbreadths above the base of the patella. This transition can be felt as a clearly raised border when palpating from the inferior side, and this can be confirmed by tensing the muscle as if to extend the knee.

## Vastus Lateralis Muscle (Fig. 9.8)

This muscle is covered in part by the iliotibial tract. The muscle–tendon junction is located about 2 to 3 fingerbreadths lateral and superior to the patella.

The terminal tendon is separated from the lateral margin of the rectus muscle by a small gap. Its insertion is approximately 1 to 1.5 cm wide and is located at the superolateral margin of the patella.

### Pathology

**Swelling of the Knee**

Swelling of the capsule is typically an annular extension directly above the patella and suggests inflammation of the fibrous layer. This type of swelling is softly compressible but cannot be displaced into the joint.

A *joint effusion*, on the other hand, can be shifted within the joint. *Dancing patella:* By compressing the anterior recess and extending the knee, the fluid accumulates under the patella. When pressure is applied to the patella, it sinks, but then it springs back into its previous position when it is released.

▷ See Chapter 9.3, Knee Joint, and Fig. 9.63

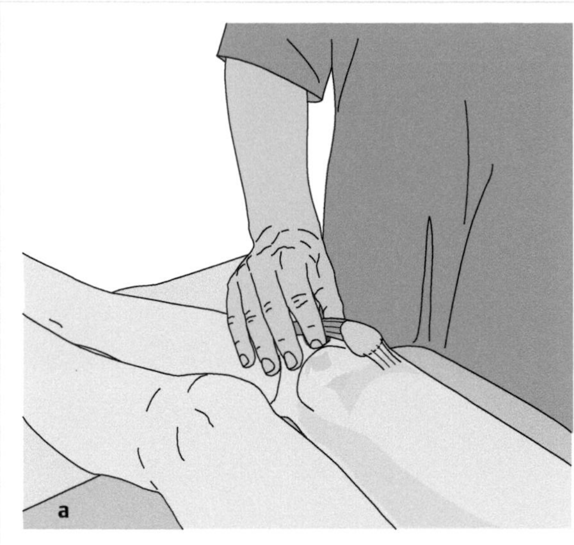


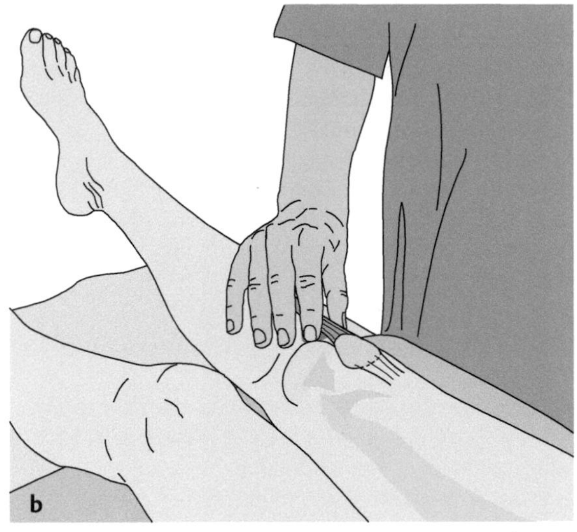


**Fig. 9.5** Palpation of the fat pad. **(a)** In flexion. **(b)** In extension.

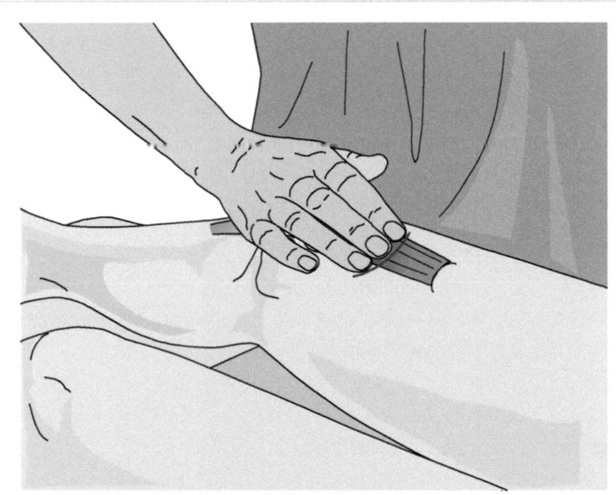

**Fig. 9.6** Palpation of the superior edge of the suprapatellar bursa.

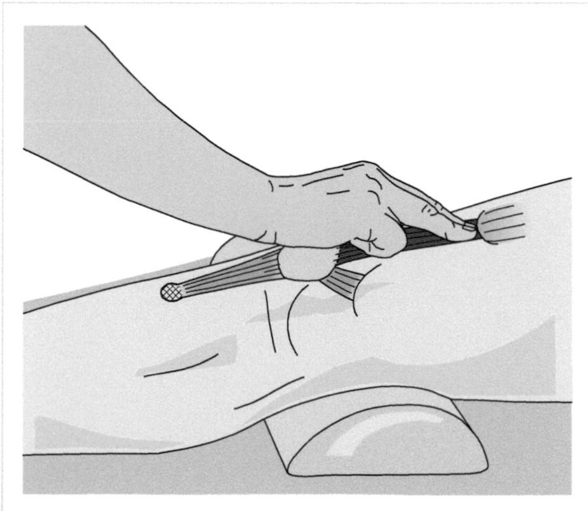

**Fig. 9.7** Palpation of the muscle–tendon junction of the rectus femoris muscle.

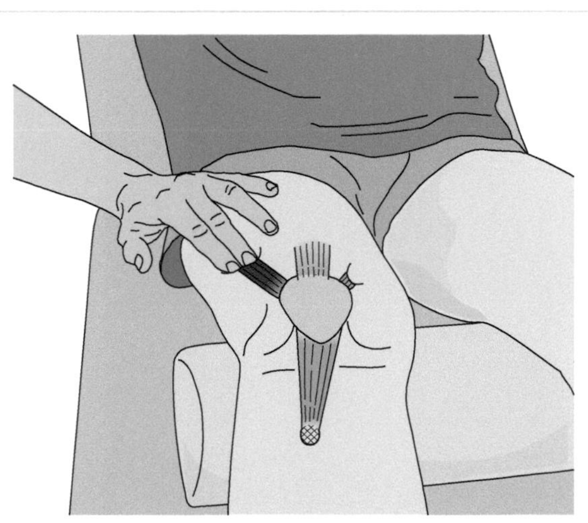

**Fig. 9.8** Palpation of the muscle–tendon junction of the vastus lateralis muscle.

## Vastus Medialis Muscle (Fig. 9.9)

The vastus medialis muscle is located medially on the distal thigh. At the end of its course, it bulges outward. The lower fibers have an almost horizontal course, so that palpation across the muscle orientation must be performed from superior to inferior.

At 0.5 to 1 cm, its terminal tendon is the shortest, and it is separated from the medial border of the rectus muscle by a gap. The insertion is located at the superomedial patellar margin.

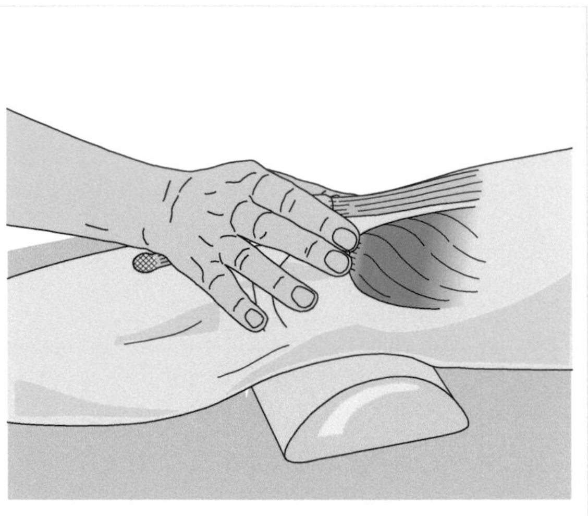

**Fig. 9.9** Palpation of the muscle–tendon junction of the vastus medialis muscle.

### Practical Tip

The rectus and vastus lateralis muscles have a greater proportion of tonic fibers and tend to shorten, which is felt as increased tone on palpation.

The vastus medialis muscle, on the other hand, has a higher proportion of phasic fibers, which is why it tends toward having reduced tone. The typical position of comfort for the knee joint is slight flexion. Since the vastus medialis muscle becomes active primarily near the end of its range of motion, it atrophies very quickly. This is visible and palpable, because a noticeable concavity develops superomedial to the patella. When comparing the right and left sides on palpation, a clear difference in the tension can be noted.

This atrophy can be considered to be the first sign of a knee problem, even though no severe symptoms may yet be present.

## 9.1.2 Palpation of Medial Knee Structures

### Medial Joint Space (Fig. 9.10)

Immediately medial to the patellar ligament is a depression that is bordered superiorly by the medial femoral condyle and inferiorly by the tibial plateau. The joint space is located deep in this area. It can be well palpated here since only the capsule covers the joint, and the anterior horn of the meniscus lies further toward the interior of the joint. This changes further medially, where the retinaculum and a ligament pass over it, and the meniscus fills the space.

In addition, it is a good idea to move the joint while resting the fingers on it so that any friction or disharmony in the movement can be evaluated.

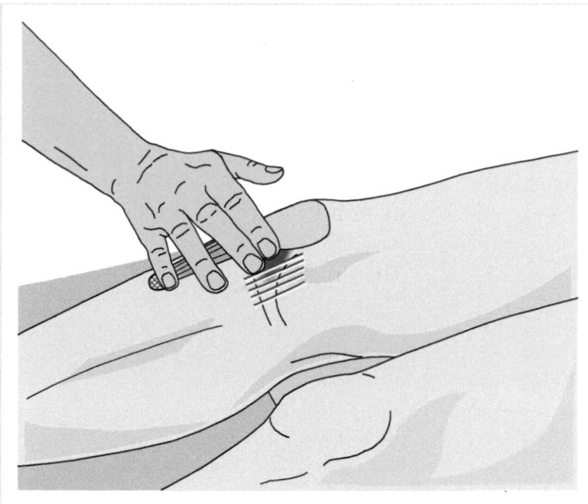

Fig. 9.10 Palpation of the medial joint space.

### Medial Meniscus (Fig. 9.11)

At 90° of flexion, the weight of the leg pulls the joint space apart slightly, making it more easily accessible for palpation.

With one hand, alternately rotate the lower leg externally and internally, while the thumb or index finger of the other hand palpates the joint space to feel the anterior horn of the meniscus as it retracts and advances. It moves away from palpating finger during external rotation of the tibia, and presses against it during internal rotation.

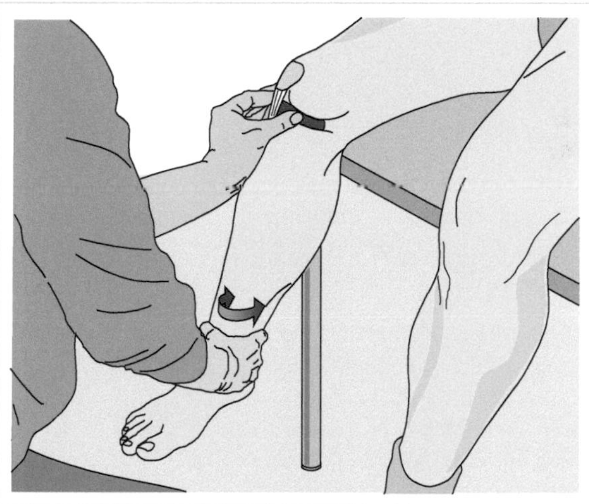

Fig. 9.11 Palpation of the medial meniscus.

**Practical Tip**

Tenderness in the joint space may indicate a meniscal lesion. However, this pain can also be found with a recent rupture of the cruciate ligament. Therefore a further diagnostic evaluation of the meniscus must be carried out.

## Retinacula

The retinacula are flat structures that consist of deep and superficially running fibers.

### Medial Transverse Patellar Retinaculum (Fig. 9.12)

- *Patellofemoral part:* Trace the transversely running retinaculum from the medial patellar margin to the medial epicondyle. The insertion on the patella can be brought under tension by tipping the lateral side of the patella outward, so that it can be better differentiated from the surrounding structures.
- *Patellotibial part:* This tracks diagonally from the side of the patella in an inferomedial direction and runs under the longitudinal fibers, which is why it cannot always be clearly palpated.

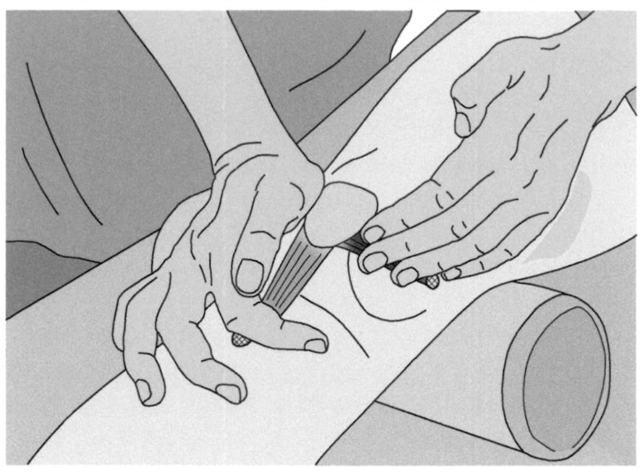

**Fig. 9.12** Palpation of the patellofemoral part of the medial transverse patellar retinaculum.

> **Practical Tip**
>
> The *patellar glide test* toward the lateral side gives an indication of the tenseness of the transverse retinaculum. Using both thumbs, displace the patella laterally and compare the right and left sides. Proviso: the quadriceps muscle must be completely relaxed (**Fig. 9.13**).

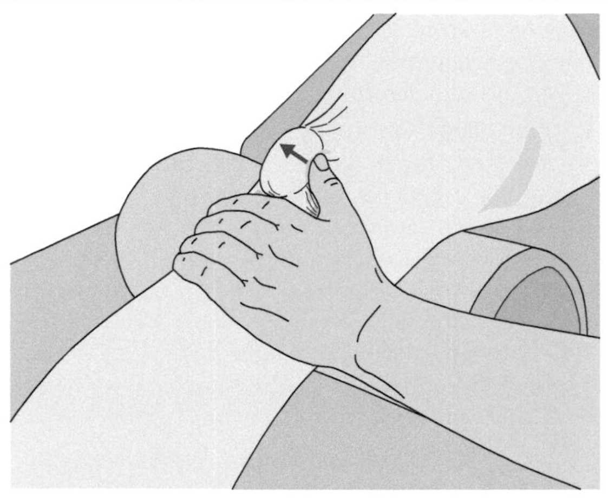

**Fig. 9.13** Patellar glide test.

### Medial Longitudinal Patellar Retinaculum (Fig. 9.14)

The palpation of this longitudinally running retinaculum proceeds from the medial border of the patellar ligament high in the joint space. Approximately 1 cm further medially, the edge of the retinaculum can be felt as a small bulge. The only other structure that can be palpated between the ligament and the retinaculum is the capsule, which is significantly softer.

Starting from this point, palpate the retinaculum across its fiber orientation superiorly toward the vastus medialis muscle, and inferiorly to the tibial border and from there approximately 1 to 1.5 cm further distally.

Follow the width of the retinaculum further medially over the joint space to the collateral ligament.

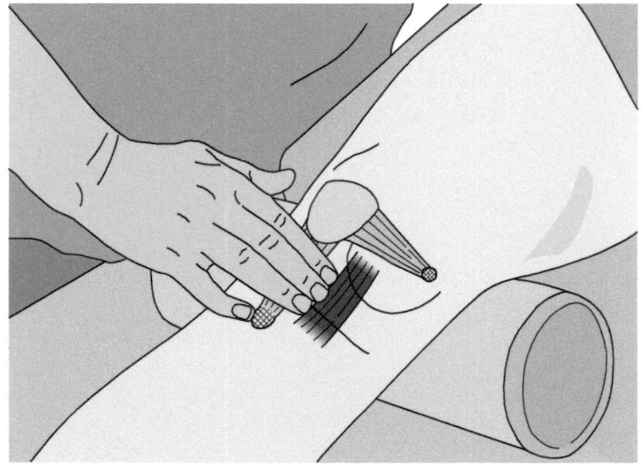

**Fig. 9.14** Palpation of the anterior edge of the medial longitudinal patellar retinaculum.

## Tibial Collateral Ligament (Fig. 9.15)

A small elevation can be palpated approximately 2 cm further medial to the retinaculum. This border tracks diagonally over the joint space from posterosuperior to anteromedial, and represents the longitudinal fiber bundles of the collateral ligament. It can be followed superiorly to the medial femoral epicondyle and inferomedially to the tibia. The insertion on the tibia is overlain by the pes anserinus.

At the level of the joint space, palpate further posteriorly to identify the short fibers. However, the posterior margin is difficult to discern because it is covered by parts of the pes anserinus.

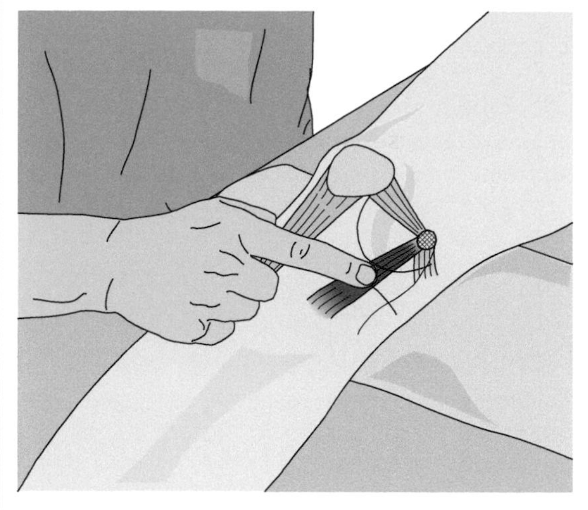

**Fig. 9.15** Palpation of the tibial collateral ligament.

## Superficial Pes Anserinus (Fig. 9.16)

Use the tibial tuberosity as an orientation guide—a soft pad can be palpated somewhat inferomedial to it. This extends three fingerbreadths from proximal to distal, and two fingerbreadths from medial to lateral. The following procedure provides an aid to palpation: with the flat of the hand over the medial aspect of the lower leg, use a little pressure while sliding it up the leg. In the proximal third, the leading lateral edge of the index finger encounters a clearly defined thickening that extends in a posterosuperior direction—this represents the muscles of the pes anserinus.

The individual muscle insertions (sartorius, gracilis, and semitendinosus) cannot be identified here. This only becomes possible further toward the popliteal fossa.

The anserine bursa, which lies between the tendon and the tibia, can only be palpated when swollen.

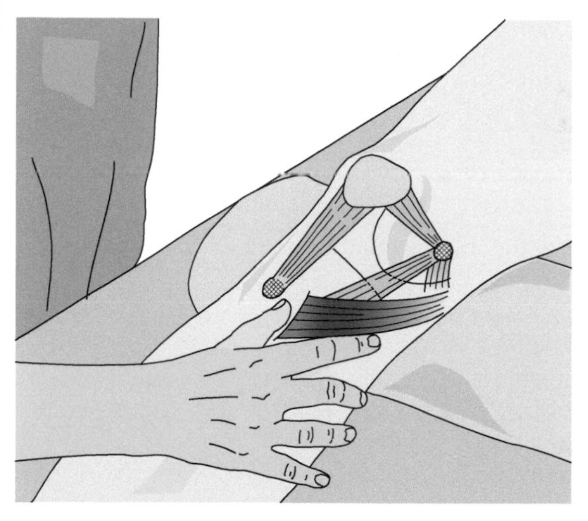

**Fig. 9.16** Help in palpating the superficial pes anserinus.

## Adductor Tubercle (Fig. 9.17)

At the posterior end of the medial femoral condyle is the adductor tubercle. Trace the edge of the condyle superiorly from the anterior joint space. At about the level of the base of the patella, a bony elevation can be palpated. The tendon of the adductor magnus inserts here as a firm, round cord, which is easy to find by tensing the muscle as if to adduct the hip.

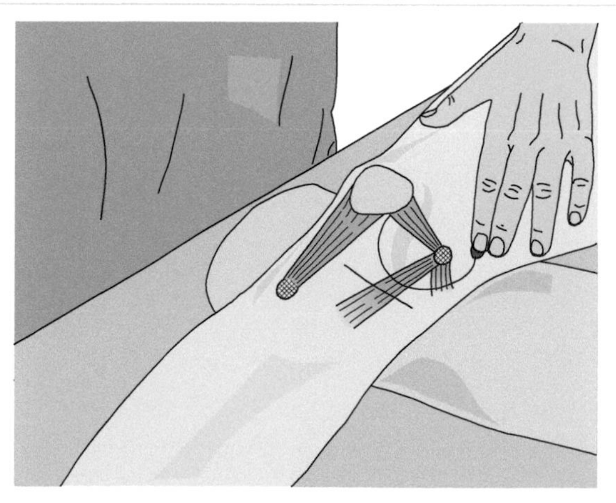

**Fig. 9.17** Palpation of the adductor tubercle.

## 9.1.3 Palpation of Lateral Knee Structures

### Lateral Joint Space (Fig. 9.18)

The lateral border of the patellar ligament helps with orientation. Superolaterally from here is the lateral femoral condyle, and in an inferolateral direction is the tibial plateau. Both these structures border the joint space, which is located immediately adjacent to the patellar ligament deep in a small depression.

Feeling further, the meniscus lies with its wide base between the tibia and femur, making palpation there more difficult.

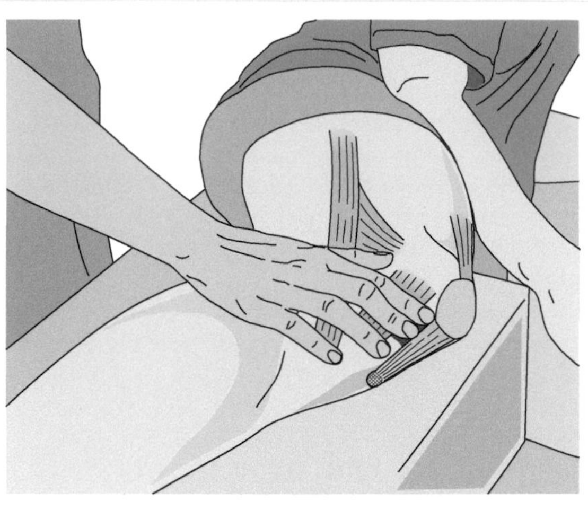

Fig. 9.18 Palpation of the lateral joint space.

### Retinacula

### Lateral Transverse Retinaculum (Fig. 9.19)

- A connection from the lateral border of the patella toward the lateral epicondyle represents the course of the *patellofemoral part*. The transversely running fibers are easy to palpate only adjacent to the patella; further toward the epicondyle, they lie under the longitudinal retinaculum.
- The *patellotibial part* tracks obliquely anterolaterally and is best palpated at the inferolateral edge of the patella.

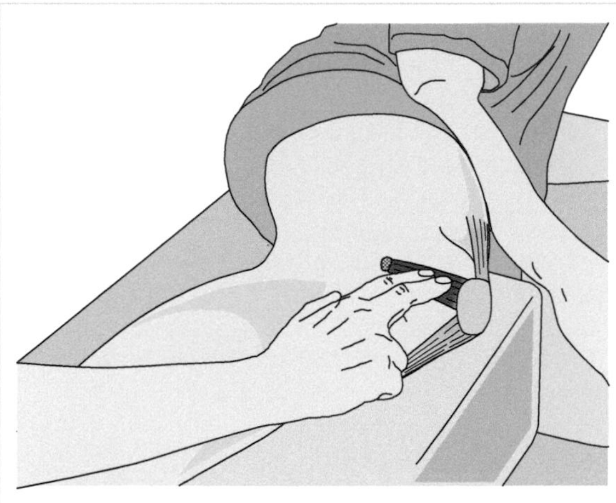

Fig. 9.19 Palpation of the patellofemoral part of the lateral transverse patellar retinaculum.

### Lateral Longitudinal Patellar Retinaculum (Fig. 9.20)

The border of this longitudinally running retinaculum can be felt about ½ to 1 fingerbreadth from the lateral border of the patellar ligament at the level of the joint space. Its edge is softer than that of the patellar ligament. A small gap lies between them.

Feeling further at the level of the joint space, palpate the obliquely running iliotibial tract with light pressure. Here these two structures combine, which is why the border of the retinaculum cannot be located.

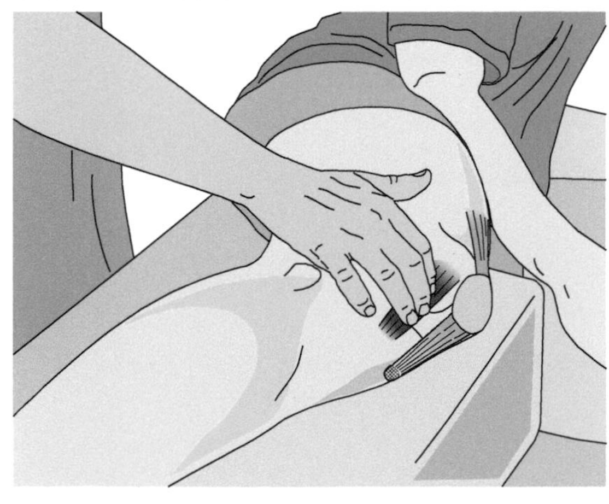

Fig. 9.20 Palpation of the anterior edge of the lateral longitudinal patellar retinaculum.

## Iliotibial Tract (Fig. 9.21)

The edge of the tract can be palpated as a well-defined, flat structure approximately one fingerbreadth lateral to the longitudinal retinaculum. Its fibers run obliquely from posterolateral to anteromedial. They end primarily on the protruding *Gerdy's tubercle* (the tubercle for the iliotibial tract), which is located about two fingerbreadths superior and lateral to the tibial tuberosity on the lateral tibial condyle.

The taut fibers can be followed superiorly to the tensor fasciae latae muscle.

## Fibular Collateral Ligament (Fig. 9.22)

Immediately lateral to the tract is the fibular collateral ligament. This is a round, pencil-thick strand that runs from the lateral epicondyle to the fibular head, obliquely from superoanterior to inferoposterior.

When assuming the figure 4 position, with the hip and knee flexed and the hip at maximal external rotation, the ligament is tightly stretched and therefore very easy to palpate.

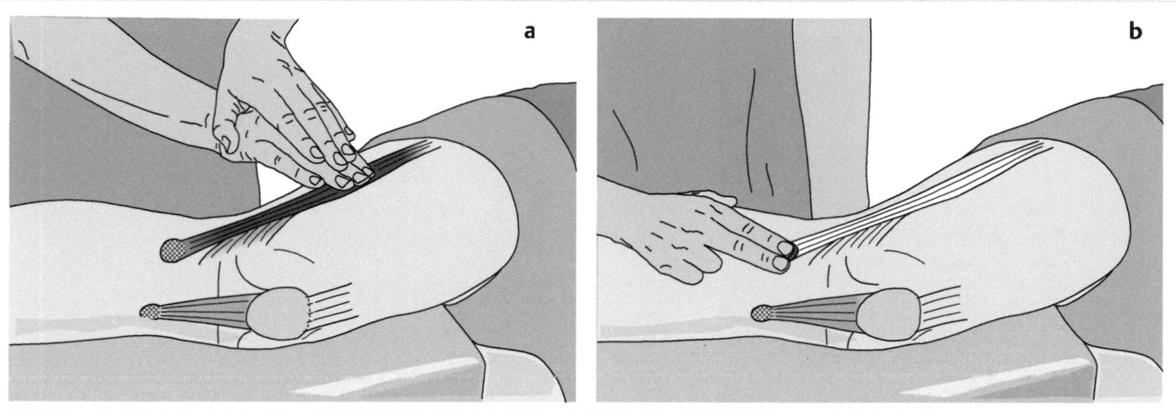


**Fig. 9.21** Palpation. **(a)** Iliotibial tract. **(b)** Gerdy's tubercle.

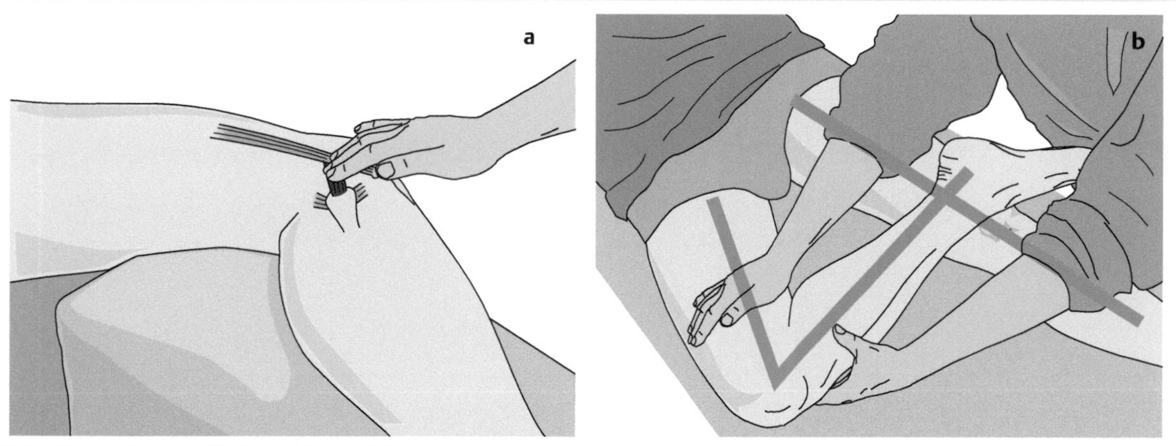


**Fig. 9.22** Palpation of the fibular collateral ligament. **(a)** Slight flexion. **(b)** Adopting a figure 4 position to stretch the ligament.

## Head of the Fibula (Fig. 9.23)

The bony outline of the head of the fibula can be found about 2 to 3 fingerbreadths inferior to the posterolateral knee joint space. The collateral ligament tracks into it from anterosuperior and the biceps femoris muscle from posterosuperior, so that these two structures form a "V."

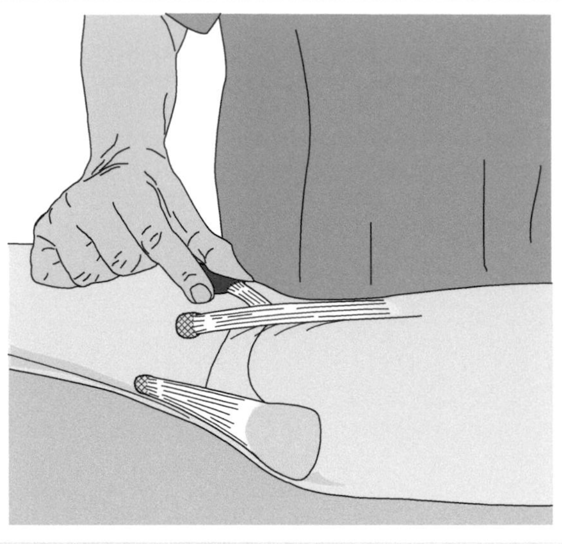

**Fig. 9.23** Palpation of the head of the fibula.

## Anterior Ligament of the Fibular Head (Fig. 9.24)

This short ligament runs horizontally from the head of the fibula to the tibia. Palpate it across the fiber orientation, immediately anterior to the fibular head.

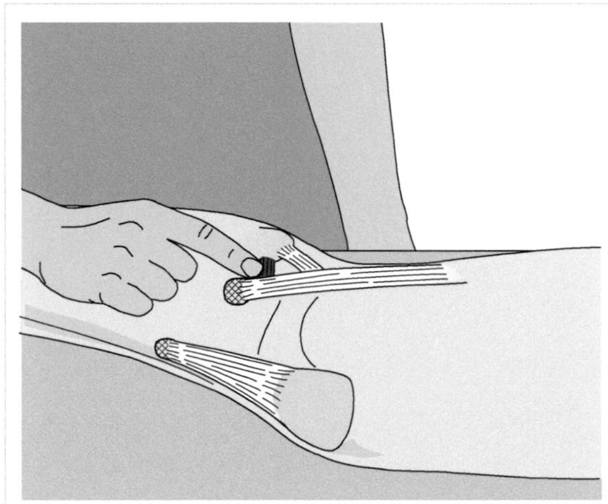

**Fig. 9.24** Palpation of the anterior ligament of the fibular head.

## Arcuate Popliteal Ligament (Fig. 9.25)

Palpate deeply for this ligament, starting from the posterior edge of the fibular head and moving in a superior and slightly medial direction. Since it is so deep, only its origin from the fibular head can be well felt. Its further course cannot be traced because of the overlapping lateral head of the gastrocnemius muscle.

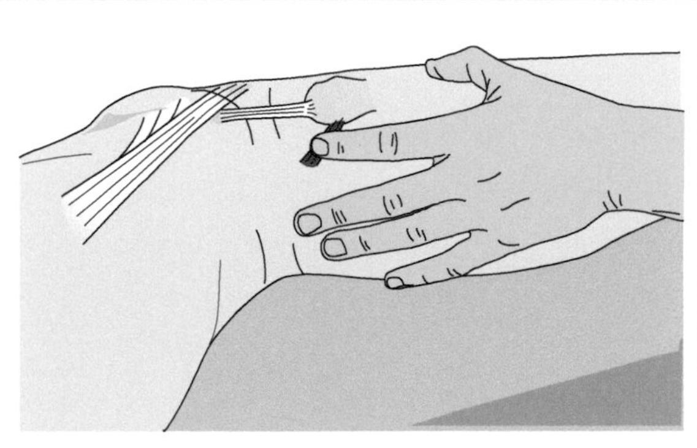

**Fig. 9.25** Palpation of the arcuate popliteal ligament.

## Popliteus Muscle (Fig. 9.26)

The site of origin lies immediately anteroinferior to the insertion of the collateral ligament on the lateral femoral condyle. It then tracks under the collateral ligament in a posteroinferior direction and can first be felt as a broad tendon directly inferior to the biceps femoris tendon. The head of gastrocnemius prevents palpation to its insertion.

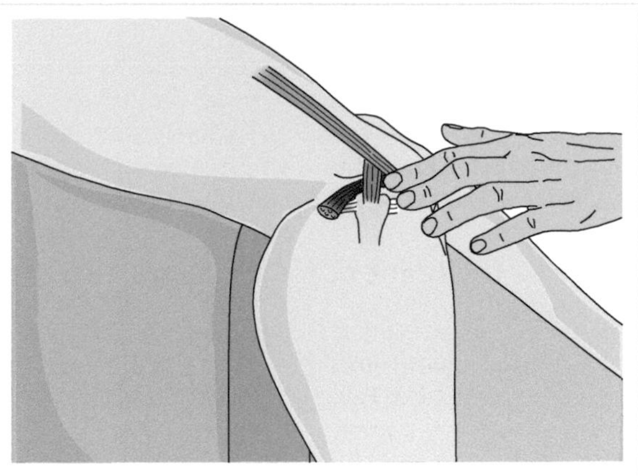

**Fig. 9.26** Palpation of the origin of the popliteus muscle on the lateral femoral condyle.

## Common Fibular Nerve (Fig. 9.27)

Palpate the nerve at the superior margin of the biceps tendon as a longitudinally running, very solid, thin strand in the popliteal fossa. It can be traced to the head of the fibula and then further, taking a superficial course around the head anteriorly.

### Pathology

Because of its superficial course around the neck of the fibula, the common fibular nerve can be easily compressed, for example by a tight bandage or by crossing the legs, leading to unpleasant sensations and temporary foot drop.

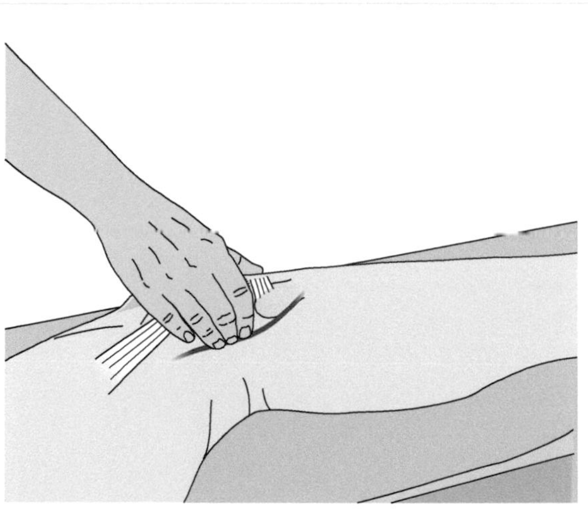

**Fig. 9.27** Palpation of the common fibular nerve.

## Biceps Femoris Muscle (Fig. 9.28)

The tendon can be easily palpated in the superolateral area of the knee. The parts of the muscle that track to the fibular head are especially easy to identify, while those to the tibia are not as easily identified. Tensing the muscle as if to flex the knee brings the tendon out even more prominently.

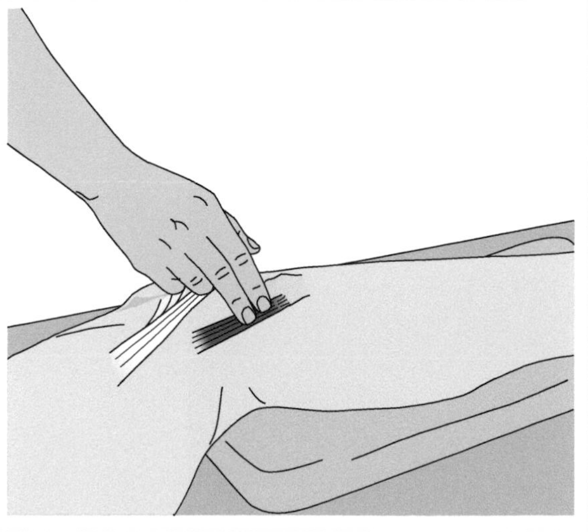

**Fig. 9.28** Palpation of the biceps femoris muscle.

### Lateral Meniscus (Fig. 9.29)

By placing the index and middle fingers in the anterior joint space immediately lateral to the patellar ligament while passively moving the lower leg toward internal rotation, the anterior horn of the meniscus can be palpated as it draws back into the joint.

During external rotation, it moves out against the palpating finger. An alternative is to alternately passively extend and flex the leg at the knee; in extension, the anterior horn moves out against the finger, and in flexion it draws back into the joint.

**Practical Tip**

**Lesions of the Meniscus**

Pain that moves anteriorly during extension and posteriorly during flexion suggests a meniscal lesion. To confirm the diagnosis, more tests should be performed on the meniscus.

## 9.1.4 Palpation of Posterior Knee Structures

### Semitendinosus Muscle (Fig. 9.30)

When tensing the muscle toward knee flexion, the tendon of the semitendinosus muscle jumps out as a superficial strand in the medial popliteal area. It tracks anteromedially and can be palpated up to its insertion on the anterior tibia.

### Semimembranosus Muscle (Fig. 9.31)

This muscle can be palpated both medial and lateral to the semitendinosus tendon in the fossa, but at a deeper level. The medial edge (pointing toward the medial side of the knee) is narrow and firm, since it is the tendinous part. In contrast, the lateral edge (the muscular part) is soft and wide. The muscle becomes more prominent when tensed as if to flex the knee.

### Gracilis Muscle (Fig. 9.32)

Moving further medially from the tendon of the semimembranosus muscle, the tendon of the gracilis muscle lies deep in the tissue of the medial knee area. It is a firm, thin strand that can be tracked further distally.

### Sartorius Muscle (Fig. 9.33)

The tendon of the sartorius muscle is broad and superficial. It is palpable as a flat strand anteromedial to the gracilis tendon.

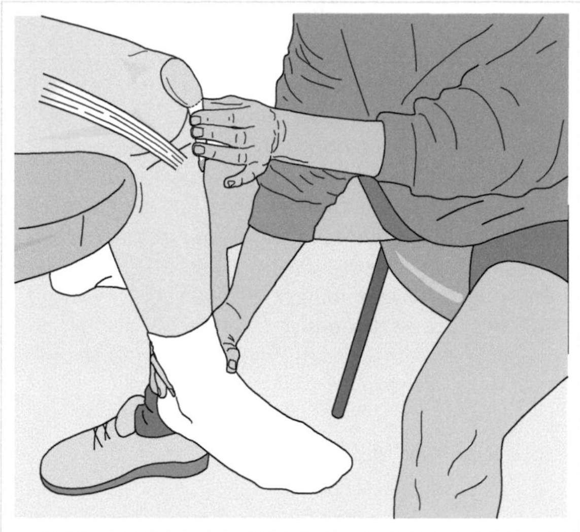

**Fig. 9.29** Palpation of the lateral meniscus.

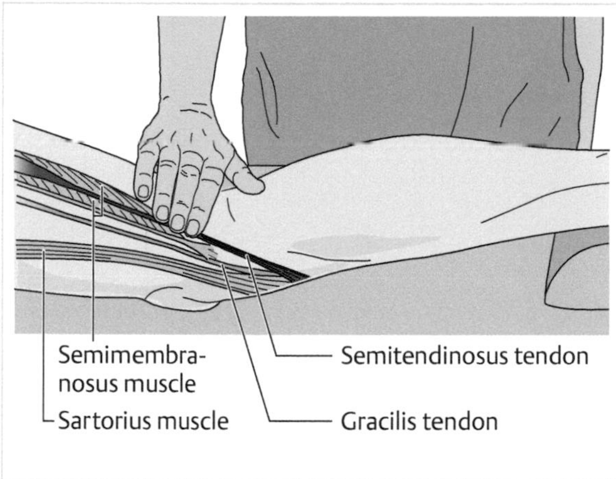


**Fig. 9.30** Palpation of the semitendinosus tendon.

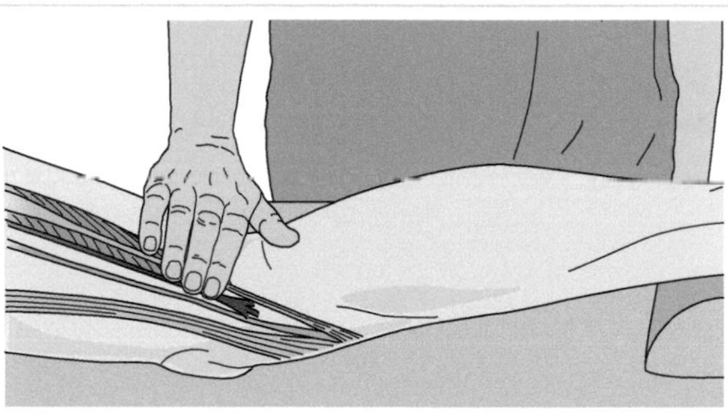

**Fig. 9.31** Palpation of the semimembranosus tendon.

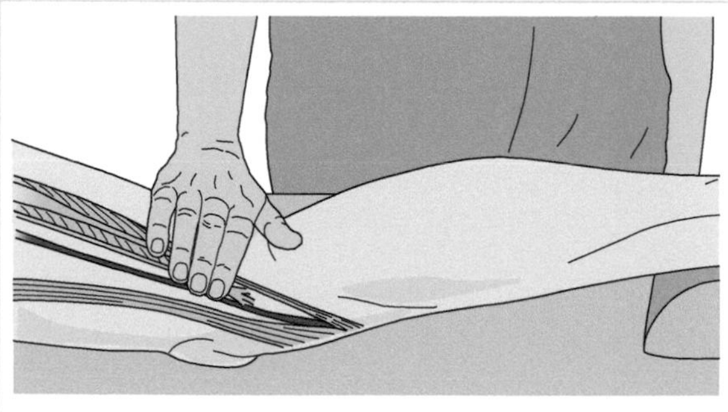

**Fig. 9.32** Palpation of the gracilis muscle.

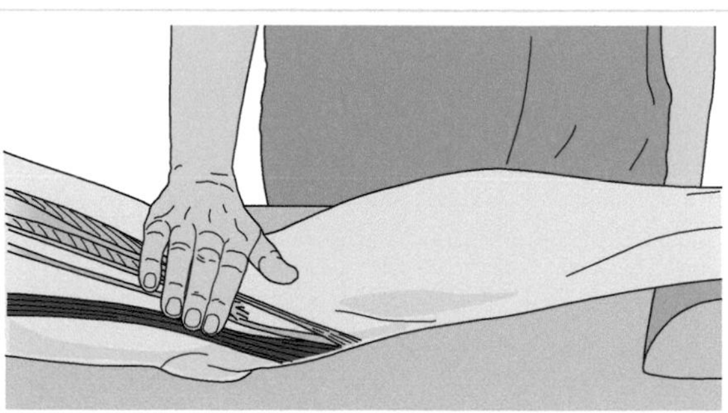

**Fig. 9.33** Palpation of the sartorius muscle.

## Gastrocnemius Muscle (Fig. 9.34)

The two heads of the gastrocnemius can be palpated only when the knee is significantly flexed because the fascia of the popliteal fossa is taut when the knee is extended.

Place the tips of the index and middle finger immediately adjacent to the tendon of the biceps femoris at the level of the popliteal crease, and only then place the knee in maximum flexion. Tensing the foot in plantarflexion will now cause the fleshy area of origin of the lateral head of the gastrocnemius muscle to bulge out clearly just proximal to the superior part of the lateral condyle. Find the medial head in the same way, but using the semimembranosus tendon for orientation instead.

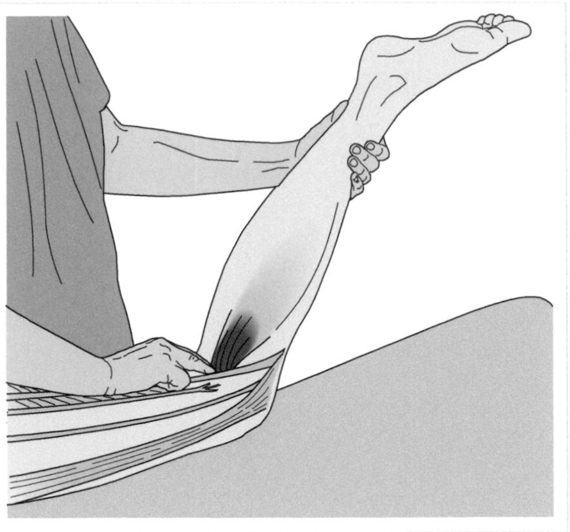

**Fig. 9.34** Palpation of the medial head of the gastrocnemius muscle.

## Tibial Nerve (Fig. 9.35)

The nerve can be felt as a cord-like structure in the center of the popliteal fossa. Place the knee in flexion for this procedure as well.

## Popliteal Artery (Fig. 9.35)

The artery lies alongside the nerve, but deeper. To feel the pulse, the knee should be flexed to at least 90°. Deep palpation is necessary.

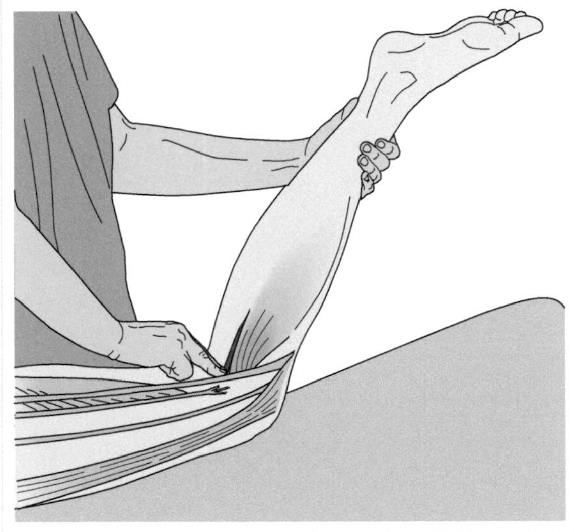

**Fig. 9.35** Palpation of the tibial nerve and the popliteal artery in the popliteal fossa.

# 9.2 X-Ray of the Knee

## 9.2.1 Anteroposterior View

### Normal Findings (Fig. 9.36)

- *Joint space width:* 3 to 5 mm, with the medial knee joint space slightly wider than the lateral.
- *Lateral condyle:* displays a small groove laterally in which the tendon of the popliteus muscle runs.
- *Intercondylar eminence:* the medial intercondylar tubercle is higher than the lateral.
- *Medial tibial joint surface*: overall, at a higher level than the lateral.
- *Fibular head:* about one-third hidden by the tibial condyle.
- *Patella:* contour projected as a faint shadow on the femoral condyles. Its shape varies considerably.
- Assessment of *patellar position:* centered = normal; pushed laterally = subluxation.
- *Fabella:* a sesamoid bone, which is located in the lateral head of the gastrocnemius and is projected as a compact, round area on the lateral femoral condyle.

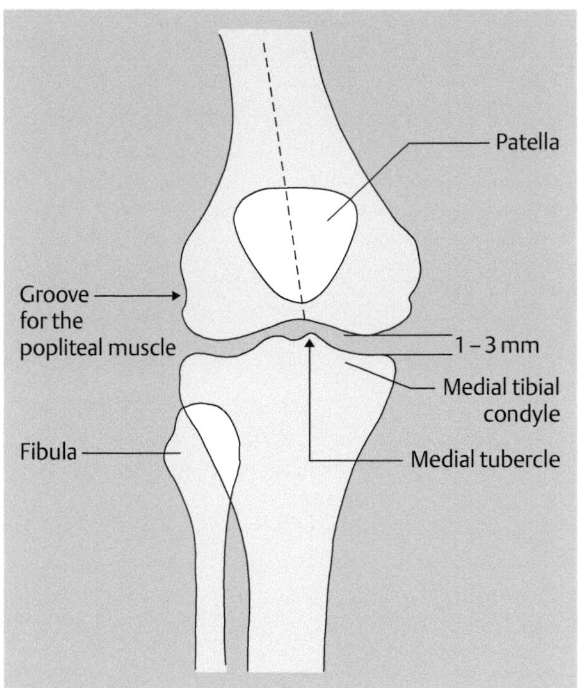


**Fig. 9.36** X-ray image: anteroposterior view.

## Pathology

### Injuries

Fractures, avulsion of ligament from bone, osteochondral fractures, and dislocations (e.g., of the head of the fibula or of the patella) can be detected.

### Degenerative Changes (Fig. 9.37)

Osteophytes and exostoses.

Loose bodies in osteochondritis dissecans, with a sclerotic border to the medial femoral condyle.

Flattening of the condyle with mild subchondral thickening as a sign of osteonecrosis.

Calcifications at the origin of the ligaments in the popliteus tendon, in the infrapatellar fat pad (Hoffa's fat pad), and in the suprapatellar and deep infrapatellar bursae.

Bone cysts.

Rauber's sign: periosteal deposition on the corresponding edge of the tibial plateau as a result of a meniscus lesion (consolidation with bone spur development).

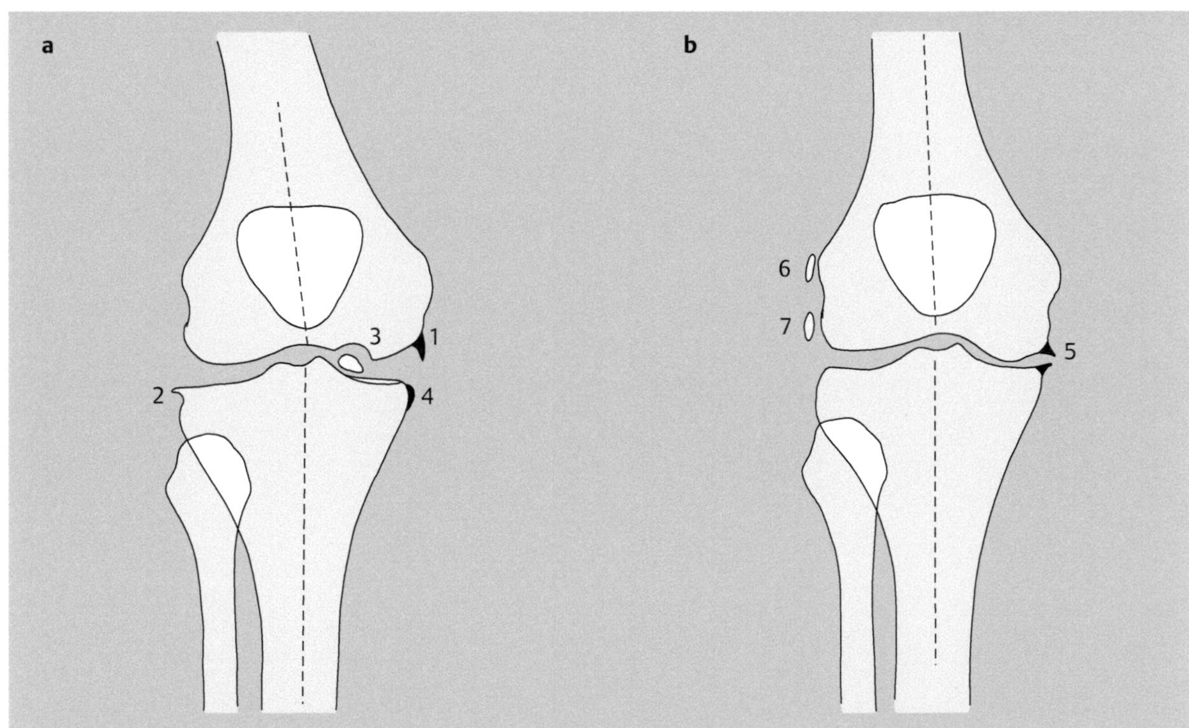


**Fig. 9.37 (a,b)** X-ray image: degenerative changes in anteroposterior view.
1 = Osteophytes
2 = Pressure erosion with a sclerotic rim at the lateral tibial plateau
3 = Osteochondritis dissecans
4 = Rauber's sign
5 = Osteophytes with joint space narrowing
6 = Calcification in the ulnar collateral ligament
7 = Calcification in the popliteus tendon

## 9.2.2 Lateral View (Profile; Fig. 9.38)

Positioning: 30° flexion in the lateral decubitus position; lateral projection.

### Normal Findings

- Condyles further from the X-ray film cassette have blurred margins.
- *Marginal grooves* on the medial and lateral condyle appear as small uniform indentations—the medial one is located in the superior third of the femoral condyle, and the lateral in the middle third.
- The *medial tibial plateau* has a concave shape, and the end of the plateau has a sharp drop-off onto the posterior aspect of the tibia.
- The *lateral tibial plateau* runs over onto the posterior aspect of the tibia in a convex arc.
- *Blumensaat's line* (roof of the intercondylar fossa), recognizable as a compression line, inclines at an angle of 40° from the axis of the femoral shaft.
- *Position of the patella:* The apex of the patella lies at approximately the same level as the extension of Blumensaat's line.
- *Patellofemoral joint* space width: 3 to 5 mm.
- The *femoral surface* of the patellar is concave. Because of the superposition of the medial and lateral facet margins, two discernible boundary lines can be seen.

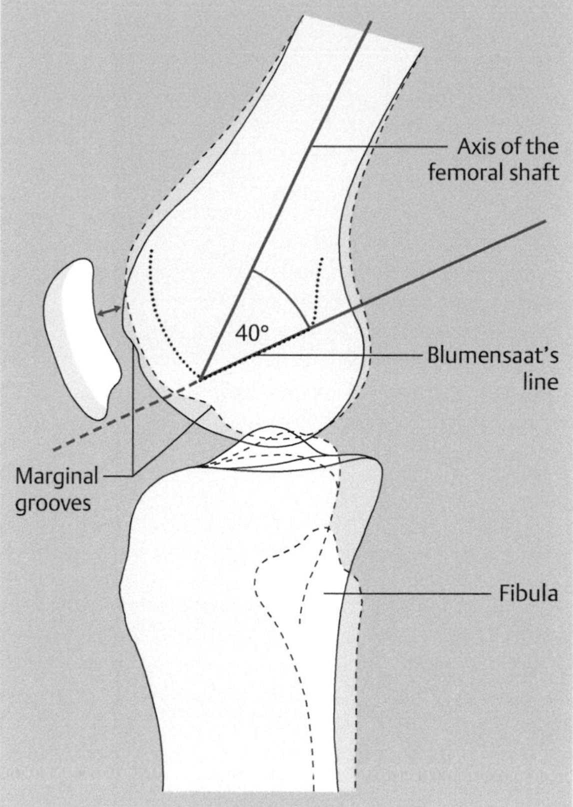


**Fig. 9.38** X-ray of the knee: lateral view.

**Pathology**

(**Fig. 9.39**)
*Highly developed marginal grooves* suggest a problem with the cruciate ligament, since the normal rolling–sliding motion is disturbed and movements (e.g., extension) end abruptly.
*Calcifications* occur within various structures such as the infrapatellar fat pad, the course of the cruciate ligaments, and the dorsal capsular area (oblique popliteal and arcuate popliteal ligaments).
*Fibro-ostosis* at the insertions of the quadriceps tendons (spur of the upper patella), the insertion of the patellar ligament on the apex of the patella (spur of the lower patella), and the tibial tuberosity (Osgood–Schlatter's disease).

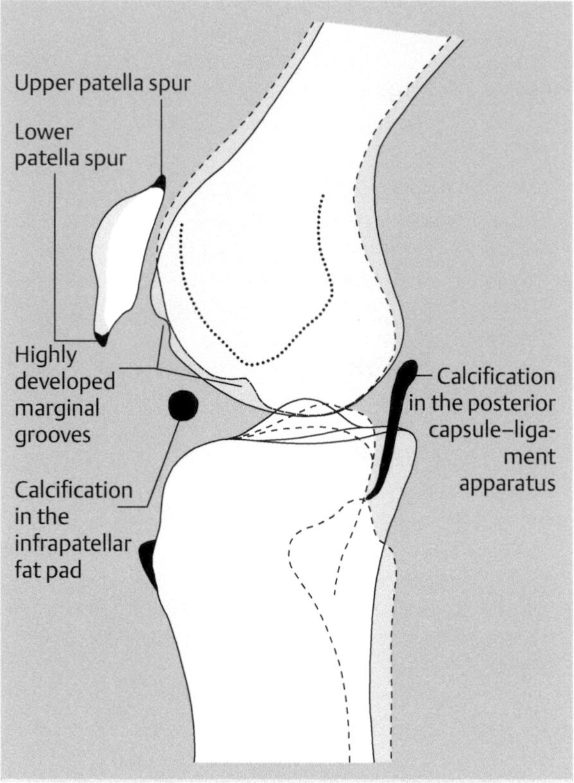


**Fig. 9.39** X-ray image: degenerative changes in the lateral view.

## 9.2.3 Tangential View

The tangential view (sunrise or défilé view) shows the patella and its corresponding femoral trochlear groove (patellar surface of the femur) in horizontal section. Dysplasias, centering of the patella, and arthritic changes can be assessed using this view.

Positioning: supine position, 60° of knee flexion, with the X-ray beam parallel to the posterior surface of the patella from in an inferior to superior direction.

### Assessment of the Patella

### Normal Findings (Fig. 9.40)

- The lateral facet is longer than the medial one and has a flatter course. Determination of the *patellar articular surface index* (*Brattström*) provides an accurate measurement: the ratio of the lateral facet length to the medial facet length = 1.7:1.
- The depth of the patella is ascertained by measuring the *patellar depth index* (*Ficat*): the ratio of segments AB:CD = 3.5–4.3.
- Facet angle: 130° ± 10°.

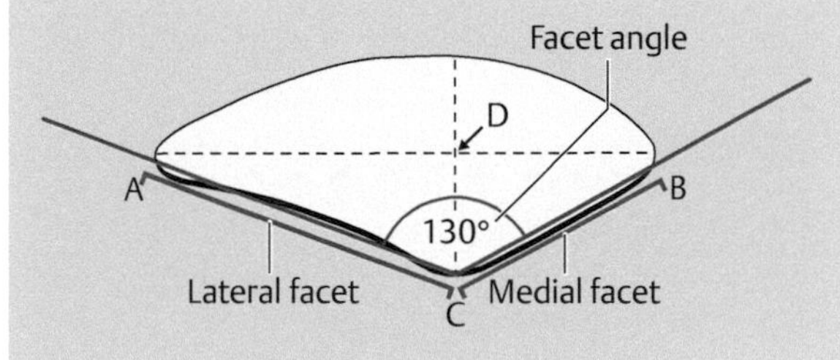


**Fig. 9.40** X-ray image: patella in the tangential view.

## Assessment of the Trochlea (Patellar Surface of the Femur)

### Normal Findings (Fig. 9.41)

- The lateral condyle is slightly higher than the medial condyle.
- The *intercondylar sulcus* is a channel-like structure located centrally to slightly medially.
- *Sulcus angle* (Brattström): 140° ± 5°.
- Depth of the sulcus from measuring the condylar depth index (Ficat): the ratio of EF:GH = 5.3 ± 1.2.

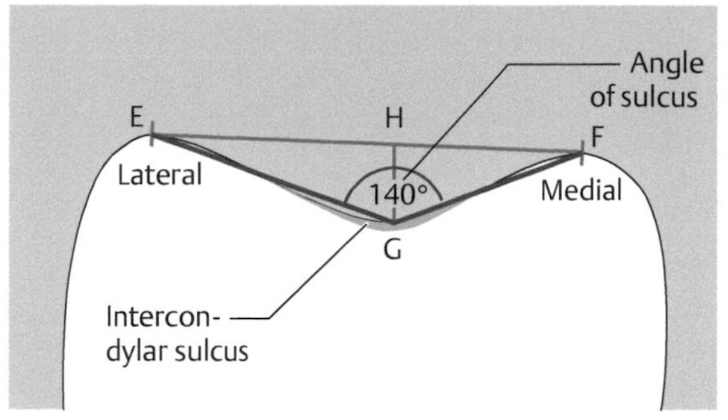


**Fig. 9.41** X-ray image: femoral trochlea in the tangential view.

## Assessment of the Patella Relative to the Trochlea

### Normal Findings (Fig. 9.42)

- The patella, together with the lateral cheeks of the condyles, forms a harmonious curve, the *patellofemoral arc*.
- There is a symmetrical gap from the patellar facets to the trochlea.

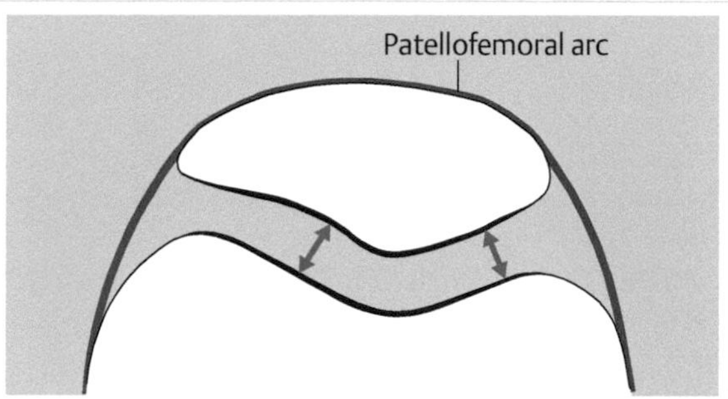


**Fig. 9.42** X-ray image: position of the patella in relation to the trochlea in the tangential view.

### Pathology

(**Fig. 9.43**)

**Degenerative Changes**

Narrowing of part of the joint space.

Increased subchondral sclerosis as a result of excess loading.

**Hypoplasia and Dysplasia**

Hypoplasia of the trochlea with flattening of the *intercondylar sulcus* and the lateral condylar cheeks, and possibly even absence of the sulcus.

Lateral misalignment of the patella as a result of a flat patellar surface of the lateral femoral trochlea, thus interrupting the patellofemoral arc. The misalignment can assume the proportions of patellar luxation.

*Patellar dysplasia*, such as a Jägerhut (hunter's hat) patella, with a very steep medial patella facet, or a bipartite patella (divided patella).

Medial *hypoplasia* of the patella, with a very short and convex medial facet and a facet angle of 90 to 100°, for example.

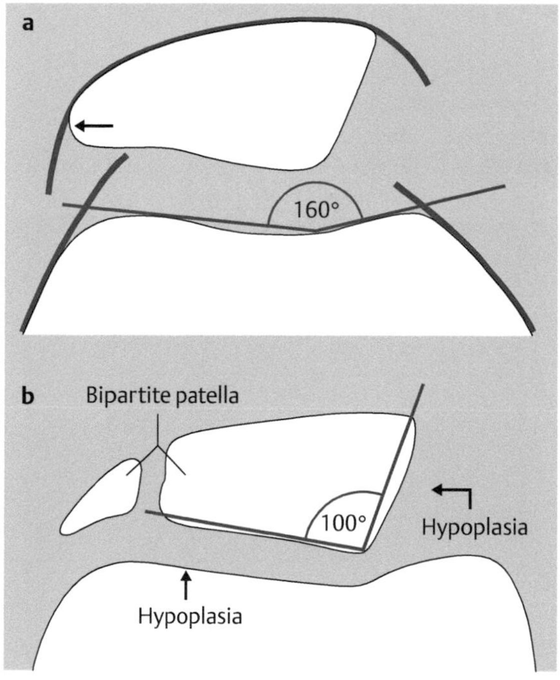


**Fig. 9.43** X-ray image: pathologic changes. **(a)** Jägerhut patella deformity with misalignment laterally. **(b)** Hypoplasia of the lateral femoral condyle and the medial facet of the patella, and an example of a bipartite patella.

# 9.3 Knee Joint

## 9.3.1 Bony Structure and Joint Surfaces

### Femur (Figs. 9.44 and Fig. 9.45)

#### Medial and Lateral Condyle

- The distal end of the femur widens into the medial and lateral femoral condyles.
- In the posterior region, they are separated by a deep wide groove, the *intercondylar fossa*.
- On the lateral surfaces of the condyles, there are small projections, the *medial and lateral epicondyles*.
- At the end of the medial condyle is the adductor tubercle, the insertion site of the adductor magnus muscle.
- In the frontal view, the medial condyle is slightly longer than the lateral condyle. Thus, in the standing position, there is an offset angle (the angle that the axis of the femoral shaft forms with the longitudinal line of the leg) of 6°.
- In the transverse view, the lateral condyle is shorter and wider than the medial condyle.

#### Popliteal Surface

- This is formed by the medial and lateral lips of the linea aspera, which move apart from each other in an inverted V shape toward the epicondyles.
- The inferior border is a ridge that connects the condyles together—the *intercondylar line*.

#### Femoral Trochlea (Patellar Surface of the Femur)

- Anteriorly, the condyles end in the patellar surface, which in the transverse view is somewhat heart-shaped with a vertical, broad groove in its center.
- The lateral borders are called *condylar cheeks*. The lateral cheek is more prominent than the medial.

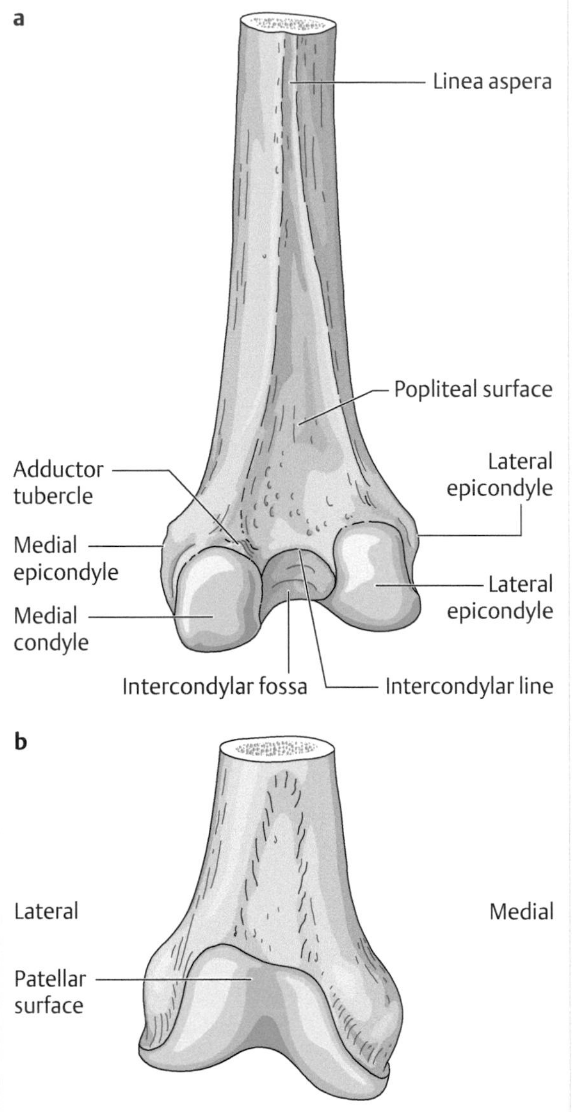


**Fig. 9.44** Distal femur. **(a)** Posterior view. **(b)** Anterior view.

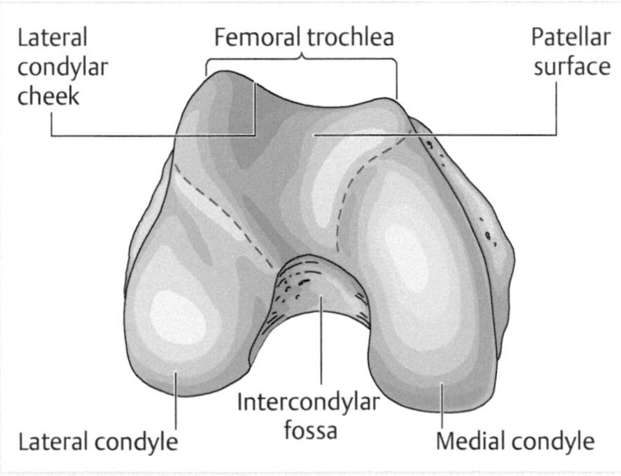


**Fig. 9.45** Distal femur (transverse view).

## Evolute (Fig. 9.46)

A representation of the condyles in profile shows that the diameter of its curvature decreases moving posteriorly. For example, the radius of the medial condyle decreases from 38 mm anteriorly to 17 mm posteriorly, and that of the lateral condyle from 60 mm to 12 mm.

The contour line of the condyles is like a spiral, but with multiple centers. The curved line formed by the centers of curvature is called the evolute. The epicondyles coincide approximately with the anterior end of the evolute, while the posterior end is at the level of the intercondylar fossa.

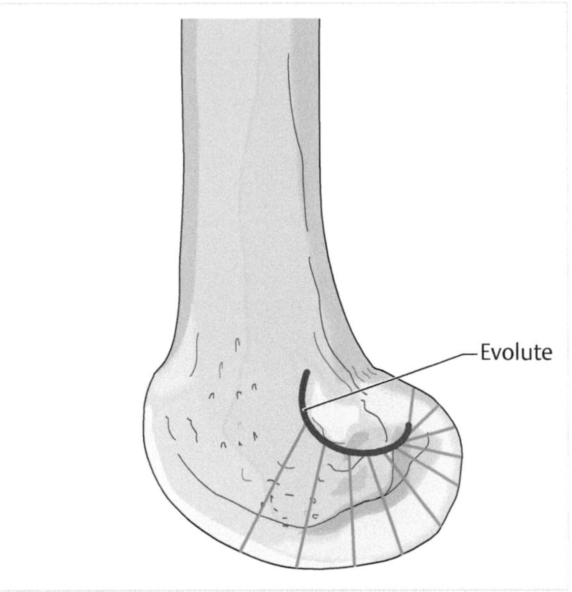


**Fig. 9.46** Evolute.

## Cartilage-Covered Joint Surfaces (Fig. 9.47)

The two condyles have an equally thick cartilage coating of 5 to 7 mm.

The patellar surface of the femur forms the sliding surface for the patella. At the transition between the condyles and the patellar surface, small elevations, the *medial and lateral condylopatellar lines*, are visible. These are also referred to as marginal grooves. They develop from the marginal pressure of the anterior horn of the meniscus at maximum extension. The medial condylopatellar line extends more proximally than the lateral line.

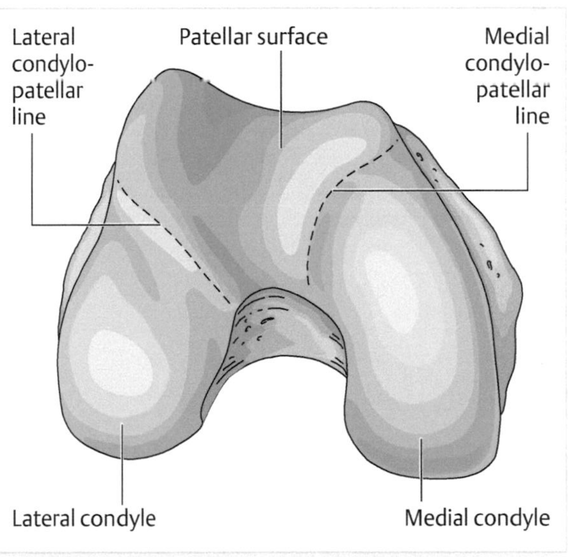


**Fig. 9.47** Cartilage-covered joint surfaces in the distal femur.

**Pathology**

### Osteochondritis Dissecans

This is aseptic necrosis of the subchondral cartilage that particularly occurs on the inner side of the medial condyle.

There is a softening and possibly detachment of a small piece of bone and cartilage (loose body). This leaves a corresponding defect in the femoral condyle. The loose body can potentially cause locking of the joint.

The cause of osteochondritis dissecans is partly increased biomechanical stress on the knee joint. This increased load may be due to recurrent microtrauma or malposition. Other possible causes include genetic and hormonal factors.

# Tibia

## Tibial Plateau (Figs. 9.48 and 9.49)

- The superiorly directed portion of the tibia is called the tibial plateau.
- It is inclined 9° posteriorly;
- The joint surface on the plateau is the *superior articular surface* and is divided into the lateral and medial joint surfaces.
- It is divided by an area that is not covered with cartilage, the *intercondylar eminence*.
- The intercondylar eminence is a clear elevation that is flatter anteriorly and posteriorly in the *anterior and posterior intercondylar areas*.
- Elevations at the transition from the facet to the eminence—the *medial and lateral intercondylar tubercles*—are particularly pronounced.
- Both joint facets have an oval shape; the medial facet is concave in both the sagittal and frontal planes; the lateral facet is concave in the frontal view and convex in the sagittal view.

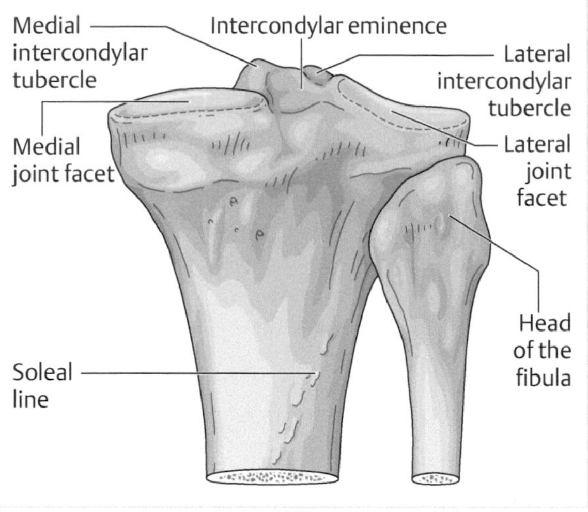


**Fig. 9.48** Proximal tibia (posterior view).

## Medial and Lateral Condyles (Fig. 9.50)

- The proximal tibia is formed into condyles on its medial and lateral sides.
- *Gerdy's tubercle*, clearly protruding from the anterior part of the lateral condyle, is the insertion site for the iliotibial tract.
- The *tibial tuberosity*, located further inferior from Gerdy's tubercle and toward the middle of the tibia, is the insertion for the patellar ligament.
- The fibular articular facet is located posterolaterally under the lateral tibial condyle. It is a slightly convex joint surface for the fibular head.

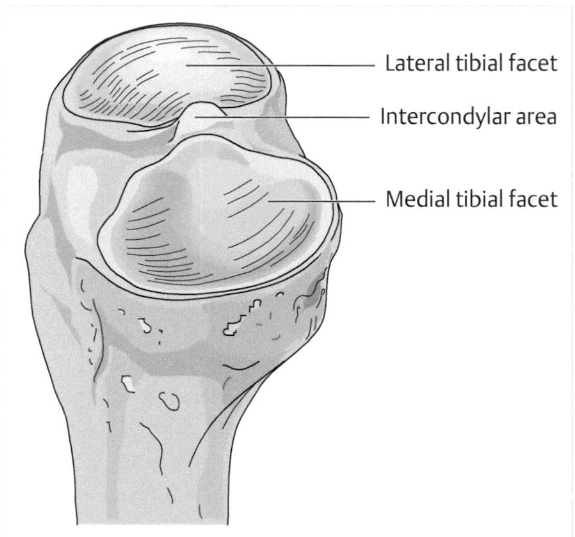


**Fig. 9.49** Articular facets of the tibia (medial view).

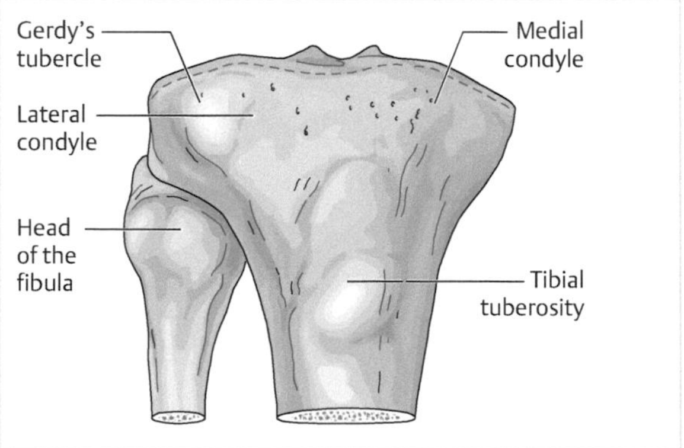


**Fig. 9.50** Proximal tibia (anterior view).

## Cartilage-Covered Joint Surfaces on the Tibia (Fig. 9.51)

The tibial articular surface on the tibial plateau is up to 5 mm thick. The cartilaginous covering is somewhat thicker on the lateral than on the medial facet.

Posteriorly, a lighter layer of joint cartilage extends posteriorly and distally over the edge of the plateau. If the lateral meniscus is displaced superiorly during knee flexion, the posterior horn glides over this part of the plateau.

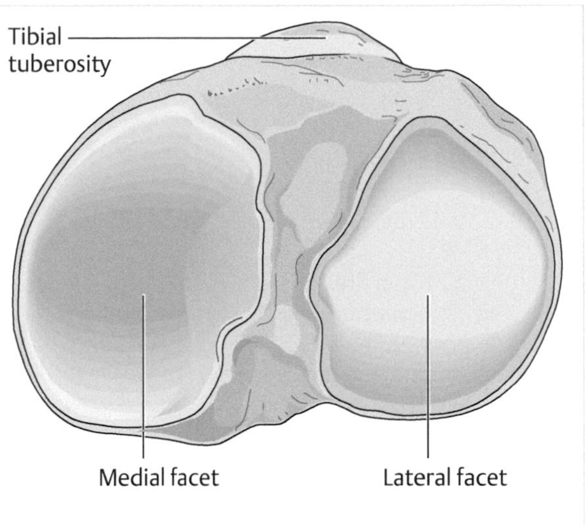


**Fig. 9.51** Cartilage-covered joint surfaces on the tibia (superior view).

## Patella (Fig. 9.52)

- This is the largest sesamoid bone of the human skeleton.
- Its shape varies considerably from oval to round or heart-shaped.
- It is proximally wider (*base of the patella*) and usually comes to a point inferiorly (*apex of the patella*).
- Approaching from proximally, the quadriceps muscle tracks to the base, and a few of its long fibers run onward over it. Its continuation is the *patellar ligament*, which tracks from the apex of the patella to the tibial tuberosity.

### Anterior Surface

- The anterior surface is slightly convex in all views.
- It has a rough surface with vertically running recesses formed by radiations of the rectus tendon; in addition, it is traversed by many blood vessels.

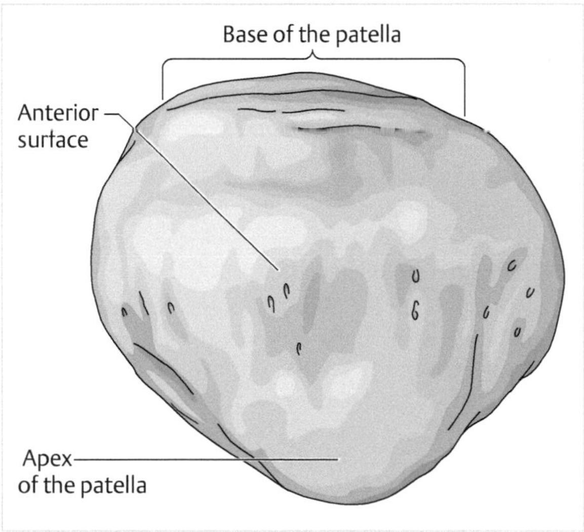


**Fig. 9.52** Patella: anterior surface of the patella.

## Articular Surface of the Patella (Fig. 9.53)

- This is also called retropatellar articular surface.
- It is the patellar joint surface for the patellofemoral joint.
- It has a vertical ridge that divides it into a broad lateral half and a narrow medial half. The *lateral facet* is concave, and the *medial facet* is concave or slightly convex.

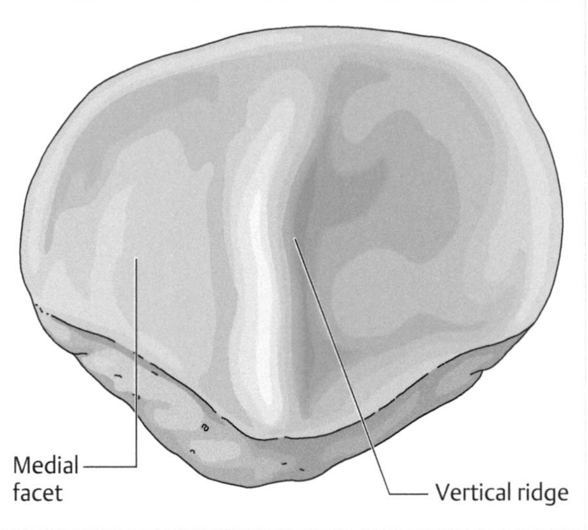


**Fig. 9.53** Patella: articular surface of the patella.

## Transverse View of the Patella (Fig. 9.54)

- The patellar has a triangular shape with the tip pointing into the joint.
- The lateral edges are of varying thicknesses, with the medial edge significantly more strongly built than the lateral. The lateral part, however, extends further.
- The angle between the medial and lateral facets (*facet angle* or *patellar opening angle*) is 120 to 140°.
- The patella is well centered if the ridge of the posterior patellar surface lies within the groove of the patellar surface of the femur.

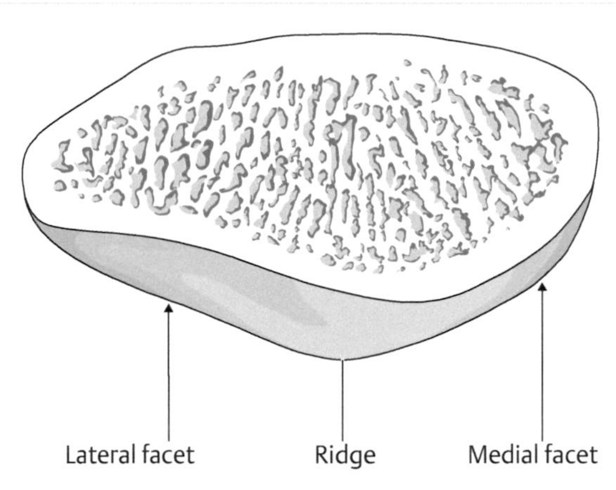


**Fig. 9.54** Transverse view of the patella.

## Cartilage-Covered Joint Surfaces

The middle region has the thickest hyaline cartilage layer, at approximately 6 mm, whereas the apex is not covered with cartilage. The retropatellar surface of the patella and the patellar surface of the femur together form the patellofemoral joint.

**Pathology**

### Patellar Luxation

Dysplasia of the patella and the patellar surface of the femur leads to instability of the patella with repeated lateral subluxation or luxation of the patella. This results in a pressure overload of the joint surfaces of the lateral patellar surface of the femur and, later, femoropatellar arthritis. The patients describe that the knee "gives way" with sudden movements. Usually, the luxation corrects itself spontaneously right after the occurrence.

Treatment: improving patellar balance within the trochlear groove (patellar surface of the femur) to prevent progression of the degenerative changes. Thus, any existing muscle imbalance should be corrected. Surgical correction involves division of the lateral retinaculum with medial capsular tightening.

## Architecture of Cancellous (Trabecular) Bone

### Distal Femur (Fig. 9.55)

Two lines of trabeculae can be identified: some compression trabeculae run almost vertically into the cortical bone of the condyles, and these are crossed by the weaker traction trabeculae that extend from medial to lateral.

### Proximal Tibia (Fig. 9.55)

In the tibial plateau region, compression trabeculae run vertically from the tibial plateau in an inferior direction. In addition, a few trabeculae extend inferiorly from the intercondylar eminence in a slightly curved path.

These are crossed by horizontally extending traction trabeculae, which run from the medial tibial condyle to the lateral condyle. These are significantly less developed than the compression trabeculae.

### Patella (Fig. 9.56)

In sagittal section, the direction of pull of the quadriceps tendon forms corresponding bundles of strong, curved traction trabeculae. In addition, on the retropatellar joint surface, compression trabeculae can be seen running toward the surface.

A transverse section demonstrates transversely aligned traction trabeculae and, perpendicular to the patellofemoral joint, compression trabeculae.

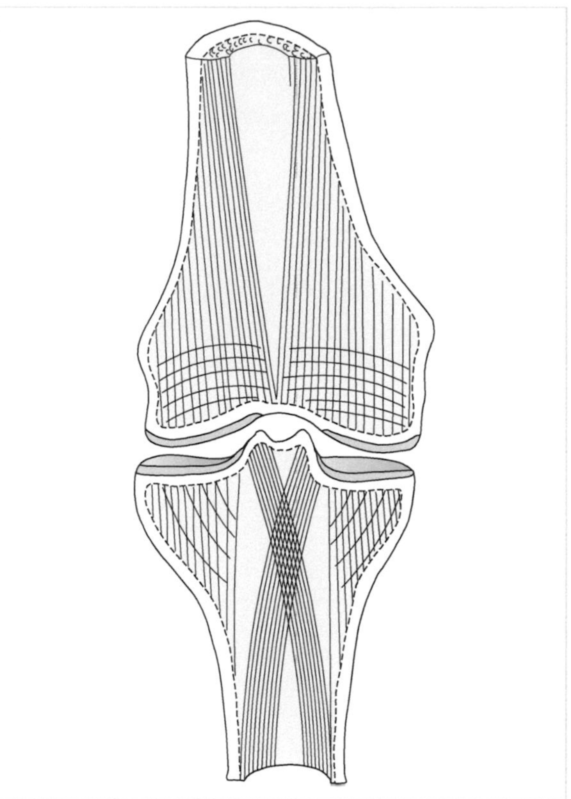

**Fig. 9.55** Architecture of the cancellous bone of the femur and tibia in frontal section.

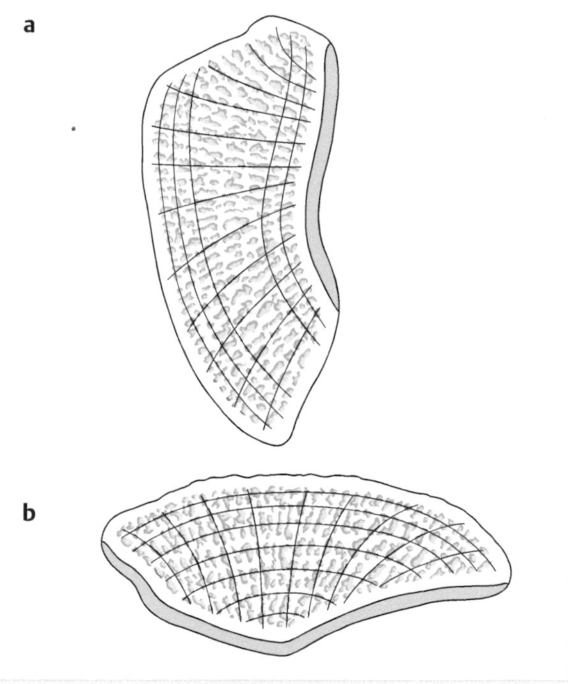


**Fig. 9.56** Architecture of the cancellous bone of the patella. **(a)** Sagittal section. **(b)** Horizontal section.

## 9.3.2 Joint Capsule

### Synovial Membrane (Figs. 9.57 and 9.58)

The synovial membrane is richly vascularized and demonstrates numerous recesses.

On the *femur*, its insertion is close to the bone–cartilage interface. Anterosuperiorly, it inserts approximately 1 cm proximal to the patellar surface and forms the suprapatellar bursa. From there, the capsule goes to the upper margin of the patella. From the bone–cartilage junction of the medial and lateral condyles, the synovial membrane passes to the lateral edges of the patella. From the lower patellar margin, it extends over the fat body to the upper edge of the anterior horn of the meniscus.

Posteriorly, the line of insertion passes around the proximal edge of the condyles just below the origins of the gastrocnemius muscle, forming recesses, the *polar caps*.

Medially, laterally, and anteriorly on the tibia, the synovial membrane inserts on the bone–cartilage interface of the tibial plateau. Posteriorly, the insertion line extends along the bone–cartilage junction of the medial and lateral tibial facets in an anterior direction and bends around the intercondylar area. In evolutionary terms, the cruciate ligaments migrated into the knee joint from posteriorly. Thus, they are covered by the synovial membrane only on the anterior side, and are therefore extrasynovial.

From the tibial plateau, the membrane moves to the lower edge of the menisci. It continues from the upper margin of the meniscus proximally and inserts on the femoral condyles.

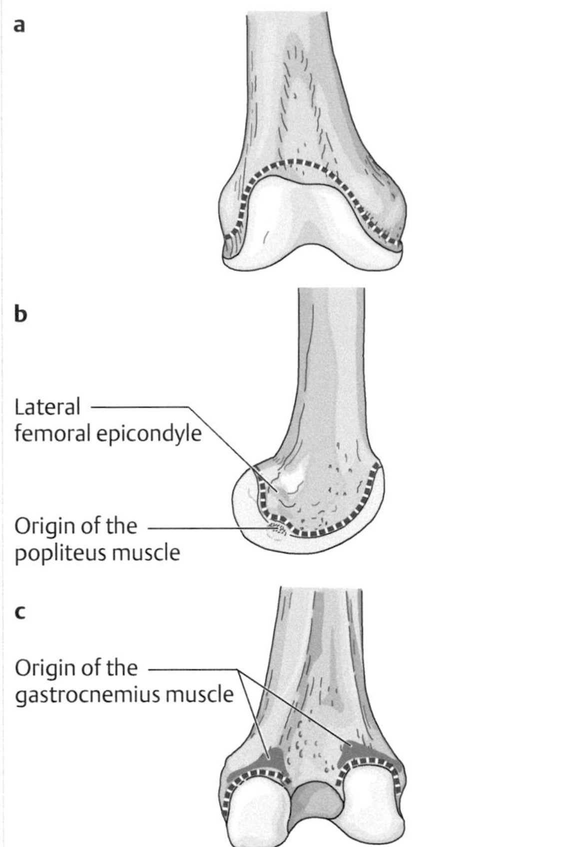


**Fig. 9.57** Insertions of the synovial membrane on the femur. **(a)** Anterior femoral region. **(b)** Lateral femoral region. **(c)** Posterior femoral region.

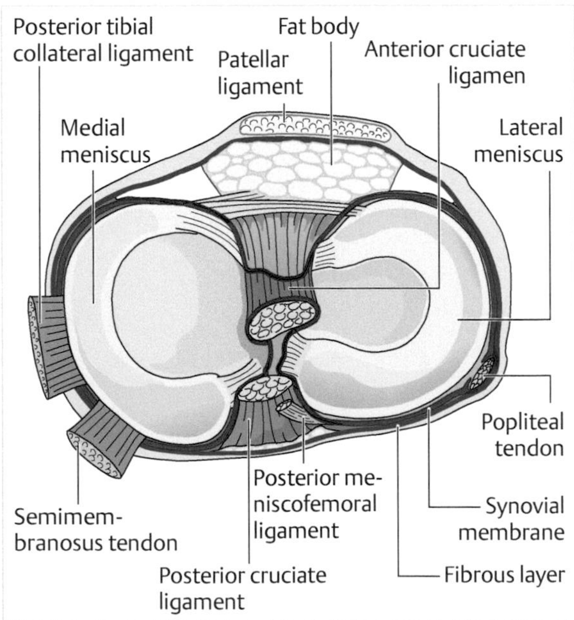


**Fig 9.58** Course of the joint capsule on the tibial plateau. Red line: synovial membrane; brown line: fibrous layer.

## Fibrous Layer (Fig. 9.59)

The fibrous capsule layer inserts along with the synovial membrane in almost all areas, with the following exceptions:

- On the tibial plateau, the insertion line runs approximately 1 cm distal to the edge of the plateau.
- Posteriorly, it bridges the intercondylar area and therefore does not follow the synovial membrane anteriorly.
- From the insertion on the lateral condyles, the fibers of the fibrous layer track to the upper outer edge of the bases of the menisci. From the tibial insertion, they extend from inferiorly to the lower outer edge of the bases, so that the menisci are embedded within the fibrous layer.

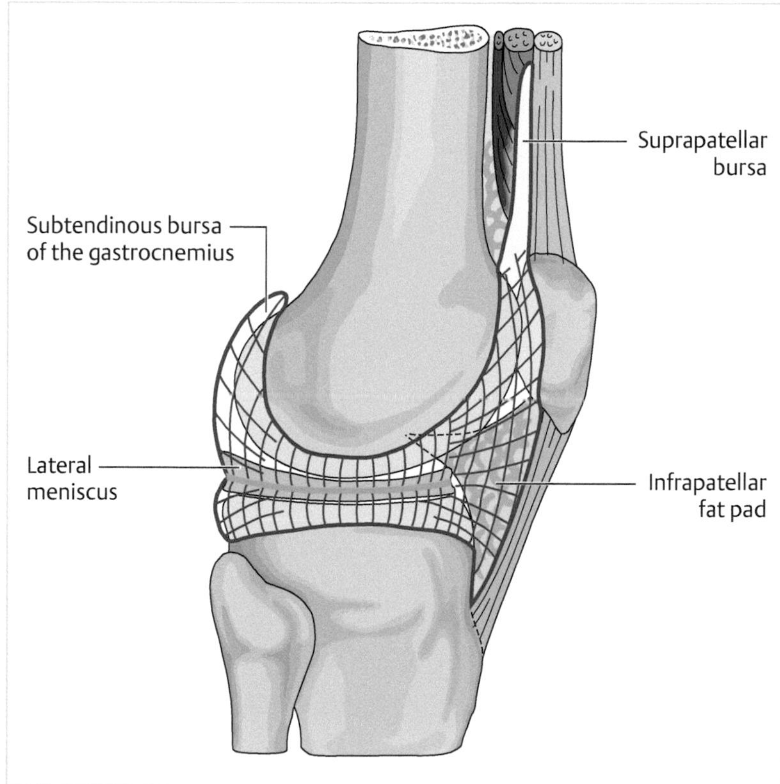


**Fig. 9.59** Insertions of the fibrous layer (lateral view).

## Recesses (Fig. 9.60)

The capsule forms recesses in various locations. This means that there is a reserve space for the capsule to carry out maximum movements without areas of the capsule being torn.

### *Parapatellar Recess*

The capsule forms small recesses between the lateral bone–cartilage borders on the femur and the lateral patellar surfaces.

### *Subpopliteal Recess*

A bursa under the tendon of origin of the popliteus muscle cushions it from the edges of the bone. This bursa always communicates with the joint cavity and is therefore referred to as a recess.

### *Subtendinous Bursa of the Gastrocnemius Muscle*

The capsule forms outpouchings between the heads of the gastrocnemius muscle and the femoral condyles—the "polar caps."

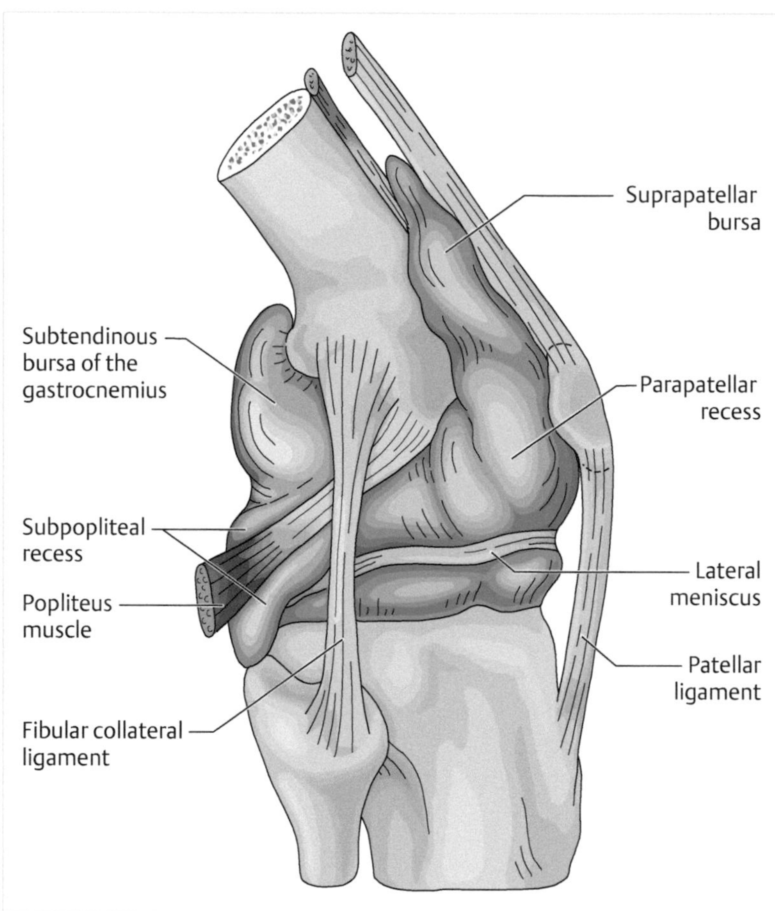


**Fig. 9.60** Recesses of the joint capsule (inflated knee joint, lateral view).

*Suprapatellar Bursa (Fig. 9.61)*

Anterior and superior to the patella, the capsule forms the largest recess. Starting at the proximal part of the patellar surface of the femur, the deep layer of the recess tracks in a superior direction. Approximately 10 to 12 cm above the base of the patella, it turns inferiorly and then forms the superficial layer, which is fixed to the base of the patella.

The recess is located directly under the rectus tendon, to which it is attached. In the distal section, fatty connective tissue is found between the lower layer and the femur. Proximal to this, the fibers of the articular muscle of the knee, which splits off from the quadriceps, insert into the recess. That means that the quadriceps has a direct effect on the movement of the recess: contraction or relaxation of the muscle causes the two layers of the recess to slide against each other.

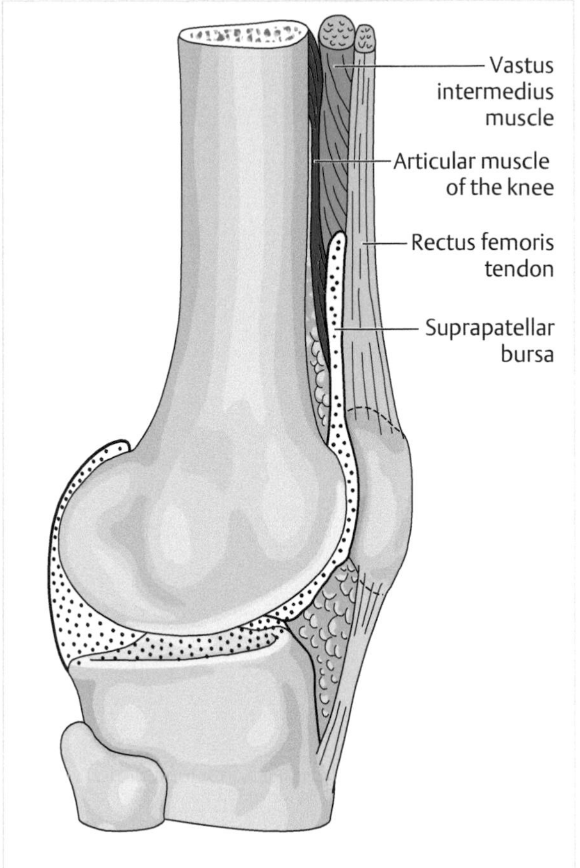


**Fig. 9.61** Suprapatellar bursa.

*The unfolding of the suprapatellar bursa* (**Fig. 9.62**): Up to 80° of flexion, the state of tension of the recess does not change very much. From that point on, however, it is necessary for the upper layer to be able to slide against the lower layer. The recess must be completely expandable to achieve maximum flexibility.

Pathology

### Joint Effusion

Due to improper loading and other inflammatory stimuli, the synovial membrane produces more liquid, thereby forming a joint effusion. The consequences of effusion are overstretching of the capsule and consequent compression of the capillaries within the joint. In addition, as a result of synovitis, leukocytes enter the joint and release lysosomal enzymes, which attack the cartilage and lead to its destruction.

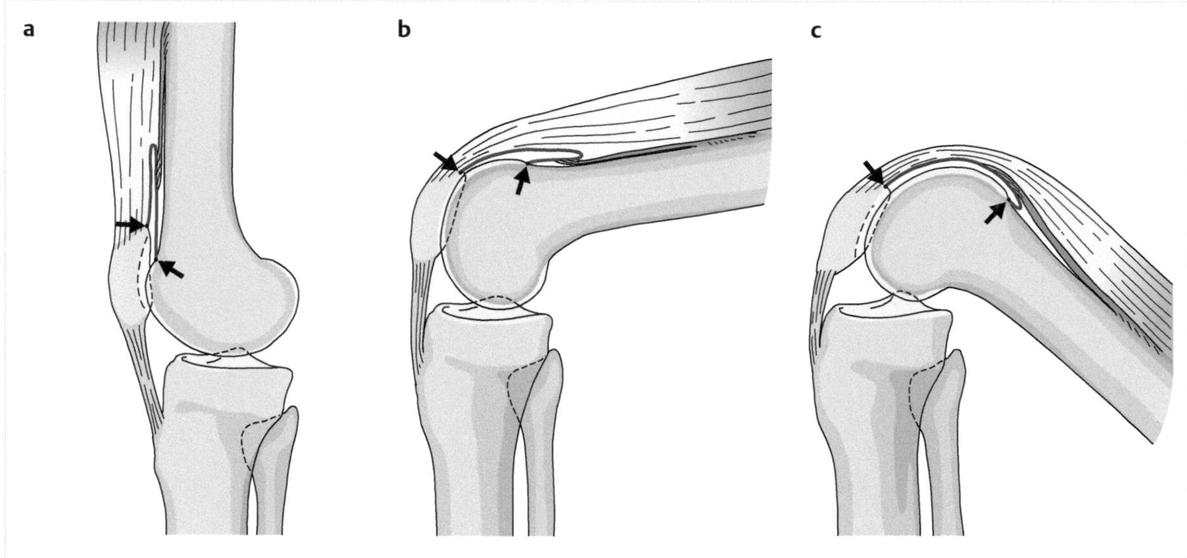


**Fig. 9.62** Unfolding the suprapatellar bursa. **(a)** In the neutral position (0°), the point of fixation of the recess at the bone–cartilage interface is opposite to the proximal third of the patella. **(b)** During the first 80° of flexion, this fixed point moves only slightly from the proximal border of the patella, and the recess has to unfold only minimally. **(c)** With further flexion up to 135°, this point moves significantly away from the proximal border of the patella, so that the recess has to extend to its full length.

## Practical Tip

### Inspection

When an effusion is present, the leg is kept in a slightly flexed position in order to relax the capsule, thus exposing the intra-articular fluid to the least pressure. With movement, the fluid shifts, depending on the position of the knee joint. By passively stretching during extension, the head of the gastrocnemius muscle presses the polar caps, forcing the liquid anteriorly into the parapatellar bursa. In flexion, the liquid shifts posteriorly, because the quadriceps muscle stretches, thus smoothing out the suprapatellar bursa.

### Dancing Patella (Fig. 9.63)

The migration of the synovial fluid can be used to check if an effusion is present. Press the leg into maximum extension and then shift the fluid from the superior and inferior recesses into the area under the patella. This will cause the patella to rise up. By applying pressure to the patella, it will sink, but then it will spring back into its previous position when released.

### Restricted Mobility

Significant unfolding of the suprapatellar bursa is required only when flexion is greater than 80°. If the bursa becomes adherent, flexion is therefore restricted to 80°.

Starting movement early in a postoperative rehabilitation program is a means of preventing, or at least decreasing, the adherence of the anterior and posterior layers of the bursa.

### Effects of the Quadriceps Muscle

Tensing exercises for the quadriceps muscle act to shift the deep layer of the recess over the articular muscle of the knee against the superficial layer, thus preventing adherence.

In addition, the quadriceps muscle exerts external pressure on the fluid-filled recess. The pumping action results in displacement of the fluid into the surrounding soft tissues, where the fluid is absorbed more quickly.

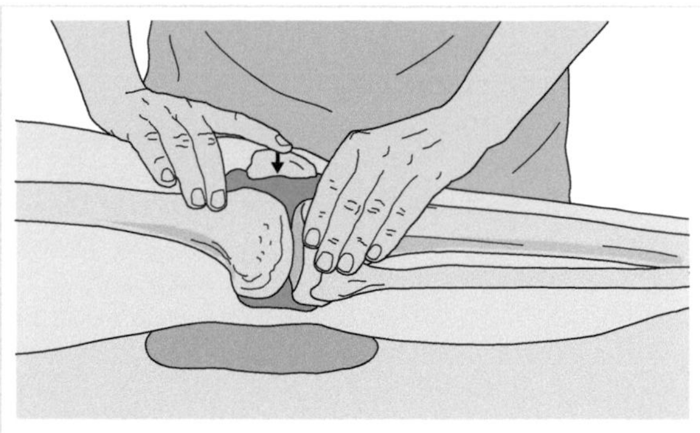

**Fig. 9.63** Test for a dancing patella.

## 9.3.3 Central Functional Complex

### Menisci (Figs. 9.64 and 9.65)

The menisci are **C**-shaped or nearly annular fibrocartilage wedges whose outer areas are thick and inner areas are thinner. Each meniscus is divided into the anterior and posterior horns. The meniscus has an inner portion in the articular cavity, and a base, which faces outward. The superiorly directed surface is concave and is in contact with the femoral condyles. The inferior surface is almost flat and lies on the respective tibial plateau. The menisci divide the joint between the femur and the tibia into the femoromeniscal and meniscotibial parts.

Both anterior meniscal horns establish a connection to the side surfaces of the patella by way of the patellomeniscal ligament.

The *transverse ligament of the knee* connects the anterior horns and also extends to the infrapatellar fat pad.

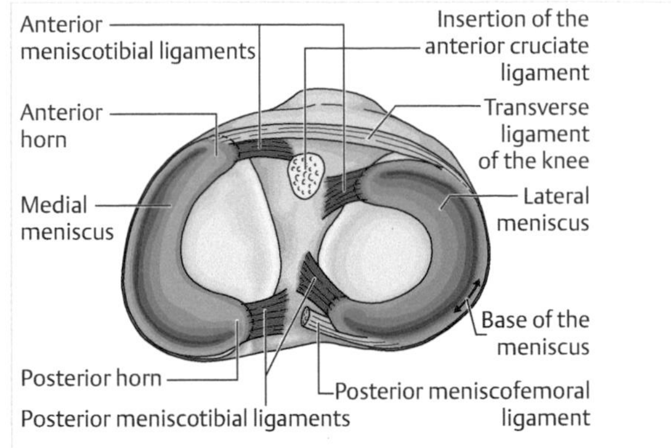


**Fig. 9.64** Medial and lateral menisci.

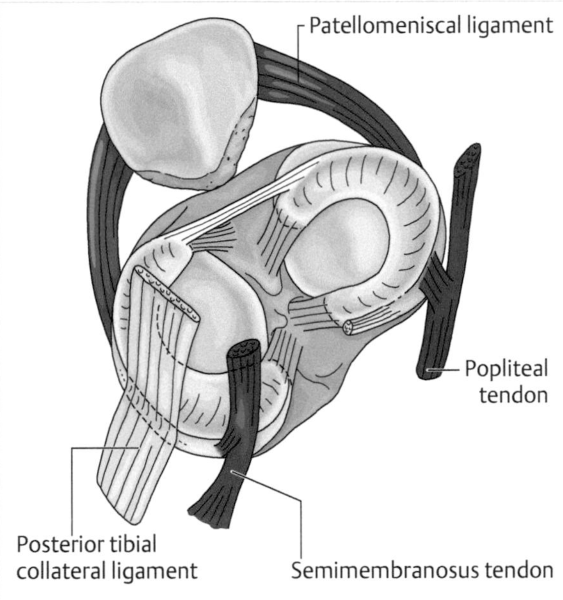


**Fig. 9.65** Connections of the menisci.

### Medial Meniscus

The medial meniscus is **C**-shaped. Its anterior horn is fixed to the anterior intercondylar area by the *anterior meniscotibial ligament*, and the posterior horn is fixed to the posterior intercondylar area by the *posterior meniscotibial ligament*.

In the middle third, *bands of capsular fibers* track from above and below to the base of the meniscus, where they intertwine with the outermost layer of the meniscus. In the posteromedial area, the *posterior tibial collateral ligament* tracks into the meniscus and the *semimembranosus muscle* into the posterior horn.

### Lateral Meniscus

The lateral meniscus is annular. As with the medial meniscus, its anterior and posterior horns attach to the middle of the tibial plateau by way of the *anterior and posterior meniscotibial ligaments*. Here, too, there are bands of capsular fibers that track to its base.

The *posterior meniscofemoral ligament* tracks from the posterior horn of the lateral meniscus to the inside of the medial condyle and thus runs parallel to the posterior cruciate ligament. The *popliteus muscle* forms a connection to the posterior horn.

## Histology (Fig. 9.66)

The menisci are composed primarily of type I collagen fibers and only a very few elastic fibers. Cartilage cells are embedded between the collagen fibrils.

In the scanning electron microscope representation, the following three layers can be distinguished:

- First layer: A network of thin fibrils covers the meniscal surface.
- Second layer: The arrangement of the lamellar fiber bundles is like a lattice, with the fibers crossing each other at various angles.
- Third layer: This thickest layer consists of circularly arranged bundles of fibrils. At the base of the meniscus, the connective tissue of the joint capsule tracks into the third layer and intertwines with it.

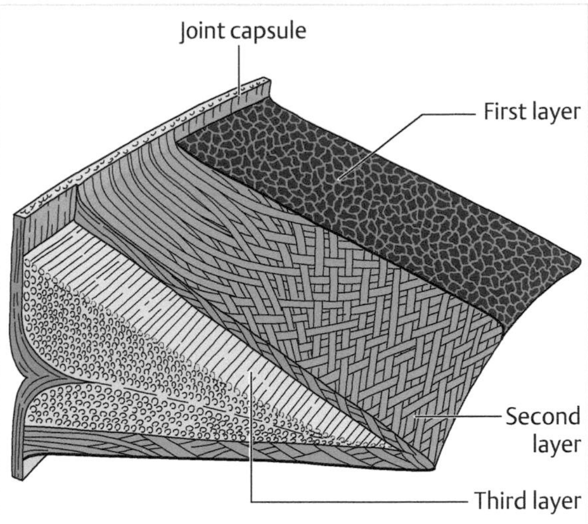


**Fig. 9.66** Histologic composition of the meniscus.

## Nutrition of the Menisci (Fig. 9.67)

In terms of nutrition, the menisci can be divided into three different zones:

- Synovial fluid nourishes two-thirds of the meniscus (the inner portion) by diffusion.
- Blood vessels from the fibrous layer supply the base of the meniscus. With the medial meniscus, further blood vessels reach the base by way of the tibial collateral ligament.
- Blood vessels from the surrounding structures enter approximately 2 mm into the margin. The density of vessels in the meniscus is significantly lower than it is in the capsule.
- Both the anterior and posterior horns receive vascularization over the meniscotibial ligaments on the tibial plateau.
- The central parts of the meniscus are the furthest away from sources of nutrition and thus have the worst nutritional status. Therefore this area is most prone to dysfunction.

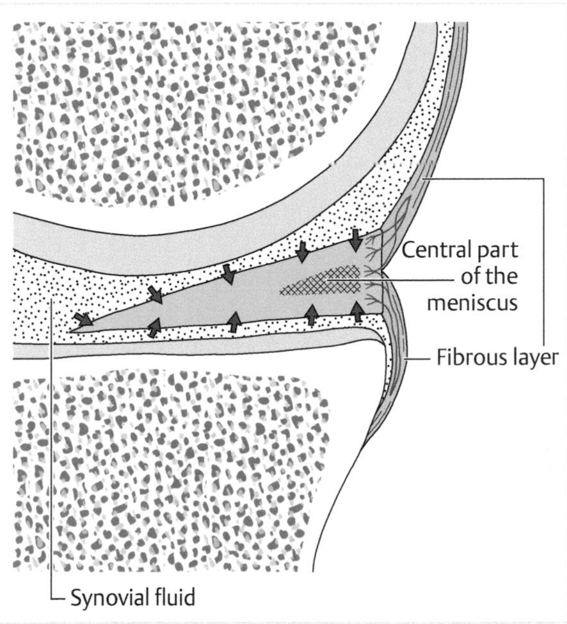


**Fig. 9.67** Blood supply to the menisci.

## Receptors in the Menisci

Proprioceptors and free nerve endings occur in the third of the meniscus near the base and in the anterior and posterior horns. The posterior horns, in particular, contain a high density of proprioceptors.

*Pacini's corpuscles* are responsible for the transmission of information on movement and speed. *Golgi's bodies* transmit changes in tension; they trigger afferent type Ib nerves that inhibit the motor neurons to ensure a smoothly controlled motion sequence.

The *free nerve endings* discern chemical stimuli. To effect a reaction, the concentration of the chemical signaling substance (e.g., products released by inflammation) must be very high.

## Displacement of the Menisci during Movement

### *Flexion (Fig. 9.68)*

The femoral condyles push the menisci posteriorly. Active factors in this movement are the semimembranosus muscle on the medial side and popliteus muscle on the lateral side.

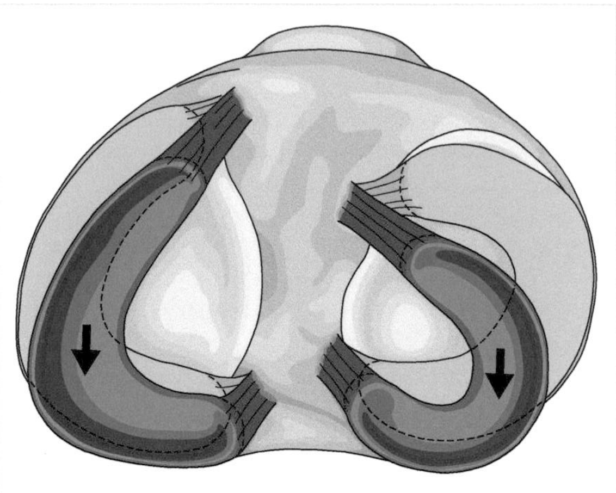

**Fig. 9.68** Displacement of the menisci during flexion.

### *Extension*

The femoral condyles push them anteriorly on the tibial plateau.

In all, the medial meniscus travels a distance of 6 mm; the lateral meniscus, being less secured, travels approximately twice that distance. Due to the fixation of the horns and the mobility of the remaining parts, the menisci deform during movement.

**Pathology**

**Blockage of Extension**

A common symptom of meniscal injury is a painful limitation of stretching. Here, part of a torn meniscus jams into the femorotibial joint space and causes the joint to lock. The extent of the extension deficit varies. Shaking or moving often clears the entrapment.

The semimembranosus and popliteus muscles can also cause a blockage of knee extension; they slacken during this movement, allowing the menisci to shift anteriorly.

*Rotation (Fig. 9.69)*

The menisci follow the movements of the femoral condyles. For example, during internal rotation of the tibia, the medial meniscus shifts anteriorly on the tibial plateau while the lateral meniscus shifts posteriorly. During external rotation of the tibia, the reverse occurs.

**Functions of the Menisci:**

- The menisci compensate for the mismatch between the condyles and the tibial plateau and increase the stability of the joint.
- They absorb peak loads by reducing the point contact stress and transform the compressive forces into circular tensile stresses; i.e., they absorb shock.
- The anterior and posterior horns of the meniscus limit excessive flexion and extension, and slow rotational movements.
- They distribute the synovial fluid and thus improve the nutrition of the articular cartilage.
- They influence muscle tension by way of their proprioceptors.

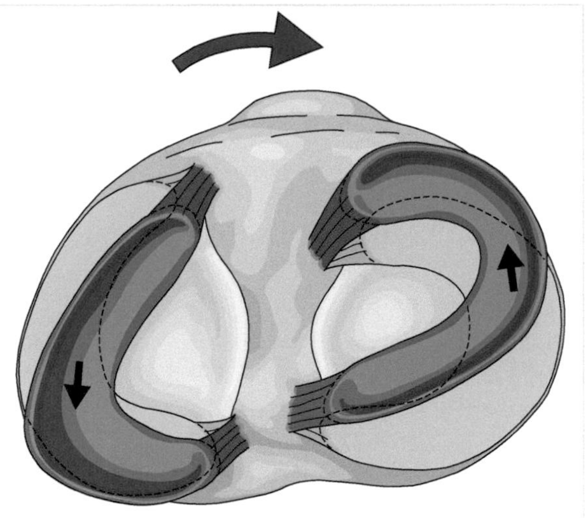

**Fig. 9.69** Displacement of the menisci during external rotation of the tibia.

## Pathology

### Meniscal Ganglion Cyst

Ganglion-like structures form at the meniscal base due to nutritional disorders or overuse; these can grow outward and become palpable. The lateral meniscus is more frequently affected than the medial. Treatment involves resection of the ganglion, and sometimes the removal of a part of the meniscus to prevent recurrences.

### Meniscal Injury (Fig. 9.70)

Numerous tests are available to test for a meniscal lesion, but, by themselves, these are not accurate enough. Only a combination of several studies can provide a reliable diagnosis.

Meniscal injuries take various forms, such as *longitudinal*, *horizontal*, and *radial tears* or ruptures; others are named according to their location, such as a *tear of the anterior or posterior horn flap*.

Bucket-handle tear: The critical load zone lies at the junction between the middle third of the meniscus and the posterior horn; it must absorb a lot of pressure with posterior shifts. Longitudinal tears develop at this point, which can expand anteriorly. The result is a large hole in the meniscus, so that the inner portion (bucket-handle) can dislocate.

Posterior horn flap tear: This also evolves from a longitudinal tear in the critical zone and tears further toward the inner part of the joint.

### Meniscectomy

Since the functions of the menisci are now recognized as being very important, the meniscus-preserving techniques such as meniscal repair or partial resection have come to the fore. The potential for recovery is best in the vascularized zones. Numerous studies have also established that osteoarthritis occurs less often after a partial meniscectomy than a total resection.

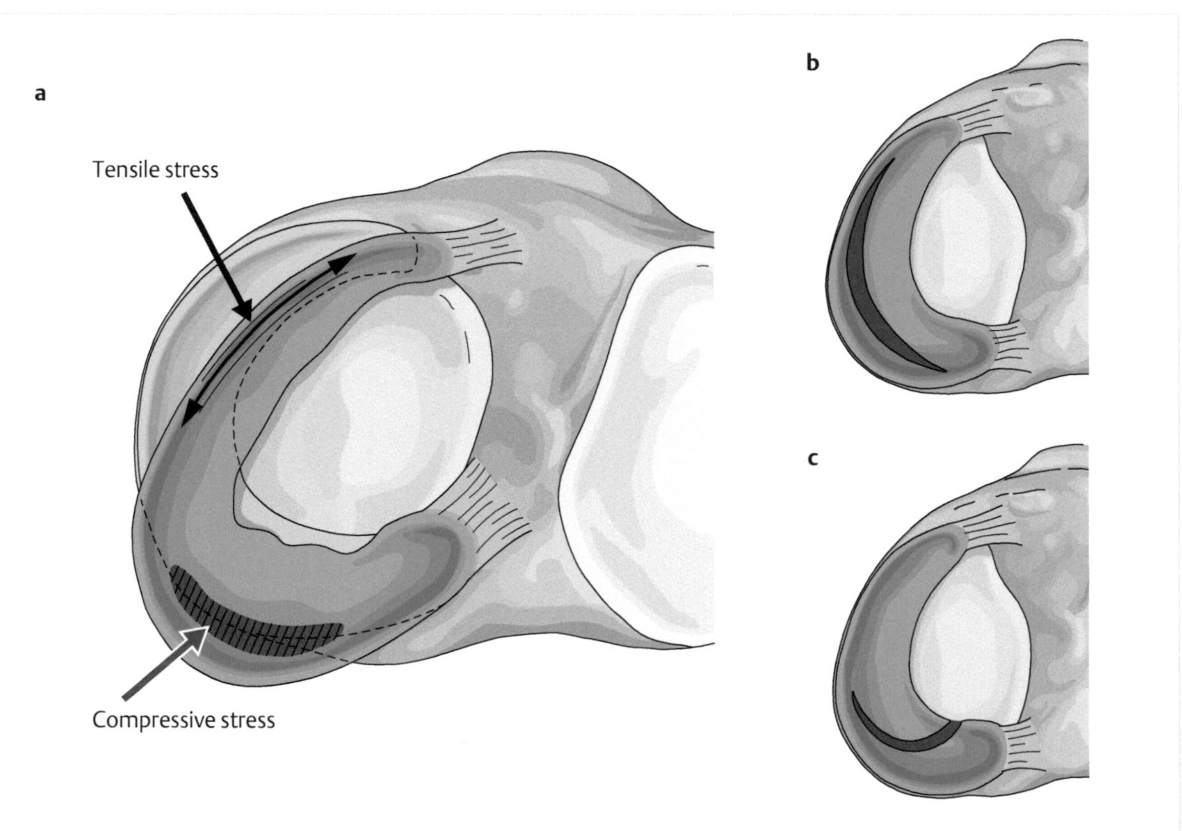


**Fig. 9.70** **(a)** Critical zones for injuries of the medial meniscus. **(b)** Bucket-handle tear. **(c)** Posterior horn flap tear.

## Anterior Cruciate Ligament (Figs. 9.71 and 9.72)

The anterior cruciate ligament has an oval area of origin on the posterior, inner lateral femoral condyle which is approximately 1.5 to 2 cm long. It runs in a distal-anteromedial direction, parallel to the roof of the intercondylar fossa. Toward its insertion, it becomes ever wider, so that its triangular insertion site—just before the medial intercondylar tubercle of the anterior tibial intercondylar area —is wider than any other cross-section of the ligament.

The fibers of the ligament vary in terms of their length and strength. Functionally, there are two bands of fibers to differentiate: the ***anteromedial bundle*** and the ***posterolateral bundle.*** The anteromedial bundle originates the furthest superiorly and inserts anteromedially on the tibial plateau. The posterolateral part arises inferiorly and inserts posteriorly. The fiber bundles grow together and twist around each other. The posterolateral fibers are shorter than the anteromedial fibers. The anterior fiber components connect to the anterior meniscotibial ligament of the medial meniscus.

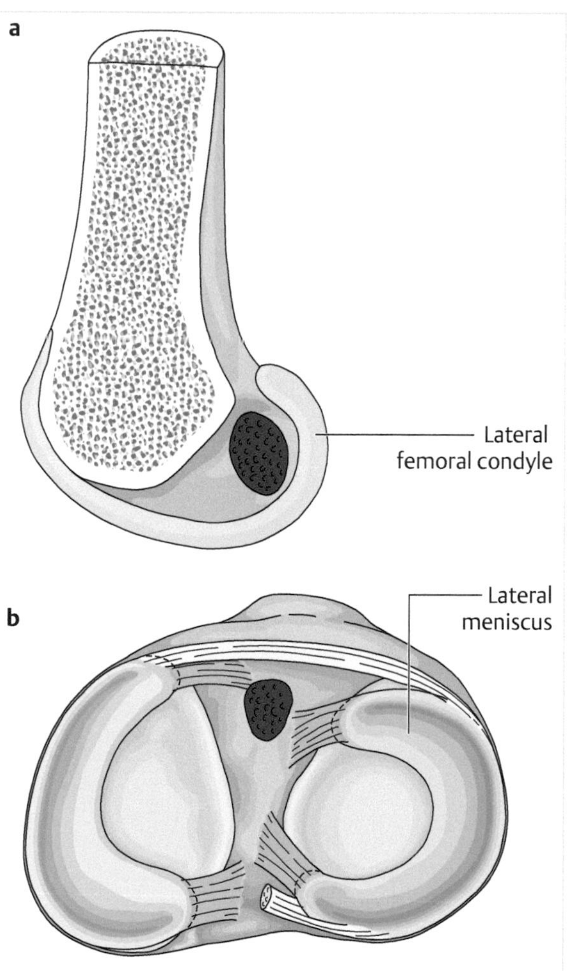


**Fig. 9.71** Insertions of the anterior cruciate ligament. **(a)** Lateral femoral condyle (view from within). **(b)** Tibial plateau.

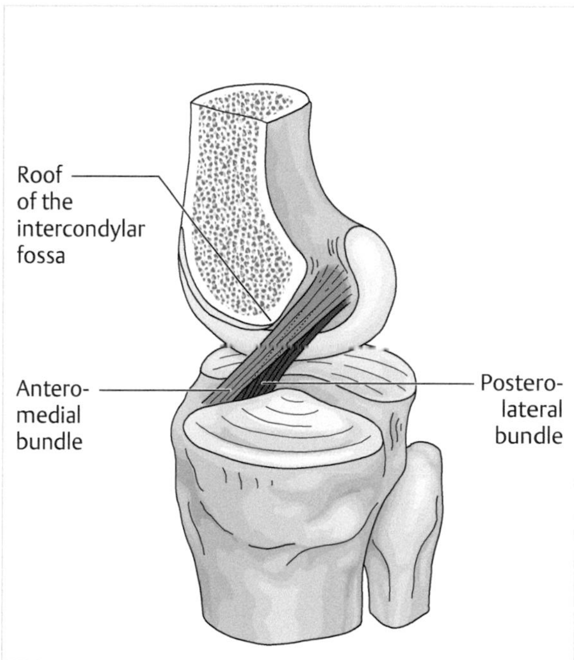


**Fig. 9.72** Course of the anterior cruciate ligament.

## Functions

*Limitations of Movement (Fig. 9.73)*

The anteromedial bundle is taut in extension because it is pressed against the bony roof of the intercondylar fossa (or notch of the femur).

During substantial flexion, the fibers twist around each other because the posterolateral fibers deflect anteriorly under the anteromedial bundle. This happens because the flexion movement shifts the insertion region of these fibers anterosuperiorly on the femur. Through this twisting of the cruciate ligament fibers, a round strand emerges from the previously flat and diverse fiber arrangement, and the ligament becomes tense.

In addition, the anterior cruciate ligament tenses during internal rotation as it loops around the posterior cruciate ligament. By hitting against the intercondylar roof, it is also stretched during maximum external rotation.

*Stabilization*

The ligament prevents anterior subluxation of the tibia, i.e., it prevents the femur from sliding posteriorly on the tibia. Together with the posterior cruciate ligament, it supports the medial and lateral stability of the knee (as a secondary stabilizer) if the primary stabilizers (the collateral ligaments) fail.

*Coordination of the Rolling–Sliding Movement*

Together with the posterior cruciate ligament, the anterior cruciate ligament participates in coordination of the rolling–sliding motion.

▷ See Chapter 9.3.10, Axes and Motion and Movements

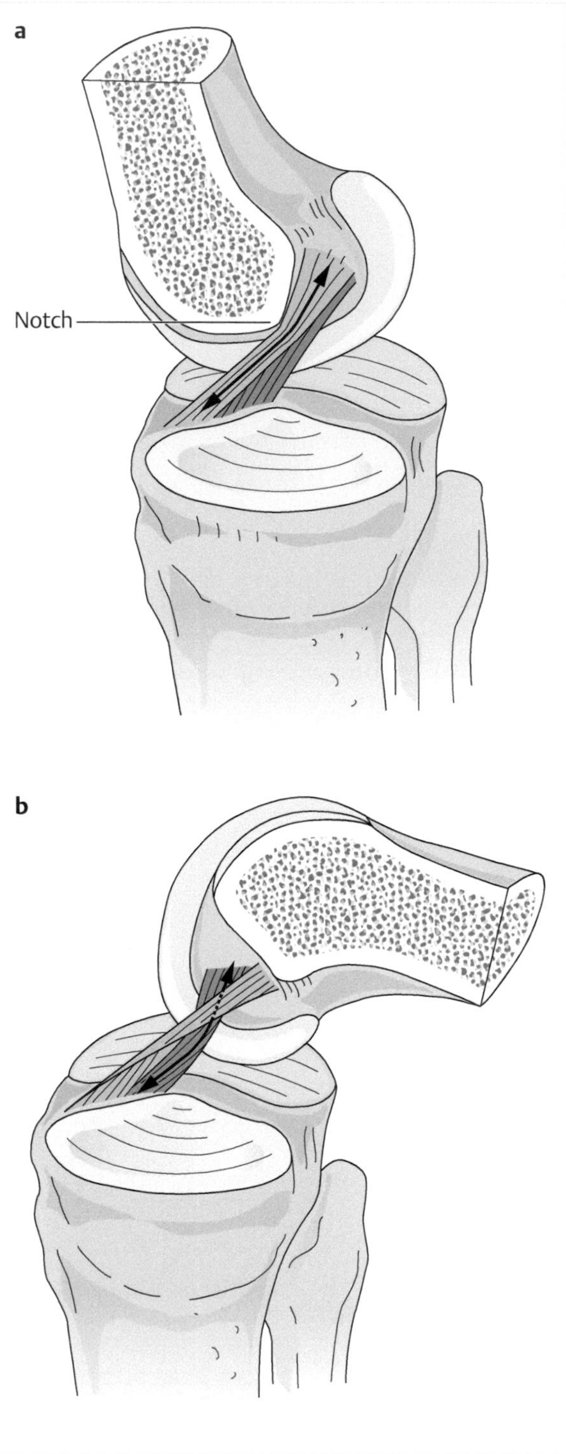


**Fig. 9.73** Anterior cruciate ligament. **(a)** In extension. **(b)** In flexion.

Pathology

### Injury to the Anterior Cruciate Ligament and its Consequences (Fig. 9.74)

A tear in the anterior cruciate ligament results in instability called the "anterior drawer," because the tibia displaces anteriorly. This means that the rolling–sliding motion is altered. Disintegration of the predominant rolling movement occurs, leading to pathologic backward displacement of the femoral support point in both the medial and lateral parts of the knee joint. The anterior sliding movement of the femur no longer takes place in conjunction with the rolling motion, but is replaced by a jerky, catch-up motion. The posterior horns of the menisci are used to slow down the rolling motion and, with time, become overstressed.

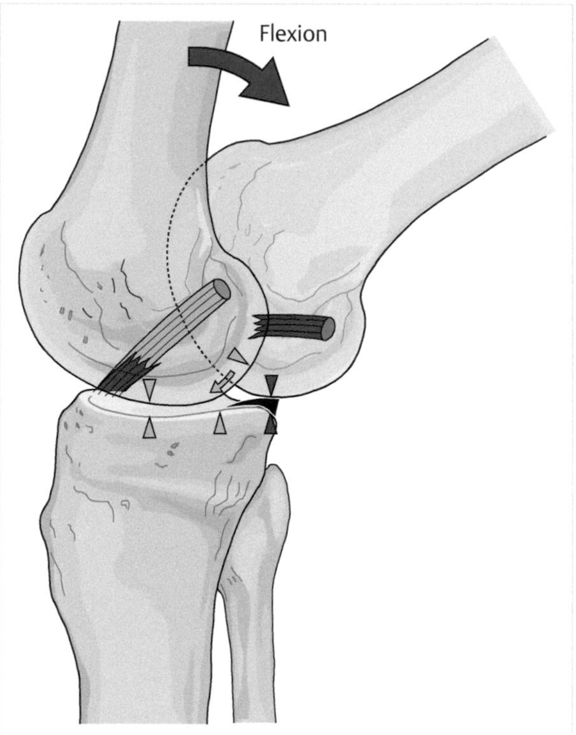


**Fig. 9.74** Disintegration of the rolling–sliding movement when the anterior cruciate ligament is ruptured.

Practical Tip

### Tests for Ruptured Anterior Cruciate Ligament (Figs. 9.75–9.76)

*Lachman's test* (**Fig. 9.75**): This test screens for instability of the anterior cruciate ligament. In a position of mild knee flexion, the tibia can be displaced anteriorly (anterior drawer sign). (continued)

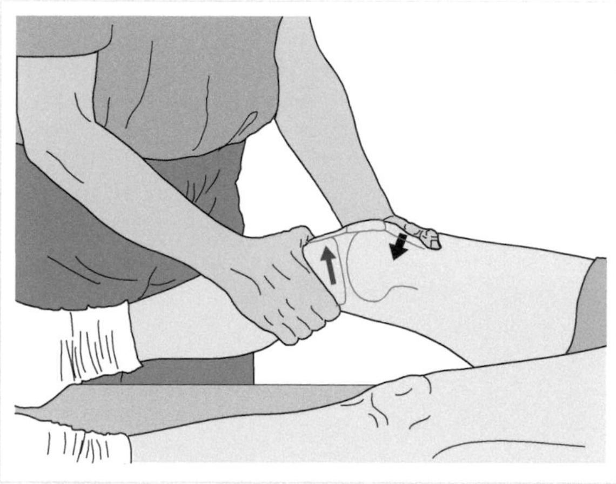

**Fig. 9.75** Lachman's test.

*Lateral pivot shift test* (**Fig. 9.76**): In this test, the mismatch between rolling and sliding in anterior cruciate ligament insufficiency becomes clear:

- In the neutral position, no displacement of the tibia is visible (**Fig. 9.76a**).
- With increasing flexion, the femur rolls increasingly posteriorly and the tibia stays in the anterior drawer position. The iliotibial tract runs anterior to the transverse flexion axis (**Fig. 9.76b**).
- At about 40° of flexion, the tract slips behind the flexion axis and pulls the tibia back to the femur with a jerk from its displaced position to the normal position **(Fig. 9.76c).**

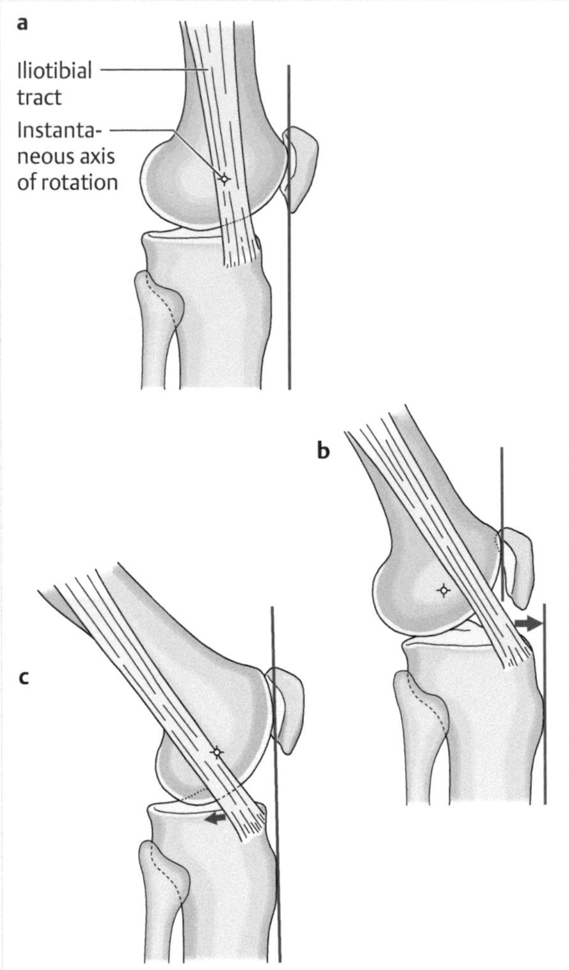


**Fig. 9.76** Testing for stability of the anterior cruciate ligament: lateral pivot shift. **(a)** Neutral position (0°). **(b)** 20° flexion. **(c)** 40° flexion.

Pathology

### Cruciate Ligament Surgery (Fig. 9.77)

The anterior cruciate ligament is often reconstructed using the middle third of the patellar tendon. The prerequisite for optimal functioning of the ligament in terms of joint stability and mobility is the calculation of the insertion points. It is best if parts of the ligament are still present, because the ligament's course must correspond to the anatomical conditions. Even a small change in the drill hole in the femoral area has significant influence on the state of tension of the anterior cruciate ligament.

### Notchplasty

Depending on the positioning of the drill hole, the roof of the intercondylar fossa (notch) may have to be chiseled off to prevent impingement of the graft on the roof. In general, very good resistance to tearing can be expected immediately after surgery. After 6 weeks, however, this is clearly reduced through remodeling, and only after a year does the anterior cruciate ligament reach 90 % of its normal load-bearing capacity.

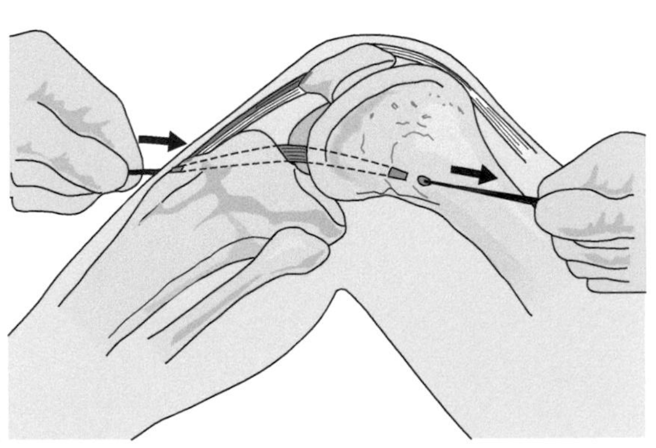

**Fig. 9.77** Cruciate ligament reconstruction with the central third of the patellar tendon.

## Posterior Cruciate Ligament (Figs. 9.78 and 9.79)

The posterior cruciate ligament arises from the inner surface of the medial femoral condyle. In the neutral position, its area of origin has a horizontal orientation. It runs obliquely in a distal-lateral-posterior direction, and inserts on the posterior intercondylar area of the tibia and the posterior tibial border. It crosses the anterior cruciate ligament at an angle of 90°. Its length is only about three-fifths of the length of the anterior cruciate ligament. It is the strongest ligament of the knee joint and is known as the "central stabilizer of the knee joint."

The posterior cruciate ligament consists of two main bands: a *posteromedial* bundle and an *anterolateral* bundle. The posteromedial bundle inserts the furthest posteriorly in the posterior intercondylar area of the tibia; the anterolateral bundle inserts laterally in the intercondylar area, near the lateral meniscus.

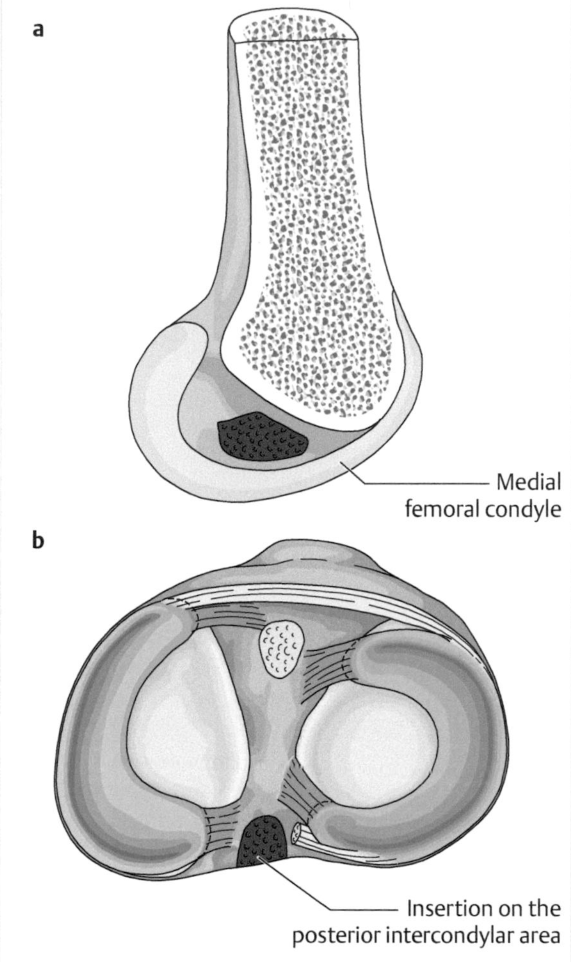


**Fig. 9.78** Insertions of the posterior cruciate ligament. **(a)** Medial femoral condyle (view from within). **(b)** Tibial plateau.

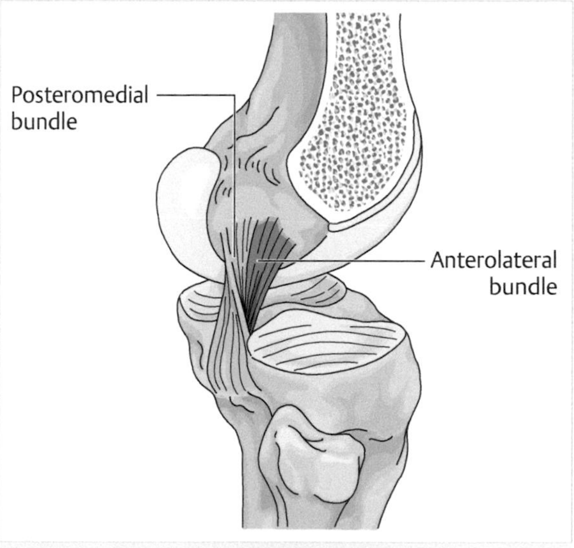


**Fig. 9.79** Course of the posterior cruciate ligament.

## Functions

*Limitation of Movement*

There are differences in tension between the two fiber bundles; the posteromedial bundle comes under tension primarily in extension. In flexion, the fibers twist around each other leading to an increase in tension (**Fig. 9.80**). Together with the anterior cruciate ligament, it limits internal rotation.

*Stabilization*

The posterior cruciate ligament prevents displacement of the tibial plateau posteriorly. Conversely, it prevents anterior slippage of the femur relative to the fixed tibia during the stance phase.

*Coordination*

This ligament helps to coordinate the rolling–sliding motion.

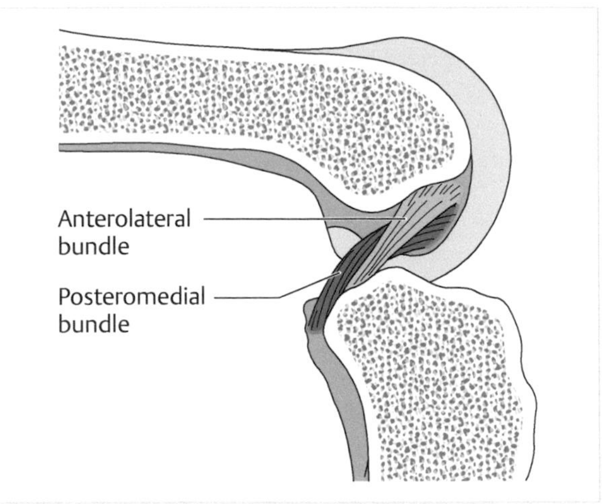


**Fig. 9.80** Posterior cruciate ligament in flexion.

### Practical Tip

**Rupture of the Posterior Cruciate Ligament**

A tear of the posterior cruciate ligament leads to a *posterior drawer*, which can be triggered, for example, by traction from the hamstring muscles while sitting. The tibia becomes decentered. The result is an early termination of extension by hard contact with the anterior horns of the meniscus and a limited displacement of the meniscus anteriorly.

The *gravity-sign test* (**Fig. 9.81**) provides information on the stability of the posterior cruciate ligament. To perform this test, the patient lies supine with both knees flexed at 90° and the feet placed on the mat. The result is a spontaneous posterior drawer sign, which can be seen by comparing the positions of the two tibial tuberosities, since the tibial plateau on the affected side sinks back slightly. If this is the case, there is reasonable suspicion of posterior cruciate ligament rupture.

**Consequences of an Injury to the Posterior Cruciate Ligament**

The anterior position of the femur can affect the anterior cruciate ligament, which becomes slack, because its attachment points on the femur and tibia end up closer together. The ligament now lacks the tension required to optimally perform the rolling-gliding motion when the knee is flexed from the extended position.

The constant tension on the fibular collateral ligament because of the anterior position of the femur can cause pain at the fibular head. A provocative test of the ligament can confirm this. The tension in the ligament may displace the ligament anteriorly.

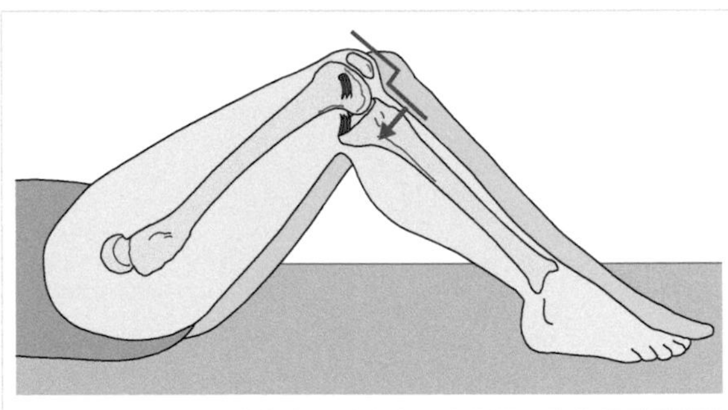

**Fig. 9.81** Stability test for the posterior cruciate ligament: gravity sign

## Course of the Cruciate Ligaments

### *Sagittal View (Fig. 9.82)*

Each cruciate ligament has a unique, variously inclined course:

- In extension, they are inclined only slightly from the horizontal. The anterior cruciate ligament forms an angle of inclination of approximately 40° with respect to the horizontal; the posterior cruciate ligament forms an angle of approximately 20°.
- In flexion, the orientation of the posterior cruciate ligament changes significantly. It becomes vertical, whereas the anterior cruciate ligament is only slightly more inclined than before.

### *Frontal View*

Viewed from anteriorly with the knee in extension and a midposition of rotation, the ligaments cross each other. This becomes even clearer with internal rotation of the tibia, because they tense and literally wrap around each other. In this way, the tibial and femoral articular surfaces also approach each other.

In external rotation, however, the ligaments are positioned parallel to each other.

### *Horizontal View (Fig. 9.83)*

In the horizontal view, the cruciate ligaments run parallel to each other.

The points of fixation of the cruciate ligaments on the tibia are located in the sagittal plane, whereas the femoral attachment points approximate the frontal plane.

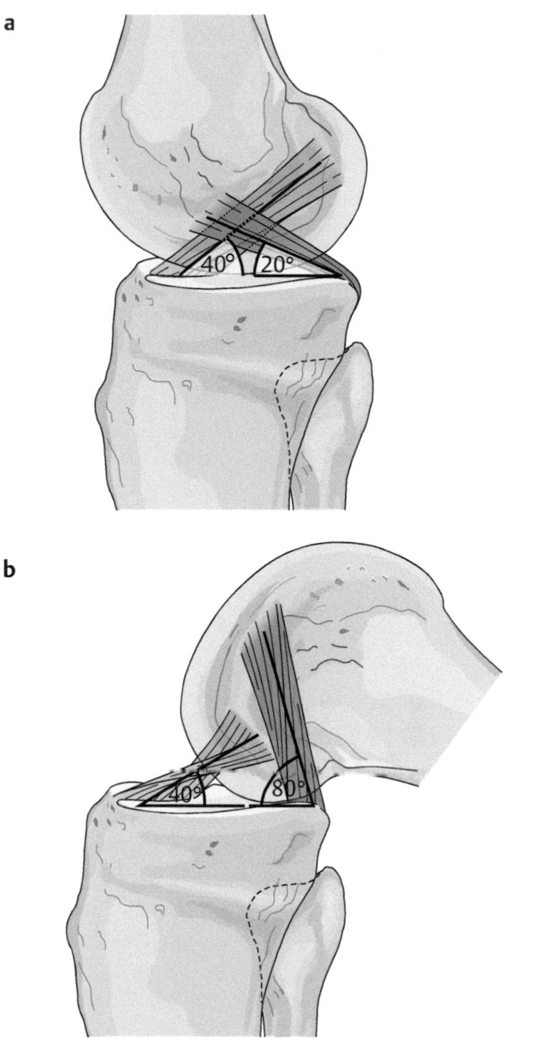


**Fig. 9.82** Course of the cruciate ligaments in the sagittal view. **(a)** In extension. **(b)** In flexion.

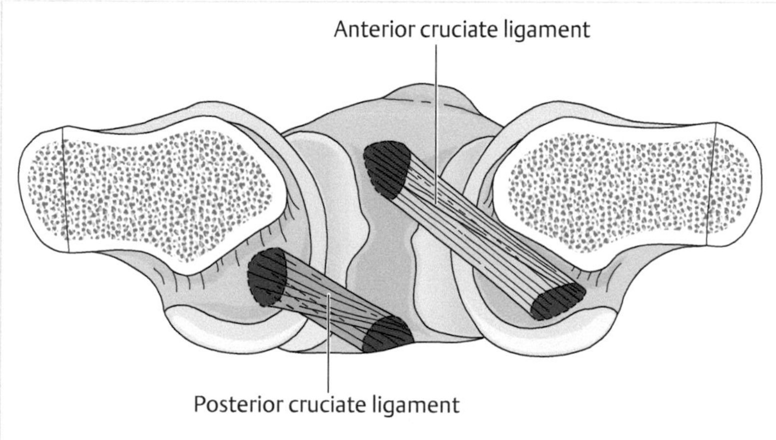


**Fig. 9.83** Course of the cruciate ligaments in the horizontal view (the distal femur is divided longitudinally and spread apart).

## 9.3.4 Anterior Functional Complex

### Patella (Fig. 9.84)

Many structures connect with the patella and thus determine its position:

- From superiorly, the rectus femoris muscle tracks to the base of the patella, with some fibers crossing over the patella. These fibers continue into the patellar ligament, the bulk of which establishes a connection between the tibial tuberosity and the apex of the patella.
- The vastus muscles approach the patella from superomedial and superolateral.
- From the lateral and medial borders, the transverse retinacula move into the epicondyles and the tibia. Laterally, fibers of the iliotibial tract can be found.
- As a second, deeper layer under the retinaculum, the patellomeniscal ligaments establish a connection between the patellar borders and the menisci.

The aggregate of forces of this bracing system determines the position of the patella. Only when the patella is centered can it carry out optimal movements.

**Functions** (**Fig. 9.85**). The patella has a stabilizing effect since it reduces the displacement of the femoral condyles during flexion, thus relieving the stress on the posterior cruciate ligament and the structures of the posterior capsular.

Because of its location, it improves the torque in the extensor mechanism by increasing the lever arm of the quadriceps muscle and thus its torque. This is especially apparent when calculating the change in the lever action that occurs after a patellectomy. Moreover, the patella protects the rectus tendon from excessive friction.

Because of the thick hyaline cartilage layer in combination with the lubricating function of the synovial fluid, the friction in the patellofemoral joint is substantially reduced.

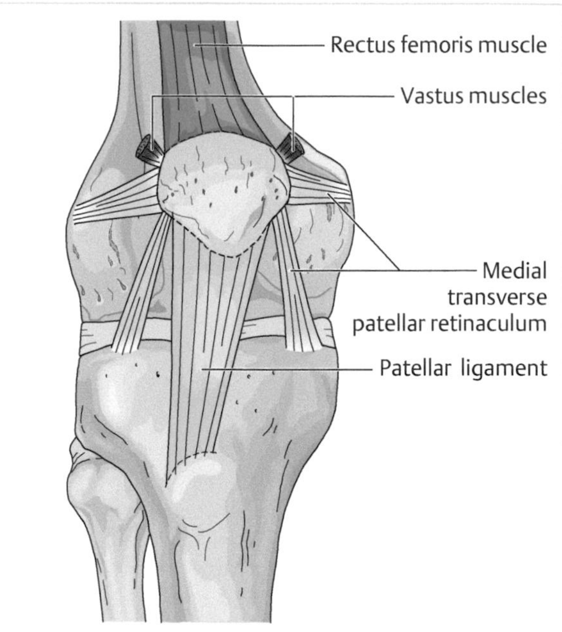


**Fig. 9.84** Patellar connections.

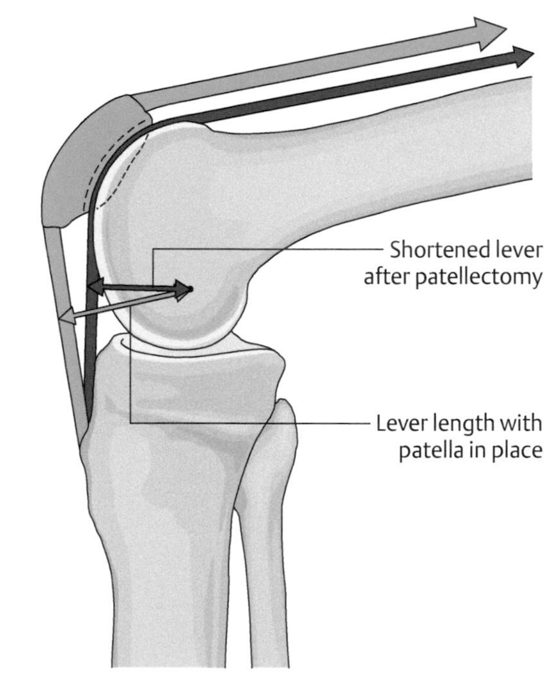


**Fig. 9.85** Changes of the lever arm of the quadriceps muscle after patellectomy.

## Patellar Ligament (Fig. 9.86)

This ligament tracks from the apex of the patella to the tibial tuberosity, a distinct protrusion of bone located about 3 to 4 fingerbreadths distal to the apex of the patella.

The ligament is approximately 5 mm thick, 3 cm wide proximally, and 2 cm wide distally. It tracks obliquely from proximal-medial to distal-lateral. The lateral part of the fiber tract sits about 2 cm deeper than the medial.

The deep infrapatellar bursa lies between the patellar ligament, the tibia, and Hoffa's fat pad (infrapatellar fat pad). Another bursa, the subcutaneous infrapatellar bursa, lies anteriorly, superficial to the ligament.

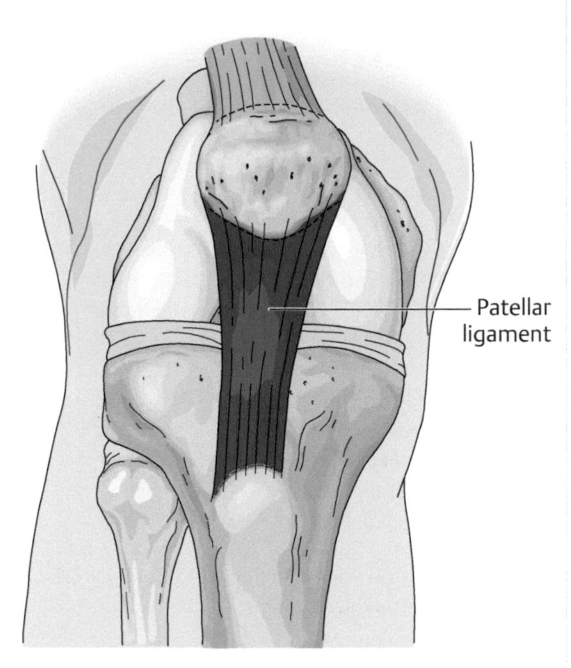


**Fig. 9.86** Patellar ligament.

### Pathology

**Osgood–Schlatter's Disease**

This aseptic necrosis of the bone builds up bony material in the area of the tibial tuberosity, which becomes considerably thicker.

It usually affects boys, who complain of stress-related pain, especially after stair-climbing or other similar stresses on the knee joint.

**Lateral Patellar Compression Syndrome**

In this syndrome, there is a lateral shift of the patella. The cause is usually a muscle imbalance, such as a high degree of tension in the iliotibial tract and atrophy of the vastus medialis muscle. The patients report pain when walking downhill and after prolonged sitting.

### Practical Tip

The treatment of lateral compression syndrome involves eliminating the muscular imbalance by, for example, stretching the lateral structures and rehabilitating the vastus medialis muscle. In addition, the patella can be brought medially using the McConnell's taping technique.

## Quadriceps Femoris Muscle (Figs. 9.87 and 9.88)

The quadriceps muscle, with its five parts (as follows), covers the entire anterior thigh.

### Rectus Femoris Muscle

Because of its site of insertion, this part of the quadriceps forms a connection between the pelvis and the knee joint. It lies in a groove on the vastus intermedius muscle; laterally, it is framed by the other vastus muscles.

Its terminal tendon is very flat and it is the longest of this complex. The largest part of the tendon tracks to the base of the patella, while some superficial fibers extend over the patella and continue on to the tibial tuberosity.

The anterior leaf of the suprapatellar bursa is adherent to the rectus tendon and shifts when the muscle relaxes or contracts.

The muscle has endurance performance to safeguard the leg as a postural support column, contains a predominance of slow-twitch fibers and tends toward "shortening."

### Vastus Intermedius Muscle

This part forms the deepest layer of the quadriceps complex. Its fiber components are connected to the deep layer of the suprapatellar bursa. The other parts track together with the tendon of the rectus to the base of the patella.

### Articular Muscle of the Knee

This muscle is fused with the deep layer of the suprapatellar bursa. Its fibers derive in part from the vastus intermedius muscle and are partly independent fibers with an origin on the anterior femur a few centimeters above the capsular fold (see **Fig. 9.61**).

### Vastus Lateralis Muscle

This is the largest of the quadriceps muscles. At its origin on the lateral lip of the linea aspera, it combines with fibers of the gluteus maximus muscle to form the *vastogluteal muscle sling*. In addition, fibers arise from the iliotibial tract, which covers the muscle laterally.

Its terminal tendon starts about four fingerbreadths superolateral to the base of the patella. Most of the fibers end on this border of the patella, but other fiber components continue into the lateral longitudinal patellar retinaculum. A third division of fibers tracks further medially and distally, crosses over the patella and the fibers of the vastus medialis muscle, and inserts onto the medial tibial condyle.

### Vastus Medialis Muscle

This is a muscle that functions with speed and strength, has a predominance of fast-twitch fibers and tends toward "slackening."

The muscle is formed primarily of muscle fibers that track steeply in a distal direction and insert at the superomedial patellar margin. Some fibers track into the patellar retinaculum, thereby forming a connection all the way to the medial tibial condyle. Some thinner fiber components track obliquely, partially over the patella, and laterally to the insertion site of the iliotibial tract.

The lowest transverse fiber bundles are called the *vastus medialis oblique muscle*. This muscle has no extensor function but pulls the patella medially, working against the laterally directed forces, and thus centers the patella within the femoral trochlear groove (patellar surface of the femur). Atrophy of the vastus medialis muscle reduces its ability to hold the patella in place, with the result that the vastus lateralis muscle overbalances it, leading to increased lateralization of the patella.

In addition, the vastus medialis muscle gives off some fibers to the joint capsule.

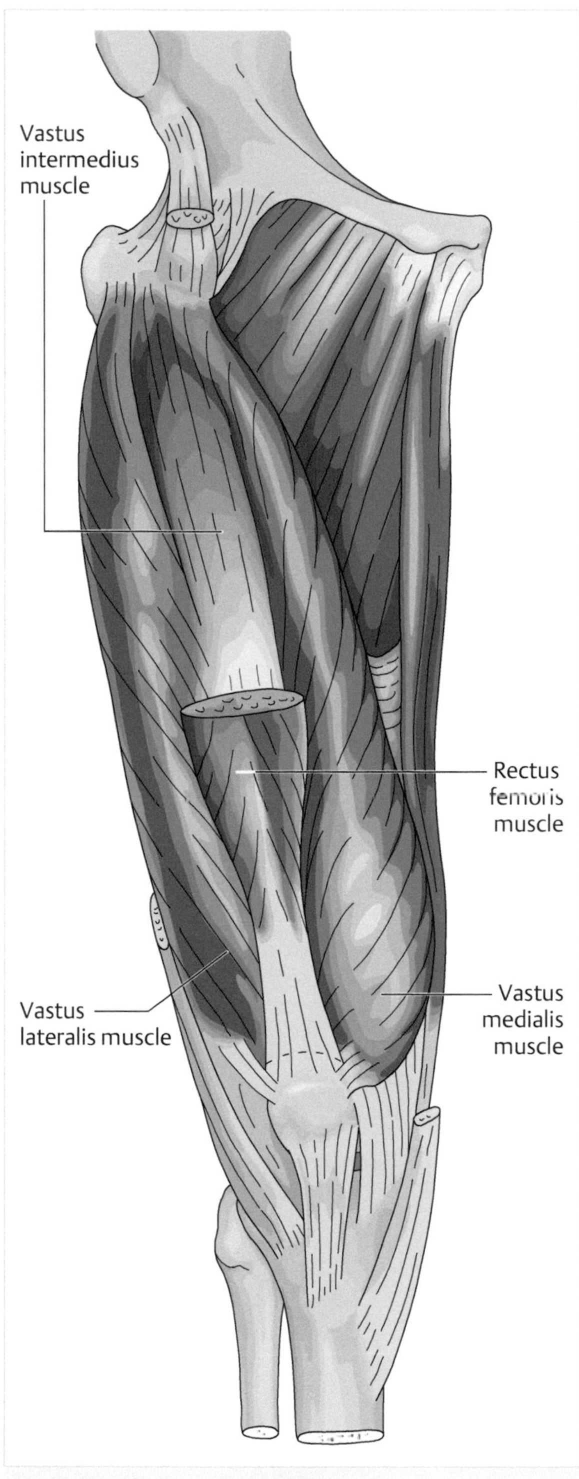


**Fig. 9.87** Quadriceps femoris muscle.

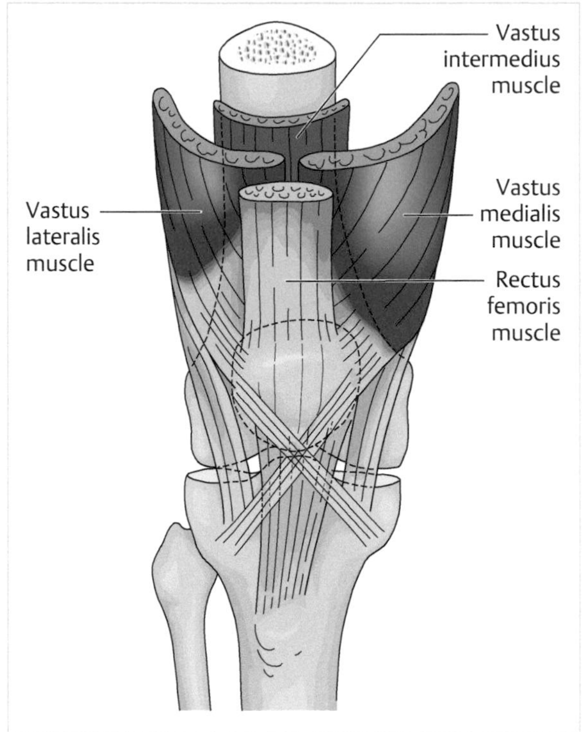


**Fig. 9.88** Connections of the vastus muscles.

**Function.** Functioning in an open-chain state, the quadriceps muscle moves the tibial lever anteriorly, which corresponds to knee extension. It also causes the tibia to glide anteriorly.

Functioning in a closed-chain state, it slows knee flexion by eccentric contraction, as in undertaking a knee bend from standing, and thus prevents kinking.

With increasing flexion of the knee while standing on one leg, the femoral condyles glide anteroinferiorly because of the plane of downhill force, since the tibial plateau slopes downward toward the front. The quadriceps muscle counteracts this thrust tendency; its resultant force pushes the femoral condyles in a posterior direction. In addition, the patella is pressed into its corresponding trochlear groove (patellar surface) of the femur. This compacting pressure is particularly high in the flexed position (**Fig. 9.89**).

*Innervation*: femoral nerve.

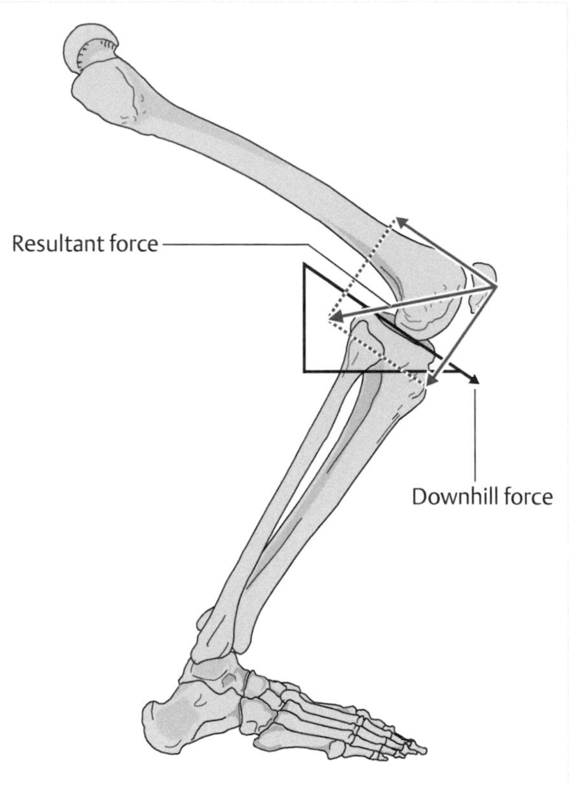


**Fig. 9.89** Effect of the quadriceps in flexion.

## Practical Tip

### Inspection

Atrophy of the quadriceps muscle is always seen in injuries that linger for some time, even after the discomfort has gone. It is a sign of disturbance of the proprioceptive feedback mechanism, and it protects the joint.

During the time the joint must be protected after an injury, it certainly makes sense to inhibit the quadriceps muscle, because its activity places stress on the joint. For example, at approximately 40° of flexion, it pulls the tibia anteriorly. This position should be avoided, especially after lesions of the anterior cruciate ligament.

### Training the Quadriceps

A coordinated, closed kinetic chain exercise program has a major influence on the proprioceptors, and thus on position sense, motion sense, and sense of force.

Movement is limited, for example, to protect a graft or postoperative meniscus. The following closed-chain exercises (fixed end distal) may be performed, among others: knee bends to 30° of flexion with the upper body tilted in various ways, while using two sets of scales to assess the weight distribution; and stabilization exercises on two small rocker balance boards, a wobble board, or a balance platform.

The gains made using closed-chain exercises are those typical of walking, and therefore adapted to the stresses of everyday life.

## Q Angle of the Knee (Fig. 9.90)

This angle is formed between the inferior extension of a straight line connecting the anterior inferior iliac spine to the middle of the patella, and the straight line from the patella to the tibial tuberosity. In men, the angle is approximately 10°; in women, it is 15° ± 5°.

Because of this angle, the patella has a tendency to dislocate laterally. The prominent lateral cheek of the patellar surface of the femur and the direction of pull of the vastus medialis oblique muscle counteract this tendency.

### Pathology

In genu valgum, the Q angle is larger, because the tibial tuberosity is located further laterally. As a result of this change, the laterally directed force components are larger, and the demands on the lateral condylar cheek increase.

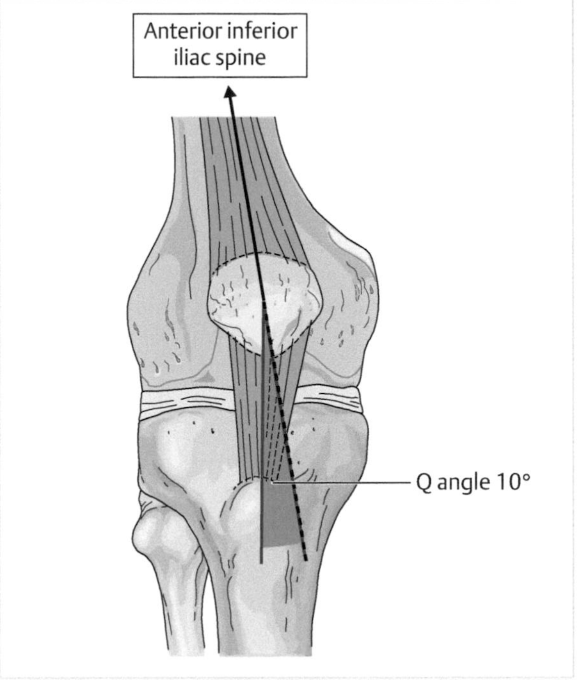


**Fig. 9.90** Q angle.

## Fat Pad and Synovial Folds

### Infrapatellar Fat Pad (Fig. 9.91)

The space between the anterior intercondylar area and the inside of the patellar ligament is occupied by a large fat pad. This fat pad, also called Hoffa's fat pad, has the shape of a four-sided pyramid with its base on the inner side of the patellar ligament. The side of the fat pad facing the joint has a synovial coating.

The fat pad consists of balls of fat with loose strands of connective tissue. It is well perfused, and its vessels, together with those of the retinaculum, provide for perfusion of the patellar ligament and the anterior cruciate ligament. Therefore, it plays a role in the revascularization of an autologous graft after ligament reconstruction. It has proprioceptors and is thus integrated into the controlling mechanism of the knee joint. It also serves to equalize the pressure within the knee.

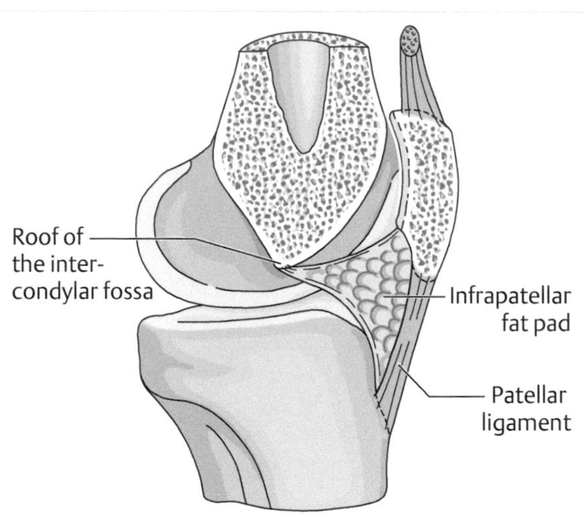


**Fig. 9.91** Infrapatellar fat pad.

**Pathology**

**Hoffa's Disease**

Enlargement of the fat pad is associated with various knee disorders such as meniscal injury or inflammation. The swelling usually recedes when the underlying disease process has healed.

When the knee is immobilized, it is to be expected that the fat pad will proliferate. It can fibrose and scar, thus losing its mobility and plasticity. Because of the important functions of the fat pad, total removal is very unfavorable for the joint. Thus, partial resection is preferable.

**Practical Tip**

**Findings in Hypertrophy of Hoffa's Fat Pad**

Patients describe pain that is resistant to therapy, pain with hyperextension, and occurrences of entrapment. Swelling alongside the patellar ligament is visible in knee flexion and can be tender to palpation.

## Synovial Folds (Fig. 9.92)

These folds are rudiments of fetal septa that divided the knee joint. They are septa in the synovium surrounding the fat body.

### *Suprapatellar Synovial Fold*

This is a synovial fold that follows a crescent-shaped course from medial to lateral along the upper border of the patella. It can form a septum that separates the suprapatellar bursa from the rest of the joint space. In this case, the joint capsule ends approximately 2 cm above the base of the patella.

### *Mediopatellar Synovial Fold*

This is a vertically running synovial fold on the medial side of the patella that has a meniscoid function for the patellofemoral joint and merges into the synovial lining of the infrapatellar fat pad.

### *Infrapatellar Synovial Fold*

Strengthening the surface of the fat pad, this fibrous strand tracks from the apex of the patella into the depth of the intercondylar fossa, where it is fixed. Anteriorly, it is adherent to the synovial membrane of the cruciate ligaments.

### *Alar Folds*

These have their origin on the lateral surfaces of the patella and form the border of the fat body laterally.

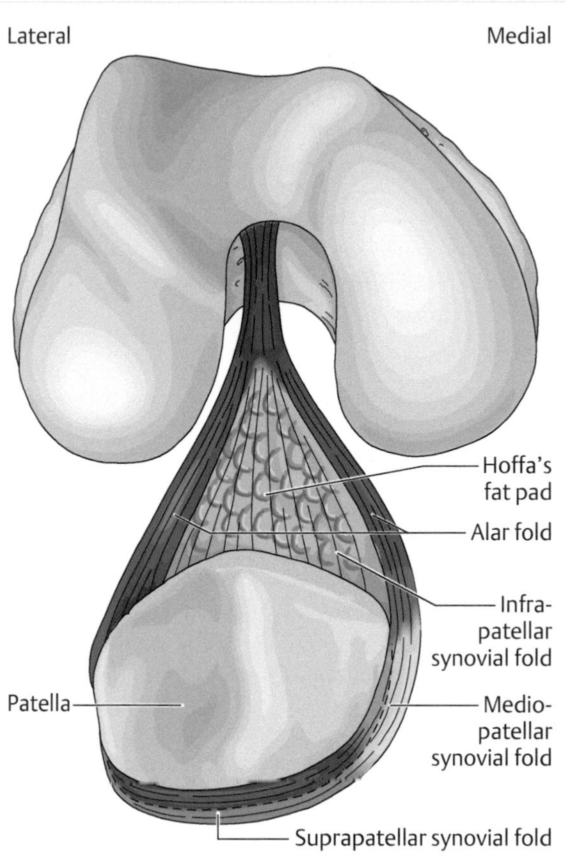


**Fig. 9.92** Synovial folds.

**Pathology**

**Plica Syndrome**

Plica syndrome, or *medial shelf syndrome*, is hypertrophy of the synovial folds. It occurs more frequently in competitive swimmers, which is why it is also known as "breaststroker's knee." Those affected claim that kicking causes the symptoms, especially in the medial knee complex, leading to thickening and scarring of the structures. During knee flexion, the mediopatellar synovial fold can tighten like a bowstring and become jammed under the medial facet of the patella. This results in pressure damage to the cartilage. Patients complain of a painful snapping with movement. Treatment consists of arthroscopic transection of the synovial fold or its resection.

## 9.3.5 Medial Functional Complex

### Tibial Collateral Ligament (Fig. 9.93)

The ligament has fibers of varying lengths extending in different directions.

A longitudinal fiber bundle arises from the medial epicondyle and tracks obliquely in a distal, anterior direction to the medial surface of the tibia. It is 9 to 11 cm long and is covered by the superficial pes anserinus at its insertion site on the tibia. Anteriorly, the fibers join with the longitudinal retinaculum.

Mixed among the long fibers are short parts of the ligament, which run from the epicondyle to the medial meniscus and from the meniscus to the tibia. Accordingly, these are referred to as the *meniscofemoral and meniscotibial parts* of the ligament.

In addition, there are bands of fibers that are part of the collateral ligament that track from the posterior part of the femoral epicondyle, near the adductor tubercle, obliquely in a distal and posterior direction to the posterior horn of the medial meniscus and to the capsule. From inferiorly, fibers running obliquely from the tibia in a proximal and superior direction also form a connection to the meniscus and to the capsule. These parts of the ligament are known as the *posterior tibial collateral ligament*. They establish a connection to the tendon of the semimembranosus muscle and are involved in the oblique popliteal ligament.

At the area of origin, fibers of the adductor magnus muscle track into the collateral ligament.

**Function.** The ligament is an important stabilizer and counteracts valgus and external rotational stresses. In extension, all parts of the ligament are taut. In flexion, the anterior, long fibers relax, while the posterior tibial collateral ligament continues to be tensed. This is due to its connections to the meniscus, which it displaces posteriorly, and to the tendon of the semimembranosus muscle, which pulls the meniscus during flexion.

The meniscofemoral and meniscotibial portions relax only during flexion. However, with increasing flexion, they come under tension, since the ligament's origin moves further from its insertion, and the meniscus is displaced posteriorly.

In extension, its stabilizing function is supported by the pes anserine group and the semimembranosus muscle.

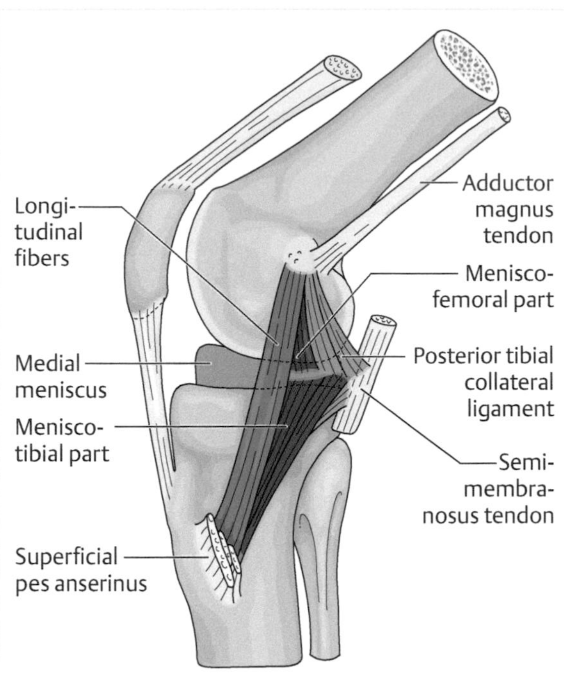


**Fig. 9.93** Tibial collateral ligament.

**Practical Tip**

**Testing the Stability of the Ligament**

When applying a valgus stress to the knee in extension, there should be no medial gapping of the joint.

**Testing the Ligament when Extension is Limited**

When applying a valgus stress with the knee flexed at approximately 20° and with slight external rotation, elastic gapping should be present. If this is not the case, the cause of the limited extension may lie in reduced elasticity of the ligament.

## Medial Patellar Retinaculum (Fig. 9.94)

- One can distinguish a superficial fibrous layer, a longitudinally extending layer, and a deeper, transverse layer:
  - The *medial longitudinal patellar retinaculum* is the distal extension of the vastus medialis aponeurosis. The fibers originate on the medial tibial condyle and track in part under the pes anserinus. They reinforce the anterior capsule between the patellar ligament and the collateral ligament.
  - The *medial transverse patellar retinaculum* divides into the *medial patellofemoral ligament*, which extends to the medial epicondyle, and the *medial patellotibial ligament*, which tracks to the anterior surface of the medial tibial condyle and gives off fibers to the anterior horn of the medial meniscus.
- *Function:* It is located in front of the flexion–extension axis and therefore acts as an anterior stabilizer, but its stabilizing force is not very pronounced.

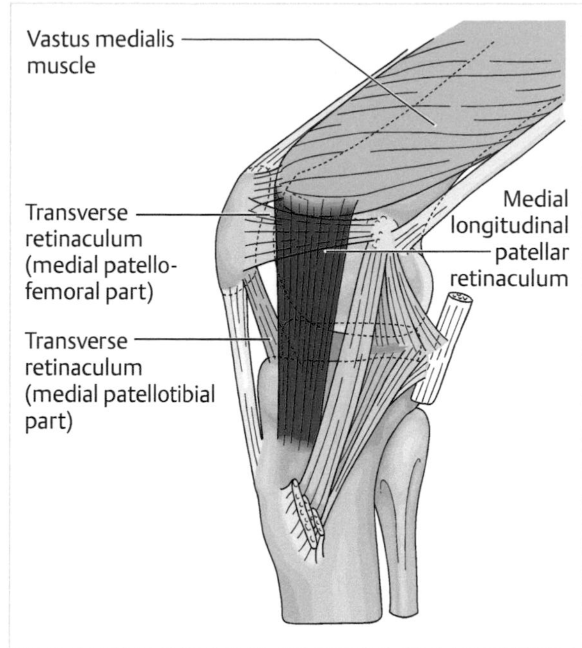


**Fig. 9.94** Medial patellar retinaculum.

## Pes Anserinus (Fig. 9.95)

### Sartorius Muscle

- At the insertion site, this forms the superficial part of the pes anserine group.
- The *subtendinous bursa of the sartorius muscle* lies between its insertion and that of the other tendons.

*Innervation:* femoral nerve.

### Gracilis Muscle

- Its tendon lies between the sartorius and semitendinosus muscles.
- Its muscle–tendon junction lies at the level of the lower third of thigh.
- *Innervation*: obturator nerve.

### Semitendinosus Muscle

- This runs within a groove formed in the semimembranosus muscle.
- Its muscle–tendon junction is at the level of the mid-thigh.
- At the insertion site, it forms the lowest part of the pes anserinus.
- *Innervation*: tibial nerve.

The anserine bursa lies between the pes anserinus and the tibial collateral ligament. Some fibers of the pes anserinus radiate into the deep fascia of the leg.

**Functions of the pes anserinus (Fig. 9.96):**

- Knee flexion/internal rotation of the tibia.
- Stabilization: In the neutral position, the tendons lie directly over the collateral ligament, and they can reinforce the ligament in counteracting valgus stress. In flexion, they change their course and move to a position almost at right angles to the tibia. Thus, they move the medial tibia posteriorly when the fixed end is on the pelvis. In this way, they are synergists of the anterior cruciate ligament. They also stabilize external rotation of the tibia.

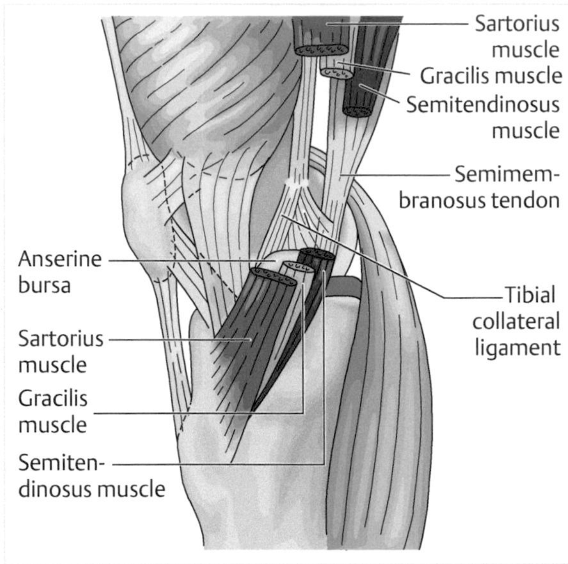


**Fig. 9.95** Superficial pes anserinus.

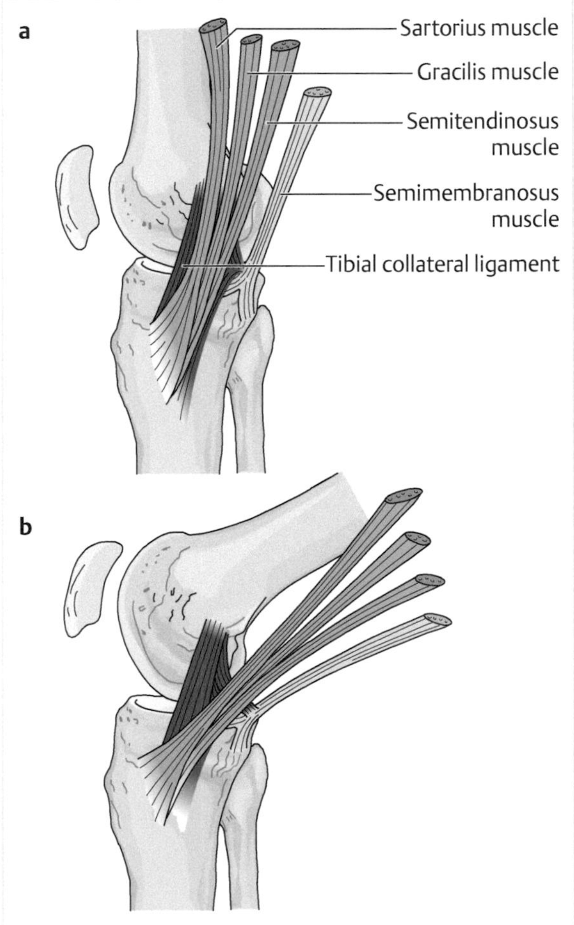


**Fig. 9.96** Course of the tendons of the pes anserinus. **(a)** In extension. **(b)** In flexion.

## Semimembranosus Muscle (Fig. 9.97)

- The insertion divides into five bands:
  1. Fibers running to the posterior capsule, to the posterior horn of the medial meniscus, and to the medial capsular ligament.
  2. Fibers with a direct insertion on the medial border of the tibia.
  3. Fibers orientated parallel to the long fibers of the collateral ligament that track anteroinferiorly to the tibia.
  4. Fibers that radiate into the aponeurosis of the popliteus muscle.
  5. Fibers tracking to a lateral insertion, which participate in the formation of the oblique popliteal ligament.
- *Functions:* Its main function is stabilization:
  - With the knee extended, the largest part of the tendon runs parallel to the collateral ligament and the pes anserinus group. Thus, it is a stabilizing muscle of the posteromedial corner.
  - Through its radiation into the collateral ligament and the medial meniscus, it spans the posteromedial portion of the joint in various flexed positions, even when the collateral ligament is relaxed.
  - In flexion, it is positioned at right angles to the tibia and prevents extreme external rotation.
  - It is a synergist to the anterior cruciate ligament in holding the tibia posterior.
- Movements: flexion/internal rotation.
- *Innervation:* tibial nerve.

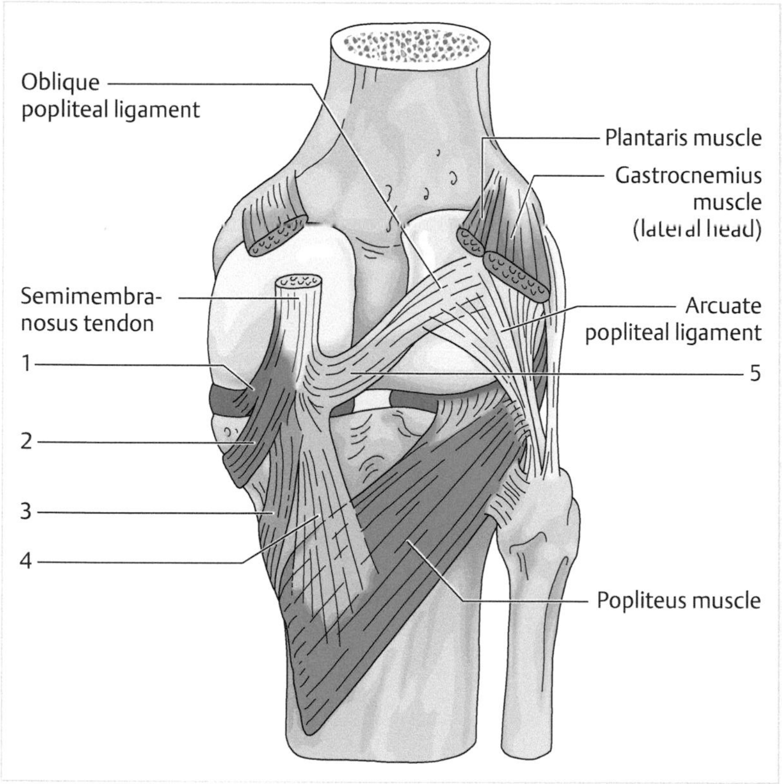


**Fig. 9.97** Insertions of the semimembranosus muscle.

## 9.3.6 Lateral Functional Complex

### Fibular Collateral Ligament (Fig. 9.98)

This ligament tracks from the lateral femoral epicondyle distally and posteriorly to the fibular head. A gap of approximately 1 cm, which contains connective tissue, blood vessels, the tendon of the popliteus muscle, and a small bursa, lies between the ligament and the capsule.

The posterior fiber components connect to the arcuate popliteal ligament and are referred to as the short fibular collateral ligament.

**Function.** Together with the iliotibial tract, the popliteus tendon, part of the biceps tendon, and the arcuate popliteal ligament, it prevents varus instability.

It is tensed during knee extension. From about 20° of flexion, it relaxes, and the dynamic stabilizers become increasingly more important.

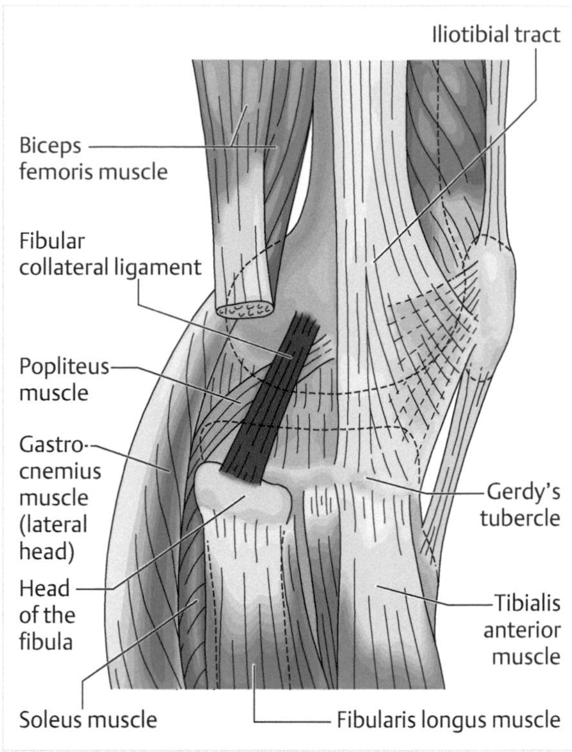


**Fig. 9.98** Fibular collateral ligament.

### Course of the Collateral Ligaments in Terms of Their Rotational Stabilization (Fig. 9.99)

In the neutral position, the longitudinal fibers of the tibial collateral ligament track inferiorly and anteriorly, while those of the fibular collateral ligament track inferiorly and somewhat posteriorly, so that they cross each other when viewed from the side.

During external rotation of the tibia, the tibial insertions move further away from those on the femur, and the ligaments become tensed. That means that the collateral ligaments provide rotational stability when the knee is in a position in which the cruciate ligaments are relaxed.

During internal rotation, the courses of the ligaments are almost parallel. They are relaxed, and the stabilization is provided by the cruciate ligaments.

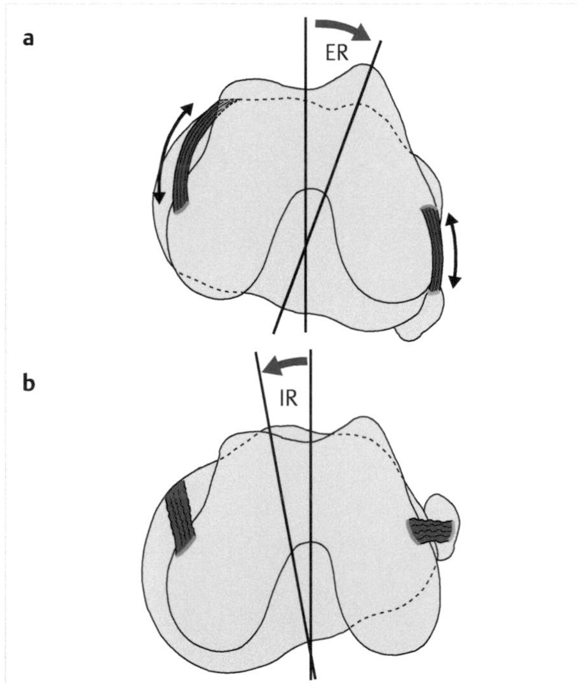


**Fig. 9.99** Course of the collateral ligaments in the horizontal view. **(a)** External rotation. **(b)** Internal rotation.

## Lateral Patellar Retinaculum (Fig. 9.100)

- This consists of a superficial fibrous layer and a deep fibrous layer:
  - The *lateral longitudinal retinaculum* is composed of fibers of the vastus lateralis muscle and the iliotibial tract. The insertion is located on the anterior part of the lateral tibial condyle, adjacent to Gerdy's tubercle.
  - The *lateral transverse retinaculum* consists of the *lateral patellofemoral ligament*, which runs from the lateral patella to the epicondyle, and the *lateral patellotibial ligament*. This extends inferolaterally to the anterior tibial condyle and inserts directly under and adjacent to the longitudinal fibers. Some fibers pass to the anterior horn of the lateral meniscus.
- *Function:* It helps with anterolateral stabilization of the knee joint.

**Pathology**

**Lateralization of the Patella**

The laterally lying structures tend toward increased tension, and, through their connections to the patella, pull it laterally. This malalignment presses the patella against the lateral condylar cheek, increasing the retropatellar pressure. Over time, this causes cartilage damage. If physical therapy cannot correct this imbalance, the lateral area can be relieved surgically by procedures such as division of the longitudinal retinaculum (lateral release).

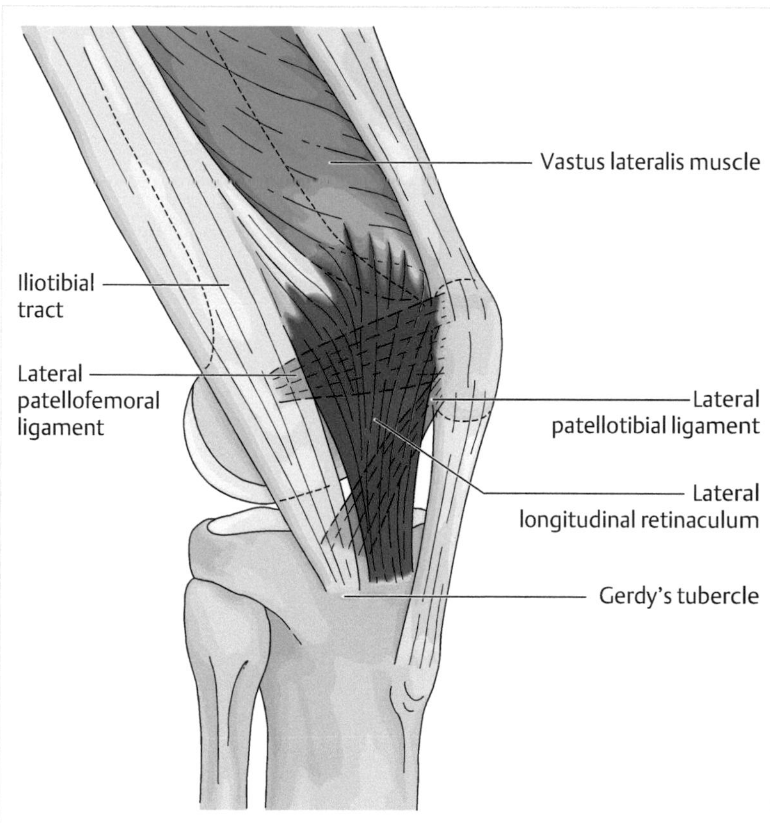


**Fig. 9.100** Lateral patellar retinaculum.

## Iliotibial Tract (Fig. 9.101)

This tract gives off fibers to the lateral capsule. Anteriorly, it forms a broad connection with the vastus lateralis aponeurosis and the lateral retinaculum. Posteriorly, it joins with the biceps femoris muscle.

Most of the fibers track to *Gerdy's tubercle* (tubercle of the iliotibial tract). From there, a few fibers run further into the aponeurosis of tibialis anterior. At the level of the base of the patella, other fibers track into the longitudinal retinaculum and to the lateral patellar margin.

**Function.** The iliotibial tract is an important stabilizer in the anterolateral area. In a knee position of 0–40°, it lies anterior to the flexion–extension axis and impedes flexion. With further flexion, it moves behind the axis and prevents anterior displacement of the tibia. It also prevents the lateral tibial plateau from shifting anteriorly. In this way, it stabilizes internal rotation.

## Biceps Femoris Muscle (Fig. 9.101)

- Its insertion site is divided into the following three parts:
  - Its superficial part has its primary insertion area on the head of the fibula.
  - The middle layer runs anteriorly directly over the collateral ligament to the lateral condyle of the tibia.
  - The deep layer consists of short fibers that track posteromedially from the collateral ligament to the tibia.
- The common fibular nerve runs right at the medial edge of the muscle. See Chapter 9.4, Neural Structures.
- *Functions:*
  - Working synergistically with the anterior cruciate ligament, it stabilizes the posterolateral area of the knee and prevents anterior displacement of the tibia.
  - It inhibits internal rotation.
  - Dynamically, it causes knee flexion and external rotation of the knee.
- *Innervation*: tibial portion of the sciatic nerve.

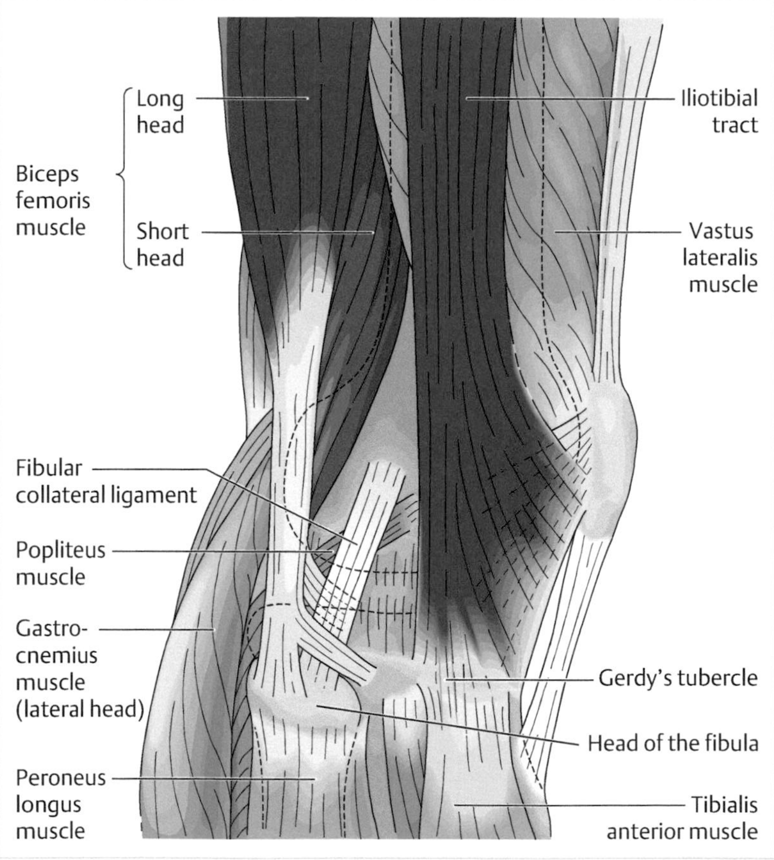


**Fig. 9.101** Course of the iliotibial tract and the biceps femoris muscle.

## 9.3.7 Posterior Functional Complex

### Oblique Popliteal Ligament (Fig. 9.102)

This ligament tracks from the medial corner of the insertion of the semimembranosus muscle to the inner side of the lateral femoral condyle. A few fibers run in an obliquely superior direction to just below the origin of the gastrocnemius muscle.

The ligament has numerous openings for vessels and nerves to pass through. It is an important reinforcement of the posterior capsule, with which it merges in many places. It is taut in extension and relaxed in flexion.

### Arcuate Popliteal Ligament (Fig. 9.102)

This spreads out into two sections in the posterolateral area of the joint, extends from the head of the fibula over the tendon of the popliteus muscle to the posterolateral capsule, and intertwines with the oblique popliteal ligament.

If a fabella (sesamoid bone) is present, located in the origin area of the lateral head of the gastrocnemius muscle in the condylar capsule, then a narrow band, the fabellofibular ligament, splits off from the arcuate popliteal ligament to the sesamoid bone and the capsular part.

The ligament stabilizes the posterolateral knee area and protects it, primarily from hyperextension.

**Pathology**

**Genu Recurvatum**

Hyperextension of the knee puts the posterior capsule–ligament apparatus under tensile stress. In contrast, the anterior horns of the menisci are subject to compressive force. The cause of this may lie in a general weakness of the ligaments.

However, if the joint is hyperextensible on only one side, further tests for stability of the posterior cruciate ligament should be performed because its rupture could be responsible for the genu recurvatum.

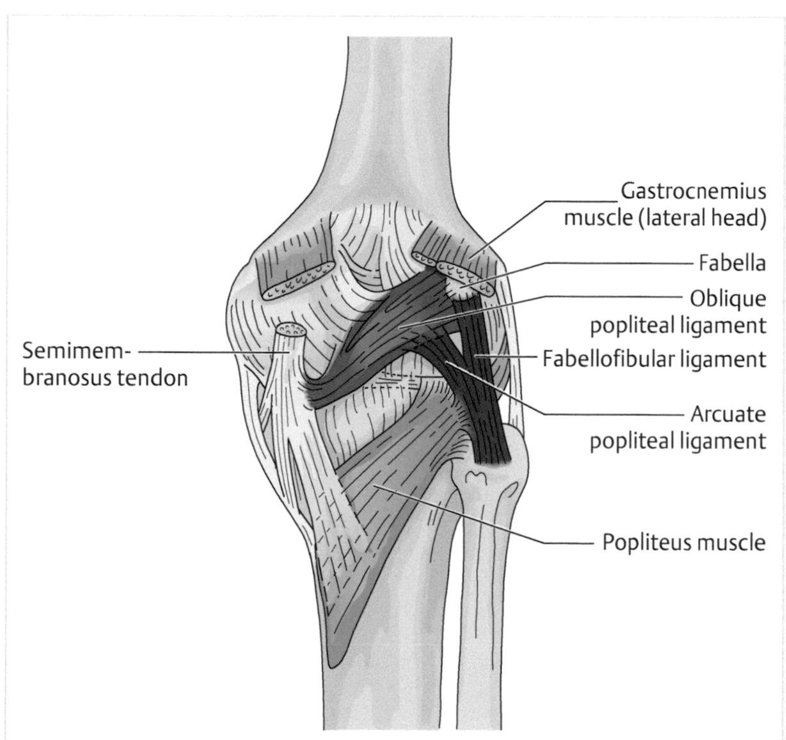


**Fig. 9.102** Oblique and arcuate popliteal ligaments.

## Popliteus Muscle (Figs. 9.103 and 9.104)

- *Popliteal tendon:*
  - Origin: inferior and anterior to the insertion of the fibular collateral ligament on the femoral epicondyle.
  - Connection to the joint capsule: the origin is located in part within the capsule.
  - Course: within a groove around the lateral condyle, crossing under the fibular collateral ligament. A small bursa is located between the ligament and the tendon.
  - It tracks in an inferoposterior direction over the edge of the tibia.
  - A small bursa, the subpopliteal recess, lies between the tendon and the tibial condyle, and communicates with the joint.
- *Popliteomeniscal fibers:*
  - Form a connection from the popliteal aponeurosis to the lateral meniscus.
  - The fascicle is 2 to 2.5 cm wide.
  - The main part extends to the joint capsule and the posterior horn.
  - A small offshoot runs anterior to the tendon of the popliteus muscle to the lateral base of the meniscus.
  - The connection between the joint capsule and the subpopliteal recess occurs between these two parts.
- *Popliteofibular fibers:*
  - 2 cm long and wide.
  - It is divided into two parts: one part inserts on the posteromedial fibular head and at this point lies below the arcuate popliteal ligament.
  - The larger part runs anteriorly, inserts medially on the fibular head, and has a few fibers that track to the tibia.
- Just distal to the joint, the popliteus muscle has a connection to the arcuate popliteal ligament.
- The muscle runs obliquely distally and medially in the depths of the popliteal fossa and is covered by the gastrocnemius muscle.
- *Functions:*
  - The popliteus muscle is the most important posterolateral stabilizer of the knee joint, as it prevents the femur from sliding forward during flexion, and it prevents varus joint gapping.
  - It limits the external rotation of the tibia. With the thigh fixed and the lower leg free, it internally rotates the tibia. When the tibia is fixed by anchoring the foot on the ground, it rotates the femur externally.
  - Prevents hyperextension.
- *Innervation:* tibial nerve.

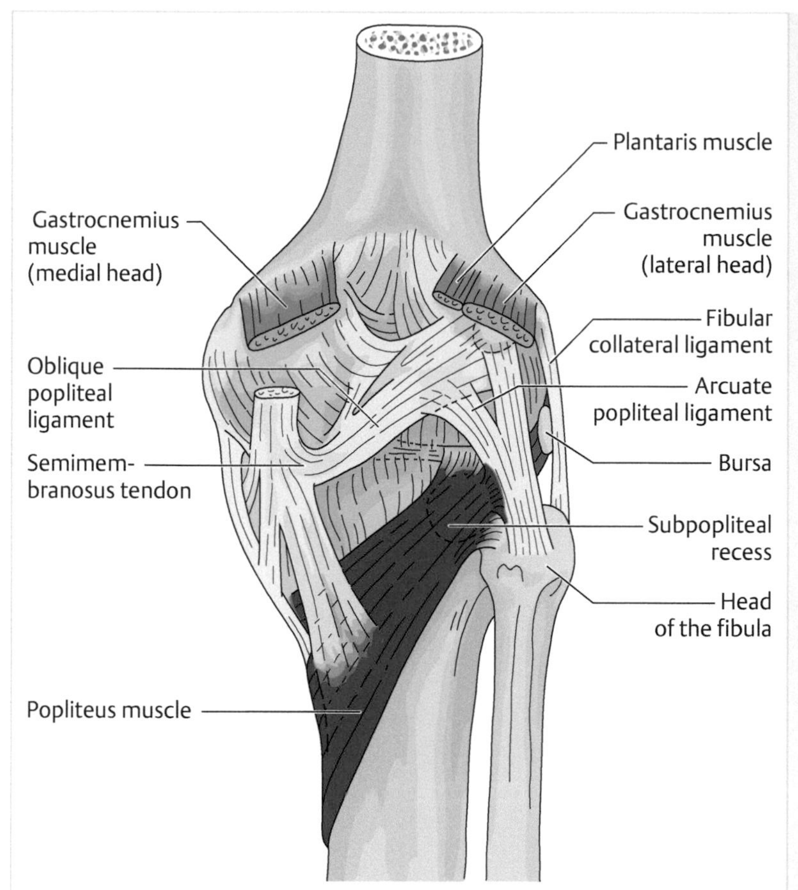


**Fig. 9.103** Popliteus muscle.

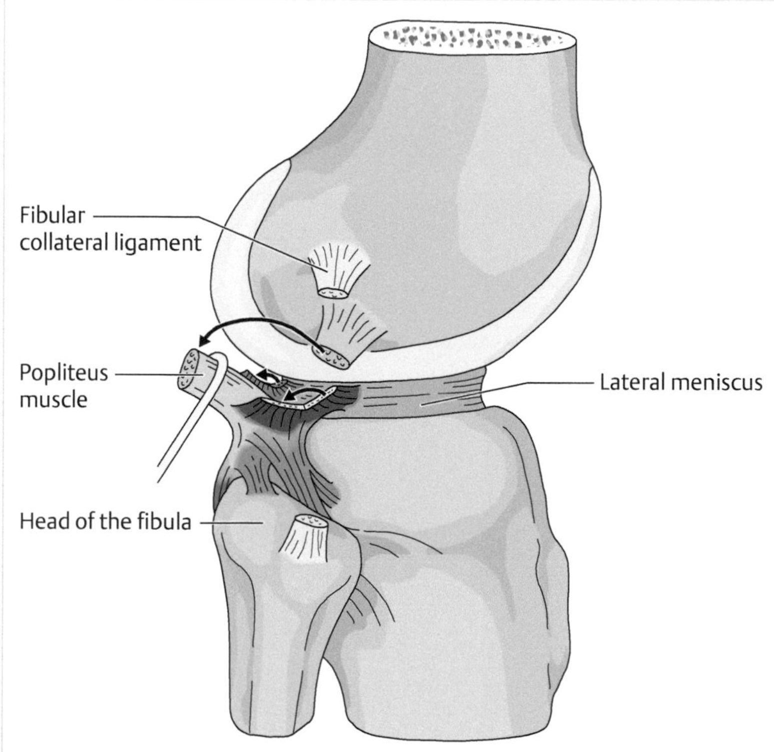


**Fig. 9.104** Popliteus muscle connections in the posterolateral corner (tendons divided and folded back—indicated by the black arrows).

## Gastrocnemius Muscle (Fig. 9.105)

- This consists of two heads: the lateral head and the medial head.
- At its origin, it adheres to the capsule proximal to the posterior end of the femoral condyles.
- Along with the soleus and plantaris muscles, the two heads of gastrocnemius unite with the triceps surae muscle and end at the calcaneus as the Achilles tendon.
- The muscle–tendon junction is located approximately in the middle of the lower leg, with the medial head somewhat deeper than the lateral head.
- *Functions:*
  - Stabilization: tenses the posterior capsule and is therefore an important stabilizer of the back of the knee. Together with the popliteus muscle, it prevents hyperextension.
  - Knee joint: flexion.
  - Upper ankle joint: plantarflexion; in the standing position, with the fixed end at the forefoot, it can raise the heel with help from the soleus muscle.
- This is the reference muscle for S1 spinal cord segment.
- *Innervation:* tibial nerve.

### Fabella

This is a sesamoid bone, just beneath the tendon of origin of the lateral head of the gastrocnemius muscle, that is found in one-fifth of all knee joints, especially in women with hyperextended knees. The function of the gastrocnemius muscle as a stabilizer of extension is disturbed by its unfavorable lever arm. The fabella improves the lever arm.

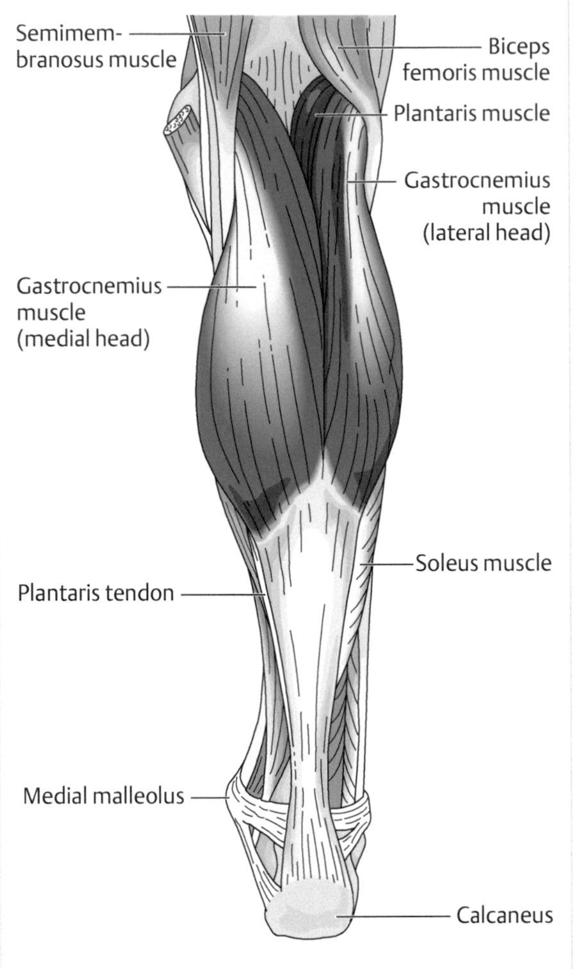


**Fig. 9.105** Gastrocnemius muscle.

## Plantaris Muscle (Fig. 9.105)

- This has a short, narrow muscle belly, which transitions into its long terminal tendon while still within the popliteal fossa.
- *Functions:*
  - Flexion.
  - Prevents the vessels from being pinched or kinked too much during flexion.
- *Innervation:* tibial nerve.

## 9.3.8 Vascular Supply

### Popliteal Artery (Figs. 9.106 and 9.107)

- The popliteal artery is the continuation of the femoral artery below the adductor hiatus.
- In its course through the popliteal fossa, it gives off the following five major branches for the knee joint:
  - *Superior and inferior medial genicular arteries.*
  - *Superior and inferior lateral genicular arteries.*
  - *Middle genicular artery.*
- The medial and lateral genicular arteries form the genicular and patellar anastomoses to supply the patellar ligament and the patella.
- The middle genicular artery divides into anterior and posterior branches, which enter into the interior of the joint and supply the anterior and posterior horns, as well as the insertions of the menisci and the areas of insertion of the cruciate ligaments on the tibial plateau.

All the vessels of the knee joint are connected by numerous anastomoses. These form vascular networks that guarantee adequate perfusion of the capsule–ligament structures.

On the other hand, in spite of numerous small anastomoses, there are many arterial branches that are functionally end-arteries. That means a reduced blood supply, and therefore poor chances of recovery. For example, the middle genicular artery, an end-artery, supplies the anterior cruciate ligament, making it difficult to repair a lesion with a primary reconstruction of the ligament.

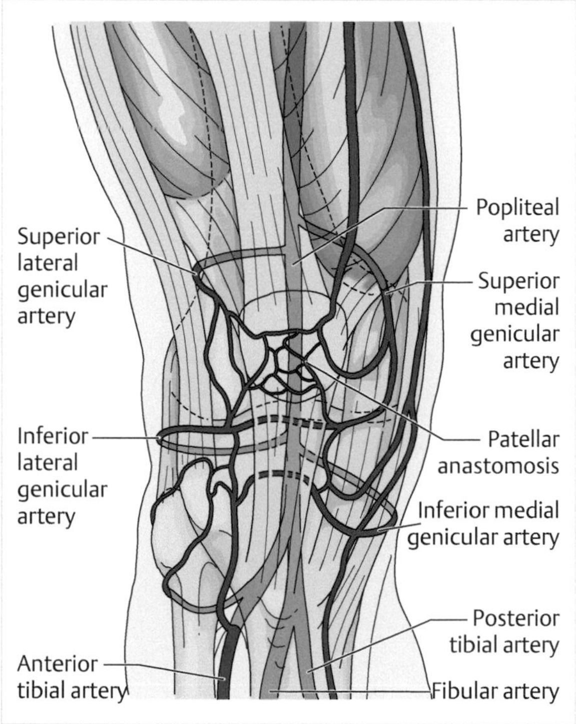


**Fig. 9.106** Vascular supply to the knee region (anterior view).

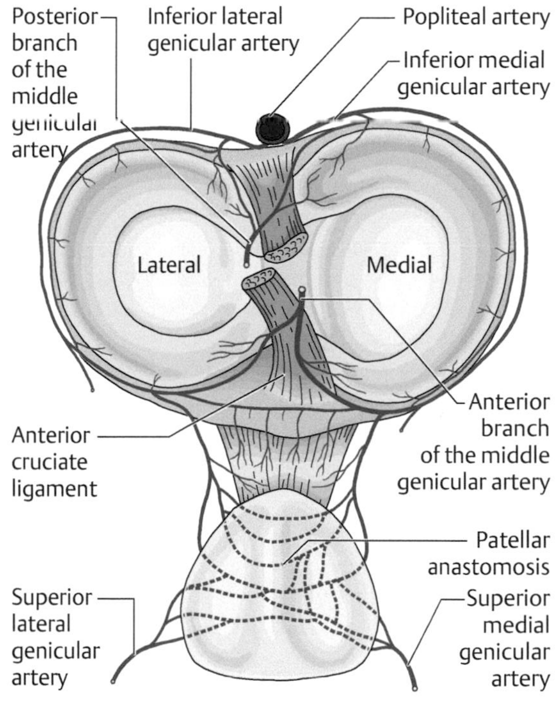


**Fig. 9.107** Vascular supply of the knee region (horizontal view; patella folded down).

## Branching of the Popliteal Artery in the Popliteal Fossa (Fig. 9.108)

- Course: in the depths of the popliteal fossa over the capsule, accompanied by the popliteal veins and popliteus muscle.
- It splits into the *anterior tibial artery, fibular artery (peroneal artery)*, and *posterior tibial artery* just distal to its passage through the tendinous arch of the soleus muscle.
- Further course of the *anterior tibial artery* in the extensor compartment: at the level of the malleoli, it transitions into the dorsalis pedis artery.
- Course of the fibular artery in the deep flexor compartment toward the foot: distal to the superior fibular retinaculum, it divides into the calcaneal divisions.
- Further course of the *posterior tibial artery*: running posterior to the tibia, under the triceps surae muscle, and behind the medial malleolus, and branching into the plantar arteries.

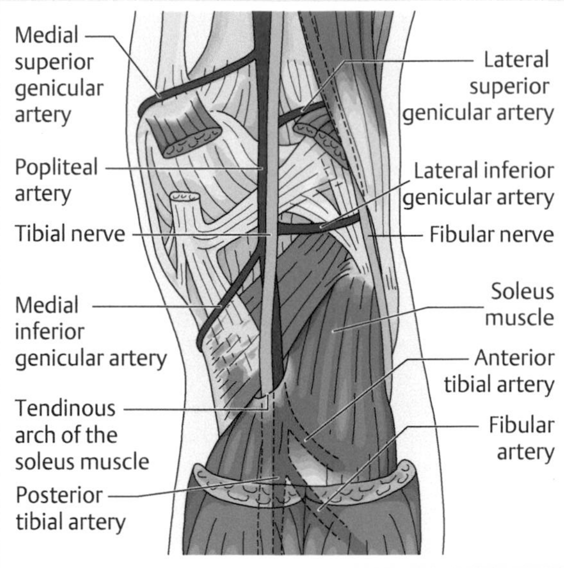


**Fig. 9.108** Branching of the popliteal artery in the popliteal fossa.

## Course of the Vessels and Nerves in the Fascial Compartments the Lower Leg (Fig. 9.109)

Laterally, the deep fascia of the leg tracks deep in the leg with both the anterior and posterior muscular septa, each of which is fixed to the fibula. This forms four osteofibrotic compartments:

- The first compartment is for the fibular muscles and the superficial fibular nerve.
- The second compartment is the extensor compartment, in which the anterior tibial vessels and the deep fibular nerve run. It lies directly on the interosseous membrane, between the tibialis anterior and extensor hallucis longus muscles.
- The third compartment is the superficial flexor compartment for the triceps surae muscle.
- The fourth compartment is the flexor compartment, which is separated from the superficial compartment by part of the deep fascia of the leg. In it run the fibular vessels, the posterior tibial vessels, and the tibial nerve. The flexor digitorum longus and brevis muscles and the tibialis posterior muscle lie in this compartment.

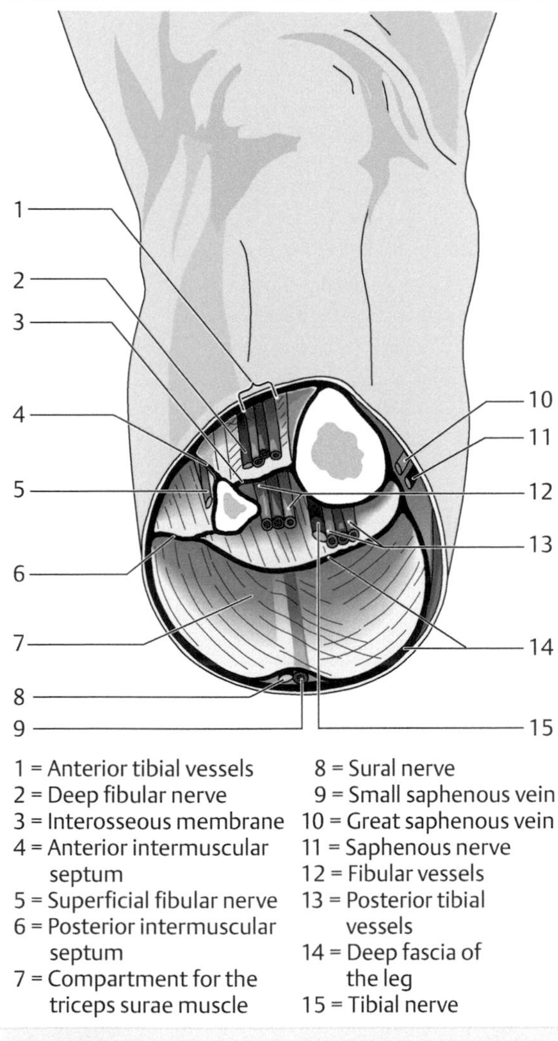


**Fig. 9.109** Course of the vessels and nerves in the fascial compartments of the proximal lower leg.

## 9.3.9 Innervation

### Articular Branches (Figs. 9.110 and 9.111)

- Articular branch from the posterior branch of the obturator nerve.
- Articular branches of the tibial nerve: Several branches supply the inferomedial area of the knee and, with two branches, the posterior capsule–ligament apparatus. Plexus-like branches supply the medial knee region.
- Articular branches of the common fibular nerve: Some branches supply the dorsolateral area of the knee, and some the anterolateral knee area.
- Articular branches arise from the femoral nerve for the periosteum of the patella and the anterior, medial, and lateral capsule–ligament sections.
- A small articular branch from the saphenous nerve supplies the medial capsular area.

### Sensory Innervation of the Knee

#### *Ruffini's Corpuscles*

These send signals on the extent and speed of movements and any increases in the intracapsular pressure. They are located primarily in the fibrous layer.

#### *Pacini's Corpuscles*

These gather information quickly and pass it on (e.g., when movements are delayed or accelerated). These bodies are found predominately in the fibrous layer, the fat pad, and the vascularized areas of the menisci.

#### *Golgi's Bodies*

These bodies measure the tension in the tissues and protect the affected structures by inhibiting motor neurons, thereby preventing a further buildup of tension. Golgi's bodies are found in the menisci and ligaments, and at the points where the ligaments and tendons connect to the capsule.

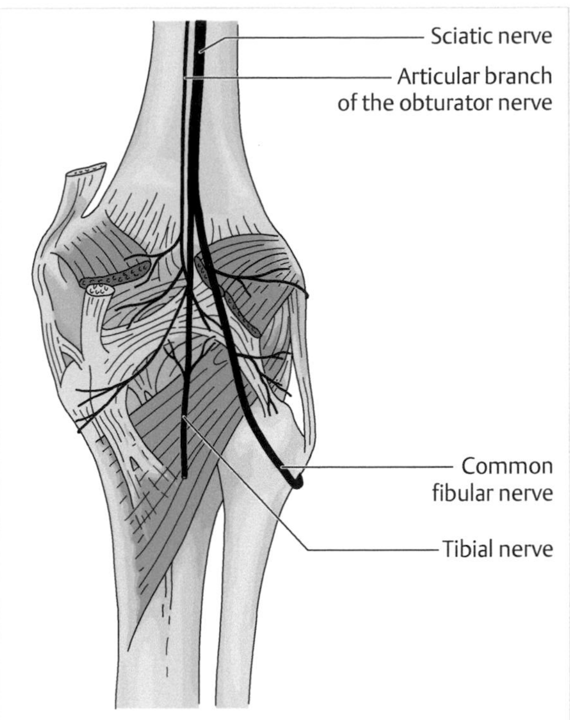


**Fig. 9.110** Innervation of the posterior region of the knee.

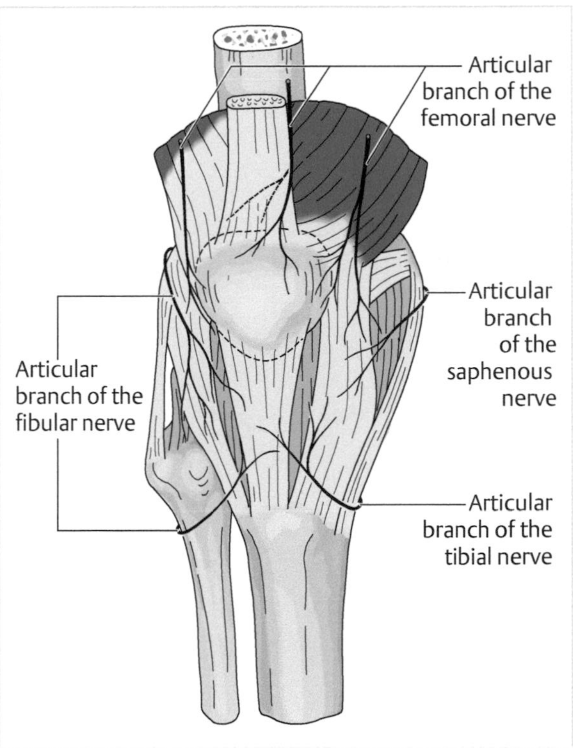


**Fig. 9.111** Innervation of the anterior region of the knee.

## 9.3.10 Axes of Motion and Movements

### Axes

#### Flexion/Extension Axis (Fig. 9.112)

The movements of flexion and extension occur around the frontal axis. This corresponds to the instantaneous point of intersection of the cruciate and collateral ligaments. It is not constant but shifts with movement. In extension, it is about one fingerbreadth inferior to the medial femoral epicondyle, and it migrates posteriorly in an arc during flexion.

#### Rotational Axis (Fig. 9.113)

This axis passes through the medial tubercle of the intercondylar eminence.

### Movements of the Knee Joint

#### Flexion/Extension (Figs. 9.114–9.116)

Active: 140°/10°, respectively, from neutral.
Passive: 160°/15°, respectively, from neutral.
Knee flexion has a wider range of motion when combined with hip flexion than it does with hip extension. The rectus femoris muscle is stretched by knee flexion but does allow maximum movement. If the muscle experiences further stretching by added hip extension, the range of motion in the knee joint is reduced. During functional examination for flexion, this means that the range of motion is expected to be different in the supine position and the prone position.

A slight rotational component can be seen at the end of motion in both flexion and extension—flexion inevitably entails internal rotation of the lower leg; extension entails external rotation. This means that, for maximum flexion and extension movements to occur, freedom of rotational movement must be guaranteed.

##### *Rolling–Sliding Motion (Fig. 9.117)*

During flexion and extension movements, the knee is subject to a motion sequence that is controlled by the interaction of the cruciate and collateral ligaments as a rolling–sliding motion.

In flexion, there are the same number of contact points on both joint surfaces. With increasing flexion, these move posteriorly. Since the distance on the femur is much greater than that on the tibia, there must be a sliding movement in addition to the rolling movement. Therefore, the distances between the contact points on the femur are greater than they are on the tibia. At the beginning of flexion, the rolling–sliding motion corresponds to a ratio of 1:2, meaning that the path on the femur is almost twice as long as that on the tibia. Toward the end of flexion, the path on the femur is approximately four times greater than that of the tibia, which corresponds to a ratio of 1 : 4.

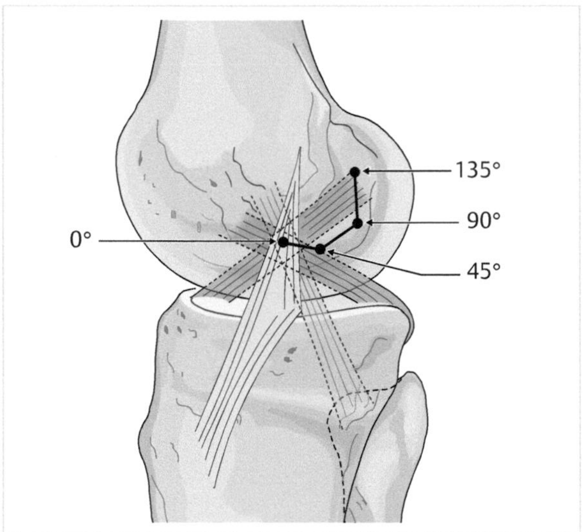


Fig. 9.112 Frontal axis in various knee positions.

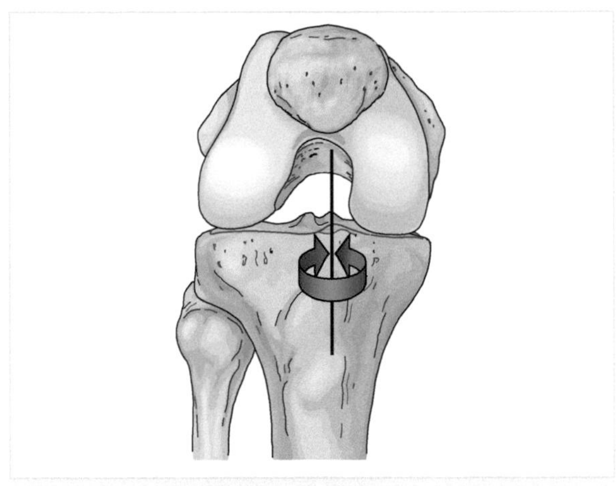

Fig. 9.113 Axis of rotation.

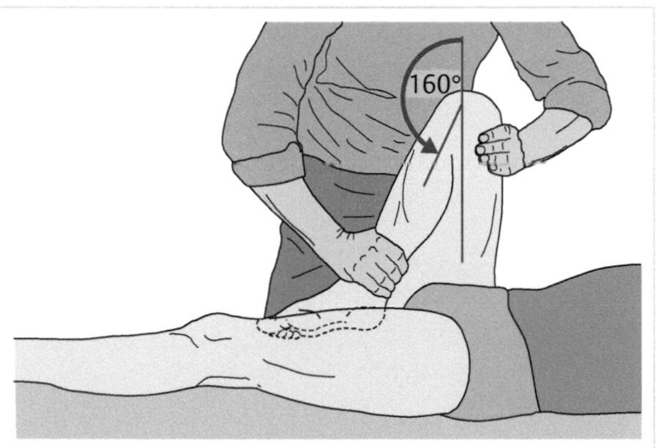


Fig. 9.114 Passive flexion in the supine position.

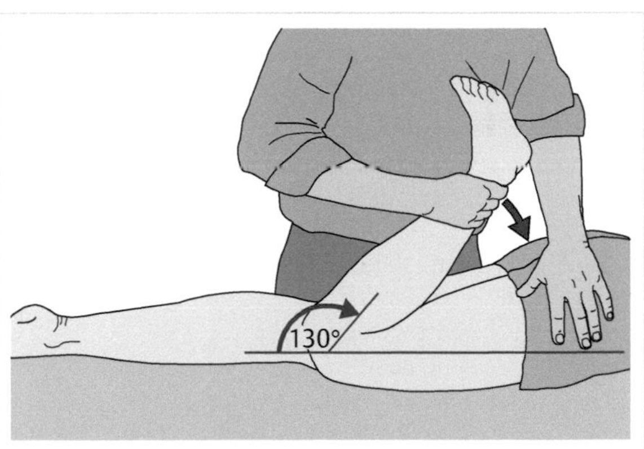


Fig. 9.115 Passive flexion in the prone position.

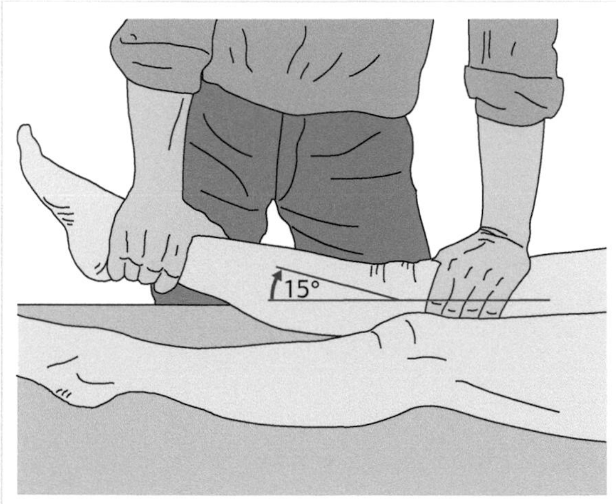


Fig. 9.116 Passive extension.

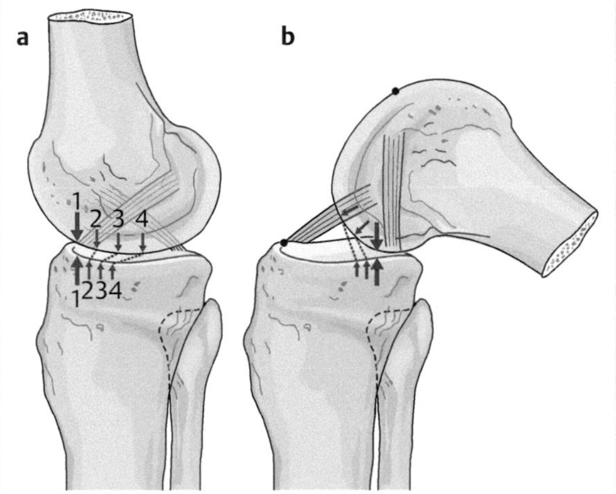


Fig. 9.117 Rolling–sliding motion. (a) At the beginning of flexion. (b) At the end of flexion.

## External Rotation/Internal Rotation (Fig. 9.118)

Active: 45°/30°, respectively, from neutral.

Passive: 50°/35°, respectively, from neutral.

Rotational movements of the knee joint are possible only in flexion. The main reason for this is the tension of the capsule and ligaments in the extended position. Rotation occurs primarily in the meniscotibial component of the joint. The collateral ligaments inhibit the movement of external rotation, with the medial ligament inhibiting it more than the lateral. The cruciate ligaments are primarily responsible for limiting internal rotation.

The lateral condyle covers more distance during rotation because the lateral meniscus is more mobile. In external rotation, the lateral condyle of the tibia moves posteriorly under the meniscus. The medial condyle shifts a shorter distance anteriorly. The reason for this reduced shift lies in the fact that the medial intercondylar tubercle is higher than the eminence, and thus represents a kind of buffer for the motion of the medial condyle.

During rotation, the patella is held in place within its sliding groove, while the tibial tuberosity clearly shifts toward rotation.

Rotation is an important movement in adapting to uneven terrain and maintaining equilibrium.

## Terminal Rotation (Fig. 9.119)

Terminal rotation occurs automatically at the end of extension. Here, the tibia externally rotates about 5° on the fixed femur. It revolves around a rotation axis that goes approximately through the insertion of the anterior cruciate ligament on the medial intercondylar area. The lateral condyle of the tibia clearly turns posteriorly about this axis. The medial condyle of the tibia turns anteriorly only minimally.

The terminal rotation is due in part to the differences in shape of the articulating surfaces (the medial condyle being longer than the lateral) and to the tension of the anteromedial bundle of the anterior cruciate ligament. Through this, the medial tibial plateau is drawn toward the lateral femoral condyle, resulting in external rotation of the lower leg.

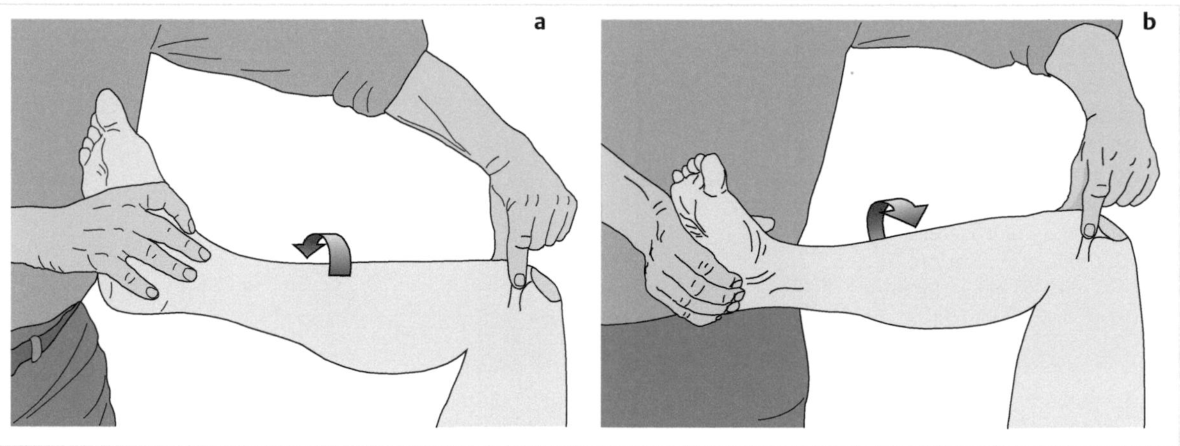


Fig. 9.118 Testing passive movement. (a) External rotation. (b) Internal rotation.

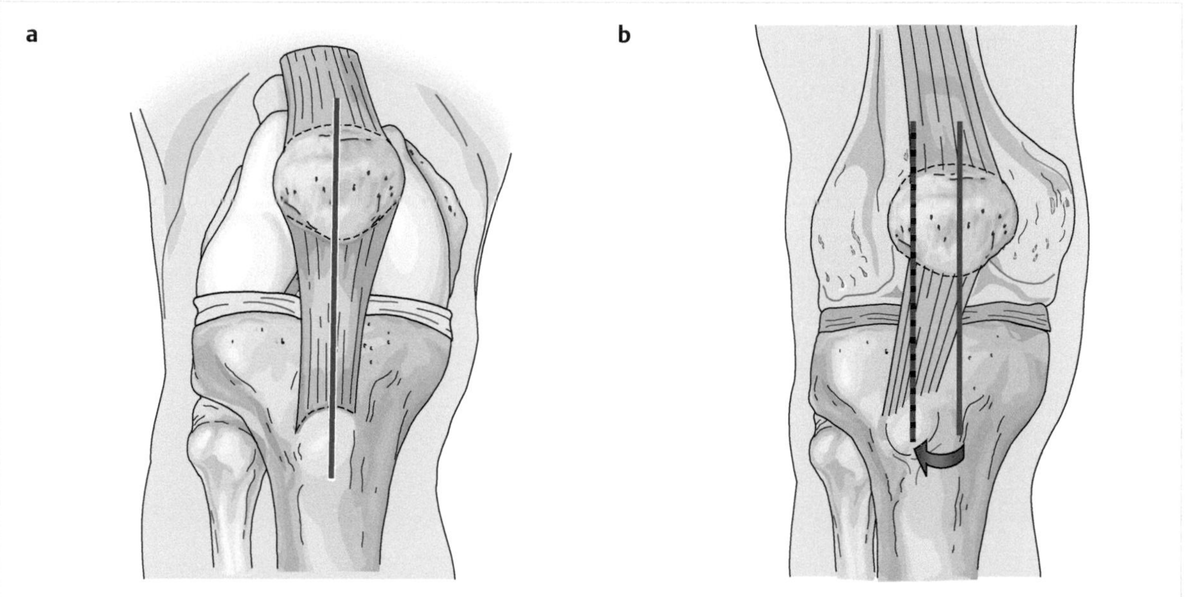


Fig. 9.119 A vertical line through the tibial tuberosity. (a) In flexion. (b) Displacement of the tibial tuberosity in extension = terminal rotation.

## Movements in the Patellofemoral Joint

The patella moves in six different degrees of freedom of motion and is the mobile end, while the femur is the fixed end. The movements are divided into translational and rotational movements.

### Translational Movements (Fig. 9.120)

Translational movements have to do with displacement in a superior/inferior direction. For example, while standing with the knee extended, the patella is at a low point when the quadriceps muscle is relaxed. When the quadriceps tenses, the patella shifts superiorly approximately 1 to 1.5 cm.

The other patellar displacements run in medial/lateral and anterior/posterior directions.

When passively testing the extent of translational shifts, it is important to compare the two sides, using the healthy side as the norm, because the shift varies between individuals. Average values of displacement are: superiorly: 1 cm; inferiorly: 2 to 3 cm; medially: 1 cm; laterally: 2 cm; and anteriorly: 0.5 cm. The test for posterior displacement is performed during movement or as a compression test against the patellar surface of the femur.

### Rotational Movements (Fig. 9.121)

With rotational movements, the movements take place around the *sagittal axis*, which passes through the middle of the patella. The base of the patella rotates around it in a medial direction while the apex rotates laterally, and vice versa.

The second axis has a *longitudinal* course, around which the patella rotates posterolaterally and posteromedially.

The third axis is the *frontal axis*, around which the base of the patella moves posteriorly, while the apex of the patella moves anteriorly, and vice versa. The degree of rotational movement is minimal. Carry out the testing for these movements during knee flexion and extension.

These movements do not occur in isolation but as coupled movements. During flexion, the patella slides distally over the patellar surface of the femur between the condyles and travels a distance of approximately 8 cm. This path requires the suprapatellar and deep infrapatellar bursae to unfold. In addition, minimal lateralization and rotation around the sagittal axis takes place, and the base of the patella approaches the condyles.

**Practical Tip**

**Testing Function (Fig. 9.122)**

Palpate the movements of the patella during knee flexion and extension. While doing this, watch for evasive movements such as abnormal translational and rotational movements. Test the translational movements against the patellar surface of the femur: proximal-distal, medial-lateral and anterior-posterior. These tests reveal something about both the ability of the joint to slide and the state of tension of the muscles and tendons attached to the patella, because these can affect the position of the patella and also its quality of movement.

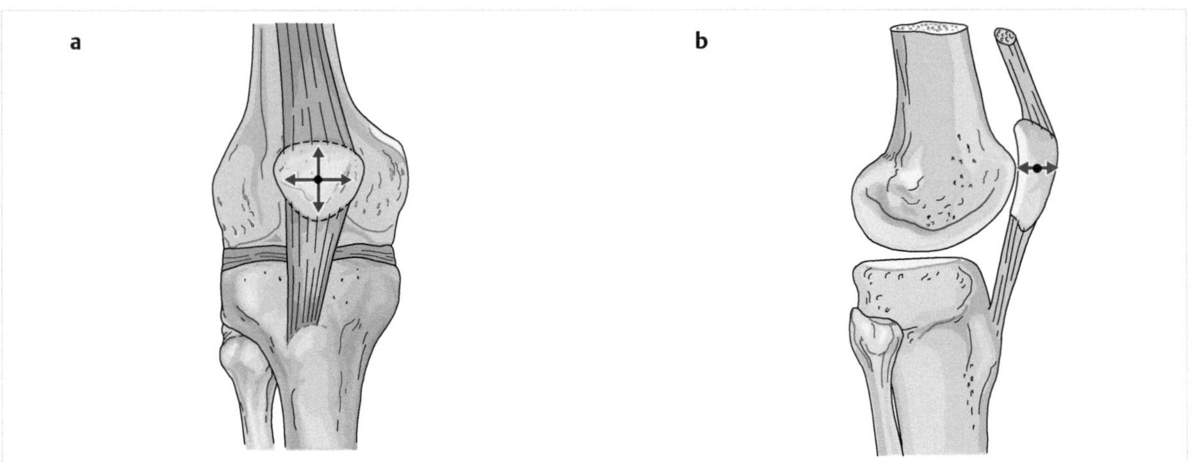


**Fig. 9.120** Translational movements of the patella. **(a)** Shifting superior-inferior and medial-lateral. **(b)** Shifting anteriorly and posteriorly.

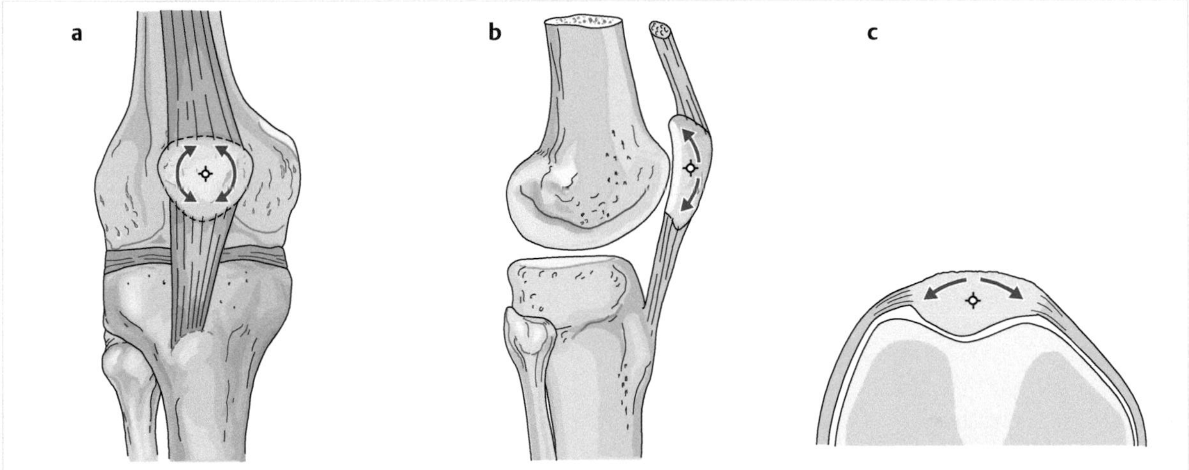


**Fig. 9.121** Rotational movements of the patella. **(a)** Sagittal axis. **(b)** Frontal axis. **(c)** Longitudinal axis.

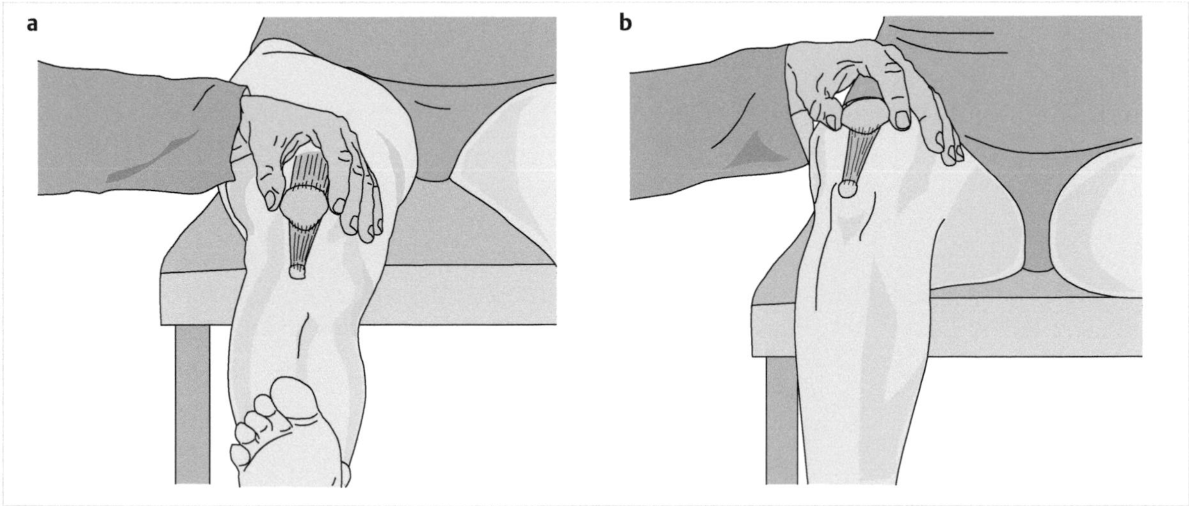


**Fig. 9.122** Palpation of patellar movements. **(a)** From maximum extension. **(b)** To maximum flexion.

## 9.3.11 Biomechanics

### Axes of the Leg

#### In the Sagittal Plane

The line of gravity passes through the center of the greater trochanter (trochanter point), through an area just posterior to the middle of the knee joint, and through an area just anterior to the upper ankle joint.

**Pathology**

**Genu Recurvatum**

The line of gravity is displaced anteriorly. In the end position, the femoral condyles show an increased posterior sliding component, in keeping with instability in the direction of an anterior tibial drawer.

#### In the Frontal Plane (Fig. 9.123)

The mechanical longitudinal line of the leg passes through the centers of the hip, knee, and the upper ankle joints. The axis of the femoral shaft deviates 6° laterally from the longitudinal line of the leg. In the lower leg, the longitudinal line and the axis of the tibial shaft coincide.

The femoral shaft axis forms an angle (*femur–tibia angle*) of 174° with the tibial shaft axis.

If the course of the longitudinal line of the leg corresponds to the norm, the articular cartilage is loaded evenly and the tension in the ligaments is also normal. In addition, the stabilizing muscles are in equilibrium.

**Pathology**

**Genu Varum (Fig. 9.124a)**

The knee joint lies lateral to the longitudinal line of the leg, and the femur–tibia angle increases. The medial joint complex is compressed, resulting in destruction of the medial articular surfaces. In the lateral joint complex, the condyles no longer have closure, and the fibular collateral ligament and the lateral part of the capsule come under stress. The iliotibial tract and the biceps femoris muscle become strained. The line of gravity falls on the medial border of the foot, leading to a decrease in the arch of the foot.

**Genu Valgum (Fig. 9.124b)**

The knee joint is medial to the longitudinal line of the leg and the femur–tibia angle becomes smaller. The lateral joint complex is overloaded. The tibial collateral ligament, medial part of the capsule, and pes anserinus group are stretched. The line of gravity falls on the lateral border of the foot, which becomes overloaded.

**Practical Tip**

The main principle in treating genu varum consists of shifting the knee toward the load line (medially) through a training program to build up the tensor fascia latae muscle and the biceps femoris muscles. In addition, alteration of the arch of the foot is significant because an increased load on the inner foot exerts more pressure on the medial knee region. Correction of this deformity is therefore approached both proximally and distally.

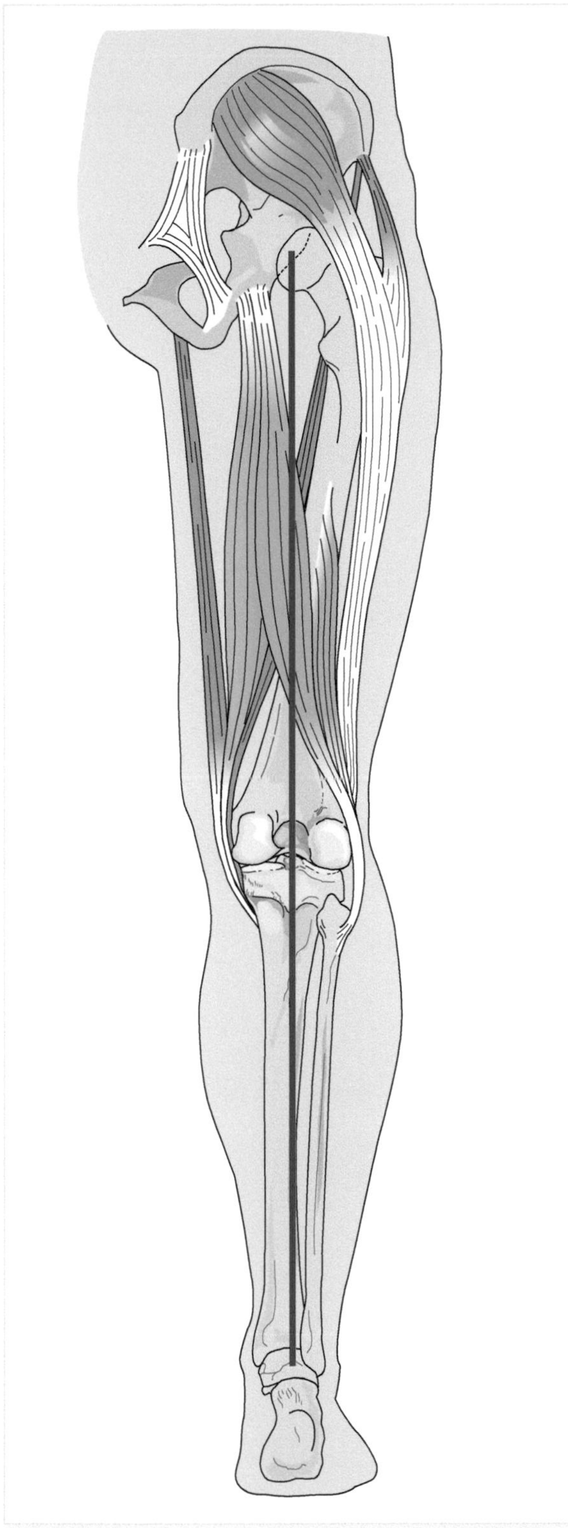

**Fig. 9.123** Normal course of the longitudinal line of the leg.

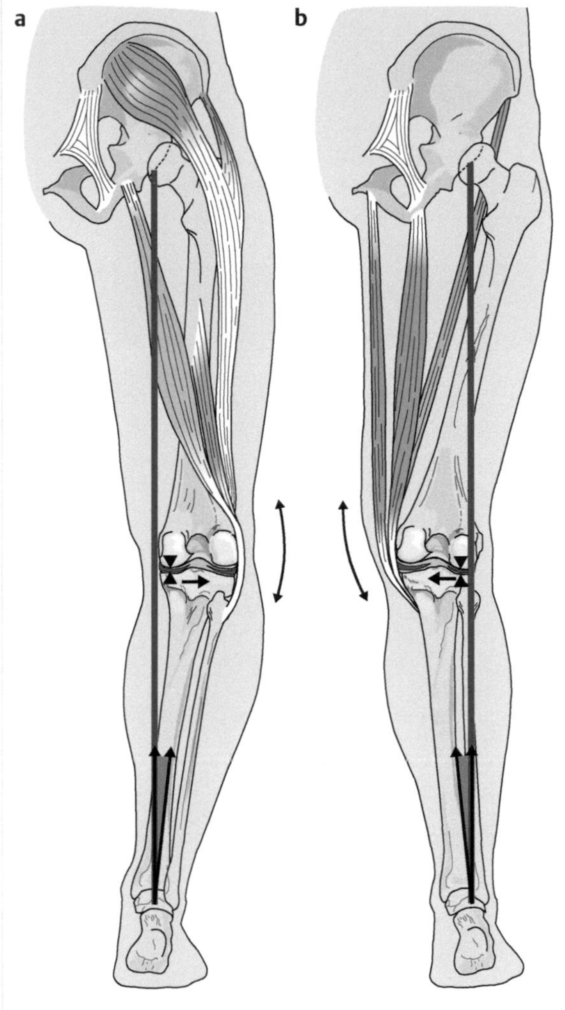


**Fig. 9.124** Deviations from the normal longitudinal line. **(a)** Genu varum. **(b)** Genu valgum.

## In the Transverse Plane (Fig. 9.125)

The transverse axes of the proximal and distal tibia are evaluated by their relationship to each other. They form an angle of 30°. This can be observed at the foot, where the anatomical longitudinal axis of the foot extends approximately 30° externally from the sagittal plane. This angle is formed by the tibial torsion, which is directed outward and occurs primarily within the proximal tibia.

### Practical Tip

Increased external tibial torsion causes a pronounced outward orientation of the functional longitudinal axis of the foot. The gait pattern of those affected shows very strong external rotation. If evaluation of the position of the patella shows it to be anterior, increased external tibial torsion may be the cause. Push-off of the foot occurs over the medial edge of the big toe, which over time becomes overused and painful.

Compensation typically occurs by internally rotating the hip joint. This in turn exposes the knee to a shear force as the thigh turns inward and the lower leg turns outward. Here again, overload and pain are the result.

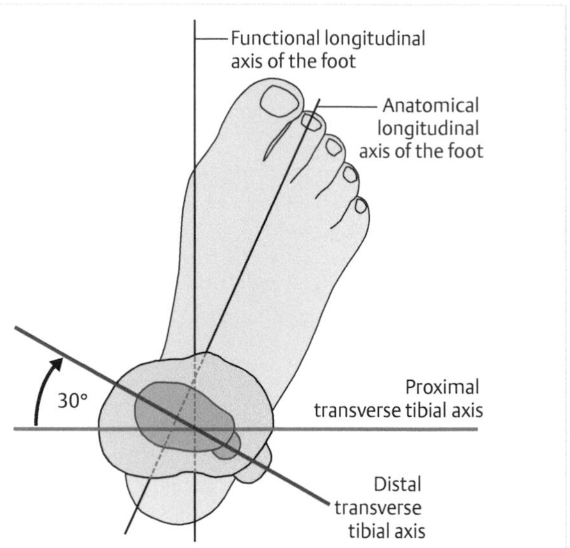


**Fig. 9.125** Tibial torsion: relationship of the transverse tibial axes to each other.

## Retropatellar Pressure

The loading force on the patellofemoral joint is made up of the vector sum of the muscle–ligament force and the force of gravity. That means that, in addition to body weight, the lever arms of the various forces as well as the vertical and horizontal tensile forces play a role. Thus, all the structures that attach to the patella have an influence on the joint pressure.

### With Movement (Fig. 9.126)

The contact pressure of the patella on the patellar surface of the femur is minimal during knee extension and increases during flexion.

While squatting, the following occurs:

- With slight flexion (10–50°), there is a steep increase in retropatellar force, but the pressure does not reach its peak value.
- With increasing flexion, the pressure becomes greater. If the center of gravity lies quite far posteriorly, the load arm lengthens, a greater force is expended, and the pressure can add up to 10 times the body weight.
- This is significantly alleviated by the anterior displacement of the center of gravity, which shortens the load arm.

At 50° of flexion, with the center of gravity acting posteriorly, the pressure can amount to 2400 N. As soon as the center of gravity shifts anteriorly, this is reduced to 860 N.

A healthy patella can tolerate such a high pressure. However, variations in the shape of the patella, unfavorable height adjustments, and changes in direction of the tensile forces of the structures acting on the patella may adversely affect the pressure.

**Pathology**

**Patellofemoral Pain Syndrome**

Anatomical changes of the patella such as dysplasia, leg axis malalignment, ligamentous laxity, and muscle imbalance can lead to disproportionate stress on the patellofemoral joint. The symptoms are tenderness on palpation of the patellar facet, deep joint pain, especially when climbing stairs, in the squatting position, and after prolonged sitting, and the symptom of "giving way," in which the knee can buckle when stressed.

**Chondromalacia**

Wear of the cartilage that is not treated, and in which no load reduction is to be expected, can lead to chondromalacia. To the symptoms of the patellofemoral pain syndrome previously described are added recurrent joint effusions, as decomposition products from necrosis of the cartilage produce synovitis. Thus the following vicious cycle occurs: an unfavorable rise in pressure → softening of the cartilage → breakdown products of cartilage necrosis in the joint → chronic synovitis → changes in composition of the synovial fluid → disturbance of cartilage nutrition → death of the chondrocytes.

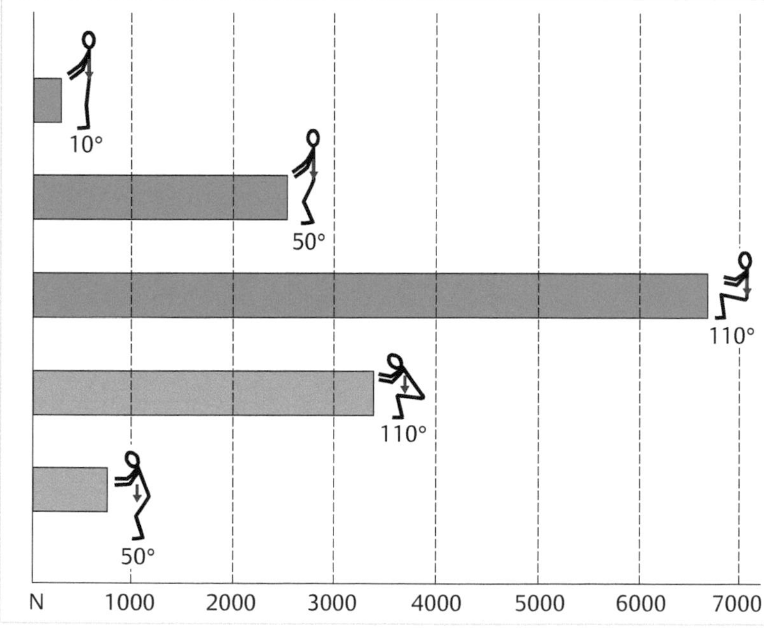


**Fig. 9.126** Changes in retropatellar pressure. Red bars: center of gravity acting posteriorly; gray bars: center of gravity acting anteriorly.

## Force-absorbing Surfaces (Fig. 9.127)

Both the patella and part of the patellar surface of the femur are available to absorb force. The force-absorbing surface is slightly smaller than the actual contact area, and which part of the joint surface is used for the transmission of force depends on the position of the joint.

### *Contact Surfaces during Movement*

- In the neutral position, only a small distal portion of the patella, just proximal to the apex, has contact with the patellar surface of the femur.
- With increasing flexion, the retropatellar contact area migrates superiorly, while the contact area on the femur moves inferiorly. At 90° flexion, this contact surface is located transversely over the base of the patella, and at the distal end of the patellar surface of the femur.
- Beyond 90° of flexion, the patella bridges over the intercondylar fossa. Only the outermost parts of the patellar facets have contact with the condyles, and the ridge extends into the intercondylar fossa.

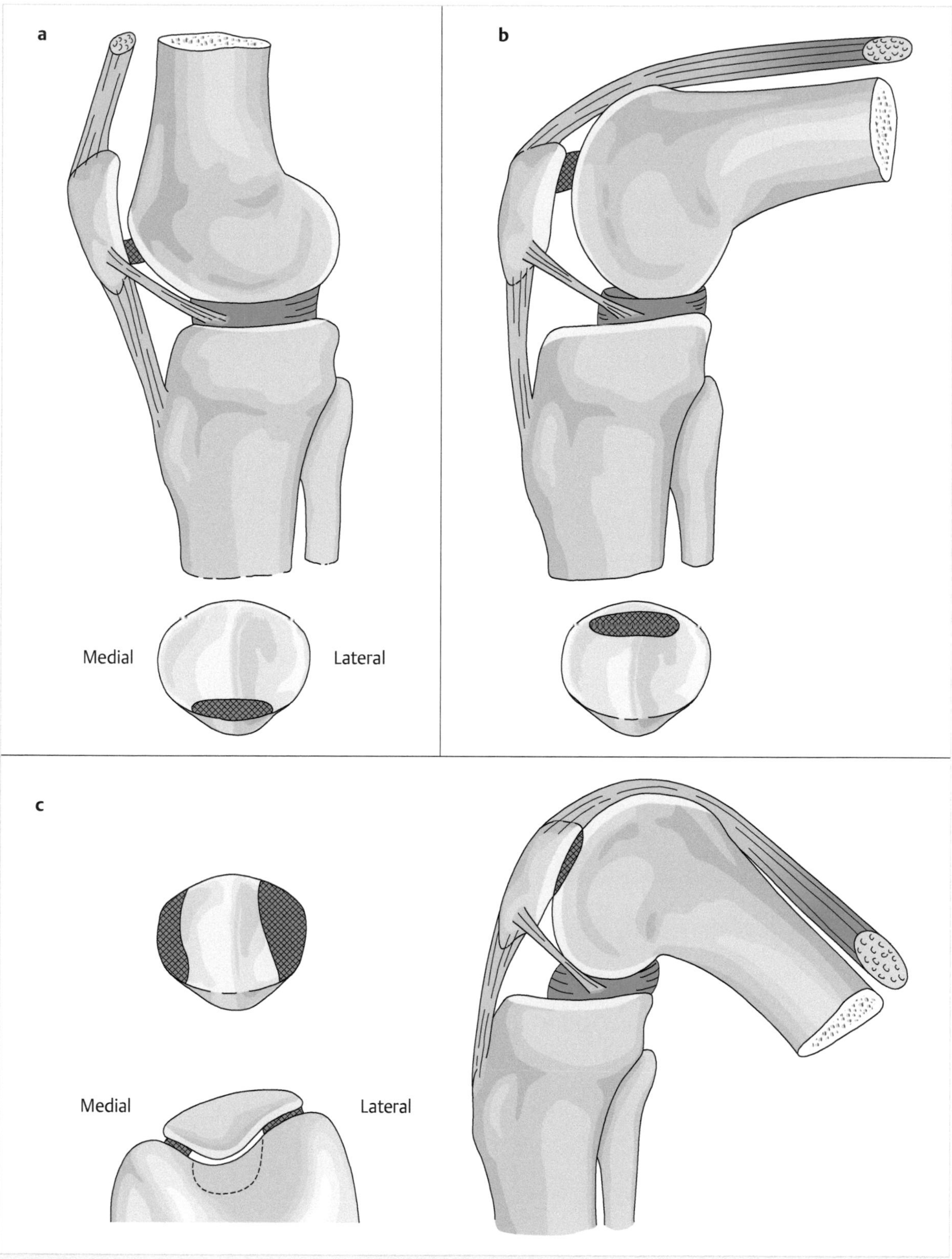


**Fig. 9.127** Retropatellar force-absorbing surfaces. Hatched red areas = contact surfaces. **(a)** Neutral position (0°). **(b)** 90° Flexion. **(c)** 120° Flexion.

# 9.4 Neural Structures

## 9.4.1 Terminal Branches of the Sciatic Nerve

- In the superior region of the popliteal fossa, the sciatic nerve runs between the semimembranosus and biceps muscles.
- In the fossa, the nerve makes its final division into its two terminal branches, the common fibular nerve and the tibial nerve, although both are already bundled far proximally in the nerve trunk of the sciatic nerve.

### Common Fibular Nerve (L4–S2; Fig. 9.128)

- This tracks distally along the medial border of the biceps muscle and superficially around the fibular head in an anterior direction.
- After this turn, it extends into the lateral compartment of the leg, which is located between the two origins of the peroneus longus muscle.
- This compartment borders the flexor group through the posterior intermuscular septum of the leg and the extensor group through the anterior intermuscular septum.
- Within this compartment, the nerve divides into the deep and superficial fibular nerves.

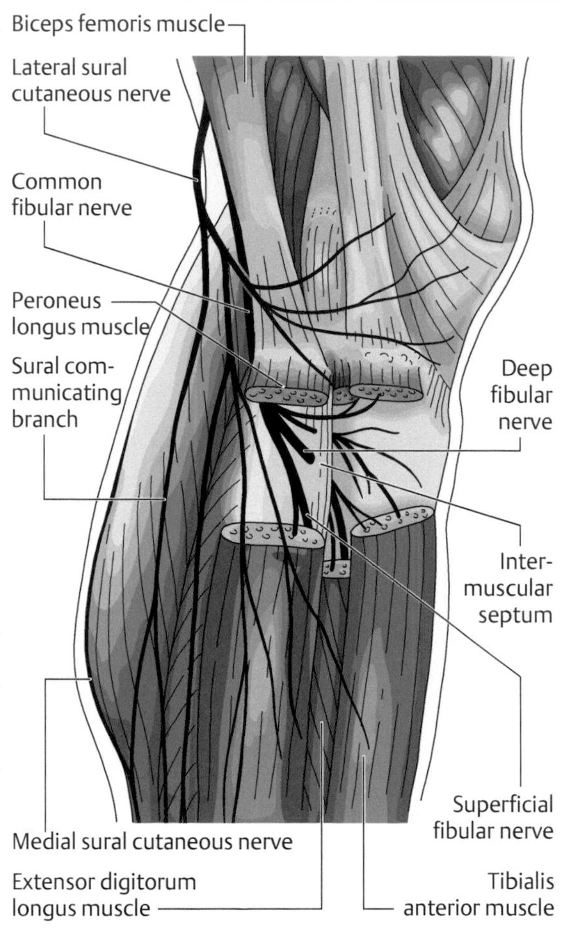


**Fig. 9.128** Branching of the common fibular nerve.

**Pathology**

**Fibular Nerve Paresis from Pressure Damage**

The most common cause of isolated fibular palsy is pressure damage to the nerve at the fibular head. Here it lies directly on the bone and can therefore be easily damaged. Crossing the legs, inept positioning of an unconscious or physically handicapped person, positioning on the operating table, or the pressure from a splint or cast is sufficient to cause this damage.

In fibular nerve palsy, sensation is disturbed on the lateral lower leg and the dorsum of the foot. Motor deficits include failure of all the dorsiflexors of the foot (foot drop), the long toe extensors, and the fibular muscles. The foot droops, and since it can no longer be actively pulled up, a *high-stepping gait* (foot-drop gait) develops.

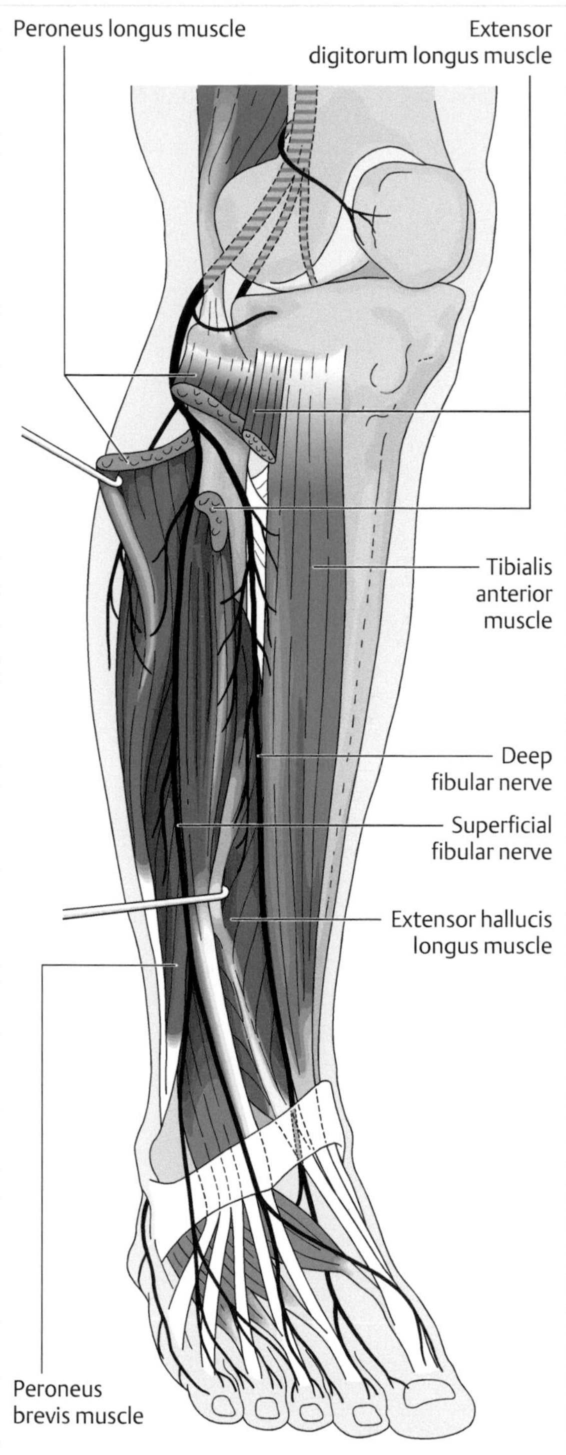


**Fig. 9.129** Course of the superficial fibular and deep fibular nerves.

## Deep Fibular Nerve (Figs. 9.129 and 9.130)

- This is a motor nerve supplying the extensor muscle group of the lower leg, which it reaches after piercing the anterior intermuscular septum.
- It extends distally on the interosseous membrane between the tibialis anterior and extensor hallucis longus muscles.
- It then passes under the superior extensor retinaculum and divides here into a lateral and medial branch.
- The nerve innervates the toe and foot extensors and only a small area of skin between the big toe and the second toe.

## Superficial Fibular Nerve (Figs. 9.129 and 9.130)

- This passes between the extensor digitorum longus and peroneus longus muscles.
- A handbreadth above the lateral malleolus, it divides into the *medial dorsal cutaneous nerve*, which runs toward the medial dorsum of the foot, and the *intermediate dorsal cutaneous nerve*, which tracks to the lateral dorsum of the foot.
- It innervates the fibular muscles and large areas of skin on the anterior lower leg and the dorsum of the foot.

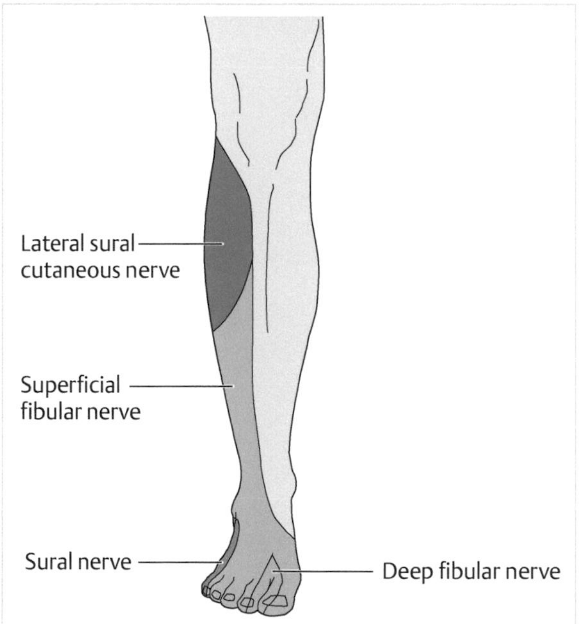


**Fig. 9.130** Cutaneous innervation by the fibular nerves.

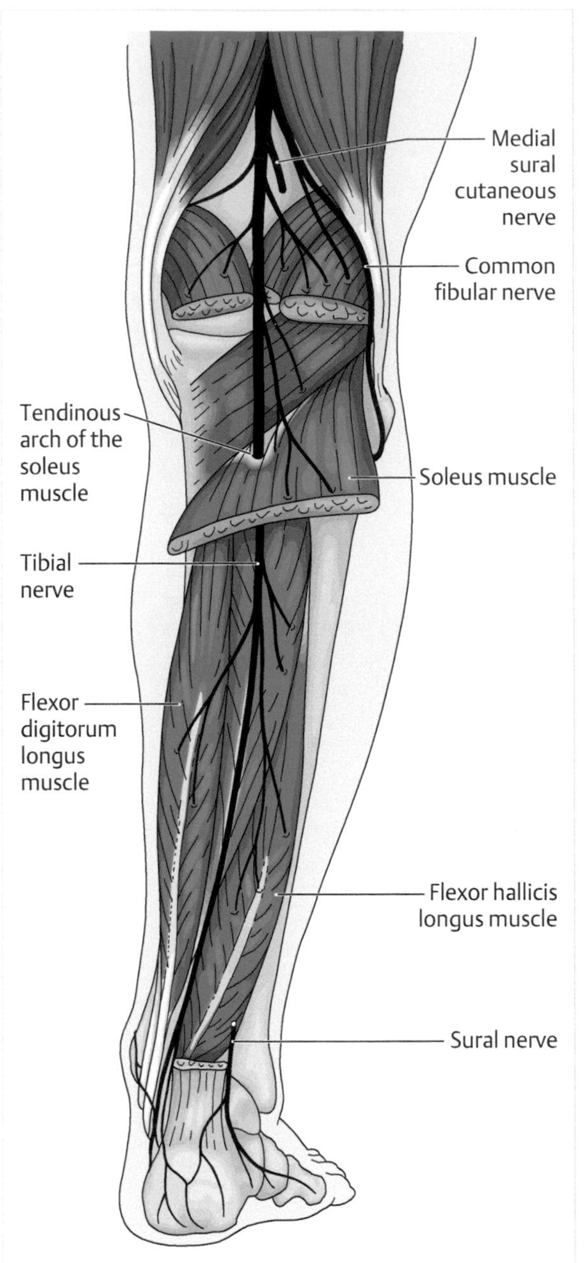


**Fig. 9.131** Course of the tibial nerve.

## Tibial Nerve (L4–S3; Figs. 9.131 and 9.132)

- The nerve tracks longitudinally through the popliteal fossa.
- Within the fossa, it divides into the muscular branches to innervate the gastrocnemius and soleus muscles, and the medial sural cutaneous nerve.
- It courses further under the heads of the gastrocnemius muscle to the tendinous arch of the soleus muscle; here it transitions into the deep flexor compartment of the leg, where it runs between the flexor digitorum longus and flexor hallucis longus muscles.
- It extends along with these tendons further toward the medial malleolus, around which it bends posteriorly.
- Distal to the malleolus, it divides into the medial and lateral plantar nerves.
- It innervates the triceps surae muscle, the tibialis posterior muscle, and the two long flexors, as well as the areas of the skin in the heel area and a large part of the sole of the foot.

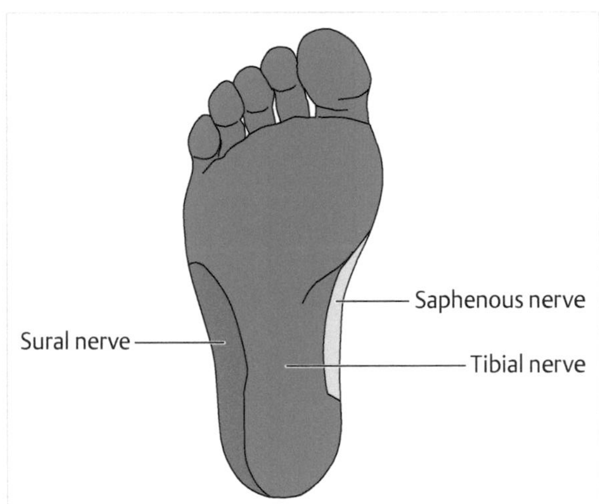


**Fig. 9.132** Innervation of the plantar surface of the foot.

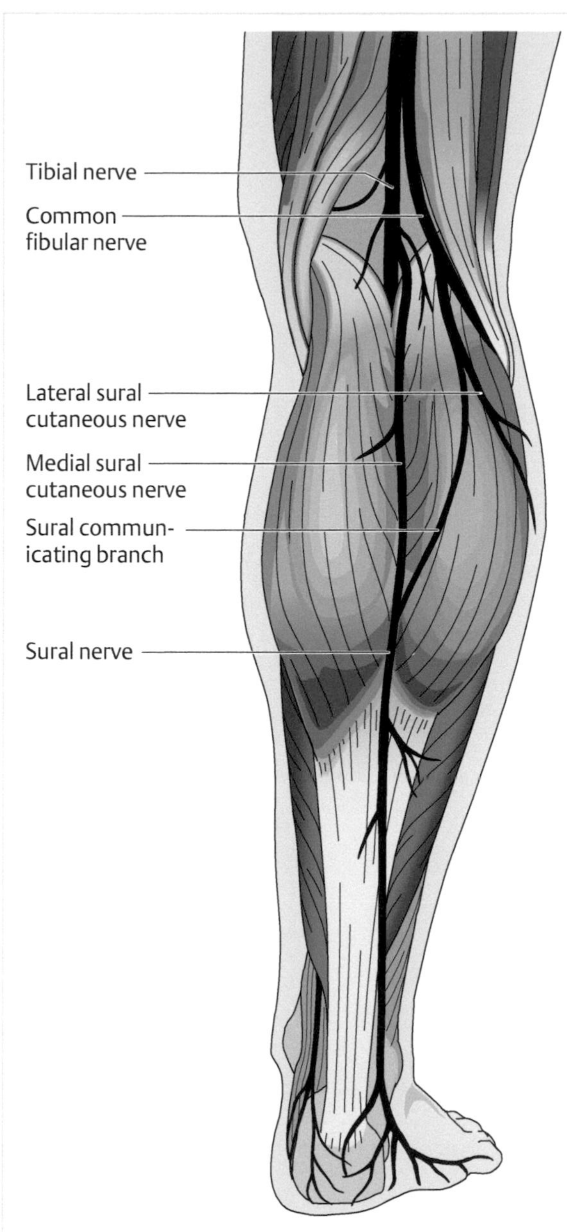


**Fig. 9.133** Course of the sural nerve.

## Sural Nerve (Figs. 9.132–9.134)

- In the popliteal fossa, the tibial nerve gives off a sensory branch, the *medial sural cutaneous nerve*, which runs distally superficially between the two heads of the gastrocnemius muscle.
- In the popliteal fossa, the common fibular nerve gives off the *lateral sural cutaneous nerve*, which tracks along the lateral surface of the lower leg to the lateral malleolus.
- The lateral sural cutaneous nerve joins with the medial sural cutaneous nerve by way of the *sural communicating branch* to form the *sural nerve* at the level of the Achilles tendon.
- It then runs further along the lateral edge of the Achilles tendon to the lateral border of the foot.
- It innervates areas of skin on the dorsolateral lower leg and the lateral border of the foot.

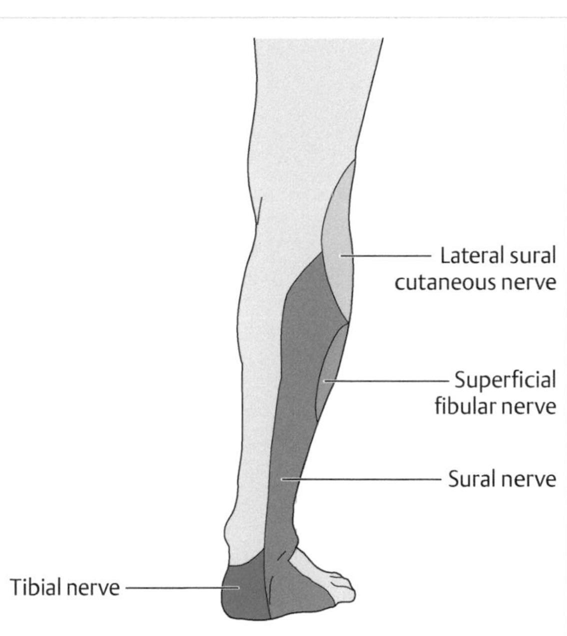


**Fig. 9.134** Cutaneous innervation by the sural nerve.

# Chapter 10

## Foot and Ankle

# 10 Foot and Ankle

The student will note that there are differences in nomenclature when it comes to the ankle joint. While anatomists agree, for the most part, on the structure and function of the individual joints, it is important to understand that there is a difference in how they view the ankle as a functional unit. Many American anatomists think of the *ankle joint* simply as the *talocrural joint*, involved essentially in dorsiflexion and plantarflexion, and consider other movements to be a function of the other joints in the foot (Moore et al 2014).

In contrast, the concept held by German anatomists—and used in this book—visualizes the ankle functionally as the *upper ankle joint* and the *lower ankle joint* (Graumann 2004). The *upper ankle joint* is the *talocrural joint*, equivalent to the *ankle joint* proper as noted above. This is discussed in Chapter 10.3. The *lower ankle joint* consists of posterior and anterior parts, the *subtalar joint* (*talocalcaneal joint*) and the *talocalcaneonavicular joint*, respectively. These will be discussed in detail in Chapter 10.5, Talotarsal Joint. There is some advantage in using this model to visualize the complex combined movements of the foot and ankle (Graumann 2004, Kelikian and Sarrafian 2011, Moore 2014).

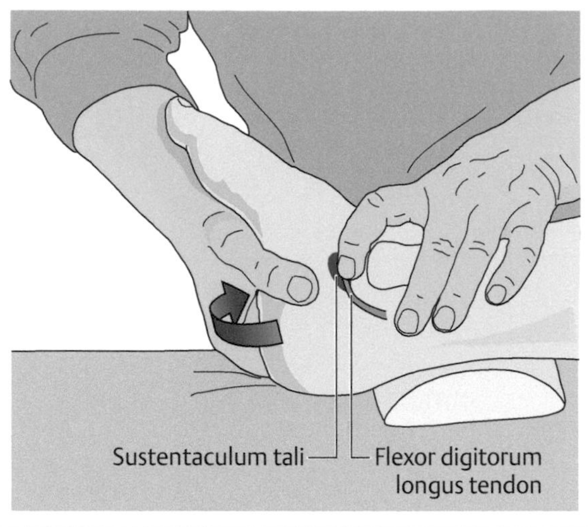


**Fig. 10.1** Palpation of the sustentaculum tali.

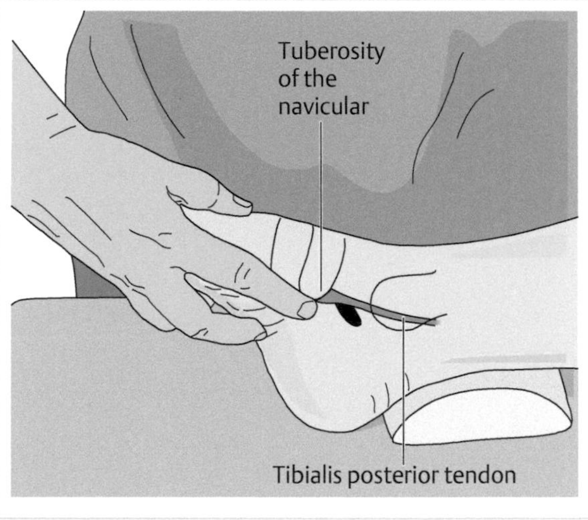


**Fig. 10.2** Palpation of the tuberosity of the navicular.

## 10.1 Palpation of the Structures of the Foot and Ankle

### 10.1.1 Medial Region of the Foot and Ankle

#### Medial Malleolus

This is the most distinct, protruding bony point in the medial foot area and serves as an important guide in locating palpable structures.

#### Sustentaculum Tali (Fig. 10.1)

The sustentaculum tali of the calcaneus lies about 1½ fingerbreadths below the tip of the malleolus. The talar joint space is located on its upper edge. By passively tilting the foot medially and laterally, one can better localize the joint space, because the gap gapes open when tilted laterally. The sustentaculum tali has a longitudinally running groove in which the tendon of the flexor digitorum longus lies.

#### Navicular Bone (Fig. 10.2)

Starting from sustentaculum and moving in a distal and inferior direction, one can palpate a distinct hump, the *navicular tuberosity*. The tendon of the tibialis posterior muscle tracks to it from posterosuperiorly, making it useful as a guide. The navicular bone is about a fingerbreadth wide.

## Talocalcaneonavicular Joint (Fig. 10.3)

Between the tendon of the tibialis anterior muscle and the medial malleolus, and a good fingerbreadth anterior to the lower leg, one can palpate the proximal border of the navicular bone. Using passive inversion and eversion movements, the examiner can feel the joint space distinctly.

## Cuneonavicular Joint (Fig. 10.4)

At the distal border of the navicular bone is the joint space to the medial cuneiform. This is best palpated from an inferomedial approach while simultaneously tilting the cuneiform medially.

## First Tarsometatarsal Joint (Fig. 10.5)

Moving distally, the base of the first metatarsal is the next salient point for orientation. The joint space to the medial cuneiform is located proximally from it. The joint space widens when traction is applied to the first metatarsal, making it easier to palpate.

The course of the tendon of the tibialis anterior muscle aids in palpation of the joint because the tendon runs right to the joint space.

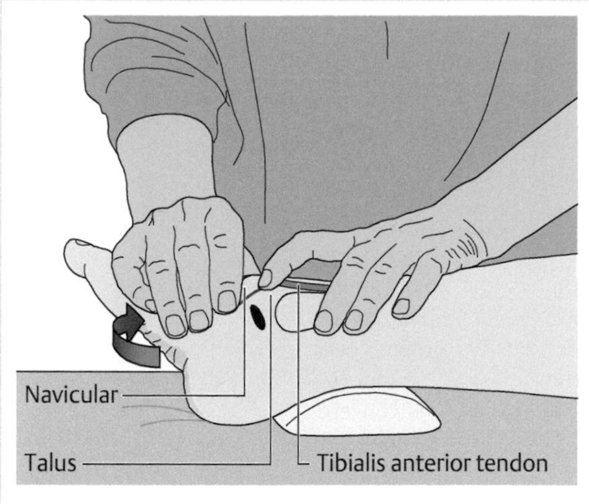


**Fig. 10.3** Palpation of the joint space between the navicular bone and the head of the talus.

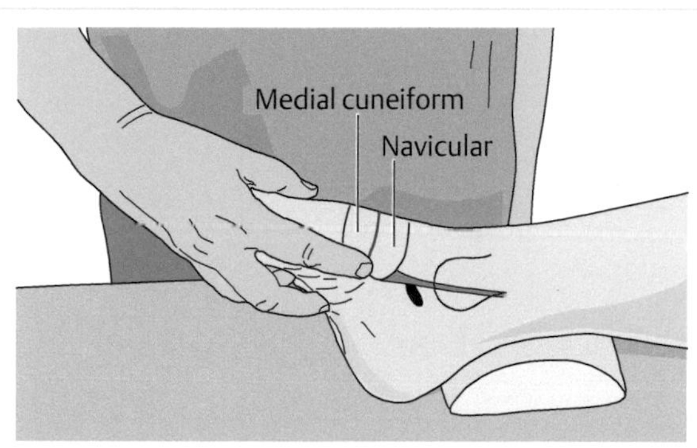


**Fig. 10.4** Palpation of the joint space between the navicular and the medial cuneiform.

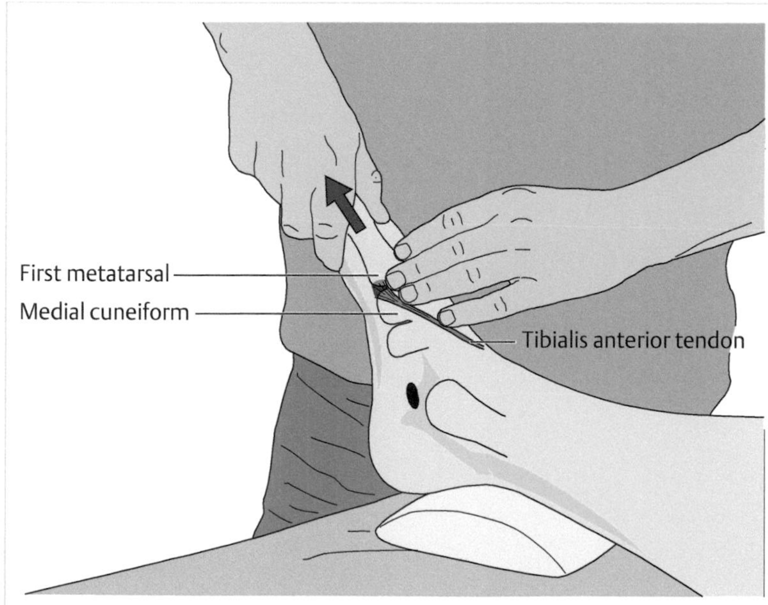


**Fig. 10.5** Palpation of the joint space between the medial cuneiform and the base of the first metatarsal.

## First Metatarsophalangeal Joint (Fig. 10.6)

Palpate the joint space between the first metatarsal and the first proximal phalanx approximately 1 cm proximal to the toe crease that is produced by extension.

By grasping the toe distally and applying traction, the examiner can now better identify the widened joint space between the two parts of the joint.

### *Orientation Guide for the Medial Ankle Region (Fig. 10.7)*

After passively bringing the foot to maximum dorsiflexion, place the index, middle, and ring fingers across the dorsum of the foot just in front of the ankle mortise. The ring finger corresponds to the width of the talar head, the middle finger to the navicular bone, and the index finger to the medial cuneiform.

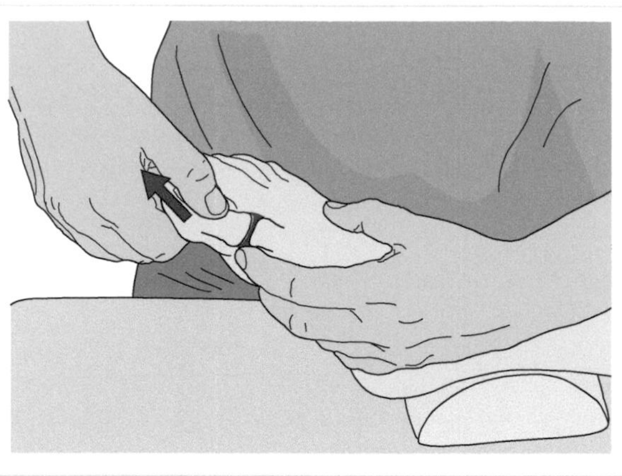

**Fig. 10.6** Palpation of the joint space between the first metatarsal and the first proximal phalanx.

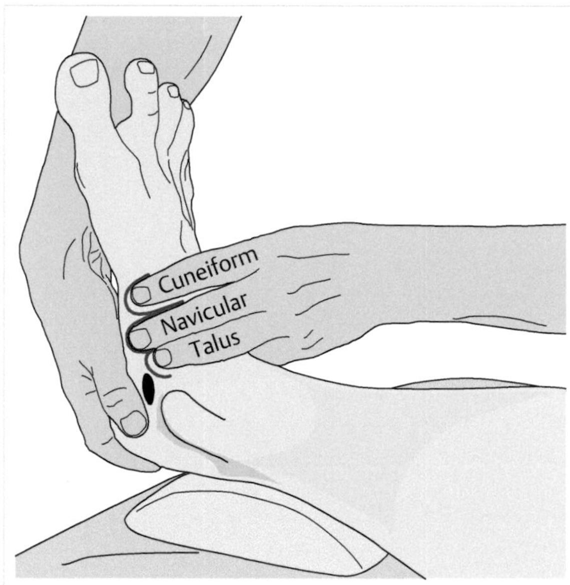


**Fig. 10.7** Orientation guide for the medial tarsal bones.

## Plantar Calcaneonavicular Ligament (Fig. 10.8)

This ligament runs from the sustentaculum anteriorly to the inferior border of the navicular bone, and is also known as the *spring ligament*. Only its firm medial border can be palpated.

## Deltoid Ligament (Fig. 10.9)

This ligament spreads out like a fan and can be well palpated only in part because of its location under the retinaculum. It consists of four sections: two extend to the talus, one forms a connection to the navicular, and runs one to the calcaneus.

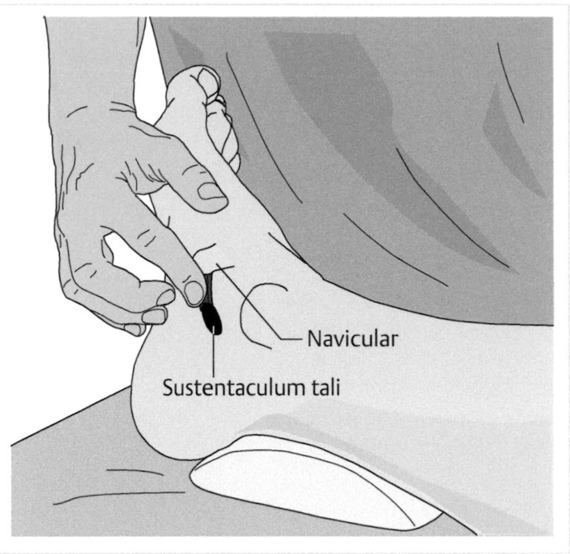


**Fig. 10.8** Palpation of the plantar calcaneonavicular ligament.

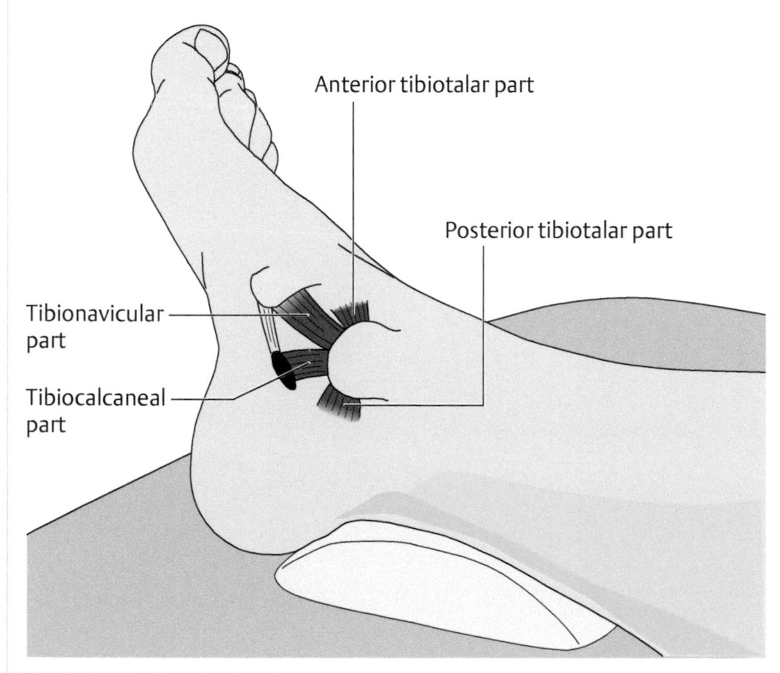


**Fig. 10.9** Palpation of the deltoid ligament.

## Anterior Tibiotalar Part (Fig. 10.10)

This ligament tracks anteriorly from the malleolus to the neck of the talus. Passively plantarflex the foot to tense the ligament and thus facilitate palpation.

## Tibionavicular Part (Fig. 10.11)

This part of the ligament tracks to the dorsal surface of the navicular and toward the navicular tuberosity. It lies directly beneath the tibialis posterior muscle. Palpation is facilitated by passive eversion because the ligament becomes taut in this position.

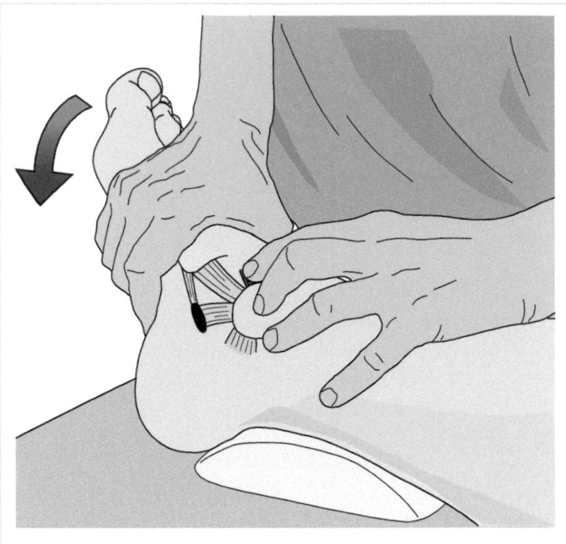

**Fig. 10.10** Palpation of the anterior tibiotalar part of the deltoid ligament.

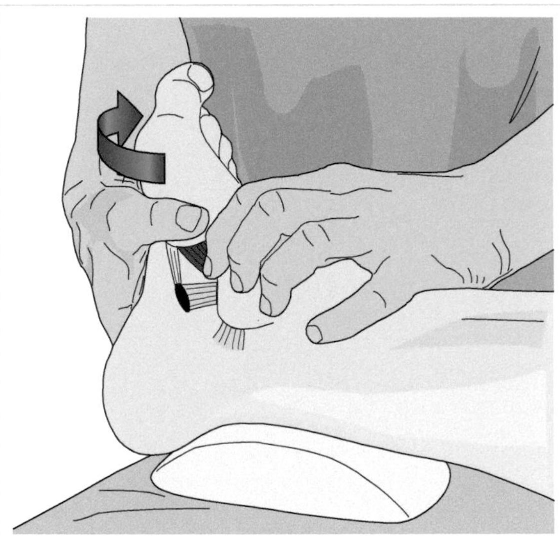

**Fig. 10.11** Palpation of the tibionavicular part of the deltoid ligament.

### Tibiocalcaneal Part (Fig. 10.12)

This ligament tracks to the sustentaculum tali and is fully covered by the flexor retinaculum. Passive eversion causes it to become taut, making it more amenable to palpation.

### Posterior Tibiotalar Part (Fig. 10.13)

The posterior part of the deltoid ligament extends to the medial tubercle of the posterior talar process. It is short and has an almost horizontal course. It is tightened by passive dorsiflexion.

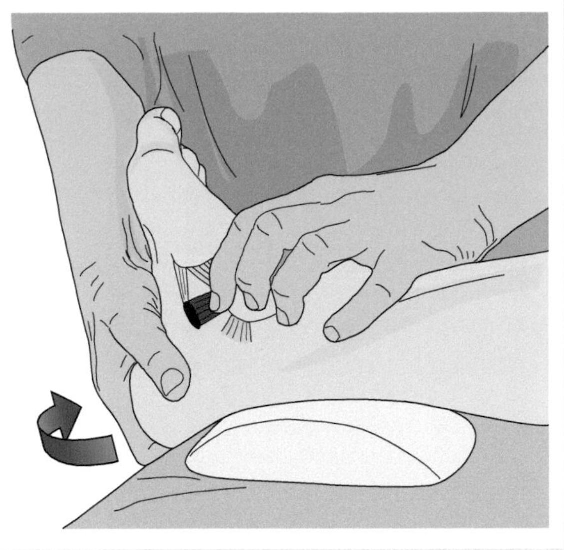

**Fig. 10.12** Palpation of the tibiocalcaneal part of the deltoid ligament.

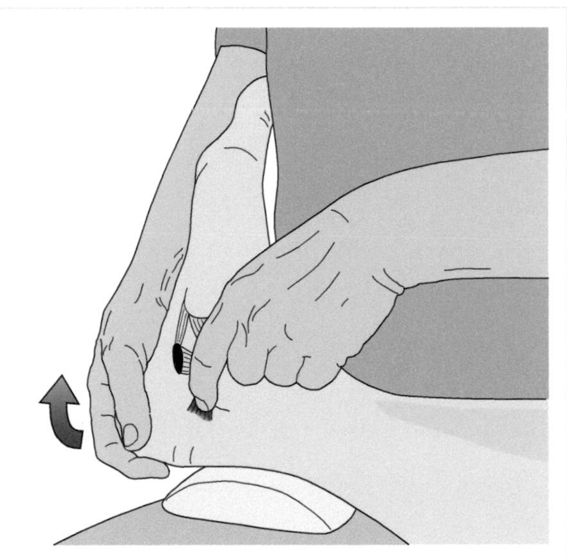

**Fig. 10.13** Palpation of the posterior tibiotalar part of the deltoid ligament.

## Tibialis Posterior Muscle (Fig. 10.14)

The tendon of this muscle lies on the posterior aspect of the medial malleolus and from there turns in an anterior direction. It runs superior to the sustentaculum toward the navicular tuberosity. Tensing toward plantarflexion and supination causes the tendon to stand out very clearly, making it accessible for palpation.

Its further course in the sole of the foot cannot be traced because of the overlying structures.

## Flexor Digitorum Longus Muscle (Fig. 10.15)

The tendon runs behind the malleolus and then turns anteriorly below it. The sustentaculum has a longitudinally running groove for the tendon. It can be easily identified by tensing the toes toward flexion.

Palpation further distally cannot identify the tendon because its course lies deeper within the sole of the foot.

## Flexor Hallucis Longus Muscle

The tendon of the flexor hallucis longus muscle runs in the depths beneath the sustentaculum. Therefore it can be palpated only with difficulty in this area

Better palpation is possible at the level of the malleolus. By tensing the big toe toward flexion, the tendon can be identified here as the most posteriorly extending structure.

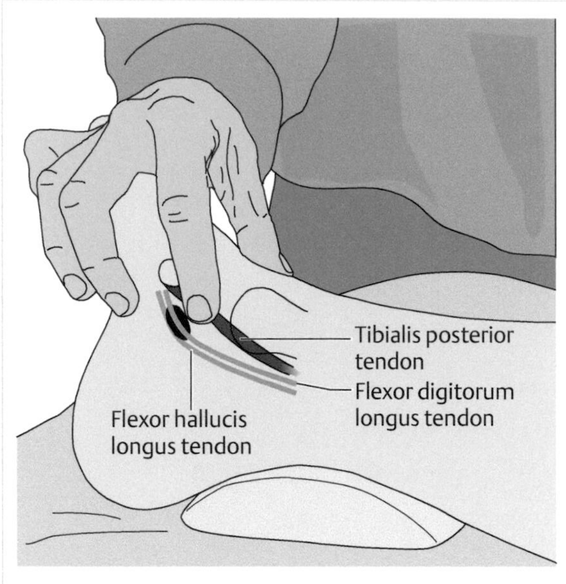


**Fig. 10.14** Palpation of the tibialis posterior muscle.

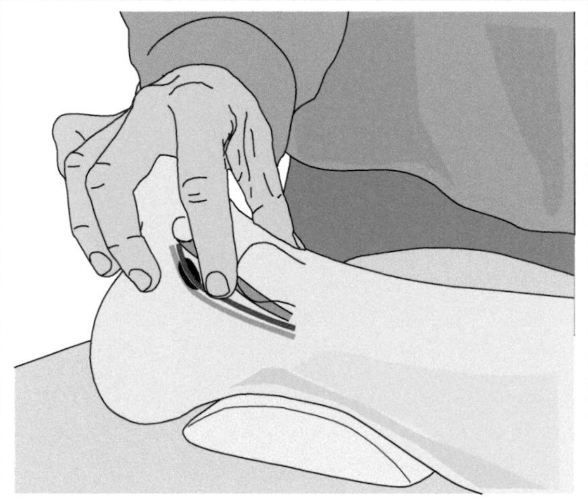

**Fig. 10.15** Palpation of the flexor digitorum longus muscle.

### Posterior Tibial Artery

The examiner can palpate the pulse of the posterior tibial artery between the posterior edge of the malleolus and the Achilles tendon. The artery runs between the tendons of the flexor digitorum and hallucis longus muscles.

A mnemonic to help learn the tendons in the area of the malleolus, from anterior to posterior, is as follows (adapted from Dos Winkel; **Fig. 10.16**):

- *Tom* = tibialis **po**sterior **m**uscle.
- *Dick* = flexor **di**gitorum longus muscle.
- *and* = posterior tibial **a**rtery, tibial **n**erve.
- *Harry* = flexor **ha**llucis longus muscle.

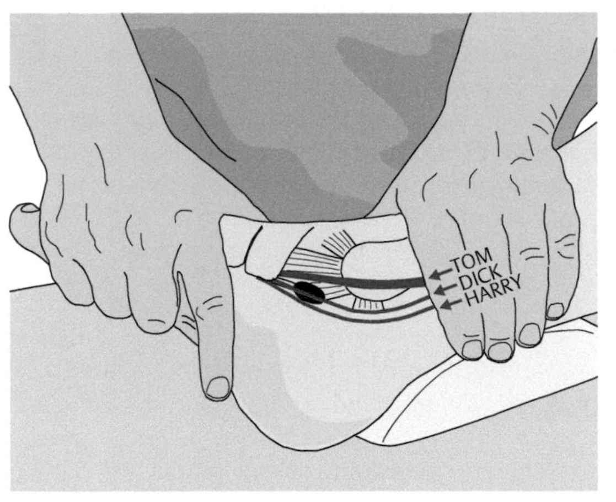


**Fig. 10.16** Palpation: mnemonic to help learn the courses of the tendons in the malleolar area.

## 10.1.2 Dorsum of the Foot

### Joint Space of the Ankle Joint (Fig. 10.17)

Approaching from proximally, place the fingertips right in front of the edge of the tibia. While passively moving the foot in plantarflexion, the broad trochlea of the talus moves distinctly against the palpating finger, only to disappear again during dorsiflexion.

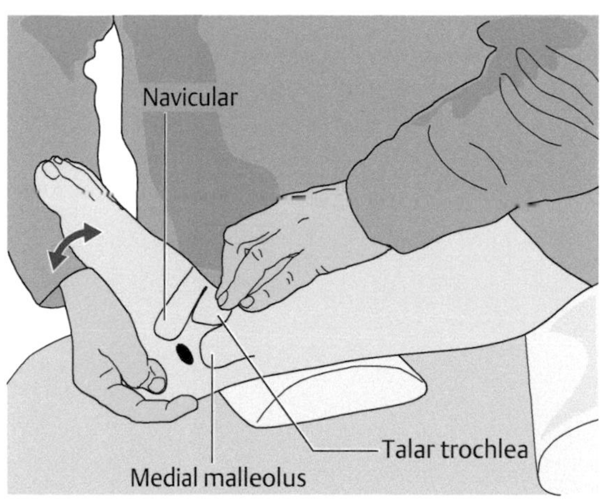


**Fig. 10.17** Palpation of the joint space of the upper ankle joint (talocrural joint).

## Tibialis Anterior Muscle (Fig. 10.18)

Its tendon is the most distinctly projecting tendon on the medial aspect of the dorsum of the foot. It tracks to the joint space of the first tarsometatarsal joint and can be easily identified. Tension in the direction of dorsiflexion and supination brings it out clearly for palpation.

## Extensor Hallucis Longus Muscle (Fig. 10.19)

Its tendon can be palpated just lateral to the tendon of the tibialis anterior muscle. It can be very well seen and palpated when tensed in the direction of extension of the big toe.

## Dorsalis Pedis Artery (Fig. 10.20)

The artery lies between the tendons of the extensor hallucis longus and extensor digitorum longus. It is subcutaneous, so the pulse is easily felt.

It may be absent in 12 to 15% of cases.

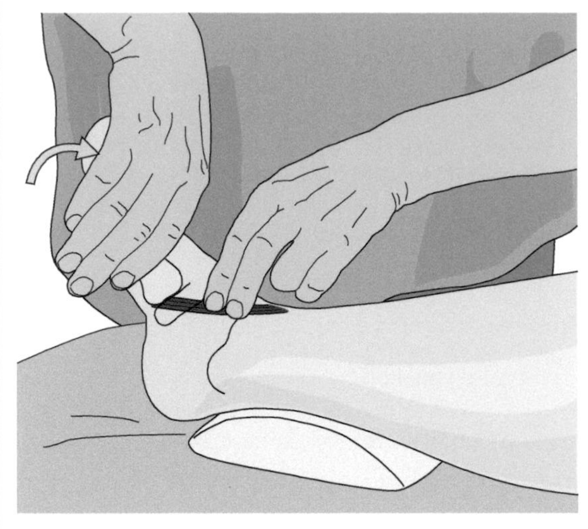

**Fig. 10.18** Palpation of the tibialis anterior tendon.

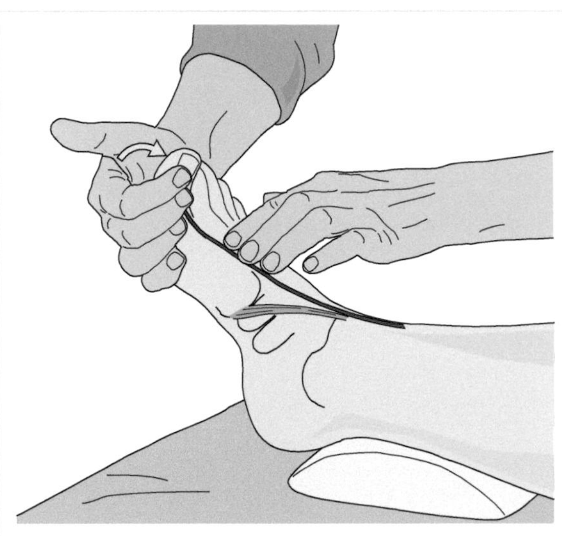

**Fig. 10.19** Palpation of the extensor hallucis longus tendon.

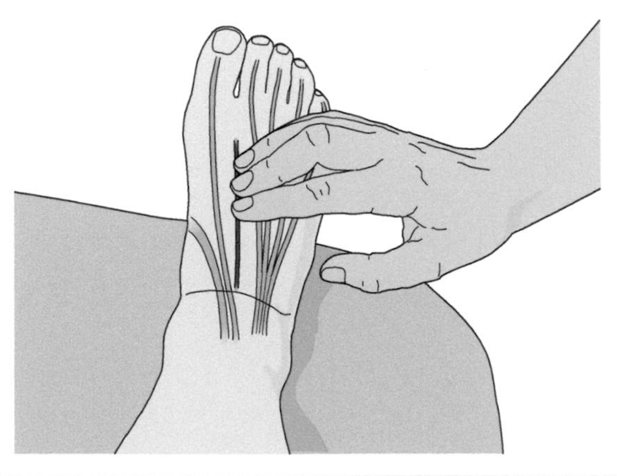

**Fig. 10.20** Palpation of the dorsalis pedis artery.

## Extensor Digitorum Longus Muscle (Fig. 10.21)

Its tendon lies the furthest laterally. Under the extensor retinaculum, it divides into its four bands, which lead to the distal phalanges. If resistance is applied to toe extension, the individual components stand out distinctly.

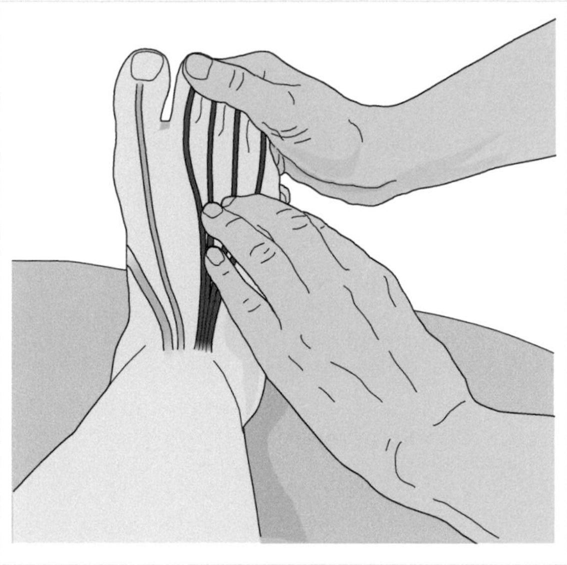

Fig. 10.21 Palpation of the extensor digitorum longus tendon.

## Further Articulations (Fig. 10.22)

Articulations in the dorsum of the foot are very difficult to palpate. Therefore, help with orientation is needed:

- The articular connection between the medial and intermediate cuneiform can be found by following the space between the first and second metatarsal further proximally. The intermediate cuneiform is substantially smaller than the medial or lateral cuneiform, because the second metatarsal is longer.
- The space between the second and third metatarsals serves as a guide to find the articulation of the intermediate and lateral cuneiforms.
- Extend the line through the space between the third and fourth metatarsals to find the joint space between the navicular and cuboid bone, and that between the lateral cuneiform and the cuboid.
- Find the tarsometatarsal joints by palpating along the metatarsals from distal to proximal. The joint space with the tarsal bones is located immediately proximal to the projecting bases of the metatarsals. Applying traction on the metatarsal makes the joint space wider and thus easier to palpate.

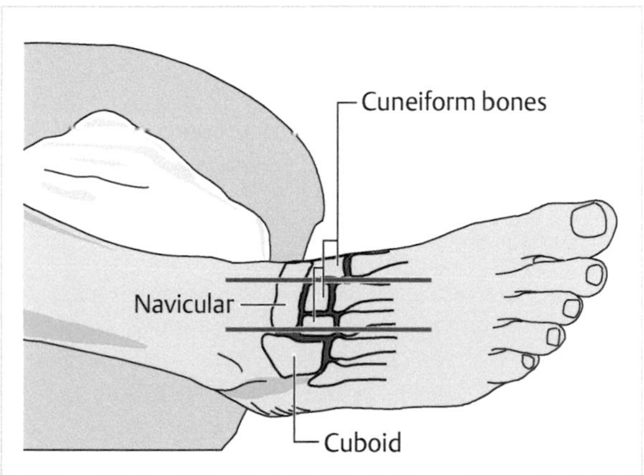


Fig. 10.22 Palpation of the articulations in the midfoot.

## 10.1.3 Lateral Region of the Foot and Ankle

### Lateral Malleolus

The lateral malleolus is located further posterior than the medial malleolus and extends further distally. Thus, there is an inclination of the ankle mortise of 15° inferolaterally. This is particularly evident when the examiner grasps both malleoli between the thumb and index finger and draws an imaginary line between the two.

### Tarsal Sinus (Fig. 10.23)

There is a recess that lies anterior to the malleolus and lateral to the neck of the talus.

Distally, this sinus contains the extensor digitorum brevis muscle. Proximally, the calcaneus can be well palpated here. The joint line between the calcaneus and cuboid runs inferiorly and slightly distally.

Part of the bifurcate ligament extends over the dorsal part of this joint space (**Fig. 10.24**). The ligament is easier to palpate if it is tensed by tilting the cuboid upward. The other part of the ligament tracks to the navicular bone, so that the palpating finger only needs to be shifted slightly toward the medial dorsum of the foot.

The lateral side of the talar neck is located medial to this. Deep in this area is the talocalcaneal interosseous ligament, which is very difficult to palpate.

### Cuboid Bone

It should be noted that the base of the fifth metatarsal extends very far laterally, and only about one-third of it has contact with the cuboid. Another aid in orientation is the extensor digitorum brevis with its surrounding gliding tissue, which is seen as a distinct thickening over the lateral dorsum of the foot and often has a bluish sheen. Palpate the cuboid bone under this cushion.

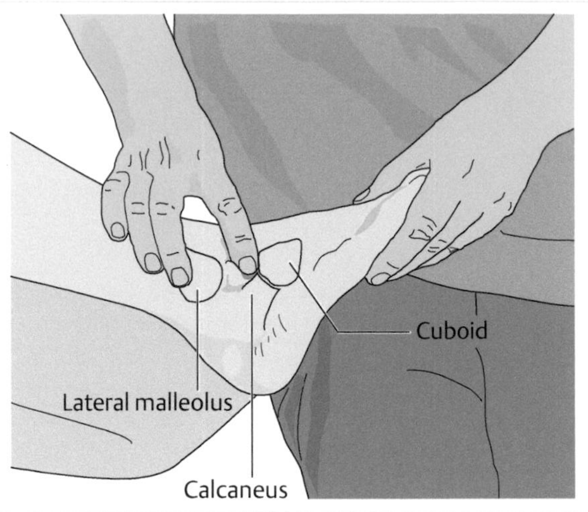


**Fig. 10.23** Palpation of the tarsal sinus.

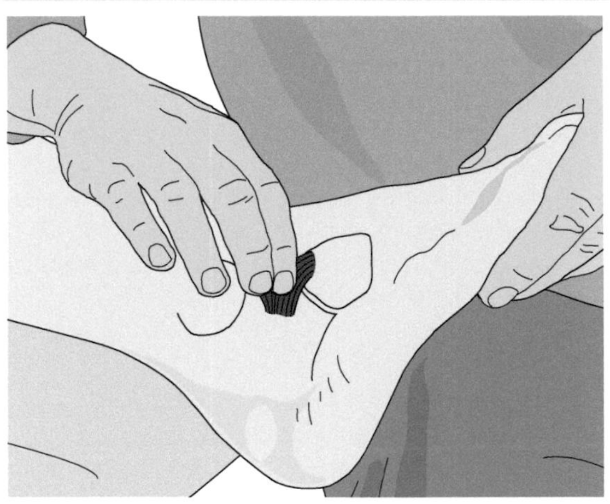

**Fig. 10.24** Palpation of the bifurcate ligament.

## Anterior Talofibular Ligament (Fig. 10.25)

This ligament can be palpated just anterior to the lateral malleolus. It tracks to the neck of the talus. Plantarflexion coupled with inversion tenses it, making it easier to palpate.

## Calcaneofibular Ligament (Fig. 10.26)

Inferior to the tip of the malleolus, the ligament extends posteriorly and slightly inferiorly to the calcaneus. It comes under tension through passive inversion.

## Posterior Talofibular Ligament (Fig. 10.27)

With a horizontal course, the ligament extends from the malleolus to the lateral tubercle of the posterior talar process. Dorsiflexion combined with inversion puts the ligament under tension.

### Practical Tip

By putting these ligamentous structures under stress while examining them, an unstable ligament is conspicuous due to excessive gapping. In addition, there is lack of tautness on palpation. In contrast, when a ligament is torn, one searches in vain for a structure that connects the malleolus with the corresponding tarsal bone.

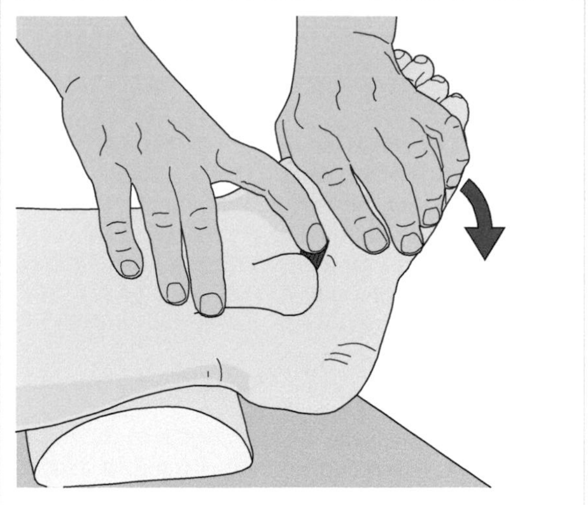

**Fig. 10.25** Palpation of the anterior talofibular ligament.

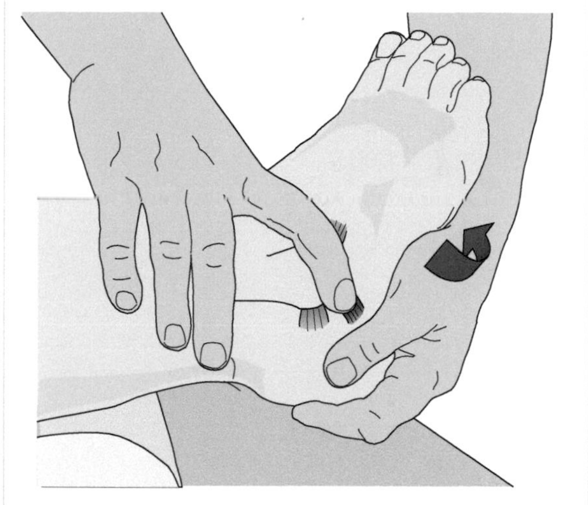

**Fig. 10.26** Palpation of the calcaneofibular ligament.

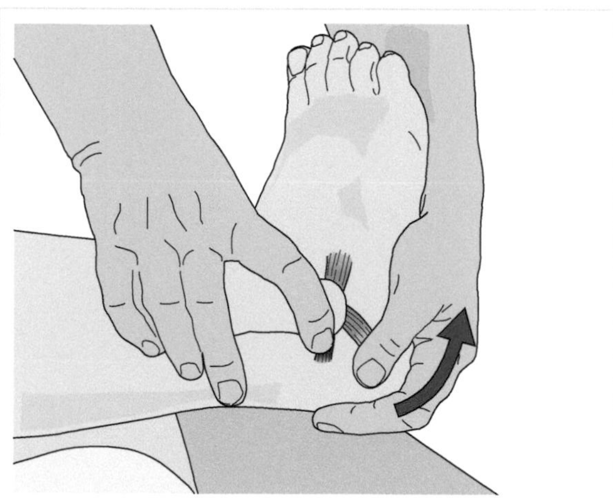

**Fig. 10.27** Palpation of the posterior talofibular ligament.

## Fibular Trochlea (Fig. 10.28)

A bony elevation can be palpated on the calcaneus inferior and slightly anterior to the lateral tip of the malleolus.

This trochlea separates the two fibular tendons. The tendon of the fibularis brevis muscle passes above the trochlea, while that of the fibularis longus muscle passes below it. A retinaculum holds them to the trochlea, and, in addition, they are enveloped in a tendon sheath. Therefore, the tendons are not as easy to palpate in this area as they are during their course before and after it.

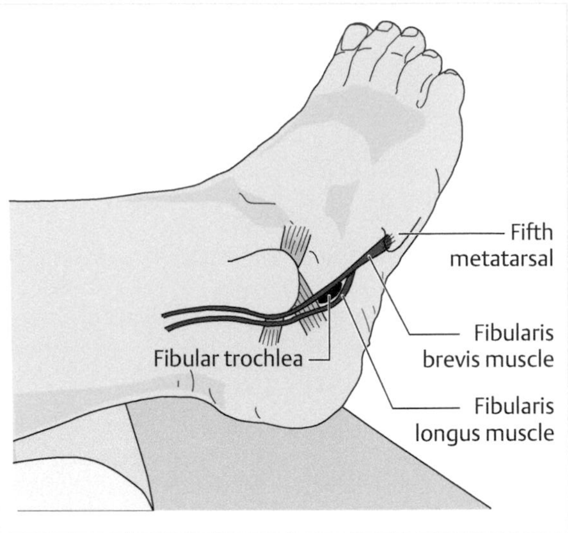


**Fig. 10.28** Palpation of the fibular trochlea and the course of the fibular muscle tendons.

## Fibularis Brevis Muscle (Fig. 10.29)

In the area of the malleolus, the tendon of the fibularis brevis muscle runs in a groove, which it uses as a fulcrum as it turns anteriorly. From here on, its further course is superficial as it runs toward the tuberosity of the fifth metatarsal bone.

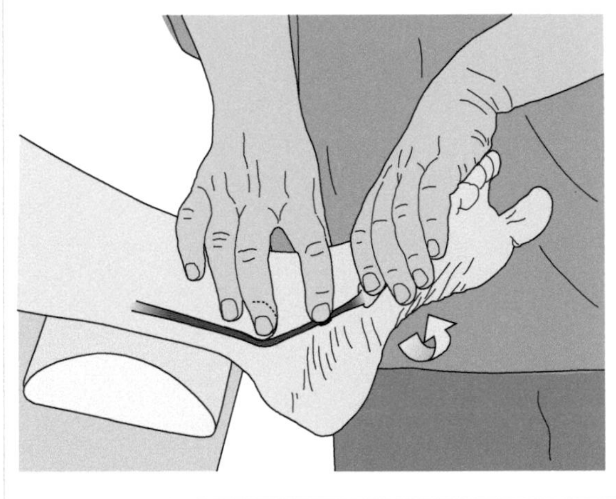

**Fig. 10.29** Palpation of the fibularis brevis tendon.

## Fibularis Longus Muscle (Fig. 10.30)

In its course around the malleolus, the tendon lies superior to that of the fibularis brevis muscle. Its further course inferior to the trochlea and its turn under the cuboid bone to the sole of the foot are easy to palpate. It is not possible to palpate its insertions on the plantar metatarsal bases and on the cuneiform because of the overlying soft tissues.

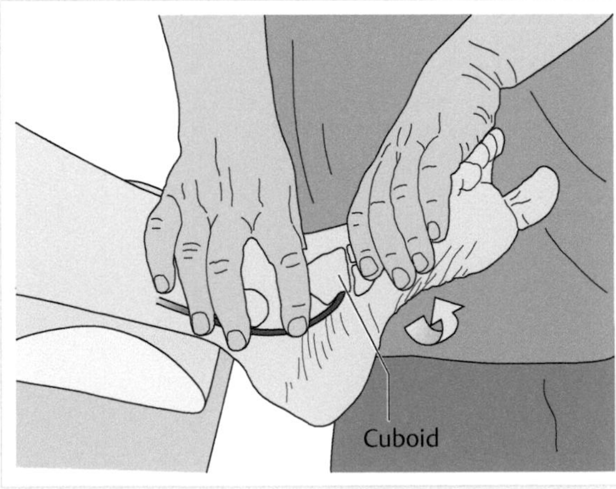


**Fig. 10.30** Palpation of the fibularis longus tendon.

## 10.1.4 Heel

### Achilles Tendon (Figs. 10.31 and 10.32)

The Achilles tendon is palpated in various positions:

- Palpation begins proximally at the musculotendinous junction at about the middle of the lower leg. Palpate this part transverse to the fiber orientation. Tensing the muscle toward plantarflexion brings out the transition area more clearly.
- The next area to palpate is approximately 2 to 3 fingerbreadths proximal to the insertion on the calcaneal tuberosity. Examine this area transverse to the fiber orientation and longitudinally along the tendon tissue, looking for roughness, indentations, and tenderness. This is the area of the Achilles tendon that is prone to tears.

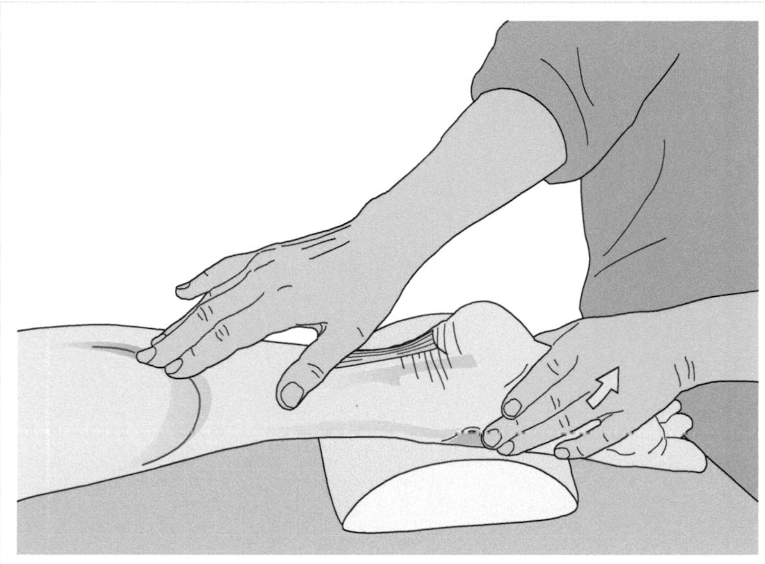

**Fig. 10.31** Palpation of the musculotendinous junction of the gastrocnemius muscle.

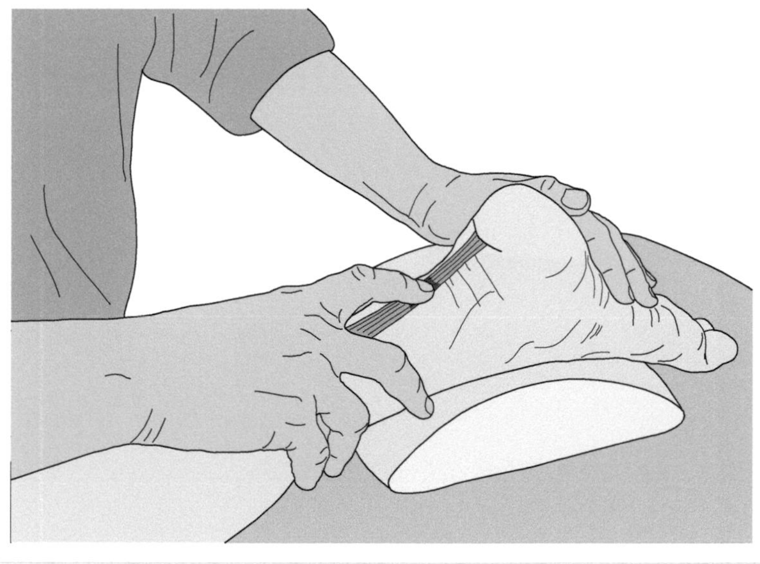

**Fig. 10.32** Palpation of the area of the Achilles tendon that is prone to injury.

- Check longitudinally along the medial and lateral borders of the Achilles tendon (**Fig. 10.33**).
- The insertion on the calcaneal tuberosity, however, should be palpated across the fiber orientation.

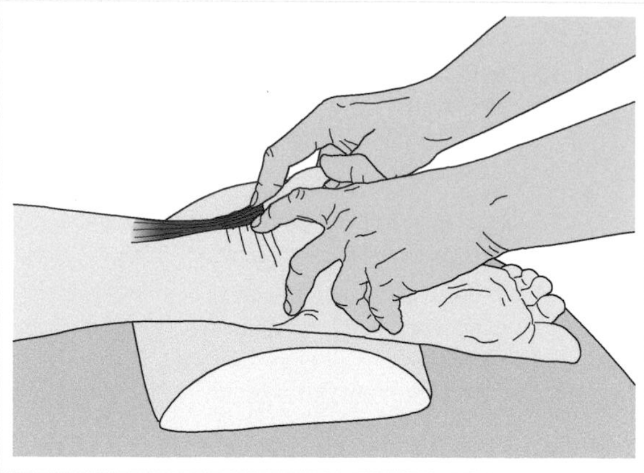

**Fig. 10.33** Palpation of the medial and lateral borders of the Achilles tendon.

**Practical Tip**

**Rupture**

When partial or complete rupture of the Achilles tendon occurs, the torn surfaces are not smooth to palpation, but much more likely demonstrate significant fraying of the tendon parts. In addition, the defect is painful on palpation.

Patients who sustain a complete rupture of the tendon describe it as a blow to the calf, associated with pain and a popping noise. The immediate deficit in the calf muscle is striking.

## Calcaneal Bursae

There are two bursae in the immediate vicinity of the insertion. The *bursa of the calcaneal tendon* lies between the Achilles tendon and the calcaneus. The *subcutaneous calcaneal bursa* lies between the skin and the tendon.

**Pathology**

**Bursitis**

Both bursae can become inflamed by tight shoes, hard heel counters, kick injuries, or other similar causes.

## 10.1.5 Plantar Surface (Fig. 10.34)

The formation of calluses on the sole of the foot indicates whether or not an individual rolls off the foot normally.

These calluses are visible on inspection. On palpation, they appear as coarse areas of induration in the skin.

### Calcaneal Tuberosity

There are two bony prominences on the plantar aspect of the calcaneal tuberosity: the medial and lateral processes. It is important to palpate these because the origins of the plantar fascia and the toe abductors are located here.

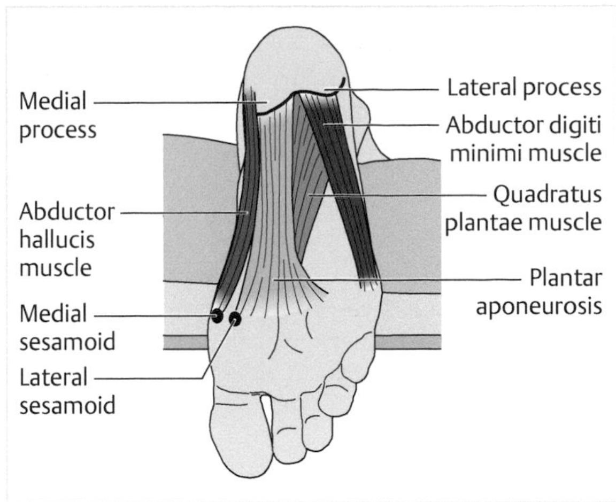


**Fig. 10.34** Palpation of the plantar surface.

### Plantar Aponeurosis (Fig. 10.35)

This is a tough fascial plate that is very firm to palpation in the center of the plantar surface, but becomes softer as one moves medially and laterally. It spreads out in a V shape as it moves toward the toes.

Palpate the entire surface lengthwise and crosswise looking for warts, bumps, and tender points. Likewise, evaluate for changes in tonicity in both the relaxed and tensed states.

> **Pathology**
>
> **Warts**
>
> Plantar warts are palpated as small circumscribed, pin-head-sized keratotic areas. They develop preferentially on areas of the plantar surface exposed to increased weight-bearing, and are very painful on weight-bearing.

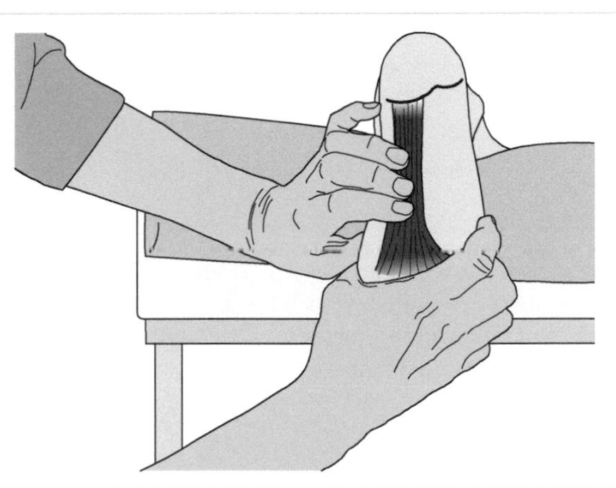

**Fig. 10.35** Palpation of the plantar aponeurosis.

### Abductor Hallucis Muscle (Fig. 10.36)

The belly of the muscle can be palpated at the medial border of the foot, immediately adjacent to the plantar aponeurosis, especially while abducting the big toe against resistance.

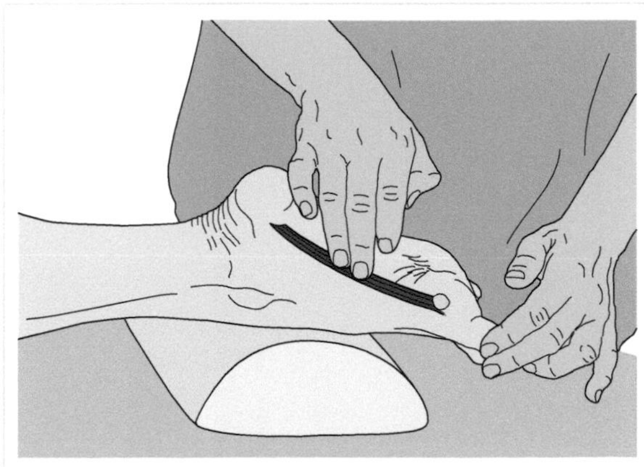

**Fig. 10.36** Palpation of the abductor hallucis muscle.

## Abductor Digiti Minimi Muscle (Fig. 10.37)

This borders the lateral edge of the foot and runs immediately adjacent to the plantar aponeurosis. The narrow muscle belly can be easily located by splaying the toes apart.

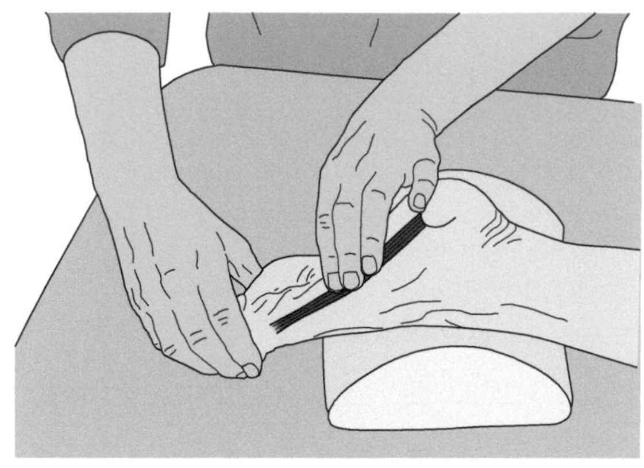

**Fig. 10.37** Palpation of the abductor digiti minimi muscle.

## Metatarsal Heads (Fig. 10.38)

Evaluate the plantar surfaces of the metatarsal heads for callous formation and painfulness.

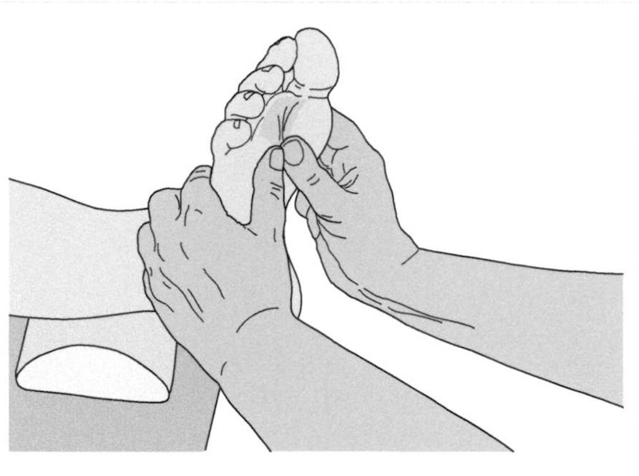

**Fig. 10.38** Palpation of the second and third metatarsal heads.

### Pathology

**Splayfoot**

In splayfoot, palpation can demonstrate significant thickening and hardening over the heads of the second and third metatarsals. Because the transverse arch sags, the heads have too much contact with the ground, and are thus subject to too much pressure, leading to callous formation.

The most prominent area—the first metatarsal head and first metatarsophalangeal (MTP) joint—is where hallux valgus occurs.

## Sesamoid Bones

These thickenings in the plantar area of the first metatarsal head are normal. They are the two sesamoid bones that are embedded in the medial and lateral heads of the flexor hallucis brevis muscle.

### Pathology

**Sesamoiditis**

Load-dependent pressure sensitivity over the sesamoid bones suggests a disorder caused by overstressing the tendons leading to the sesamoid bones (sesamoiditis). To relieve the sesamoid bones during the process of pushing-off, an insert is made with a padded recess for the sensitive area.

**Splayfoot**

Splaying of the metatarsals can cause swelling on the medial side of the metatarsal head. As a result of pressure and friction, bursitis can develop here, which is extremely painful.

**Morton's Neuroma (Fig. 10.39)**

This is a scar tissue thickening of the third proper plantar digital nerve that is entrapped between the third and fourth metatarsal heads. As a result of pressure, microtraumatization of the nerve develops. A neuroma develops in response to repeated lesions. Complaints occur primarily when walking in tight shoes because the metatarsal heads are pressed together. As a provocation test, compress the forefoot together from side to side, which causes piercing pain.

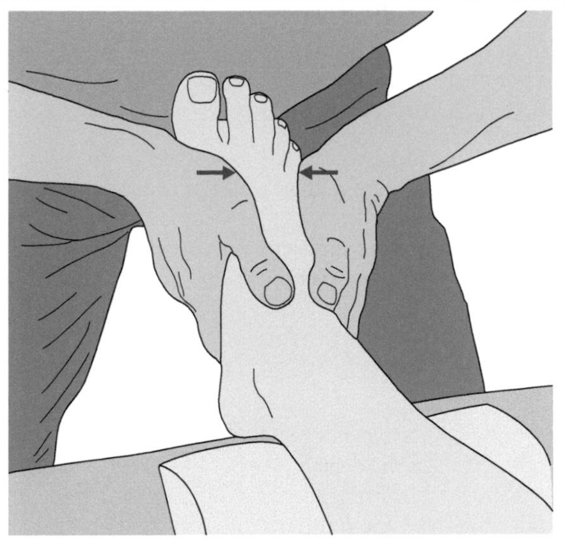

**Fig. 10.39** Compression of the metatarsal heads for suspected Morton's neuroma.

▷ See Chapter 10.15, Neural Structures of the Foot and Ankle

# 10.2 X-Ray Image

## 10.2.1 Anteroposterior View (Fig. 10.40)

The standard radiographs are performed in the neutral position, i.e., with the patient standing or sitting with the foot forward on the floor.

This anteroposterior view of the ankle provides a good overview of the position of the talus in the ankle mortise. Because of the superposition of the subtalar bones, evaluation further distally is not possible.

To assess the joint position, the following angles are determined:

- *Lateral distal tibial angle*: approximately 92°. The angle is formed by the axis of the tibial shaft and a line that is placed on the top of the talar trochlea. It is close to a right angle.
- *Tibial angle:* 50–65°. The trochlea line forms an angle with a line along the tibial malleolar articular surface, which is open inferiorly.

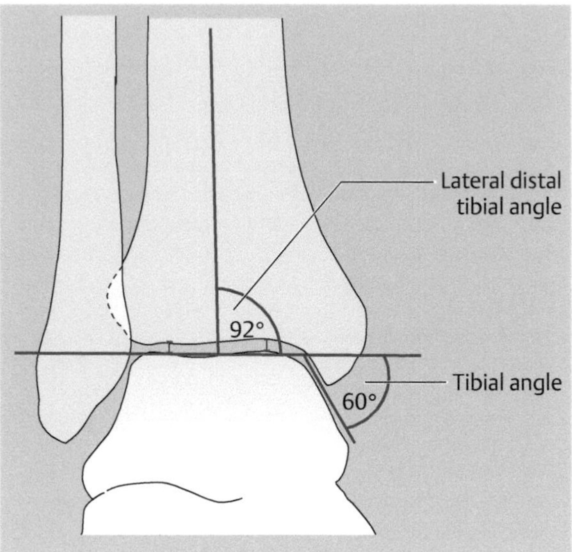


**Fig. 10.40** X-ray image: anteroposterior view.

### *Further Evaluation*

- *Joint space width* of the ankle joint: uniform width of approximately 3 mm.
- *Configuration of the ankle mortise:* The tip of the fibula protrudes approximately 1 to 1.5 cm further distally than the tibia.
- The articulating joint surfaces are smooth and sharply defined.
- There is a normal arrangement of the trabeculae.

## 10.2.2 Lateral View (Fig. 10.41)

### *Evaluation*

- *Upper ankle joint* (talocrural joint):
  - Joint space width: 3 to 4 mm.
  - Contours of the talar trochlea and the distal tibia: smooth and uniform.
- *Position of the talus:* talus–floor angle: 20 to 25°. Extend the longitudinal axis through the talar neck and head anteriorly down to the floor; the angle formed opens posteriorly.
- *Lower ankle joint* (subtalar and talocalcaneonavicular joints):
  - Inspection of the tarsal canal: round or oval shape.
  - Joint space between the talus and navicular: approximately 2 mm.
- *Position of the calcaneus:*
  - Calcaneus–floor angle: approximately 40°. The longitudinal axis of the calcaneus forms an angle with the floor that opens anteriorly.
  - Tuberosity–joint angle: 30 to 40°. This angle, open posteriorly, is formed between the tangent that is placed on the upper edge of the calcaneal tuberosity and a line that goes through the subtalar joint space.

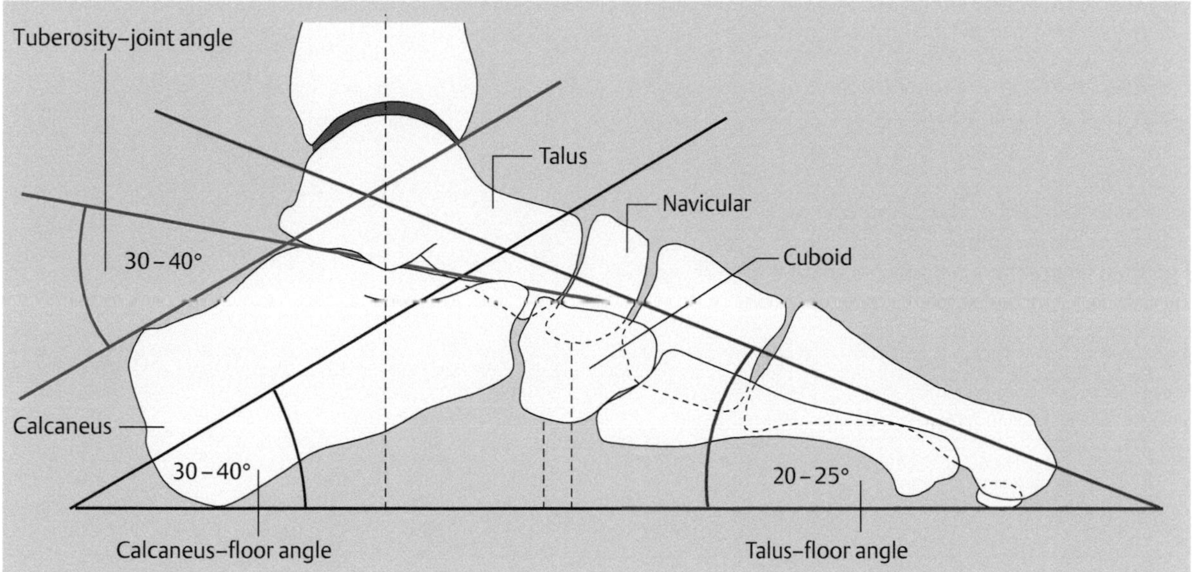


**Fig. 10.41** X-ray image: lateral view.

## 10.2.3 Dorsal-Plantar View (Fig. 10.42)

This view displays the midfoot and toe regions very well.

The following angles provide information about the positions of the bones in relation to each other:

- Angle between the *axis of the talus* and the *axis of the calcaneus:* 20 to 30°. The talar neck axis forms an angle with the longitudinal axis of the calcaneus, which is open distally.
- *Intermetatarsal angle:* less than 8°. The longitudinal axes of the first and second metatarsals together form an angle that should not be greater than 8° (see **Fig. 10.147**).
- *Valgus angle of the first MTP joint:* less than 20°. A distally open angle is formed between the longitudinal axis of the first metatarsal and the longitudinal axis of the first proximal phalanx.

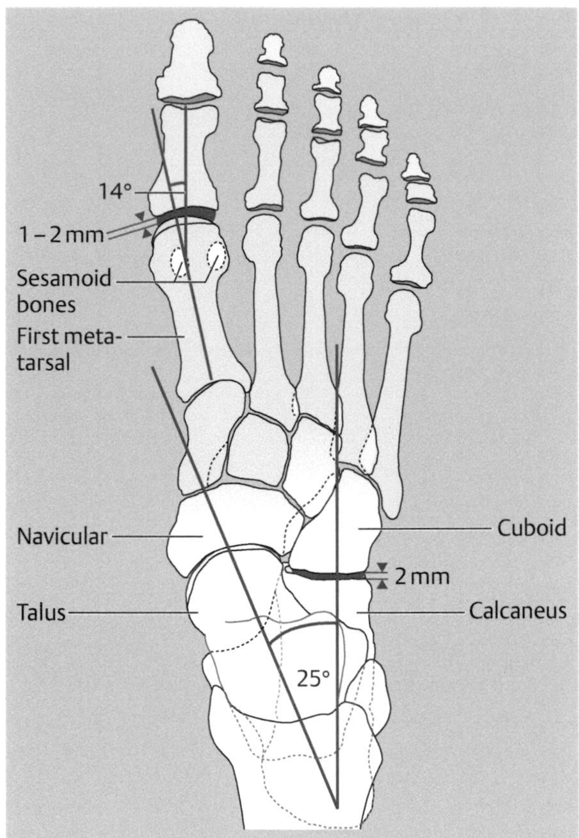


**Fig. 10.42** X-ray image: dorsal-plantar view.

### *Further Evaluation*

- *Joint space widths* of the intertarsal, metatarsal, tarsometatarsal, MTP, and interphalangeal joints: 1.5 to 2.5 mm.
- *Sesamoid bones* present as compressed oval areas at the level of the metatarsal heads. The medial sesamoid is shifted slightly more to the middle. The lateral sesamoid lies away from the longitudinal axis.

## 10.2.4 Stress Views (Figs. 10.43 and 10.44)

If a ruptured ligament is suspected, the degree of gapping of the upper ankle joint is determined using stress views.

This technique has recently been utilized less and less because ultrasound and magnetic resonance imaging places significantly less stress on the affected structures.

### *Assessment of Talar Tilt*

In the anteroposterior view, placing the lower leg in slight internal rotation presents an improved view of the ankle mortise. The examiner fixes the heel, and thus the talus as well, in supination, and then pushes the distal lower leg laterally to observe the tilt between the talus and lower leg.

*Normal tilt angle:* 5°. This is increased with hypermobility, so that a side-to-side comparison is important.

**Pathology**

The magnitude of the angle of tilt can provide information on whether only the anterior talofibular ligament is torn, in which case the angle is about 10°. If the tilt angle is 15° or more, the calcaneofibular ligament and possibly the posterior talofibular ligament are injured as well. The tilting of the talus is also evident in an increased fibulotalar distance.

### *Assessment of Anterior Stability*

For the lateral view, support the heel on a small footstool and put anterior pressure on the tibia so that it moves posteriorly. On the X-ray, assess the advance of the talus in relation to the tibia in the lateral view, thus measuring the distance from the posterior border of the tibia to the trochlea.

*Normal displacement:* 2 to 4 mm bilaterally. Here again, the separation is more apparent if there is weakness of the connective tissue.

**Pathology**

(**Figs. 10.44–10.46**)

1. Talar displacement of over 7 mm for 30 seconds, using a stress force of 150 N, suggests rupture of a ligament.

2. *Syndesmosis separation* with possible medial dislocation of the talus is visible at the medial part of the joint space because this enlarges to significantly greater than 3 mm. (continued)

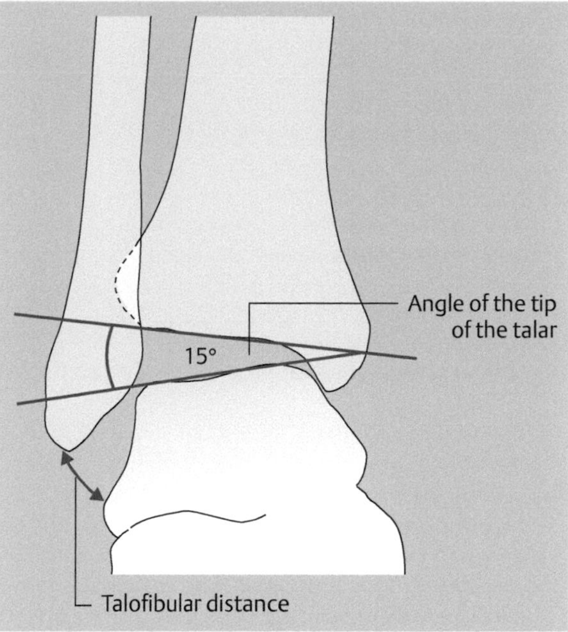


**Fig. 10.43** X-ray image: anteroposterior stress view.

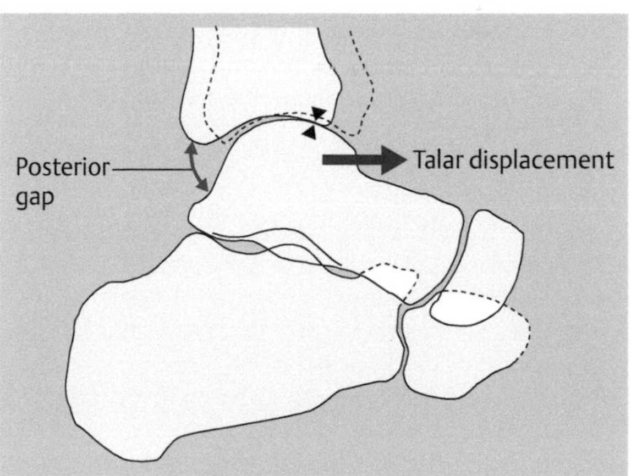


**Fig. 10.44** X-ray image: lateral stress view.

3. *Fractures:*

- *Fracture of the calcaneus* (**Fig. 10.45**): changes the tuberosity–joint angle, which can become smaller or negative by collapse of the calcaneus.
- *Weber's fracture classification:* fracture line at the level of the joint space (Weber B); fracture line above the syndesmosis (Weber C).
- *Fracture of the talar neck:* fracture line through the neck of the talus. Because of the poor blood supply and therefore an increased difficulty in fracture healing, this fracture has an unfavorable prognosis.
- Metatarsal fracture as a march fracture.
- Avulsion of the base of the fifth metatarsal, which can sometimes occur with severe distortion injuries.
- Toe fractures.

4. *Chronic polyarthritis.* Radiologic signs include joint space narrowing, marginal cortical erosions, and subchondral cysts, with late findings of deformities toward talipes valgus and hallux valgus. This primarily affects the metatarsal heads, the fifth MTP joint, and the first interphalangeal joint.

5. *Hallux valgus* (**Fig. 10.46**). The valgus angle of the first phalanx is more than 20°. The intermetatarsal angle of the first and second metatarsals is above 10°, which reflects their divergence. The first metatarsal head is displaced medially in relation to the sesamoid bones.

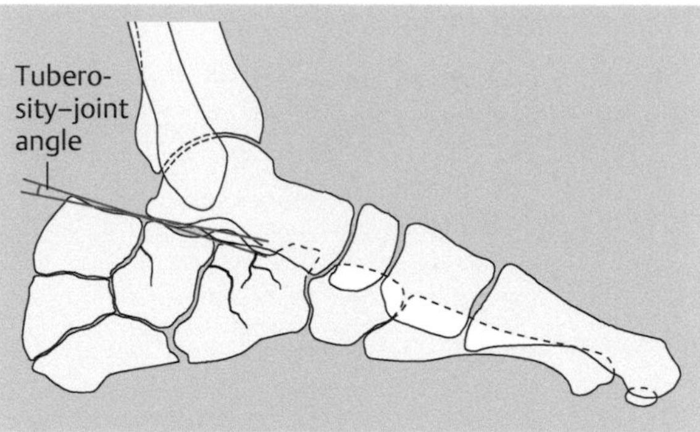


**Fig. 10.45** X-ray image: change of the tuberosity–joint angle in a calcaneal fracture.

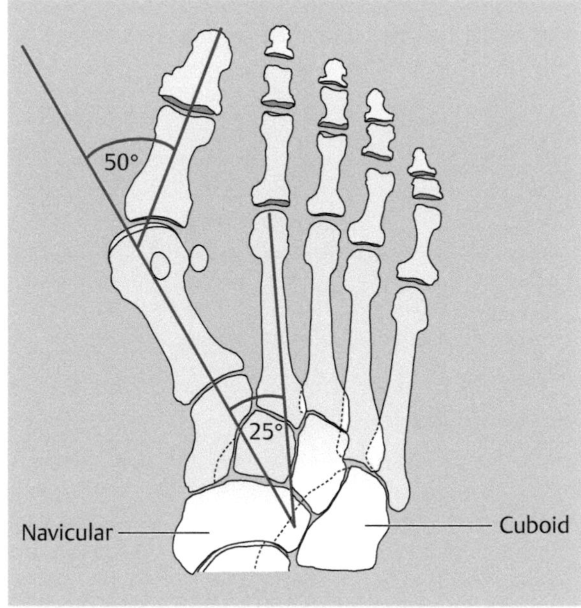


**Fig. 10.46** X-ray image: changes in hallux valgus.

### *Accessory Tarsal Bones*

These are usually partially developed ossification centers. They are inconstant and must be differentiated from fractures. Examples include:

- Accessory navicular bone (os tibiale externum): on the medial side of the navicular bone.
- Os trigonum: on the posterior process of the talus.
- Os perineum: on the dorsal-lateral edge of the cuboid bone.

## 10.2.5 MRI (Fig. 10.47)

Magnetic resonance imaging as a modern imaging technique plays a large role not only in evaluating ligamentous lesions, but also in detecting osteochondral lesions (flake fractures), since they cannot be demonstrated by conventional radiologic techniques.

Ligament injuries show up as discontinuities and thickenings and may not always be represented.

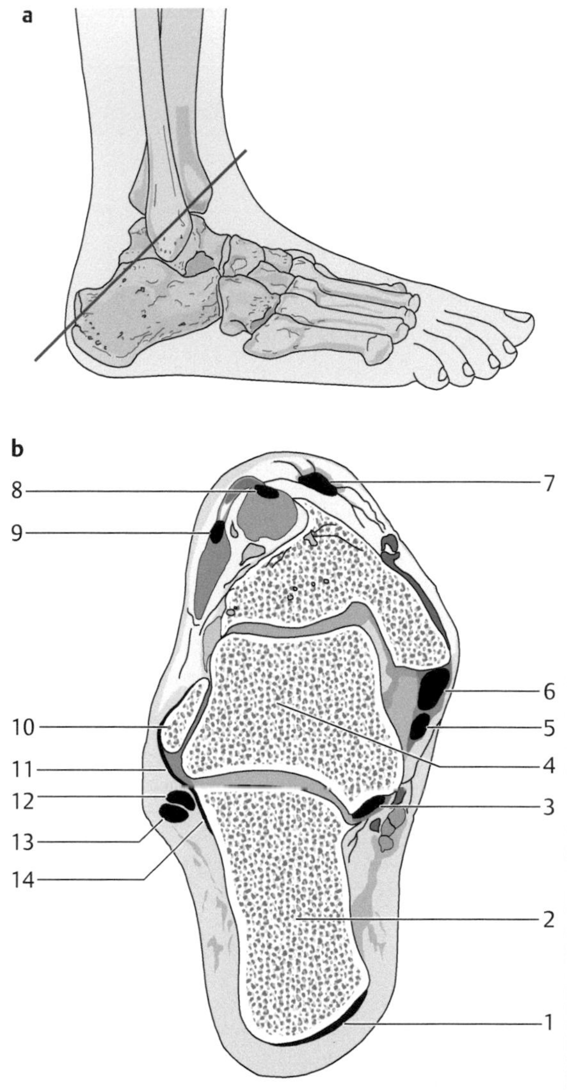


**Fig. 10.47** Magnetic resonance imaging. **(a)** Oblique axial cut. **(b)** View at the level of the calcaneofibular ligament.
1 Calcaneal (Achilles) tendon
2 Calcaneus
3 Flexor hallucis longus tendon
4 Talus
5 Flexor digitorum longus tendon
6 Tibialis posterior tendon
7 Tibialis anterior tendon
8 Extensor hallucis longus tendon
9 Extensor digitorum longus tendon
10 Lateral malleolus
11 Calcaneofibular ligament (proximal part)
12 Fibularis brevis muscle tendon
13 Fibularis longus muscle tendon
14 Calcaneofibular ligament (distal part)

# 10.3 Ankle Joint (Talocrural Joint)

## 10.3.1 Bony Structures and Joint Surfaces

### Talus (Figs. 10.48–10.50)

#### Body of the Talus

- The *talar trochlea* is located on the superior aspect of the body of the talus. It is approximately 0.5 cm wider anteriorly than posteriorly. It has three joint surfaces:
  - The *superior facet of the talar trochlea* articulates with the tibia, and is convex in shape. In the center, it features a groove that extends slightly obliquely from posteromedially to anterolaterally. The lateral border runs medially as an arc and is longer than the medial border.
  - The *medial malleolar facet* is almost flat. It articulates with the malleolar articular surfaces of the tibia. The joint plane is inclined 30° superolaterally to the sagittal plane.
  - The *lateral malleolar facet* articulates with the fibula, is concave, and has a triangular shape with the point facing inferiorly. Orientation of the articular surface: the upper section is in the sagittal plane; the inferior section is almost horizontal and lies on the *lateral process.*
  - On the posterior edge of the lateral malleolar facet is a small ridge that divides the surface into another facet, the *facet of Fawcett*, which develops as a contact point for the *posterior tibiofibular ligament*. See Chapter 10.4, Tibiofibular Joint.
- *Posterior process of the talus:* the posterior end of the body of the talus. The groove for the tendon of the flexor hallucis longus divides it into the medial intercondylar tubercle and the lateral tubercle.

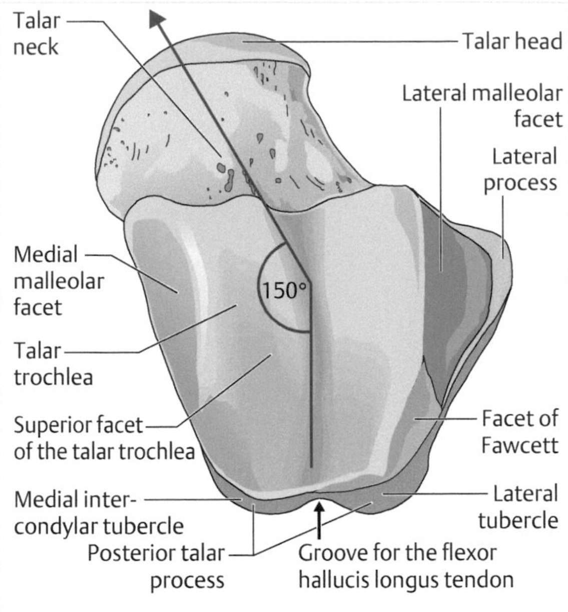


**Fig. 10.48** Talus, talar neck angle (superior view).

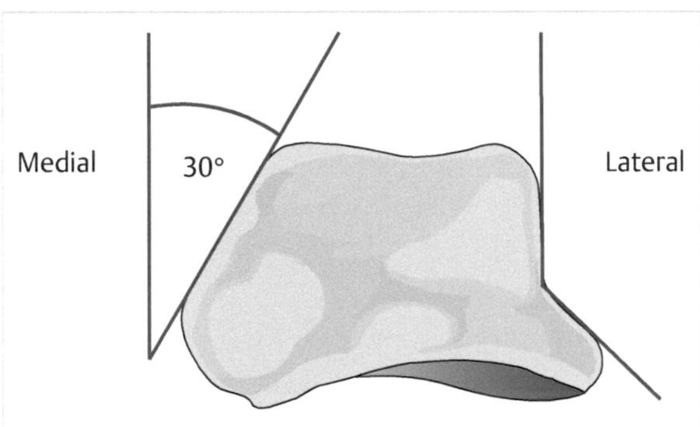


**Fig. 10.49** Position of the articular surface of the malleolar facet on the right talus (posterior view).

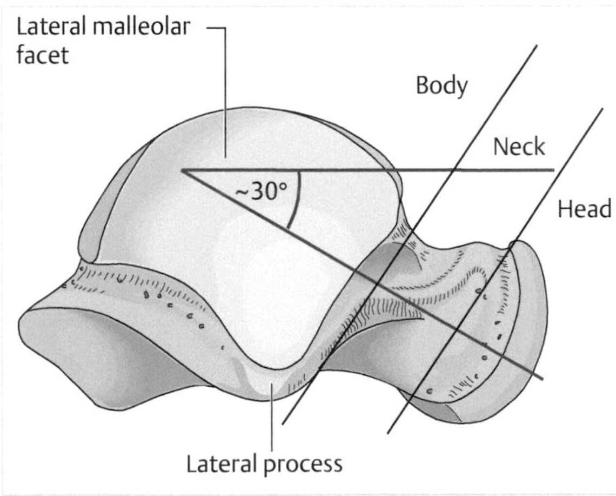


**Fig. 10.50** Talar angle of inclination (lateral view).

## Neck of the Talus

- The axis through the talar neck is directed anteromedially and forms a medial angle of 150° with the trochlear groove.
- The neck of the talus is inclined 30° inferiorly relative to a horizontal line through the body (*angle of inclination*).
- On its plantar side, it features the sulcus tali, which, together with the calcaneal sulcus, forms the tarsal canal (see **Fig. 10.78**).

## Head of the Talus

This is completely covered with cartilage and forms the articular surfaces for the navicular and calcaneus bones.

▷ See Chapter 10.5, Talotarsal Joint

### Pathology

**Osteochondritis Dissecans (Fig. 10.51)**

The most common site of this on the talus is peripherally on the medial margin. The symptoms are swelling, painful blockages, and snapping sounds in the joint with movement. In milder cases, the treatment is conservative, with immobilization and stress reduction. In more severe grades of injury, such as loose body formation, treatment is surgical—excision of the damaged area with subsequent curettage of the subchondral bone.

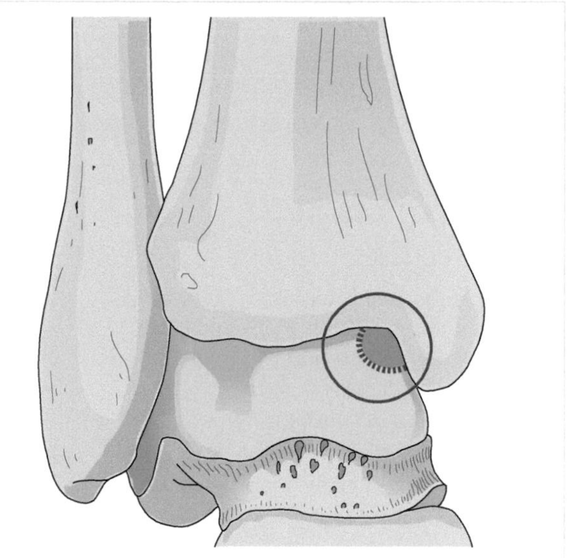

**Fig. 10.51** Osteochondritis dissecans of the talus.

## Tibia (Figs. 10.52 and 10.53)

### *Articular Facet of the Medial Malleolus*

- This is located on the inside of the medial malleolus.
- It articulates with the medial malleolar facet on the talus.
- It is inclined 30° inferomedially, corresponding to the joint surface of the talus.
- The articular surface is slightly concave to planar.
- Superiorly, the facet merges into the adjacent cartilage-covered surface of the tibia, over the talus.

### *Inferior Articular Surface of the Tibia*

- This articulates with the superior facet of the talar trochlea and is about one-third smaller.
- It has a quadrilateral, concave shape.
- A ridge in the center corresponds to the groove on the trochlea.

### *Malleolar Groove*

- This is a longitudinally running groove on the posterior side.
- It forms the floor for an osseofibrous channel in which the tendons of the tibialis posterior, flexor digitorum longus, and flexor hallucis longus muscles run.

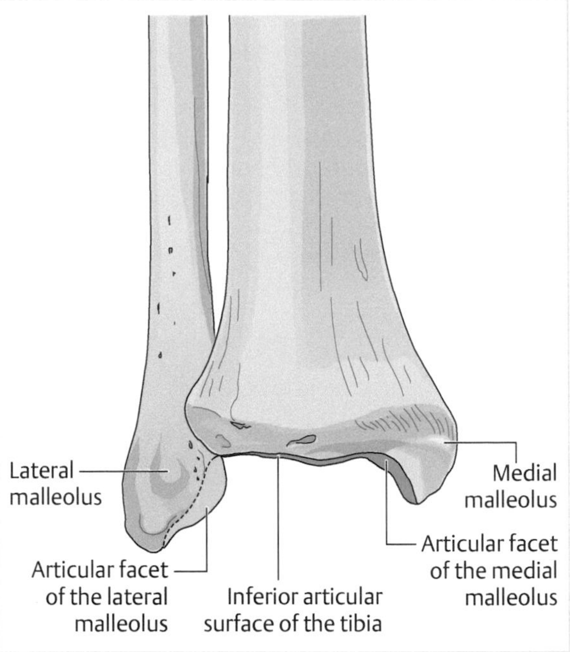


**Fig. 10.52** Distal end of the tibia and fibula (anterior view).

## Fibula (Figs. 10.52 and 10.53)

### *Articular Facet of the Lateral Malleolus*

- It is located on the inner side of the lateral malleolus.
- It articulates with the talus.
- The facet has a triangular shape; at first, it is sagittally oriented, and inferiorly almost horizontal.

### *Lateral Malleolar Fossa*

- This is a depression posterior to the articular facet of the lateral malleolus.
- It acts as the origin for the posterior talofibular ligament and the capsule.

### *Groove for the Fibular Muscle Tendons*

- This is located on the outer surface of the lateral malleolus and carries for the tendons of the fibular muscles.
- It has a cartilage-covered surface at the point where the tendons bend around.

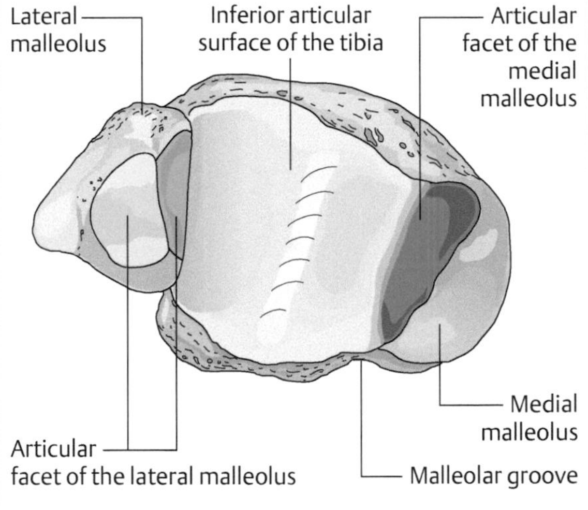


**Fig. 10.53** Articular surfaces on the distal tibia and fibula (inferior view).

## 10.3.2 Architecture of Cancellous (Trabecular) Bone (Fig. 10.54)

Posterior ***tibial trabeculae*** form a slightly concave arch extending anteriorly. The trabecular arch continues through the body, neck, and head of the talus, as well as the navicular and cuneiform bones and the first to third metatarsals.

The anterior tibial trabeculae follow a slightly concave curve that continues toward the dorsal part of the talar body and the calcaneal tuberosity.

In the *calcaneus*, compression trabeculae run from the tarsal sinus obliquely in an anteroinferior direction toward the cuboid bone.

Traction trabeculae caused by the Achilles tendon arise on the posteroinferior part of the calcaneal tuberosity.

In addition, because of the traction effect of the long plantar ligament, there are resultant trajectories extending obliquely in a posterosuperior direction, and, from the plantar region, trabeculae extending in an anterior and slightly superior direction into the cuboid bone and the fourth and fifth metatarsals.

A small zone in the midcalcaneal area remains free of trabeculae.

In the *midfoot area*, bundles run laterally from the navicular and medial cuneiform bones and cross the longitudinal bands.

The *metatarsal bones* have three trabecular pathways:

- Longitudinal.
- In both the bases and heads of the metatarsal bones, oblique, criss-crossing bundles that extend from medial-proximal to lateral-distal and from medial-distal to proximal-lateral.
- A few transverse bands running in the base area.

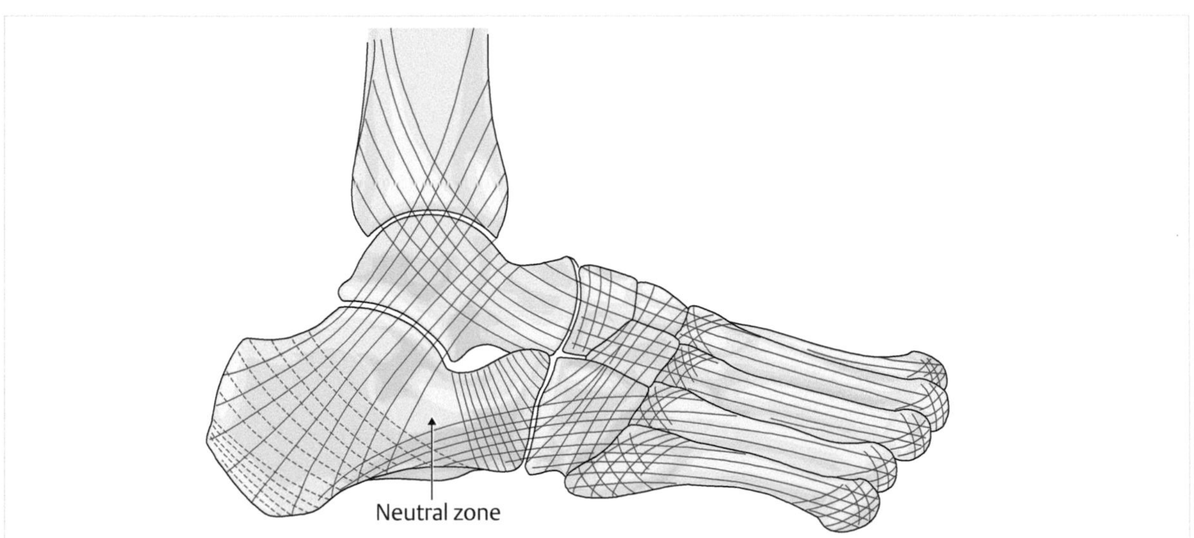


**Fig. 10.54** Course of the trabeculae. Solid lines: compression trabeculae; dashed lines: traction trabeculae.

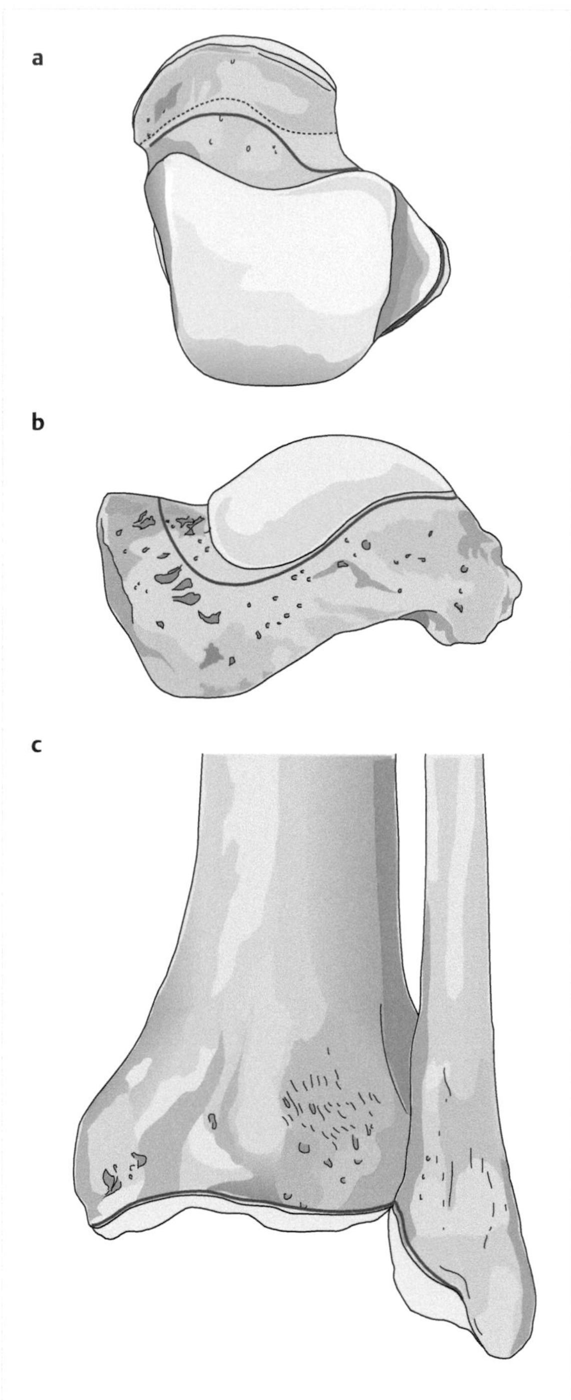


Fig. 10.55 Joint capsule insertions. (a) Talus: superior view. (b) Talus: medial view. (c) Distal end of the tibia and fibula: posterior view.

## 10.3.3 Joint Capsule (Figs. 10.55 and 10.56)

Both the synovial membrane and the fibrous layer of the joint capsule insert into the area of the bone–cartilage interface. An exception is the insertion on the neck of the talus, because here the insertion of both parts of the capsule occurs somewhat further distally.

In its anterior, posterior, posteromedial, and dorsolateral sections, the synovial membrane forms folds that protrude into the joint cavity—the *synovial folds.*

The capsule demonstrates, especially in the anterior area, a recess that is, for the most part, covered by the tendon sheaths of the extensors and by the inferior extensor retinaculum. The fibrous layer is thicker posteriorly than anteriorly.

The collateral ligaments track into the medial and lateral parts of the capsule.

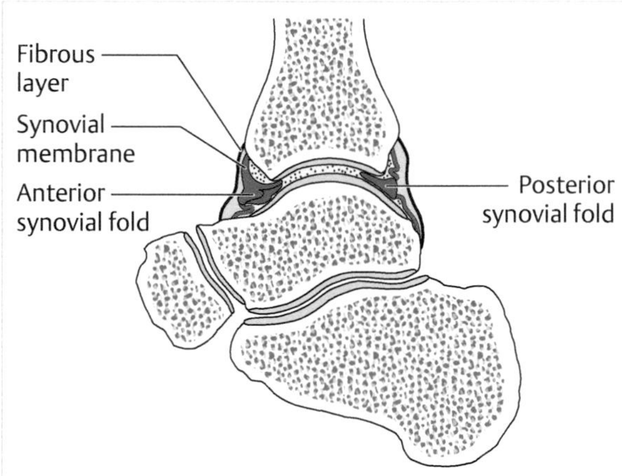


Fig. 10.56 Synovial folds in the upper ankle joint.

Pathology

**Effusion (Fig. 10.57)**

An effusion of the upper ankle (talocrural joint) can be recognized by a distinct bulge in the anterior region adjacent to the extensor tendons. The contours of the malleoli are no longer sharp, but diffuse.

Practical Tip

An effusion fills the entire joint space and stretches the capsule. Because of this, when a ligament is injured, the joint may appear to be stable even when it is not. For this reason, and also because of the great pain, stability testing is not feasible at this stage. Therefore measures such as performing small muscular movements and elevating the leg should be taken to reduce the swelling and allow the effusion to regress, so that the examination can be carried out 48 hours later.

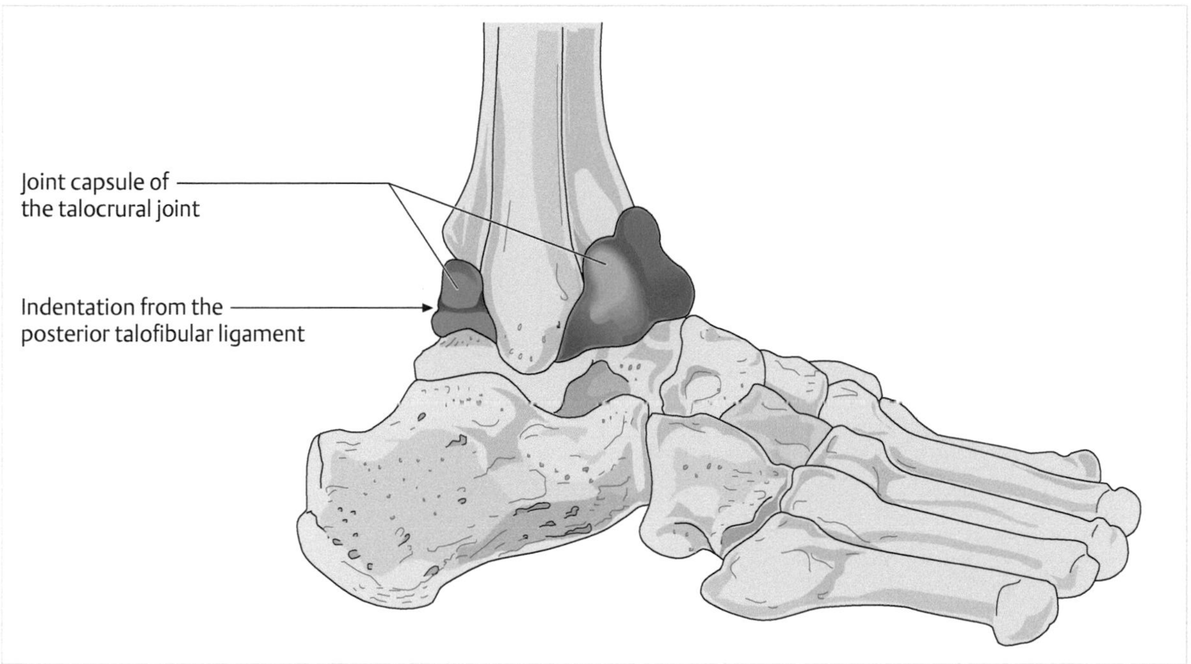


**Fig. 10.57** Bulging of the joint capsule due to upper ankle joint effusion.

## 10.3.4 Ligaments

### Medial Ligament of the Ankle Joint (Figs. 10.58 and 10.59)

Because of its shape, this ligament is called the *deltoid ligament*. It consists of four fiber tracts that partially overlap. The ligament's connections to the calcaneus and navicular bones pass over both the upper (talocrural) and the lower (subtalar and talocalcaneonavicular) ankle joints. The tibiotalar connections only stabilize the upper ankle joint.

### Tibiocalcaneal Part of the Deltoid Ligament

This ligament extends from the tip of the medial malleolus to the sustentaculum tali and connects to the plantar calcaneonavicular ligament. It has a vertical course and is the strongest component of the superficial ligaments. It is wider inferiorly (1 cm at the malleolus and 1.5 cm at the insertion) and is approximately 2 to 3 cm long and 3 mm thick.

### Tibionavicular Part of the Deltoid Ligament

This extends from the anterior edge of the medial malleolus to the superior and medial surface of the navicular bone. In addition, fibers track into the plantar calcaneonavicular ligament. The anterior fiber components almost completely overlie the deeper lying anterior tibiotalar part.

### Anterior Tibiotalar Part of the Deltoid Ligament

Deep fiber components lie directly over the capsule and merge with it. They extend almost horizontally from the anterior part of the malleolus to the posterior talar neck, next to the insertion line of the capsule.

The superficial fibers, in contrast, track more steeply inferiorly to the medial talar neck.

### Posterior Tibiotalar Part of the Deltoid Ligament

The deep fiber components extend in an inferoposterior direction from the posterior surface of the medial malleolus and insert next to the capsule on the medial tu-

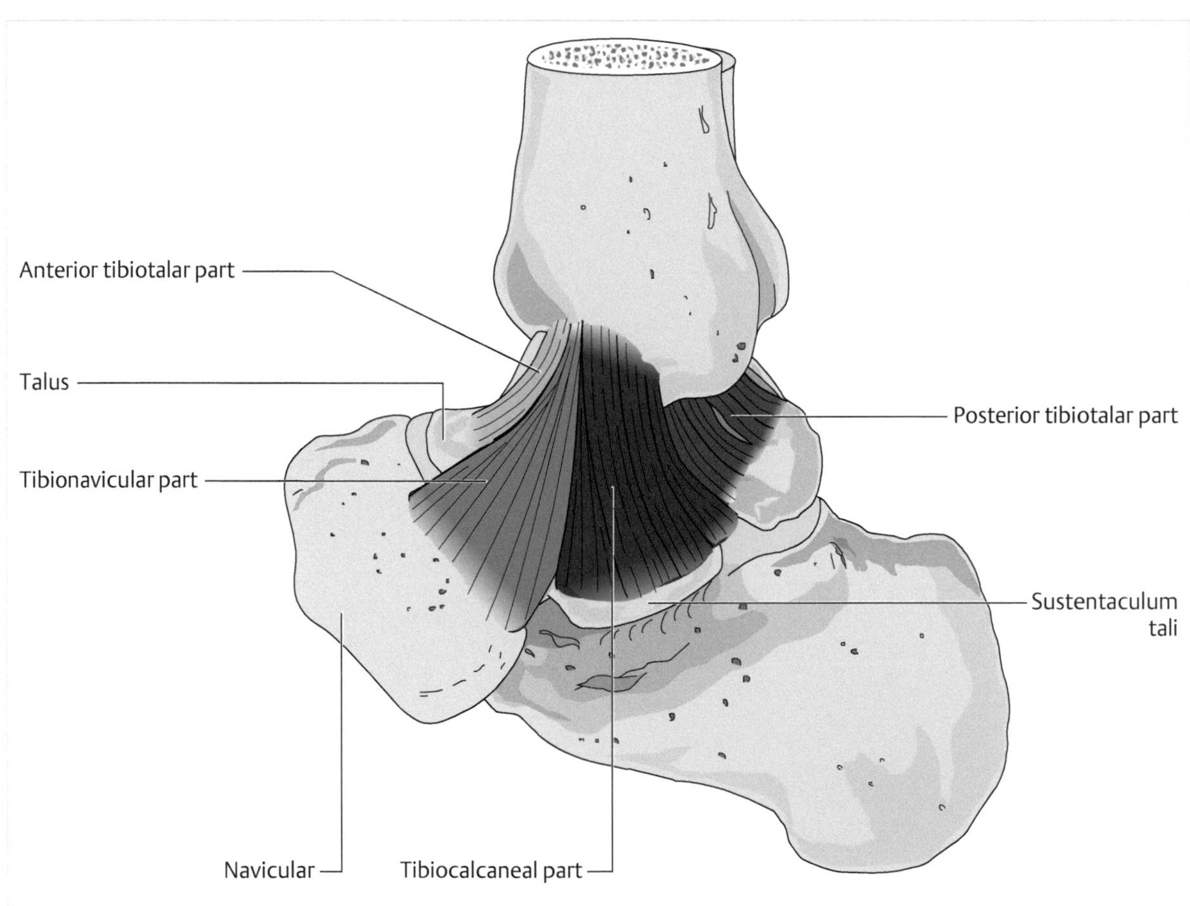


**Fig. 10.58** Tibial collateral ligament.

bercle of the posterior talar process. They lie directly on the capsule and are approximately 1.5 cm in length and width. With a thickness of 1 cm, this is the thickest ligament and the strongest part of the entire medial ligament complex.

The superficial ligamentous bands, on the contrary, are not as thick, but they are longer because they extend to the posterior end of the medial intercondylar tubercle.

**Function of the ligaments.** These stabilize the medial side and prevent a lateral shift of the talus. The anterior and posterior parts of the ligaments limit the movement of the talus anteriorly and posteriorly.

Deep portions of the posterior tibiotalar ligament and tibiocalcaneal parts of the deltoid ligament limit dorsiflexion. Superficial parts of the anterior tibiotalar and tibionavicular ligaments limit plantarflexion, and the tibiocalcaneal part of the deltoid ligament limits eversion of the calcaneus.

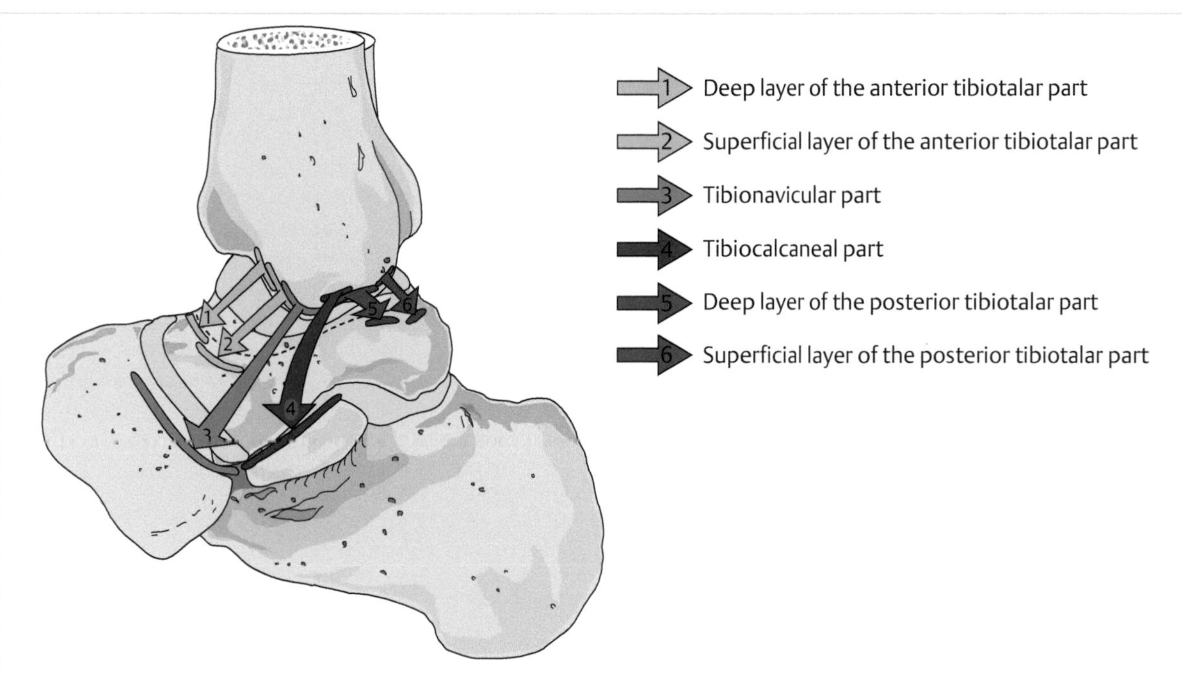


**Fig. 10.59** Insertions of the tibial collateral ligament.

## Lateral Ligament of the Ankle (Figs. 10.60–10.63)

The lateral ligament is of great clinical interest because it is especially prone to injury.

### Anterior Talofibular Ligament (Fig. 10.60)

The ligament is approximately 1.5 to 2 cm long. The upper band of fibers is larger and stronger than the lower band. Small blood vessels run through the gap between the two parts.

The ligament arises anteroinferior to the articular facet of the lateral malleolus. The superior part has a connection to the anterior tibiofibular ligament, and the inferior part a connection to the calcaneofibular ligament.

The insertion of the ligament lies on the body of the talus, immediately adjacent to the insertion of the capsule, with which it merges.

In the neutral position, it has an almost horizontal course. It is stretched by plantarflexion, and takes on an oblique orientation from superior-lateral-posterior to inferior-medial-anterior.

### Calcaneofibular Ligament (Fig. 10.61)

The ligament is approximately 3 cm long and 3 mm thick. It arises from the inferior edge of the articular facet of the lateral malleolus and extends posteroinferiorly to a roughened area on the outer side of the calcaneus (*tuberosity for the calcaneofibular ligament*). This tuberosity lies distinctly posterior and somewhat superior to the fibular trochlea.

The tendons of the fibular muscles cross over the ligament. There is a sliding surface between the muscle and ligament. A few fibers entwine the tendon sheath, which is why this ligament undergoes increased tension when the fibular muscles are tensed.

The calcaneofibular ligament crosses over the talotarsal joint and is separated from it by the lateral talocalcaneal ligament, which runs over the joint. Fatty tissue is found between the two ligaments.

The ligament is tensed by a valgus position of the calcaneus, by eversion, and by dorsiflexion.

### Posterior Talofibular Ligament (Fig. 10.62)

This is a very strong ligament that expands from the fibula to its insertion on the talus. It takes a horizontal course and is approximately 3 cm long and 5 to 8 mm thick. The site of origin on the fibula is inferior and posterior on the malleolar fossa. Its fibers have varying courses. Short fibers insert in a small groove located adjacent to the lateral malleolar facet of the talus. Long fibers insert on the lateral tubercle of the posterior process of the talus. From there, superiorly running superficial fibers extend toward the medial side of the foot, connecting with longer fibers of the posterior tibiotalar part of the deltoid ligament to form a type of sling. Inferior fibers form the floor of the tunnel for the tendon of the flexor hallucis longus muscle.

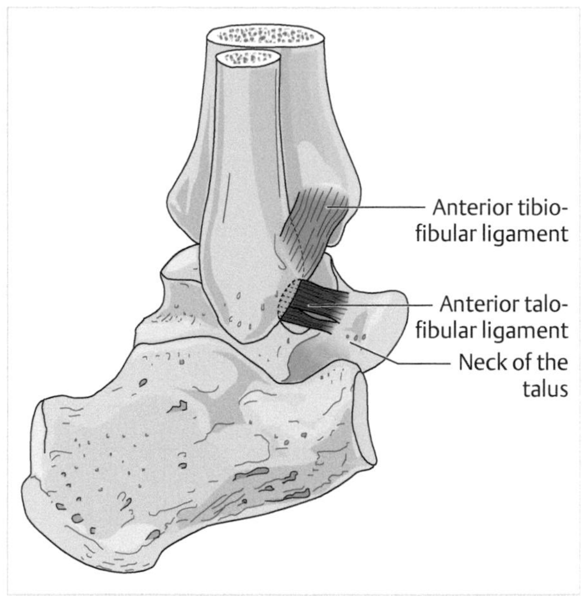


**Fig. 10.60** Anterior talofibular ligament.

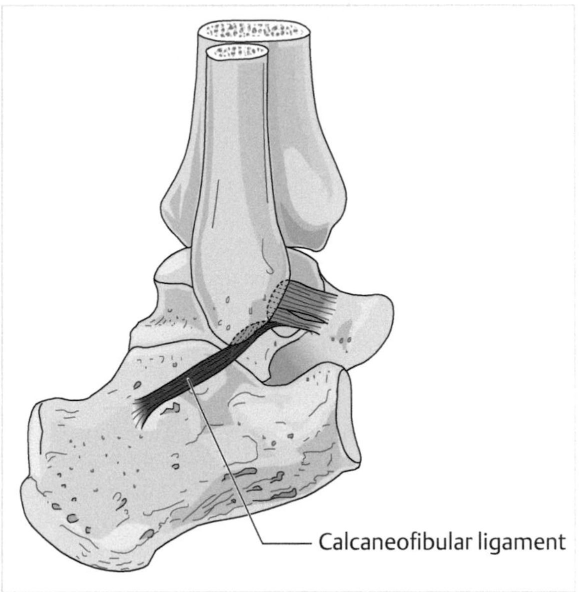


**Fig. 10.61** Calcaneofibular ligament.

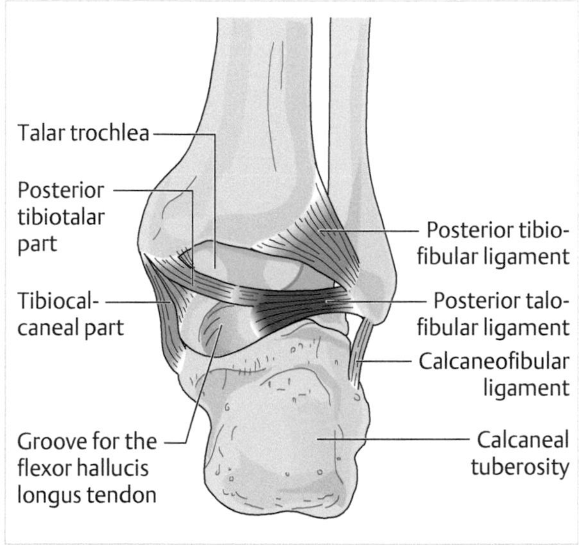


**Fig. 10.62** Posterior talofibular ligament.

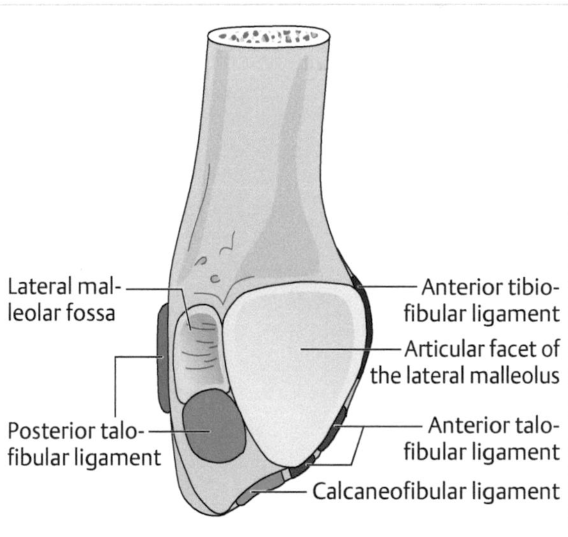


**Fig. 10.63** Insertions of the ligaments on the inner side of the distal fibula.

**Functions of the ligaments:**

- The *anterior talofibular ligament* is tensed by plantarflexion. In particular, it stabilizes standing on tiptoes in that it prevents the talus from tilting medially and from extreme anterior displacement. With its fixed end placed distally, it prevents posterior displacement and external rotation of the fibula.
- The *posterior talofibular ligament* becomes tensed in dorsiflexion, and it slows the posterior displacement of the talus and thus the anterior displacement of the lower leg. In addition, it limits internal rotation of the fibula.
- The *calcaneofibular ligament* stabilizes both the upper and lower ankle joints on the lateral side. It becomes taut with dorsiflexion, and relaxed in plantarflexion and in the varus position. In the valgus position of the calcaneus, both this ligament and the medial connection between the tibia and the calcaneus tighten. This occurs because the valgus tilt causes the insertion site of the calcaneofibular ligament on the calcaneus to shift medially, and the insertion site of the tibiocalcaneal part of the deltoid ligament on the sustentaculum tali to shift inferiorly (**Fig. 10.64**).

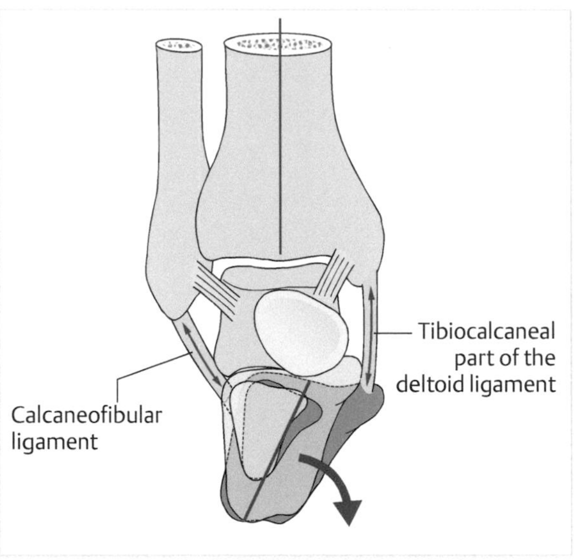


**Fig. 10.64** Tightening the ligaments by placing the calcaneus in a valgus position (anterior view of the right foot).

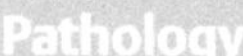

Pathology

### Supination Trauma (Fig. 10.65)

In distortion trauma, which almost always occurs in supination, the anterior talofibular ligament is the first to be torn. With severe overstretching, the calcaneofibular ligament is also involved, often combined with tearing of the tendon sheaths of the fibular tendons. The talus tilts medially, and the calcaneus moves inferomedially, clearly separating from the tip of the fibula. In addition, compression develops between the sustentaculum tali and the talus, and this convergence causes the tibiocalcaneal part of the deltoid ligament to relax.

Treatment is conservative with an Aircast splint or a special shoe, which prevents supination and the associated joint gapping. Surgically, the ligaments can be repaired by suturing. If this is not possible, tenodesis using the fibularis brevis muscle tendon can be performed. During the repair, the surgeon attempts to replicate the natural course of the ligaments being replaced.

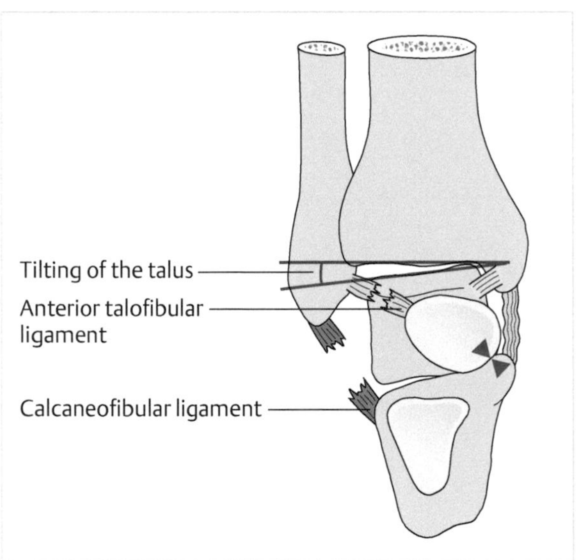


**Fig. 10.65** Tilting of the talus in rupture of the lateral ligaments with compression in the medial region.

▷ See Chapter 10.6, Stabilization of the Ankle Joints

## Practical Tip

### Examination of the Ligaments

In the case of ruptured tendons, test the joint gapping of the talus by fixing the ankle mortise and tilting the talus medially. In performing this test, it is important to compare the right and left sides, because, in terms of tensing and loosening the ligaments, individuals vary significantly in the distance that the talus can be tilted.

A further test provides information about the ability of the talus to move anteriorly (or the lower leg to move posteriorly). In a rupture of the anterior talofibular ligament, the lower leg can be shifted posteriorly, and this can be seen expecially well when the right and left sides are compared (**Fig 10.66**).

### Treatment of Supination Trauma

In the treatment of this condition, building up the strength of the fibular muscles is paramount because these muscles can inhibit supination. The emphasis here is on coordination therapy, with, for example, mobile support surfaces such as wobble boards.

▷ See Chapter 10.6, Stabilization of the Ankle Joints, and Chapter 10.15, Neural Structures of the Foot and Ankle

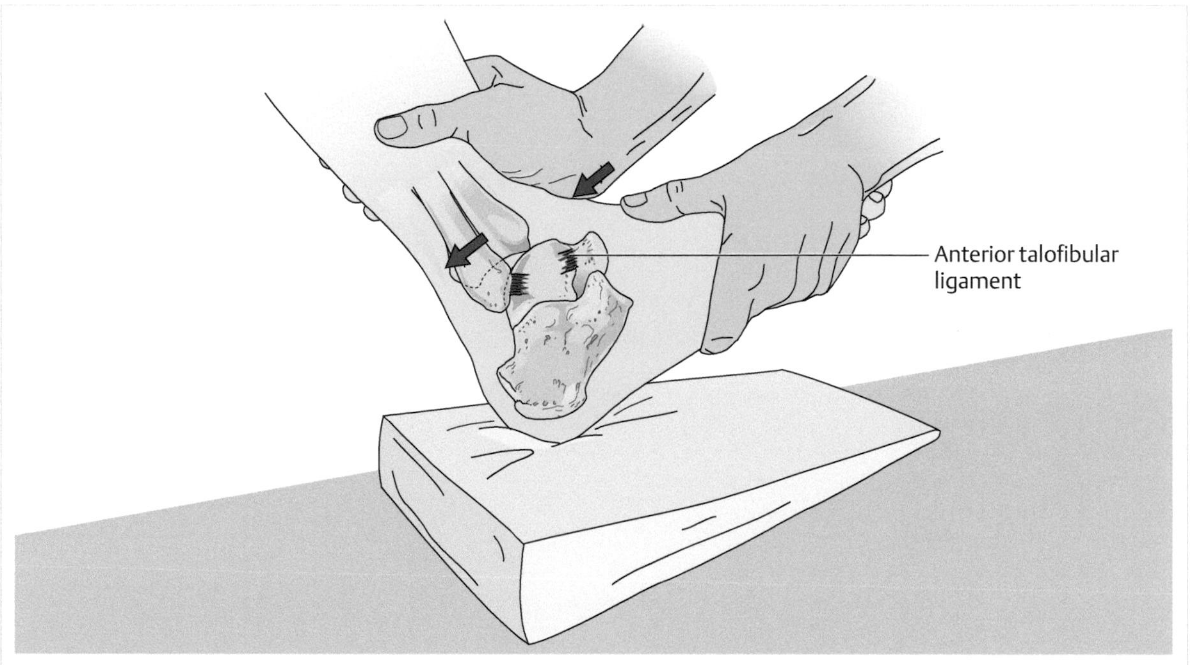


**Fig. 10.66** Stability test for the anterior talofibular ligament.

## 10.3.5 Axes of Motion and Movements

### Axes

Movement at the talocrural joint can be described using a multitude of momentary axes. However, there are many differences that depend on the type of foot.

The compromise axis (**Fig. 10.67**) that suffices for clinical purposes lies in the talus, approximately 5 mm inferior to the tip of the medial malleolus, and 3 mm inferior and 8 mm anterior to the tip of the lateral malleolus.

It runs from anterior-medial-distal to posterior-lateral-distal and therefore has an oblique orientation. In the frontal plane, it forms an angle of 80 to 82° with the tibial shaft axis (**Fig. 10.68**).

In the transverse view, it forms an angle of 20° with the frontal plane that is open medially.

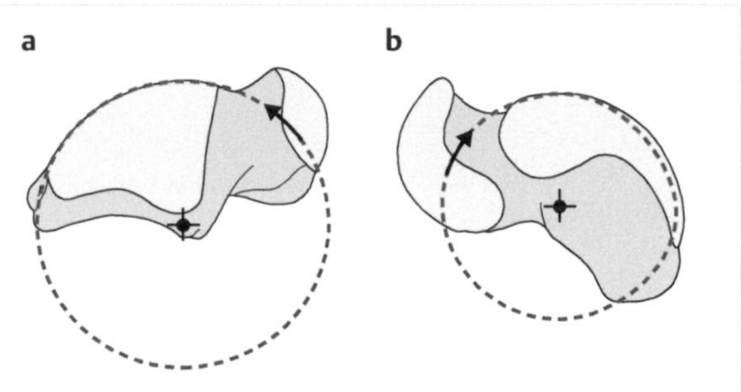


**Fig. 10.67** Movement axis of the talocrural (upper ankle) joint in the sagittal plane in dorsiflexion. **(a)** Lateral view. **(b)** Medial view.

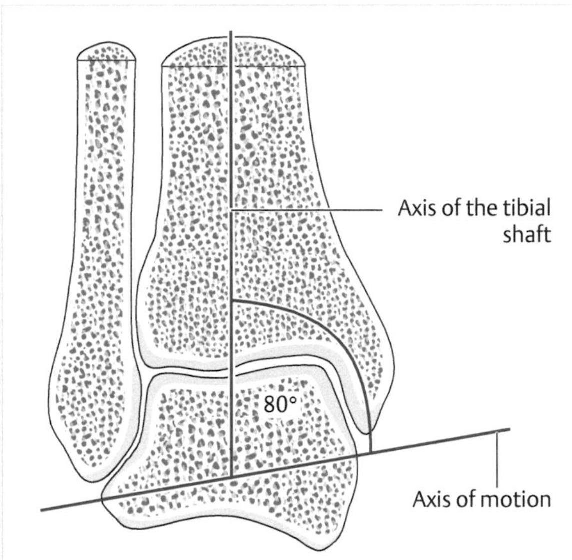


**Fig. 10.68** Orientation of the movement axis of the talocrural joint in the frontal plane.

## Movements

### *Dorsiflexion/Plantarflexion (Fig. 10.69)*

Active: 20°/40°, respectively, from neutral.

In dorsiflexion, the talus glides posteriorly in an arc; in plantarflexion, it glides anteriorly.

When considering the foot as a whole during dorsiflexion and plantarflexion, the movements appear to be more extensive. The values represented here relate only to movements between the talus and the lower leg, and are therefore significantly less than the combined movement of the entire foot.

Passive: 30°/50°, respectively, from neutral (**Fig. 10.70**).

With the fixed end of the foot on the floor, the mobility is increased at least 10° in each direction.

The elasticity at the end of both movements is firm because the movements are limited by ligaments.

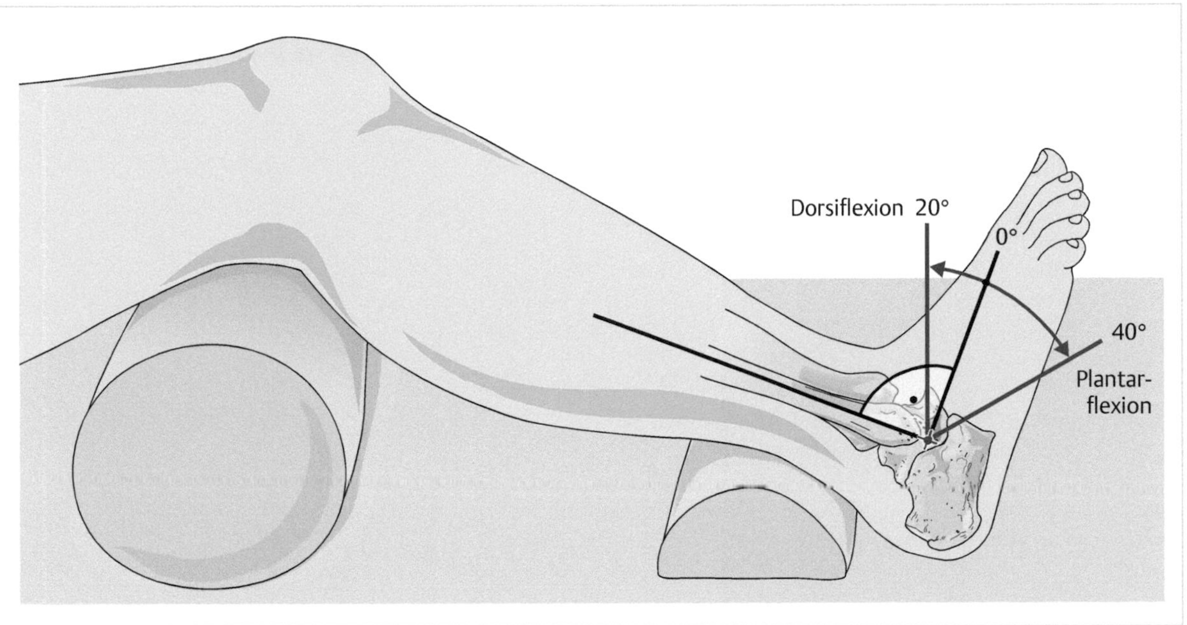


**Fig. 10.69** Movements of the upper ankle joint (talocrural joint): dorsiflexion, plantarflexion.

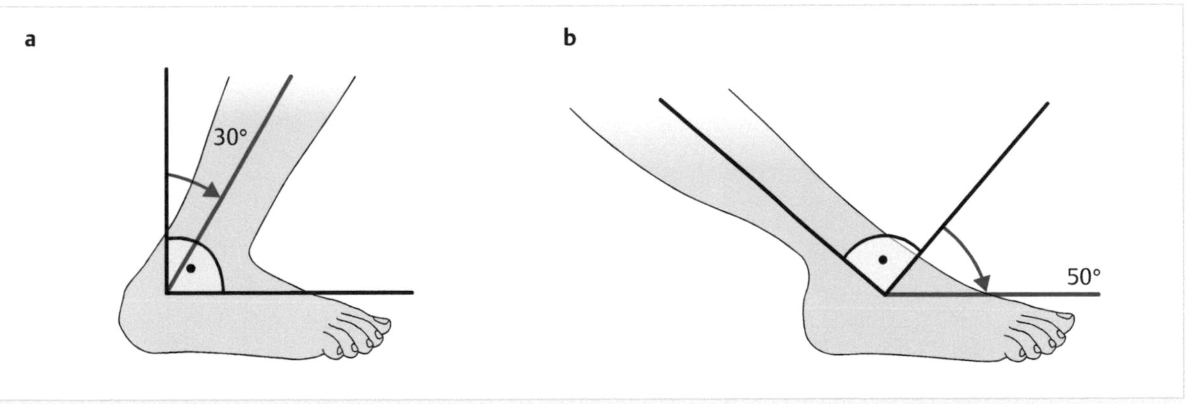


**Fig. 10.70** Passive movements of the talocrural joint with the fixed end distally. **(a)** Dorsiflexion. **(b)** Plantarflexion.

> **Practical Tip**
>
> **Measurement of Dorsiflexion**
>
> When measuring dorsiflexion, the limitation of mobility caused by stretching the gastrocnemius muscle must be taken into account. Therefore measurement of the ankle joint should be carried out with the knee flexed, thus shortening the muscle.
>
> **Combined Movements**
>
> The radius of curvature of the lateral roll edge of the talar trochlea generates a circle. The medial edge demonstrates a smaller radius of curvature anteriorly than superiorly. The talar trochlea thus forms a cone with the tip pointing medially (**Fig. 10.71**). Because of its anatomical configuration, the lateral part of the talar trochlea moves farther than the medial.
>
> However, the movements are coupled with a small rotatory component. In dorsiflexion, the talus turns outward by approximately 5° in relation to the lower leg. In plantarflexion, it turns inward.

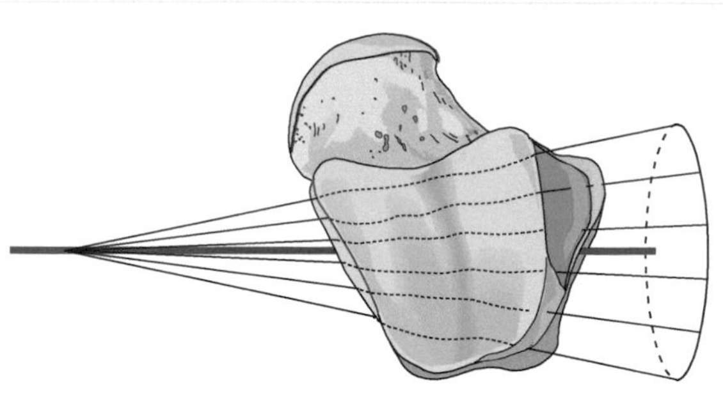

**Fig. 10.71** Representation of the talar trochlea in the form of a cone.

### *Locked Position*

The *close-packed position* is dorsiflexion, in which the broad anterior part of the trochlea wedges between the sides of the ankle mortise. Through this, the malleoli are forced apart, and the ligamentous connections to the talus are brought under stress, as is the syndesmosis area.

### *Resting Position*

The most relaxed position for the upper ankle joint (talocrural joint) and its surrounding structures is at approximately 10° of plantarflexion.

# 10.4 Tibiofibular Joint

## 10.4.1 Bony Structures and Joint Surfaces of the Tibiofibular Syndesmosis

- This forms the distal connection between the tibia and the fibula.
- The *fibular notch* on the tibia establishes the syndesmotic connection to the fibula. It is not cartilage-covered and is slightly concave.
- Between the two bones lies a synovial fold of the upper ankle joint (talocrural joint).
- The fibula does not have a surface corresponding to the fibular notch, which thus has contact with a small section of the fibular diaphysis.

## 10.4.2 Ligaments of the Tibiofibular Syndesmosis (Fig. 10.72)

### Anterior Tibiofibular Ligament

This is a rectangular ligament that runs obliquely from superomedial to inferolateral. It extends over the anterior edge of the trochlea of the talus, possibly forming a small joint facet there.

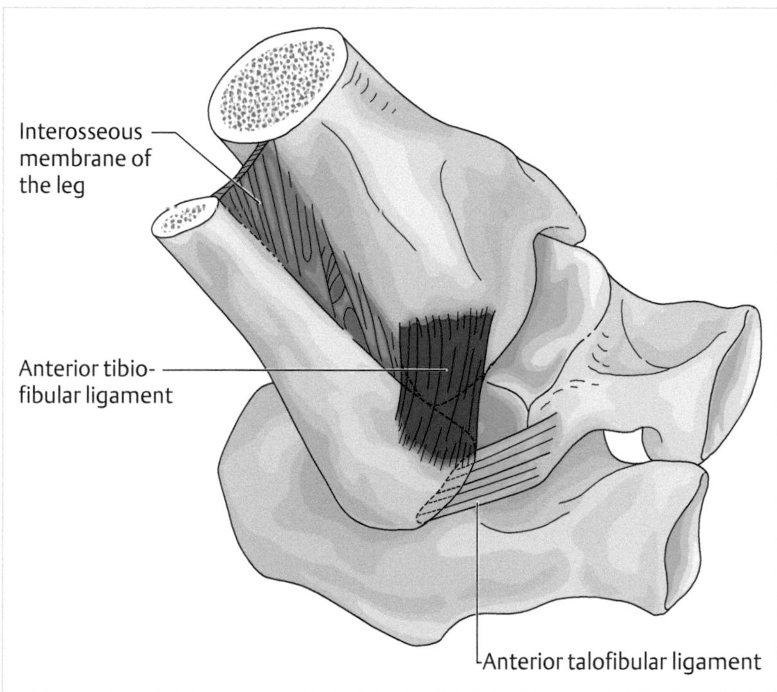


**Fig. 10.72** Anterior tibiofibular ligament (superolateral view).

### Posterior Tibiofibular Ligament (Fig. 10.73)

This is divided into deep and superficial fibers. Some of the deep fibers run horizontally, while others run obliquely from superomedial to inferolateral, or, more precisely, from the posteroinferior border of the fibular notch to the posteroinferior part of the lateral malleolar fossa. The deepest parts have contact with the posterolateral edge of the trochlea of the talus, where there is a triangular facet, the *facet of Fawcett*.

Superficial fibers run slightly obliquely from the posterosuperior border of the fibular notch to the posterior edge of the lateral malleolus. These fibers connect distally with the capsule of the upper ankle joint (talocrural joint) and the upper part of the posterior talofibular ligament.

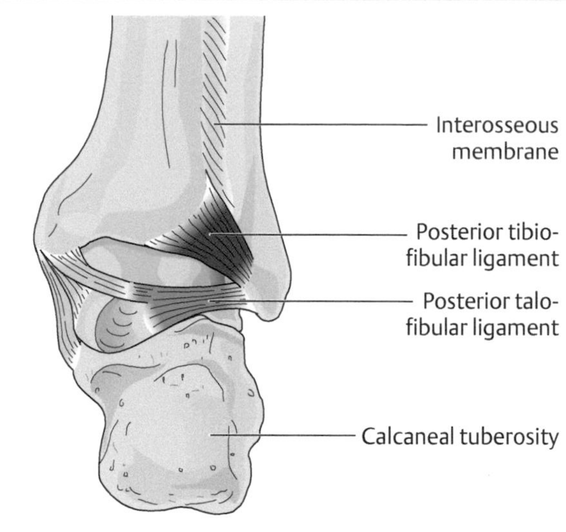


**Fig. 10.73** Posterior tibiofibular ligament, superficial fibers (posterior view).

## 10.4.3 Interosseous Membrane of the Leg (Fig. 10.74)

The membrane consists of taut bands of connective tissue that primarily extend from the interosseous border of the tibia obliquely in a distal direction to the corresponding border of the fibula. Other fibers run across these bands in the opposite direction.

In the superior portion, there is a large opening for the anterior tibial vessels, which here run from posterior to anterior. A narrow opening in the distal portion allows branches from the posteriorly running fibular vessels to pass through.

The membrane has an important stabilizing function in that it holds the two lower leg bones together. It also serves as the site of origin for many muscles of the foot.

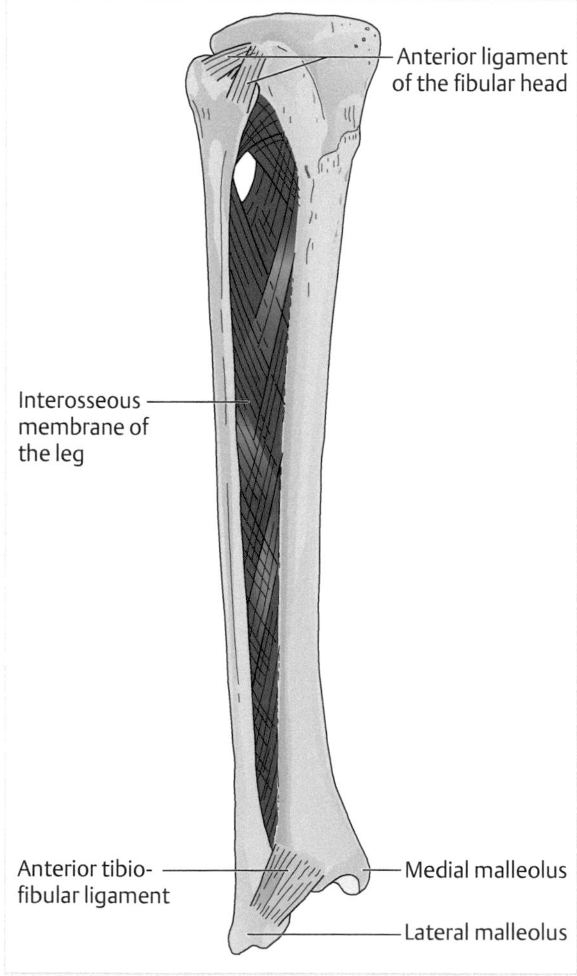


**Fig. 10.74** Interosseous membrane of the leg (anterolateral view).

## 10.4.4 Bony Structures and Joint Surfaces of the Superior Tibiofibular Joint (Fig. 10.75)

### Proximal Tibia

- The *fibular articular facet of the tibia* is slightly convex.
- The articular surface faces in a posterior-lateral-inferior direction.
- It lies beneath the lateral tibial plateau.

### Proximal Fibula

- The *articular facet of the fibula* is slightly concave.
- The joint surface faces in a superior-medial-anterior direction, so that the joint surfaces for the sliding movements are at a 60° angle to the sagittal plane, opening posteriorly.

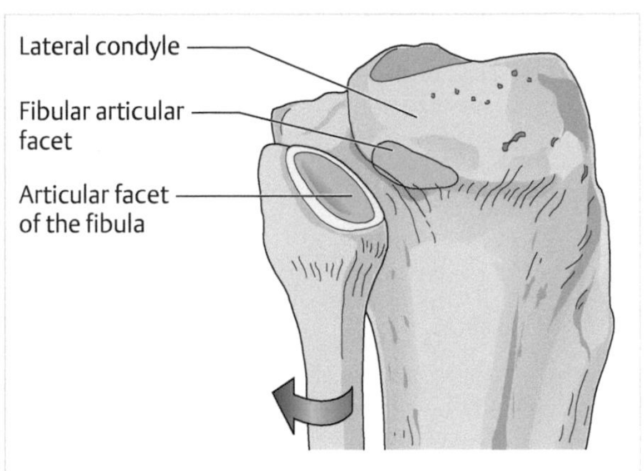


**Fig. 10.75** Superior tibiofibular joint (posterolateral view, fibula turned outward).

## 10.4.5 Joint Capsule of the Superior Tibiofibular Joint

The capsule is taut and has no recesses. The capsule communicates with the subpopliteal recess, via which there is a connection with the knee joint.

▷ See Chapter 9.3, Knee Joint

## 10.4.6 Ligaments of the Superior Tibiofibular Joint (Fig. 10.76)

### Anterior Ligament of the Fibular Head

The ligament is divided into two parts. The proximal fibers are short and merge with the capsule of the knee joint. They run from the tip of the fibula roughly horizontally to the tibia. A few fibers of the popliteus muscle track into the proximal part of the ligament.

Longer fibers extend from the tibia obliquely in an inferolateral direction and insert on the anteroinferior head of the fibula.

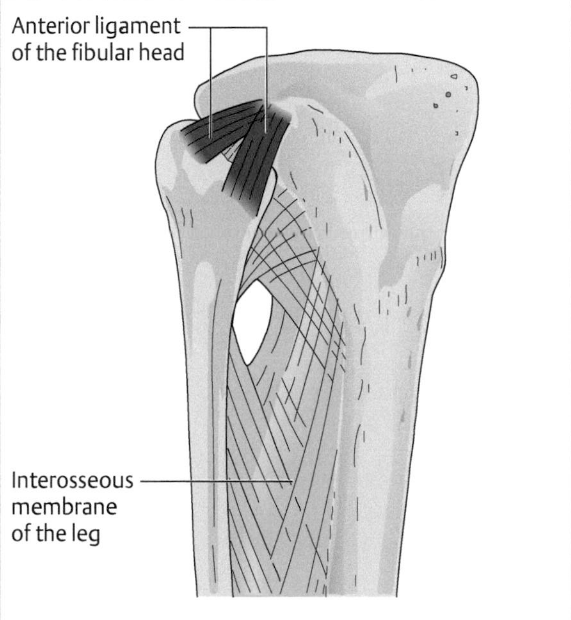


**Fig. 10.76** Anterior ligament of the fibular head.

### Posterior Ligament of the Fibular Head

This ligament is thin and extends from the posterior head of the fibula obliquely in a superomedial direction to the lateral tibial condyle.

## 10.4.7 Axis of the Superior Tibiofibular Joint

An axis of movement cannot be determined here. Sliding movements in this joint occur in the superomedial, anterolateral, posterosuperior, and inferior directions.

## 10.4.8 Mechanics of the Tibiofibular Connections

The tibiofibular connections must be considered as a joint complex because a shift can only occur in the syndesmosis if a movement also occurs in the proximal articulation. A movement of the foot causes a compulsive three-dimensional combination of movements to occur.

During dorsiflexion, the following components can be observed in the distal tibiofibular articulation (**Fig. 10.77**):

- *Lateral fibular translation*, because the shape of the talus pushes the ankle mortise wide apart.
- *Superior fibular translation:* Likewise, the broad anterior talar trochlea causes the fibula to be displaced proximally. A purely proximal displacement would lead to compression in the proximal joint because the tibia projects above the fibula like a roof. Therefore proximal movement always occurs in combination with posterior translation.
- *Posterior fibular translation* in the form of the fibula turning inward: Because the anterior tibiofibular ligament inserts on the outer side of the fibula, and the deep, strong parts of the posterior tibiofibular ligament on the inner side, the fibula turns inward when there is tightening of the ligaments.

The extent of the fibular translations is minimal—only 1 to 2 mm. In comparison, the change in width of the ankle mortise has been noted to be 1.4 mm (Seiler 1999).

In *plantarflexion*, the reciprocal movements take place.

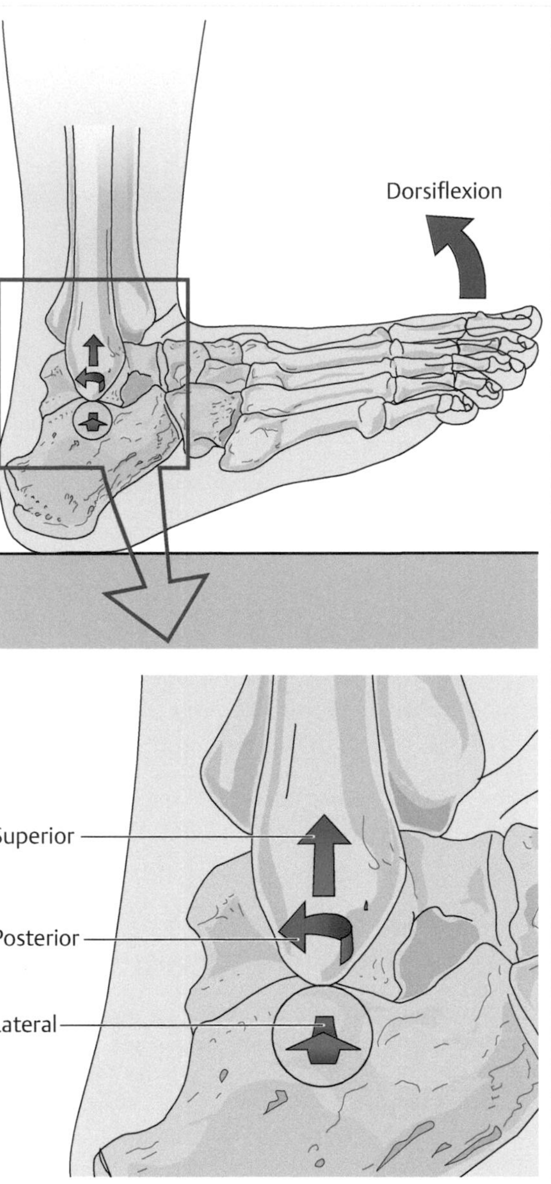


**Fig. 10.77** Fibular translation movements in dorsiflexion.

# 10.5 Talotarsal Joint

Anatomically, the lower ankle joint consists of two separate joints, known as the *posterior and anterior chambers.* The two chambers are completely separated from each other by the joint capsule as well as the tarsal sinus and the tarsal canal. However, they form a functional unit.

## 10.5.1 Bony Structures and Joint Surfaces of the Subtalar Joint

The subtalar joint forms the posterior chamber of the lower ankle joint.

### Talus (Fig. 10.78)

- The *posterior calcaneal articular facet* is located on the inferior body of the talus.
- The joint surface is distinctly concave in an anterior-posterior orientation. In a medial-lateral orientation, it is flat, which is why it appears somewhat like a saddle.
- The longitudinal axis through the joint surface points in an anterolateral direction and forms an angle of 30 to 40° with the anterior border of the trochlea.
- The anterior edge of the joint surface represents the posterior border of the *sulcus tali.*

### Calcaneus (Fig. 10.79)

- The *posterior talar articular surface* articulates with the talar facet.
- The joint surface, with its very distinct convexity in the anteroposterior orientation, appears somewhat saddle-like.
- The longitudinal axis through the joint surface runs the same as that of the talus—from posteromedial to anterolateral.
- The posterior joint surface has an inclination of 65 to 75° to the superior surface of the calcaneus (see **Fig. 10.81**).
- Immediately anterior to the joint surface lies the *calcaneal sulcus.* This runs obliquely in an anterolateral direction and forms the floor of the tarsal canal, which ends laterally as the *tarsal sinus.*

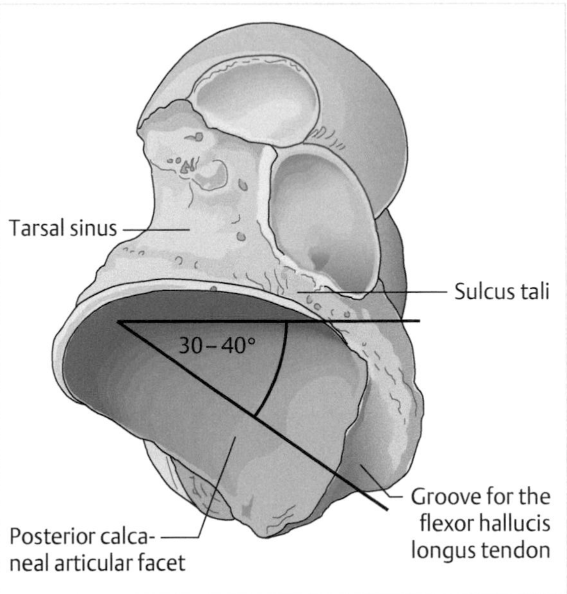


**Fig. 10.78** Subtalar joint: articular surfaces on the talus (inferior view of the right talus).

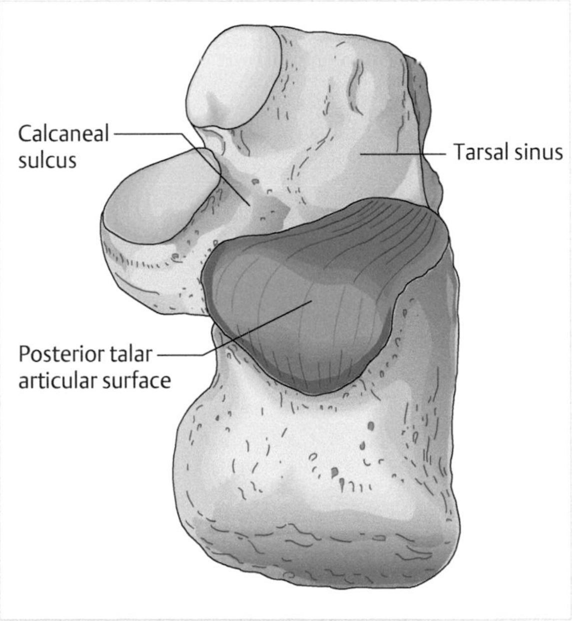


**Fig. 10.79** Subtalar joint: articular surfaces on the calcaneus (superior view of the right calcaneus).

## 10.5.2 Bony Structures and Joint Surfaces of the Talocalcaneonavicular Joint

This joint forms the anterior chamber of the lower ankle joint. Here the talus, calcaneus, and navicular bones as well as the plantar calcaneonavicular ligament (spring ligament) articulate with each other.

### Talus (Fig. 10.80)

- The *middle facet for the calcaneus* on the inferior neck of the talus articulates with the calcaneus and is slightly convex.
- The *anterior facet for the calcaneus* on the anteroinferior head of the talus articulates with the calcaneus and is convex in both orientations, although not as distinctly as the articular surface for the navicular bone.
- The *articular surface for the navicular bone* lies anteriorly on the talar head. This articulates with the navicular bone, and an inferior part articulates with the spring ligament. Its surface is convex in both orientations.

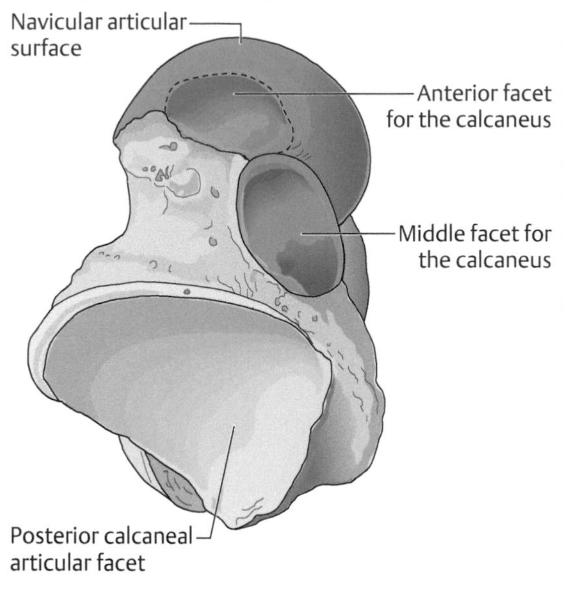


**Fig. 10.80** Articular surfaces on the right talus (inferior view).

### Calcaneus (Fig. 10.81)

- This is the largest tarsal bone.
- Its longitudinal axis is oriented anteriorly and slightly superiorly and laterally.
- The *anterior talar articular surface* lies anterosuperiorly and is concave.
- The *middle talar articular surface* on the sustentaculum tali is a balcony-like projection on the medial side of the calcaneus:
  - It is concave.
  - The posterolateral border of the joint surface forms the anteromedial border of the calcaneal sulcus.
- The cartilage-covered surface becomes narrower in the transition area between these two joint surfaces. Often it is completely missing, so that, in the superior view, the cartilage covering looks like the sole of a shoe.

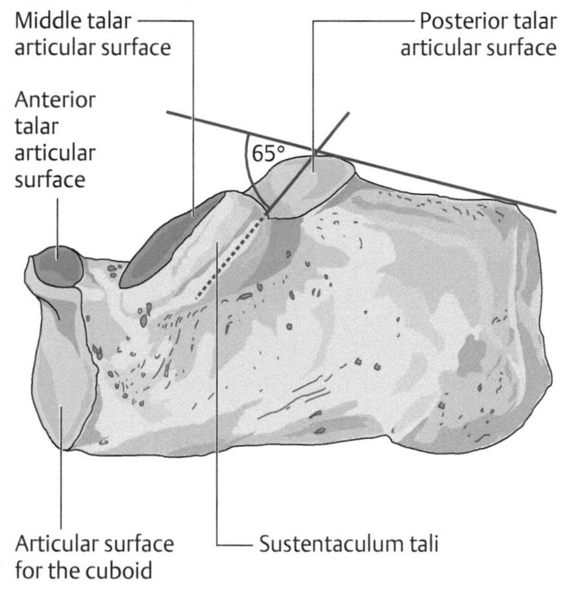


**Fig. 10.81** Articular surfaces on the right calcaneus, and the angle of inclination (medial view).

## Navicular Bone (Fig. 10.82)

- The *navicular tuberosity* is a projection on the medial margin of the bone that projects inferiorly. It serves as insertion site for the tibialis posterior muscle.
- The *posterior articular surface of the navicular* (for the talus) is an oval, prominent joint surface that is concave in both orientations. It is narrower than the corresponding articular surface on the talus.

## Plantar Calcaneonavicular Ligament (Spring Ligament; Fig. 10.82)

This ligament extends from the anterior edge of the sustentaculum tali to the plantar surface of the navicular bone and is shaped like a trapezoid. It is also known as the *spring ligament*. It is coated with a thick layer of cartilage, which serves as a joint surface for the inferior part of the head of the talus. A fat pad covered by a synovial membrane lies on the anterolateral part of the ligament.

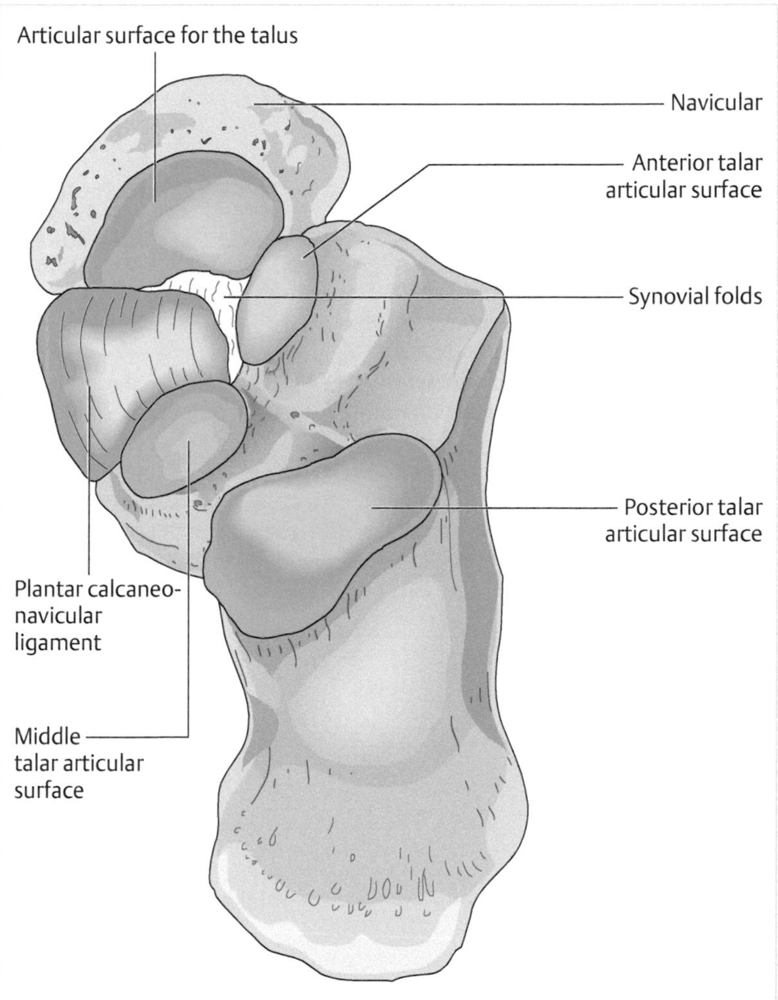


**Fig. 10.82** Joint surfaces of the right lower ankle joint (superior view with talus removed).

## Lateral Talocalcaneal Ligament (Fig. 10.87)

The ligament is short and flat. It extends from the lateral process of the talus obliquely in a posteroinferior direction to the outer side of the calcaneus, immediately adjacent to the capsule insertion, and runs roughly parallel to the calcaneofibular ligament.

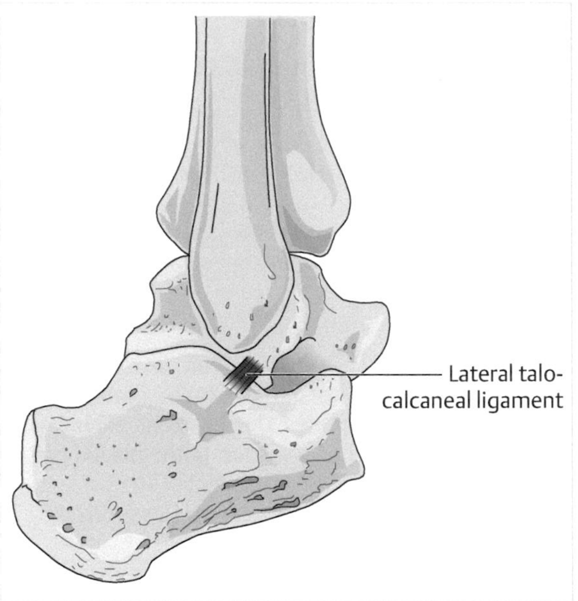


Fig. 10.87 Lateral talocalcaneal ligament.

## Medial Talocalcaneal Ligament (Fig. 10.88)

This is a short, strong ligament that extends from the medial tubercle of the posterior talar process anteroinferiorly to the superior edge of the sustentaculum tali.

## Posterior Talocalcaneal Ligament (Fig. 10.88)

This short, flat ligament extends from the medial tubercle of the posterior talar process to the superomedial surface of the calcaneal tuberosity.

Deeper fibers join with the fibrous roof of the flexor hallucis longus tunnel. At the talar insertion, the fibers join with the posterior talofibular ligament.

**Functions of the ligaments:**

- *Talocalcaneal interosseous ligament:* Both parts tense in both inversion and eversion movements. During tensing, the tarsal canal ligament limits eversion more, while the ligament of the talar neck limits inversion more.
- The *lateral talocalcaneal* ligament, together with the calcaneofibular ligament, limits lateral tilting of the calcaneus.
- The *medial talocalcaneal ligament* blocks medial tilting of the tarsal canal.
- The *posterior talocalcaneal ligament* stabilizes the posterior joint complex and becomes tensed with dorsiflexion.

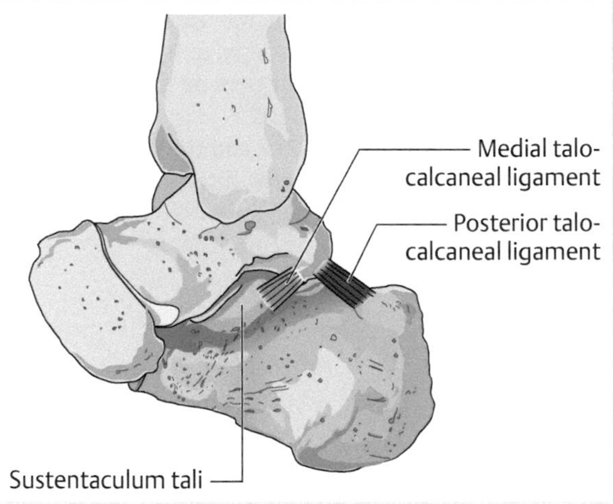


Fig. 10.88 Medial and posterior talocalcaneal ligaments.

## 10.5.5 Axes and Movements

### Axes

The course of the axes of movement in the lower ankle joint arises from the joint contours of the articulating joint surfaces, their orientation, and the stabilizing ligaments. Localizing an axis is very problematic due to this complex joint structure. By a more exact analysis of the above considerations, three secondary axes can be established:

### Longitudinal Axis (Figs. 10.89 and 10.90)

This axis goes longitudinally through the calcaneus. Supination and pronation movements take place around it.

### Vertical Axis (Fig. 10.89 and 10.90)

This runs perpendicular to the joint surface. Abduction and adduction movements take place around it.

### Frontal Axis (Fig. 10.89 and 10.90)

It extends from medial to lateral through the calcaneus. The movements of extension and flexion take place around this axis.

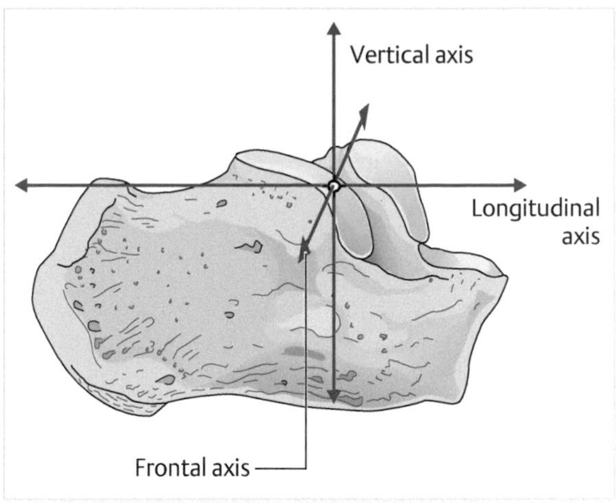


**Fig. 10.89** Axes of the subtalar joint in lateral view.

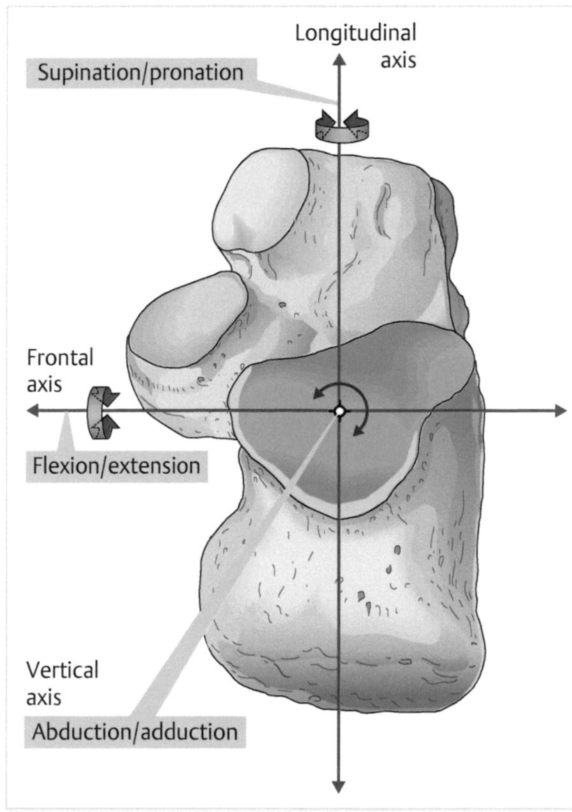


**Fig. 10.90** Axes of the subtalar joint in superior view.

### Inversion/Eversion Axis (Figs. 10.91 and 10.92)

The basic axis is composed from a combination of the three above-named axes. It extends through the posterolateral corner of the calcaneus, crosses the tarsal canal in the medial area, and pierces the neck of the talus in the superomedial area.

Its course is therefore from posterior-lateral-inferior to anterior-medial-superior. It forms an angle of 40° ± 10° to the horizontal plane and an angle of 23° ± 10° to the sagittal plane.

Movements around this axis are designated *eversion* and *inversion*. The navicular and the calcaneus rotate around the axis opposite to the talus.

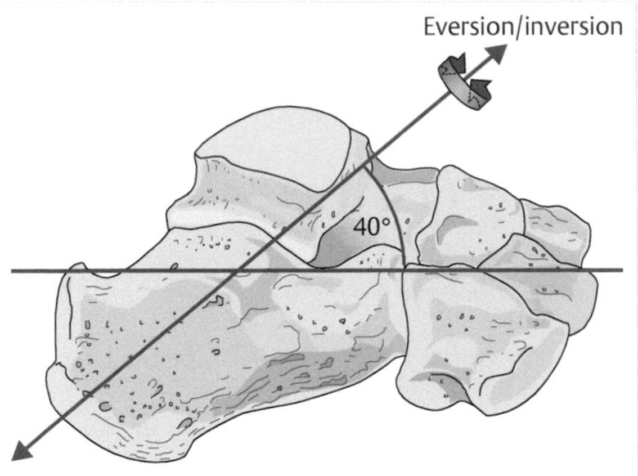


**Fig. 10.91** Primary axis of the subtalar joint (lateral view).

## Movements

The anterior and posterior chambers of the lower ankle form a functional unit. Every movement is a combination of three components in the following configuration:

- *Flexion/adduction/supination = inversion:* This combination movement of the calcaneus on the one side and the talus on the other is similar to that of a right-handed screw. It equates to varus position of the heel.
- *Extension/pronation/abduction = eversion:* This movement combination equates to valgus position of the heel.

These combination movements are necessary for the foot to adapt to uneven ground during locomotion. All the joints of the foot take part in twisting movements of the foot.

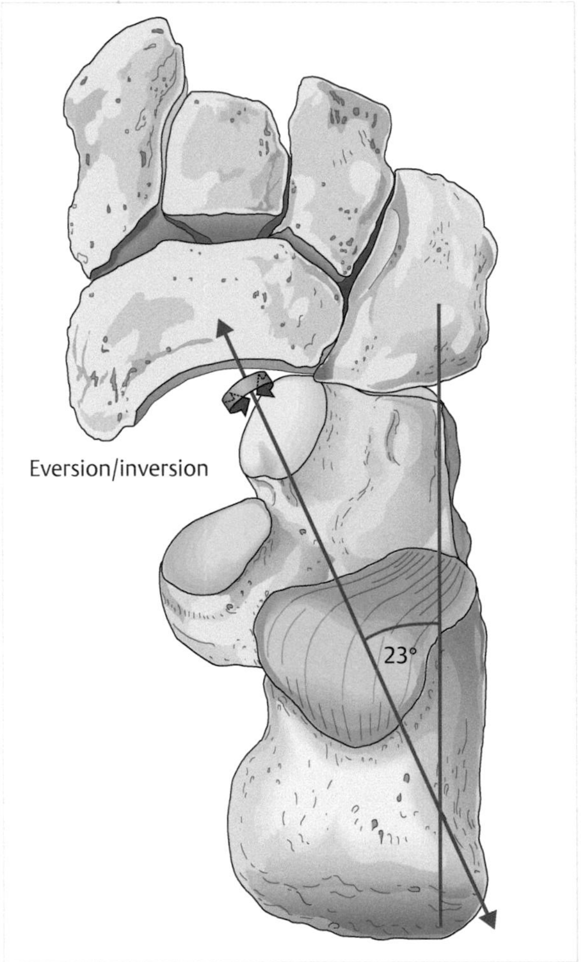


**Fig. 10.92** Primary axis of the subtalar joint (superior view).

## Inversion (Figs. 10.93 and 10.94)

*Range of motion:* 20 to 30°.

In particular, the following movement components take place:

- The calcaneus glides anteroinferiorly, which equates to the movement of flexion.
- The calcaneus turns medially, equating to adduction.
- The calcaneus turns superomedially, equating to the movement of supination.
- The navicular moves in a similar way, resulting in an arc-shaped movement in an inferomedial direction.

### *Factors that Limit Inversion*

Inversion is limited by structures lying lateral to the axis, for example the calcaneofibular ligament and the lateral part of the talocalcaneal interosseous ligament.

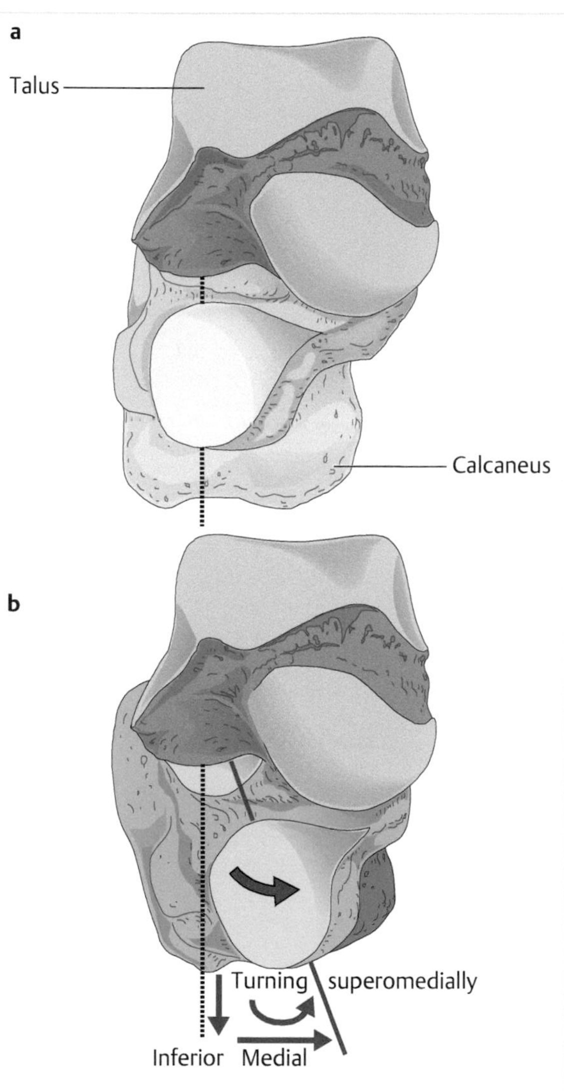


**Fig. 10.93** Position of the calcaneus opposite from the talus. **(a)** In the neutral position (0°). **(b)** In inversion.

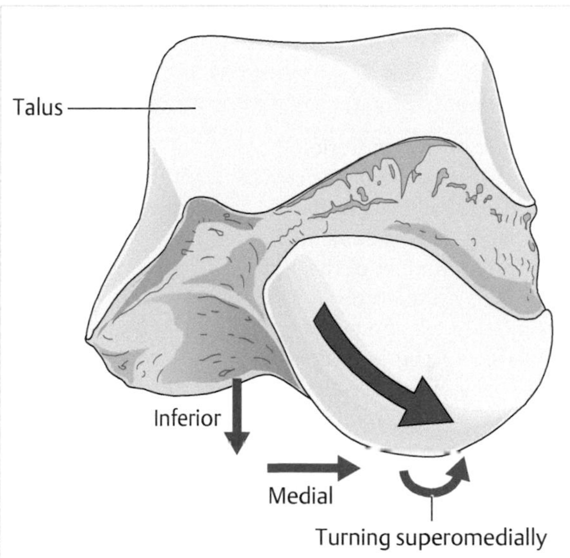


**Fig. 10.94** Sliding movement of the navicular bone opposite from the talus in inversion.

## Eversion (Figs. 10.95 and 10.96)

*Range of motion:* 10 to 20°.

In particular, the following movement components occur:

- The calcaneus glides in a posterosuperior direction, equating to extension.
- The calcaneus turns laterally (abducts).
- The calcaneus turns superolaterally—this is the pronation component.
- The navicular bone moves in a similar way, resulting in an arched movement in a superolateral direction.

### *Factors that Limit Eversion*

Eversion is limited by the structures that lie medial to the axis, such as the tarsal canal ligament and the tibionavicular and tibiocalcaneal sections of the deltoid ligament.

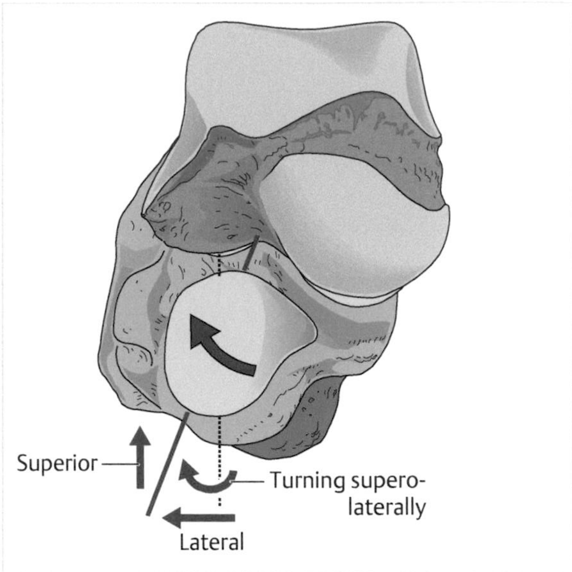


**Fig. 10.95** Eversion of the calcaneus opposite from the talus.

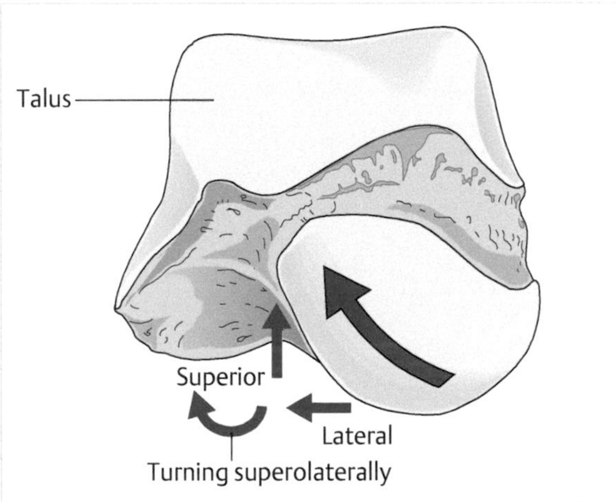


**Fig. 10.96** Sliding movement of the navicular opposite from the talus in eversion.

# 10.6 Stabilization of the Ankle Joints

Both parts of the ankle joint are stabilized by passive and dynamic factors.

## 10.6.1 Passive Stabilization

### Side-to-Side Stability (Fig. 10.97)

Side-to-side stability is ensured by the extensive bony structure of the ankle mortise in conjunction with the tibiofibular ligaments.

The collateral ligaments offer effective support in that the parts of the ligaments that connect the malleoli and the talus stabilize the upper (talocrural) ankle joint. The upper and lower ankle joints are both supported by the ligamentous connections between the tibia and calcaneus and those between the fibula with the calcaneus, as well as the tibionavicular part of the deltoid ligament. The ligaments that span between the talus and calcaneus only stabilize the lower ankle joint. In this regard, the powerful talocalcaneal interosseous ligament plays the biggest role.

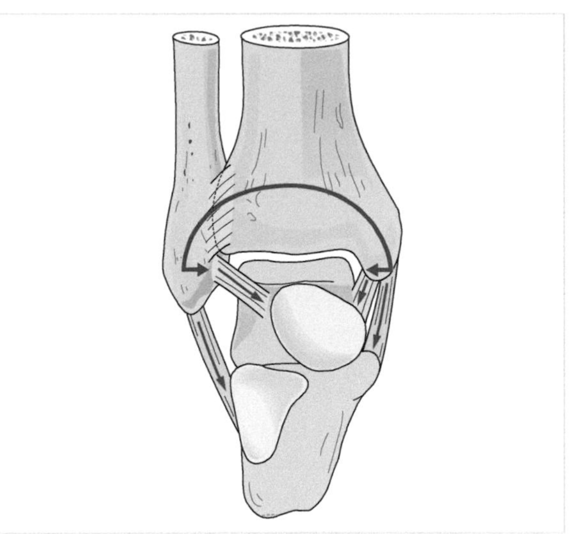

**Fig. 10.97** Passive side-to-side stability of the ankle joints.

### Anterior-Posterior Stability (Fig. 10.98)

The most unstable area in terms of anterior and posterior displacement is the upper ankle joint. Since there are no bony structures to support stabilization, the ligaments assume this role. The anterior and posterior talofibular ligaments and the anterior and posterior tibiotalar parts of the deltoid ligament are called upon as stabilizers. The anterior malleolar connections to the talus impede any anterior shift of the talus (or posterior shift of the lower leg).

The posterior connections prevent the talus from shifting posteriorly (and the lower leg from shifting anteriorly).

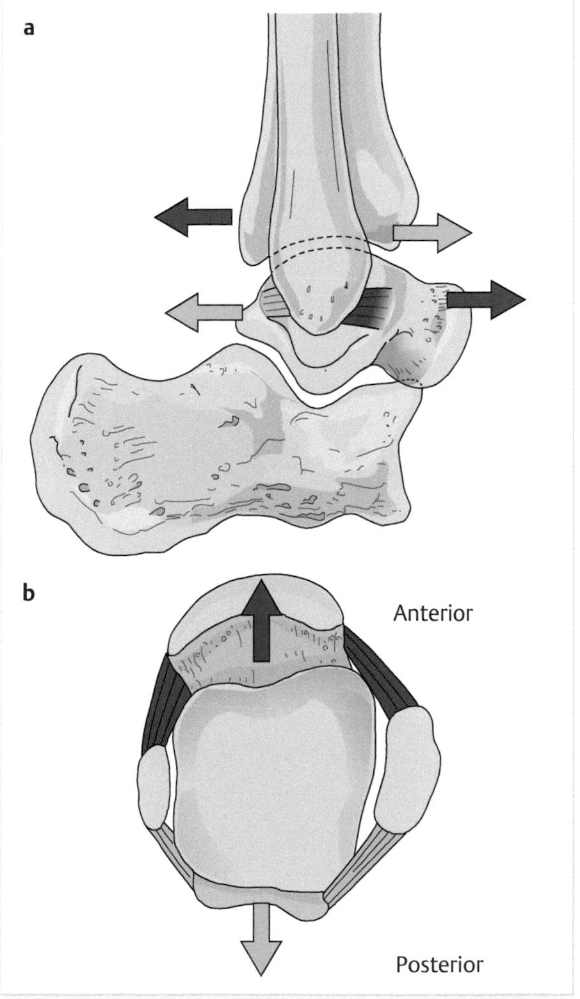


**Fig. 10.98** Stability of the upper ankle joint (talocrural joint) in the anterior-posterior direction. **(a)** Lateral view. **(b)** Posterior view.

## 10.6.2 Dynamic Stabilization

Dynamic stabilization of the upper ankle joint (talocrural joint) is ensured by the load (e.g., weight transfer while walking) and by various muscular activities. The coordination of muscular activity can only function, however, if the reflex mechanism in the joint capsule and the ligaments is intact.

### Posteromedial Stabilization

#### Tibialis Posterior Muscle (Fig. 10.99)

- This runs distally deep within the posterior aspect of the lower leg on the interosseous membrane.
- It crosses under the flexor digitorum longus muscle above the medial malleolus (*chiasma crurale*).
- Its tendon runs on the posterior part of the malleolus and then bends around in an anteroinferior direction.
- It extends over the tibiotalar and tibiocalcaneal parts of the deltoid ligament and, somewhat further distally, over the insertion of the plantar calcaneonavicular ligament.
- It then runs over the sustentaculum tali, where the flexor retinaculum spreads widely over the tendon.
- Shortly before reaching the navicular bone, it divides into its three insertions:
  - The *anterior fibers* form the strongest direct continuation of the previous course of the tendon, and insert on the navicular tuberosity and the plantar aspect of the medial cuneiform bone. In addition, fibers track into the capsule of the cuneonavicular joint.
  - The *middle fibers* run deep in the sole of the foot, insert on the intermediate and lateral cuneiform bones, and extend with a few parts to the cuboid bone and possibly to the base of the fourth and fifth metatarsal bones.
  - The *posterior fibers insert* on the anterior border of the sustentaculum tali.

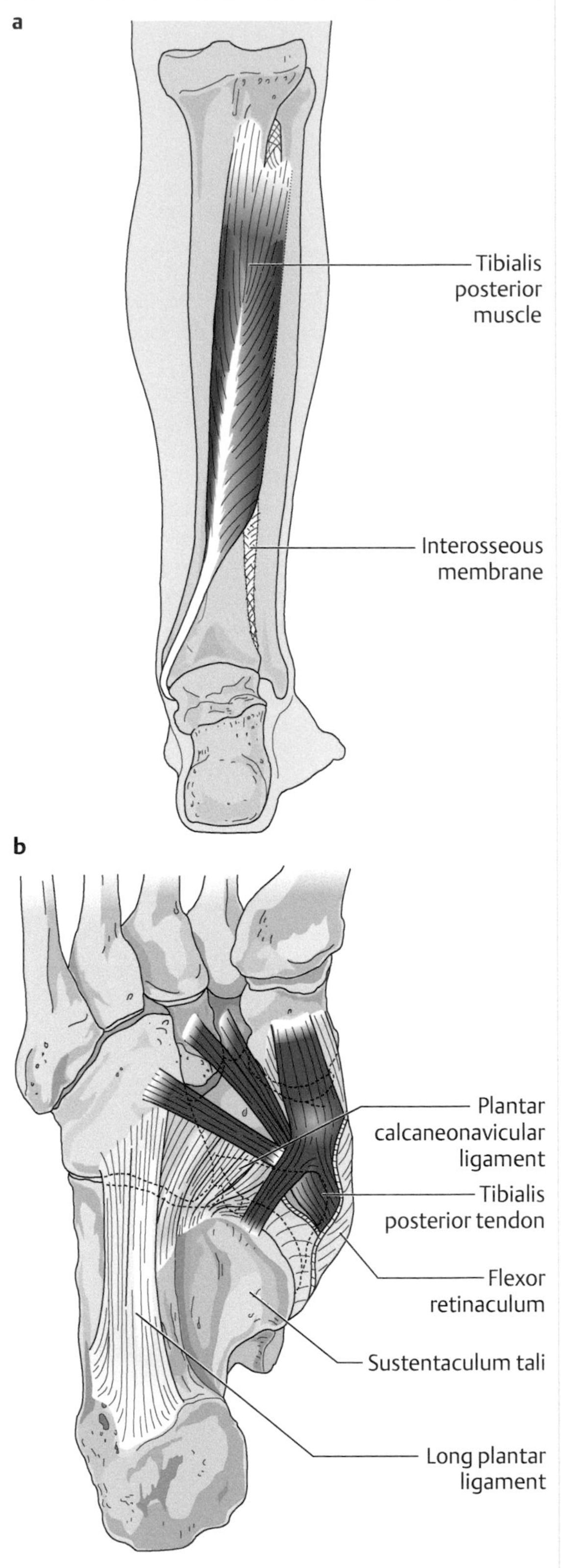


**Fig. 10.99** Course of the tibialis posterior muscle. **(a)** In the lower leg area. **(b)** In the plantar area.

## Flexor Digitorum Longus Muscle (Fig. 10.100)

- Its tendon crosses the tendon of the tibialis posterior (*chiasma crurale*) above the medial malleolus.
- It extends further over the posterior area of the talus and over the subtalar joint.
- It then runs over the sustentaculum tali, which has a groove here, and then bends inferolaterally to the sole of the foot.
- At the medial margin of the foot, it crosses over the tendon of the flexor hallucis longus muscle (*chiasma plantare*).
- Shortly thereafter, it divides into the four individually running terminal tendons.
- In this area where the tendon separates, it also connects with the flexor hallucis longus muscle (*junctura tendineum*). Thus, the movements of both flexor muscles are coupled.
- In the plantar area, the most lateral part of the tendon serves as the insertion site for the quadratus plantae muscle.
- Further distally, the four tendon parts function as sites of origin for the lumbrical muscles.
- In the plantar area, the tendons run together with the flexor digitorum brevis muscle, which extends superficially.
- At the level of the proximal phalanx, the tendons of the flexor digitorum longus muscle penetrate the tendons of the flexor digitorum brevis muscle and insert on the bases of the distal phalanges.

## Flexor Hallucis Longus Muscle (Fig. 10.100)

- The tendon crosses the subtalar joint posteriorly and passes under the sustentaculum tali.
- Soon after, it crosses under the tendon of the flexor digitorum muscle as the *chiasma plantare*.
- It remains in the medial plantar area through the remainder of its course.
- The tendon ends at the base of the distal phalanx.

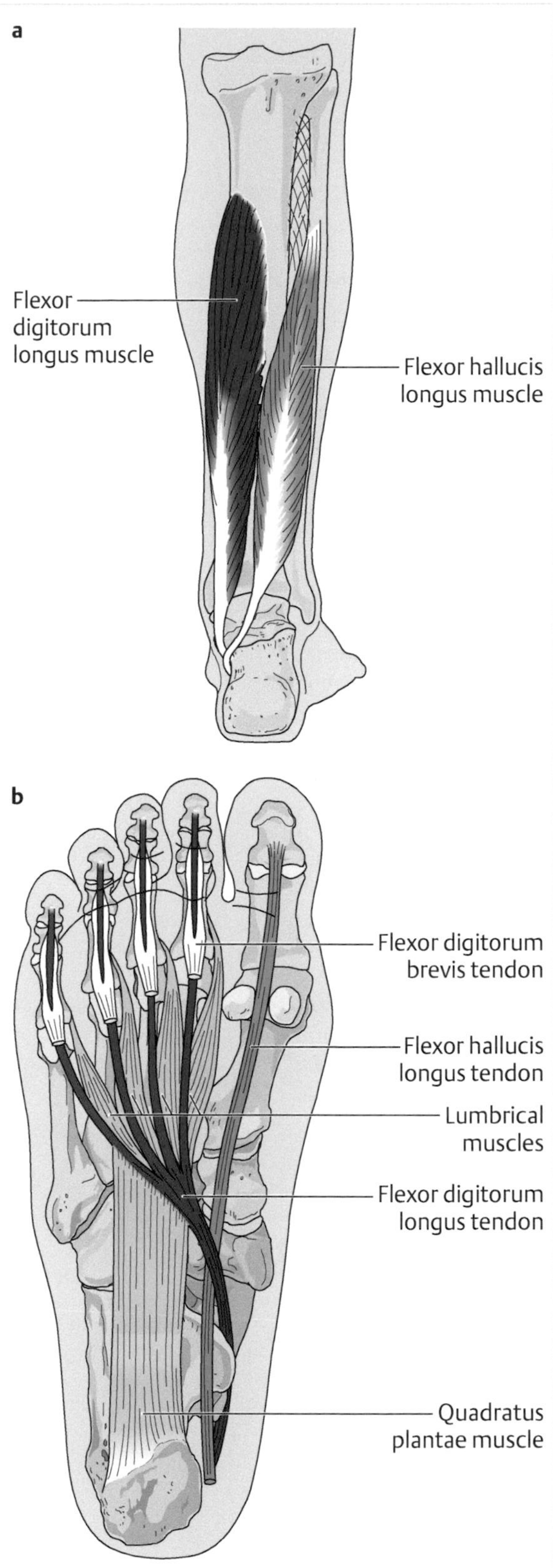


**Fig. 10.100** Course of the flexor digitorum and hallucis longus muscles. **(a)** In the lower leg area. **(b)** In the plantar area.

*Course of the Tendons in the Bone Area (Fig 10.101)*

The malleolar canal is divided by connective tissue septa into several compartments, with a tendon running in each of these. The sequence from anterior to posterior is as follows: tibialis posterior muscle, flexor digitorum longus muscle, and flexor hallucis longus muscle.

The tendon of the tibialis posterior muscle passes by the closest to the malleolus. The flexor hallucis tendon describes the largest posteriorly extending arch around the malleolus. The groove for the flexor hallucis longus tendon is found on the posterior talus. At this point, the tendon turns sharply anteriorly.

Tendon sheaths surround all three tendons. The tendinous sheath of the tibialis posterior begins far above the malleolus and ends shortly before the insertion on the navicular tuberosity. The tendinous sheath of the flexor digitorum longus, like that of the flexor hallucis longus muscle, begins shortly above the malleolus and extends to the chiasma plantare.

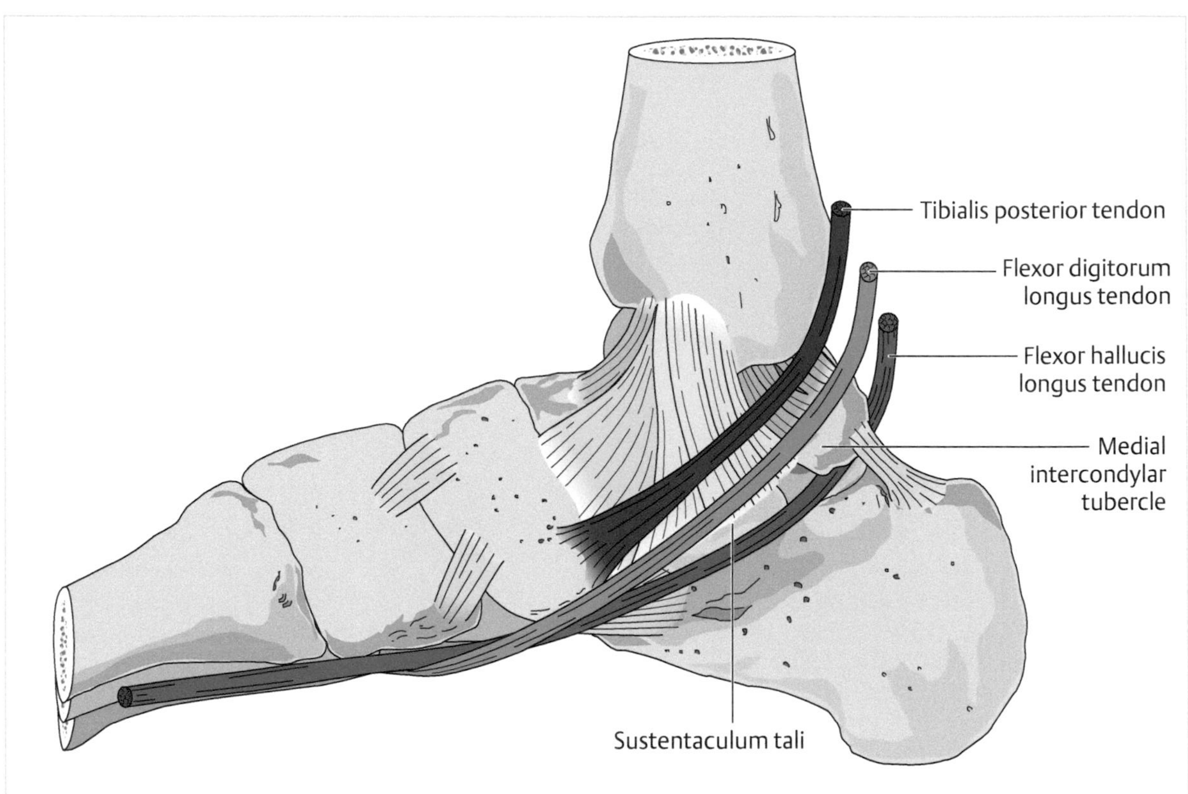


**Fig. 10.101** Course of the tendons of the tibialis posterior, flexor digitorum longus, and flexor hallucis longus muscles.

*Flexor Retinaculum (Fig. 10.102)*

This involves a guidance device for the flexor tendons, the tibialis posterior muscle, and the neurovascular bundle. The retinaculum is a component of the deep fascia of the leg. Its superficial layer is strengthened and fans out toward the Achilles tendon between the medial tibial surface and the calcaneal tuberosity.

The deep layer is shorter. It extends from the medial malleolus to the medial surface of the talus and encloses the tendons of the tibialis posterior and flexor digitorum longus muscles. Further fibrous parts track from the inner surface of the talus to the medial calcaneus and enclose the tendon of the flexor hallucis longus muscle.

The two layers form the malleolar canal, in which the above-named tendons and a strand of vessels and nerves extend distally.

**Functions of the muscles:**

- Stabilization of the posteromedial area of the foot.
- Stabilization of the arch of the foot. See Chapter 10.13, Biomechanics.
- Plantarflexion.
- Adduction and supination of the foot.
- Flexion of the toes at the distal joint by the flexor muscles.

*Innervation* of the posteromedial stabilizers: tibial nerve.

## Posterolateral Stabilization

### Fibularis Longus Muscle (Fig. 10.103)

- This runs in the lateral area of the lower leg.
- At the transition to the lower third of the lower leg, it merges into its long terminal tendon; at this point, it lies on top of the fibularis brevis muscle.
- The first narrow point occurs behind the malleolus, because here the *superior fibular retinaculum* forms a type of tunnel in which both fibular tendons run. The lateral malleolus forms a groove here, which serves as the floor of the tunnel.
- Shortly after the retinaculum, the tendon first changes its direction, making an almost right-angle turn anteriorly.
- Shortly thereafter, it runs into a second tunnel formed by the *inferior fibular retinaculum.*
- This retinaculum is fixed to the fibular trochlea, a bony projection on the lateral calcaneus. The trochlea separates the two fibularis muscles from each other, so that the tendon of the fibularis longus muscle runs inferior to it.
- At the level of the cuboid bone, the tendon changes direction for a second time. It turns medially toward the plantar area and runs here in a sulcus (*groove for the tendon of fibularis longus*), which runs anteromedially. Here it passes through overlying ligamentous structures, such as the long plantar ligament, to an osteofibrotic canal.

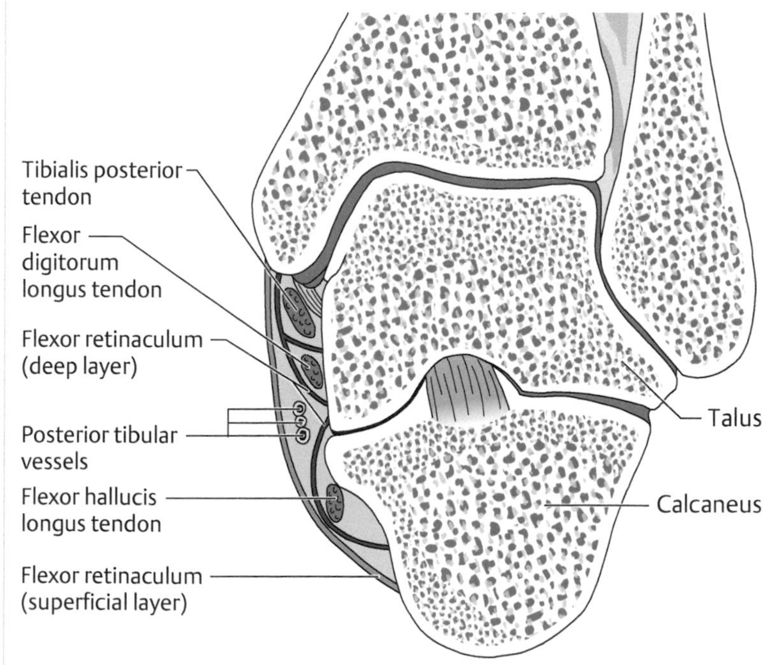


**Fig. 10.102** The retinaculum and course of the nerves in the medial malleolar canal.

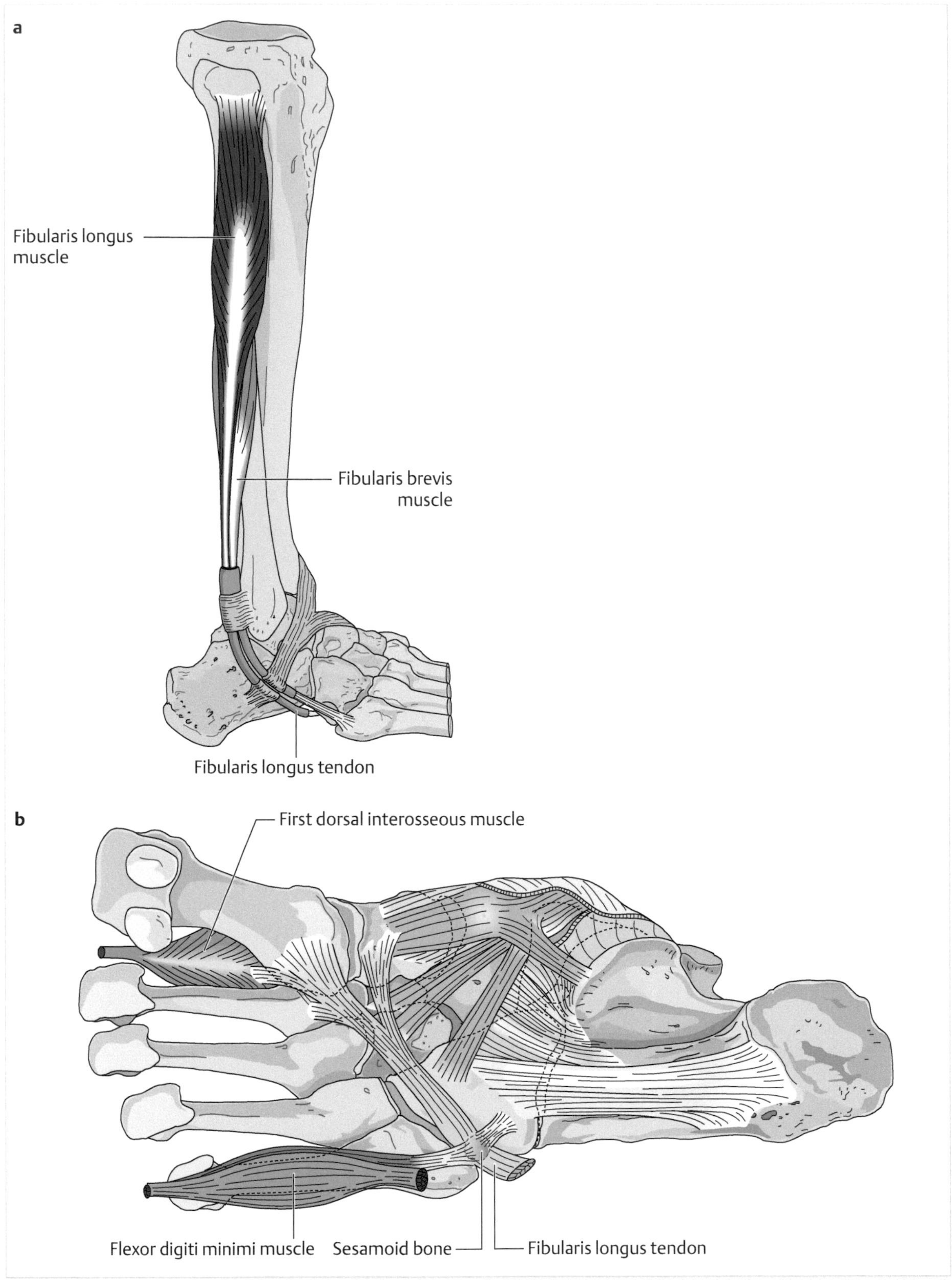


**Fig. 10.103** Course of the fibularis longus muscle. **(a)** In the lower leg. **(b)** In the plantar area.

- Proximal to the sulcus, the *cuboid tuberosity*, which is covered with a layer of cartilage, serves as an abutment for the tendon.
- At the point where it turns, a sesamoid bone is sometimes embedded in the tendon. If it is, the sesamoid is fixed with small ligaments to the cuboid bone and to the base of the fifth metatarsal. There it merges with the flexor digiti minimi muscle.
- The insertions lie very far medially on the medial cuneiform bone and on the base of the first and second metatarsal bones. In addition, the most medial part of the tendon merges with the first dorsal interosseous muscle.

## Fibularis Brevis Muscle (Fig. 10.104)

- This lies below the fibularis longus muscle and forms a groove for its tendon.
- Its terminal tendon begins shortly before the superior fibular retinaculum.
- Together with the fibularis longus muscle tendon, it turns anteriorly around the lateral malleolus, where both tendons cross the calcaneofibular ligament.
- Its tendon runs superior to the fibular trochlea and ends on the base of the fifth metatarsal.

**Functions of the muscles:**
- Stabilization of the posterior and lateral regions of the foot.
- Dynamic protection from inversion.
- Plantarflexion, abduction, and pronation.
- Tensing of the longitudinal and transverse arches through the tendon of the fibularis longus muscle. See Chapter 10.13, Biomechanics.

*Innervation:* superficial fibular nerve.

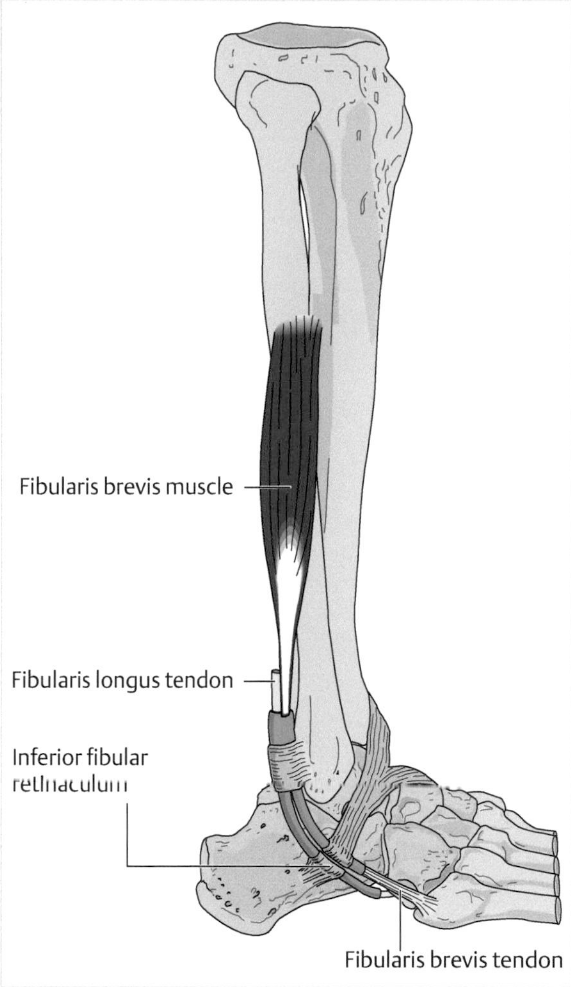


**Fig. 10.104** Fibularis brevis muscle.

**Pathology**

### Inversion Trauma

Inversion trauma damages the receptors, resulting in a proprioceptive deficit. The result is a functionally unstable joint. The fibular tendon usually provides protection from sudden inversion. Abrupt overstretching during trauma causes microtraumatization in the tendon and in the surrounding tendon sheath so they are no longer fully capable of functioning. For example, their reaction time is prolonged, so that they cannot be stabilized when faced with repeat trauma.

### Luxation of the Fibular Tendons

This occurs because the malleolar groove in which the tendons run in the posterior region is too shallow. If they are jerked, they can be displaced anteriorly within the fixed retinaculum. This usually occurs during dorsiflexion and pronation.

### *Tendon Sheaths (Fig. 10.105)*

The two fibular tendons are surrounded by tendon sheaths in the malleolar area. Proximal to the malleolus, the sheaths surround both tendons together, but they separate under the malleolus into two separate synovial sheaths, which continue on to the cuboid bone.

### *Superior and Inferior Fibular Retinacula (Fig. 10.105)*

These form guidance channels for the tendons. Proximal to the lateral malleolus, there is a common chamber for both tendons. The *superior fibular retinaculum* is a firm aponeurotic ring that is attached to the superolateral surface of the fibula. Superiorly, it is sometimes joined with the flexor retinaculum, which comes from the medial side.

Distal to the malleolus, *the inferior fibular retinaculum* forms two separate tendon channels. Posteriorly it is fixed to the calcaneus, attaches to the fibular trochlea between the two fibular tendons, and then attaches to the outermost edge of the tarsal sinus. There it forms a connection to the inferior extensor retinaculum, which approaches from over the dorsum of the foot.

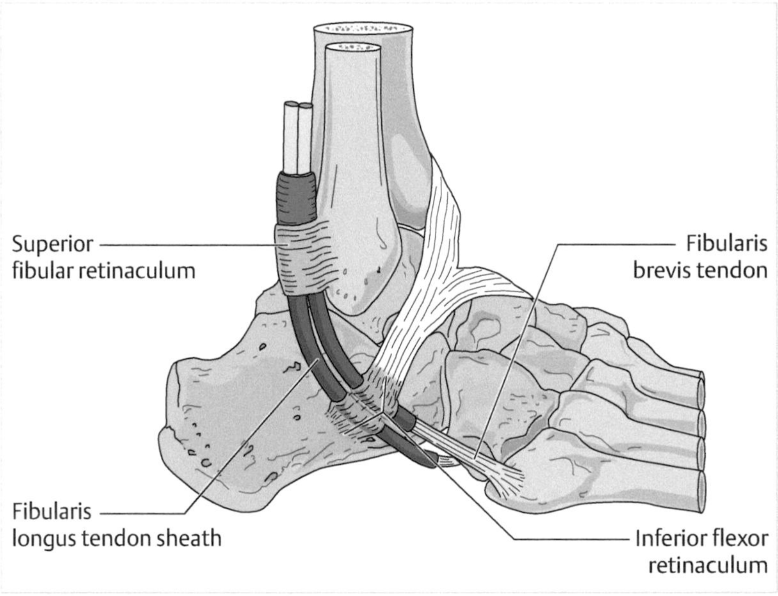


**Fig. 10.105** Tendon sheaths and retinacula of the fibular muscles.

## Posterior Stabilization

### Gastrocnemius Muscle (Fig. 10.106)

▷ See Chapter 9.3, Knee Joint

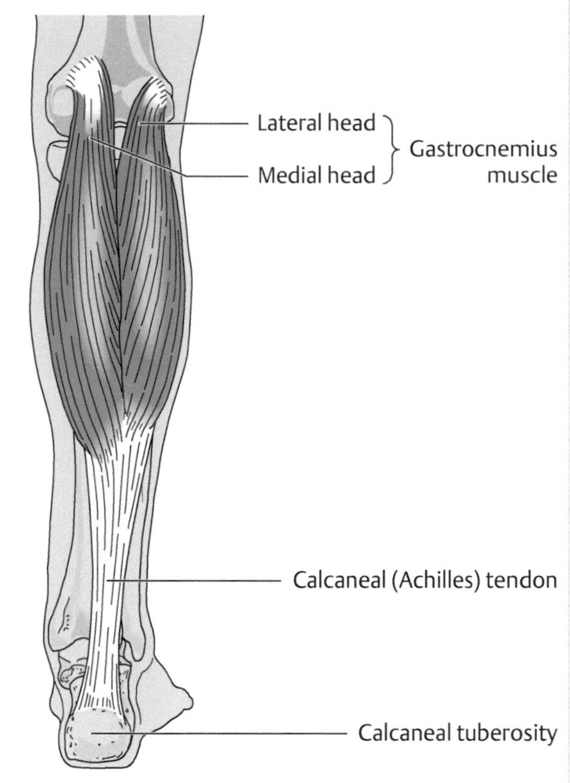


**Fig. 10.106** Gastrocnemius muscle.

### Soleus Muscle (Fig. 10.107)

- This lies beneath the gastrocnemius muscle.
- It has a broad site of origin.
- From its dual origin points on the head of the fibula and the medial edge of the tibia, it forms a fibrous arch, the *tendinous arch of soleus muscle*, through which the posterior tibial artery and the tibial nerve pass into the deep flexor compartment.
- On the medial and lateral sides of the muscles, the transition into the Achilles tendon occurs significantly further distally than in the midmuscle area, i.e., about a handbreadth above the insertion of the Achilles tendon onto the calcaneus.

### Plantaris Muscle (Fig. 10.107)

- The tendon courses under the gastrocnemius muscle and, in the inferior third of the lower leg, medial to the Achilles tendon.
- Together with the Achilles tendon, it inserts on the medial calcaneal tuberosity.

▷ See Chapter 9.3, Knee Joint

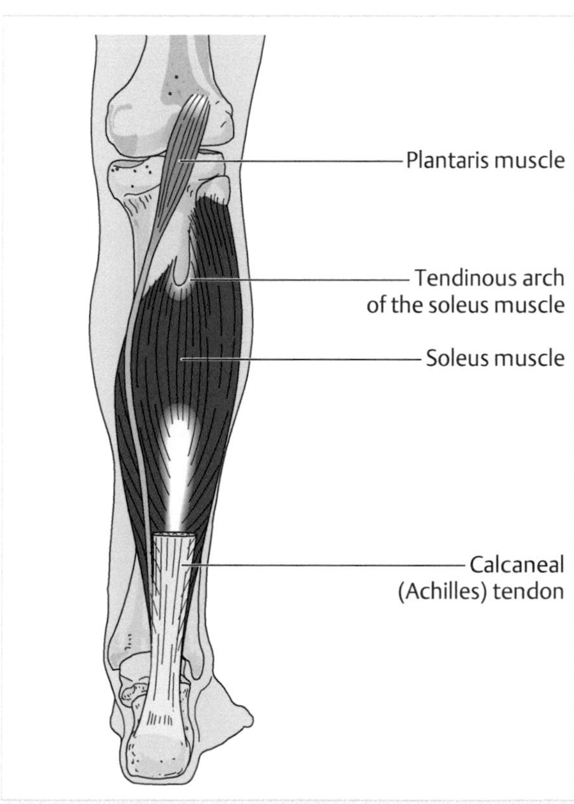


**Fig. 10.107** Soleus muscle and plantaris muscle.

*Calcaneal (Achilles) Tendon*

- This is the common terminal tendon of the triceps surae muscle.
- It becomes significantly narrower at the level of the malleoli, and then wider again at its insertion.
- At its insertion site, it is 2 cm wide.
- The fibers of the gastrocnemius muscle run posteriorly within the tendon while those of the soleus muscle run anteriorly.
- At a point 12 to 15 cm above the insertion, the fibers twist around, so that the medially running fibers insert laterally on the calcaneal tuberosity, and a few lateral fibers track medially. In addition, in the process, fibers from posterior switch to anterior, and vice versa.
- The *bursa of the calcaneal tendon* lies between the inner side of the tendon and the upper edge of the tuberosity. Another bursa, the *subcutaneous calcaneal bursa*, is located in the insertion area between the tendon and skin (**Fig. 10.108**).

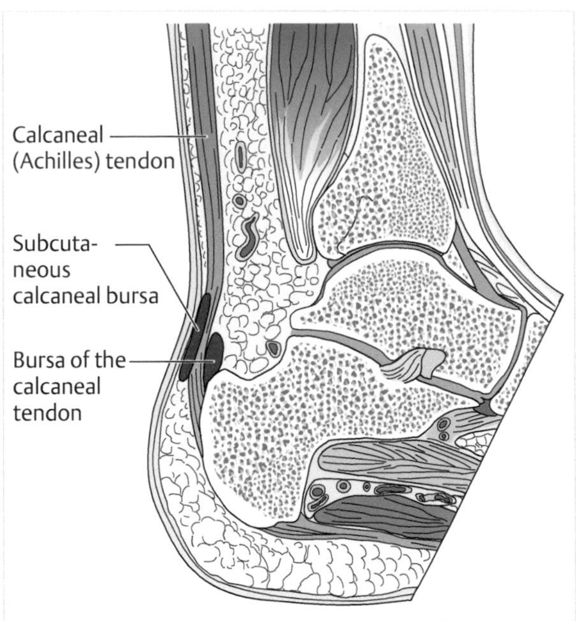


**Fig. 10.108** Calcaneal bursae.

**Functions of the triceps surae muscle:**

- With its three powerful parts, it prevents the body from tipping forward over the upper ankle joint.
- Plantarflexion: For instance, it raises the entire body weight while on tiptoes.
- It produces inversion because its insertion mostly lies superomedial to the axis. See Chapter 9.3, Knee Joint.

*Innervation* of the triceps surae muscle: tibial nerve.

**Pathology**

### Achilles Tendon Rupture (Fig. 10.109)

The most common site for tears lies approximately 2 to 6 cm above the insertion of the tendon. In terms of perfusion, this is a critical area because it is the border zone between vascular systems coming from above and below. In addition, this area experiences the greatest strain when walking. Repeated microtrauma causes tissue destruction, and then sudden dorsiflexing or pushing off with the foot causes the tendon to finally tear.

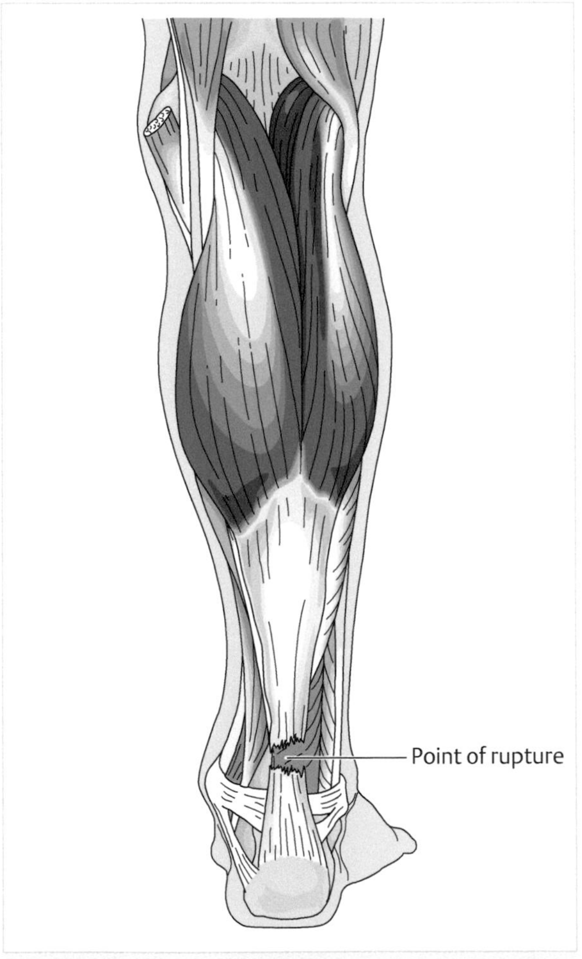


**Fig. 10.109** Achilles tendon rupture.

## Anterior Stabilization

### Tibialis Anterior Muscle (Fig. 10.110)

- The muscle passes under the superior extensor retinaculum in the medial region, and under the inferior extensor retinaculum further distally.
- It extends distally toward the medial edge of the foot.
- At a point 1 to 2 cm before the first tarsometatarsal joint, it divides into two tendon slips, one of which extends to the medial and plantar surfaces of the base of the metatarsal, and the other to the medial surface of the medial cuneiform bone;
- At the level of the joint, the tendon parts bend around almost vertically and here merge with the capsule.

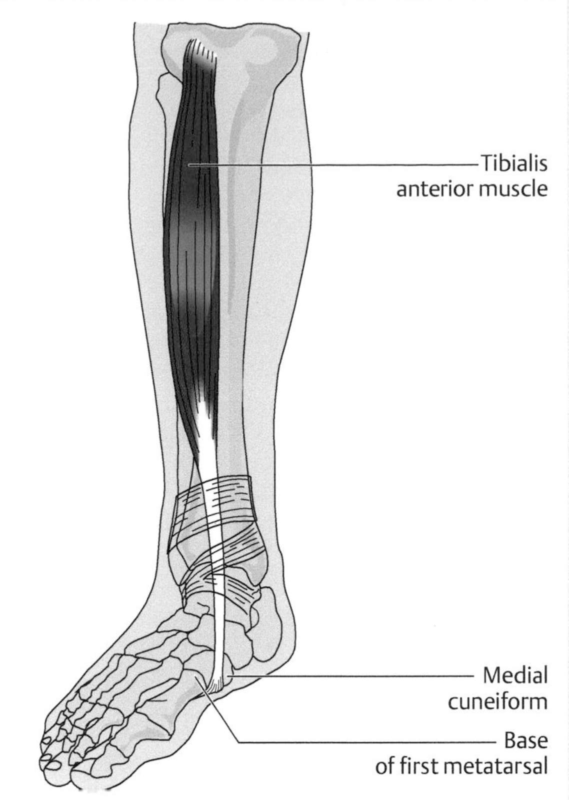


**Fig. 10.110** Tibialis anterior muscle.

### Extensor Hallucis Longus Muscle (Fig. 10.111)

- At the level of the malleoli, its tendon passes deep under the superior extensor retinaculum and lateral to the tibialis anterior muscle.
- The tendon has its own separate compartment under the inferior extensor retinaculum.
- After that, it extends superficially on the dorsum of the foot distally and medially toward the distal phalanx of the big toe.
- There is often a small medial offshoot to the base of the proximal phalanx.

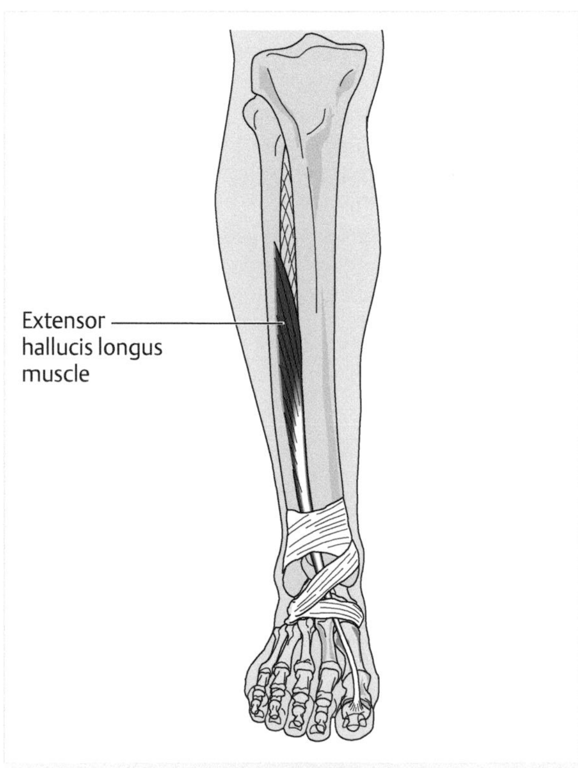


**Fig. 10.111** Extensor hallucis longus muscle.

## Extensor Digitorum Longus Muscle (Fig. 10.112)

- This passes under the superior and inferior extensor retinacula.
- Under the superior retinaculum, the tendon divides into two parts, each of which in turn divides into two parts under the inferior retinaculum, so that there are four terminal tendons to identify.
- At the level of the proximal phalanx, the tendons of the extensor digitorum brevis muscle extend from laterally to join with these tendons.
- It ends with the dorsal aponeurosis (**Fig. 10.113**), which covers the proximal phalanx. From here, a middle part of the tendon extends to the middle phalanx, and two outer tendon slips extend to the dorsal base of the distal phalanx, where they join together in a common insertion.
- Through the dorsal aponeurosis, the extensor digitorum longus muscle has a connection with interosseous muscles.
- An offshoot can extend as a fifth terminal tendon to the base of the fifth metatarsal = *fibularis tertius muscle.*

**Functions of the extensor group:**

- These muscles support the ligaments in *anterior stabilization* of the upper ankle joint (talocrural joint).
- *Dorsiflexion:* In the swing phase of ambulation, for example, the fixed end is proximal, and the muscles pull the foot into dorsiflexion. Conversely, in the stance phase, the fixed end is the foot and the muscles extend the lower leg, resulting in dorsiflexion of the foot.
- Tibialis anterior tendon: This produces *supination*, since its insertion lies medial to the longitudinal axis. In this, it is supported by the extensor hallucis longus muscle.
- On the other hand, most of the parts of the extensor digitorum longus muscle support pronation.
- The toe extensors cause *extension* in all the toe joints. They also have a stabilizing effect on the longitudinal arch of the foot in that they exert tension on the plantar aponeurosis by extending the toes. See Chapter 10.13, Biomechanics.

*Innervation* of the extensors: deep fibular nerve.

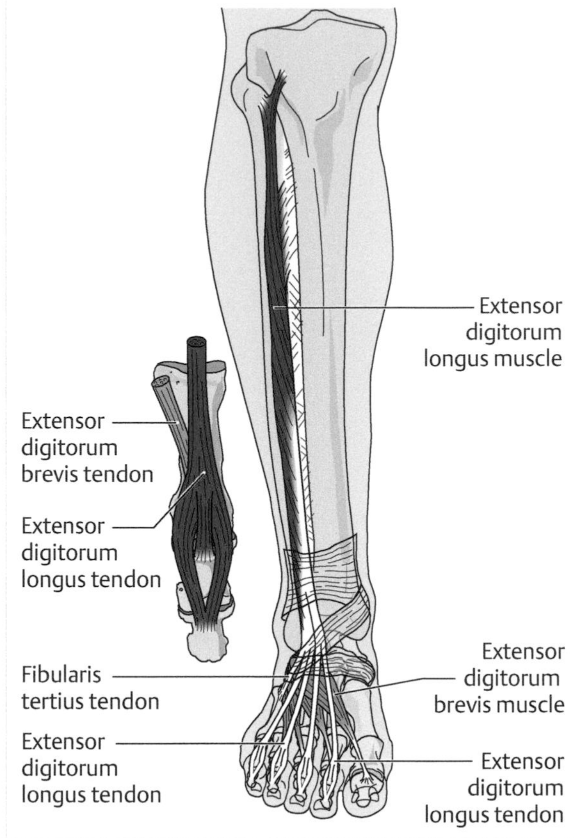


**Fig. 10.112** Extensor digitorum longus muscle.

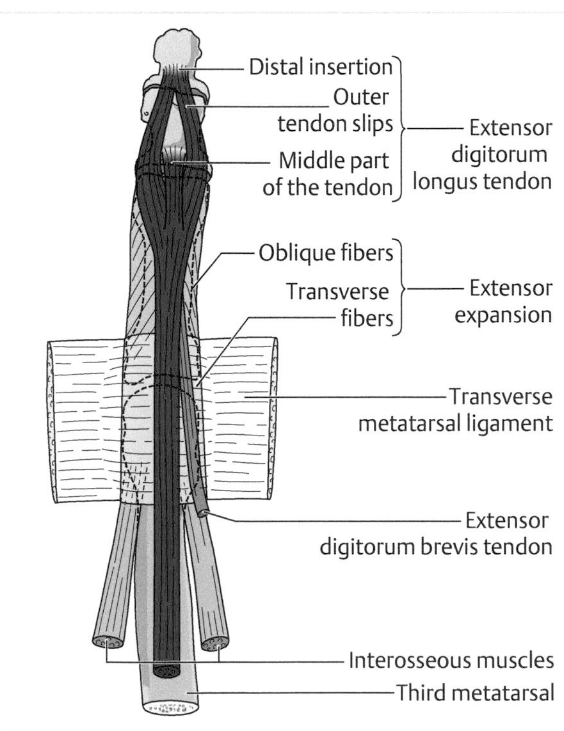


**Fig. 10.113** Terminal tendon of the extensor digitorum longus muscle.

### *Superior and Inferior Extensor Retinacula (Fig. 10.114)*

The *superior extensor retinaculum* begins about one handbreadth proximal to the malleoli and is about three fingerbreadths wide. It extends from the medial side of the tibia to the anterior surface of the fibula. It secures the long extensors and the tibialis anterior muscle on the lower leg.

The *inferior extensor retinaculum* is laid out as a cross and consists of two main parts. The proximal part comes from the medial malleolus and extends obliquely inferolaterally to the tarsal sinus with a small offshoot to the lateral malleolus. The distal part joins the navicular tuberosity with the tarsal sinus. An additional small part runs from the medial cuneiform bone to the second metatarsal. All these parts serve as a retaining band for the tendons.

### *Tendon Sheaths*

The tendons run in a tibial, middle, and fibular compartment under the retinacula and are surrounded by synovial sheaths. They are of various lengths. For example, the tibialis anterior muscle begins proximal to the superior retinaculum and ends distal to the upper portion of the inferior extensor retinaculum. The tendon sheath of the extensor hallucis longus muscle, on the other hand, is very long and runs on to the level of the base of the first metatarsal.

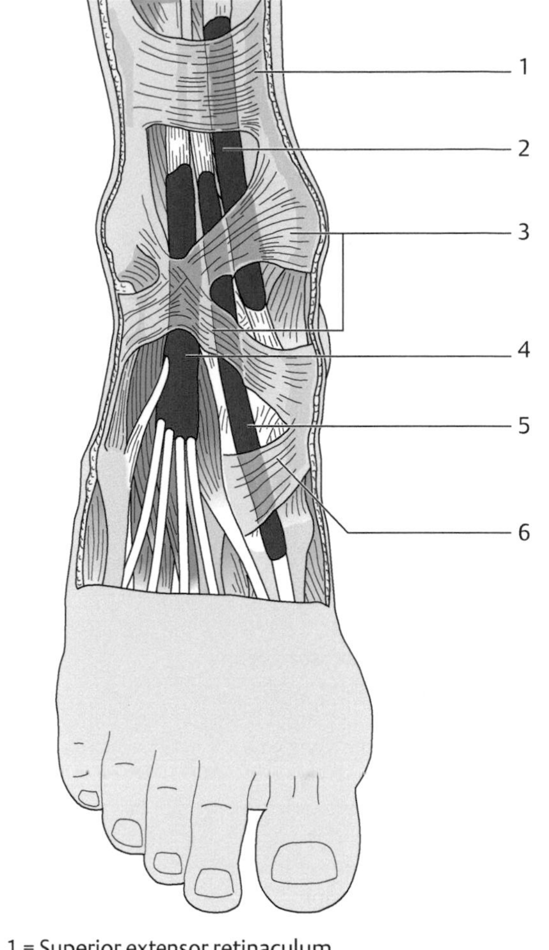


1 = Superior extensor retinaculum
2 = Tendon sheath of tibialis anterior
3 = Inferior extensor retinaculum
4 = Tendon sheath of extensor digitorum longus
5 = Tendon sheath of extensor hallucis longus
6 = Offshoot of the inferior extensor retinaculum

**Fig. 10.114** Retinacula and tendon sheaths of the dorsum of the foot.

Pathology

#### Anterior Tibial Syndrome (Anterior Compartment Syndrome)

This involves a compression syndrome of the anterior compartment, in which the tendons of the tibialis anterior muscle runs. The compartment is bounded by bones and the extensor retinaculum, so that distension of the enclosed tendon is not possible. For example, overuse can cause inflammation with development of edema. The capillaries supplying the area can be compromised, leading to ischemic necrosis of the muscles in the tibial compartment.

Patients complain of intense pain in the pretibial area and weakness of dorsiflexion.

# 10.7 Ankle Joint during Ambulation

## 10.7.1 Electromyographic Muscle Activity during Ambulation

Mechanical receptors in the capsules and ligaments coordinate the activity of the muscles of the lower leg and foot, which stabilizes the foot on uneven ground.

**Fig. 10.115** gives an overview of the muscular activities that are required to walk without difficulty (Sarrafian 1993).

## 10.7.2 Range of Motion

The range of motion utilized in walking does not reach the maximal possible movements of the joint. As a rule, only 50 % is used.

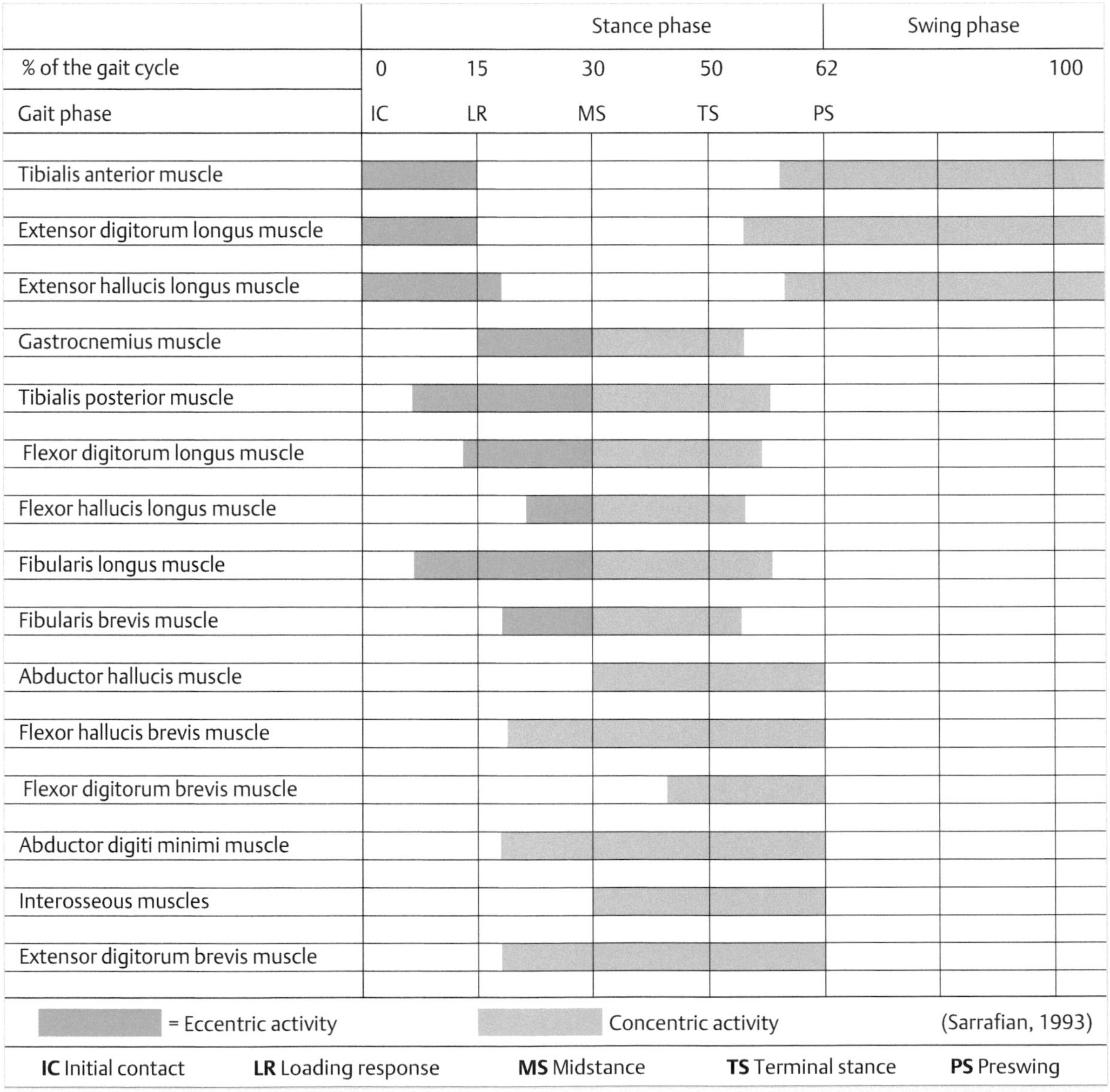

| | Stance phase | | | | Swing phase | |
|---|---|---|---|---|---|---|
| % of the gait cycle | 0 | 15 | 30 | 50 | 62 | 100 |
| Gait phase | IC | LR | MS | TS | PS | |
| Tibialis anterior muscle | | | | | | |
| Extensor digitorum longus muscle | | | | | | |
| Extensor hallucis longus muscle | | | | | | |
| Gastrocnemius muscle | | | | | | |
| Tibialis posterior muscle | | | | | | |
| Flexor digitorum longus muscle | | | | | | |
| Flexor hallucis longus muscle | | | | | | |
| Fibularis longus muscle | | | | | | |
| Fibularis brevis muscle | | | | | | |
| Abductor hallucis muscle | | | | | | |
| Flexor hallucis brevis muscle | | | | | | |
| Flexor digitorum brevis muscle | | | | | | |
| Abductor digiti minimi muscle | | | | | | |
| Interosseous muscles | | | | | | |
| Extensor digitorum brevis muscle | | | | | | |

= Eccentric activity  Concentric activity  (Sarrafian, 1993)

**IC** Initial contact **LR** Loading response **MS** Midstance **TS** Terminal stance **PS** Preswing

**Fig. 10.115** Activity of the lower leg muscles while walking.

> **Practical Tip**
>
> **Gait Analysis (Fig. 10.116)**
>
> When evaluating the joint position, keep in mind that a patient, when walking, will not be able to utilize the improvements in range of motion right away, even though intensive therapy has improved the significant movement deficit that the patient had.
>
> *Example:* Plantarflexion is measured at 10°, and during preswing, the patient uses only 7 to 10°. In spite of this, he or she cannot optimally carry out this phase, and compensates by advancing the knee. The reasons for this are undoubtedly multifactorial, but it is certain that the patient requires a certain movement tolerance—here perhaps +7°—to initiate the necessary range of motion while walking.

a

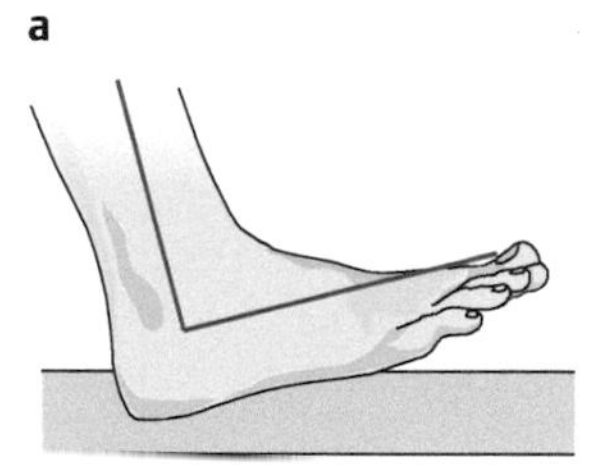

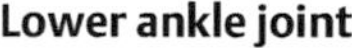

**Initial contact**

**Upper ankle joint**

Dorsiflexion 0 – 3°

**Lower ankle joint**

Inversion 3 – 4°

b

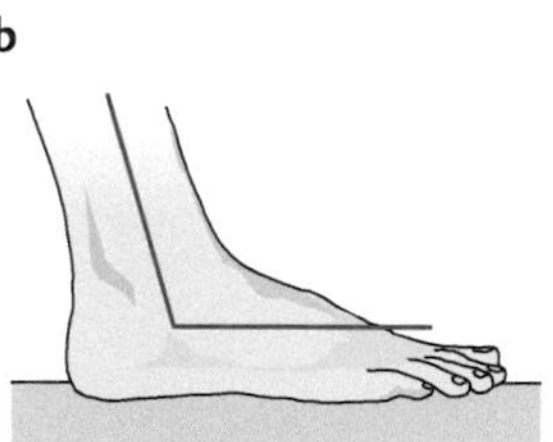

**Loading response**

Plantarflexion 7 – 10° (controlled by the eccentrically working dorsiflexors)

Eversion to 7°

c

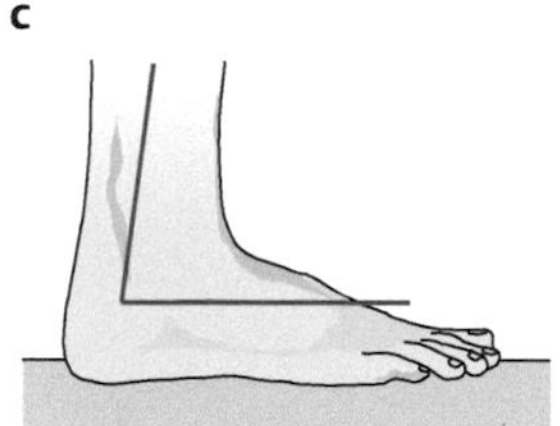

**Midstance**

Increasing dorsiflexion (the lower leg moves anteriorly over the talus)

Goes into inversion of 2 – 3°

d

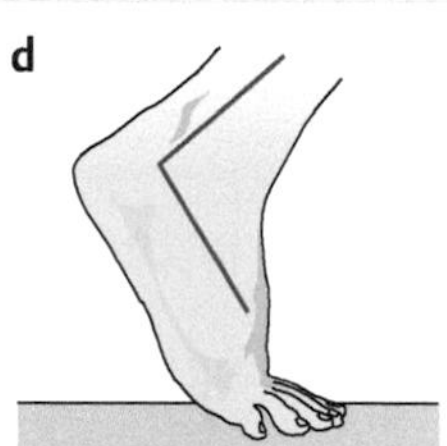

**Preswing**

Plantarflexion 10 – 15° (concentric work by the calf muscles)

Inversion 4°

e

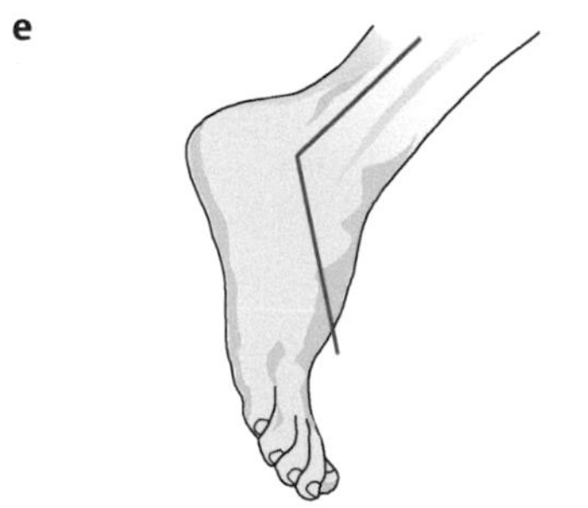

**Initial swing**

**Upper ankle joint**

Plantarflexion 10 – 15°

f

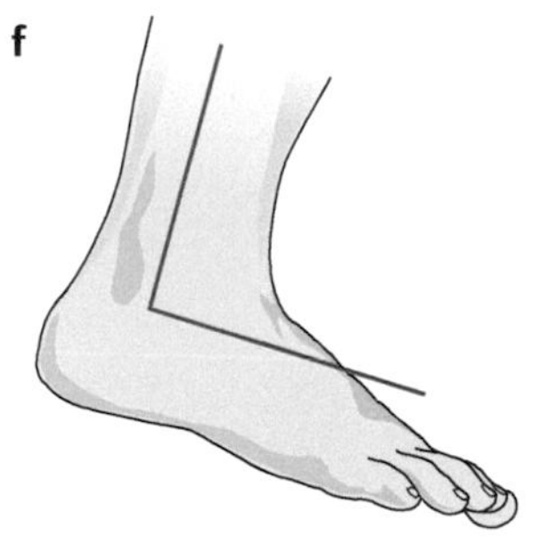

**Midswing**

0°

(active stabilization by dorsiflexors)

g

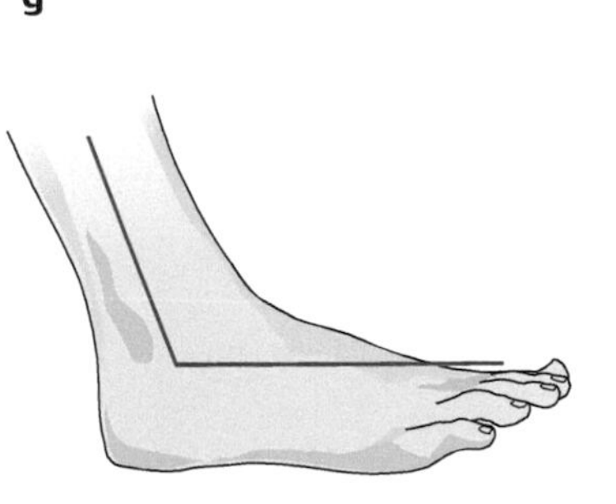

**Terminal swing**

Plantarflexion 0 – 10°

(active stabilization by dorsiflexion)

**Fig. 10.116** Range of motion of the ankle joints. **(a–d)** In the stance phase. **(e–g)** In the swing phase.

# 10.8 Calcaneocuboid Joint

## 10.8.1 Bony Structure and Joint Surfaces

### Calcaneus (Fig. 10.117)

- Anteriorly, the bone is somewhat funnel-shaped. The superior part protrudes distally like a down-sloping roof. Somewhat further medially on this roof is the anterior talar articular surface.
- The *articular surface for the cuboid* is found on the anterior surface.
- The joint surface is shaped somewhat like a saddle—convex in the medial-lateral orientation, and concave in the vertical orientation.

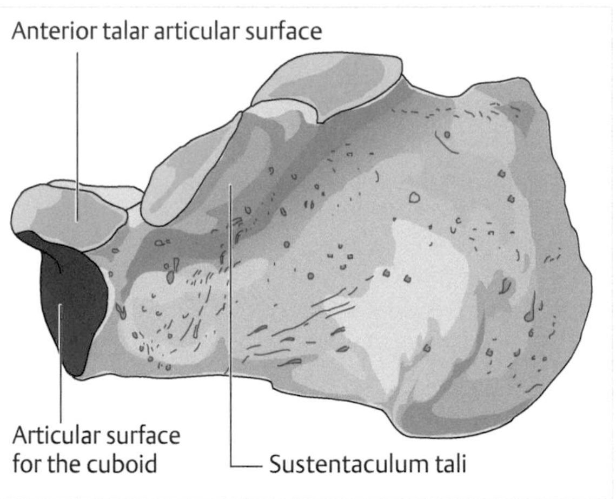


**Fig. 10.117** Right calcaneus, medial view.

### Cuboid Bone (Fig. 10.118)

- This is located on the lateral side of the foot, distal to the calcaneus.
- It has a triangular shape with a broad medial part and a short lateral part.
- The *calcaneal articular surface* on the proximal cuboid bone articulates with the calcaneus.
- This articular surface exhibits a somewhat saddle-like shape to match the corresponding joint surface on the calcaneus.

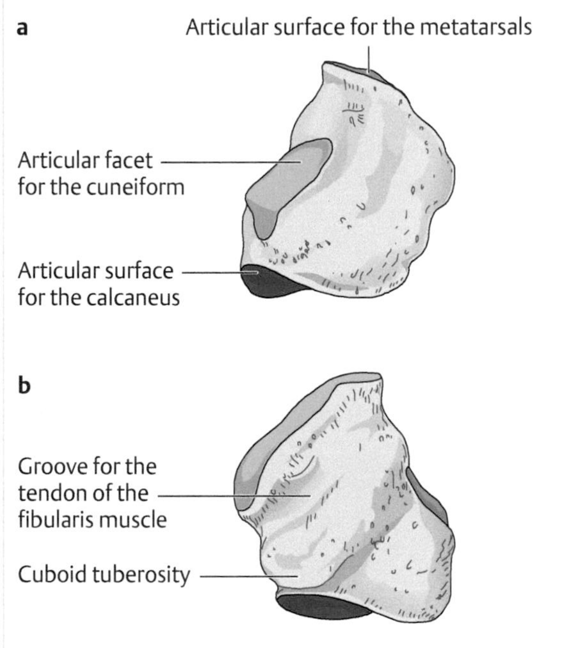


**Fig. 10.118** Right cuboid bone. **(a)** Superior view. **(b)** Inferior view.

## 10.8.2 Joint Capsule

The joint capsule inserts right at the bone-cartilage border and merges with all the ligaments that run immediately over it.

## 10.8.3 Ligaments

### Bifurcate Ligament (Fig. 10.119)

This unites the navicular bone, the cuboid bone, and the calcaneus into a functional unit and is therefore designated as the key ligament of Chopart's joint.

The ligament consists of the following two parts, which move apart from each other in a V-shaped form.

#### Lateral Calcaneonavicular Ligament

This ligament arises on the anteromedial corner of the tarsal sinus, immediately lateral to the anterior talar articular surface. The insertion is approximately 1 cm wide. It extends superiorly, anteriorly, and medially, and inserts on the posterior navicular.

The ligament is 2 to 2.5 cm long. The deeper lying fibers are shorter, and the more superficial fibers are longer. It is 1 cm wide.

#### Calcaneocuboid Ligament

This forms the lateral shank of the "**V**." It is 1 cm long and 0.5 cm wide. The ligament inserts immediately lateral to the insertion of the calcaneonavicular ligament and extends medially and almost horizontally to the lateral cuboid bone.

### Lateral Calcaneocuboid Ligament (Fig. 10.120)

This ligament is usually split, so that superior and inferior parts can be differentiated. The superior part is narrow. The inferior part is very wide and reaches to the plantar side. The ligament strengthens the capsule on the lateral side of the joint.

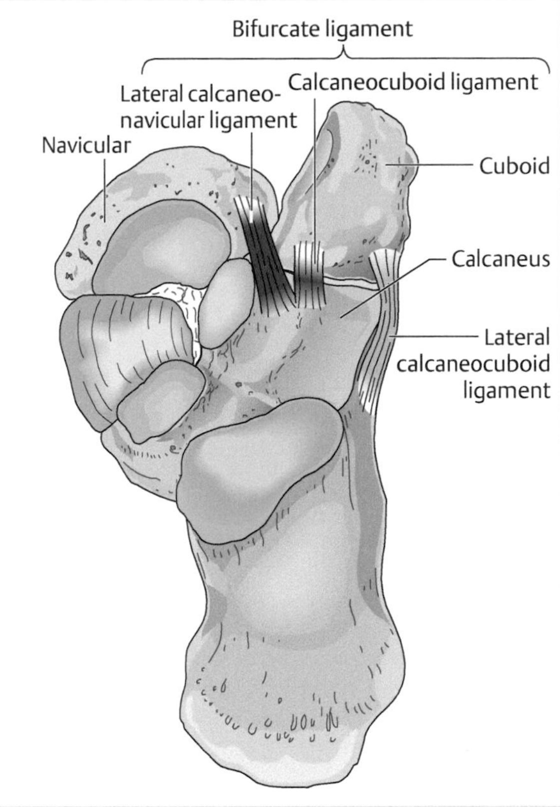


**Fig. 10.119** Bifurcate ligament.

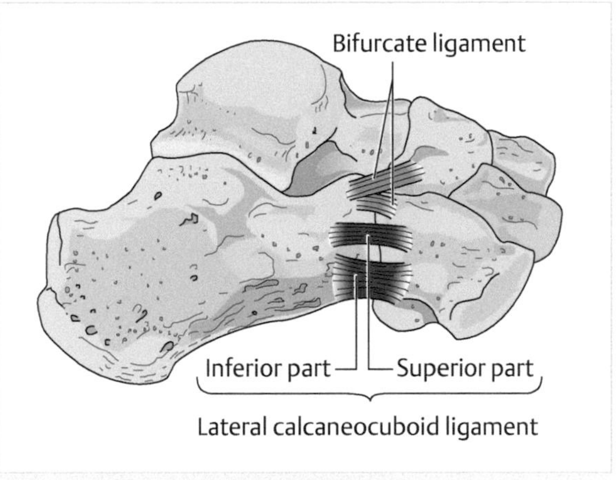


**Fig. 10.120** Lateral calcaneocuboid ligament.

## Plantar Calcaneocuboid Ligament (Fig. 10.121)

Long, superficial fibers spread out from the medial and lateral processes of the calcaneal tuberosity to the cuboid bone and the base of the metatarsals. There they track into the capsule–ligament apparatus of the second to fifth tarsometatarsal joints. The fibers run straight from posterior to anterior and distally cross over the tendon of the fibularis longus muscle, and are known as the *long plantar ligament*.

Short fibers of the ligament lie under the long plantar ligament. They connect with the capsule and run directly over the joint space between the calcaneus and the cuboid. This part spreads out like a fan from proximal to distal. It represents the continuation of the plantar calcaneonavicular ligament laterally.

**Functions of the ligaments:**

- Pronation movements tense the *bifurcate ligament*.
- The *calcaneocuboid ligament* prevents lateral gapping of the joint, as occurs, for example, with adduction.
- The *plantar calcaneocuboid ligament* tenses with supination of the cuboid bone, or, conversely, with pronation of the calcaneus. It also plays a large role in stabilizing the arch of the foot.

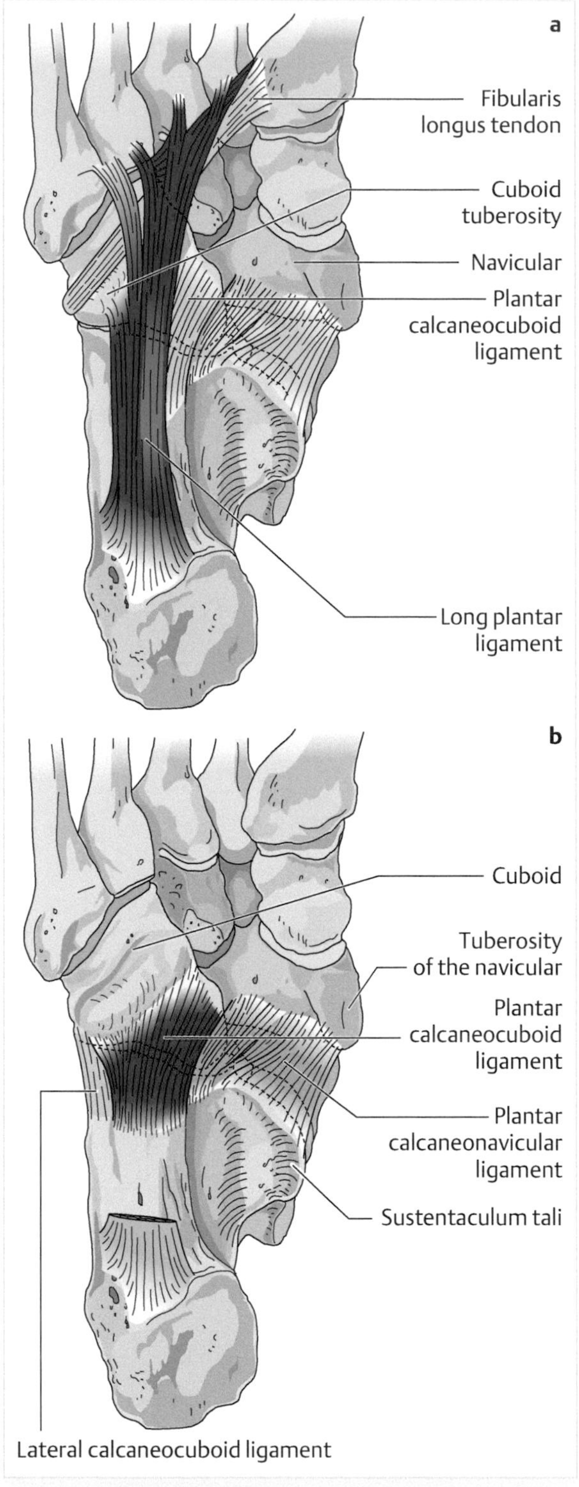


**Fig. 10.121** Plantar calcaneocuboid ligament. **(a)** Long plantar ligament, superficial fibers. **(b)** Deep fibers.

## 10.8.4 Axes and Movements

### Longitudinal Axis (Fig. 10.122)

This axis extends diagonally through the calcaneus and the "nose" of the cuboid bone (a protruding area of the plantar-medial aspect of the bone). The orientation of this axis is from posterior-inferior-lateral to anterior-superior-medial, with an inclination of 15° to the horizontal plane and 9° to the sagittal plane. The movements of pronation and supination take place around this axis. The extent of the movement can be substantial, because this is where the forefoot and hindfoot twist against each other (**Fig. 10.142**).

### Oblique Axis (Fig. 10.122)

This axis runs steeply and obliquely from superomedially to inferolaterally and extends through the navicular bone and the nose of the cuboid bone. It forms an angle of about 50° with the horizontal. Around it, combination movements in the direction of extension/abduction and flexion/adduction are possible.

### Movements

A type of spiral movement combination takes place around both axes, like a screw, but opposite to the subtalar joint. The composition of the movements is as in the ankle joints—extension/abduction/pronation and flexion/adduction/supination.

The calcaneocuboid joint laterally and the talocalcaneonavicular joint medially form a joint that appears somewhat like an "S" when viewed from above—*Chopart's joint* (transverse tarsal joint). Together, they form a functional unit.

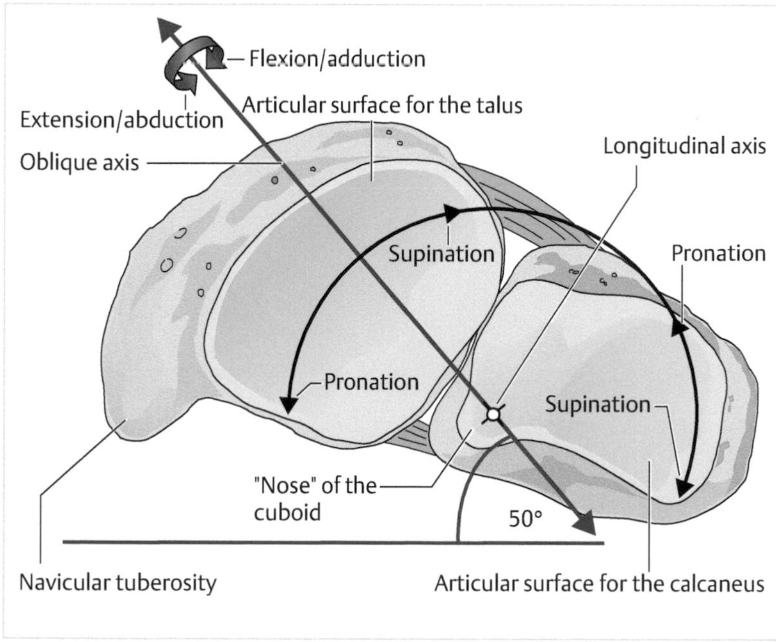


**Fig. 10.122** Axes of motion and movements of Chopart's joint.

# 10.9 Tarsal Joints

## 10.9.1 Bony Structures and Joint Surfaces of the Cuneonavicular and Cuboideonavicular Joints

### Medial Cuneiform Bone (Fig. 10.123a)

- Synonym: *first cuneiform.*
- This is the largest of the three cuneiform bones.
- It is only slightly wedge-shaped, with a broad, flat base.
- On the proximal surface, there is a concave joint facet for the navicular bone.

### Intermediate Cuneiform Bone (Fig. 10.123b)

- Synonym: *second cuneiform bone.*
- It is the smallest of the three cuneiform bones.
- It exhibits a distinct wedge shape, with the base at the dorsum of the foot and the point toward the plantar surface.
- Consistent with its wedge shape, it demonstrates a triangular joint facet with a plantar surface at the proximal end.

### Lateral Cuneiform Bone (Fig. 10.123c)

- Synonym: *third cuneiform bone.*
- This also exhibits a wedge shape.
- On the proximal surface, there is a concave joint facet for the navicular bone.

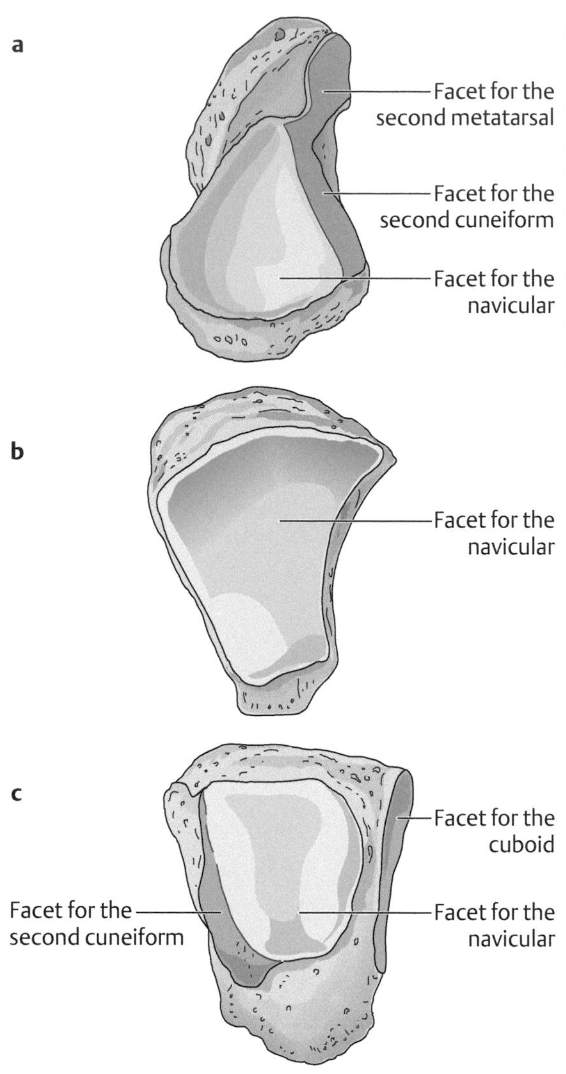


**Fig. 10.123** Proximal joint facets. **(a)** First cuneiform. **(b)** Second cuneiform. **(c)** Third cuneiform.

## Navicular Bone (Fig. 10.124)

- Distally, this demonstrates three joint facets that are divided by vertically running ridges.
- The medial facet represents the largest part of the joint surface. It is almost rectangular and is convex.
- The middle facet is triangular with the point toward the plantar surface. It is the least convex of the facets.
- An oval facet lies on the lateral border and is also convex.
- A small facet for the cuboid bone lies on the lateral surface.

## Cuboid Bone (Fig. 10.125)

- This has a small facet is on the medial, proximal side for the navicular bone.
- Distal to that lies the facet for the third cuneiform bone.

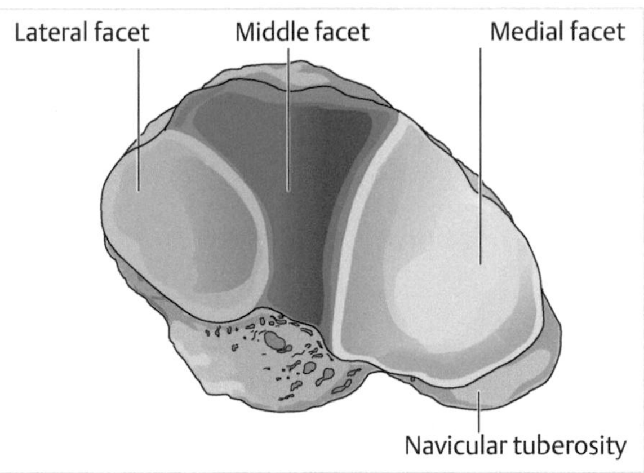


**Fig. 10.124** Distal joint surfaces on the navicular bone.

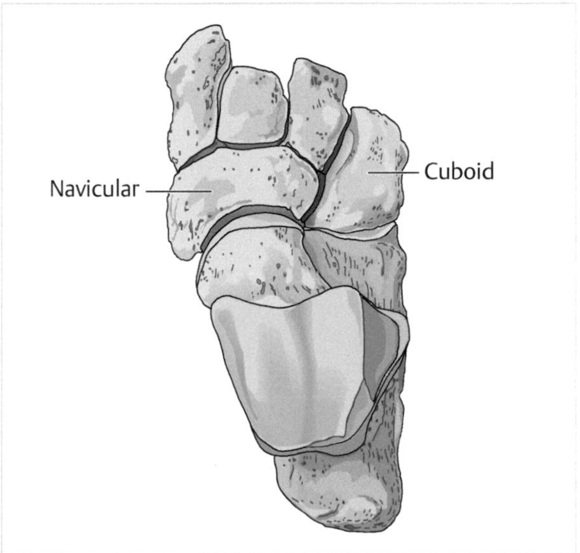


**Fig. 10.125** Cuboideonavicular joint.

## 10.9.2 Joint Capsule and Ligaments of the Cuneonavicular and Cuboideonavicular Joints

The capsule insertions are found at the bone–cartilage border of the respective joint surfaces. The capsule is tightly knit with the surrounding ligaments. The joint cavity of the cuneonavicular joint often communicates with that of the intercuneiform joints.

### Dorsal and Plantar Cuneonavicular Ligaments (Figs. 10.126 and 10.127)

Each cuneiform bone connects to the navicular bone by means of a dorsal and a plantar ligament, which intertwine with the joint capsule. The dorsal ligaments are very thin. The medial ligament is the strongest of the three.

The medial plantar ligament has very short fibers and is also the strongest. The lateral ligament has an oblique course and contains the longest fibers. Some of the fibers combine with the tendon of the tibialis posterior muscle.

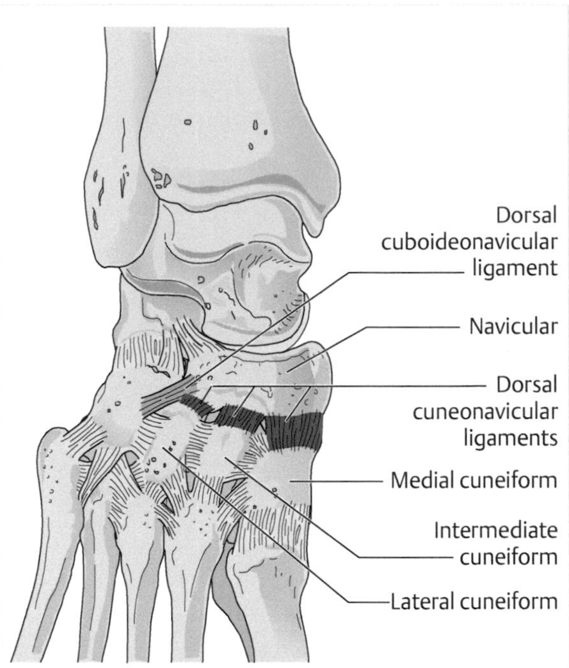


**Fig. 10.126** Dorsal cuneonavicular ligaments and dorsal cuboideonavicular ligament.

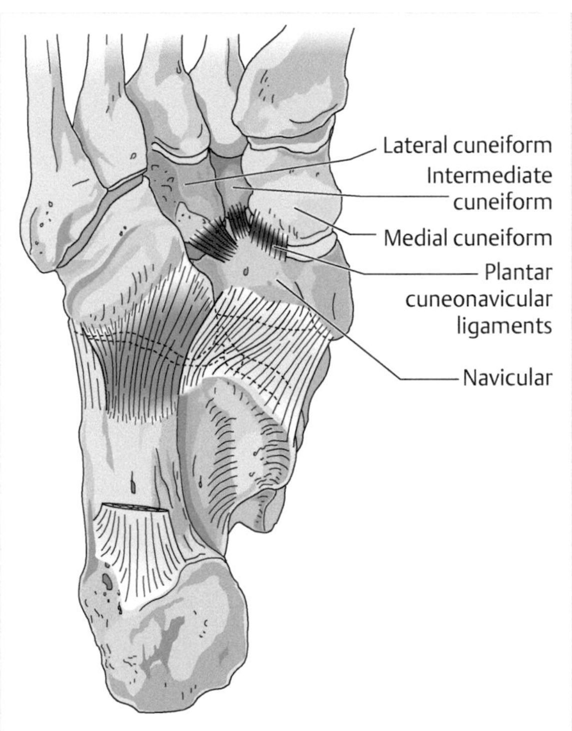


**Fig. 10.127** Plantar cuneonavicular ligaments.

## Dorsal and Plantar Cuboideonavicular Ligaments (Figs. 10.126 and 10.128)

The dorsal ligamentous connection is very narrow. It runs anteriorly in front of the bifurcate ligament.

The plantar ligamentous bands spread out in an approximate fan shape with a broad base on the navicular, becoming narrower as they approach the cuboid.

**Function of the ligaments.** Arising from a multitude of joints, they form a stable framework. At the same time, these ligaments, especially the plantar ligaments, support the construction of the arches of the foot.

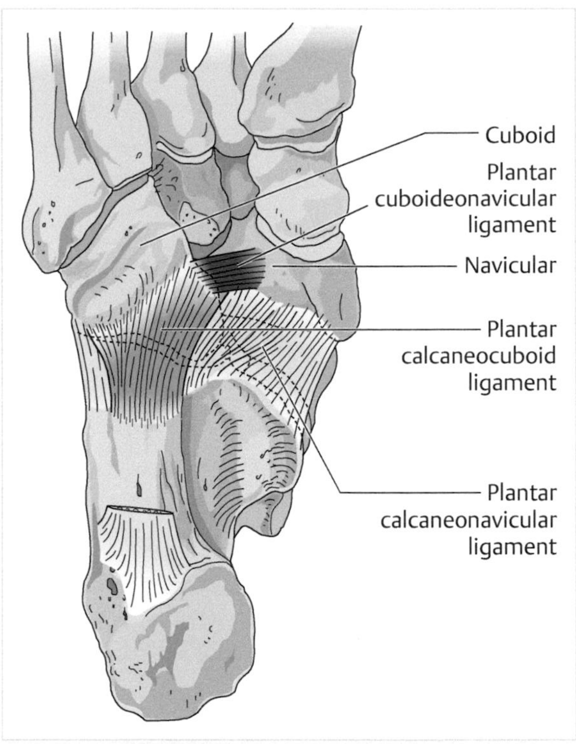


**Fig. 10.128** Plantar cuboideonavicular ligament.

## 10.9.3 Axes and Movements of the Cuneonavicular and Cuboideonavicular Joints

▷ See Chapter 10.10, Tarsometatarsal and Intermetatarsal Joints

## 10.9.4 Bony Structures and Joint Surfaces of the Cuneocuboid and Intercuneiform Joints

### Lateral Cuneiform Bone (Figs. 10.129a and 10.130)

- This demonstrates a large lateral joint surface, three-quarters of which articulates with the cuboid bone and one-quarter with the base of the fourth metatarsal.
- Because of the diagonal arch formed by the tarsal bones, the cuneiform bone lies on top of the cuboid bone, which is why the course of the joint line is oblique from dorsolateral to plantar-medial.

### Cuboid Bone (Fig. 10.129b)

The joint facet for the third cuneiform bone is located on the medial side.

### Cuneiform Bones (Fig. 10.130)

- These exhibit cartilage-covered joint facets on the surfaces facing each other.
- The course of the joint surfaces between the first two cuneiform bones goes from dorsal to plantar. Between the second and third cuneiform bones, the direction is more oblique because of the transverse arch of the foot.

> **Practical Tip**
>
> **Glide Mobilization**
>
> In the mobilization of the cuboid bone on the navicular and the third cuneiform, the direction must be consistent with the course of the joint surfaces. For example, gliding in a plantar direction is, more accurately speaking, in a plantar-medial direction.

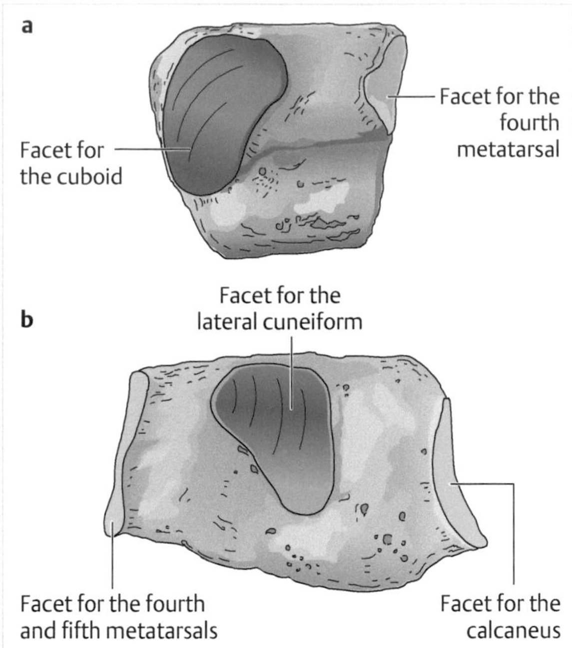


**Fig. 10.129** Joint surfaces of the cuneocuboid joint. **(a)** On the lateral cuneiform. **(b)** On the cuboid bone.

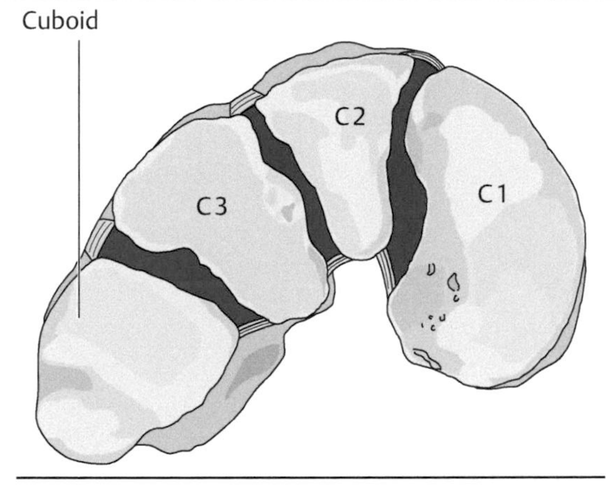


**Fig. 10.130** Cuneocuboid and intercuneiform joints

## 10.9.5 Joint Capsules and Ligaments of the Cuneocuboid and Intercuneiform Joints

The joint capsules of the intercuneiform joints are very taut and, together with the ligaments, allow hardly any movement. Therefore this joint unit is designated as an *amphiarthrosis.*

### Dorsal and Plantar Cuneocuboid Ligaments (Figs. 10.131 and 10.137)

The dorsal connection spreads out like a fan from the cuneiform bone to the cuboid.

The plantar ligament strengthens the capsule and is short.

### Cuneocuboid Interosseous Ligament

Its origin lies distal to the joint facet for the cuboid bone, and it inserts on the roughened, medial side of the cuboid.

### Dorsal and Plantar Intercuneiform Ligaments (Figs. 10.131 and 10.137)

The ligaments join the cuneiform bones together on the dorsal and plantar sides of the foot.

### Intercuneiform Interosseous Ligaments

These represent a transverse connection between the cuneiform bones. They insert immediately distal and proximal to the facing joint facets.

## 10.9.6 Axes and Movements of the Cuneocuboid and Intercuneiform Joints

▷ See Chapter 10.10, Tarsometatarsal and Intermetatarsal Joints

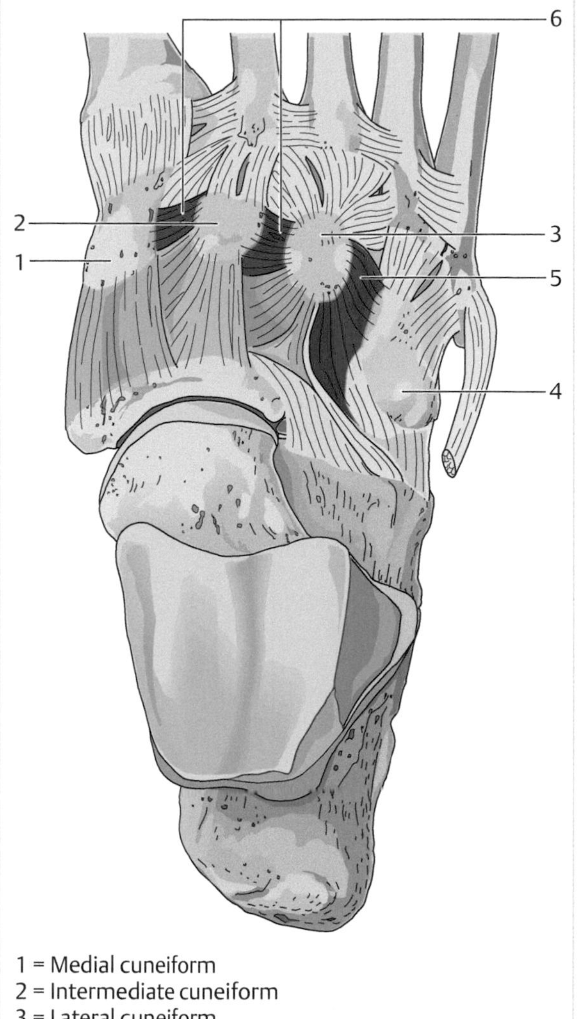


**Fig. 10.131** Dorsal cuneocuboid and intercuneiform ligaments.

# 10.10 Tarsometatarsal and Intermetatarsal Joints

## 10.10.1 Bony Structures and Joint Surfaces

### Cuboid Bone (Fig. 10.132)

- Distally, this has two joint facets.
- The lateral facet has a triangular shape and is larger than the medial facet. It articulates with the base of the fifth metatarsal.
- The medial facet articulates with the fourth metatarsal.
- Its shape is slightly convex.

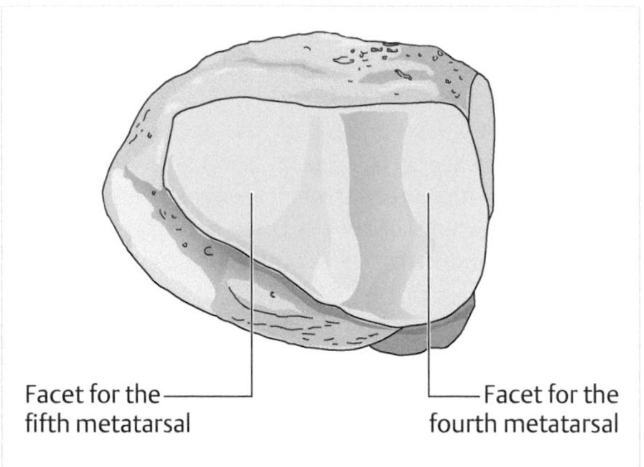


**Fig. 10.132** Distal joint surfaces on the cuboid bone.

### Cuneiform Bones (Fig. 10.133)

- The medial cuneiform bone has a distal facet for the first metatarsal and a small lateral facet for the second metatarsal.
- The intermediate cuneiform articulates with the base of the second metatarsal.
- The lateral cuneiform bone has a distal facet for the base of the third metatarsal. The lateral facet is in contact with the fourth metatarsal and the cuboid bone. The medial facet contacts the intermediate cuneiform and the second metatarsal bone.

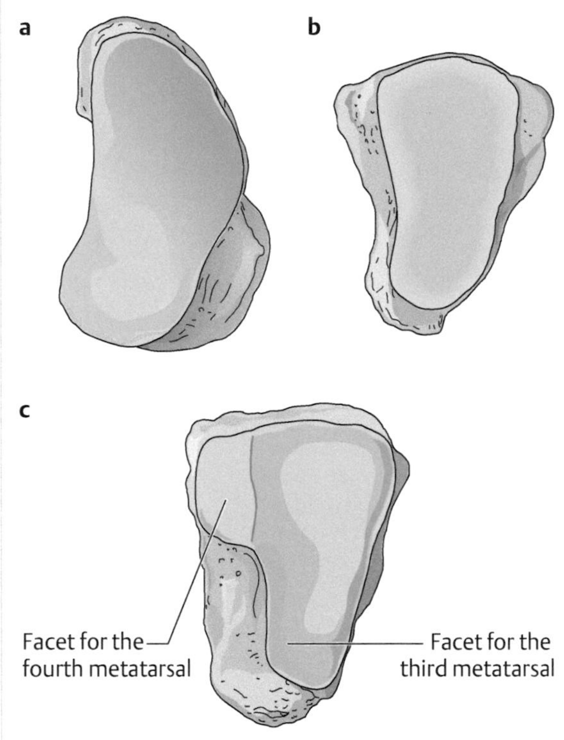


**Fig. 10.133** Distal joint surfaces. **(a)** On the medial cuneiform. **(b)** On the intermediate cuneiform. **(c)** On the lateral cuneiform.

## Metatarsal Bones (Figs. 10.134 and 10.135)

- The first metatarsal bone is shorter than the second metatarsal.
- The bases of the second, third, and fourth metatarsals are wedge-shaped.
- The first to third metatarsals form proximal joint surfaces for the cuneiform bones.
- The fourth and fifth metatarsals articulate with the cuboid bone.
- The base of the second metatarsal is tightly wedged in between the medial cuneiform bone on one side, the lateral cuneiform bone on the other side, and the intermediate cuneiform proximally.
- Because of this interlocking system, the second metatarsal is the most stable of the midfoot bones.
- From a superior view, the joint line between fifth metatarsal and the cuboid bone demonstrates an oblique course from proximal-lateral to distal-medial.
- If a line is drawn along the first metatarsal joint and connected to the line representing the fifth metatarsal joint, the point of intersection lies between the second and third metatarsals.
- Except between the first and second metatarsal bones, the sides of the metatarsal bases have joint surfaces for the intermetatarsal joints.
- The base of the first metatarsal has a tubercle on the inferomedial edge for the insertion of the tibialis anterior muscle.

### Practical Tip

When applying traction to the metatarsal joints, the oblique course of the joints must be taken into consideration. For example, traction on the first tarsometatarsal joint should be carried out by pulling the base of the first metatarsal in a distal-medial direction.

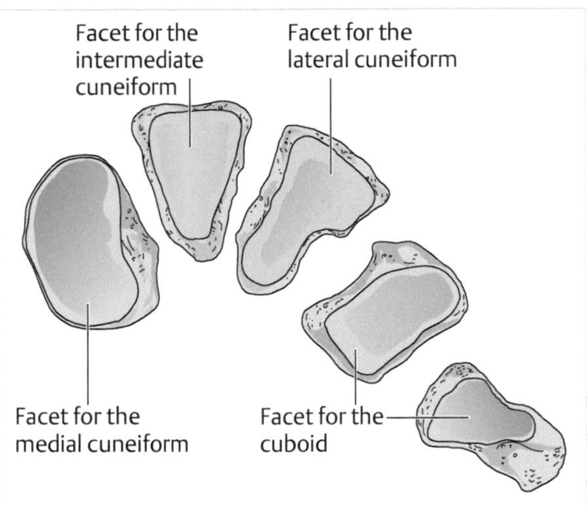


**Fig. 10.134** Joint surfaces at the bases of the first through fifth metatarsals.

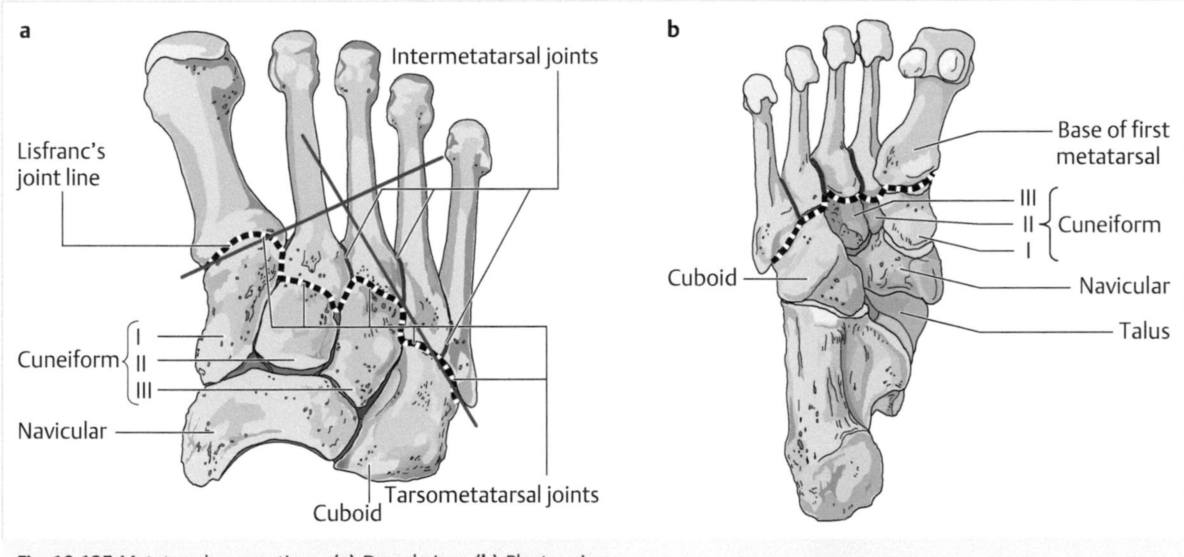


**Fig. 10.135** Metatarsal connections. **(a)** Dorsal view. **(b)** Plantar view.

## 10.10.2 Joint Capsules and Ligaments

The tarsometatarsal joints form three discrete joints, each enclosed by a capsule. Of these, the second and third tarsometatarsal joints form a joint cavity, as do the fourth and fifth. The first, third, and fourth intermetatarsal joints have connections to the corresponding tarsometatarsal joints. The surrounding capsule is taut, since no distinct movements are possible.

### Dorsal and Plantar Tarsometatarsal Ligaments (Figs. 10.136 and 10.137)

These ligamentous connections strengthen the capsules on the dorsal and plantar sides.

The medial dorsal ligamentous connection is the strongest, and that of the second metatarsal the broadest, in that its fibers extend to the medial, intermediate, and lateral cuneiform bones. From the fourth metatarsal, parts of the ligament run to the lateral cuneiform bone as well as to the cuboid bone.

On the plantar side, parts of the tendon of the tibialis posterior muscle and fibers of the long plantar ligament combine with the ligaments.

### Dorsal and Plantar Metatarsal Ligaments (Figs. 10.136 and 10.137)

The joint connections between the bases of the metatarsals are stabilized by plantar and dorsal ligamentous structures. The plantar ligaments are constructed more strongly than the dorsal.

### Cuneometatarsal Interosseous Ligament (Fig. 10.138)

This is also called *Lisfranc's ligament*. The first ligament runs on the plantar side between the medial cuneiform bone and the second metatarsal. The insertions lie on the lateral surface of the cuneiform bone and on the medial plantar surface of the second metatarsal.

Further interosseous ligaments run between the intermediate and lateral cuneiform bones and the second and third metatarsals.

### Metatarsal Interosseous Ligaments

These are three very short ligaments that connect the metatarsal bones to each other in the immediate area of the joint surfaces. They are important for the stability of the joints.

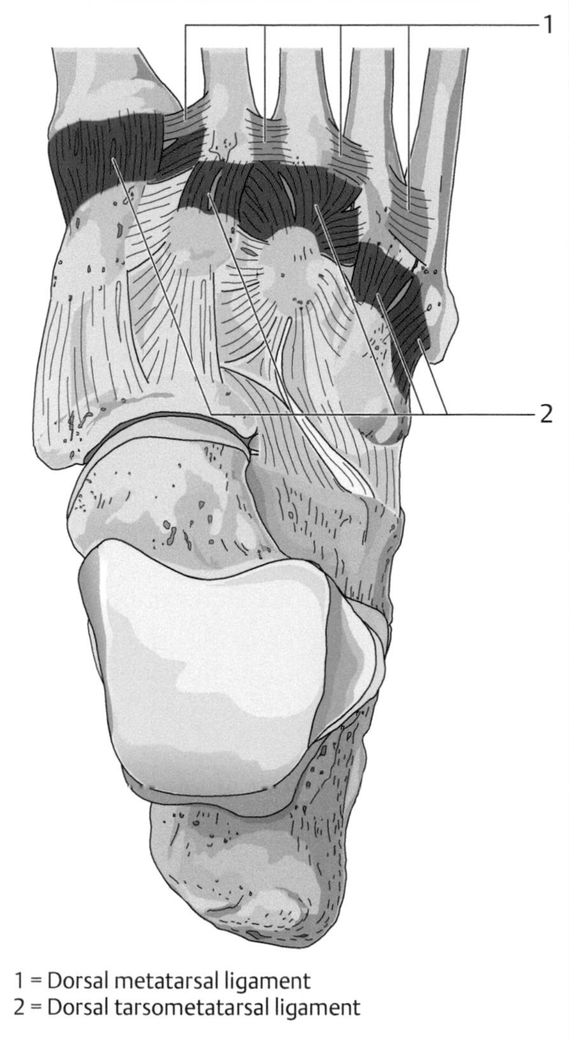


**Fig. 10.136** Dorsal tarsometatarsal and metatarsal ligaments.

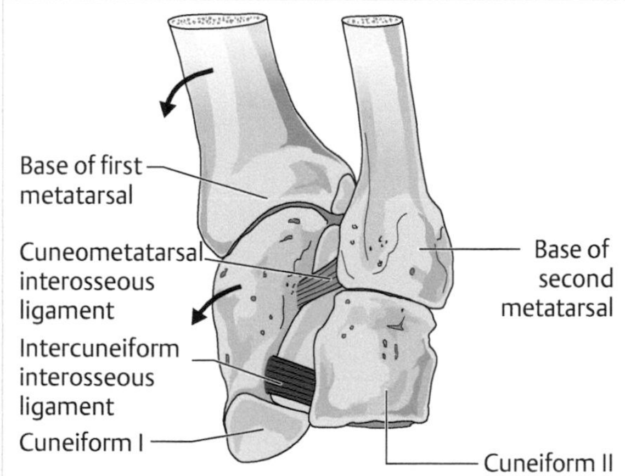


**Fig. 10.138** Cuneometatarsal and intercuneiform interosseous ligaments. (The first metatarsal and the medial cuneiform have been tilted outward; plantar view.)

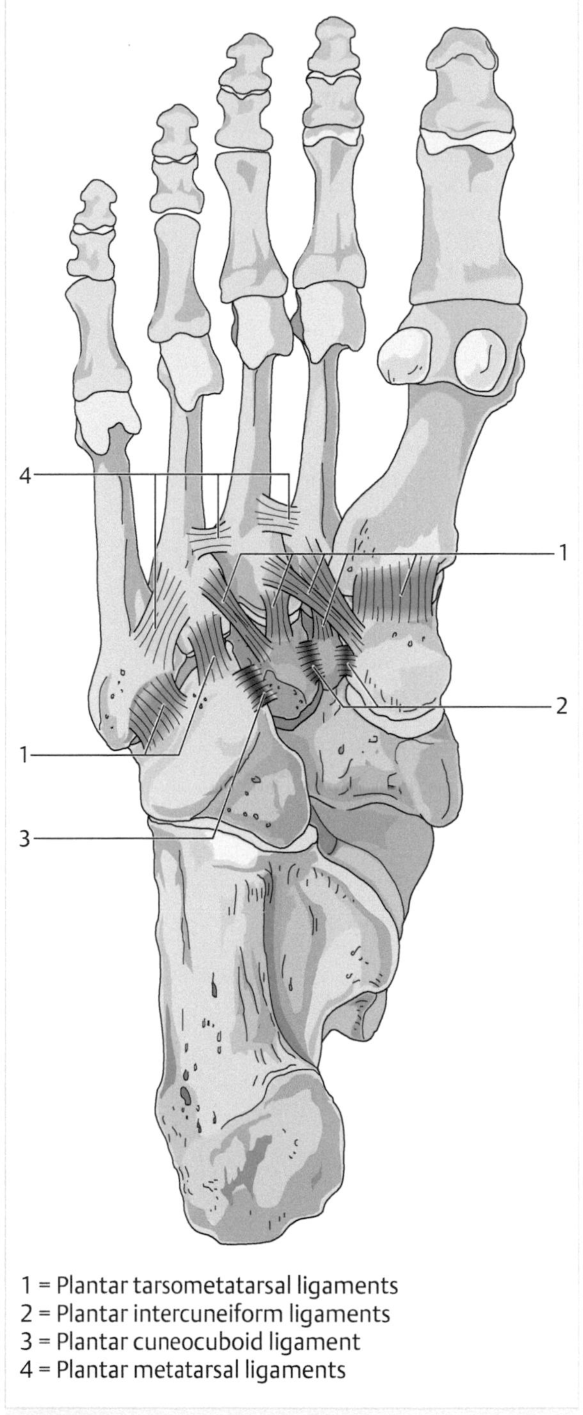


**Fig. 10.137** Plantar ligamentous connections in the tarsometatarsal region.

## 10.10.3 Axes and Movements of the Tarsal and Tarsometatarsal Joints

In this joint complex as well, the axes cannot be precisely established. Here only compromise axes can be given.

### Longitudinal Axis (Fig. 10.139)

This axis corresponds approximately to the midline of the foot, running between the second and third metatarsals. Extended posteriorly, it runs through the middle of the heel. The movements of pronation and supination take place around this axis.

### Sagittal Axes

There is an axis for each individual joint, around which the movements of flexion and extension take place.

In spite of limited mobility—as the joints involved are amphiarthroses—the sum of the movements contributes to changing the foot shape toward supination/adduction/flexion and pronation/abduction/extension, thereby allowing the foot to adapt to the surface of the ground during ambulation.

### Supination/Pronation (Fig. 10.140)

*Range of Motion*

Active: 40°/25°, respectively, from neutral.

Passive: +10°.

To obtain precise information concerning the twisting motion of the forefoot in comparison with the hindfoot, fixate the calcaneus. Then, to evaluate pronation motion, raise the outer edge of the foot. For supination, raise the inner edge (**Fig. 10.140**).

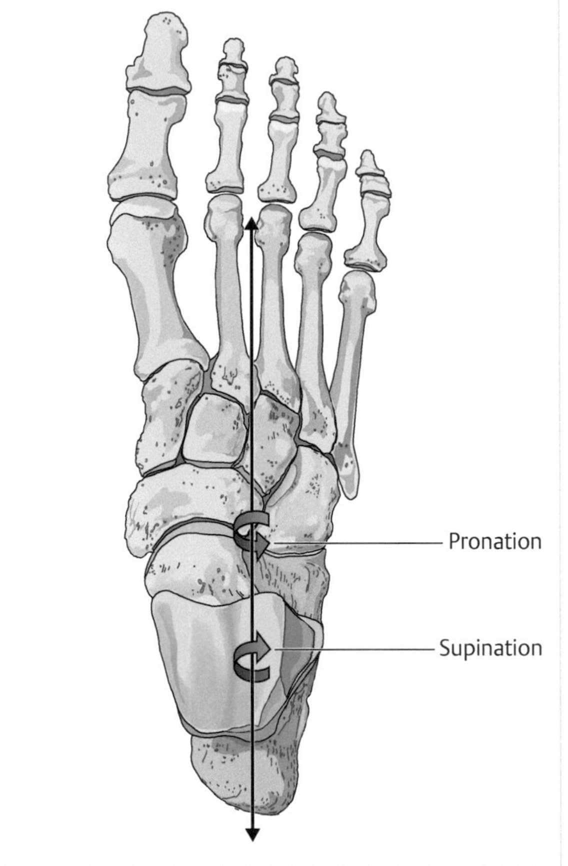


**Fig. 10.139** Pronation and supination axis.

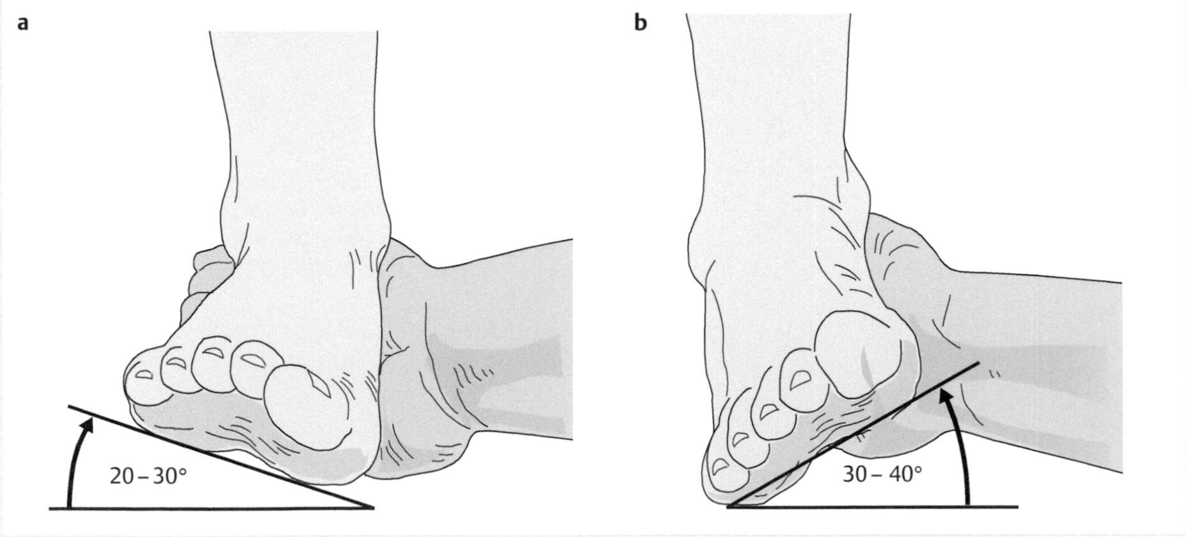


**Fig. 10.140** Movements in the tarsal joints. **(a)** Active pronation with fixed calcaneus. **(b)** Active supination with fixed calcaneus.

Twisting motions of the foot can be observed particularly well if the patient is standing on tiptoes. Here the forefoot is fixed, and the entire base of the foot pivots over it, which is especially well seen in the calcaneus (**Fig. 10.141**).

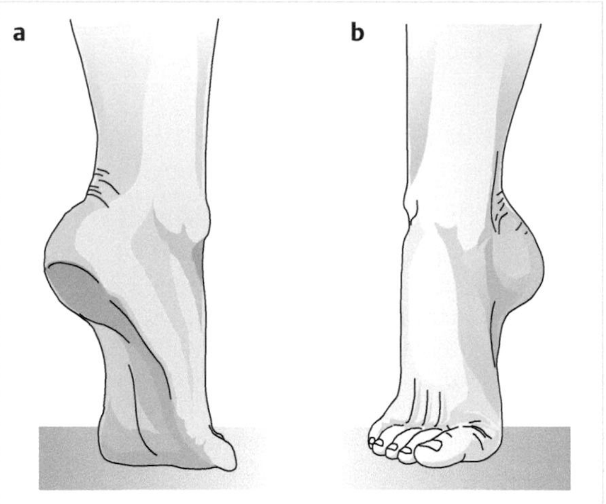


**Fig. 10.141 (a, b)** Pivoting the hindfoot on the forefoot while standing on tiptoe.

## Flexion/Extension

The movements of the upper ankle joint (talocrural joint) proceed distally and add up to plantarflexion of 80° and dorsiflexion of 30 to 40°.

### *Range of Motion (Fig. 10.142)*

The range of motion of each individual joint subsection is not measurable. The data given in **Fig. 10.142** come from an analysis by Ouzounian and Shereff (1989). The values are mean values that were statistically derived.

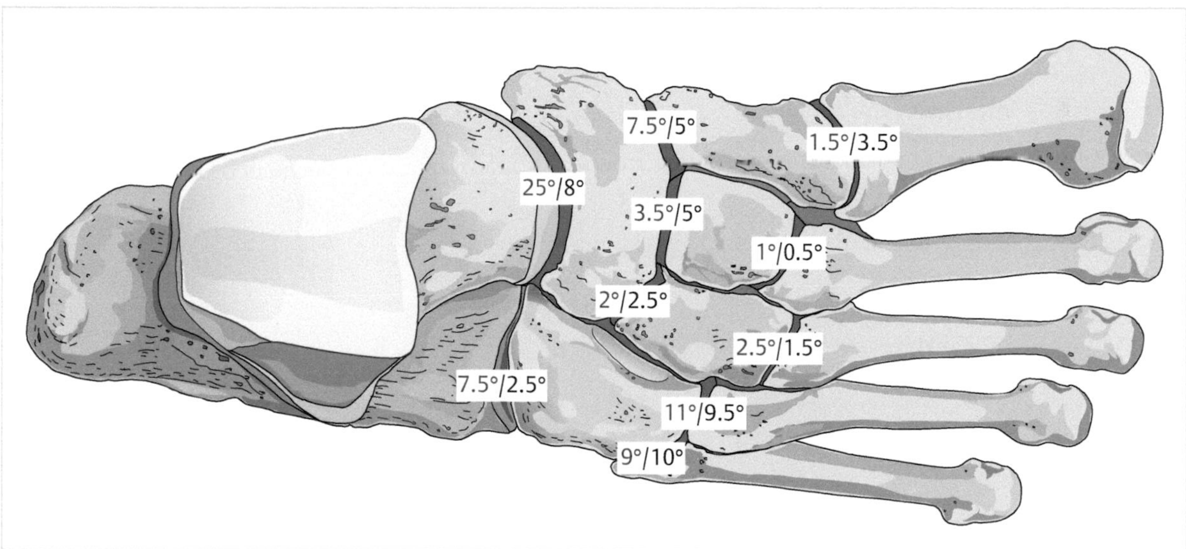


**Fig. 10.142** Range of motion of the tarsal joints. Red: pronation and supination; black: flexion and extension.

# 10.11 Metatarsophalangeal and Interphalangeal Joints

## 10.11.1 Bony Structures and Joint Surfaces of the Metatarsophalangeal and Interphalangeal Joints

### Metatarsal Bones (Fig. 10.143)

- The head of the metatarsal bone has a convex, cylindrical joint surface that extends in a plantar direction.
- The first metatarsal head has two plantar grooves in which the two sesamoid bones can glide.
- Between the MTP joints lie small bursae. On the medial edge of the foot, there is a bursa over the first metatarsal head.

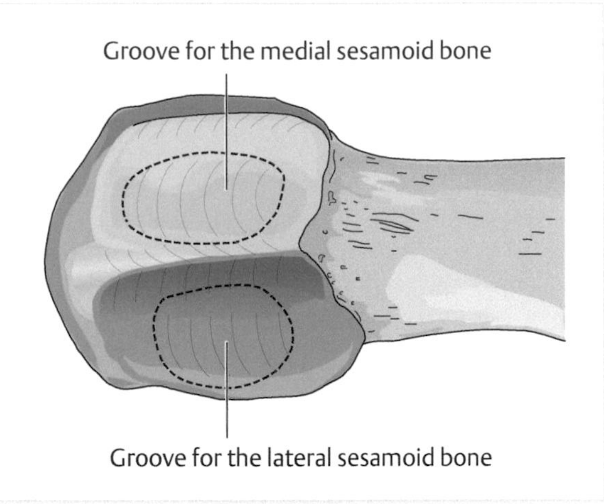


**Fig. 10.143** Head of the first metatarsal bone (plantar view).

### Sesamoid Bones (Fig 10.144)

- These are attached on the sides of the joint capsule and the collateral ligaments of the first MTP joint.
- The *medial sesamoid bone* is embedded in the tendon of the abductor hallucis muscle and the medial head of the flexor hallucis brevis muscle.
- The medial sesamoid bone is offset from the longitudinal axis of the first metatarsal bone.
- The lateral head of the flexor hallucis brevis muscle and the adductor hallucis muscle track to the *lateral sesamoid bone*.
- The tendon of the flexor hallucis longus muscle runs between the two sesamoid bones.
- The sesamoids travel a path of almost 50° between the movements of flexion and extension, which corresponds to a distance of 1 to 1.5 cm. In flexion, the sesamoid bones are near the transition between the head and neck of the first metatarsal bone. In extension, they shift distally.

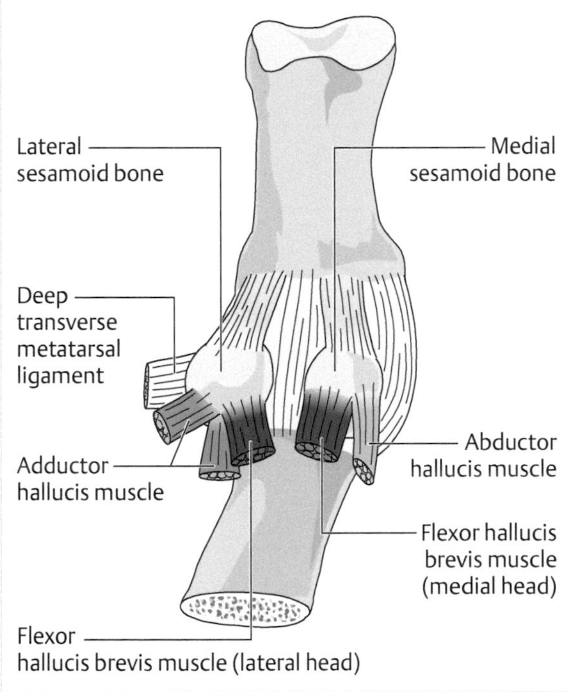


**Fig. 10.144** Connections to the sesamoid bones.

## Phalanges (Fig. 10.145)

- The bases of the proximal phalanges demonstrate joint facets for the metatarsal heads.
- The joint surfaces are slightly concave in shape.
- The oval joint sockets of the bases of the proximal phalanges are broadened by fibrocartilaginous plates (see **Fig. 10.149**).
- The spool-shaped joint surfaces on the head of each phalanx are convex in shape.
- There is a slight groove on the plantar surface in the middle of the head of the phalanx, which in flexion has contact with the base of the next phalanx.
- At the base, there is a corresponding protruding, wedge-shaped joint surface that fits into the groove and is concave in shape.
- The head of the distal phalanx demonstrates a mushroom-shaped enlargement.
- The big toe has only one interphalangeal joint.

### *Angle of Inclination (Fig. 10.146)*

The longitudinal axis of the first metatarsal forms an angle of 18 to 25° with the ground. The inclination decreases toward the fifth metatarsal, so that the angle there measures only 5°.

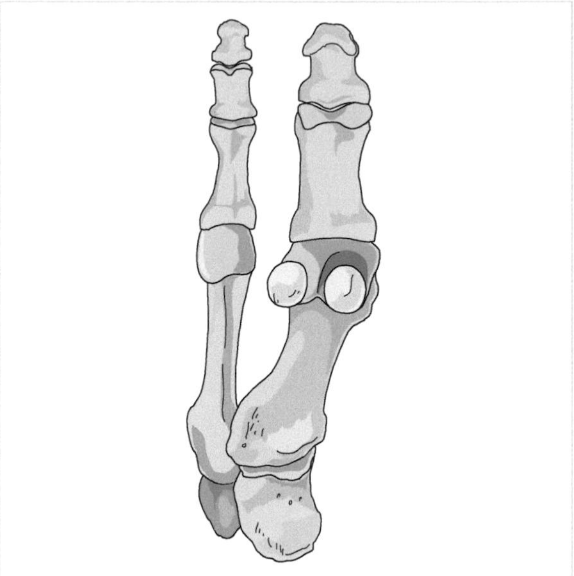

**Fig. 10.145** Joint surfaces of the phalangeal joints (plantar view).

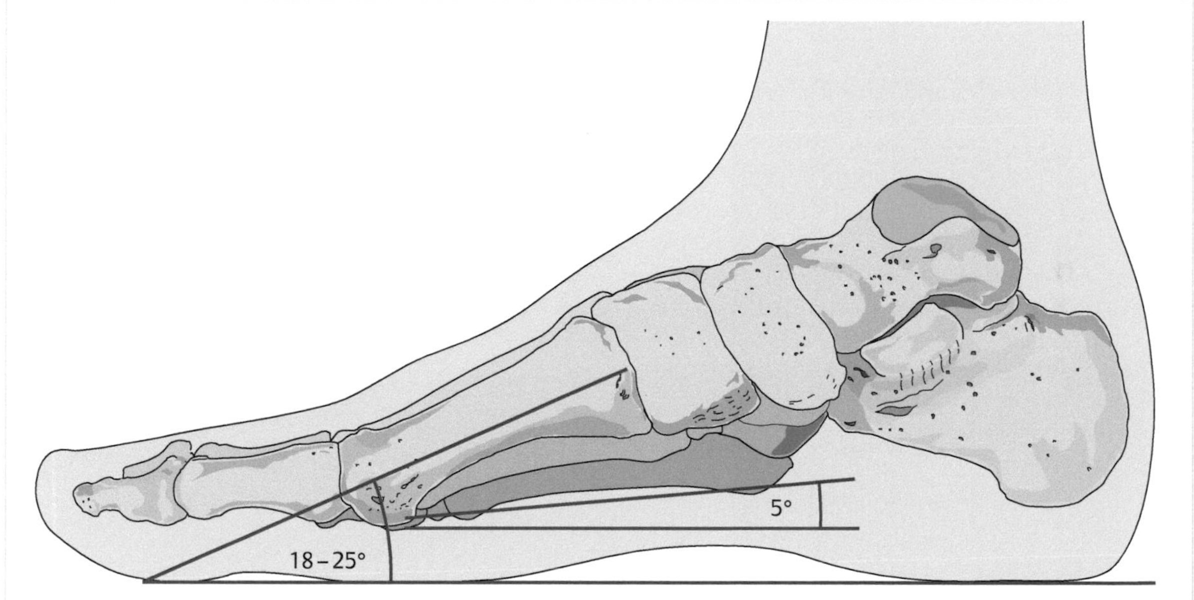


**Fig. 10.146** Angle of inclination of the metatarsal bones.

## Intermetatarsal Angle (Fig. 10.147)

The neutral position of the first metatarsal with respect to the big toe in the transverse plane is of vital importance, because this is where the most frequent alteration of the forefoot occurs—the *splayfoot*. The longitudinal axes through the first and second metatarsals form an angle with each other that should be less than 8°.

## Valgus Angle of the First Metatarsophalangeal Joint (10.147)

This is determined using the angle between the longitudinal axis of the metatarsal and the longitudinal axis through the proximal phalanx. It should not be more than 10 to 20°.

### Pathology

#### Hallux Valgus (Fig. 10.148)

This involves a deviation of the axis of the big toe laterally in the form of a subluxation of the first MTP joint. The diagnosis becomes clear by measuring the valgus angle of the first phalanx, which is more than 20° in this condition. See Chapter 10.13, Biomechanics.

#### Splayfoot

The enlargement of the intermetatarsal angle, on the other hand, is an expression of splayfoot, which often precedes hallux valgus.

Because the metatarsals spread apart, the head of the first metatarsal bulges out badly on the medial side and is constantly exposed to pressure from footwear. The result is repeated irritation of the subcutaneous bursa of the first metatarsal head, which swells and can be very painful. See Chapter 10.13, Biomechanics.

#### March or Fatigue Fracture

This pertains to a subtle crack in the metatarsal shaft that divides the bone transversely or obliquely. The second metatarsal bone is most often affected due to the large bending stress on it. This fracture is noted after prolonged marches on foot.

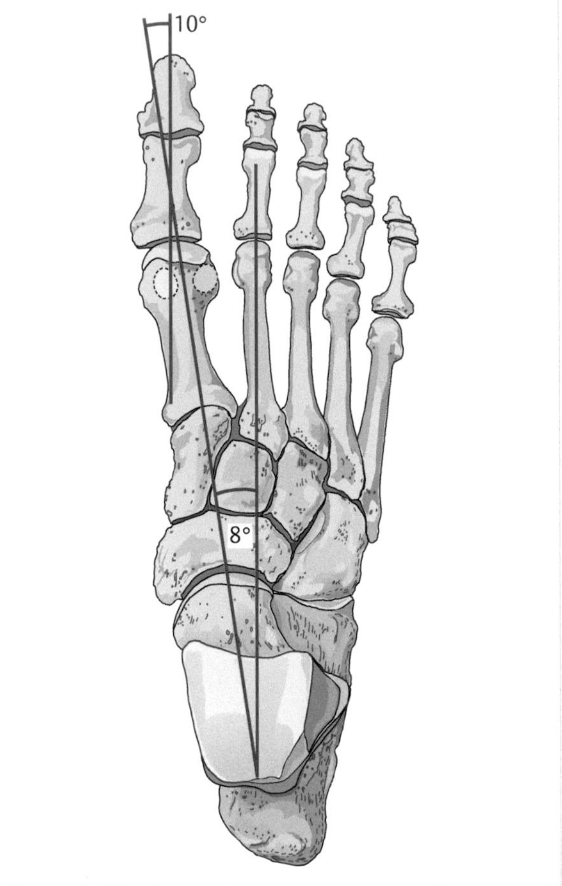


**Fig. 10.147** Intermetatarsal angle and valgus angle of the first metatarsophalangeal joint.

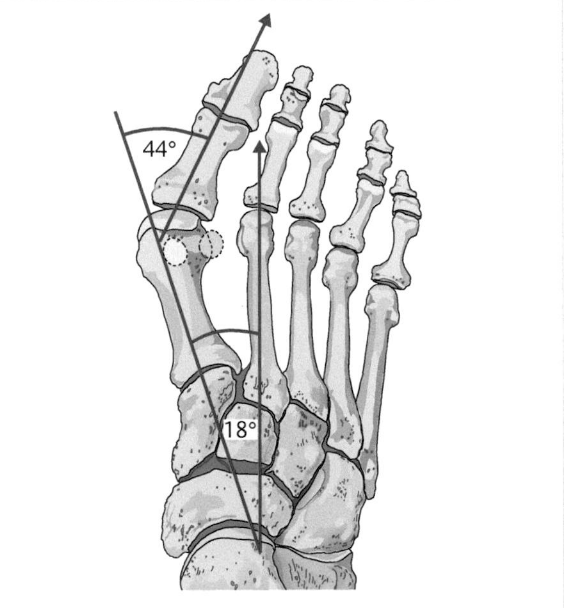


**Fig. 10.148** Change in the intermetatarsal angle and the valgus angle of the first metatarsophalangeal joint in hallux valgus.

## 10.11.2 Joint Capsules and Ligaments of the Metatarsophalangeal and Interphalangeal Joints

The joint capsules are relatively wide and allow extensive movements. They are strengthened on the plantar side, by the fibrocartilaginous plates, and dorsally and on the sides by the dorsal digital aponeurosis and the collateral ligaments.

### Lateral and Medial Collateral Ligaments (Fig. 10.149)

The course of these ligaments is oblique from proximal-dorsal to distal-plantar in each case. Therefore they are tensed in flexion and relaxed in extension.

### Plantar Ligament (Figs. 10.149 and 10.150)

This ligament lies on the fibrocartilaginous plate on the plantar side of the joint. In each case, it is fixed to the base of the phalanx and merges with the joint capsule. There is also a connection to the flexor tendons.

### Deep Transverse Metatarsal Ligament (Fig. 10.150)

This strong ligament runs between the metatarsal heads; each of its segments is fixed to the plantar ligaments. The transverse head of the adductor hallucis muscle arises in part from it.

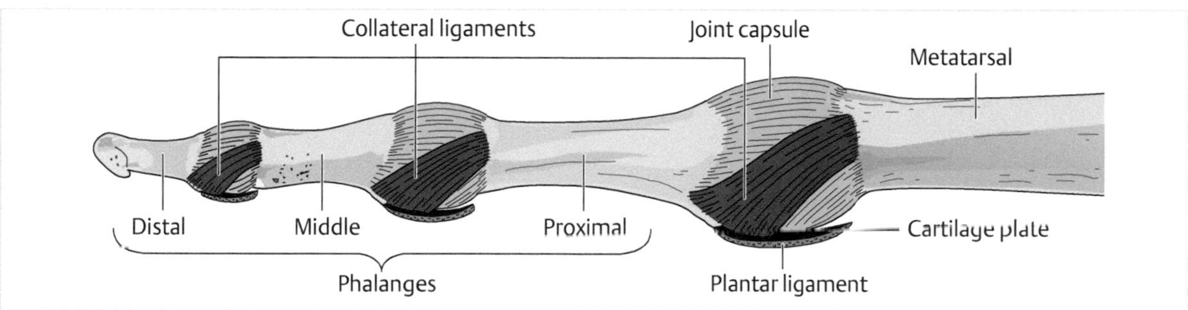


**Fig. 10.149** Collateral and plantar ligaments (medial view of the second toe).

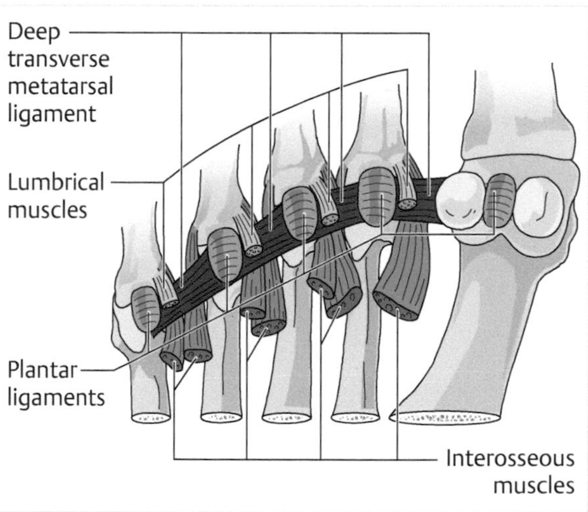


**Fig. 10.150** Deep transverse metatarsal ligament and plantar ligaments (plantar view).

## 10.11.3 Axes and Movements

In each joint segment, the axes of motion lie in the proximal joint partner and extend in the frontal plane for the movements of flexion and extension, and in the vertical plane for the movements of abduction and adduction.

At the MTP joints, flexion, extension, and side-to-side motions are possible.

The interphalangeal joints are hinge joints that can only perform the movements of flexion and extension:

- *MTP* joint of the big toe (**Fig. 10.151**):
  - Flexion/extension: 45°/70° from neutral; active.
  - Abduction/adduction: 10°/5° from neutral; active.
- *Interphalangeal joint* (big toe): Flexion/extension: 60°/5°; active.
- *MTP* joint of the other toes (**Fig. 10.152**):
  - Flexion/extension: 40°/70°; active.
  - Abduction/adduction: minimal.
- *Proximal interphalangeal joint:* Flexion/extension: 35°/0°; active.
- *Distal interphalangeal joint:* Flexion/extension: 60°/30°; active.

*Movements of the Toes when Walking (Fig. 10.153)*

In the phase between heel-off and toe-off, the toes are pushed into maximal extension from proximal outward. The big toe thus reaches its greatest range of motion of 90°.

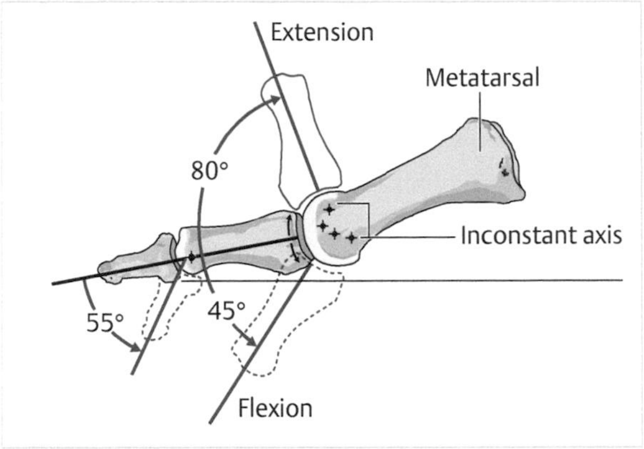


**Fig. 10.151** Extent of flexion and extension of the big toe.

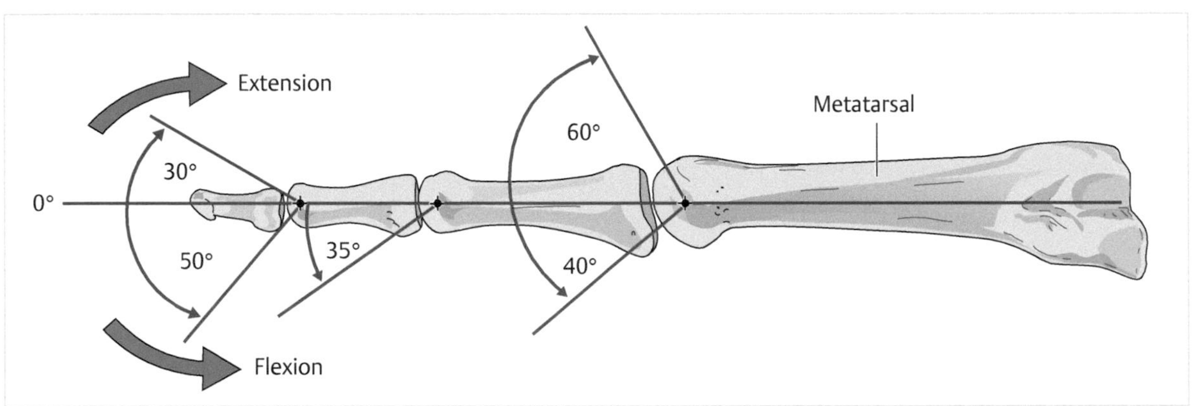


**Fig. 10.152** Extent of flexion and extension of the toes.

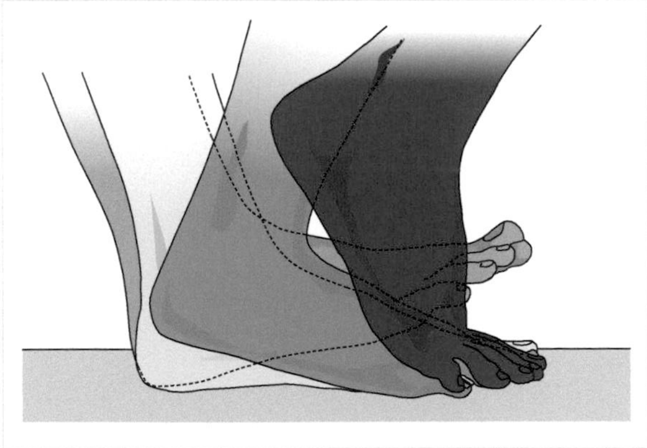

**Fig. 10.153** Movements of the toes when walking.

# 10.12 Musculature

## 10.12.1 Dorsiflexors (Fig. 10.154)

- Tibialis anterior muscle.
- Extensor digitorum longus muscle.
- Extensor hallucis longus muscle.
- (Fibularis tertius muscle).

▷ See Chapter 10.6, Stabilization of the Ankle Joints

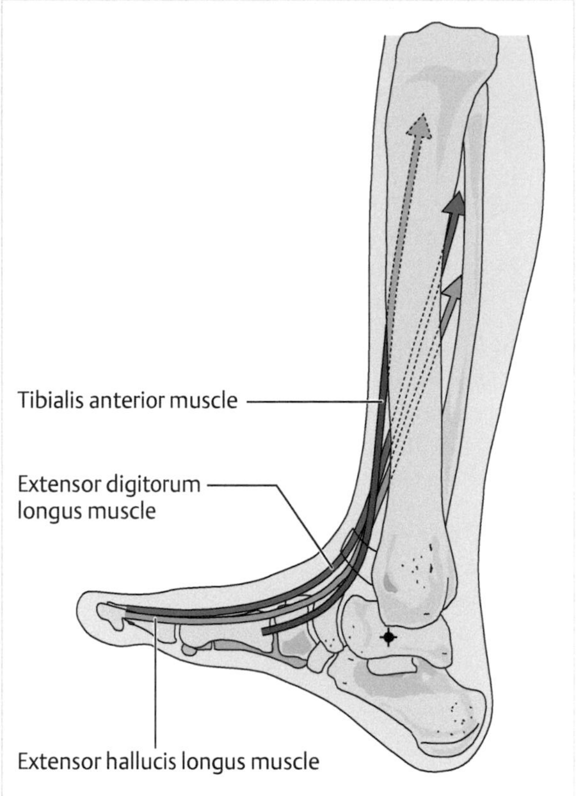


**Fig. 10.154** Dorsiflexors.

## 10.12.2 Plantarflexors (Fig. 10.155)

- Triceps surae muscle.
- Tibialis posterior muscle.
- Flexor digitorum longus muscle.
- Flexor hallucis longus muscle.
- Fibularis longus muscle.
- Fibularis brevis muscle.

▷ See Chapter 10.6, Stabilization of the Ankle Joints

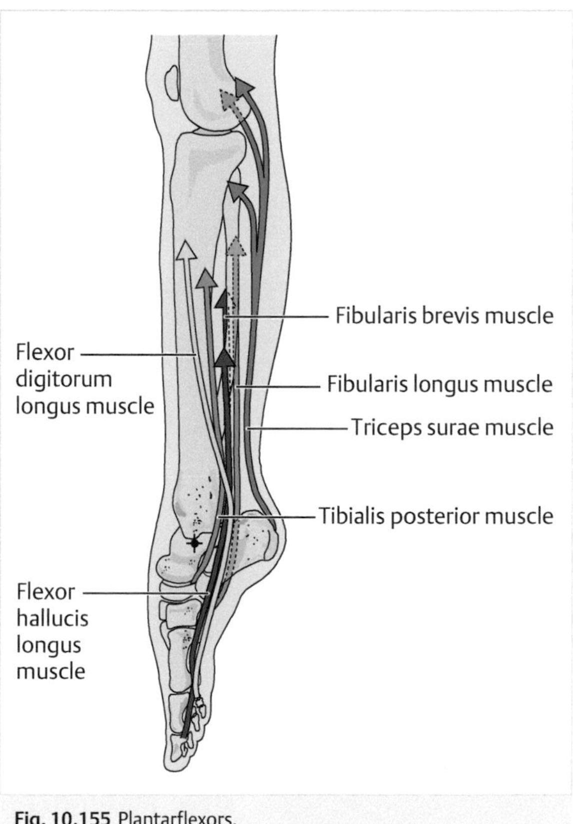


**Fig. 10.155** Plantarflexors.

## 10.12.3 Pronators/Abductors (Fig. 10.156)

### *Fibularis Brevis Muscle*

The fibularis brevis muscle causes abduction of the forefoot with simultaneous elevation of the fifth metatarsal and thus the outer edge of the foot. The fifth metatarsal takes the cuboid bone with it, and finally, the navicular bone and the calcaneus. The calcaneus shifts posteriorly, during which the tarsal sinus narrows.

### *Fibularis Longus Muscle*

The fibularis longus muscle also guides the forefoot laterally and lowers the medial margin of the foot through its connection to the medial cuneiform bone and the first metatarsal.

### *Extensor Digitorum Longus Muscle*

Both of the above muscles are supported by most parts of the extensor digitorum longus muscle.

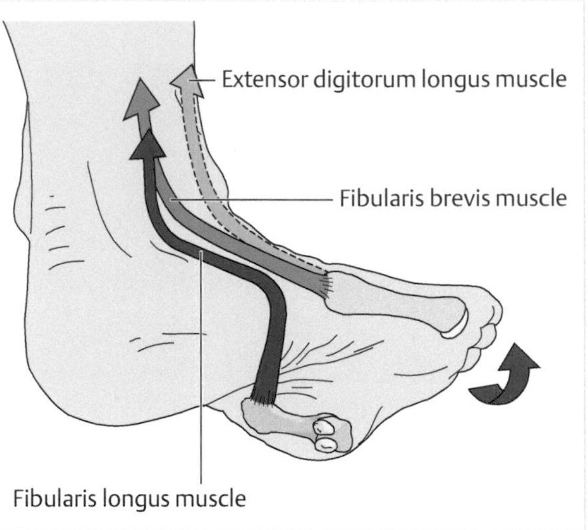


**Fig. 10.156** Pronators/abductors of the foot.

## 10.12.4 Supinators/Adductors (Fig. 10.157)

### *Tibialis Anterior Muscle*

The tibialis anterior muscle pulls the foot into adduction and raises the inner margin of the foot through its connection with the medial cuneiform bone and first metatarsal. The forefoot follows this movement.

### *Tibialis Posterior Muscle*

The tibialis posterior muscle primarily supports the adductor component in that it pulls the navicular bone medially. The navicular bone takes the cuboid with it, and finally the calcaneus, which displaces medially, as a result of which the tarsal sinus widens.

### *Triceps Surae Muscle*

This supports supination from the hindfoot. Because of the slight valgus position of the heel, most of the muscle lies medial to the supination–pronation axis.

### *Flexor Digitorum Longus and Flexor Hallucis Longus Muscles*

These muscles support the movements of adduction and supination from the forefoot.

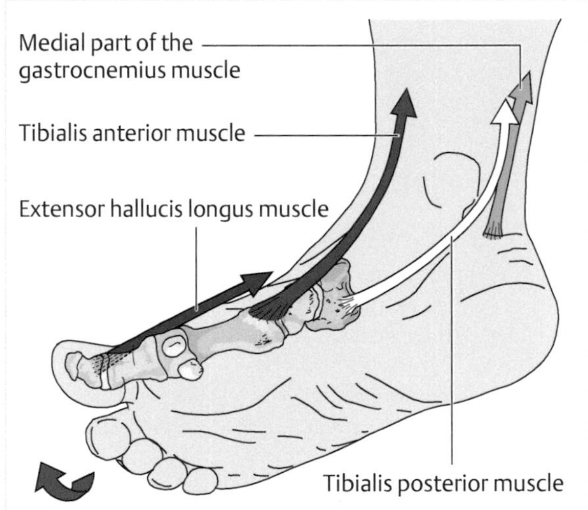


**Fig. 10.157** Supinators/adductors of the foot.

## 10.12.5 Muscles of the Dorsum of the Foot

### Extensor Digitorum Brevis Muscle (Fig. 10.158)

- The site of origin is in the tarsal sinus in close relationship to that of the ligaments and the inferior extensor retinaculum.
- Going forward, it develops a powerful muscle belly, which forms a soft tissue arch over the lateral dorsal area.
- It transitions into three terminal tendons in the mid-metatarsal area.
- Approaching from the lateral side, the three tendons radiate into the tendons of the extensor digitorum longus muscle.

### Extensor Hallucis Brevis Muscle (Fig. 10.158)

- This is a part of the extensor digitorum brevis muscle.
- At its origin, it has a connection with the talocalcaneal interosseous ligament.
- It tracks into the extensor hallucis longus muscle tendon and connects to the dorsal digital expansion.
- *Function:* It brings about extension of all the toe joints.
- *Innervation:* deep fibular nerve.

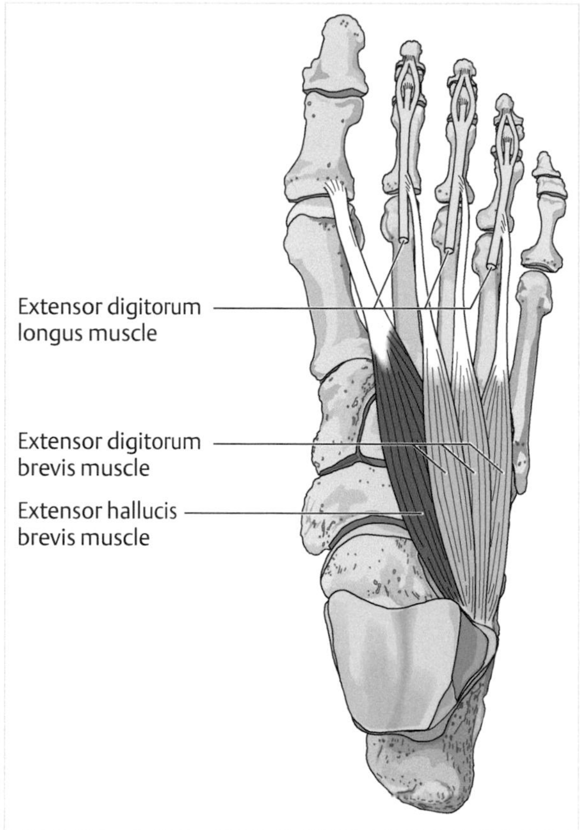


**Fig. 10.158** Extensor digitorum brevis and extensor hallucis brevis muscles.

## 10.12.6 Plantar Muscles of the Foot

### Flexor Digitorum Brevis Muscle (Fig. 10.159)

- This lies directly under the plantar aponeurosis.
- It runs in the central muscle compartment.
- It connects the calcaneal tuberosity with the middle phalanges.
- The muscle comprises four thick bellies that transition into terminal tendons at the level of the metatarsal bases.
- At the level of the proximal phalanx, each tendon generates a slit through which the corresponding tendon of the long flexors runs to the distal phalanx, while it itself tracks onto the middle phalanx (see **Fig. 10.100b**).
- *Function:* flexion of the toes at the proximal and middle phalanges, and tensing of the longitudinal arch.
- *Innervation:* medial plantar nerve.

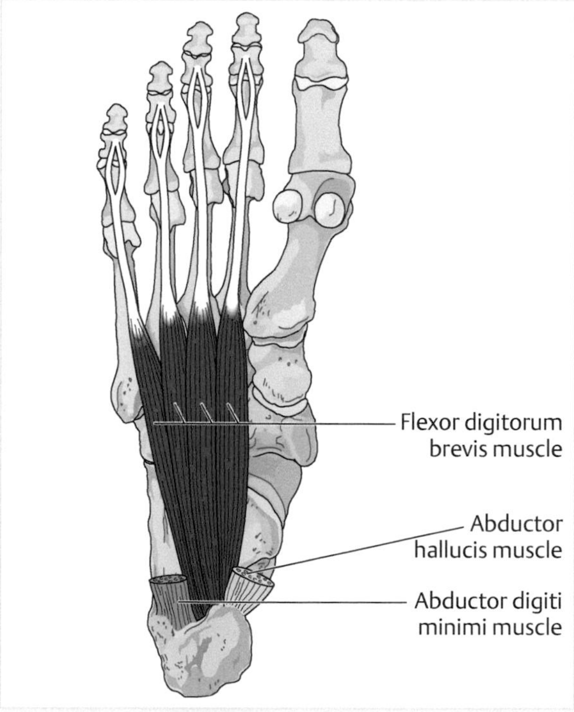


**Fig. 10.159** Flexor digitorum brevis muscle.

## Quadratus Plantae Muscle (Fig. 10.160)

- This lies under the flexor digitorum brevis muscle.
- It has a broad origin on the calcaneus and in part from the long plantar ligament.
- Having no bony insertion, it attaches to the lateral aspect of the tendons of the flexor digitorum longus muscle.
- *Function:* It supports the flexor digitorum longus muscle in flexing the toes. In this, it improves the effect of the longus muscle by pulling the obliquely running parts of the tendon into a longitudinal direction.
- *Innervation:* lateral plantar nerve.

## Lumbrical Muscles (Fig. 10.160)

- Four muscles arise from the medial sides of the four terminal tendons of the flexor digitorum longus muscle.
- At the level of the deep transverse metatarsal ligament, there are bursae between the ligament and the muscles.
- The lumbrical muscles form connections to the joint capsules of the MTP joints and course further to the dorsal digital expansion.
- *Function:* flexion of the MTP joints, and weak extension of the other toe joints.
- *Innervation:* first and second lumbrical muscles: medial plantar nerve; third and fourth lumbricals: lateral plantar nerve.

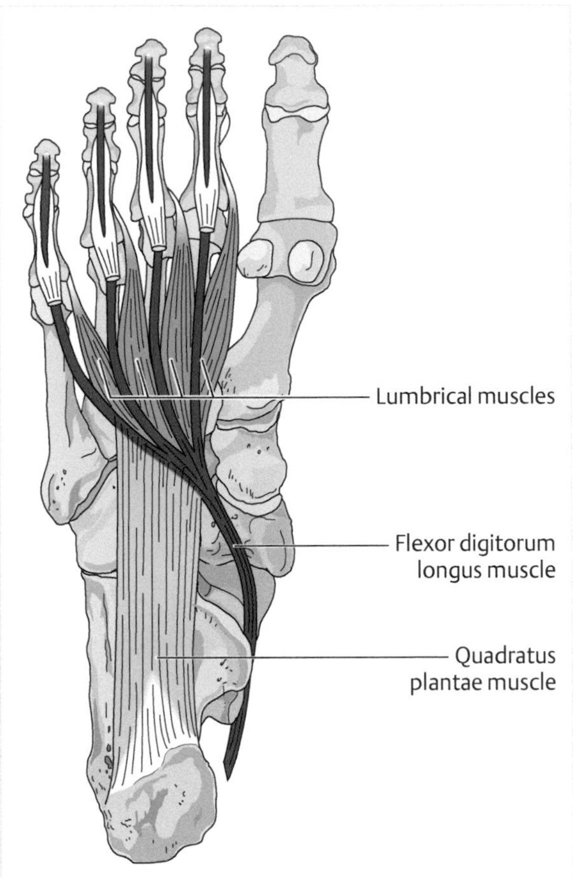


**Fig. 10.160** Quadratus plantae muscle and lumbrical muscles.

## Dorsal and Plantar Interosseous Muscles (Fig. 10.161)

- These belong to the deepest layer and lie in the intermetatarsal spaces.
- They originate from the sides of the metatarsal bones and the plantar ligaments, and extend into the dorsal digital expansion and the side edges of the proximal phalanges.
- There are three plantar and four dorsal muscle heads.
- *Function:* flexion at the MTP joints: The plantar muscles guide the toes toward the second toe (adduction). The dorsal muscle splays the toes.
- *Innervation:* lateral plantar nerve.

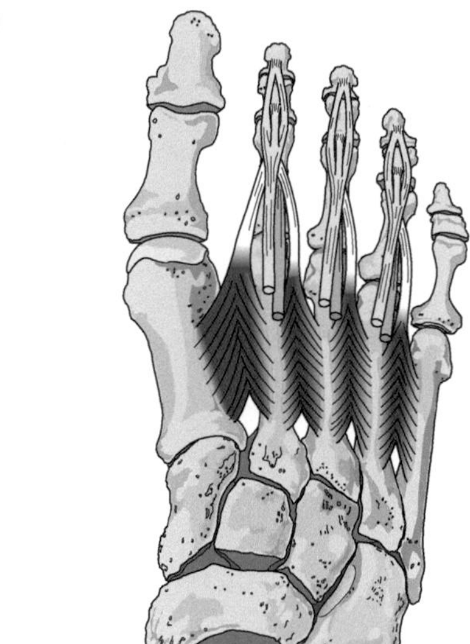


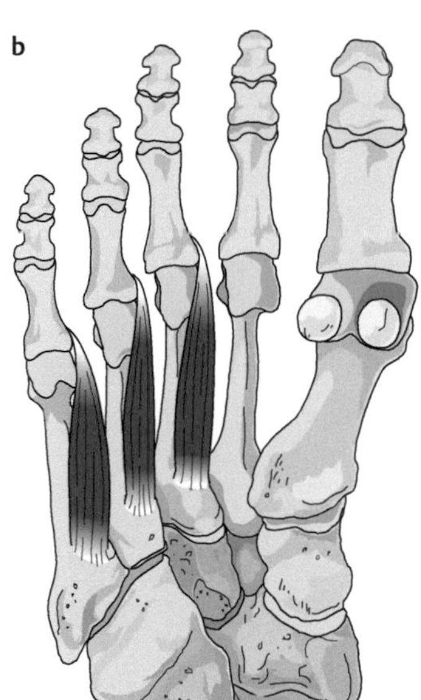


**Fig. 10.161 (a)** Dorsal interosseous muscles. **(b)** Plantar interosseous muscles.

## 10.12.7 Muscles of the Big Toe

### Abductor Hallucis Muscle (Fig. 10.162)

- This belongs to the superficial layer.
- It runs on the medial border of the foot and here forms the border of the plantar aponeurosis.
- The medial sesamoid bone is embedded in its insertion tendon.
- It connects to the capsule–ligament apparatus of the MTP joint of the big toe and inserts on the proximal phalanx.
- *Function:* abduction of the big toe, flexion of the MTP joint of the big toe, and tensing of the longitudinal arch.
- *Innervation:* medial plantar nerve.

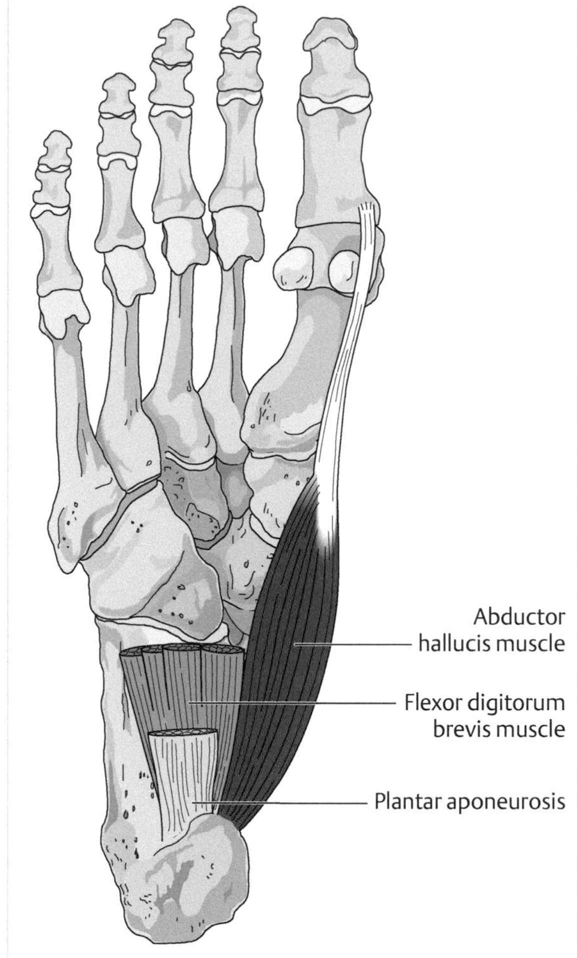


**Fig. 10.162** Abductor hallucis muscle.

### Flexor Hallucis Brevis Muscle (Fig. 10.163)

- This belongs to the third layer of foot muscles.
- It is covered in part by the adductor and abductor hallucis muscles.
- It divides into two heads. The *medial head* extends to the medial sesamoid bone, and the *lateral head* to the lateral sesamoid.
- The muscle inserts on the proximal phalanx and merges with the joint capsule of the MTP joint of the big toe.
- The terminal tendon of the flexor hallucis longus muscle runs between the two insertion tendons.
- *Function:* flexion of the first MTP joint and tensing of the longitudinal arch of the foot.
- *Innervation:* medial head of the medial plantar nerve and lateral head of the lateral plantar nerve.

### Adductor Hallucis Muscle (Fig. 10.163)

- This lies under the flexor digitorum longus and brevis muscles.
- It divides into two heads. The *oblique head* comes from the cuboid bone and runs longitudinally. The *transverse head* establishes a transverse connection from the third, fourth, and fifth metatarsal heads to the first MTP joint.
- Both heads connect to the lateral sesamoid bone and to the capsule–ligament apparatus of the first MTP joint.
- *Function:* adduction of the big toe. The oblique head helps with flexion of the MTP joint. The transverse head plays a large role in tensing the transverse arch.
- *Innervation:* lateral plantar nerve.

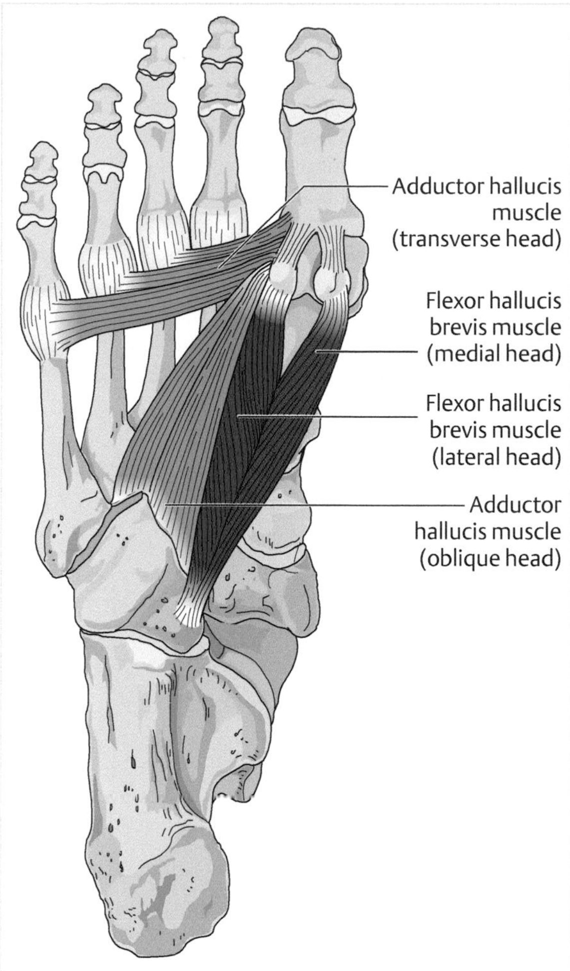


**Fig. 10.163** Flexor hallucis brevis and adductor hallucis muscles.

## 10.12.8 Muscles of the Little Toe

### Abductor Digiti Minimi Muscle (Fig. 10.164)

- This runs superficially on the lateral border of the foot and combines there with the plantar aponeurosis.
- It extends from the lateral process of the calcaneal tuberosity to the base of the fifth proximal phalanx.
- *Function:* abduction of the little toe, flexion of the MTP joint of the little toe, and tensing of the longitudinal arch.
- *Innervation:* lateral plantar nerve.

### Flexor Digiti Minimi Muscle (Fig. 10.165)

- This forms a connection between the base of the metatarsal and the base of the fifth proximal phalanx.
- It has a connection to the long plantar ligament.
- *Function:* flexion of the MTP joint of the fifth toe.
- *Innervation:* lateral plantar nerve.

### Opponens Digiti Minimi Muscle (Fig. 10.165)

- It connects the fifth metatarsal base with the proximal phalanx.
- It runs lateral to the flexor digiti minimi muscle and is intertwined with it.
- *Function:* it pulls the fifth metatarsal in a plantar-medial direction.
- *Innervation:* lateral plantar nerve.

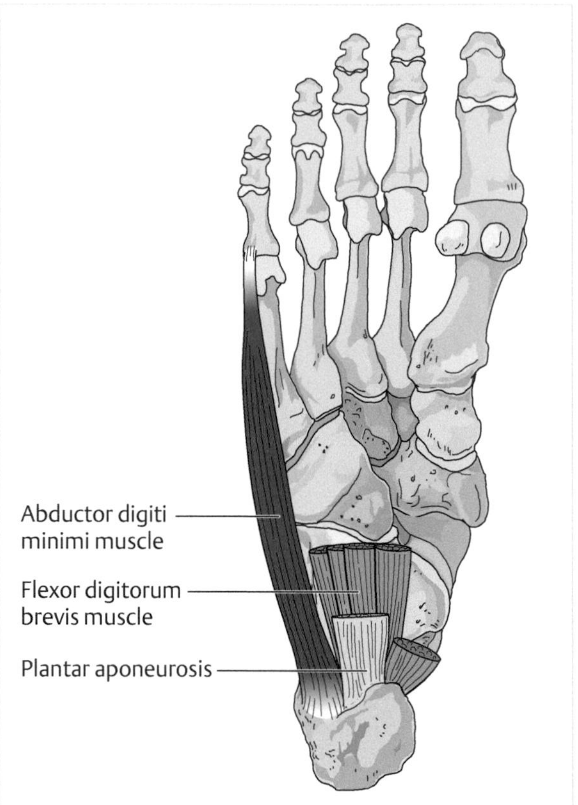


**Fig. 10.164** Abductor digiti minimi muscle.

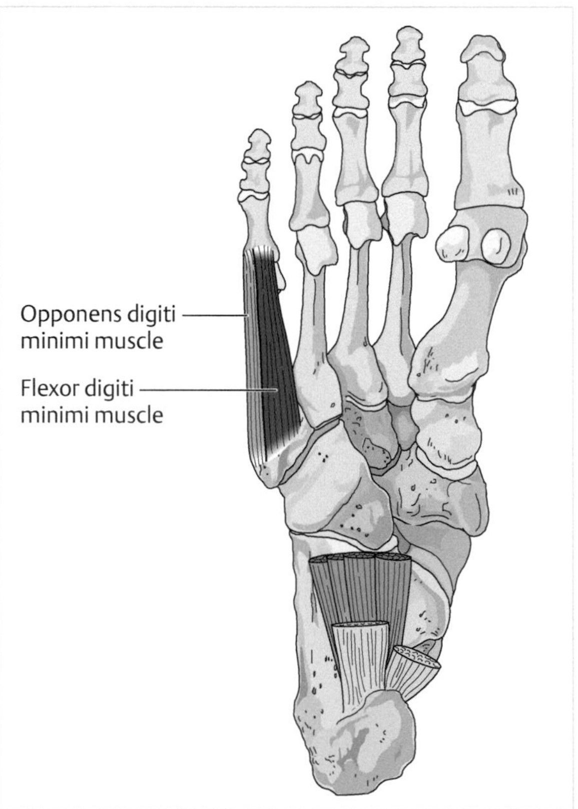


**Fig. 10.165** Flexor digiti minimi and opponens digiti minimi muscles.

# 10.13 Biomechanics

## 10.13.1 Arches of the Foot

### Longitudinal Arch (Fig. 10.166)

In the medial area of the arch, the head of the first metatarsal and medial process of the calcaneus have contact with the ground. The navicular bone, at 1.5 to 2 cm, is at the greatest distance from the ground.

The posterior contact point of the outer border of the foot is the lateral process of the calcaneus, and the anterior contact point is the fourth and fifth metatarsal heads. The cuboid bone, at approximately 5 mm, is at the greatest distance from the ground. However, this space is taken up with soft tissue, on which the bone is supported.

The weight of the body pressing down on the foot has a tendency to press the contact surfaces of the arch of the foot apart from each other. Minimal flattening is physiologic. The structures running under the arch (on the plantar side) in particular, prevent further flattening of the arch.

### Tensing the Longitudinal Arch

*Plantar Ligaments (Fig. 10.167)*

The ligaments bear the greatest responsibility for stabilizing the arch because only the ligamentous structures have the ability to withstand the constant load.

All the ligaments in the plantar area that join the tarsal bones together act to tense the longitudinal arch. The plantar calcaneonavicular ligament and the plantar calcaneocuboid ligament, whose longer fibers (the long plantar ligament) tense the arch over a longer distance, have a particular importance here.

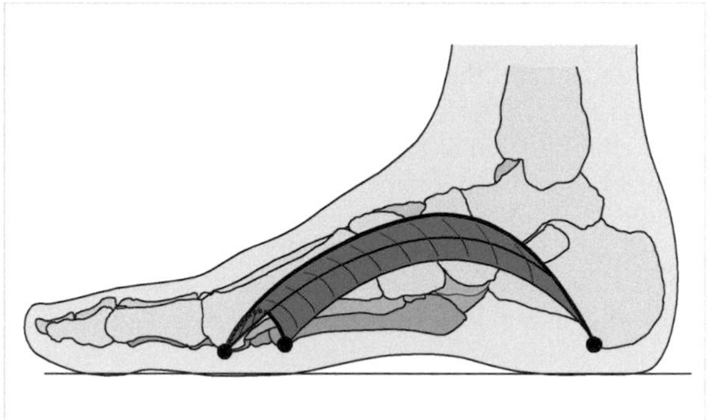

**Fig. 10.166** Longitudinal arch of the foot.

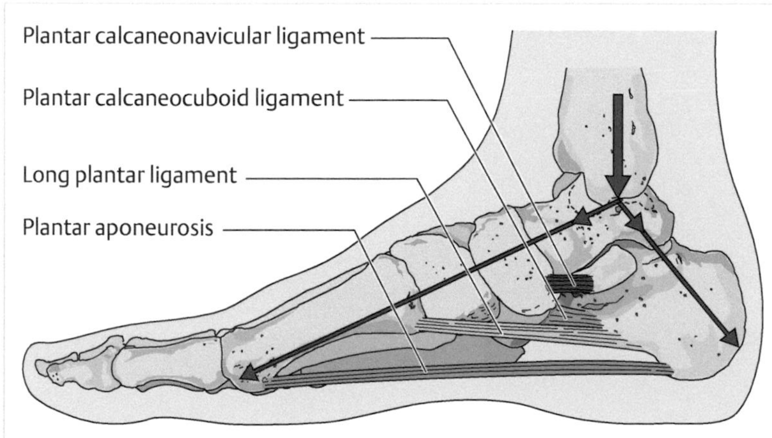


**Fig. 10.167** Plantar ligaments.

### *Plantar Aponeurosis (Fig. 10.168)*

This is a taut fascial plate that is divided into central, medial, and lateral sections.

The *central section* is the thickest and firmest. Its proximal fixation lies on the medial process of the calcaneal tuberosity. The aponeurosis broadens as it moves distally. At the level of the metatarsals, it ends in the ***longitudinal fascicles***, which diverge into four sections and extend into the superficial transverse metatarsal ligament. At the midmetatarsal level, the transversely running ***transverse fascicles*** connect with the longitudinal fibers. Along with a few of the deeper lying parts, they form an annular ligament for the tendons of the flexor digitorum longus muscle.

Intermuscular septa extend deeply from the edges of the central section of the aponeurosis and form compartments in which the muscles run distally. In the central compartment are the flexor digitorum brevis muscle, quadratus plantae, and adductor hallucis muscles, and the tendon of the flexor digitorum longus muscle.

The *lateral section* is thick in the proximal area and becomes thinner as it runs distally. It arises laterally on the medial process of the calcaneal tuberosity, extends toward the cuboid bone, and fans out distally to the base of the fifth metatarsal bone. This section forms the lateral compartment for the flexor, opponens, and abductor digiti minimi muscles.

The *medial section* is thin proximally and becomes thicker distally. It forms the fascia overlying the abductor hallucis muscle and the medial compartment, in which it and the flexor hallucis brevis muscle run.

Between the three sections are grooves, the *lateral and medial plantar sulci*. The lateral sulcus is larger and is covered by a few superficial fibers from the central section. The neurovascular bundle runs in a distal direction within this groove.

**Functions:**

- It tenses the arch of the foot.
- It stabilizes the chambered fat pads in the plantar region by tightening the septa surrounding them.
- It protects the muscles running within the compartments.

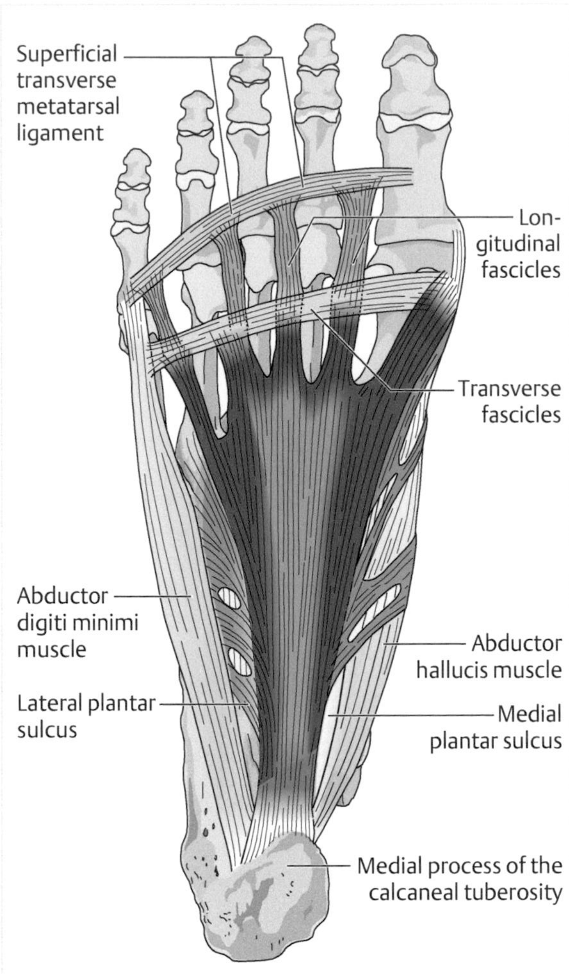


**Fig. 10.168** Plantar aponeurosis.

### *Muscles Running in the Plantar Region*

The short plantar foot muscles—*flexor digitorum brevis, hallucis brevis, abductor hallucis, and abductor digiti minimi muscles*—help to tense the longitudinal arch of the foot. The tibialis posterior muscle, flexor hallucis and digitorum longus muscles, and fiblularis brevis and longus muscles also help to tense the arch.

### *Tibialis Posterior Muscle (Fig. 10.169)*

This inserts on the plantar side of the navicular bone and thereby on the tarsal bone that is at the greatest distance from the ground. Therefore it raises the *keystone* of the arch.

Considering the further course of the terminal tendon in the plantar region, Tillmann (1977) noted that the forces of its terminal course can be broken down into longitudinal and transverse components, with the longitudinal force component being greater than the transverse component.

### *Toe Extensors (Fig. 10.170)*

The extensor digitorum and hallucis longus and brevis muscles have an indirect effect on the stability of the longitudinal arch. For example, the extensors of the big toe create a deflection—by raising the big toe, tension is placed on the metatarsal insertion of the plantar aponeurosis. Thus, the arch tenses and rises. Because of this effect, the longitudinal arch is stabilized in the *terminal stance* and *preswing* phases of gait.

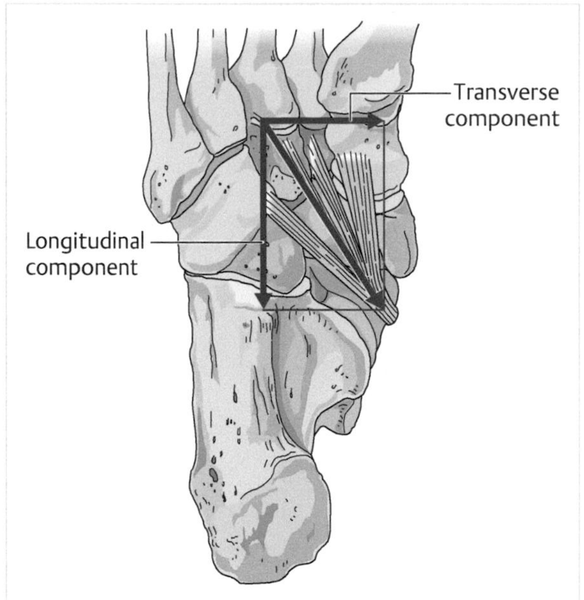


**Fig. 10.169** Breakdown of the forces on the terminal tendon of the tibialis posterior muscle in view of its stabilizing components.

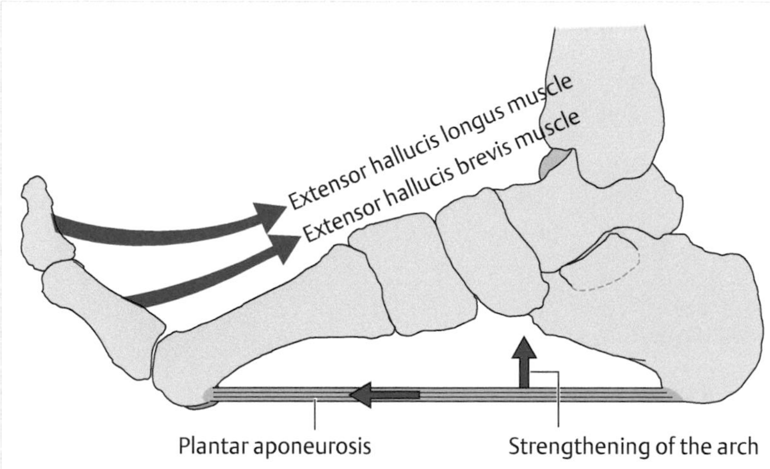


**Fig. 10.170** Effect of the toe extensors on the longitudinal arch.

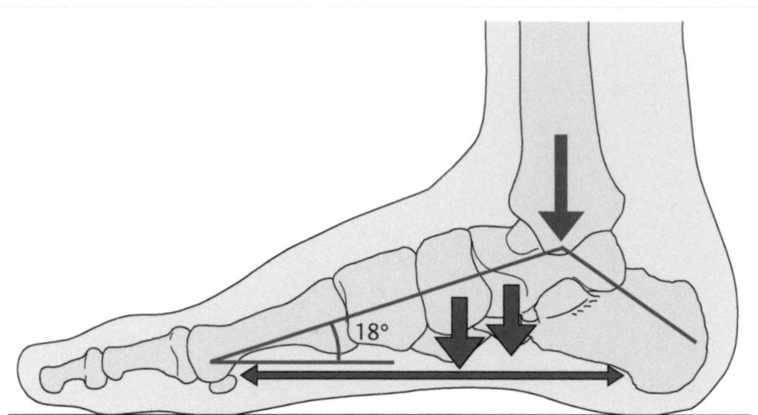


Fig. 10.171 Fallen longitudinal arch (flat foot deformity).

## Practical Tip

### Fallen Longitudinal Arch (Flat Foot Deformity) (Fig. 10.171)

The following are found in flat foot deformity:

- The angle of inclination of the metatarsal bone decreases significantly—instead of being 25°, it amounts to less than 18° in the medial area of the foot (see **Fig. 10.146**).
- The navicular bone is conspicuously displaced in a plantar direction—instead of two fingerbreadths, only one fits between the bone and the ground. Because the navicular bone sinks, the calcaneus and first metatarsal shift away from each other. The plantar calcaneonavicular ligament, the plantar aponeurosis, and the long plantar ligament are tensed. They are very sensitive to palpation.
- The talus shifts in a plantar and medial direction. Because of this, the hindfoot assumes a tilted position. The plumb line of the leg meets the ground at the medial calcaneus instead of in the middle of the calcaneus. The hindfoot is in the valgus position (**Fig. 10.172**).
- As a result of the displacement of the talus medially, the forefoot deviates into abduction. Normally, the talar neck axis continues on in a longitudinal direction as a line within the first metatarsal bone. In *pes abductus*, there is an angle between the two lines (**Fig. 10.173**).
- As a result of the talar deviation, there is internal rotation of the ankle mortise proximally.

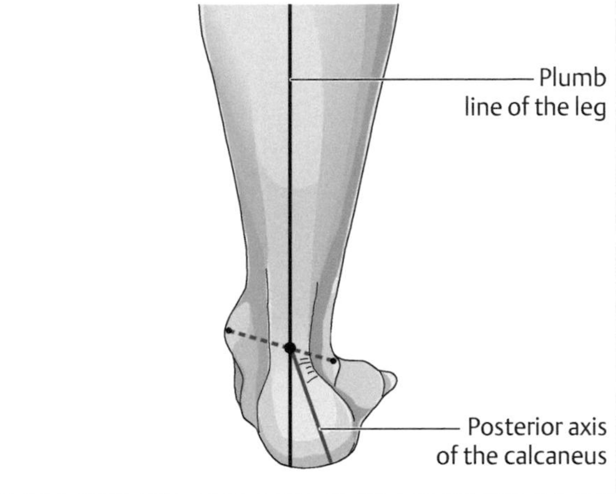


**Fig. 10.172** Tilted position of the hindfoot in pes planovalgus (dorsal view of right foot).

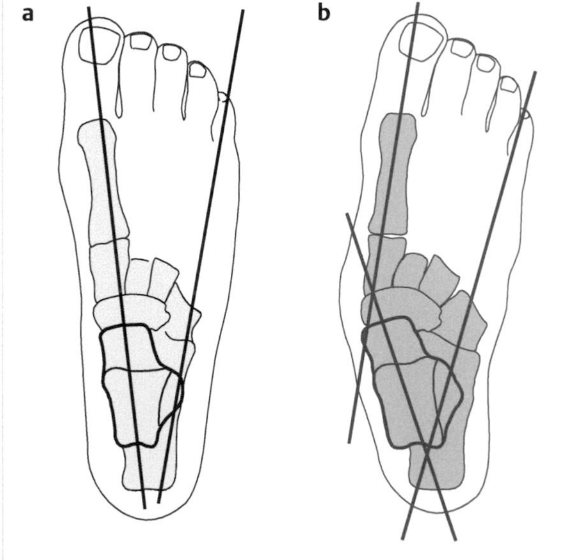


**Fig. 10.173** Forefoot position. **(a)** Normal relationship of the axes. **(b)** Abduction deviation in pes valgus/flat foot.

## Transverse Arches

The bony structures form arches in the form of a segmented beam construction. They are secured by ligaments that run in plantar and transverse directions.

### Midfoot Arch (Fig. 10.174)

The construction of the arch in the midfoot area can be clearly seen at the level of the cuneiform bones, because these are wedge-shaped and thus constitute a proper arch. The keystone here is the intermediate cuneiform bone. However, this arch has contact with the ground only laterally through the cuboid bone and the underlying soft tissues.

Somewhat further proximally, the navicular bone forms the medial part of the arch instead of the cuneiform bones.

The plantar ligaments (e.g., cuneocuboid ligament, cuboideonavicular ligament, and intercuneiform ligaments) tense the arch. The plantar interosseous ligaments have a particular stabilizing effect because they bind the tarsal bones together in close proximity to the joint surfaces, sometimes even within the joint.

The *fibularis longus muscle* is the most important stabilizing muscle for this area. It has both a longitudinal and a transverse component through the course of its plantar terminal tendon. Because of the distribution of the forces, the transverse component represents a somewhat larger force than the longitudinal component (**Fig. 10.175**).

The tibialis posterior muscle, approaching from medially, supports the arch, especially at the level of the navicular bone, but its effect supports transverse tension less than longitudinal tension.

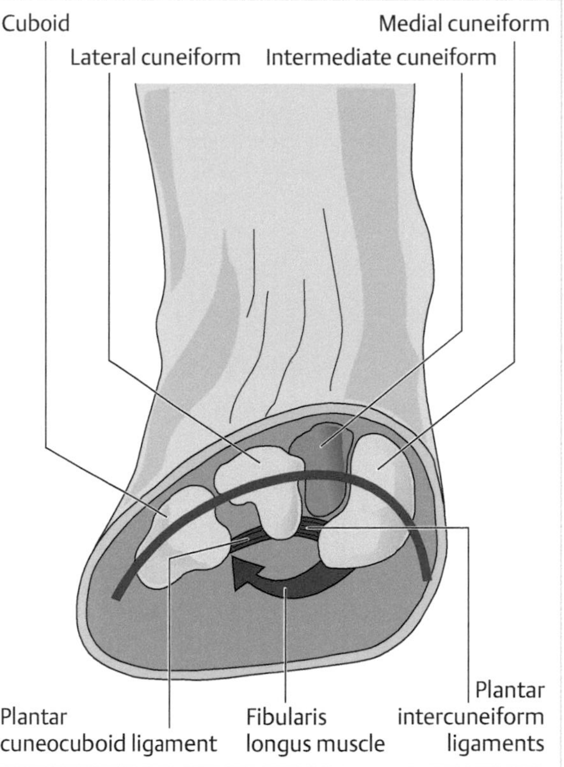


**Fig. 10.174** Transverse arches of the foot: midfoot arch.

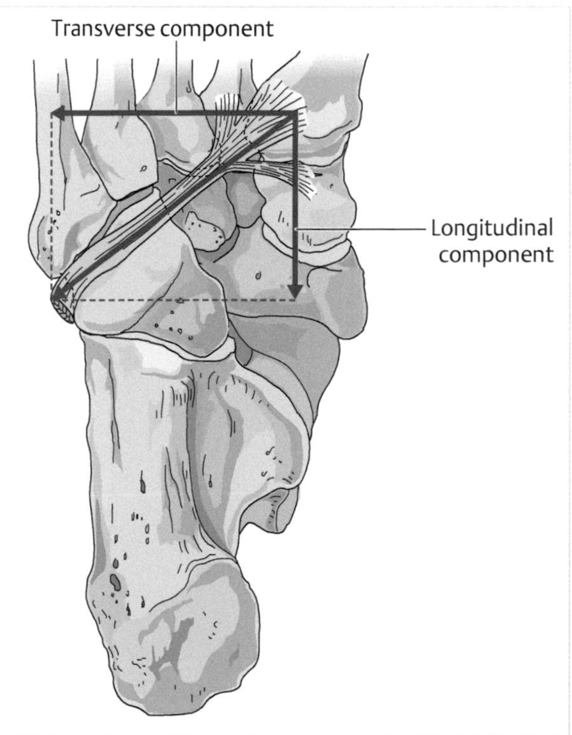


**Fig. 10.175** Breakdown of the forces on the terminal tendon of the fibularis longus muscle in view of its stabilizing components.

## Forefoot Arch (Fig. 10.176)

In the forefoot area, the arch is no longer as high as in the midfoot. Slightly proximal to the metatarsal heads, it can be seen that the head of the second metatarsal is the farthest from the ground. The padded heads of the first and fifth metatarsals provide side support for the arch.

The ligaments again bear the responsibility for tensing this arch, although here they are not as strong as in the midfoot. In this, the transverse fascicles of the plantar aponeurosis support the deep transverse metatarsal ligament.

The most important muscular stabilizer of the transverse arch is the transverse head of the adductor hallucis muscle. The fibers that most clearly tense the arch are those that extend medially from the fifth metatarsal.

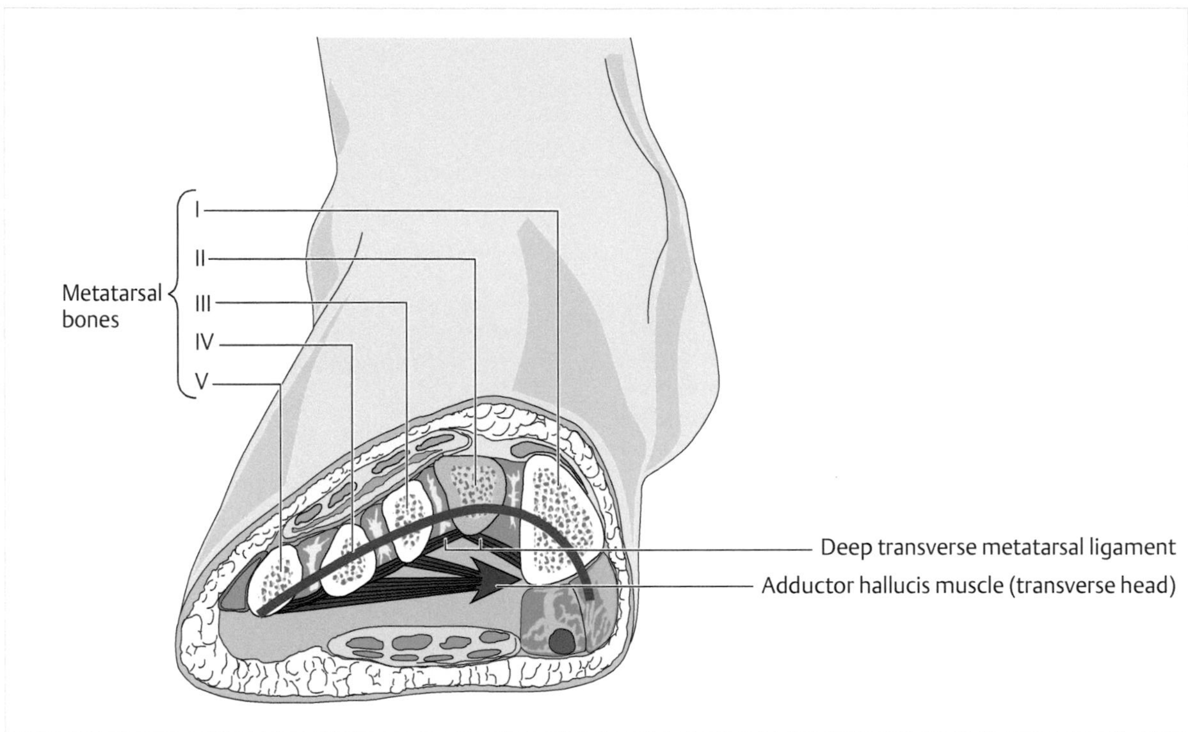


**Fig. 10.176** Transverse arches of the foot: forefoot arch.

## Pathology

### Splayfoot (Fig. 10.177)

Splayfoot involves a static deformity resulting from constitutional weakness of connective tissue in combination with being overweight and the use of inappropriate footwear.

The transverse metatarsal arch sags in the mid-arch area. The metatarsals splay apart—the first and fifth are especially prominent. Because of this, the forefoot broadens, and the shoes put stress on the metatarsal heads on the inside and outside of the foot. An increased buildup of callous occurs at these spots and on the plantar surface under the second and third metatarsal heads.

Because of the compression of the MTP joints, they become irritated and inflamed (*metatarsalgia*). The pain from the pressure load is especially bad during push-off.

### Hallux Valgus (Fig. 10.178)

This is the lateral subluxation of the big toe at the MTP joint, usually combined with splayfoot.

Contingent on the axis deviation of the first metatarsal in terms of adduction, there is a disturbance in the muscular equilibrium—the direction in which the tendon insertions pull on the toes changes. The abductor muscle shifts laterally in relation to the abduction axis and thus becomes an adductor. The flexor and extensor tendons also relocate laterally to a significant degree, and thus reinforce the lateral shift at the MTP joint.

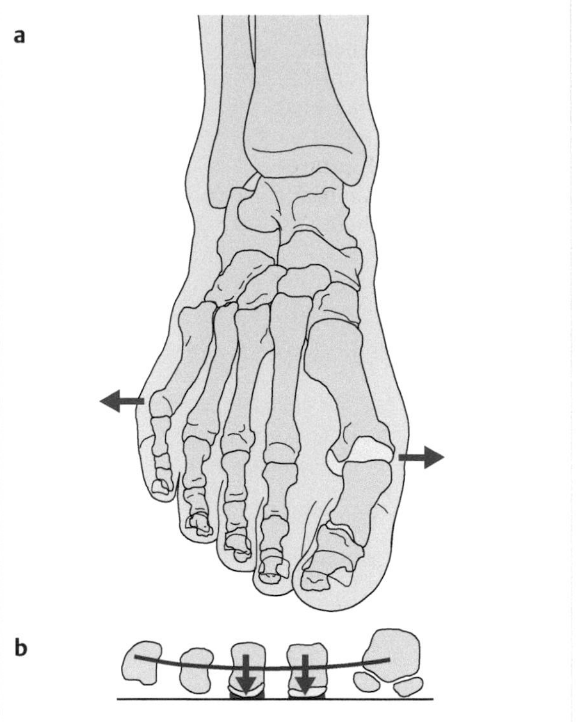


**Fig. 10.177** Splayfoot. **(a)** Widening of the forefoot. **(b)** Compressive stress on the second and third metatarsal heads.

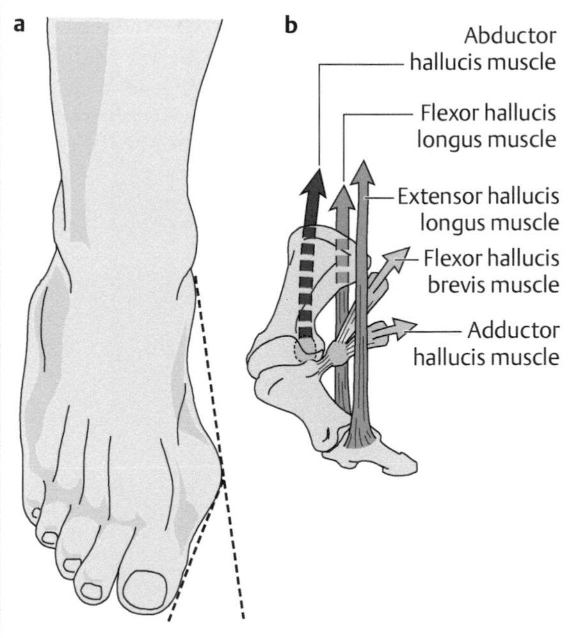


**Fig. 10.178** Hallux valgus. **(a)** Lateral deviation of the right big toe. **(b)** Altered direction of pull of the muscles of the left big toe.

## 10.13.2 Statics of the Foot

### Distribution of Pressure in the Standing Position

The body weight is distributed to the right and left ankle joints (talocrural joints), then on each side to the talus, posteriorly toward the calcaneal tuberosity, and anteriorly toward the forefoot. The heel thus receives approximately 60% of the body weight, the midfoot 8%, and the forefoot 32%.

A more precise measurement of plantar pressure is possible using a sensor-equipped pedal force measurement platform. With the help of a computer, the pressure is represented in various shades of color or by lines similar to those on a topographical map. The measurements confirm the high pressure values in the heel and forefoot areas (**Fig. 10.179**).

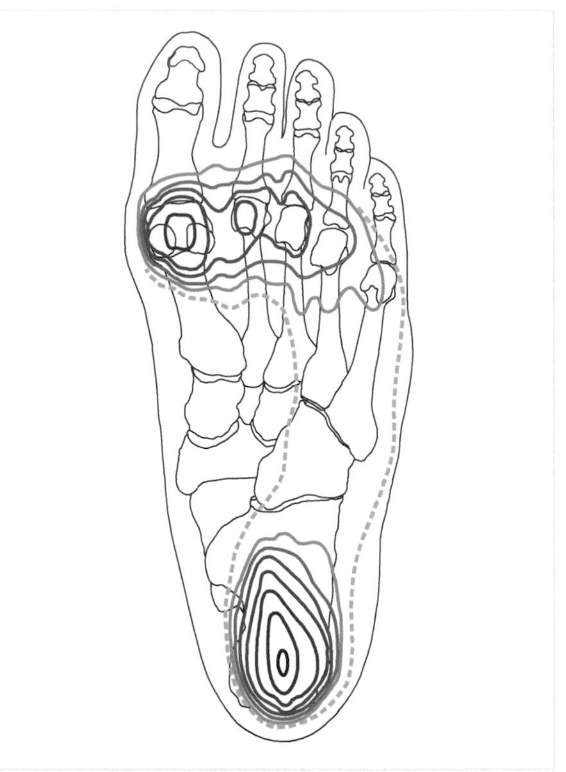

**Fig. 10.179** Weight-bearing diagram of a normal right foot.

### Weight-bearing Surfaces (Fig. 10.180)

It is possible to obtain evidence on the extent of the weight-bearing surface on the sole of the foot by means of a *podogram*, which is a graphic representation of the load. One method is to place the underside of a rubber mat that has been covered with stamp-pad ink on a sheet of paper, and then ask the patient to place the whole foot on it. As a result of the weight transfer, the paper is colored on the support area, with the heavily weighted points more heavily colored than those less heavily weighted.

The examiner can now evaluate the relationship between the width of the heel print and the width of the forefoot. The *isthmus width* is the narrowest loaded area of the foot. With help from the podogram, one can diagnose pathologic foot shapes. For instance, the flat foot has a widened isthmus, the high-arched foot has a very narrow or absent isthmus, and the splayfoot demonstrates widening of the forefoot.

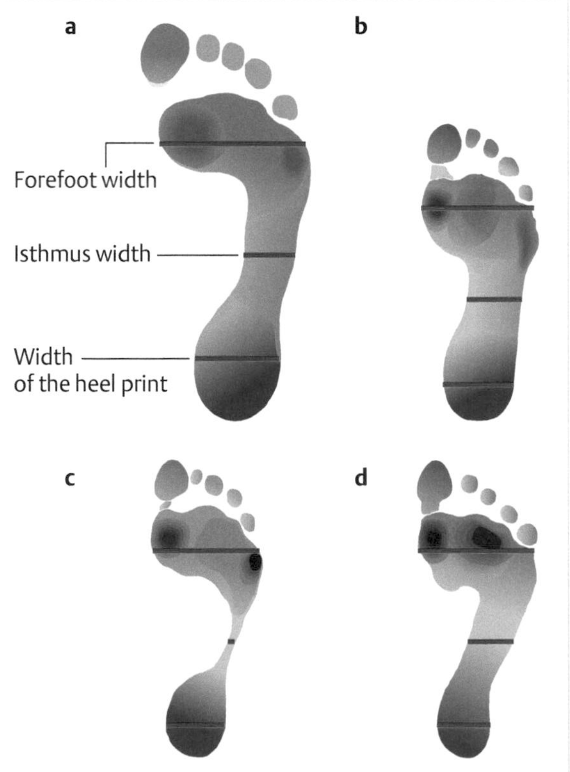


**Fig 10.180** Podogram. **(a)** Normal foot. **(b)** Flat foot. **(c)** High-arched foot. **(d)** Splayfoot.

## Body Center of Gravity (Fig. 10.181)

In the standing position, the vertical projection of the center of gravity lies approximately 1 to 2 cm in front of the navicular bone between the feet. It is subject to vacillations, which shift in all directions within an area of 4 mm around this point. These vacillations are obvious when first standing still, but later become smaller and more constant in direction.

Positional changes in the center of gravity are sensed through the visual, vestibular, and proprioceptive systems, which are interdependent and regulated centrally. For example, the extent of vacillation is greater when the eyes are closed.

Stability increases from childhood on and decreases again in old age. The amplitude of vacillation also becomes larger in patients with pareses.

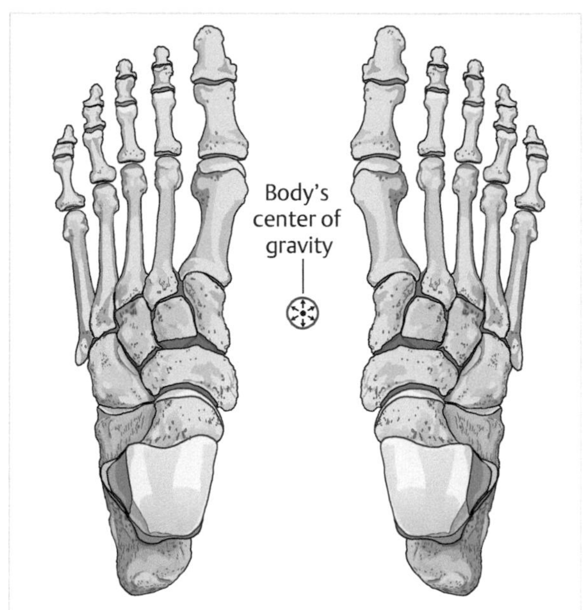


**Fig. 10.181** Projection of the body's center of gravity.

### *Equilibrium and Muscle Activities*

Muscle action is required to establish a state of equilibrium. With a medial or lateral shift, the first reaction occurs in the hip area and involves the adductors and abductors. In the foot region, however, the fibular muscles—especially the fibularis brevis muscle—play a role.

Okada (1983) found, by means of electromyographic measurements, that there is an interdependence of muscle activity in terms of the projection of the center of gravity. If the center of gravity shifts posteriorly, the tibialis anterior muscle activates. If, however, it shifts anteriorly, there is increasing activity in the gastrocnemius, soleus, and abductor hallucis muscles.

## Distribution of Force during Ambulation

Ultrasonography shows that the longitudinal arch of the foot changes only slightly when under pressure (Hennig 1985). As a result of the load, the talus turns inward, which leads to eversion, and because of this the arch, if anything, appears to decrease.

During walking, the individual peak loads can be recognized by way of a graphic representation. The highest values measured in the gait cycle occur in the heel area on initial contact and in the forefoot area in the terminal stance phase (**Fig. 10.182**). In the last phase of gait, however, pressure is put on the big toe. Here measurement of compressive loads reaches 48% of body weight.

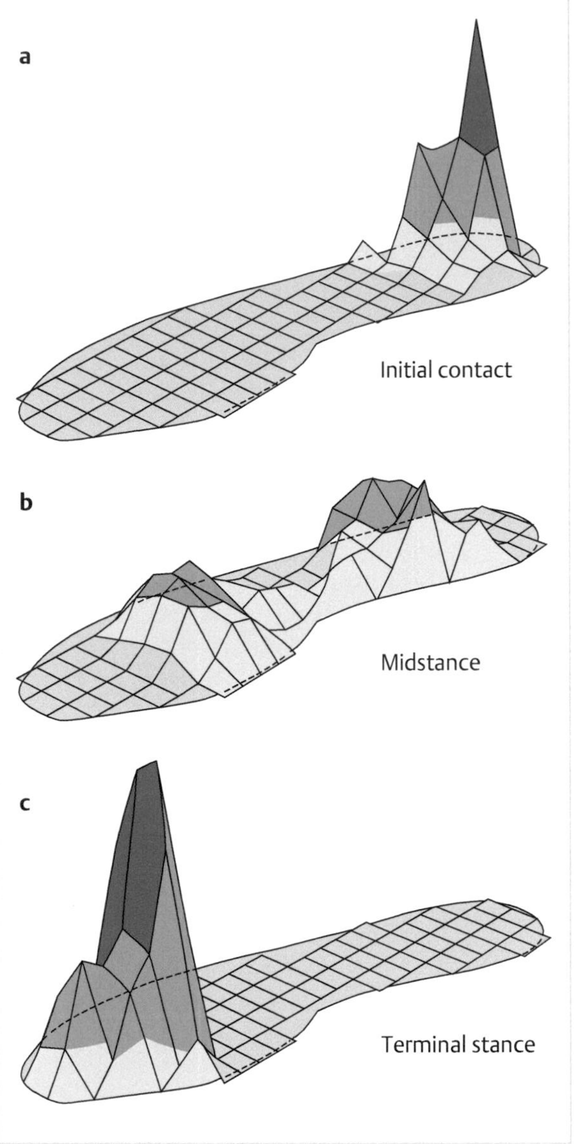


**Fig. 10.182** Graphic representation of pressures on the foot while rolling from heel to toe. **(a)** At initial contact. **(b)** In midstance. **(c)** At terminal stance.

## Pressure on the Sole of the Foot

### Construction of the Sole of the Foot (Fig. 10.183)

The subcutaneous layer is approximately 1.8 to 2 cm thick. The outer layer is fibrous, with many collagen fibers and a thick network of vessels. Strong connective tissue septa cross through the subcutaneous layer and form chambers that hold the fat tissue together. These septa are in part arranged in a **U**-shaped or spiral form. They connect fascial and skeletal points of the foot with the skin. Further inward, the chambers become larger and the fibers more elastic.

With pressure, the sole of the foot presses together to half its usual thickness, i.e., to 0.9 to 1 cm. It has a special cushioning property in that the tissue becomes increasingly firmer when placed under pressure.

**Functions:**

- Because of the special construction of the sole of the foot, forces acting on a loaded skeletal point distribute over an extended contact area.
- The chambers contribute to the absorption of shock because they deform and yield elastically, and because the fat masses shift within them.
- As a result of the firm chambering, the heel achieves a high mechanically stability.

In infants, the fat pads on the sole are particularly pronounced, but they disappear in early childhood.

Africans who go barefoot have a particularly thick cushion in the medial foot area of 2.5 to 3 cm. Because of this, they appear to have flat feet, but on X-ray, the arch construction is completely normal.

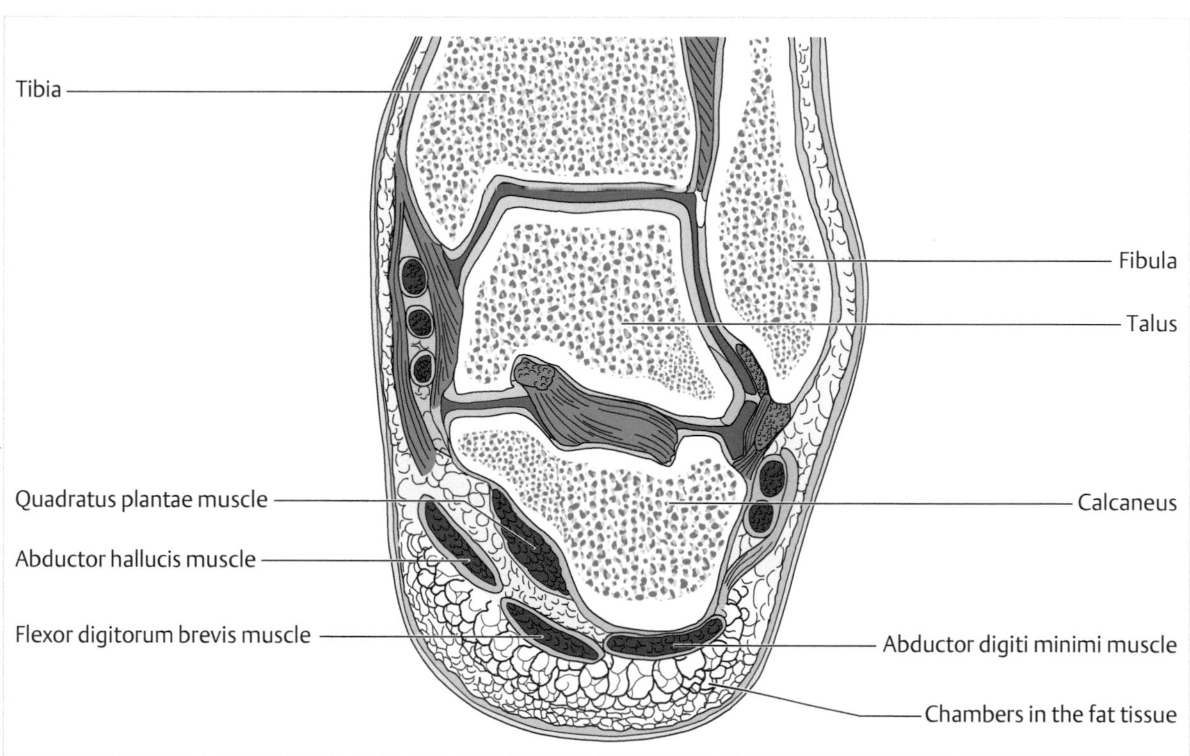


**Fig. 10.183** Cushion of the sole of the foot in the heel area (frontal section through the right hindfoot, posterior view).

## 10.14 Vascular Supply

Inferior to the popliteal fossa, the popliteal artery divides into the posterior tibial artery and the anterior tibial artery.

### Posterior Tibial Artery (Fig. 10.184)

- This artery runs in the posterior lower leg.
- It extends through the tendinous arch of the soleus muscle into the deep flexor compartment.
- The artery then runs between the tibialis posterior and flexor digitorum longus muscles along the posterior side of the tibia.
- At the level of the medial malleolus, it gives off the *medial malleolar branches.*
- It runs inferior to the medial malleolus toward the plantar surface.
- There it forms the *deep plantar arch* from the *lateral plantar artery* running within the lateral plantar sulcus, and from the *medial plantar artery* running within the medial plantar sulcus.
- It ends in the *plantar digital arteries* for the toes.
- The artery supplies the gastrocnemius muscle and all the muscles of the sole of the foot, as well as the plantar part of the lower ankle joint (subtalar and talocalcaneonavicular joints) and the other joints of the foot.

### Fibular Artery (Fig. 10.184)

- This arises from the posterior tibial artery about one handbreadth inferior to the popliteal fossa.
- It runs on top of the posterior fibula between the tibialis posterior and flexor hallucis longus muscles.
- It ends with the *lateral malleolar branch,* which supplies the lateral malleolus and the lateral parts of the upper (talocrural) and lower ankle joints.
- It also supplies the deep flexors and the fibular muscles.

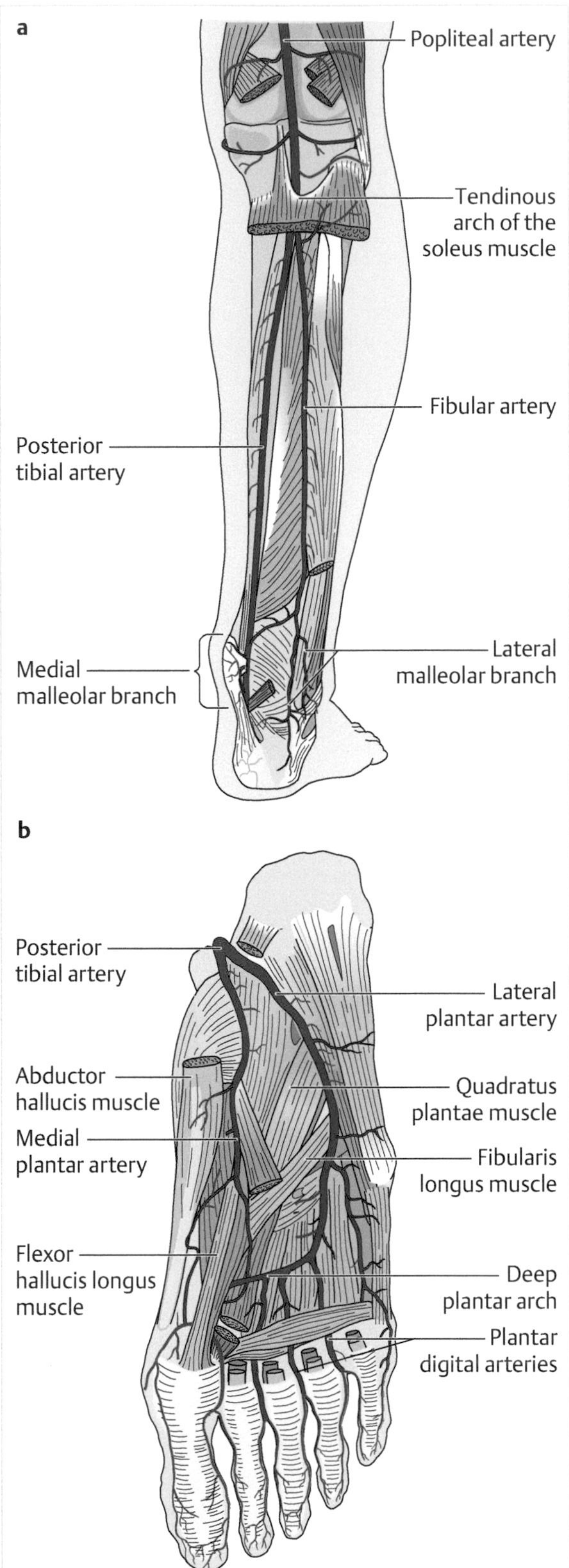


**Fig. 10.184** Posterior tibial and fibular arteries. **(a)** Course in the posterior lower leg. **(b)** Course in the plantar area.

## Anterior Tibial Artery (Fig. 10.185)

- This extends through the proximal hiatus of the interosseous membrane.
- It runs further distally in the extensor compartment.
- Between the superior and inferior extensor retinacula, it gives off *anterior malleolar arteries* to the medial and lateral malleoli.
- After the retinacula, it divides into the *lateral tarsal artery* and the *dorsalis pedis artery*, which runs superficially distally over the dorsum of the foot between the extensor hallucis longus muscle and the tibialis anterior muscle.
- On the dorsum of the foot at the level of the metatarsal bases, it forms the *arcuate artery*, which joins with the lateral tarsal artery.
- It ends as the *dorsal digital arteries* at the toes.
- It supplies the extensors of the lower leg and provides branches to the dorsal side of all the joints of the foot.

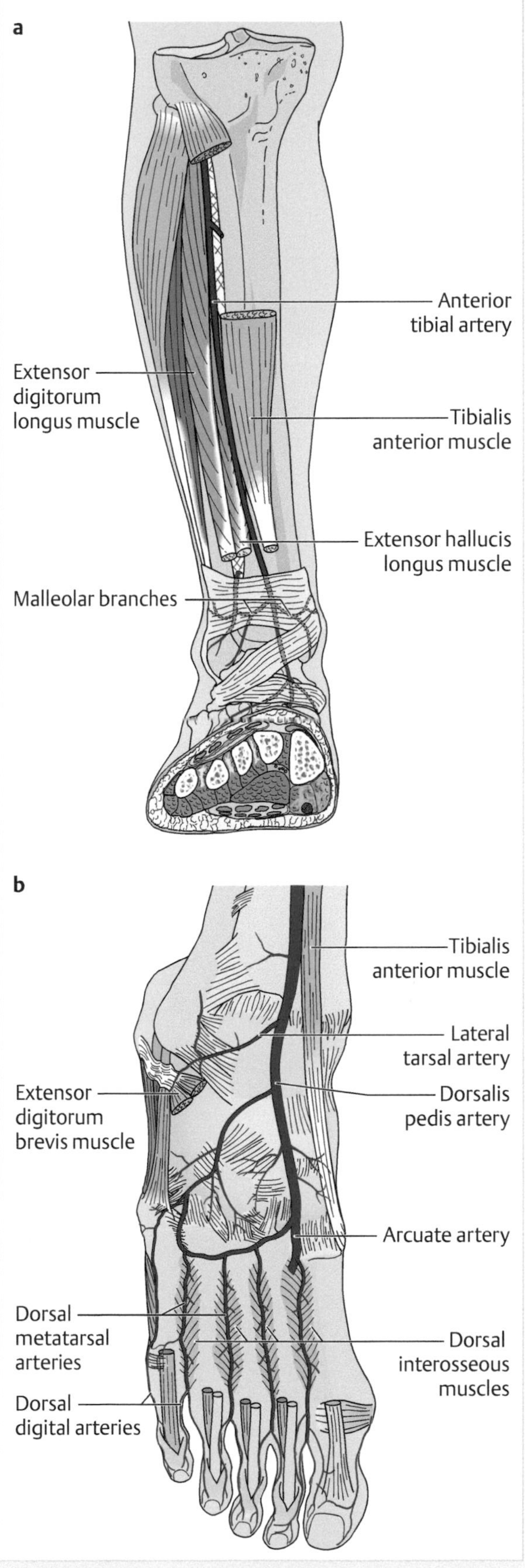


**Fig. 10.185** Course of the anterior tibial artery. **(a)** In the lower leg area. **(b)** On the dorsum of the foot.

# 10.15 Neural Structures of the Foot and Ankle

## 10.15.1 Innervation of the Joints of the Foot and Ankle

### Talocrural and Talotarsal Joints (10.186)

- The *saphenous nerve* supplies a part of the medial side of the upper ankle joint (talocrural joint) with its articular branches.
- The *sural nerve* extends with its branches to the posterior parts of the joint and inferolaterally to the lower ankle joint (subtalar and talocalcaneonavicular joints). It also supplies the tarsal sinus.
- At the level of the malleoli, the *deep fibular* nerve divides into its articular branches to the posterior and lateral parts of the joint as well as anteriorly to the navicular bone.
- The *tibial nerve* divides into the articular branches anteriorly and medially.

The remaining parts of the joints, including the capsules and the ligaments of the foot on the plantar side, are supplied by branches of the medial and lateral plantar nerves, and the dorsum of the foot by branches of the superficial and deep fibular nerves.

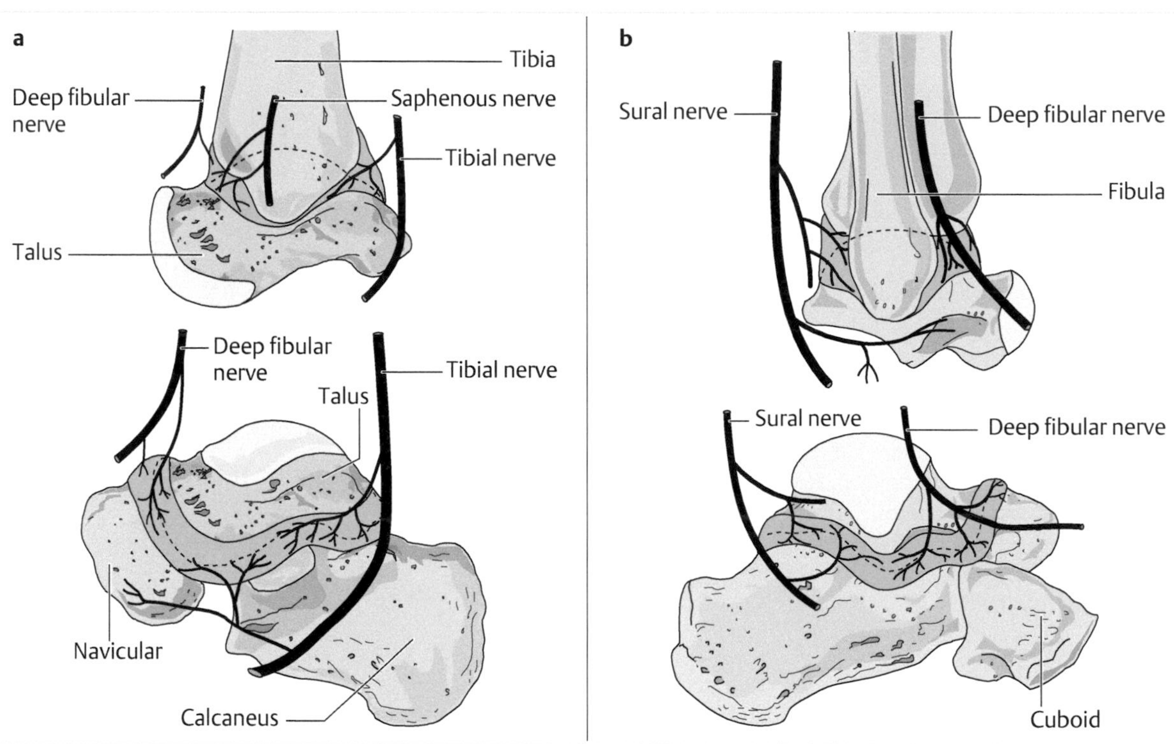


**Fig. 10.186** Innervation. **(a)** Upper and lower ankle joint (medial view). **(b)** Upper and lower ankle joint (lateral view).

## 10.15.2 Courses of the Nerves in the Foot and Ankle

### Deep Fibular Nerve (Figs. 10.187 and 10.188)

- This nerve pierces the anterior intermuscular septum.
- It runs distally between the tibialis anterior and extensor hallucis longus muscles on the interosseous membrane.
- Its further course extends inferiorly parallel to the anterior tibial artery, under the extensor retinaculum toward the medial aspect of the dorsum of the foot.
- It ends with branches to the skin to provide sensory innervation to the space between the first and the second toes.
- It innervates the extensor group of the lower leg, the extensor hallucis brevis muscle, and the extensor digitorum brevis muscle.

### Superficial Fibular Nerve (Figs. 10.187 and 10.188)

- This lies under the fibularis longus muscle.
- Further distally, it runs along the anterior border of the fibularis brevis muscle.
- It gives off muscular branches to the fibular muscles and cutaneous branches to the lower leg.
- Above the lateral malleolus, it divides into two branches:
  - The *medial dorsal cutaneous nerve* extends over the extensor retinaculum toward the dorsum of the foot, which it supplies, and goes on to supply the medial surface to the big toe and, with a further branch, the space between the second and third toes.
  - The *intermediate dorsal cutaneous nerve* extends over the extensor retinaculum to the lateral aspect of the dorsum of the foot and innervates the skin here and the lateral half of the third toe, the entire fourth toe, and the medial half of the fifth toe.

### Sural Nerve

This accompanies the small saphenous vein lateral to the Achilles tendon in the malleolar groove. From there, it gives off cutaneous branches to the lateral surface of the heel, the lateral edge of the foot, and the outer surface of the small toe.

▷ See Chapter 9.4, Neural Structures

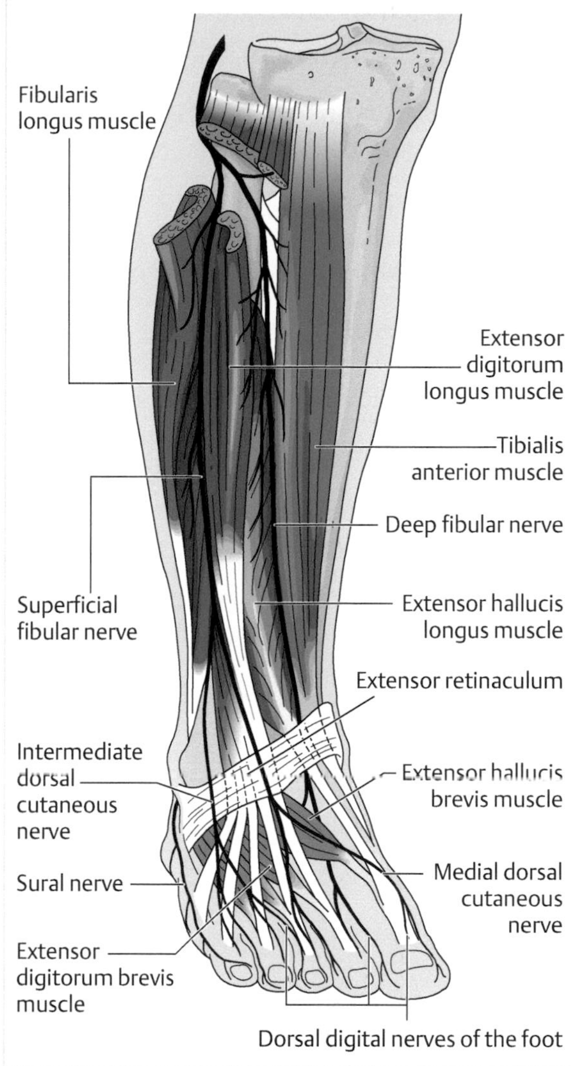


**Fig. 10.187** Deep and superficial fibular nerves.

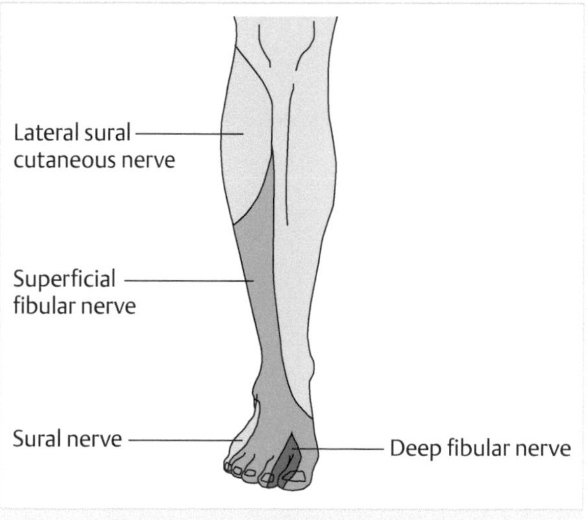


**Fig. 10.188** Cutaneous innervation by the fibular nerves.

Practical Tip

**Supination Trauma**

When the lateral edge of the foot twists medially, as occurs in supination trauma, the superficial fibular nerve is rapidly overstretched and thus traumatized. This results in retardation of the nerve conduction velocity, which must be remembered when performing proprioceptive exercises. It is possible for repeated twist injuries to occur, because the ability to react to threatened stabilization is severely impaired. It is absolutely necessary to take these facts into consideration during the training program.

Pathology

**Anterior Tarsal Tunnel Syndrome**

This syndrome occurs because of a narrow spot under the extensor retinaculum. Here the deep fibular nerve extends distally on the dorsum of the foot.

Patients complain of pain and hypesthesia over the first interosseous metatarsal space. Paresis of the extensor digitorum brevis muscle may occur.

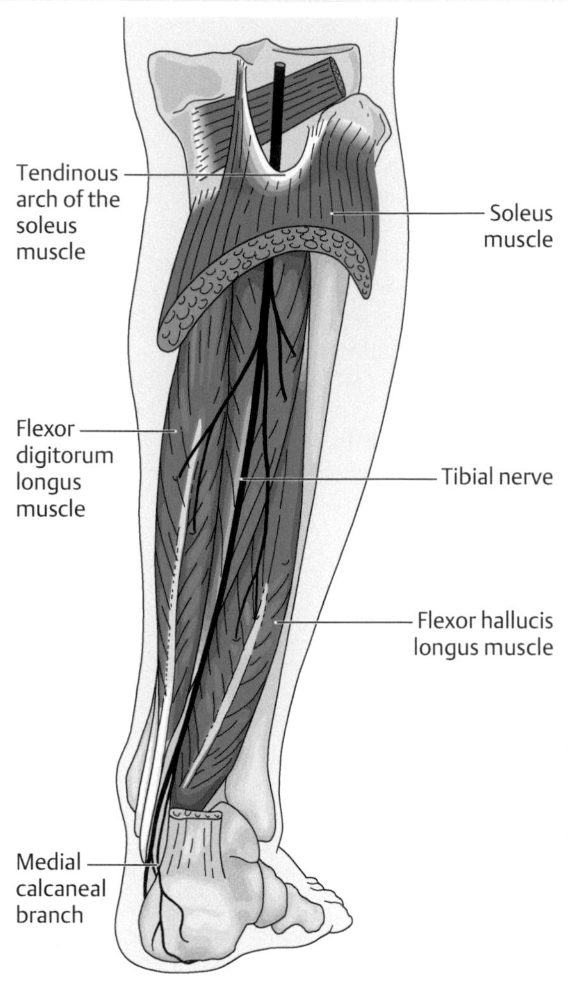


**Fig. 10.189** Course of the tibial nerve in the lower leg.

## Tibial Nerve (L4–S3; Figs. 10.189–10.191)

- This runs under the gastrocnemius muscle between the flexor digitorum longus and the flexor hallucis longus muscles and innervates these muscles as it passes distally.
- It extends further with these tendons toward the medial malleolus.
- It gives off the medial calcaneal branch above the malleolus, which provides sensory innervation to the heel and posterior parts of the sole of the foot, and motor innervation for the flexor digitorum brevis.
- It then runs under the flexor retinaculum and bends around the medial malleolus toward the sole of the foot.
- Together with the long toe flexors, it extends toward the plantar surface under the abductor hallucis muscle in an osteofibrotic canal, where it divides into two large branches.

*Lateral Plantar Nerve (Figs. 10.190 and 10.191)*

- This runs between the flexor digitorum brevis muscle and the quadratus plantae muscle toward the lateral edge of the foot.
- With its *deep branch*, it supplies the third and fourth lumbrical muscles and the quadratus plantae muscle.
- With its superficial branch, it innervates the interosseous muscles, the adductor hallucis muscle, and the short small toe muscles.
- It also supplies sensory innervation to the lateral region of the sole of the foot and the plantar surface of half of the fourth toe and the entire fifth toe.

*Medial Plantar Nerve (Figs. 10.190 and 10.191)*

- This tracks distally between the abductor hallucis muscle and the tendons of the flexor digitorum longus muscle.
- It divides into four branches, which spread out to the first to fourth toes.
- It supplies motor innervation for the first and second lumbrical muscles and the small muscles of the big toe up to the adductor, and sensory innervation to the middle and medial area of the sole and the plantar surfaces of the first to fourth toes.

## Compartments

A strand of neurovascular tissue, consisting of the posterior tibial artery and vein and the tibial nerve, runs distally in the deep flexor compartment of the leg, along with the tendons. In the lower leg, this neurovascular bundle lies between the flexor hallucis longus and the flexor digitorum longus muscles. Their course is superficial in the retromalleolar area.

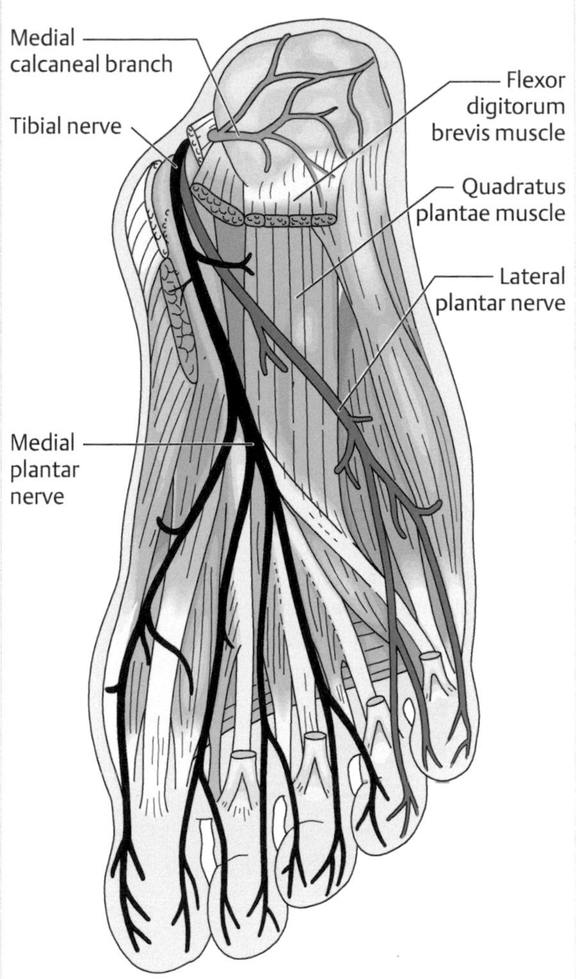


**Fig. 10.190** Course of the tibial nerve in the plantar area.

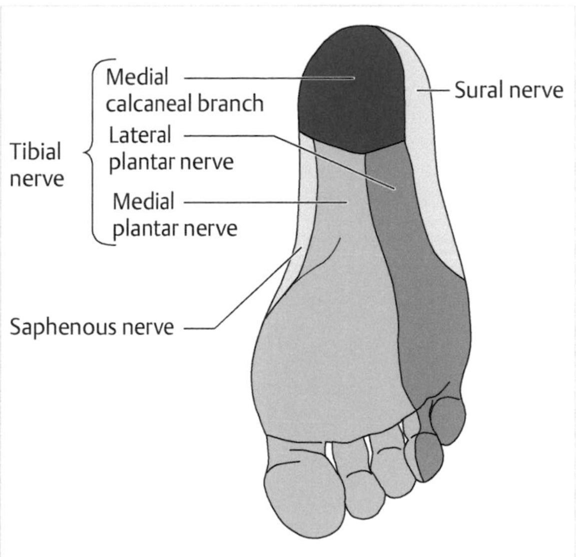


**Fig. 10.191** Innervation of the skin in the plantar area.

## Pathology

### Posterior Tarsal Tunnel Syndrome

This syndrome occurs because of compression of the tibial nerve behind the malleolus under the flexor retinaculum. The cause can be a traumatic lesion in the joint area, for example from a sprain. An increased proliferation of tissue under the retinaculum in the form of a pseudoneuroma is another possible cause. Patients complain of painful paresthesias on the sole of the foot and dysesthesias in the distribution area of the plantar nerves. During examination, sensitivity to pressure is apparent over the course of the tibial nerve. In some cases, passive extension of the toes or forcible pronation of the foot can provoke the symptoms. Paresis of the short plantar muscles with intact toe flexors may possibly occur, resulting in a claw position of the toes. Electrophysiologically, there is delay in the conduction speed of the sensory nerve, and prolonged distal latency occurs.

Treatment consists of division of the retinaculum posterior to the medial malleolus.

### Morton Neuroma

This is isolated damage to an interdigital sensory terminal branch of the tibial nerve. Splayfoot is most often cited as the cause.

Patients complain of a burning pain in the midplantar section at the level of the metatarsals with radiation to the third and fourth toes. At first, this occurs only with weight-bearing, but later it becomes persistent. During examination, the pain is reproducible by pressing the metatarsals together. Sensation is impaired in the distribution area of the second and third digital nerves.

Therapeutically, the splayfoot is treated with an orthotic insert with retrocapital support. Non-weight-bearing may be required temporarily. If the symptoms are not relieved in this manner, the neuroma must be excised. See Chapter 10.1.5, Plantar Surface, and **Fig. 10.39**.

# Bibliography


[1] American Academy of Craniomandibular Disorders. Craniomandibular Disorders: Guidelines for Evaluation, Diagnosis and Management. Chicago, IL: Quintessence Publishing Co. Inc.; 1990

[2] Andersson G, McNeill T. Lumbar Spine Syndromes. Heidelberg, Germany: Springer; 1989

[3] Arlen A. Biometrische Röntgenfunktionsdiagnostik der HWS. Manuelle Medizin; vol 5. Heidelberg: Fischer; 1979:123

[4] Bankart ASB. The pathology and treatment of recurrent dislocation of the shoulder joint. Br J Surg 26:23–39

[5] Basmajian JV. Muscles Alive. Baltimore, MD: Williams & Wilkins; 1974

[6] Benzel EC. The Cervical Spine. Philadelphia, PA: Lippincott Williams & Wilkins; 2012

[7] Bergmann G, Deuretzbacher G, Heller M, et al. Hip contact forces and gait patterns from routine activities. J Biomech 2001;34:859–871

[8] Bergmann G, Graichen F, Rohlmann A. Hip joint loading during walking and running, measured in two patients. J Biomech 1993;26:969–990

[9] Bigliani LV, Ticker JB, Flatow EL, Soslowsky LJ, Mow VC. The relationship of acromial architecture to rotator cuff disease. Clin Sport Med 1991;10:823–838

[10] Bogduk N. Clinical and Radiological Anatomy of the Lumbar Spine. Edinburgh, UK: Churchill Livingstone; 2012

[11] Bogduk N, Marstand A. The cervical zygapophysial joints as a source of neck pain. Spine 1988;13:610–617

[12] Brown BJ, Tatlow WF. Radiographic studies of the vertebral arteries in cadavers. J Radiol 1963;81:80–88

[13] Brügger A. Die Erkrankungen des Bewegungsapparates und seines Nervensystems. Munich, Germany: Urban & Fischer; 1977

[14] Butler DS. Mobilisation of the Nervous System. Oxford, UK: Elsevier; 1991

[15] Carl HD, Swoboda B. Effectiveness of arthroscopic synovectomy in rheumatoid arthritis. Z Rheumatol 2008;67:485–490

[16] Chaitow L. Palpation and Assessment Skills. Edinburgh, UK: Churchill Livingstone; 2009

[17] Chaitow L, DeLany J. The Upper Body. Edinburgh, UK: Elsevier Churchill Livingstone; 2008. Clinical Application of Neuromuscular Techniques; vol 1

[18] Chaitow L, DeLany J, Donnerholt J. The Lower Body. Edinburgh, UK: Churchill Livingstone; 2011. Clinical Application of Neuromuscular Techniques; vol 2

[19] Cole BJ, Sekiya JK. Surgical Techniques of the Shoulder, Elbow, and Knee in Sports Medicine. Philadelphia, PA: WB Saunders; 2013

[20] Cook CE, Hegedus EJ. Orthopedic Physical Examination Tests: An Evidence-Based Approach. Upper Saddle River, NJ: Prentice Hall; 2011

[21] Davies AM, Grainger AJ, James SJ, eds. Imaging of the Hand and Wrist. Berlin, Germany: Springer; 2013

[22] De Klejn A, Nienwenhuyse AC. Schwindelanfälle und Nystagmus bei einer bestimmten Stellung des Kopfes. Acta Otolaryngol (Stockh) 1917;11:155

[23] DeStefano L. Greenman's Principles of Manual Medicine. Philadelphia, PA: Lippincott-Raven Publishers; 2010

[24] Di Giacomo G, Pouliart N, Costantini A, de Vita A, eds. Atlas and Functional Shoulder Anatomy. Berlin, Germany: Springer; 2008

[25] Doyle JR. Anatomy of the finger flexor tendon sheath and pulley system. J Hand Surg 1988;13:473–484

[26] Drake R, Vogl W, Mitchell A. Anatomy for Students. Philadelphia, PA: Elsevier; 2005

[27] Dvorak J, Panjabi MM. Functional anatomy of the ligaments. Spine 1987;12:183–189

[28] Ellmann H. Diagnosis and treatment of incomplete rotator cuff tears. Clin Orthop Relat Res 1990;354:64–74

[29] Fabrizius J, Davidsen HG, Hanset AT. Cardiac function in funnel chest. Dan Med Bull 1957;4:251–257

[30] Fagerson TL. The Hip Handbook. Boston, MA: Butterworth-Heinemann Ltd; 1998

[31] Fielding JW. Normal and selected abnormal motion of the cervical spine from the second to the seventh cervical vertebra based on cineroentgenography. J Bone Joint Surg 1964;46a:1779–1781

[32] Fortin JD, Kissling RO, O'Connor BL, Vilensky JA. Sacroiliac joint innervation and pain. Am J Orthop 1999;28:687–690

[33] Frisch H, Wagner M. Systematic Musculoskeletal Examination. Berlin, Germany: Springer; 2012

[34] Froimson HJ. Keyhole tenodesis of biceps origin at the shoulder. Clin Orthop 1975;112:245–249

[35] Genda E, Horii E. Theoretical stress analysis in wrist joint – neutral position and functional position. J Hand Surg 2000;25:292–295

[36] Genda E, Horii E, et al. Load transmission through the wrist in the extended position. J Hand Surg 2008;33:182–188

[37] Giles LGF. Clinical Anatomy and Management of Thoracic Spine Pain. Vol 2. Oxford, UK: Elsevier; 2000

[38] Giles LGF, Singer K. Clinical Anatomy and Management of Cervical Spine Pain. Oxford, UK: Elsevier; 1998

[39] Gobbi A, Espregueira Mendes J, Nakamura N, eds. The Patellofemoral Joint. Berlin, Germany: Springer; 2014

[40] Gould JS. The Handbook of Foot and Ankle Surgery: An Intellectual Approach to Complex Problems. London, UK: JP Medical Ltd; 2013

[41] Graumann W, Sasse D. Bewegungsapparat. Stuttgart: Schattauer; 2004. Compact Lehrbuch Anatomie in 4 Bändern; vol 2

[42] Gray H. Anatomy for Students. Edinburgh, UK: Churchill Livingstone; 2004

[43] Gray H. Gray's Anatomy of the Human Body. Edinburgh, UK: Churchill Livingstone; 2008

[44] Greenman PE. Principles of Manual Medicine. 3rd ed. Philadelphia, PA: Lippincott Williams & Wilkins; 2004

[45] Greenspan A. Orthopedic Imaging: A Practical Approach. Philadelphia, PA: Lippincott Williams & Wilkins; 2004

[46] Gschwend N, Raemy H, Nittner H, Ivosević-Radovanović D. Long-term results of endoprosthetic joint replacement and synovectomy. Handchir Mikrochir Plast Chir 1986;18:135–149

[47] Gyot J. Atlas of Human Limb Joints. Berlin, Germany: Springer; 1981

[48] Hanke P. Das Hanke-Konzept, Physiotherapeutische Behandlung auf entwicklungsphysiologischer Grundlage. Schwartbuck, Germany: Verlag für Vitaltherapien; 2001

[49] Hall JE. Guyton and Hall: Textbook of Medical Physiology. London, UK: WB Saunders; 2010

[50] Harden RN, Swan M, King A, Costa B, Barthel J. Treatment of complex regional pain syndrome: functional restoration. Clin J Pain 2006;5:420–424

[51] Hawkins RJ, Bokor DJ. Clinical evaluation of shoulder problems. The Shoulder 1990;149–177

[52] Helsmoortel J, Hirth T, Wührl P. Visceral Osteopathy: The Peritoneal Organs. Seattle, WA: Eastland Press; 2010

[53] Hicks JH. The mechanics of the foot II. The plantar aponeurosis and the arch. J Anat (Lond) 1954;88:25–31

[54] Hill HA, Sachs MD. The grooved defect of the humeral head: a frequently unrecognized complication of dislocation of the shoulder joint. Radiol 1940;35:690–700

[55] Hill JA. Epidemiologic perspective on shoulder injuries. Clin Sports Med 1983;2:241–246

[56] Hollister A, Giurintono DJ. Thumb movements, motions and moments. J Hand Ther 1995;8:106–114

[57] Hoppenfeld S. Physical Examination of the Spine and Extremities. Upper Saddle River, NJ: Prentice Hall; 1976

[58] Iannotti J, Parker R. The Netter Collection of Medical Illustrations: Musculoskeletal System. Vol 6. London, UK: WB Saunders; 2013

[59] Idler RS. Anatomy and biomechanics of the digital flexor tendons. Hand Clin 1985;1:3–12

[60] Inman VT. The Joints of the Ankle. Baltimore, MD: Williams & Wilkins; 1976

[61] Irnich D. Myofascial Trigger Points: Comprehensive Diagnosis and Treatment. Edinburgh, UK: Churchill Livingstone; 2013

[62] Isberg A. Temporomandibular Joint Dysfunction. London, UK: Taylor & Francis Ltd; 2001

[63] Jayson M. The Lumbar Spine and Back Pain. Edinburgh, UK: Churchill Livingstone; 1992
[64] Kahle W, Frotscher M. Nervous System and Sensory Organs. Stuttgart: Thieme; 2010. Color Atlas and Textbook of Human Anatomy; vol 3
[65] Kaltenborn F, Vollowitz E. Extremities. Orthopedic Physical Therapy & Rehabilitation; 2014. Manual Mobilisation of the Joints; vol 1
[66] Kaltenborn F, Vollowitz E. The Spine. Orthopedic Physical Therapy & Rehabilitation; 2012. Manual Mobilisation of the Joints; vol 2
[67] Kapandji IA. The Spinal Column, Pelvic Girdle and Head. Edinburgh, UK: Churchill Livingstone; 2008. Physiology of the Joints; vol 3
[68] Kapandji IA, Hoebke J. Funktionelle Anatomie der Gelenke. Stuttgart: Thieme; 2009
[69] Kaufmann RA, Pfaeffle HJ, Blankenhorn BD, Stabile K, Robertson D, Goitz R. Kinematics of the midcarpal and radiocarpal joint in flexion and extension: an in vitro study. J Hand Surg 2006;31:1142–1148
[70] Kelikian A, Sarrafian S. Sarrafian's Anatomy of the Foot and Ankle. Philadelphia, PA: Lippincott, Williams & Wilkins; 2011
[71] Klein-Vogelbach S. Therapeutic Exercises in Functional Kinetics: Analysis and Instruction of Individually Adaptable Exercises. Berlin, Germany: Springer; 1991
[72] Kostopoulos D, Rizopoulos K. The Manual of Trigger Point and Myofascial Therapy. Thorofare, NJ: Slack Inc; 2001
[73] Krämer J. Intervertebral Disk Disease: Causes, Diagnosis, Treatment and Prophylaxis. Stuttgart: Thieme; 2008
[74] Lang J. Clinical Anatomy of the Cervical Spine. Stuttgart: Thieme; 1993
[75] Lefèvre S, Knedla A, Tennie C, et al. Synovial fibroblasts spread rheumatoid arthritis to unaffected joints. Nat Med 2009;15:1414–1420
[76] Leroux JL, Codine P, Thomas E, Pocholle M, Mailhe D, Blotman F. Isokinetic evaluation of rotational strength in normal shoulders and shoulders with impingement syndrome. Clin Orthop Relat Res 1994;(304):108–115
[77] Leroux JL, Thomas E, Bonnel F, Blotman F. Diagnostic value of clinical tests for shoulder impingement syndrome. Rev Rhum Engl Ed 1995;62:423–428
[78] Lysell E. Motion in the cervical spine. Acta Orthop Scand 1969;123:5–61
[79] Magee D. Orthopedic Physical Assessment. Philadelphia, PA: Elsevier Saunders; 2014
[80] Mameren H van. Motion Patterns in the Cervical Spine [thesis]. Maastricht, The Netherlands: University of Maastricht;1988
[81] Matthews LS. Load bearing characteristics of the patella-femoral joint. Acta Orthop Scand 1977;48:511–516
[82] Maquet P. Biomechanics of the Knee. Berlin, Germany: Springer; 1976
[83] McKenzie R, May S. The Lumbar Spine: Mechanical Diagnosis and Therapy. Waikanae, New Zealand: Spinal Publications; 2003
[84] Milne N. Composite motion in cervical disc segments. Clin Biomech 1993;8:193–202
[85] Moeller T, Reif E. Pocket Atlas of Radiographic Anatomy. Stuttgart: Thieme; 2010
[86] Moeller T, Reif E. Head and Neck. Stuttgart, Germany: Thieme; 2013. Pocket Atlas of Sectional Anatomy; vol 1
[87] Moeller T, Reif E. Thorax, Heart, Abdomen and Pelvis. Stuttgart, Germany: Thieme; 2013. Pocket Atlas of Sectional Anatomy; vol 2
[88] Moeller T, Reif E. Spine, Extremities, Joints. Stuttgart, Germany: Thieme; 2007. Pocket Atlas of Sectional Anatomy; vol 3
[89] Moore K, Dalley A, Agur A. Clinically Oriented Anatomy. Baltimore, MD: Lippincott, Williams & Wilkins; 2014
[90] Morrey BF. The Elbow and its Disorders. Oxford, UK: Elsevier Ltd; 2008
[91] Moseley IF, Goldie I. The arterial pattern of the rotator cuff of the shoulder. J Bone Joint Surg 1963;45:780–789
[92] Müller W. The Knee: Form, Function and Ligament Reconstruction. Berlin, Germany: Springer; 2012
[93] Mumenthaler M, Mattle M. Fundamentals of Neurology. Stuttgart, Germany: Thieme; 2006
[94] Nachemson A. The load on lumbar discs in different positions of the body. Clin Orthop 1966;45:107
[95] Nachemson A. Lumbar intradiscal pressure. In: Jayson, M. The Lumbar Spine and Back Pain. London, UK: Pitman; 1985
[96] Nakamura R, Linscheid RL, Miura T, eds. Wrist Disorders. Berlin, Germany: Springer; 2013
[97] Nash LL Jr, Moe JH. In vivo measurements of intradiscal pressure. J Bones Joint Surg 1964;46:1077–1092
[98] Nash LL Jr, Moe JH. A study of vertebral rotation. J Bone Joint Surg 1969;51:223–229
[99] Neer CS II. Shoulder Reconstruction. Philadelphia, PA: WB Saunders; 1990:73–77
[100] Netter FH. Atlas of Human Anatomy. Philadelphia, PA: WB Saunders; 2014
[101] Nordin M, Frankel V. Basic Biomechanics of the Musculoskeletal System. Philadelphia, PA: Wolters Kluwer Health; 2014
[102] Oatis C. Kinesiology: The Mechanics and Pathomechanics of Human Movement. Philadelphia, PA: Lippincott Williams & Wilkins; 2008
[103] Özkaya N, Nordin, M., Goldsheyder, D., Leger, D. Fundamentals of Biomechanics. Berlin, Germany: Springer; 2012
[104] Palmer AK, Werner FW. The triangular fibrocartilage complex of the wrist; anatomy and function. J Hand Surg 1981;6:153–162
[105] Panjabi MM. Three-dimensional movements of the upper cervical spine. Spine 1988;13:726
[106] Pauwels F. Atlas zur Biomechanik der gesunden und kranken Hüfte. Berlin, Germany: Springer 1973
[107] Pécina M, Krmpotić-Nemanić J, Markwietz AD. Tunnel Syndromes: Peripheral Nerve Compression Syndromes. Boca Raton, FL: CRC Press Inc; 2001
[108] Perry J. Anatomy and biomechanics of the shoulder in throwing, swimming, gymnastics, and tennis. Clin Sports Med 1983;2:247–270
[109] Perry J. Anatomy and biomechanics of the foot and function in the sacroiliac joint in throwing, swimming, gymnastics, and tennis. Spine 1983;15:130–136
[110] Pitkin J. Biomechanics of Life. Berlin, Germany: Springer; 2011
[111] Platzer W. Locomotor System. Stuttgart: Thieme; 2008. Color Atlas and Textbook of Human Anatomy; vol 1
[112] Porter RW. Lumbar Spine Disorders. Singapore: World Scientific Publishing Ltd; 1995
[113] Rockwood CA, Matsen FA, eds. The Shoulder. Vol 1 and 2. Philadelphia, PA: Saunders; 2009
[114] Rohlmann A, Graichen F, Weber U, Bergmann G. Monitoring in vivo implant loads with a telemeterized internal spinal fixation device. J Spine 2000;25:2981–2986
[115] Rohlmann A, Neller S, Bergmann G, Graichen F, Claes L, Wilke HJ. Effects of an internal fixator and a bone graft on intersegmental spinal motion and intradiscal pressure in the adjacent regions. J Eur Spine 2001;10:301–308
[116] Rothmann RH, Parker WW. The vascular anatomy of the rotator cuff. Clin Orthop 1965;41:176–186
[117] Sahrmann S. Movement System Impairment Syndromes of the Extremities, Cervical and Thoracic Spines. CV St. Louis, MO: Mosby Co; 2010
[118] Schildt-Rudloff K. Thoraxschmerz. Berlin, Germany: Ullstein & Mosby; 1994
[119] Schmidt HM, Lanz U. Chirurgische Anatomie der Hand. Stuttgart, Germany: Thieme; 2003
[120] Schmidt HM, Lanz U. Surgical Anatomy of the Hand. Stuttgart, Germany: Thieme; 2011
[121] Schünke M, Schulte E, Ross LM. Thieme Atlas of Anatomy. Head and Neuroanatomy. Stuttgart, Germany: Thieme; 2010
[122] Schünke M, Schulte E, Schumacher U, Ross LM. Thieme Atlas of Anatomy. General Anatomy and Musculoskeletal System. Thieme Atlas of Anatomy. General Anatomy and Musculoskeletal System. Stuttgart, Germany: Thieme; 2010
[123] Schünke M, Schulte E, Ross LM. Thieme Atlas of Anatomy. Neck and Internal Organs. Stuttgart, Germany: Thieme; 2010
[124] Shacklock M. Clinical Neurodynamics: A New System of Neuromusculoskeletal Treatment. Philadelphia, PA: Elsevier Saunders; 2005
[125] Shen FH, Smartzis D, Fessler RG. Textbook of Cervical Spine. Philadelphia, PA: Saunders; 2014
[126] Sherk H. The Cervical Spine. Philadelphia, PA: Lippincott-Raven Publishers; 1994

[127] Shibutani N. Three dimensional architecture of the acetabulum labrum – a scanning electron microscopic study. J Jpn Orthop Assoc 1988;62:321–329

[128] Short WH, Werner FW, Green JK, Masaoka S. Biomechanical evaluation of the ligamentous stabilizers of the scaphoid and lunate. J Hand Surg 2002;27:991–1002

[129] Skirven TM, Osterman AL, Fedorczyk J, Amardio PC. Rehabilitation of the Hand and Upper Extremity. Elsevier Mosby, Philadelphia; 2011

[130] Snyder SJ, Karzel RP, Del Pizzo W, Ferkel RD, Friedman MJ. SLAP lesions of the shoulder. Arthroscopy 1990;6:274–279

[131] Sohier R. La Kinésithérapie de la hanche. La Hestre, Belgium: Kiné-Sciences; 1974

[132] Sokolow C, Saffar P. Anatomy and histology of the scapholunate ligament. J Hand Clin 2001;17:77–81

[133] Stoller DW. Stoller's Orthopedics and Sports Medicine: The Shoulder. Philadelphia, PA: Lippincott William & Wilkins; 2014

[134] Strobel M, Stedtfeld H-W. Diagnostic Evaluation of the Knee. Berlin, Germany: Springer; 1990

[135] Taylor JR. The development and adult structure of lumbar intervertebral discs. J Man Med 1990;5:43–47

[136] Taylor TK, Little K. Intercellular matrix of the intervertebral disk in ageing and in prolapse. Nature 1965;208–384

[137] Thompson JC, et al. Netter's Concise Orthopaedic Anatomy. Philadelphia, PA: Saunders WB; 2009

[138] Travell J, Simons D. The Upper Extremities. Philadelphia, USA: Lippincott William & Wilkins; 1998. Myofascial Pain and Dysfunction: The Trigger Point Manual; vol 1

[139] Travell J, Simons D. The Lower Extremities. Philadelphia, USA: Lippincott William & Wilkins; 1998. Myofascial Pain and Dysfunction: The Trigger Point Manual; vol 2

[140] Trumble T, Budoff J, Cornwall R. Core Knowledge in Orthopaedics: Hand, Elbow, Shoulder. Philadelphia, PA: Mosby & Elsevier; 2006

[141] Upledger JE. Craniosacral Therapy. Seattle, WA: Eastland Press; 1983

[142] Van den Berg F. Das Bindegewebe des Bewegungsapparates verstehen und beeinflussen. Stuttgart, Germany: Thieme; 1999. Angewandte Physiologie; vol 1

[143] Vleeming A, et al. Relation between form and function in the sacroiliac joint. Spine 1990;15:130–136

[144] White A, Panjabi MM. The basic kinematics of the human spine. A review of post and current knowledge. Spine 1978;3:12–20

[145] White A, Panjabi MM. Clinical Biomechanics of the Spine. Philadelphia, PA: Lippincott-Raven Publishers; 1990

[146] Wiberg G. Roentgenographic and anatomic studies on the patellar joint. Acta Orthop Scand 1974;12:319–410

[147] Wilke HJ, et al. Biomechanical comparison of calf and human spines. J Orthop Res 1996;14:500–503

[148] Wilke HJ, et al. New in vivo measurements of pressures in the intervertebral disc in daily life. Spine 1999;24(8):755–762

# Index

Page numbers in *italics* refer to illustrations; those in **bold** refer to tables

## D



## E



## F

## I

## Q



## R

## S

## T

## U



## V



## W



## X



## Z